A Reference Guide to Fetal and Neonatal Risk

DRUGS IN PREGNANCY AND LACTATION

third edition

A Reference Guide to Fetal and Neonatal Risk

DRUGS IN PREGNANCY AND LACTATION

third edition

Gerald G. Briggs, B.Pharm.

Clinical Pharmacist, Women's Hospital
Memorial Hospital of Long Beach, California
Assistant Clinical Professor of Pharmacy University of California, San Francisco
Assistant Clinical Professor of Pharmacy University of Southern California,
Los Angeles

Roger K. Freeman, M.D.

Medical Director, Women's Hospital
Memorial Hospital of Long Beach, California
Professor of Obstetrics and Gynecology University of California, Irvine

Sumner J. Yaffe, M.D.

Director, Center for Research for Mothers and Children
National Institute of Child Health and Human Development
National Institutes of Health Bethesda, Maryland

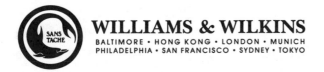

WILLIAMS & WILKINS
BALTIMORE · HONG KONG · LONDON · MUNICH
PHILADELPHIA · SAN FRANCISCO · SYDNEY · TOKYO

Editor: John P. Butler
Associate Editor: Marjorie Kidd Keating
Copy Editor: Deborah Tourtlotte
Designer: Bob Och
Production Coordinator: Anne Stewart Seitz
Cover Designer: Dan Pfisterer

Copyright © 1990
Williams & Wilkins
428 East Preston Street
Baltimore, Maryland 21202, USA

Accurate indications, adverse reactions, and dosage schedules for drugs are provided in this book, but it is possible that they may change. The reader is urged to review the package information data of the manufacturers of the medications mentioned.

Printed in the United States of America

First Edition, 1983
Second Edition, 1986
ISSN: 0897-6112

91 92 93 94

2   3   4   5   6   7   8   9   10

Foreword

This book was written to be used by the clinician who deals with pregnant patients. Every day in an obstetric, pediatric, or other medical practice, one encounters frequent questions about the use of drugs in pregnancy and lactation. These questions may involve the use of a drug for therapy of an associated condition, an inquiry about some drug a patient has already taken and then decides to ask about, or the determination of whether an untoward pregnancy outcome or an adverse effect observed in the infant was caused by the patient's consumption of some therapeutic agent. Other health professionals, such as nurses and pharmacists, also are often confronted with questions concerning drug usage in the pregnant or breast-feeding woman.

Of course, this book of necessity lacks absolute answers on most drugs in question because experience in humans is not easy to gather. One seldom knows, even when the drug history is thought to be realistic, whether there is an actual cause-effect relationship between a specific drug and an adverse pregnancy outcome. Because the answers are generally inconclusive, physicians caring for pregnant patients should counsel their patients accordingly either when answering a question about some drug already ingested or when explaining the cost:benefit ratio to a patient who is being considered for some specific drug therapy.

For the breast-feeding patient, the risks from a particular drug are usually much clearer, although there are frequent examples where the risk must be inferred from related drugs. Unfortunately, many drugs have not been studied during nursing so the effects on the infant, if any, are completely unknown. A good rule to follow is if the drug can safely be given directly to the infant, it is generally safe to give to the mother during lactation.

This book allows the clinician to have at his or her fingertips an up-to-date summary of available data bearing on specific drugs. It is easy to read and organized in a logical manner to save the busy clinician time.

Roger K. Freeman, M.D.
Medical Director
Women's Hospital
Long Beach Memorial Medical Center
Long Beach, California
Professor of Obstetrics and Gynecology
University of California, Irvine

Preface

Many of the monographs in this third edition of *Drugs in Pregnancy and Lactation* have been extensively revised. For example, cocaine, indomethacin, isotretinoin, valproic acid, the antineoplastic agents, and most of the vitamin products, to name a few, have all undergone major revisions. Some of these, along with the other revisions and the addition of new drugs, were published in UPDATES during 1988 and 1989. UPDATES, a quarterly newsletter, has provided us a vehicle to disseminate new information to our readers in a much more timely fashion. Even then, some of the revisions published in UPDATES have been further revised in this edition as additional information became available.

Of course, the fetus and nursing infant are the ones who ultimately benefit from this explosion of information. As we gain new insights into how drugs and chemicals affect the products of human conception, we are better able to counsel and advise the parents on how they can protect their offspring during these vulnerable periods.

As with the previous editions, we have been fortunate to have the able assistance of the Long Beach Memorial Medical Center Medical Library staff and volunteers. Their continued support is invaluable, and we offer a special thank you to the Director, Marion Sabella, and her staff, Emi Wong (Medical Librarian), Mori Lou Higa (Library Technician), Barbara Malinofsky (Clerk), and the four hard-working volunteers, George Treadway, Griff Meade, Eva Florsheim, and Ann Fishman. Our thanks also go to those in the Memorial Pharmacy Department and Drug Information Service who either helped us directly with selected references, or provided us with time, space, and encouragment to work on this edition. In particular, we want to acknowledge Drs. Bill Smith, Byron Schweigert, Phil Towne, and Brian Moore.

We wish to acknowledge the assistance on some of the monographs of two of our former students: Doris Sue, Pharm.D., and Florence Wong, Pharm.D.

Gerald G. Briggs, B.Pharm.

Contents

Introduction

Sumner J. Yaffe, M.D.

The birth of a normal infant is the expectation of the parents when pregnancy is considered. Normality is not limited to the time of birth but includes the achievement of full potential in adulthood. Today advances in medical knowledge and delivery have made this aspiration more readily achievable than ever before. However, there is a threat to the fulfillment of the prospective parents' dreams resulting from the very advances that contributed to better health. Indeed, modern technology poses a risk to the fetus and lactating infant from the drugs used in obstetric practice and from the increasing numbers of chemicals in the environment. New social, cultural, and ecologic conditions have modified the experiences of today's pregnant woman.

Studies are needed to clarify their specific impact and to facilitate the development of preventive and/or curative strategies. This knowledge must be transferred rapidly to all interested parties—physicians, midwives, nurses, mothers-to-be, and the public at large—because an informed individual will be more inclined to seek and follow medical advice.

Every day physicians and midwives usher newborns into the world with the full expectation that their advice and prescribed medications will be adhered to by the new mothers and will result in healthy infants. In addition, if they so wish, new mothers are ready to nurse their baby.

Special responsibilities are vested in the partnership between the pregnant woman and her physician. The physician has the responsibility to provide all the medical knowledge and skills available to him or her. The pregnant woman is expected to follow the physician's advice and prescriptions.

This has been the established arrangement since physicians began attending childbirth. The primary difference between those early times and today is what is expected of the physician. Hippocrates, Soranus, Aetios, and Avicenna, whose time ranged from the 4th century before the common era through the 1st millenium AD, maintained highly authoritative positions within their communities and provided their ministrations in a categorical fashion.

Soranus of Ephesus (1), representing the consummate thinking of the time (2nd century AD), wrote in a threatening autocratic manner, "Even if a woman transgresses some or all of the rules mentioned (re: administration of drugs, sternutatives, pungent substances, and drunkenness, especially during the first trimester) and yet miscarriage of the fetus does not take place, let no one assume that the fetus has not been injured at all. For it has been harmed: it is weakened, becomes retarded in growth, less well nourished, and in general, more easily injured and susceptible to harmful agents; it becomes misshapen and of ignoble soul."

Drugs in Pregnancy

Today's physician does not have the authoritative luxury of yesterday's practitioner. In particular, the present-day obstetrician has suffered a diminution of confidence because of the thalidomide catastrophe.

In 1941 Gregg (2) demonstrated that rubella infection in the mother could result in anatomic malformation in the fetus. This raised the concept that environment could affect fetal outcome. In spite of this, physicians continued to practice their profession with little concern to the empirical observations.

Because of its sedative and hypnotic effects, physicians administered thalidomide to the pregnant woman for her discomfort. Thalidomide had been evaluated for safety in several animal species, had been given a clean bill of health, and had come to be regarded as a good pharmacologic agent. Yet the catastrophic and distinct embryopathic effects resulting from thalidomide administration to the human mother during early pregnancy are well known.

It is important to note that even though thalidomide induces a distinct cluster of anatomic defects that are virtually pathognomonic for this agent, it required several years of thalidomide use and the birth of many thousands of grossly malformed infants before the cause-effect relationship between thalidomide administration in early pregnancy and its harmful effects was recognized. This serves to emphasize the difficulties that exist in incriminating drugs and chemicals that are harmful when administered during pregnancy. Hopefully, we will never have another drug prescribed for use during pregnancy whose teratogenicity is as potent as thalidomide (about one-third of women taking this agent during the first trimester gave birth to infants with birth defects).

Concern about the safety of foreign compounds administered to pregnant women has been increasingly evident since thalidomide. It was the direct response to this misadventure that led to the promulgation of the drug regulations of 1962 in the United States. According to these regulations, a drug must be demonstrated to be safe and effective for the conditions of use prescribed in its labeling. The regulations concerning this requirement state that a drug should be investigated for the conditions of use specified in the labeling, including dosage levels and patient populations for whom the drug is intended. In addition, appropriate information must be provided in the labeling in cases in which the drug is prescribed. The intent of the regulations is not only to ensure adequate labeling information for the safe and effective administration of the drug by the physician but also to ensure that marketed drugs have an acceptable benefit:risk ratio for their intended uses.

It is clear that any drug or chemical substance administered to the mother is able to cross the placenta to some extent unless it is destroyed or altered during passage. Placental transport of maternal substrates to the fetus and of substances from the fetus to the mother is established at about the 5th week of fetal life. Substances of low molecular weight diffuse freely across the placenta, driven primarily by the concentration gradient. It is important to note, therefore, that almost every substance used for therapeutic purposes can and does pass from the mother to the fetus. Of greater importance is whether the rate and extent of transfer are sufficient to result in significant concentrations within the fetus. We must discard the concept that there is a placental barrier.

Experiments with animals have provided considerable information concerning the teratogenic effects of drugs. Unfortunately, these experimental findings cannot be extrapolated from species to species, or even from strain to strain within the same species, much less from animals to humans. Research in this area and the prediction of toxicity in the human are further hampered by a lack of specificity between cause and effect.

Traditionally, teratogenic effects of drugs have been noted as anatomic malformations. It is clear that these are dose and time related and that the fetus is at great risk during the first 3 months of gestation. However, it is possible for drugs and chemicals to exert their effects upon the fetus at other times during pregnancy. Functional and behavioral changes are much more difficult to identify as to cause and effect. Consequently, they are rarely recognized. A heightened awareness on the part of health providers and recipients will make this task easier.

This was also understood by Hippocrates who, in the Corpus (3), maintained the 2nd trimester as a safe stage of fetal development for the administration of drugs. In the Aphorisms, that collection of short medical truths, he prescribed, "Drugs may be administered to pregnant women from the fourth to the seventh month of gestation. After that period, the dose should be less."

The mechanisms of teratogenic agents are poorly understood, particularly in the human. Drugs may affect maternal tissues with indirect effects upon the fetus or they may have a direct effect on the embryonic cells and result in specific abnormalities. Drugs may affect the nutrition of the fetus by interfering with the passage of nutrients across the placenta. Alterations in placental metabolism influence the development of the fetus since placental integrity is a determinant of fetal growth.

Administration of a drug to a pregnant woman presents a unique problem for the physician. Not only must maternal pharmacologic mechanisms be taken into consideration when prescribing a drug but also the fetus must always be kept in mind as a potential recipient of the drug.

Recognition of the fact that drugs administered during pregnancy can affect the fetus should lead to decreased drug consumption. Nonetheless, studies conducted in the past few years indicate that drug consumption during pregnancy is increasing. This may be due to several reasons. Most people in the Western world are unaware of their drug and chemical exposure. Many are uninformed as to the potentially harmful effects of drugs on the fetus. Also, there are some who feel that many individuals in modern society are overly concerned with their own comfort.

Whatever the reasons, exposure to drugs, both prescribed and over-the-counter, among mothers-to-be continues unabated throughout pregnancy. It is possible that this exposure to drugs and chemicals may be responsible for the large numbers of birth defects that are seen in the newborn infant and in later development.

It is crucial that concern also be given to events beyond the narrow limits of congenital anatomic malformations; evidence exists that intellectual, social, and functional development also can be adversely affected. There are examples that toxic manifestations of intrauterine exposure to environmental agents may be subtle, unexpected, and delayed.

Concern for the delayed effects of drugs, following intrauterine exposure, was first raised following the tragic discovery that female fetuses exposed to diethylstilbestrol (DES) are at an increased risk for adenocarcinoma of the vagina. This type of malignancy is not discovered until after puberty. Additional clinical findings indicate that male offspring were not spared from the effects of the drug. Some have abnormalities of the reproductive system, such as epididymal cysts, hypotrophic testes, capsular induration, and pathologic semen.

The concept of long-term latency has been confirmed by investigations conducted in the research laboratories. Researchers found that when the widely used hypnotic-sedative agent phenobarbital was administered to pregnant rats it resulted in the birth of offspring that were significantly smaller than normal and that experienced delays in vaginal opening. Sixty percent of the females of these animals were infertile (4).

Investigators in a laboratory at Children's Hospital of Philadelphia reported their research results with male animals (5). They found lower than normal testosterone levels in the brain and bloodstream of male rats whose mothers were given low doses of phenobarbital late in pregnancy. Even at 120 days of age, these male rats showed abnormal testosterone synthesis. It is felt by the investigators that phenobarbital exposure in fetal life may alter brain programming, resulting in permanent changes in sexual function. Phenobarbital is an old drug that is widely prescribed. It is also a component of many multi-ingredient pharmaceuticals whose use does not abate during pregnancy. The clinical significance of these experiments in animals is admittedly unknown, but the striking effects upon reproductive function warrant careful scrutiny of the safety of these agents during human pregnancy before prescribing them.

The physician is confronted with two imperatives in treating the pregnant woman: Alleviate maternal suffering, and do not harm the fetus. Until now the emphasis has been on the amelioration of suffering, but the time has come to concentrate on not harming the fetus. The simple equation to be applied here is weighing the therapeutic benefits of the drug to the mother against its risk potential to the developing fetus.

When one considers that more than 1.2 billion drug prescriptions are written each year, that there is unlimited self-administration of over-the-counter drugs, and that approximately 500 new pharmaceutical products are introduced annually, the need for prudency in the administration of pharmaceuticals has reached a critical point. Pregnancy is a symptom-producing event. Pregnancy has the potential of causing women to increase their intake of drugs and chemicals, with the potential being that the fetus will be nurtured in a sea of drugs.

In today's society the physician cannot stand alone in the therapeutic decision-making process. It now has become the responsibility of each woman of childbearing age to consider carefully her use of drugs. In a pregnant woman, the decision to administer a drug should be made only after a collaborative appraisal between the woman and her physician of the benefits:risk ratio.

Breast Feeding and Drugs

Between 1930 and the late 1960s there was a dramatic decline in the percentage of American mothers who breast fed their babies. This was accompanied by a reduction in the length of breast feeding for those who did nurse. The incidence of breast feeding declined from approximately 80% of the children born between

1926–1930 to 49% of children born some 25 years later. For children born between 1966–1970, 28% were breast fed. As data have become available for the 1970s, it is clear the decline has been reversed (6). By 1975, the percentage of first-born babies who were breast fed rose to 37%. At the present time in the United States, a number of surveys indicate that more than 50% of babies discharged from the hospital are breast fed, and the number is increasing.

Any number of hypotheses can be made regarding the decline and recent increase in breast feeding in this country. A fair amount of credit can be given to biomedical research of the past 15 years that has demonstrated the benefits of breast feeding.

Breast milk is known to possess nutritional and immunologic properties superior to those found in infant formulas (6–9). An American Academy of Pediatrics position paper emphasizes breast feeding as the best nutritional mode for infants for the first 6 months of life (6). In addition to those qualities, some studies also suggest significant psychologic benefits of breast feeding for both the mother and the infant.

The upswing in breast feeding, together with a markedly increased concern about health needs on the part of parents, has led to increased questioning of the physician, pharmacist, and other health professionals about the safety and potential toxicity of drugs and chemicals that may be excreted in breast milk. Answers to these questions are not very apparent. Our knowledge concerning the long- and short-term effects and safety of maternally ingested drugs on the suckling infant is meager. We know more now than Soranus did in 150 AD when he admonished wet nurses to refrain from the use of drugs and alcohol lest it have an adverse effect on the nursing infant. We must know more! The knowledge to be acquired should be specific with respect to dose administered to the mother, amount excreted in breast milk, and amount absorbed by the suckling infant. In addition, effects on the infant should be determined (both acute and chronic).

It would be easy to recommend that the medicated mother not nurse, but it is likely that this recommendation would be ignored by the mother in discomfort and may well offend many health providers as well as their patients on both psychosocial and physiologic grounds.

It must be emphasized that virtually all investigations concerned with milk secretion and synthesis have been carried out in animals. The difficulty in studying human lactation using histologic techniques and the administration of radioactive isotopes is obvious. There are considerable differences in the composition of milk in different species. Some of these differences in composition would obviously bring about changes in drug elimination. Of great importance in this regard are the differences in the pH of human milk (pH usually >7.0) as contrasted to the pH of cow's milk (pH usually <6.8) where drug excretion has been extensively studied.

Human milk is a suspension of fat and protein in a carbohydrate-mineral solution. A nursing mother easily makes 600 ml of milk/day containing sufficient protein, fat, and carbohydrate to meet the nutritional demands of the developing infant. Milk proteins are fully synthesized from substrates delivered from the maternal circulation. The major proteins are casein and lactalbumin. The role of these proteins in the delivery of drugs into milk has not yet been completely elucidated. Drug excretion into milk may be accomplished by binding to the proteins or onto the surface of the milk fat globule.

There also exists the possibility for drug binding to the lipid as well as to the protein components of the milk fat globule. It is also possible that lipid-soluble drugs may be sequestered within the milk fat globule. In addition to lipids and protein, carbohydrate is entirely synthesized within the breast. All of these nutrients achieve a concentration in human milk that is sufficient for the needs of the human infant for the first 6 months of life.

The transport of drugs into breast milk from maternal tissues and plasma may proceed by a number of different routes. In general, however, the mechanisms that determine the concentration of a drug in breast milk are similar to those existing elsewhere within the organism. Drugs traverse membranes primarily by passive diffusion, and the concentration achieved will be dependent not only on the concentration gradient but also on the intrinsic lipid solubility of the drug and its degree of ionization as well as binding to protein and other cellular constituents.

A number of reviews (10–12) give tables of the concentration of drugs in breast milk. Many times these tables also give the milk:plasma ratio. Most of the values from which the tables are derived consist of a single measurement of the drug concentration. Important information—such as the maternal dose, the frequency of dose, the time from drug administration to sampling, the frequency of nursing, and the length of lactation—is not given.

What these concentrations mean to the physician concerned about the infant is that the drug is present in the milk. This fact is apparent since, with few exceptions, all drugs that are present in the maternal circulation will be transferred to milk. Because the drug in the nursing infant's blood or urine is not measured, we have little information about the amount that is actually absorbed by the infant from the milk and, therefore, have no way of determining the possible pharmacologic effects on the infant. In fact, a critical examination of the tables that have been published reveals that much of the information was gathered decades ago when analytic methodology was not as sensitive as it is today. Since the discipline of pharmacokinetics was not developed until recently, many of the studies quoted in the tables of the review articles do not look precisely at the time relationship between drug administration and disposition.

Certain things are clear with regard to drugs administered during lactation. It is clear that physicians will have to become aware of the results of animal studies in this area and of the potential risk of maternal drug ingestion to the suckling infant. It is clear that a great many other drugs employed at this time need to be thoroughly studied in order to assess their safety during lactation. It is clear that if the mother needs the drugs for therapeutic purposes, then she should consider not nursing. The ultimate decision must be individualized according to the specific illness and the therapeutic modality. It is clear that nursing should be avoided following the administration of radioactive pharmaceuticals that are usually given to the mother for diagnostic purposes.

The situation with the excretion of drugs into human breast milk might well be considered analogous to the prethalidomide era when the effects on the fetus from maternally ingested drugs were recognized only as a result of a catastrophe. Objective evaluation of the efficacy and safety of drugs in breast milk must be undertaken. Until such data are available, the physician should always weigh the risk:benefit ratio when prescribing any maternal medication. It is also obligatory upon the nursing mother to become aware of the same factors and apply a measure of self-control before ingesting over-the-counter drugs. As stated before, it is quite evident that nearly all drugs will be present in breast milk following maternal ingestion. It is prudent to minimize maternal exposure, although very few drugs are currently known to be hazardous to the suckling child. If, after examining the benefit:risk factor, the physician decides that maternal medication is necessary, drug exposure to the infant may be minimized by scheduling the maternal dose just after a nursing period. More often than not, drugs are prescribed to the nursing mother for the relief of symptoms that do not require drug therapy. If mothers were apprised by their physicians of the potential risk to their infants, most would probably endure the symptoms rather than take the drug and discontinue breast feeding.

Conclusions

Two basic situations are dealt with throughout this book: (a) risk potential to the fetus of maternal drugs ingested during the course of pregnancy and (b) risk potential to the infant of drugs taken by the mother while nursing.

The obvious solution to fetal and nursing infant risk avoidance is maternal abstinence. However, from a pragmatic standpoint, that would be impossible to implement. Another solution is to disseminate knowledge, in an authoritative manner, to all those involved in the pregnancy and breast-feeding processes: physician, mother, midwife, nurse, father, and pharmacist.

This book helps to fill a communication/information gap. We have carefully evaluated the research literature, animal and human, applied and clinical. We have established a risk factor for each of the more than 500 drugs, in keeping with the Food and Drug Administration guidelines, that may be administered during pregnancy and lactation. We feel that this book will be helpful to all concerned parties in developing the benefit:risk decision.

This is but a beginning. It is our fervent hope that the information gained from the use of this book will cause the concerned parties to be more trenchant in their future decision making, either before prescribing or before ingesting drugs during pregnancy and lactation.

References

1. Soranus. *Gynecology* (translation). Baltimore: Johns Hopkins University Press, 1956.
2. Gregg NM. Congenital cataract following German measles in the mother. Trans Ophthalmol Soc Aust 1941;3:35–41.
3. Chadwick J, Mann WN. *The Medical Works of Hippocrates*. Springfield, IL:Charles C Thomas, 1935.
4. Gupta C, Sondwane BR, Yaffe SJ, Shapiro BH. Phenobarbital exposure in utero: alterations in female reproductive functions in rats. Science 1980;208:508–10.
5. Gupta C, Yaffe SJ, Shapiro BH. Prenatal exposure to phenobarbital permanently decreases testosterone and causes reproductive dysfunction. Science 1982;216:640–2.
6. Nutrition Committee of the Canadian Pediatric Society and the Committee on Nutrition of the American Academy of Pediatrics. Breast feeding. Pediatrics 1978;62:591–601.
7. Fomon SJ. *Infant Nutrition*, 2nd ed. Philadelphia:WB Saunders, 1974:360–70.
8. Jelliffe DB, Jelliffe EFP. Breast is best: modern meanings. N Engl J Med 1977;297:912–5.
9. Applebaum RM. The obstetrician's approach to the breasts and breast feeding. J Reprod Med 1975;14:98–116.
10. Knowles JA. Excretion of drugs in milk: a review. J Pediatr 1965;66:1068–82.
11. Hervada AR, Feit E, Sagrames R. Drugs in breast milk. Perinatal Care 1978;2:19–25.
12. O'Brien TE. Excretion of drugs in human milk. Am J Hosp Pharm 1974;31:844–854.

Instructions for Use of the Reference Guide

The Reference Guide is arranged so that the user can quickly locate a monograph. If the American generic name is known, go directly to the monographs, which are listed in alphabetical order. If only the trade or foreign name is known, refer to the Index for the appropriate American generic name. Foreign trade names have been included in the Index. To the best of our knowledge, all trade and foreign generic names are correct as shown, but since these may change, the reader should check other reference sources if there is any question as to the identity of an individual drug. Combination products are generally not listed in the Index. The user should refer to the manufacturer's product information for the specific ingredients and then use the Reference Guide as for single entities.

Each monograph contains six parts:
Generic name (United States)
Pharmacologic Class
Risk Factor
Fetal Risk Summary
Breast Feeding Summary
References (omitted from some monographs)

Fetal Risk Summary

The Fetal Risk Summary is a brief review of the literature concerning the drug. The intent of the Summary is to provide clinicians and other individuals with sufficient data to counsel patients and to arrive at conclusions on the risk:benefit ratio a particular drug poses for the fetus. Since few absolutes are possible in the area of human teratology, the reader must carefully weigh the evidence, or lack thereof, before utilizing any drug in a pregnant woman. Animal data have been excluded from most monographs unless they contribute significantly, in our opinion, to the total information. Readers who require more details than are presented should refer to the specific references listed at the end of the monograph.

Breast Feeding Summary

The Breast Feeding Summary is a brief review of the literature concerning the passage of the drug into human breast milk and the effects, if any, on the nursing infant. In many studies of drugs in breast milk, infants were not allowed to breast feed. Readers should pay close attention to this distinction (i.e., excretion into milk vs. effects on the nursing infant) when using a Summary. Those who require more details than are presented should refer to the specific references listed at the end of the monograph.

Risk Factors

Risk Factors (A, B, C, D, X) have been assigned to all drugs, based on the level of risk the drug poses to the fetus. Risk Factors are designed to help the reader quickly classify a drug for use during pregnancy. They do not refer to breast-feeding risk. Because they tend to oversimplify a complex topic, they should always be used in conjunction with the Fetal Risk Summary. The definitions for the Factors are those used by the Food and Drug Administration (Federal Register 1980;44:37434-67). Since most drugs have not yet been given a letter rating by their manufacturers, the Risk Factor assignments were usually made by the authors. If the manufacturer rated its product in its professional literature, the Risk Factor on the monograph will be shown with a subscript M (e.g., C_M). If the manufacturer and the authors differed in their assignment of a Risk Factor, our Risk Factor is marked with an asterisk and the manufacturer's rating is shown at the end of the Fetal Risk Summary. Other Risk Factors marked with an asterisk (e.g., sulfonamides, morphine, etc.) are drugs that present different risks to the fetus depending on when or for how long they are used. In these cases, a second Risk Factor will be found with a short explanation at the end of the Fetal Risk Summary. We hope this will increase the usefulness of these ratings. The definitions used for the Risk Factors are presented below.

Category A: Controlled studies in women fail to demonstrate a risk to the fetus in the first trimester (and there is no evidence of a risk in later trimesters), and the possibility of fetal harm appears remote.

Category B: Either animal-reproduction studies have not demonstrated a fetal risk but there are no controlled studies in pregnant women or animal-reproduction studies have shown an adverse effect (other than a decrease in fertility) that was not confirmed in controlled studies in women in the first trimester (and there is no evidence of a risk in later trimesters).

Category C: Either studies in animals have revealed adverse effects on the fetus (teratogenic or embryocidal or other) and there are no controlled studies in woman or studies in women and animals are not available. Drugs should be given only if the potential benefit justifies the potential risk to the fetus.

Category D: There is positive evidence of human fetal risk, but the benefits from use in pregnant women may be acceptable despite the risk (e.g., if the drug is needed in a life-threatening situation or for a serious disease for which safer drugs cannot be used or are ineffective).

Category X: Studies in animals or human beings have demonstrated fetal abnormalities or there is evidence of fetal risk based on human experience or both, and the risk of the use of the drug in pregnant women clearly outweighs any possible benefit. The drug is contraindicated in women who are or may become pregnant.

Name: **ACEBUTOLOL**

Class: **Sympatholytic (β-Adrenergic Blocker)**   Risk Factor: **B$_M$**

Fetal Risk Summary

Acebutolol, a cardioselective β-adrenergic blocking agent, has been used for the treatment of hypertension occurring during pregnancy (1–5). No fetal malformations attributable to acebutolol have been observed, but experience with the drug during the 1st trimester is lacking. In a study comparing three β-blockers, the mean birth weight of 56 newborns was slightly lower than 38 pindolol-exposed infants but higher than 31 offspring of atenolol-treated mothers (3160 g vs. 3375 g vs. 2745 g) (2). It is not known whether these differences were due to the degree of maternal hypertension, the potency of the drugs used, or a combination of these and other factors.

Acebutolol crosses the placenta producing maternal:cord ratios of 0.8 (3). The corresponding ratio for the metabolite, *N*-acetyl-acebutolol, was 0.6. Newborn serum levels of acebutolol and the metabolite were <5–244 ng/ml and 17–663 ng/ml, respectively (3). A cord:maternal ratio of 0.7 has also been reported (4).

In a comparison of 20 pregnant women treated with either acebutolol or methyldopa for mild to moderate hypertension, no differences between the drugs were found for pregnancy duration, birth weight, Apgar scores, or placental weight (5). In addition, no evidence of bradycardia, hypoglycemia, or respiratory problems was found in the acebutolol-exposed newborns. In an earlier study, however, 10 newborns exposed to acebutolol near term had blood pressures and heart rates significantly lower than similar infants exposed to methyldopa (6). The hemodynamic differences were still evident 3 days after birth. Measurements were not made after this point, so it is not known how long the β-blockade persisted. Mean blood glucose levels were not significantly lower than those of similar infants exposed to methyldopa, but transient hypoglycemia was present 3 hours after birth in four term newborns (5). The mean half-life of acebutolol in the serum of newborns has been calculated to be 10.1 hours, but the half-life based on urinary excretion was 15.6 hours (6). Therefore, newborn infants of women consuming the drug near delivery should be closely observed for signs and symptoms of β-blockade. Long-term effects of *in utero* exposure to β-blockers have not been studied but warrant evaluation.

Breast Feeding Summary

Acebutolol and its metabolite, *N*-acetyl-acebutolol, are excreted into breast milk (3, 7). Milk:plasma ratios for the two compounds were 7.1 and 12.2, respectively (3). Absorption of both compounds was demonstrated in breast-feeding infants, but no adverse effects were mentioned (3). In a study of seven nursing, hypertensive mothers treated with 200–1200 mg/day within 13 days of delivery, milk:plasma acebutolol ratios in three varied from 2.3–9.2, while similar ratios of the metabolite ranged from 1.5–13.5 (7). The highest milk concentration of acebutolol, 4123 ng/ml, occurred in a mother taking 1200 mg/day. Two to 3 days after treatment was stopped, milk:plasma ratios of acebutolol and the metabolite in the seven women were 1.9–9.8 and 2.3–24.7, respectively (7). Symptoms of β-blockade (hypotension, bradycardia, and transient tachypnea) were observed in one nursing infant, although the time of onset of the adverse effects was not given. Neonatal plasma concentrations of the drug and metabolite (specific data not given), which were already high from *in utero* exposure, rose sharply after nursing commenced. The mother was taking 400 mg/day and her milk:plasma ratios of acebutolol and metabolite during treatment were 9.2 and 13.5, respectively, the highest observed in this study. Breast-fed infants of mothers taking acebutolol should be closely observed for hypotension, bradycardia, and other signs or symptoms of β-blockade. Long-term effects of exposure to β-blockers from milk have not been studied but warrant evaluation. The American Academy of Pediatrics considers acebutolol to be compatible with breast feeding (8).

References

1. Dubois D, Petitcolas J, Temperville B, Klepper A. Beta blockers and high-risk pregnancies. Int J Biol Res Pregnancy 1980;1:141–5.
2. Dubois D, Petitcolas J, Temperville B, Klepper A, Catherine P. Treatment of hypertension in pregnancy with β-adrenoceptor antagonists. Br J Clin Pharmacol 1982;13(Suppl):375S–8S.
3. Bianchetti G, Dubruc C, Vert P, Boutroy MJ, Morselli PL. Placental transfer and pharmacokinetics of acebutolol in newborn infants. Clin Pharmacol Ther 1981;29:233–4 (Abstract).
4. Boutroy MJ. Fetal and neonatal effects of the beta-adrenoceptor blocking agents. Dev Pharmacol Ther 1987;10:224–31.
5. Williams ER, Morrissey JR. A comparison of acebutolol with methyldopa in hypertensive pregnancy. Pharmatherapeutica 1983;3:487–91.
6. Dumez Y, Tchobroutsky C, Hornych H, Amiel-Tison C. Neonatal effects of maternal administration of acebutolol. Br Med J 1981;283:1077–9.
7. Boutroy MJ, Bianchetti G, Dubruc C, Vert P, Morselli PL. To nurse when receiving acebutolol: is it dangerous for the neonate? Eur J Clin Pharmacol 1986;30:737–9.
8. Committee on Drugs, American Academy of Pediatrics. Transfer of drugs and other chemicals into human milk. Pediatrics 1989;84:924–36.

Name: **ACETAMINOPHEN**

Class: **Analgesic/Antipyretic**   Risk Factor: **B**

Fetal Risk Summary

Acetaminophen is routinely used during all stages of pregnancy for pain relief and to lower elevated body temperature. The drug crosses the placenta (1). In therapeutic doses, it is apparently safe for short-term use. However, continuous, high daily dosage in one mother probably caused severe anemia (hemolytic?) in her and fatal kidney disease in her newborn (2).

The pharmacokinetics of acetaminophen in pregnancy have been reported (3). In six healthy women who ingested a 1000-mg dose at 36 weeks' gestation and again 6 weeks after delivery, the mean serum half-lifes were similar, 3.7 hours and 3.1 hours, respectively. The absorption, metabolism, and renal clearance of the drug were similar in the pregnant and nonpregnant states.

The potential for acetaminophen-induced fetal liver toxicity following a toxic maternal dose was first suggested in 1979 (4). In 1984, a case of fetal death was described in this situation. A woman, in her 27th–28th week of pregnancy, ingested 29.5 g of acetaminophen over less than 24 hours for severe dental pain (5). Fetal movements were last felt about 23 hours after the first dose, and on presentation to the hospital 16 hours later, no fetal heart beat was heard. The mother eventually recovered, although her serum levels of acetaminophen by extrapolation were thought to exceed 300 μg/ml, a toxic level. Autopsy of the 2190-g female fetus revealed a liver acetaminophen concentration of 250 μg/g of tissue. The extensive lysis of the fetal liver and kidneys, which may have been caused by autolysis prior to delivery (approximately 3 days after the mother last felt fetal movement), prevented documentation of the characteristic lesions observed in acetaminophen overdose. In four other cases of acute overdosage, acetaminophen-induced fetal liver toxicity was apparently not observed, although such damage may have resolved prior to delivery in some cases (6–9). One woman, at 36 weeks' gestation, consumed a single dose of 22.5 g of acetaminophen producing toxic blood levels of 200 μ/ml (6). She delivered a normal infant approximately 6 weeks later. In another case, a woman at 20 weeks' gestation consumed a total of 25 g in two doses over a 10-hour period (7). She gave birth at 41 weeks to a normal infant with an occipital cephalohematoma due to birth position. At 24 hours of age, the infant developed jaundice that responded to phototherapy. No evidence of permanent liver damage was observed. The jaundice was thought to have been due to the cephalohematoma. A third case of acute maternal overdose occurred at 15.5 weeks of gestation when a mother ingested 64 g of the drug (8). Her acetaminophen level 10 hours after the ingestion was 198.5 μg/ml. Marked hepatic necrosis and adult respiratory distress syndrome (due to aspiration pneumonia) ensued and then gradually resolved. The patient was discharged home approximately 3 weeks after ingestion and subsequently delivered a healthy 2000-g male infant at 32 weeks' gestation. The infant developed physiologic hyperbilirubinemia with a peak level on the 4th day of life of 10.3 mg/100 ml, but phototherapy was not required. Follow-up evaluation at 4 months indicated normal development. The final case involved a 22-year-old woman in her 31st week of pregnancy who consumed a 15-g dose followed by a 50-g dose 1 week later (9). Fetal distress was observed 16 hours after the second overdose as evidenced by complete lack of fetal movements and breathing, a marked decrease in fetal heart rate beat-to-beat variability with no accelerations, and a falling baseline rate. Because of the fetal condition, labor was induced (cesarean section was excluded because of the mother's incipient hepatic failure). Eighty-four hours after the overdose, a healthy 2198-g female infant was delivered with Apgar scores at 1 and 5 minutes of 9 and 10, respectively. Except for hypoglycemia, mild respiratory disease, and mild jaundice, the newborn did well. Liver enzymes were always within the normal range, and the jaundice was compatible with immaturity. Acetaminophen was not detected in the cord blood. Follow-up examinations of the infant at 6 weeks and again at 6 months were normal. In each of these instances, protection against serious or permanent liver damage was probably afforded by the prompt administration of intravenous N-acetylcysteine.

The Rocky Mountain Poison and Drug Center reported the results of a nation-wide study on acetaminophen overdose during pregnancy involving 113 women (10). Of the 60 cases that had appropriate laboratory and pregnancy outcome data, 19 occurred during the 1st trimester, 22 during the 2nd trimester, and 19 during the 3rd trimester. In those cases with a potentially toxic serum level of acetaminophen, early treatment with N-acetylcysteine was statistically associated with an improved pregnancy outcome by lessening the incidence of spontaneous abortion and fetal death. Only one congenital anomaly was observed in the series and that involved a 3rd trimester overdose with nontoxic maternal acetaminophen serum levels (10). Based on these observations, neither acetaminophen nor N-acetylcysteine is a likely teratogen, although follow-up data on the infants were not available (10).

The Collaborative Perinatal Project monitored 50,282 mother-child pairs, 226 of which had 1st trimester exposure to acetaminophen (11, pp. 286–295). Although no evidence was found to suggest a relationship to large categories of major or minor malformations, a possible association, based on three cases, with congenital dislocation of the hip was found (11, p. 471). The statistical significance of this association is unknown, and independent confirmation is required. For use any-time during pregnancy, 781 exposures were recorded (11, p. 434). As with the qualifications expressed for 1st trimester exposure, possible associations with congenital dislocation of the hip (eight cases) and clubfoot (six cases) were found (11, p. 484).

A 1982 report described craniofacial and digital anomalies in an infant exposed *in utero* to large daily doses of acetaminophen and propoxyphene throughout pregnancy (12). The infant also exhibited withdrawal symptoms due to the pro-poxyphene (see also Propoxyphene). The authors speculated with caution that the combination of propoxyphene with other drugs, such as acetaminophen, might have been teratogenic. In a study examining 6509 women with live births, acetaminophen with or without codeine was used by 697 (11%) during the 1st trimester (13). No evidence of a relationship to malformations was observed.

Unlike aspirin, acetaminophen does not affect platelet function, and there is no increased risk of hemorrhage if the drug is given to the mother at term (14, 15). In a study examining intracranial hemorrhage in premature infants, the incidence of bleeding after exposure of the fetus to acetaminophen close to birth was no differ-ent than in nonexposed controls (see also Aspirin) (16).

In a prospective study of 1529 pregnant women studied in the mid-1970s, acetaminophen was used in the first half of pregnancy by 41% (17). Using a com-puterized system for stratifying on maternal alcohol and smoking histories, 421 newborns were selected for follow-up. Of this group, 43.5% had been exposed *in utero* to acetaminophen in the first half of pregnancy. After statistical control of numerous potentially confounding covariates, the data indicated that acetami-nophen was not significantly related to child IQ at 4 years of age or to attention variables (see Aspirin for opposite results). Three physical growth parameters (height, weight, and head circumference) were also not significantly related to *in utero* acetaminophen exposure.

Breast Feeding Summary

Acetaminophen is excreted into breast milk in low concentrations (18–22). A sin-gle case of maculopapular rash on a breast-feeding infant's upper trunk and face was described in 1985 (18). The mother had taken 1 g of the drug at bedtime for 2 days prior to the onset of the symptoms. The rash resolved 24 hours after discontinuing acetaminophen. Two weeks later, the mother took another 1-g dose and the rash recurred in the infant after breast feeding at 3, 8, and 12 hours postdose. Milk levels at 2.25 and 3.25 hours after the dose were 5.78/7.10 μg/ml (right/left breasts) and 3.80/5.95 μg/ml (right/left breasts), respectively. These represented milk:plasma ratios of 0.76 and 0.50, respectively.

Unpublished data obtained from one manufacturer showed that following an oral dose of 650 mg, an average milk level of 11 μg/ml occurred (personal communication, McNeil Laboratories, 1979). Timing of the samples was not provided.

In 12 nursing mothers (nursing 2–22 months) given a single oral dose of 650 mg, peak levels of acetaminophen occurred at 1–2 hours in the range of 10–15 μg/ml (19). Assuming 90 ml of milk were ingested at 3-, 6-, and 9-hour intervals after ingestion, the amount of drug available to the infant was estimated to range from 0.04–0.23% of the maternal dose. Following ingestion of a single analgesic combination tablet containing 324 mg of phenacetin, average milk levels of acetaminophen, the active metabolite, were 0.89 μg/ml (20). Milk:plasma ratios at 1 and 12 hours were 0.91 and 1.42, with a milk half-life of 4.7 hours compared to 3.0 hours in the serum. Repeated doses at 4-hour intervals were expected to result in a steady-state concentration of 2.69 μg/ml. In three lactating women, a mean milk:plasma ratio of 0.76 was reported following a single oral dose of 500 mg of acetaminophen (21). In this case, the mean serum and milk half-lives were 2.7 and 2.6 hours, respectively. Peak milk concentrations of 4.2 μg/ml occurred at 2 hours. In a more recent study, the calculated milk:plasma ratio was approximately 1.0 (22). Based on a dose of 1000 mg, the estimated maximum dose the infant could ingest was 1.85% of the maternal dose. Except for the single case of rash, no other adverse effects of acetaminophen ingestion via breast milk have been reported. The American Academy of Pediatrics considers acetaminophen to be compatible with breast feeding (23).

References

1. Levy G, Garretson LK, Soda DM. Evidence of placental transfer of acetaminophen. Pediatrics 1975;55:895.
2. Char VC, Chandra R, Fletcher AB, Avery GB. Polyhydramnios and neonatal renal failure—a possible association with maternal acetaminophen ingestion. J Pediatr 1975;86:638–9.
3. Rayburn W, Shukla U, Stetson P, Piehl E. Acetaminophen pharmacokinetics: comparison between pregnant and nonpregnant women. Am J Obstet Gynecol 1986;155:1353–6.
4. Rollins DE, Von Bahr C, Glaumann H, Moldens P, Rane H. Acetaminophen: potentially toxic metabolite formed by human fetal and adult liver microsomes and isolated fetal liver cells. Science 1979;205:1414–6.
5. Haibach H, Akhter JE, Muscato MS, Cary PL, Hoffmann MF. Acetaminophen overdose with fetal demise. Am J Clin Pathol 1984;82:240–2.
6. Byer AJ, Taylor TR, Semmer JR. Acetaminophen overdose in the third trimester of pregnancy. JAMA 1982;247:3114–5.
7. Stokes IM. Paracetamol overdose in the second trimester of pregnancy. Case report. Br J Obstet Gynaecol 1984;91:286–8.
8. Ludmir J, Main DM, Landon MB, Gabbe SG. Maternal acetaminophen overdose at 15 weeks of gestation. Obstet Gynecol 1986;67:750–1.
9. Rosevear SK, Hope PL. Favourable neonatal outcome following maternal paracetamol overdose and severe fetal distress: case report. Br J Obstet Gynaecol 1989;96:491–3.
10. Riggs BS, Bronstein AC, Kulig K, Archer PG, Rumack BH. Acute acetaminophen overdose during pregnancy. Obstet Gynecol 1989;74:247–53.

11. Heinonen OP, Slone D, Shapiro S. *Birth Defects and Drugs in Pregnancy*. Littleton:Publishing Sciences Group, 1977.
12. Golden NL, King KC, Sokol RJ. Propoxyphene and acetaminophen: possible effects on the fetus. Clin Pediatr 1982;21:752–4.
13. Aselton P, Jick H, Milunsky A, Hunter JR, Stergachis A. First-trimester drug use and congenital disorders. Obstet Gynecol 1985;65:451–5.
14. Pearson H. Comparative effects of aspirin and acetaminophen on hemostasis. Pediatrics 1978;62(Suppl):926–9.
15. Rudolph AM. Effects of aspirin and acetaminophen in pregnancy and in the newborn. Arch Intern Med 1981;141:358–63.
16. Rumack CM, Guggenheim MA, Rumack BH, Peterson RG, Johnson ML, Braithwaite WR. Neonatal intracranial hemorrhage and maternal use of aspirin. Obstet Gynecol 1981;58(Suppl):52S-6S.
17. Streissguth AP, Treder RP, Barr HM, Shepard TH, Bleyer WA, Sampson PD, Martin DC. Aspirin and acetaminophen use by pregnant women and subsequent child IQ and attention decrements. Teratology 1987;35:211–9.
18. Matheson I, Lunde PKM, Notarianni L. Infant rash caused by paracetamol in breast milk? Pediatrics 1985;76:651–2.
19. Berlin CM Jr, Yaffe SJ, Ragni M. Disposition of acetaminophen in milk, saliva, and plasma of lactating women. Pediatr Pharmacol 1980;1:135–41.
20. Findlay JWA, DeAngelis RL, Kearney MF, Welch RM, Findlay JM. Analgesic drugs in breast milk and plasma. Clin Pharmacol Ther 1981;29:625–33.
21. Bitzen PO, Gustafsson B, Jostell KG, Melander A, Wahlin-Boll E. Excretion of paracetamol in human breast milk. Eur J Clin Pharmacol 1981;20:123–5.
22. Notarianni LJ, Oldham HG, Bennett PN. Passage of paracetamol into breast milk and its subsequent metabolism by the neonate. Br J Clin Pharmacol 1987;24:63–7.
23. Committee on Drugs, American Academy of Pediatrics. Transfer of drugs and other chemicals into human milk. Pediatrics 1989;84:924–36.

Name: **ACETAZOLAMIDE**

Class: **Carbonic Anhydrase Inhibitor**   Risk Factor: **C**

Fetal Risk Summary

Despite widespread usage, no reports linking the use of acetazolamide with congenital defects have been located. A single case of a neonatal sacrococcygeal teratoma has been described (1). The mother received 750 mg daily for glaucoma during the 1st and 2nd trimesters. A relationship between the drug and carcinogenic effects in the fetus has not been supported by other reports. Retrospective surveys on the use of acetazolamide during gestation have not demonstrated an increased fetal risk (2, 3). The Collaborative Perinatal Project monitored 50,282 mother-child pairs, 12 of which had 1st trimester exposure to acetazolamide (4, p. 373). For use anytime during pregnancy, 1,024 exposures were recorded (4, p. 441). In neither case was evidence found to suggest a relationship to large categories of major or minor malformations or to individual defects.

Breast Feeding Summary

Acetazolamide is excreted into breast milk (5). A mother, 6 days postpartum, was given 500 mg (sustained release formulation) twice daily for glaucoma and breast fed her infant for the following week. Nursing was stopped after this time because of the mother's concerns over exposing the infant to the drug. However, no changes attributable to drug exposure were noted in the infant. Breast milk levels of acetazolamide on the 4th and 5th days of therapy, 1–9 hours after a maternal dose, varied between 1.3–2.1 μg/ml. A consistent relationship between concentration and time from last dose was not apparent. A milk:plasma ratio 1 hour after a dose was 0.25. Three plasma levels of acetazolamide in the infant were 0.2, 0.2, and 0.6 μg/ml. The authors estimated the infant ingested about 0.6 mg/day (i.e., 0.06% of the maternal dose) (1).

References

1. Worsham GF, Beckman EN, Mitchell EH. Sacrococcygeal teratoma in a neonate. Association with maternal use of acetazolamide. JAMA 1978;240:251–2.
2. Favre-Tissot M, Broussole P, Robert JM, Dumont L. An original clinical study of the pharmacologic-teratogenic relationship. Ann Med Psychol 1964;1:389. As cited in: Nishimura H, Tanimura T, eds. *Clinical Aspects of The Teratogenicity of Drugs*. New York:Excerpta Medica, 1976;210.
3. McBride WG. The teratogenic action of drugs. Med J Aust 1963;2:689–93.
4. Heinonen OP, Slone D, Shapiro S. *Birth Defects and Drugs in Pregnancy*. Littleton:Publishing Sciences Group, 1977.
5. Soderman P, Hartvig P, Fagerlund C. Acetazolamide excretion into human breast milk. Br J Clin Pharmacol 1984;17:599–60.

Name: **ACETOHEXAMIDE**

Class: **Oral Hypoglycemic**   Risk Factor: **D**

Fetal Risk Summary

Acetohexamide is a sulfonylurea used for the treatment of adult-onset diabetes mellitus. It is not indicated for the pregnant diabetic. When administered near term, acetohexamide crosses the placenta and may persist in the neonatal serum for several days (1). One mother, who took 1 g/day throughout pregnancy, delivered an infant whose serum level was 4.4 mg/100 ml at 10 hours of life (1). Prolonged symptomatic hypoglycemia due to hyperinsulinism lasted for 5 days. If used in pregnancy, acetohexamide should be stopped at least 48 hours before delivery to avoid this complication (2).

Although teratogenic in animals, an increased incidence of congenital defects, other than that expected in diabetes mellitus, has not been found with acetohexamide (see also Chlorpropamide, Tolbutamide) (3–5). Maternal diabetes is known to increase the rate of malformations 2- to 4-fold, but the mechanisms are not understood (see also Insulin). In spite of the lack of evidence for acetohexamide teratogenicity, the drug should not be used in pregnancy since it will not provide good control in patients who cannot be controlled by diet alone (2). The manufacturer recommends the drug not be used in pregnancy (6).

Breast Feeding Summary

No data are available (see Tolbutamide).

References

1. Kemball ML, McIver C, Milnar RDG, Nourse CH, Schiff D, Tiernan JR. Neonatal hypoglycaemia in infants of diabetic mothers given sulphonylurea drugs in pregnancy. Arch Dis Child 1970;45:696–701.
2. Friend JR. Diabetes. Clin Obstet Gynaecol 1981;8:353–82.

3. Malins JM, Cooke AM, Pyke DA, Fitzgerald MG. Sulphonylurea drugs in pregnancy. Br Med J 1964;2:187.
4. Adam PAJ, Schwartz R. Diagnosis and treatment: should oral hypoglycemic agents be used in pediatric and pregnant patients? Pediatrics 1968;42:819–23.
5. Dignan PSJ. Teratogenic risk and counseling in diabetes. Clin Obstet Gynecol 1981;24:149–59.
6. Product information. Dymelor. Eli Lilly and Company, 1985.

Name: **ACETOPHENAZINE**

Class: **Tranquilizer**   Risk Factor: **C**

Fetal Risk Summary

Acetophenazine is a piperazine phenothiazine in the same group as prochlorperazine (see Prochlorperazine). Phenothiazines readily cross the placenta (1). No specific information on the use of acetophenazine in pregnancy has been located. Although occasional reports have attempted to link various phenothiazine compounds with congenital malformations, the bulk of the evidence indicates that these drugs are safe for the mother and the fetus (see also Chlorpromazine).

Breast Feeding Summary

No data are available.

Reference

1. Moya F, Thorndike V. Passage of drugs across the placenta. Am J Obstet Gynecol 1962;84:1778–98.

Name: **ACETYLCHOLINE**

Class: **Parasympathomimetic (Cholinergic)**   Risk Factor: **C**

Fetal Risk Summary

Acetylcholine is used primarily in the eye. No reports of its use in pregnancy have been located. As a quaternary ammonium compound, it is ionized at physiologic pH and transplacental passage in significant amounts would not be expected.

Breast Feeding Summary

No data are availble.

Name: **ACETYLDIGITOXIN**

Class: **Cardiac Glycoside**   Risk Factor: **B**

Fetal Risk Summary.

See Digitalis.

Breast Feeding Summary

See Digitalis.

Name: **ACYCLOVIR**

Class: **Antiviral**   Risk Factor: **C$_M$**

Fetal Risk Summary

Acyclovir is a synthetic acyclic purine nucleoside analogue used as an antiviral agent against the herpes viruses. The drug readily crosses the placenta to the fetus (1–5). After intravenous dosing, acyclovir levels in cord blood were higher than those in maternal serum with ratios of 1.4 and 1.25 reported (1, 2).

Acyclovir has been administered orally and intravenously during all stages of pregnancy, but experience during the 1st trimester is very limited (1–22). In most cases the drug was given in the last third of pregnancy. A review published in 1989 cited a total of 274 published and unpublished cases of pregnant women treated with acyclovir (22). No adverse fetal effects attributable to acyclovir have been reported. A few infants have been followed for periods ranging up to several years. Although developmental problems have not been observed either at birth or later, the number of exposures is still too limited to assess whether long-term sequelae may occur.

Acyclovir applied topically may produce low levels of the drug in maternal serum, urine, and vaginal secretions (23). Although the antiviral agent has been used topically during pregnancy for the treatment of genital herpes, no published reports of these cases have yet appeared. The manufacturer is currently monitoring a group of these women during pregnancy, and data will be available when they deliver (personal communication, Burroughs-Wellcome, 1985). They are also aware of two women treated topically during the 3rd trimester in England who delivered normal infants (personal communication, Burroughs-Wellcome, 1985).

Breast Feeding Summary

Acyclovir is concentrated in human milk with levels usually exceeding those found in maternal serum (24, 25). A woman, breast feeding a 4-month-old infant, was treated with acyclovir 200 mg orally every 3 hours (five times daily) for presumed oral herpes (24). She had taken 15 doses of the drug prior to the study dose. Approximately 9 hours after her fifteenth dose, she was given another 200-mg dose and paired maternal plasma/breast milk samples were drawn at 0, 0.5, 1.5, 2.0, and 3.0 hours. Breast feeding was discontinued during the study interval. Milk:plasma ratios ranged from 0.6–4.1. Milk concentrations were greater than those in maternal serum at all times except at 1.5 hours, the time of peak plasma concentration (4.23 μM) (note: 1 μM = 0.225 μg/ml (22)). The initial level in the milk was 3.3 μM, reflecting the doses taken prior to the study period. The highest level measured in milk was 5.8 μM at 3.2 hours, but this was not the peak concentration because it was still rising at the time of sampling. Acyclovir was demonstrated in the infant's urine. Based on the poor lipid solubility of the drug, the pKa's, and other known pharmacokinetic parameters, the authors calculated a theoretical milk:plasma ratio of 0.15 (24). Since the actual measured ratio was much greater than this value, the authors concluded that acyclovir entered the milk by an active or facilitated process that would make it unique from any other medicinal agent (24). The maximum ingested dose, based on 750 ml of milk/day, was calculated to be 1500 μg/day, approximately 0.2 mg/kg/day in the infant, or about 1.6% of the adult dose. This was thought not to represent an immediate risk to the infant, and in fact, no adverse effects of the exposure were observed in the infant.

In a second case, a woman 1 year postpartum was treated with oral acyclovir, 200 mg five times a day, for presumed herpes zoster (25). The mean concentrations in the milk and serum were 1.06 μg/ml and 0.33 μg/ml, respectively, a milk:plasma ratio of 3.24. Detectable amounts were present in both serum and milk 48 hours after the last dose with an estimated half-life in the milk of 2.8 hours (25). The estimated amount of acyclovir ingested by the infant consuming 1000 ml/day of milk was about 1 mg.

Since acyclovir has been used to treat herpes virus infections in the neonate, and due to the lack of adverse effects in the above cases, mothers undergoing treatment with acyclovir can probably breast feed safely. The American Academy of Pediatrics considers acyclovir to be compatible with breast feeding (26).

References

1. Landsberger EJ, Hager WD, Grossman JH III. Successful management of varicella pneumonia complicating pregnancy: a report of three cases. J Reprod Med 1986;31:311–4.
2. Utley K, Bromberger P, Wagner L, Schneider H. Management of primary herpes in pregnancy complicated by ruptured membranes and extreme prematurity: case report. Obstet Gynecol 1987;69:471–3.
3. Greffe BS, Dooley SL, Deddish RB, Krasny HC. Transplacental passage of acyclovir. J Pediatr 1986;108:1020–1.
4. Haddad J, Simeoni U, Messer J, Willard D. Transplacental passage of acyclovir. J Pediatr 1987;110:164.
5. Kingsley S. Fetal and neonatal exposure to acyclovir [Abstract]. Second World Congress on Sexually Transmitted Diseases, Paris, June 1986. As cited by Haddad J, Simeoni U, Messer J, Willard D. Transplacental passage of acyclovir. J Pediatr 1987;110:164.
6. Lagrew DC Jr, Furlow TG, Hager WD, Yarrish RL. Disseminated herpes simplex virus infection in pregnancy. JAMA 1984;252:2058–9.
7. Grover L, Kane J, Kravitz J, Cruz A. Systemic acyclovir in pregnancy: a case report. Obstet Gynecol 1985;65:284–7.
8. Berger SA, Weinberg M, Treves T, Sorkin P, Geller E, Yedwab G, Tomer A, Rabey M, Michaeli D. Herpes encephalitis during pregnancy: failure of acyclovir and adenine arabinoside to prevent neonatal herpes. Isr J Med Sci 1986;22:41–4.
9. Anderson H, Sutton RNP, Scarffe JH. Cytotoxic chemotherapy and viral infections: the role of acyclovir. J R Coll Physicians Lond 1984;18:51–5.
10. Hockberger RS, Rothstein RJ. Varicella pneumonia in adults: a spectrum of disease. Ann Emerg Med 1986;15:931–4.
11. Glaser JB, Loftus J, Ferragamo V, Mootabar H, Castellano M. Varicella-zoster infection in pregnancy. N Engl J Med 1986;315:1416.
12. Tschen EH, Baack B. Treatment of herpetic whitlow in pregnancy with acyclovir. J Am Acad Dermatol 1987;17:1059–60.
13. Kundsin RB, Falk L, Hertig AT, Horne HW Jr. Acyclovir treatment of twelve unexplained infertile couples. Int J Fertil 1987;32:200–4.
14. Chazotte C, Andersen HF, Cohen WR. Disseminated herpes simplex infection in an immunocompromised pregnancy: treatment with intravenous acyclovir. Am J Perinatol 1987;4:363–4.
15. Cox SM, Phillips LE, DePaolo HD, Faro S. Treatment of disseminated herpes simplex virus in pregnancy with parenteral acyclovir: a case report. J Reprod Med 1986;31:1005–7.

16. Hankins GDV, Gilstrap LC III, Patterson AR. Acyclovir treatment of varicella pneumonia in pregnancy. Crit Care Med 1987;15:336–7.
17. Hankey GR, Bucens MR, Chambers JSW. Herpes simplex encephalitis in third trimester of pregnancy: successful outcome for mother and child. Neurology 1987;37:1534–7.
18. Leen CLS, Mandal BK, Ellis ME. Acyclovir and pregnancy. Br Med J 1987;294:308.
19. Eder SE, Apuzzio JJ, Weiss G. Varicella pneumonia during pregnancy: treatment of two cases with acyclovir. Am J Perinatol 1988;5:16–8.
20. Boyd K, Walker E. Use of acyclovir to treat chickenpox in pregnancy. Br Med J 1988;296:393–4.
21. Brown ZA, Baker DA. Acyclovir therapy during pregnancy. Obstet Gynecol 1989;73:526–31.
22. Key TC, Resnik R, Dittrich HC, Reisner LS. Successful pregnancy after cardiac transplantation. Am J Obstet Gynecol 1989;160:367–71.
23. Product information. Zovirax. Burroughs-Wellcome, 1985.
24. Lau RJ, Emery MG, Galinsky RE. Unexpected accumulation of acyclovir in breast milk with estimation of infant exposure. Obstet Gynecol 1987;69:468–71.
25. Meyer LJ, de Miranda P, Sheth N, Spruance S. Acyclovir in human breast milk. Am J Obstet Gynecol 1988;158:586–8.
26. Committee on Drugs, American Academy of Pediatrics. Transfer of drugs and other chemicals into human milk. Pediatrics 1989;84:924–36.

Name: **ALBUTEROL**

Class: **Sympathomimetic (Adrenergic)**   Risk Factor: C_M

Fetal Risk Summary

Albuterol is a β-sympathomimetic used to prevent premature labor (see also Terbutaline and Ritodrine) (1–12). In an *in vitro* experiment using perfused human placentas, 2.8% of infused drug crossed to the fetal side, but the method only used about 5% of the exchange area of the total placenta (13). Maternal serum concentrations during intravenous and oral albuterol therapy have been reported (14).

No reports linking the use of albuterol to congenital anomalies have been located. In one patient, albuterol was infused continuously for 17 weeks via a catheter placed in the right subclavian vein (10, 15, 16). A normal male infant was delivered within a few hours of stopping the drug. A 1982 report described the use of albuterol in two women with incompetent cervix from the 14th week of gestation to near term (17). Both patients delivered normal infants.

Adverse reactions observed in the fetus and mother following albuterol treatment are secondary to the cardiovascular and metabolic effects of the drug. Albuterol may cause maternal and fetal tachycardia with fetal rates exceeding 160 beats/minute (1–3, 12, 18). Major decreases in maternal blood pressure have been reported with both systolic and diastolic pressures dropping more than 30 mm Hg (2, 4, 6). Fetal distress following maternal hypotension was not mentioned. One study observed a maximum decrease in diastolic pressure of 24 mm Hg (34% decrease) but a rise in systolic pressure (18). Other maternal adverse effects associated with albuterol have been acute congestive heart failure, pulmonary edema, and death (19–27).

Like all β-mimetics, albuterol may cause transient fetal and maternal hyperglycemia followed by an increase in serum insulin (4, 28–31). Cord blood levels of insulin are about twice those of untreated controls and are not dependent on the duration of exposure, gestational age, or birth weight (30, 31). These effects are more pronounced in diabetic patients, especially in juvenile diabetics, with the occurrence of significant increases in glycogenolysis and lipolysis (18, 32, 33). Maternal blood glucose should be closely monitored and neonatal hypoglycemia prevented with adequate doses of glucose.

A group of 20 women in premature labor, treated with oral albuterol 4 mg every 4 hours for several weeks, was matched with a control group of women who were not in premature labor (34). The mean gestational ages at delivery for the treated and nontreated patients were 36.4 and 37.0 weeks, respectively. No significant differences were found between the groups for cord blood concentrations of insulin, triiodothyronine (T3), thyroxine (T4), and thyroid-stimulating hormone (TSH). However, growth hormone levels were significantly higher in the treated group than in controls, 36.5 vs. 17.4 ng/ml, respectively ($P < 0.001$). The investigators did not determine the reason for the elevated growth hormone level but speculated that it could be due either to the use of betamethasone for fetal lung maturation in some women of the albuterol group (and resulting fluctuations in fetal blood glucose and insulin levels) or to direct adrenergic stimulation of the fetal pituitary (34). Of interest, of the 12 women who received betamethasone, cord blood growth hormone levels in 11 were compared to 8 untreated controls. Although the levels in the treated patients were higher, 39.5 vs. 31.4 ng/ml, the difference was not significant.

Albuterol decreases the incidence of neonatal respiratory distress syndrome similar to other β-mimetics (35, 36). Long-term evaluation of infants exposed to *in utero* β-mimetics has been reported but not specifically for albuterol (37, 38). No harmful effects were observed in the infants.

Breast Feeding Summary

No data are available.

References

1. Liggins GC, Vaughan GS. Intravenous infusion of salbutamol in the management of premature labor. J Obstet Gynaecol Br Commonw 1973;80:29–33.
2. Korda AR, Lynerum RC, Jones WR. The treatment of premature labor with intravenous administered salbutamol. Med J Aust 1974;1:744–6.
3. Hastwell G. Salbutamol aerosol in premature labour. Lancet 1975;2:1212–3.
4. Hastwell GB, Halloway CP, Taylor TLO. A study of 208 patients in premature labor treated with orally administered salbutamol. Med J Aust 1978;1:465–9.
5. Hastwell G, Lambert BE. A comparison of salbutamol and ritodrine when used to inhibit premature labour complicated by ante-partum haemorrhage. Curr Med Res Opin 1979;5:785–9.
6. Ng KH, Sen DK. Hypotension with intravenous salbutamol in premature labour. Br Med J 1974;3:257.
7. Pincus R. Salbutamol infusion for premature labour - the Australian trials experience. Aust NZ Obstet Gynaecol 1981;21:1–4.
8. Gummerus M. The management of premature labor with salbutamol. Acta Obstet Gynecol Scand 1981;60:375–7.
9. Crowhurst JA. Salbutamol, obstetrics and anaesthesia: a review and case discussion. Anaesth Intensive Care 1980;8:39–43.
10. Lind T, Godfrey KA, Gerrard J, Bryson MR. Continuous salbutamol infusion over 17 weeks to preempt premature labour. Lancet 1980;2:1165–6.
11. Kuhn RJP, Speirs AL, Pepperell RJ, Eggers TR, Doyle LW, Hutchison A. Betamethasone, albuterol, and threatened premature delivery: benefits and risks. Study of 469 pregnancies. Obstet Gynecol 1982;60:403–8.
12. Eggers TR, Doyle LW, Pepperell RJ. Premature labour. Med J Aust 1979;1:213–6.

13. Sodha RJ, Schneider H. Transplacental transfer of β-adrenergic drugs studied by an *in vitro* perfusion method of an isolated human placental lobule. Am J Obstet Gynecol 1983;147:303–10.
14. Haukkamaa M, Gummerus M, Kleimola T. Serum salbutamol concentrations during oral and intravenous treatment in pregnant women. Br J Obstet Gynaecol 1985;92:1230–3.
15. Boylan P, O'Discoll K. Long-term salbutamol or successful Shirodkar suture? Lancet 1980;2:1374.
16. Addis GJ. Long-term salbutamol infusion to prevent premature labor. Lancet 1981;1:42–3.
17. Edmonds DK, Letchworth AT. Prophylactic oral salbutamol to prevent premature labour. Lancet 1982;1:1310–1.
18. Wager J, Fredholm B, Lunell NO, Persson B. Metabolic and circulatory effects of intravenous and oral salbutamol in late pregnancy in diabetic and non-diabetic women. Acta Obstet Gynecol Scand 1982;Suppl 108:41–6.
19. Whitehead MI, Mander AM, Hertogs K, Williams RM, Pettingale KW. Acute congestive cardiac failure in a hypertensive woman receiving salbutamol for premature labour. Br Med J 1980;280:1221–2.
20. Poole-Wilson PA. Cardiac failure in a hypertensive woman receiving salbutamol for premature labour. Br Med J 1980;281:226.
21. Fogarty AJ. Cardiac failure in a hypertensive woman receiving salbutamol for premature labour. Br Med M 1980;281:226.
22. Davies PDO. Cardiac failure in a hypertensive woman receiving salbutamol for premature labour. Br Med J 1980;281:226–7.
23. Robertson M, Davies AE. Cardiac failure in a hypertensive woman receiving salbutamol for premature labour. Br Med J 1980;281:227.
24. Crowley P. Cardiac failure in a hypertensive woman receiving salbutamol for premature labour. Br Med J 1980;281:227.
25. Whitehead MI, Mander AM, Pettingale KW. Cardiac failure in a hypertensive woman receiving salbutamol for premature labour. Reply. Br Med J 1980;281:227.
26. Davies AE, Robertson MJS. Pulmonary oedema after the administration of intravenous salbutamol and ergometrine—case report. Br J Obstet Gynaecol 1980;87:539–41.
27. Milliez, Blot Ph, Sureau C. A case report of maternal death associated with betamimetics and betamethasone administration in premature labor. Eur J Obstet Gynaecol Reprod Biol 1980;11:95–100.
28. Thomas DJB, Dove AF, Alberti KGMM. Metabolic effects of salbutamol infusion during premature labour. Br J Obstet Gynaecol 1977;84:497–9.
29. Wager J, Lunell NO, Nadal M, Ostman J. Glucose tolerance following oral salbutamol treatment in late pregnancy. Acta Obstet Gynecol Scand 1981;60:291–4.
30. Lunell NO, Joelsson I, Larsson A, Persson B. The immediate effect of a β-adrenergic agonist (salbutamol) on carbohydrate and lipid metabolism during the third trimester of pregnancy. Acta Obstet Gynecol Scand 1977;56:475–8.
31. Procianoy RS, Pinheiro CEA. Neonatal hyperinsulinism after short-term maternal beta sympathomimetic therapy. J Pediatr 1982;101:612–4.
32. Barnett AH, Stubbs SM, Mander AM. Management of premature labour in diabetic pregnancy. Diabetologia 1980;188:365–8.
33. Wager J, Fredholm BB, Lunell NO, Persson B. Metabolic and circulatory effects of oral salbutamol in the third trimester of pregnancy in diabetic and non-diabetic women. Br J Obstet Gynaecol 1981;88:352–61.
34. Desgranges M-F, Moutquin J-M, Peloquin A. Effects of maternal oral salbutamol therapy on neonatal endocrine status at birth. Obstet Gynecol 1987;69:582–4.
35. Hastwell GB. Apgar scores, respiratory distress syndrome and salbutamol. Med J Aust 1980;1:174–5.
36. Hastwell G. Salbutamol and respiratory distress syndrome. Lancet 1977;2:354.
37. Wallace RL, Caldwell DL, Ansbacher R, Otterson WN. Inhibition of premature labor by terbutaline. Obstet Gynecol 1978;51:387–92.
38. Freysz H, Willard D, Lehr A, Messer J, Boog G. A long term evaluation of infants who received a β-mimetic drug while in utero. J Perinat Med 1977;5:94–9.

Name: **ALPHAPRODINE**

Class: **Narcotic Analgesic**   Risk Factor: **C$_M$***

Fetal Risk Summary

No reports linking the use of alphaprodine with congenital defects have been located. Characteristic of all narcotics used in labor, alphaprodine may produce respiratory depression in the newborn (1–8). Tissue pO_2 and pCO_2 were determined in nine women in active labor at term given intravenous alphaprodine, 0.4 mg/kg (prepregnancy weight) (9). Peak decreases in $tcpO_2$ occurred at 5 minutes postinjection with peak increases of $tcpCO_2$ occurring at 20 minutes. Both changes were statistically significant variations from baseline values. The fetal heart rate fell from a mean predose rate of 139 beats/minute to 132 beats/minute at 20 minutes, a significant change, with a consistent loss of variability occurring at 25 minutes. No adverse effects were noted in the mother or the fetus.

In a group of 40 women treated with alphaprodine during labor, sinusoidal fetal heart rate patterns were observed in 17 fetuses (42.5%) (10). The pattern occurred about 19 minutes after administration of the narcotic and persisted for about 60 minutes. No apparent harm resulted from the abnormal patterns.

Suppression of collagen-induced platelet aggregation has been demonstrated, but specific data were not given (11). Abnormal bleeding following use of this drug has not been reported, even though the magnitude of platelet dysfunction was comparable to that found in hemorrhagic states.

[*Risk Factor D if used for prolonged periods or in high doses at term.]

Breast Feeding Summary

No data are available.

References

1. Smith EJ, Nagyfy SF. A report on comparative studies of new drugs used for obstetrical analgesia. Am J Obstet Gynecol 1949;58:695–702.
2. Hapke FB, Barnes AC. The obstetric use and effect on fetal respiration of Nisentil. Am J Obstet Gynecol 1949;58:799–801.
3. Kane WM. The results of Nisentil in 1,000 obstetrical cases. Am J Obstet Gynecol 1953;65:1020–6.
4. Backner DD, Foldes FF, Gordon EH. The combined use of alphaprodine (Nisentil) hydrochloride and levallorphan (Lorfan) tartrate for analgesia in obstetrics. Am J Obstet Gynecol 1957;74:271–82.
5. Gillan JS, Hunter GW, Darner CB, Thompson GR. Meperidine hydrochloride and alphaprodine hydrochloride as obstetric analgesic agents; a double-blind study. Am J Obstet Gynecol 1958;75:1105–10.
6. Roberts H, Kuck MAC. Use of alphaprodine and levallorphan during labour. Can Med Assoc J 1960;83:1088–93.
7. Burnett RG, White CA. Alphaprodine for continuous intravenous obstetric analgesia. Obstet Gynecol 1966;27:472–7.
8. Anthinarayanan PR, Mangurten HH. Unusually prolonged action of maternal alphaprodine causing fetal depression. Q Pediatr Bull (Winter) 1977;3:14–6.
9. Miller FC, Mueller E, McCart D. Maternal and fetal response to alphaprodine during labor. A preliminary study. J Reprod Med 1982;27:439–42.
10. Gray JH, Cudmore DW, Luther ER, Martin TR, Gardner AJ. Sinusoidal fetal heart rate pattern associated with alphaprodine administration. Obstet Gynecol 1978;52:678–81.

11. Corby DG, Schulman I. The effects of antenatal drug administration on aggregation of platelets of newborn infants. J Pediatr 1971;79:307–13.

Name: **AMANTADINE**

Class: **Antiviral/Antiparkinsonism**   Risk Factor: **C_M**

Fetal Risk Summary

A cardiovascular defect (single ventricle with pulmonary atresia) has been reported in an infant exposed to amantadine during the 1st trimester (1). The mother was taking 100 mg/day for a Parkinson-like movement disorder. The relationship between the drug and the defect is unknown. Amantadine is embryotoxic and teratogenic in animals in high doses (1, 2). Theoretically, amantadine may be a human teratogen, but the absence of reports may have more to do with the probable infrequency of use in pregnant patients than to its teratogenic potency (3).

Breast Feeding Summary

Amantadine is excreted into breast milk in low concentrations. Although no reports of adverse effects in nursing infants have been located, the manufacturer recommends the drug be used with caution in nursing mothers because of the potential for urinary retention, vomiting, and skin rash (2).

References

1. Nora JJ, Nora AH, Way GL. Cardiovascular maldevelopment associated with maternal exposure to amantadine. Lancet 1975;2:607.
2. Product Information. Symmetrel. Du Pont Pharmaceuticals, 1985.
3. Coulson AS. Amantadine and teratogenesis. Lancet 1975;2:1044.

Name: **AMBENONIUM**

Class: **Parasympathomimetic (Cholinergic)**   Risk Factor: **C**

Fetal Risk Summary

Ambenonium is a quaternary ammonium chloride with anticholinesterase activity used in the treatment of myasthenia gravis. It has been used in pregnancy, but too little information is available to analyze (1, 2). Because it is ionized at physiologic pH, it would not be expected to cross the placenta in significant amounts. McNall and Jafarnia (1) have cautioned that intravenous anticholinesterases should not be used in pregnancy for fear of inducing premature labor. Although apparently safe for the fetus, cholinesterase inhibitors may affect the condition of the newborn (1). Transient muscular weakness has been observed in about 20% of newborns whose mothers were treated with these drugs during pregnancy.

Breast Feeding Summary

Because it is ionized at physiologic pH, ambenonium would not be expected to be excreted into breast milk (3).

References

1. McNall PG, Jafarnia MR. Management of myasthenia gravis in the obstetrical patient. Am J Obstet Gynecol 1965;92:518–25.
2. Heinonen OP, Slone D, Shapiro S. *Birth Defects and Drugs in Pregnancy.* Littleton:Publishing Sciences Group, 1977:345–56.
3. Wilson JT. Pharmacokinetics of drug excretion. In Wilson JT, ed. *Drugs in Breast Milk.* Australia (Balgowlah):ADIS Press, 1981:17.

Name: **AMIKACIN**

Class: **Antibiotic**   Risk Factor: **C**

Fetal Risk Summary

Amikacin is an aminoglycoside antibiotic. The drug rapidly crosses the placenta into the fetal circulation and amniotic fluid (1–4). Studies in patients undergoing elective abortions in the 1st and 2nd trimesters indicate that amikacin distributes to most fetal tissues except the brain and cerebrospinal fluid (1, 3). The highest fetal concentrations were found in the kidneys and urine. At term, cord serum levels were one-half to one-third of maternal serum levels while measurable amniotic fluid levels did not appear until almost 5 hours postinjection (2).

No reports linking the use of amikacin to congenital defects have been located. Ototoxicity, which is known to occur after amikacin therapy, has not been reported as an effect of *in utero* exposure. However, eighth cranial nerve toxicity in the fetus is well known following exposure to other aminoglycosides (see Kanamycin and Streptomycin) and could potentially occur with amikacin.

Breast Feeding Summary

Amikacin is excreted into breast milk in low concentrations. Following 100- and 200-mg intramuscular doses, only traces of amikacin could be found over 6 hours in two of four patients (2, 5). Since oral absorption of this antibiotic is poor, ototoxicity in the infant would not be expected. However, three potential problems exist for the nursing infant: modification of bowel flora, direct effects on the infant, and interference with the interpretation of culture results if a fever workup is required.

References

1. Bernard B, Abate M, Ballard C, Wehrle P. Maternal-fetal pharmacology of Bβ-K8. Antimicrob Agents Chemother 14th Ann Conf: Abstr 71, 1974.
2. Matsuda C, Mori C, Maruno M, Shiwakura T. A. study of amikacin in the obstetrics field. Jpn J Antibiot 1974;27:633–6.
3. Bernard B, Abate M, Thielen P, Attar H, Ballard C, Wehrle P. Maternal-fetal pharmacological activity of amikacin. J Infect Dis 1977;135:925–31.
4. Flores-Mercado F, Garcia-Mercado J, Estopier-Jauregin C, Galindo-Hernandez E, Diaz-Gonzalez C. Clinical pharmacology of amikacin sulphate: blood, urinary and tissue concentrations in the terminal stage of pregnancy. J Int Med Res 1977;5;292–4.
5. Yuasa M. A study of amikacin in obstetrics and gynecology. Jpn J Antibiot 1974;27;377–81.

Name: **AMILORIDE**

Class: **Diuretic**   Risk Factor: **B$_M$**

Fetal Risk Summary

Amiloride is a potassium-conserving diuretic. Animal studies have not shown adverse effects in the fetus (1). Three reports of fetal exposure to amiloride have been located (2–4). In one case, a malformed fetus was discovered following voluntary abortion in a patient with renovascular hypertension (2). The patient had been treated during the 1st trimester with amiloride, propranolol, and captopril. The left leg of the fetus ended at midthigh without distal development and no obvious skull formation was noted above the brain tissue. The authors attributed the defects to captopril.

The second case involved a 21-year-old woman with Bartter's syndrome who was maintained on amiloride (20–30 mg/day) and potassium chloride (160–300 mEq/day) throughout pregnancy (3). Progressive therapy with the two agents was required to maintain normal potassium levels. Mild intrauterine growth retardation was detected at 30 weeks' gestation with eventual vaginal delivery at 41 weeks' gestation of a 6 pounds 2 ounces (about 2800-g) female infant. No abnormalities were noted in the infant. A normal 3500-g female infant was delivered by cesarean section at 37 weeks' gestation from a mother who had been treated throughout pregnancy with amiloride, hydrochlorothiazide, and amiodarone for severe chronic atrial fibrillation (4).

Breast Feeding Summary

No data are available.

References

1. Product Information. Midamor. Merck Sharpe & Dohme, 1985.
2. Duminy PC, Burger PT. Fetal abnormality associated with the use of captopril during pregnancy. S Afr Med J 1981;60:805.
3. Almeida OD Jr, Spinnato JA. Maternal Bartter's syndrome and pregnancy. Am J Obstet Gynecol 1989;160:1225–6.
4. Robson DJ, Jeeva Raj MV, Storey GCA, Holt DW. Use of amiodarone during pregnancy. Postgrad Med J 1985;61:75–7.

Name: **AMINOCAPROIC ACID**

Class: **Hemostatic**   Risk Factor: **C**

Fetal Risk Summary

Aminocaproic acid was used during the 2nd trimester in a patient with subarachnoid hemorrhage due to multiple intracranial aneurysms (1). The drug was given over 3 days preceding surgery (dosage not given). No fetal toxicity was observed.

Breast Feeding Summary

No data are available.

Reference

1. Willoughby JS. Sodium nitroprusside, pregnancy and multiple intracranial aneurysms. Anaesth Intensive Care 1984;12:358–60.

Name: **AMINOGLUTETHIMIDE**

Class: **Anticonvulsant/Antisteroidogenic**   Risk Factor: **D$_M$**

Fetal Risk Summary

Aminoglutethimide when given throughout pregnancy has been suspected of causing virilization (1, 2). No adverse effect was seen when exposure was limited to the 1st and early 2nd trimesters (3, 4). Virilization may be due to inhibition of adrenocortical function.

Breast Feeding Summary

No data are available.

References

1. Iffy L, Ansell JS, Bryant FS, Hermann WL. Nonadrenal female pseudohermaphroditism: an unusual case of fetal masculinization. Obstet Gynecol 1965;26;59–65.
2. Marek J, Horky K. Aminoglutethimide administration in pregnancy. Lancet 1970;2:1312–3.
3. Le Maire WJ, Cleveland WW, Bejar RL, Marsh JM, Fishman L. Aminoglutethimide: a possible cause of pseudohermaphroditism in females. Am J Dis Child 1972;124:421–3.
4. Hanson TJ, Ballonoff LB, Northcutt RC. Aminoglutethimide and pregnancy. JAMA 1974;230:963–4.

Name: **AMINOPHYLLINE**

Class: **Spasmolytic/Vasodilator**   Risk Factor: **C**

Fetal Risk Summary

See Theophylline.

Breast Feeding Summary

See Theophylline.

Name: **AMINOPTERIN**

Class: **Antineoplastic**   Risk Factor: **X**

Fetal Risk Summary

Aminopterin is an antimetabolite antineoplastic agent. It is structurally similar to and has been replaced by methotrexate (amethopterin). Several reports have described fetal anomalies when the drug was used as an unsuccessful abortifacient (1–8). The malformations included:

Meningocephalocele	Cleft lip/palate
Cranial anomalies	Low-set ears
Abnormal positioning of extremities	Hypoplasia of thumb and fibula
Short forearms	Brachycephaly
Hydrocephaly	Anencephaply
Talipes	Clubfoot
Incomplete skull ossification	Syndactyly
Mental retardation	Hypognathia or retrognathia

Use of aminopterin in the 2nd and 3rd trimesters has not been associated with congenital defects (8). Long-term studies of growth and mental development in offspring exposed to aminopterin during the 2nd trimester, the period of neuroblast multiplication, have not been conducted (9).

Breast Feeding Summary

No data are available.

References

1. Meltzer HJ. Congenital anomalies due to attempted abortion with 4–aminopteroglutamic acid. JAMA 1956;161:1253.
2. Warkany J, Beaudry PH, Hornstein S. Attempted abortion with aminopterin (4–amino-pteroyl-glutamic acid). Am J Dis Child 1959;97:274–881.
3. Shaw EB, Steinbach HL. Aminopterin-induced fetal malformation. Am J Dis Child 1968;115:477–82.
4. Brandner M, Nussle D. Foetopathic due a l'aminopterine avec stenose cogenitale de l'espace medullaire des os tubulaires ongs. Ann Radiol 1969;12:705–10.
5. Shaw EB. Fetal damage due to maternal aminopterin ingestion: follow-up at age 9 years. Am J Dis Child 1972;124:93–4.
6. Reich EW, Cox RP, Becker MH, Genieser NB, McCarthy JG, Converse JM. Recognition in adult patients of malformations induced by folic acid antagonists. Birth Defects 1978;14:139–60.
7. Shaw EB, Rees EL. Fetal damage due to aminopterin ingestion: follow-up at 17 1/2 years of age. Am J Dis Child 1980;134:1172–3.
8. Nicholson HO. Cytotoxic drugs in pregnancy; review of reported cases. J Obstet Gynaecol Br Commonw 1968;75:307–12.
9. Dobbing J. Pregnancy and leukemia. Lancet 1977;1:1155.

Name: *para*-AMINOSALICYLIC ACID

Class: **Antitubercular**   Risk Factor: **C**

Fetal Risk Summary

The Collaborative Perinatal Project monitored 50,282 mother-child pairs, 43 of which had 1st trimester exposure to *para*-aminosalicylic acid (4–aminosalicyclic acid) (1). Congenital defects were found in five infants. This incidence (11.6%) was nearly twice the expected frequency. No major category of malformations or individual defects were identified. An increased malformation rate for ear, limb, and hypospadias has been reported for 123 patients taking 7–14 g of *para*-aminosalicylic acid per day with other antitubercular drugs (2). An increased risk of congenital defects has not been found in other studies (3–5).

Breast Feeding Summary

Para-aminosalicylic acid is excreted into human breast milk. In one non-breast-feeding patient given an oral 4-g dose of the drug, a peak milk concentration of 1.1 µg/ml was measured at 3 hours with an elimination half-life of 2.5 hours (6). The peak maternal plasma concentration, 70.1 µg/ml, occurred at 2 hours.

References

1. Heinonen OP, Slone D, Shapiro S. *Birth Defects and Drugs in Pregnancy*. Littleton:Publishing Sciences Group, 1977:299.
2. Varpela E. On the effect exerted by first line tuberculosis medicines on the foetus. Acta Tuberc Scand 1964;35:53–69.
3. Lowe CR. Congenital defects among children born to women under supervision or treatment for pulmonary tuberculosis. Br J Prev Soc Med 1964;18:14–6.
4. Wilson EA, Thelin TJ, Ditts PV. Tuberculosis complicated by pregnancy. Am J Obstet Gynecol 1973;115;526–9.
5. Scheinhorn DJ, Angelillo VA. Antituberculosis therapy in pregnancy. Risk to the fetus. West J Med 1977;127;195–8.
6. Holdiness MR. Antituberculosis drugs and breast-feeding. Arch Intern Med 1984;144:1888.

Name: **AMIODARONE**

Class: **Antiarrhythmic**   Risk Factor: **C**

Fetal Risk Summary

Amiodarone is an antiarrhythmic agent used for difficult or resistant cases of arrhythmias. The drug contains about 75 mg of iodine per 200-mg dose (1–3).

Amiodarone and its metabolite, desethylamiodarone, cross the placenta to the fetus (1–6). In six infants, cord blood concentrations of the parent compound were 0.05–0.35 µg/ml, representing cord:maternal ratios of 0.10–0.28 (mean 0.14). Cord blood concentrations of the metabolite varied between 0.15–0.55 µg/ml, about one-fourth of the maternal levels.

In eight cases of amiodarone therapy during pregnancy, the antiarrhythmic was administered for maternal indications (1–4, 6, 7). One patient in the last 3 months of pregnancy was treated with 200 mg daily for resistant atrial tachycardia (1). A second woman was also treated by these investigators under similar conditions. Both infants were normal, including normal thyroid function. In another report, a woman was treated at 34 weeks' gestation when quinidine failed to control her atrial fibrillation (2). After an initial dose of 800 mg/day for 1 week, the dose was decreased to 400 mg/day and continued at this level until delivery at 41 weeks' gestation. The healthy 3220-g infant developed bradycardia during labor induction (104–120 beats/minute) and during the first 48 hours after birth. No other adverse effects were observed in the infant, who had normal thyroid and liver function tests. A woman was treated during the 37th–39th weeks of pregnancy with daily doses of 600 mg, 400 mg, and 200 mg, each for 1 week for atrial tachycardia resistant to propranolol, digoxin, and verapamil (3). No bradycardia or other abnormalities were noted in the newborn. The infant's thyroid stimulating hormone (TSH) level on the 4th day was 9 mU/L, a normal value. Goiter was not observed and the infant was clinically euthyroid. A 1985 report described the treatment of two women with amiloride for maternal heart conditions (4). One of these patients, a 31-year-old woman with atrial fibrillation, was treated with amiloride, 200 mg/day, and diuretics throughout gestation. She delivered a healthy 3500-g girl without goiter or corneal changes at 37 weeks' gestation. A cord blood thyroxine (T4) level was elevated (209 nmol/L) which was still elevated 1 week later (207 nmol/L), but TSH concentrations at these times were 3.2 mU/L and <1 mU/L (both normal), respectively. The second woman, a 27-year-old primigravida, was treated with amiodarone, 400–800 mg/day, starting at 22 weeks' gestation. Fetal bradycardia, 100–120 beats/minute, was observed at approximately 33 weeks' gestation. Spontaneous labor ensued at 39 weeks with delivery of a healthy 2900-g boy. Thyroid function studies were not reported but "all neonatal examinations were normal" (4). A woman in her 16th week of pregnancy presented with severe atrial fibrillation and was treated with amiodarone, 800 mg/day for 1 week followed by 200 mg/day for the remainder of her pregnancy (6). She delivered a 2660-g boy in the 39th week of gestation who had no goiter and whose free T4 index, serum free triiodothyronine (T3), and serum TSH concentrations were all within normal limits. Follow-up of the infant at 6 months was normal. In another case, a woman was treated with propranolol and amiodarone, 400 mg/day for 4 days each week, throughout gestation (7). A healthy 2670-g female infant was delivered, but the gestational age was not specified. No goiter or corneal microdeposits were present in the infant and clinically she was euthyroid. The T4 and TSH levels in cord blood were both normal although a total serum iodine level (290 μg/100 ml) was markedly elevated (normal 5.5–17.4 μg/100 ml) (7).

Three cases of amiodarone therapy for refractive fetal tachycardia have been described in the literature (5, 8, 9). In the first of these, a fetus at 27 weeks' gestation experienced tachycardia, 260 beats/minute, unresponsive to digoxin and propranolol (7). Lidocaine and procainamide lowered the heart rate somewhat but were associated with unacceptable maternal toxicity. Amiodarone combined with verapamil was successful in halting the tachycardia and reversing the signs of congestive heart failure. An amiodarone maintenance dose of 400 mg/day was required for control. Spontaneous labor occurred after 39 days of therapy with delivery at 33 weeks' gestation of a 2700-g male infant. Atrial flutter with a 2:1 block and a ventricular rate of 200 beats/minute were converted on the 3rd day by electrical cardioversion. No adverse effects from the drug therapy were mentioned. A fetus with supraventricular tachycardia, 220 beats/minute, showed evidence of congestive failure at 32 weeks' gestation (5). Maternal therapy with digoxin alone or in combination with sotalol (a β-blocker) or verapamil failed to stop the abnormal rhythm. Digoxin was then combined with amiodarone, 1600 mg/day for 4 days, then 1200 mg/day for 3 days, then 800 mg/day for 6 weeks. The fetal heart rate fell to 140 beats/minute after 14 days of therapy, and the signs of congestive failure gradually resolved. Neonatal thyroid indices at birth (about 38 weeks' gestation) and at 1 month were as follows (normal values are shown in parentheses): free T3 index 3.4 and 5.6 pmol/L (4.3–8.6 pmol/L); free T4 index 5.4 and 25 pmol/L (9–26 pmol/L); T3 1.7 and 2.7 nmol/L (1.2–3.1 nmol/L); T4 196 and 300 nmol/L (70–175 nmol/L); and TSH 30 and 4.12 mU/L (<5 mU/L). The elevated T4 level returned to normal at a later unspecified time. No mention was made if a goiter was present at birth. At 10 months of age, all thyroid function tests were within normal limits. The third case involved a fetus at 30 weeks of gestation with tachycardia, 220 beats/minute, with congestive heart failure that had not responded to digoxin and propranolol (9). At 32 weeks of gestation, digoxin and amiodarone lowered the rate to 110–180 beats/minute with improvement in the congestive failure. Amiodarone was given at 1200 mg/day for 3 days, then 600 mg/day until delivery 3 weeks later. The newborn had tachycardia to 200 beats/minute that was treated with digoxin, furosemide, and propranolol. Hypothyroidism was diagnosed based on the presence of a goiter and abnormal thyroid tests (normal values are in parentheses): T4 48 μg/ml (70–180 μg/ml); free T4 0.5 μg/ml (>1.5 μg/ml); and TSH >240 mU/L (<30 mu/L). The infant was treated with 10 μg/day of T4 until age 3 months, at which time his cardiac and thyroid functions were normal. Follow-up at 15 months was normal.

Investigators using amiodarone during pregnancy have been concerned about the effects of iodine, contained in each dose, on the fetal thyroid gland (see Potassium Iodide for fetal effects of iodine). However, only 1 of the 11 exposed newborns apparently had goiter (the presence or absence of a goiter was not mentioned in 2 of the remaining 10 cases), and most had normal thyroid function tests. Other abnormalities associated with amiodarone, such as corneal defects, were also absent.

Following chronic administration, amiodarone has a very long elimination half-life of 14–58 days (10). Therefore, the drug must be stopped several months before conception to avoid exposure in early gestation. Although no adverse effects other than transient bradycardia and mild reversible thyroid dysfunction have been observed, the drug should be used with caution during pregnancy due to the limited data available. A 1987 review of the management of cardiac arrhythmias during pregnancy recommends that amiodarone be restricted to refractive cases (11). Newborns exposed to amiodarone *in utero* should have thyroid function studies performed because of the large proportion of iodine contained in each dose.

Breast Feeding Summary

Amiodarone is excreted into breast milk (2, 3). The drug contains about 75 mg of iodine/200-mg dose (2–4). One woman, consuming 400 mg/day, had milk levels of amiodarone and its metabolite, desethylamiodarone (activity unknown), determined at varying times between 9–63 days after delivery (2). Levels of the two substances in milk were highly variable during any 24-hour period. Peak levels of amiodarone and the metabolite ranged from 3.6–16.4 μg/ml and 1.3–6.5 μg/ml. The milk:plasma ratio of the active drug at 9 weeks postpartum ranged from 2.3–9.1 and that of desethylamiodarone from 0.8–3.8. The authors calculated the nursing infant received about 1.4–1.5 mg/kg/day of active drug. Plasma levels of amiodarone in the infant remained constant at 0.4 μg/ml (about 25% of maternal plasma) from birth to 63 days. In a second case, a mother taking 200 mg/day did not breast feed, but milk levels of the drug and the metabolite on the 2nd and 3rd days after delivery were 0.5–1.8 μg/ml and 0.4–0.8 μg/ml, respectively (3).

Although no adverse effects were observed in the one breast-fed infant, relatively large amounts of the drug and its metabolite are available through the milk.

Amiodarone, after chronic administration, has a very long elimination half-life of 14–58 days in adults (10). Data in pediatric patients suggests a more rapid elimination, but the half-life in newborns has not been determined. The effects of chronic neonatal exposure to this drug are unknown. Because of this uncertainty and also due to the high proportion of iodine contained in each dose (see also Potassium Iodide), breast feeding is not recommended if the mother is currently taking amiodarone or has taken it chronically within the past several months.

References

1. Candelpergher G, Buchberger R, Suzzi GL, Padrini R. Transplacental passage of amiodarone: electrocardiographic and pharmacologic evidence in a newborn. G Ital Cardiol 1982;12:79–82.
2. McKenna WJ, Harris L, Rowland E, Whitelaw A, Storey G, Holt D. Amiodarone therapy during pregnancy. Am J Cardiol 1983;51:1231–3.
3. Pitcher D, Leather HM, Storey GAC, Holt DW. Amiodarone in pregnancy. Lancet 1983;1:597–8.
4. Robson DJ, Jeeva Raj MV, Storey GAC, Holt DW. Use of amiodarone during pregnancy. Postgrad Med J 1985;61:75–7.
5. Arnoux P, Seyral P, Llurens M, Djiane P, Potier A, Unal D, Cano JP, Serradimigni A, Rouault F. Amiodarone and digoxin for refractory fetal tachycardia. Am J Cardiol 1987;59:166–7.
6. Penn IM, Barrett PA, Pannikote V, Barnaby PF, Campbell JB, Lyons NR. Amiodarone in pregnancy. Am J Cardiol 1985;56:196–7.
7. Rey E, Bachrach LK, Burrow GN. Effects of amiodarone during pregnancy. Can Med Assoc J 1987;136:959–60.
8. Rey E, Duperron L, Gauthier R, Lemay M, Grignon A, LeLorier J. Transplacental treatment of tachycardia-induced fetal heart failure with verapamil and amiodarone: a case report. Am J Obstet Gynecol 1985;153:311–2.
9. Laurent M, Betremieux P, Biron Y, LeHelloco A. Neonatal hypothyroidism after treatment by amiodarone during pregnancy. Am J Cardiol 1987;60:942.
10. Sloskey GE. Amiodarone: a unique antiarrhythmic agent. Clin Pharm 1983;2:330–40.
11. Rotmensch HH, Rotmensch S, Elkayam U. Management of cardiac arrhythmias during pregnancy: current concepts. Drugs 1987;33:623–33.

Name: **AMITRIPTYLINE**

Class: **Antidepressant**   Risk Factor: **D**

Fetal Risk Summary

Limb reduction anomalies have been reported with amitriptyline (1). However, analysis of 522,630 births, 86 with 1st trimester exposure to amitriptyline, did not confirm an association with this defect (2–9). Reported malformations other than limb reduction defects include (4, 8, 9):

> Micrognathia, anomalous right mandible, left pes equinovaruus (1 case)
> Swelling of hands and feet (1 case)
> Hypospadias (1 case)

Neonatal withdrawal following *in utero* exposure to other antidepressants (see Imipramine) has been reported but not with amitriptyline. However, the potential for this complication exists due to the close similarity among these compounds.

Urinary retention in the neonate has been associated with maternal use of nortriptyline, an amitriptyline metabolite (see Nortriptyline) (10).

Breast Feeding Summary

Amitriptyline and its metabolite, nortriptyline, are excreted into breast milk (11–13). Serum and milk concentrations of amitriptyline in one patient were 0.14 and 0.15 µg/ml, respectively, a milk:plasma ratio of 1.0 (11). No drug was detected in the infant's serum. In another patient, it was estimated that the baby received about 1% of the mother's dose (13). No clinical signs of drug activity were observed in the infant.

Although levels of amitriptyline and its metabolite have not been detected in infant serum, the effects of exposure to small amounts in the milk are not known (11–14). The American Academy of Pediatrics classifies amitriptyline as a drug whose effect on the nursing infant is unknown but may be of concern (15).

References

1. McBride WG. Limb deformities associated with iminodibenzyl hydrochloride. Med J Aust 1972;1:492.
2. Australian Drug Evaluation Committee. Tricyclic antidepressants and limb reduction deformities. Med J Aust 1973;1:768–9.
3. Heinonen OP, Slone D, Shapiro S. *Birth Defects and Drugs in Pregnancy*. Littleton:Publishing Sciences Group, 1977:336–7.
4. Idanpaan-Heikkila J, Saxen L. Possible teratogenicity of imipramine/chloropyramine. Lancet 1973;2:282–3.
5. Rachelefsky GS, Glynt JW, Ebbin AJ, Wilson MG. Possible teratogenicity of tricyclic antidepressants. Lancet 1972;1:838.
6. Banister P, Dafoe C, Smith ESO, Miller J. Possible teratogenicity of tricyclic antidepressants. Lancet 1972;1:838–9.
7. Scanlon FJ. Use of antidepressant drugs during the first trimester. Med J Aust 1969;2:1077.
8. Crombie DL, Pinsent R, Fleming D. Imipramine in pregnancy. Br Med J 1972;1:745.
9. Kuenssberg EV, Knox JDE. Imipramine in pregnancy. Br Med J 1972;2:292.
10. Shearer WT, Schreiner RL, Marshall RE. Urinary retention in a neonate secondary to maternal ingestion of nortriptyline. J Pediatr 1972;81:570–2.
11. Bader TF, Newman K. Amitriptyline in human breast milk and the nursing infants serum. Am J Psychiatry 1980;137;855–6.
12. Wilson JT, Brown D, Cherek DR, Dailey JW, Hilman B, Jobe PC, Manno BR, Manno JE, Redetzki HM, Stewart JJ. Drug excretion in human breast milk. Principles, pharmacokinetics and projected consequences. Clin Pharmacokinet 1980;5:1–66.
13. Brixen-Rasmussen L, Halgrener J, Jorgensen A. Amitriptyline and nortriptyline excretion in human breast milk. Psychopharmacology (Berlin) 1982;76:94–5.
14. Erickson SH, Smith GH, Heidrich F. Tricyclics and breast feeding. Am J Psychiatry 1979;136:1483.
15. Committee on Drugs, American Academy of Pediatrics. Transfer of drugs and other chemicals into human milk. Pediatrics 1989;84:924–36.

Name: AMMONIUM CHLORIDE

Class **Expectorant/Urinary Acidifier**   Risk Factor: **B**

Fetal Risk Summary

The Collaborative Perinatal Project monitored 50,282 mother-child pairs, 365 of which had 1st trimester exposure to ammonium chloride as an expectorant in cough medications (1, pp. 378–381). For use anytime during pregnancy, 3,401 exposures were recorded (1, p. 442). In neither case was evidence found to suggest a relationship to large categories of major or minor malformations. Three possible associations with individual malformations were found but the statistical significance of these is unknown (1, pp. 478, 496). Independent confirmation is required to determine the actual risk.

Inguinal hernia (1st trimester only) (11 cases)
Cataract (6 cases)
Any benign tumor (17 cases)

When consumed in large quantities near term, ammonium chloride may cause acidosis in the mother and the fetus (2, 3). In some cases, the decreased pH and pCO_2, increased lactic acid, and reduced oxygen saturation were as severe as those seen with fatal apnea neonatorum. However, the newborns did not appear in distress.

Breast Feeding Summary

No data are available.

References

1. Heinonen OP, Slone D, Shapiro S. *Birth Defects and Drugs in Pregnancy.* Littleton:Publishing Sciences Group, 1977.
2. Goodlin RC, Kaiser IH. The effect of ammonium chloride induced maternal acidosis on the human fetus at term. I. pH, hemoglobin, blood gases. Am J Med Sci 1957;233:666–74.
3. Kaiser IH, Goodlin RC. The effect of ammonium chloride induced maternal acidosis on the human fetus at term. II. Electrolytes. Am J Med Sci 1958;235:549–54.

Name: **AMOBARBITAL**

Class **Sedative/Hypnotic**   Risk Factor: **D***

Fetal Risk Summary

Amobarbital is a member of the barbiturate class. The drug crosses the placenta, achieving levels in the cord serum similar to the maternal serum (1, 2). Single or continuous dosing of the mother near term does not induce amobarbital hydroxylation in the fetus as demonstrated by the prolonged elimination of the drug in the newborn (half-life 2.5 times maternal). An increase in the incidence of congenital defects in infants exposed *in utero* to amobarbital has been reported (3; 4, pp. 336, 344). One survey of 1,369 patients exposed to multiple drugs found 273 who received amobarbital during the 1st trimester (3). Ninety-five of the exposed mothers delivered infants with major or minor abnormalities. Malformations associated with barbiturates, in general, were:

Anencephaly
Congenital heart disease
Severe limb deformities
Cleft lip and palate
Intersex
Papilloma of the forehead
Hydrocele

Congenital dislocation of the hip
Soft-tissue deformity of the neck
Hypospadias
Accessory auricle
Polydactyly
Nevus

The Collaborative Perinatal Project monitored 50,282 mother-child pairs, 298 of which had 1st trimester exposure to amobarbital (4, pp. 336, 344). For use anytime during pregnancy, 867 exposures were recorded (4, p. 438). A possible association was found between the use of the drug in the 1st trimester and the following:

Cardiovascular malformations (7 cases)
Polydactyly in blacks (2 cases in 29 blacks)
Genitourinary malformations other than hypospadias (3 cases)
Inguinal hernia (9 cases)
Clubfoot (4 cases)

In contrast to the above reports, a 1964 survey of 187 pregnant patients who had received various neuroleptics, including amobarbital, found a 3.1% incidence of malformations in the offspring (5). This is approximately the expected incidence of abnormalities in a nonexposed population. Arthrogryposis and multiple defects were reported in an infant exposed to amobarbital during the 1st trimester (6). The defects were attributed to immobilization of the limbs at the time of joint formation, multiple drug use, and active tetanus.

[*Risk Factor B according to manufacturer—Eli Lilly & Co., 1985].

Breast Feeding Summary

No data are available.

References

1. Kraver B, Draffan GH, Williams FM, Calre RA, Dollery CT, Hawkins DF. Elimination kinetics of amobarbital in mothers and newborn infants. Clin Pharmacol Ther 1973;14:442–7.
2. Draffan GH, Dollery CT, Davies DS, Krauer B, Williams FM, Clare RA, Trudinger BJ, Darling M, Sertel H, Hawkins DF. Maternal and neonatal elimination of amobarbital after treatment of the mother with barbiturates during late pregnancy. Clin Pharmacol Ther 1976;19:271–5.
3. Nelson MM, Forfar JO. Associations between drugs administered during pregnancy and congenital abnormalities of the fetus. Br Med J 1971;1:523–7.
4. Heinonen OP, Slone D, Shapiro S. Birth Defects and Drugs in Pregnancy. Littleton:Publishing Sciences Group, 1977.
5. Favre-Tissot M. An original clinical study of the pharmacologic-teratogenic relationship. Ann Med Psychol (Paris) 1967:389.
6. Jago RH. Arthrogryposis following treatment of maternal tetanus with muscle relaxants. Arch Dis Child 1970;45:277–9.

Name: **AMOXAPINE**

Class **Antidepressant**   Risk Factor: **C$_M$**

Fetal Risk Summary

No reports linking the use of amoxapine with congenital defects have been located. Animal studies have demonstrated embryotoxicity and fetotoxicity but no teratogenic effects (1).

Breast Feeding Summary

Amoxapine and its metabolite are excreted into breast milk. A 29-year-old woman suffering from depression was treated with approximately 250 mg/day of amoxapine (2). She developed galactorrhea and oligomenorrhea. Milk samples were collected after 10 and 11 months of therapy and analyzed for amoxapine and the active metabolite, 8-hydroxyamoxapine. The levels of the parent compound at the sample collection times were both less than 20 ng/ml, but the metabolite was present in both samples, 45 minutes after the last dose at 10 months and 11.5 hours after the last dose at 11 months. Levels of the active metabolite at these times were 113 ng/ml and 168 ng/ml, respectively. A venous blood specimen obtained simultaneously with the first milk sample had concentrations of amoxapine and 8-hydroxyamoxapine of 97 ng/ml and 375 ng/ml, respectively. The American Academy of Pediatrics classifies amoxapine as a drug whose effect on the nursing infant is unknown but may be of concern (3).

References

1. Product information. Asendin. Lederle Laboratories, 1990.
2. Gelenberg AJ. Amoxapine, a new antidepressant, appears in human milk. J Nerv Ment Dis 1979;167:635–6.
3. Committee on Drugs, American Academy of Pediatrics. Transfer of drugs and other chemicals into human milk. Pediatrics 1989;84:924–36.

Name: **AMOXICILLIN**

Class: **Antibiotic**   Risk Factor: **B**

Fetal Risk Summary

Amoxicillin is a penicillin antibiotic similar to ampicillin (see also Ampicillin). No reports linking its use to congenital defects have been located. The Collaborative Perinatal Project monitored 50,282 mother-child pairs, 3,546 of which had 1st trimester exposure to penicillin derivatives (1, pp. 297–313). For use anytime during pregnancy, 7,171 exposures were recorded (1, p. 435). In neither case was evidence found to suggest a relationship to large categories of major or minor malformations or to individual defects. Amoxicillin has been used as a single 3-g dose to treat bacteriuria in pregnancy without causing fetal harm (2, 3).

Amoxicillin depresses both plasma-bound and urinary excreted estriol (see also Ampicillin) (4). Urinary estriol was formerly used to assess the condition of the fetoplacental unit, but this is now done by measuring plasma unconjugated estriol, which is not usually affected by amoxicillin.

Breast Feeding Summary

Amoxicillin is excreted into breast milk in low concentrations. Following a 1-g oral dose given to six mothers, peak milk levels occurred at 4–5 hours, averaging 0.9 μg/ml (range 0.68–1.3 μg/ml) (5). Mean milk:plasma ratios at 1, 2, and 3 hours were 0.014, 0.013, and 0.043, respectively. Although no adverse effects have been observed, three potential problems exist for the nursing infant: modification of bowel flora, direct effects on the infant (e.g., allergy/sensitization), and interference with the interpretation of culture results if a fever workup is required.

References

1. Heinonen OP, Slone D, Shapiro S. *Birth Defects and Drugs in Pregnancy*. Littleton:Publishing Sciences Group, 1977.
2. Masterton RG, Evans DC, Strike PW. Single-dose amoxycillin in the treatment of bacteriuria in pregnancy and the puerperium—a controlled clinical trial. Br J Obstet Gynaecol 1985;92:498–505.
3. Jakobi P, Neiger R, Merzbach D, Paldi E. Single-dose antimicrobial therapy in the treatment of asymptomatic bacteriuria in pregnancy. Am J Obstet Gynecol 1987;156:1148–52.
4. Van Look PFA, Top-Huisman M, Gnodde HP. Effect of ampicillin or amoxycillin administration on plasma and urinary estrogen levels during normal pregnancy. Eur J Obstet Gynaecol Reprod Biol 1981;12:225–33.
5. Kafetzis D, Siafas C, Georgakopoulos P, Papadatos C. Passage of cephalosporins and amoxicillin into the breast milk. Acta Paediatr Scand 1981;70:285–8.

Name: **AMPHETAMINE**

Class: **Central Stimulant**　　　　　　　　　　　　Risk Factor: C_M

Fetal Risk Summary

The amphetamines are a group of sympathomimetic drugs that are used to stimulate the central nervous system. Members of this group include amphetamine, dextroamphetamine, and methamphetamine. A number of studies have examined the possible relationship between amphetamines and adverse fetal outcome. Women were using these drugs for appetite suppression, narcolepsy, or illicit abuse purposes.

The question whether amphetamines are teratogenic in humans has been examined in a number of studies and single-patient case histories. Cardiac malformations and other defects were produced in mice injected with very large doses (about 200 times the usual human dose) of detroamphetamine (1). These same investigators then retrospectively and prospectively examined human infants whose mothers had ingested the drug (2). In the retrospective portion of the study, 219 infants and children under 2 years of age with congenital heart disease were compared with 153 similarly aged infants and children without heart defects. Neither maternal exposure to dextroamphetamine during pregnancy nor exposure during the vulnerable period differed statistically between the groups. However, a positive family history of congenital heart disease occurred in 31.1% of the infants with the defects compared to only 5.9% of the control group ($p = 0.001$). The prospective study compared 52 mothers with a documented exposure to dextroamphetamine during the vulnerable period to 50 nonexposed mothers. Neither group produced an infant with congenital heart disease, and the numbers of other congenital abnormalities were similar (nine vs. seven). Thus, this study found no evidence for an association between congenital heart defects and dextroamphetamine. However, in a follow-up study published 3 years later, the investigators reported a significant relationship between dextroamphetamine exposure and heart defects (3). Comparing 184 infants under 1 year of age with congenital heart disease with 108 controls, significant differences were found for maternal exposure to dextroamphetamine (18% vs. 8%, $p < 0.05$), exposure during the vulnerable period (11% vs. 3%, $p = 0.025$), and positive family history of congenital heart disease (27% vs. 6%, $p < 0.001$). Infants who were both exposed during the vulnerable period and who had a positive family history were statistically similar for the groups (5% vs. 1%).

In a fourth study by the above investigative group, 240 women were followed prospectively during their pregnancies to determine exposure to medicinal agents, radiation, and other potential teratogens (4). Thirty-one (13%) consumed an appetite suppressant (usually dextroamphetamine) during the 1st trimester and an additional 34 (14%) were exposed later in pregnancy. Eight (3.3%) babies had a major congenital defect noted at birth, which is approximately the expected incidence in the United States. Three of the affected infants had been exposed during the 1st trimester to an appetite suppressant. Although the authors identified a wide range of maternal drug consumption during the 1st trimester, no conclusions as to the etiology of the defects can be drawn from the data.

Four other reports have related various defects with amphetamine exposure (5–8). An infant with a bifid exencephalia was delivered from a mother who took 20–30 mg of dextroamphetamine daily throughout pregnancy (5). The infant died after an attempt was made at surgical correction. A second case involved a mother who ingested dextroamphetamine daily for appetite suppression and who delivered a full-term infant. The infant died 6 days later as a result of a congenital heart defect (6). Drug histories were obtained from mothers of 11 infants with biliary atresia and compared with the histories of 50 control mothers (7). Amphetamine exposure occurred in five women in the study group and in three of the controls. A 1966 report described a mother with two infants with microcephaly, mental retardation, and motor dysfunction (8). The mother had taken an appetite suppressant containing methamphetamine and phenobarbital during the 1st and 2nd trimesters of both pregnancies (pregnancies number 1 and 3). A spontaneous abortion occurred in pregnancy number 2, but no details were given of the mother's drug intake. Her fourth pregnancy, in which she did not take the appetite suppressant, resulted in the delivery of a normal child. There was no family history of developmental disorders, congenital defects, mental retardation, cerebral palsy, or epilepsy.

Fetal structural defects have been associated with maternal abuse of drugs in a large volume of literature (see also Ethanol, Cocaine, Heroin, Lysergic Acid Diethylamide [LSD], Marijuana, and Methadone). For example, in a 1972 case, multiple brain and eye anomalies were observed in an infant exposed *in utero* to amphetamines, LSD, meprobamate, and marijuana (9). In this and similar cases, the etiology of the structural abnormalities is probably multifactoral, involving drug use, life-styles, infections, poor maternal health, and other factors.

In a retrospective study, 458 mothers who delivered infants with major ($N = 175$) or minor ($N = 283$) abnormalities were compared with 911 matched controls (10). Appetite suppressants were consumed during pregnancy by significantly more mothers of infants with anomalies than by controls (3.9% vs. 1.1%, $p < 0.01$). Dextroamphetamine consumption accounted for 13 of the 18 maternal exposures in the anomaly group. During the first 56 days of pregnancy, dextroamphetamine-containing compounds were used by 10 mothers in the anomaly group (2.2%) compared to only five of the controls (0.5%) ($p < 0.05$). The abnormalities (three major/seven minor) observed in the 10 infants were urogenital system defects (four cases), congenital heart disease (one case), cleft lip (one case), severe limb deformity (one case), accessory auricles (one case), congenital dislocation of hip (one case), and pilonidal sinus (one case). Although statistically significant results were found in this study, the results must be interpreted cautiously due to the retrospective collection of drug histories and the lack of information pertaining to past and present maternal medical and obstetric histories.

A prospective study of 1824 Caucasian mothers who took anorectic drugs (primarily amphetamines) during pregnancy compared to 8989 Caucasian mothers who did not take such drugs measured rates of severe congenital defects in infants with a gestational age of at least 37 weeks of 3.7% and 3.4%, respectively (11). When children of all known gestational ages were included, amphetamine usage occurred in 85% (1694 of 1992) of the group consuming anorectic drugs. The incidence of severe congenital defects in the amphetamine group was 3.4%. Fourteen infants were exposed in the first 84 days after the last menstrual period, and except for three infants with cleft lip and/or palate, no pattern of malformations was observed.

The effects of amphetamine abuse on fetal outcome and subsequent development were described in a series of reports from Sweden (12–16). Twenty-three women who ingested amphetamine during the 1st trimester were divided into two groups: 6 who claimed they stopped use of the drug after they became aware of their pregnancy or after the 1st trimester, and 17 who continued use of the drug throughout gestation (12). Two of the infants (group not specified) had congenital defects: a stillborn infant with myelomeningocele, and an infant with extensive telangiectasis (considered to be an inherited disorder). The outcome of the infants exposed throughout gestation included six preterm (<37 weeks), three small-for-gestational-age (all with poor prenatal care), one of whom had a seizure on the 1st day, and two full-term but extremely drowsy infants. In a later report, 66 infants born to amphetamine-addicted mothers were followed during their 1st year of life (14). Except for temporary drowsiness in the first few months, all children had normal somatic and psychomotor development at 12 months of age. In the final report from these investigators, the fetal outcome of 69 amphetamine-addicted women who delivered 71 children (one delivered twice and one delivered twins) was described (15). Seventeen of the women claimed to have stopped amphetamine ingestion as previously described, and 52 continued use of amphetamines throughout pregnancy. Three women in the first group and 17 in the second group were alcoholics (16). Four infants had congenital defects: intestinal atresia (one also had hydrocephalus) (two cases—both died), congenital heart defect (one case), and epidermolysis bullosa without known heredity (one case). In one of the four cases the mother was an alcoholic, but the particular case was not specified. Drowsiness was observed in eight infants and jitteriness in 11 infants; four full-term infants required tube feedings. The four studies (12–15) were combined into a single article published in 1980 (16).

The Collaborative Perinatal Project monitored 50,282 mother-child pairs, 671 of which had 1st trimester exposure to amphetamines (17, pp. 346–347). For use anytime during pregnancy, 1898 exposures were recorded (17, p. 439). In neither case was evidence found to suggest a relationship to large categories of major or minor malformations. Two case reports failed to observe any neonatal effects from the treatment of narcolepsy with large doses of amphetamine (18, 19). A 1988 report described a mother who had used amphetamines, barbiturates, cocaine, LSD, alcohol, and marijuana during pregnancy who delivered a female infant with bilateral cerebrovascular accident and resulting porencephaly (20). The infant expired at 2.5 months of age. The fetal injury was thought to be due to cocaine (see also Cocaine).

The effects of intravenous methamphetamine abuse on the fetus were evaluated in a 1988 report (21). Maternal use of the drug was identified by self-reporting before delivery in 52 women, and an equal number of controls were selected for comparison. Although self-reporting of illegal drug use is prone to underreporting, the drug histories were validated by social worker interviews and were thought to represent actual drug use in the study population. Other drugs used in the study and control groups were tobacco (24 vs. 6), marijuana (20 vs. 1), cocaine (14 vs. 0), and one each in the study group for alcohol, lorazepam, dextroamphetamine, heroin, opium, LSD, and diazepam. No statistical differences were measured between the groups in the rate of obstetric complications (12% vs. 27%) or neonatal complications (21% vs. 17%). The latter category included meconium (10% vs. 12%), fetal heart rate decelerations (4% vs. 0) and tachycardia (2% vs. 0), tachypnea (4% vs. 2%), and withdrawal symptoms (2% vs. 0). Mean birth weight, length, and head circumference were all lower in the study infants compared to controls ($p = 0.001$). Six (12%) of the infants in the study group had a congenital defect compared to seven (14%) of the controls. Statistically, however, the investigators could only conclude that methamphetamine abuse does not cause a 12-fold or greater increase in congenital anomalies (21).

Amphetamine withdrawal has been described in newborns whose mothers were addicted to amphetamines during pregnancy (22–24). In a report of four mothers using methamphetamine, symptoms consisting of shrill cries, irritability, jerking, and sneezing were observed in two infants (22). One of the infants was evaluated at 4 months of age and appeared normal except for small size (weight 3rd percentile, head circumference 10th percentile). The author speculated that the symptoms in the newborns may have been due to hidden narcotic addiction (22). Another report of four women with methamphetamine dependence described one newborn with marked drowsiness lasting for 4 days (23). The mother had not been taking narcotics. The third report of neonatal withdrawal involved an infant delivered from a mother who was a known amphetamine addict (24). Beginning 6 hours after birth, the female infant had diaphoresis, agitation alternating with periods of lassitude, apnea with feedings, a seizure on the 6th day, vomiting, miotic pupils, and a glassy-eyed stare. Her first 3 months were marked by slow development, but at 2.5 years of age there was no evidence of neurologic disability and intelligence was considered above normal.

Methamphetamine withdrawal characterized by abnormal sleep patterns, poor feeding, tremors, and hypertonia was reported in a 1987 study (25). Infants exposed to methamphetamine or cocaine, either singly or in combination, were combined into a single group ($N = 46$) because of similar maternal and neonatal medical factors. The drug group had a significantly greater incidence of prematurity compared to drug-free controls (28% vs. 9%, $p < 0.05$), and a greater incidence of placental hemorrhage and anemia compared to narcotic-using mothers and controls (13% vs. 2% vs. 2.2%, $p < 0.05$ and 13% vs. 2% vs. 0%, $p < 0.05$). Maternal methamphetamine abuse was significantly associated with lower gestational age, birth weight, length, and occipitofrontal circumference.

Echoencephalography (ECHO) was performed within 3 days of birth on 74 term (>37 weeks) infants who had tested positive for cocaine or methamphetamine, but who otherwise had uncomplicated perinatal courses (26). The infants had no other known risk factors for cerebral injury. The 74 newborns were classified into three groups: 24 (32%) methamphetamine exposed, 32 (43%) cocaine exposed, and 18 (24%) exposed to cocaine plus heroin or methadone, or both. Two comparison groups were formed: a group of 87 term, drug-free infants studied by ECHO because of clinical concerns for hypoxic-ischemic encephalopathy, and a normal group of 19 drug-free term newborns. Both groups of comparison infants were also studied by ECHO within 3 days of birth. Only one structural anomaly, consisting of an absent septum pellucidum, was observed in the infants examined. The affected newborn, exposed to methamphetamine, was also found to have bilateral optic nerve atrophy and diffuse attenuation of the white matter. Twenty-six (35.1%) of the drug-exposed infants had cranial abnormalities detected by ultrasonography, which was similar to the 27.6% (24 of 87) incidence in the ill comparison group ($p = 0.7$). The normal controls had an incidence of 5.3% (1 of 19) ($p < 0.01$ in comparison to both of the other groups). The lesions observed in the drug-exposed infants were intraventricular hemorrhage, echodensities known to be associated with necrosis, and cavitary lesions. Lesions were concentrated in the basal ganglion, frontal lobes, and posterior fossa (26). The ECHO abnormalities were not predicted by standard neonatal clinical assessment and were believed to be consistent with those observed in adult abusers of amphetamines and cocaine (26).

In summary, the use of amphetamines for medical indications does not pose a significant risk to the fetus for congenital anomalies. Amphetamines do not appear to be human teratogens (27–29). Mild withdrawal symptoms may be observed in the newborns, but the few studies of infant follow-up have not shown long-term sequelae, although more studies of this nature are needed. Illicit maternal use of amphetamines, on the other hand, presents significant risks to the fetus and newborn, including intrauterine growth retardation, premature delivery, and the potential for increased maternal, fetal, and neonatal morbidity. These poor outcomes are probably multifactorial in origin, involving multiple drug use, life-styles, and poor maternal health. However, cerebral injuries occurring in newborns exposed *in utero* appear to be directly related to the vasoconstrictive properties of amphetamines (26).

Breast Feeding Summary

Amphetamine, the racemic mixture of levo- and dextroamphetamine, is concentrated in breast milk (19). After continuous daily dosing of 20 mg, milk concentrations ranged from 55–138 ng/ml with milk:plasma ratios varying between 2.8 and 7.5. Amphetamine was found in the urine of the nursing infant. No adverse effects of this exposure were observed over a 24-month period. In a second study, no neonatal insomnia or stimulation was observed in 103 nursing infants whose mothers were taking various amounts of amphetamine (30). The American Academy of Pediatrics considers amphetamines to be contraindicated during breast feeding (31).

References

1. Nora JJ, Trasler DG, Fraser FC. Malformations in mice induced by dexamphetamine sulphate. Lancet 1965;2:1021–2.

2. Nora JJ, McNamara DG, Fraser FC. Dextroamphetamine sulphate and human malformations. Lancet 1967;1:570–1.

3. Nora JJ, Vargo T, Nora A, Love KE, McNamara DG. Dextroamphetamine: a possible environmental trigger in cardiovascular malformations. Lancet 1970;1:1290–1.

4. Nora JJ, Nora AH, Sommerville RJ, Hill RM, McNamara DG. Maternal exposure to potential teratogens. JAMA 1967;202:1065–9.

5. Matera RF, Zabala H, Jimenez AP. Bifid exencephalia: teratogen action of amphetamine. Int Surg 1968;50:79–85.

6. Gilbert EF, Khoury GH. Dextroamphetamine and congenital cardiac malformations. J Pediatr 1970;76:638.

7. Levin JN. Amphetamine ingestion with biliary atresia. J Pediatr 1971;79:130–1.

8. McIntire MS. Possible adverse drug reaction. JAMA 1966;197:62–3.

9. Bogdanoff B, Rorke LB, Yanoff M, Warren WS. Brain and eye abnormalities: possible sequelae to prenatal use of multiple drugs including LSD. Am J Dis Child 1972;123:145–8.

10. Nelson MM, Forfar JO. Associations between drugs administered during pregnancy and congenital abnormalities of the fetus. Br Med J 1971;1:523–7.

11. Milkovich L, van den Berg BJ. Effects of antenatal exposure to anorectic drugs. Am J Obstet Gynecol 1977;129:637–42.

12. Eriksson M, Larsson G, Winbladh B, Zetterstrom R. The influence of amphetamine addiction on pregnancy and the newborn infant. Acta Paediatr Scand 1978;67:95–9.

13. Larsson G, Eriksson M, Zetterstrom R. Amphetamine addiction and pregnancy: psycho-social and medical aspects. Acta Psychiatr Scand 1979;60:334–45.

14. Billing L, Eriksson M, Larsson G, Zetterstrom R. Amphetamine addiction and pregnancy. III. One year follow-up of the children: psychosocial and pediatric aspects. Acta Paediatr Scand 1980;69:675–80.

15. Eriksson M, Larsson G, Zetterstrom R. Amphetamine addiction and pregnancy. II. Pregnancy, delivery and the neonatal period: socio-medical aspects. Acta Obstet Gynecol Scand 1981;60:253–9.

16. Larsson G. The amphetamine addicted mother and her child. Acta Paediatr Scand 1980;Suppl 278.

17. Heinonen OP, Slone D, Shapiro S. Birth Defects and Drugs in Pregnancy. Littleton:Publishing Sciences Group, 1977.

18. Briggs GG, Samson JH, Crawford DJ. Lack of abnormalities in a newborn exposed to amphetamine during gestation. Am J Dis Child 1975;129:249–50.

19. Steiner E, Villen T, Hallberg M, Rane A. Amphetamine secretion in breast milk. Eur J Clin Pharmacol 1984;27:123–4.

20. Tenorio GM, Nazvi M, Bickers GH, Hubbird RH. Intrauterine stroke and maternal polydrug abuse: case report. Clin Pediatr 1988;27:565–7.

21. Little BB, Snell LM, Gilstrap LC III. Methamphetamine abuse during pregnancy: outcome and fetal effects. Obstet Gynecol 1988;72:541–4.

22. Sussman S. Narcotic and methamphetamine use during pregnancy: effect on newborn infants. Am J Dis Child 1963;106:325–30.

23. Neuberg R. Drug dependence and pregnancy: a review of the problems and their management. J Obstet Gynaecol Br Commonw 1970;66:1117–22.

24. Ramer CM. The case history of an infant born to an amphetamine-addicted mother. Clin Pediatr 1974;13:596–7.

25. Oro AS, Dixon SD. Perinatal cocaine and methamphetamine exposure: maternal and neonatal correlates. J Pediatr 1987;111:571–8.

26. Dixon SD, Bejar R. Echoencephalographic findings in neonates associated with maternal cocaine and methamphetamine use: incidence and clinical correlates. J Pediatr 1989;115:770–8.

27. Chernoff GF, Jones KL. Fetal preventive medicine: teratogens and the unborn baby. Pediatr Ann 1981;10:210–7.

28. Kalter H, Warkany J. Congenital malformations (second of two parts). N Engl J Med 1983;308:491–7.

29. Zierler S. Maternal drugs and congenital heart disease. Obstet Gynecol 1985;65:155–65.

30. Ayd FJ Jr. Excretion of psychotropic drugs in human breast milk. Int Drug Ther News Bull 1973;8:33–40.

31. Committee on Drugs, American Academy of Pediatrics. Transfer of drugs and other chemicals into human milk. Pediatrics 1989;84;924–36.

Name: **AMPHOTERICIN B**

Class: **Antifungal Antibiotic**   Risk Factor: **B**

Fetal Risk Summary

No reports linking the use of amphotericin B with congenital defects have been located. The antibiotic crosses the placenta to the fetus with cord blood:maternal serum ratios ranging from 0.38–1.0 (1–3). In a term (42 weeks) infant whose mother was treated with amphotericin B 0.6 mg/kg every other day, cord and maternal blood levels at delivery were both 2.6 μg/ml, a cord blood:maternal serum ratio of 1.0 (1). Amniotic fluid concentration was 0.08 μg/ml at delivery. The time interval between the last dose and delivery was not specified. Concentrations in the cord blood and maternal serum of a woman treated with 16 mg of amphotericin B just prior to delivery (one-fifth of a planned total dose of 80 mg had infused when delivery occurred) were 0.12 and 0.32 μg/ml, respectively, a ratio of 0.38 (2). The woman's last dose before this time was 7 days previously when she had received 80 mg. In a third case, a mother was receiving 20 mg intravenously every other day (0.5 mg/kg) (3). The cord and maternal serum concentrations were 1.3 μg/ml and 1.9 μg/ml, respectively, a ratio of 0.68. The levels were determined 26 hours after her last dose.

The Collaborative Perinatal Project monitored 50,282 mother-child pairs, 9 of which had 1st trimester exposure to amphotericin B (4). Numerous other reports have also described the use of amphotericin B during various stages of pregnancy, including the 1st trimester (2–20). No evidence of adverse fetal effects was found by these studies. Amphotericin B can be used during pregnancy in those patients who will clearly benefit from the drug.

Breast Feeding Summary

No data are available.

References

1. McCoy MJ, Ellenberg JF, Killam AP. Coccidioidomycosis complicating pregnancy. Am J Obstet Gynecol 1980;137:739–40.
2. Ismail MA, Lerner SA. Disseminated blastomycosis in a pregnant woman. Review of amphotericin B usage during pregnancy. Am Rev Respir Dis 1982;126:350–3.
3. Hager H, Welt SI, Cardasis JP, Alvarez S. Disseminated blastomycosis in a pregnant woman successfully treated with amphotericin-B: a case report. J Reprod Med 1988;33:485–8.
4. Heinonen OP, Slone D, Shapiro S. Birth Defects and Drugs in Pregnancy. Littleton:Publishing Sciences Group, 1977:297.
5. Neiberg AD, Maruomatis F, Dyke J, Fayyad A. Blastomyces dermatitidis treated during pregnancy. Am J Obstet Gynecol 1977;128:911–2.
6. Philpot CR, Lo D. Cryptococcal meningitis in pregnancy. Med J Aust 1972;2:1005–7.
7. Aitken GWE, Symonds EM. Cryptococcal meningitis in pregnancy treated with amphotericin. A case report. Br J Obstet Gynaecol 1962;69:677–9.
8. Feldman R. Cryptococcosis (torulosis) of the central nervous system treated with amphotericin B during pregnancy. South Med J 1959;52:1415–7.
9. Kuo D. A case of torulosis of the central nervous system during pregnancy. Med J Aust 1962;1:558–60.
10. Crotty JM. Systemic mycotic infections in northern territory Aborigines. Med J Aust 1965;1:184.
11. Littman ML. Cryptococcosis (torulosis). Current concepts and therapy. Am J Med 1959;27:976–8.
12. Mick R, Muller-Tyl E, Neufeld T. Comparison of the effectiveness of Nystatin and amphotericin B in the therapy of female genital mycoses. Wien Med Wochenschr 1975;125:131–5.

13. Silberfarb PM, Sarois GA, Tosh FE. Cryptococcosis and pregnancy. Am J Obstet Gynecol 1972;112:714–20.
14. Curole DN. Cryptococcal meningitis in pregnancy. J Reprod Med 1981;26:317–9.
15. Sanford WG, Rasch JR, Stonehill RB. A therapeutic dilemma: the treatment of disseminated coccidioidomycosis with amphotericin B. Ann Intern Med 1962;56:553–63.
16. Harris RE. Coccidioidomycosis complicating pregnancy. Report of 3 cases and review of the literature. Obstet Gynecol 1966;28:401–5.
17. Smale LE, Waechter KG. Dissemination of coccidioidomycosis in pregnancy. Am J Obstet Gynecol 1970;107:356–9.
18. Hadsall FJ, Acquarelli MJ. Disseminated coccidioidomycosis presenting as facial granulomas in pregnancy: a report of two cases and a review of the literature. Laryngoscope 1973;83:51–8.
19. Daniel L, Salit IE. Blastomycosis during pregnancy. Can Med Assoc J 1984;131:759–61.
20. Peterson CW, Johnson SL, Kelly JV, Kelly PC. Coccidiodal meningitis and pregnancy: a case report. Obstet Gynecol 1989;73:835–6.

Name: **AMPICILLIN**

Class: **Antibiotic**   Risk Factor: **B**

Fetal Risk Summary

Ampicillin is a penicillin antibiotic (see also Penicillin G). The drug rapidly crosses the placenta into the fetal circulation and amniotic fluid (1–6). Fetal serum levels can be detected within 30 minutes and equilibrate with maternal serum in 1 hour. Amniotic fluid levels can be detected in 90 minutes, reaching 20% of the maternal serum peak in about 8 hours. The pharmacokinetics of ampicillin during pregnancy have been reported (7, 8).

Ampicillin depresses both plasma-bound and urinary excreted estriol by inhibiting steroid conjugate hydrolysis in the gut (9–13). Urinary estriol was formerly used to assess the condition of the fetoplacental unit, depressed levels being associated with fetal distress. This assessment is now made by measuring plasma unconjugated estriol, which is not usually affected by ampicillin. An interaction between ampicillin and oral contraceptives resulting in pregnancy has been suspected (14, 15). Two studies, however, failed to confirm this interaction and concluded that alternate contraceptive methods were not necessary during ampicillin therapy (16, 17).

The use of ampicillin in early pregnancy was associated with a prevalence ratio estimate of 3.3 (90% confidence limits 1.3–8.1, $p = 0.02$) for congenital heart disease in a retrospective study (18). A specific defect, transposition of the great arteries, had a risk of 7.7 (90% confidence limits 1.3–38) based on exposure in two of the 29 infants with the anomaly. The investigators did note, however, that the results had to be viewed cautiously since the data were subject to recall bias (drug histories were taken by questionnaire or telephone up to a year after presumed exposure) and the study could not distinguish between the fetal effects of the drug versus those of the infectious agent(s) for which the drugs were used. Others have also shared this concern (19). Other reports linking the use of ampicillin with congenital defects have not been located. The Collaborative Perinatal Project monitored 50,282 mother-child pairs, 3,546 of which had 1st trimester exposure to penicillin derivatives (20, pp. 297–313). For use anytime during pregnancy, 7,171 exposures were recorded (20, p. 435). In neither case was evidence found to suggest a relationship to large categories of major or minor malformations or to individual defects. Based on these data, it is unlikely that ampicillin is teratogenic.

Ampicillin is often used in the last half of pregnancies where either the woman or her fetus is at risk for infections because of premature rupture of the membranes or other risk factors (21–23).

Breast Feeding Summary

Ampicillin is excreted into breast milk in low concentrations. Milk:plasma ratios have been reported up to 0.2 (24, 25). Candidiasis and diarrhea were observed in one infant whose mother was receiving ampicillin (26). Other reports of this effect have not been located. Although adverse effects are apparently rare, three potential problems exist for the nursing infant: modification of bowel flora, direct effects on the infant (e.g., allergic response/sensitization), and interference with the interpretation of culture results if a fever workup is required.

References

1. Bray R, Boc R, Johnson W. Transfer of ampicillin into fetus and amniotic fluid from maternal plasma in late pregnancy. Am J Obstet Gynecol 1966;96:938–42.
2. MacAulay M, Abou-Sabe M, Charles D. Placental transfer of ampicillin. Am J Obstet Gynecol 1966;96:943–50.
3. Biro L, Ivan E, Elek E, Arr M. Data on the tissue concentration of antibiotics in man. Tissue concentrations of semi-synthetic penicillins in the fetus. Int Z Klin Pharmakol Ther Toxikol 1970;4:321–4.
4. Elek E, Ivan E, Arr M. Passage of penicillins from mother to foetus in humans. Int J Clin Pharmacol Ther Toxicol 1972;6:223–8.
5. Kraybill EN, Chaney NE, McCarthy LR. Transplacental ampicillin: inhibitory concentrations in neonatal serum. Am J Obstet Gynecol 1980;138:793–6.
6. Jordheim O, Hagen AG. Study of ampicillin levels in maternal serum, umbilical cord serum and amniotic fluid following administration of pivampicillin. Acta Obstet Gynecol Scand 1980;59:315–7.
7. Philipson A. Pharmacokinetics of ampicillin during pregnancy. J Infect Dis 1977;136:370–6.
8. Noschel VH, Peiker G, Schroder S, Meinhold P, Muller B. Untersuchungren zur pharmakokinetik von antibiotika und sulfanilamiden in der schwangerschaft und unter der geburt. Zentralbl Gynakol 1982;104:1514–8.
9. Willman K, Pulkkinen M. Reduced maternal plasma and urinary estriol during ampicillin treatment. Am J Obstet Gynecol 1971;109:893–6.
10. Boehn F, DiPietro D, Goss D. The effect of ampicillin administration on urinary estriol and serum estradiol in the normal pregnant patient. Am J Obstet Gynecol 1974;119:98–101.
11. Sybulski S, Maughan G. Effect of ampicillin administration on estradiol, estriol and cortisol levels in maternal plasma and on estriol levels in urine. Am J Obstet Gynecol 1976;124:379–81.
12. Aldercreutz H, Martin F, Lehtinen T, Tikkanen M, Pulkkinen M. Effect of ampicillin administration on plasma conjugated and unconjugated estrogen and progesterone levels in pregnancy. Am J Obstet Gynecol 1977;128:266–71.
13. Van Look PFA, Top-Huisman M, Gnodde HP. Effect of ampicillin or amoxycillin administration on plasma and urinary estrogen levels during normal pregnancy. Eur J Obstet Gynecol Reprod Biol 1981;12:225–33.
14. Dossetor J. Drug interactions with oral contraceptives. Br Med J 1975;4:467–8.
15. DeSano EA Jr, Hurley SC. Possible interactions of antihistamines and antibiotics with oral contraceptive effectiveness. Fertil Steril 1982;37:853–4.
16. Friedman CI, Huneke AL, Kim MH, Powell J. The effect of ampicillin on oral contraceptive effectiveness. Obstet Gynecol 1980;55:33–7.
17. Back DJ, Breckerridge AM, MacIver M, Orme M, Rowe PH, Staiger C, Thomas E, Tjia J. The effects of ampicillin on oral contraceptive steroids in women. Br J Clin Pharmacol 1982;14:43–8.
18. Rothman KJ, Fyler DC, Goldblatt A, Kreidberg MB. Exogenous hormones and other drug exposures of children with congenital heart disease. Am J Epidemiol 1979;109:433–9.

19. Zierler S. Maternal drugs and congenital heart disease. Obstet Gynecol 1985;65:155–65.
20. Heinonen OP, Slone D, Shapiro S. *Birth Defects and Drugs in Pregnancy*. Littleton:Publishing Sciences Group, 1977.
21. Boyer KM, Gotoff SP. Prevention of early-onset neonatal group B streptococcal disease with selective intrapartum chemoprophylaxis. N Engl J Med 1986;314:1665–9.
22. Amon E, Lewis SV, Sibai BM, Villar MA, Arheart KL. Ampicillin prophylaxis in preterm premature rupture of the membranes: a prospective randomized study. Am J Obstet Gynecol 1988;159:539–43.
23. Morales WJ, Angel JL, O'Brien WF, Knuppel RA. Use of ampicillin and corticosteroids in premature rupture of membranes: a randomized study. Obstet Gynecol 1989;73:721–6.
24. Wilson J, Brown R, Cherek D, Dailey JW, Hilman B, Jobe PC, Manno BR, Manno JE, Redetzki HM, Stewart JJ. Drug excretion in human breast milk: principles, pharmacokinetics and projected consequences. Clin Pharmacol Ther 1980;5:1–66.
25. Knowles J. Excretion of drugs in milk—a review. J Pediatr 1965;66:1068–82.
26. Williams M. Excretion of drugs in milk. Pharm J 1976;217:219.

Name: **AMRINONE**

Class: **Cardiac Agent**   Risk Factor: **C$_M$**

Fetal Risk Summary

Amrinone is a cardiac inotropic agent that also has a vasodilatory effect (1). The drug is unrelated to cardiac glycosides or catecholamines. The principal indication for amrinone is the short-term management of congestive heart failure. Amrinone is teratogenic in animals (1). No reports of the use of this drug in human pregnancy have been located. In pregnant baboons, amrinone infusion did not significantly affect uterine artery blood flow (2). As expected, the manufacturer cautions that amrinone should only be used when the potential maternal benefits justify the potential risk to the fetus.

Breast Feeding Summary

No data are available.

References

1. Product information, Inocor. Winthrop Pharmaceuticals, 1989.
2. Fishburne JI Jr, Dormer KJ, Payne GG, Gill PS, Ashrafzadeh AR, Rossavik IK. Effects of amrinone and dopamine on uterine blood flow and vascular responses in the gravid baboon. Am J Obstet Gynecol 1988;158:829–37.

Name: **AMYL NITRITE**

Class: **Vasodilator**   Risk Factor: **C**

Fetal Risk Summary

Amyl nitrite is a rapid acting, short duration vasodilator used primarily for the treatment of angina pectoris. Due to the nature of its indication, experience in pregnancy is limited. The Collaborative Perinatal Project recorded 7 1st trimester exposures to amyl nitrite and nitroglycerin plus 8 other patients exposed to other vasodilators (1). From this small group of 15 patients, 4 malformed children were produced, a statistically significant incidence (p < 0.02). It was not stated whether amyl nitrite was taken by any of the mothers of the affected infants. Although the data serve as a warning, the number of patients is so small that conclusions as to the relative safety of amyl nitrite in pregnancy cannot be made.

Breast Feeding Summary

No data are available.

Reference

1. Heinonen OP, Slone D, Shapiro S. *Birth Defects and Drugs in Pregnancy*. Littleton:Publishing Sciences Group, 1977:371–3.

Name: **ANILERIDINE**

Class: **Narcotic Analgesic**   Risk Factor: **B***

Fetal Risk Summary

No reports linking the use of anileridine with congenital defects have been located. Usage in pregnancy is primarily confined to labor. Withdrawal may occur in infants exposed *in utero* to prolonged maternal treatment with anileridine. Respiratory depression in the neonate similar to that produced by meperidine or morphine should be expected (1).

[*Risk Factor D if used for prolonged periods or in high doses at term.]

Breast Feeding Summary

No data are available.

Reference

1. Bonica J. *Principles and Practice of Obstetric Analgesia and Anesthesia*. Philadelphia:FA Davis, 1967:250.

Name: **ANISINDIONE**

Class: **Anticoagulant**   Risk Factor: **D**

Fetal Risk Summary

In an investigation of the effects of occlusive thromboaortopathy (Takayasu's disease) on pregnancy, four women of a total 27 were maintained on anisindione throughout five pregnancies (1). No neonatal complications or anomalies were observed in the five infants. (See Coumarin Derivatives.)

Breast Feeding Summary

See Coumarin Derivatives.

Reference

1. Ishikawa K, Matsuura S. Occlusive thromboaortopathy (Takayasu's disease) and pregnancy: clinical course and management of 33 pregnancies and deliveries. Am J Cardiol 1982;50:1293–1300.

Name: **ANISOTROPINE**

Class: **Parasympatholytic**   Risk Factor: **C**

Fetal Risk Summary

Anisotropine is an anticholinergic quaternary ammonium methylbromide. In a large prospective study, 2323 patients were exposed to this class of drugs during the 1st trimester, 2 of whom took anisotropine (1). A possible association was found between the total group and minor malformations.

Breast Feeding Summary

No data are available (see also Atropine).

Reference

1. Heinonen OP, Slone D, Shapiro S. *Birth Defects and Drugs in Pregnancy*. Littleton:Publishing Sciences Groups, 1977:346–53.

Name: **ANTAZOLINE**

Class: **Antihistamine**   Risk Factor: **C**

Fetal Risk Summary

No data are available. See Diphenhydramine for representative agent in this class.

Breast Feeding Summary

No data are available.

Name: **APROBARBITAL**

Class: **Sedative/Hypnotic**   Risk Factor: **C**

Fetal Risk Summary

No data are available.

Breast Feeding Summary

No data are available.

Name: **APROTININ**

Class: **Hemostatic**   Risk Factor: **C**

Fetal Risk Summary

No reports linking the use of aprotinin and congenital defects have been located. The drug crosses the placenta and decreases fibrinolytic activity in the newborn (1). The drug has been used safely in severe accidental hemorrhage with coagulation where labor was not established (2).

Breast Feeding Summary

No data are available.

References

1. Hoffhauer H, Dobbeck P. Untersuchungen uber die plactapassage des kallikrein-inhibitors. Klin Wochenschr 1970;48:183–4.
2. Sher G. Trasylol in cases of accidental hemorrhage with coagulation disorder and associated uterine inertia. S Afr Med J 1974;48:1452–5.

Name: **ASPIRIN**

Class: **Analgesic/Antipyretic**   Risk Factor: **C***

Fetal Risk Summary

Aspirin is the most frequently ingested drug in pregnancy either as a single agent or in combination with other drugs (1). The terms "aspirin" and "salicylate" are used interchangeably in this monograph unless specifically separated. In eight surveys totaling over 54,000 patients, aspirin was consumed sometime during gestation by slightly over 33,000 (61%) (2–9). The true incidence is probably much higher than this since many patients either do not remember taking aspirin or consume drug products without realizing that they contain large amounts of salicylates (2, 4, 8). Evaluation of the effects of aspirin on the fetus is thus difficult due to this common, and often hidden, exposure. However, some toxic effects on the mother and fetus from large doses of salicylates have been known since 1893 (10).

Aspirin consumption during pregnancy may produce adverse effects in the mother: anemia, antepartum and/or postpartum hemorrhage, prolonged gestation, and prolonged labor (5, 11–14). The increased length of labor and frequency of postmaturity result from the inhibition of prostaglandin synthetase by aspirin. Aspirin has been shown to delay significantly the induced abortion time in nulliparous (but not multiparous) patients by this same mechanism (15). In an Australian study, regular aspirin ingestion was also found to increase the number of complicated deliveries (cesarean sections, breech, and forceps) (5). Small doses of aspirin may decrease urinary estriol excretion (16).

Aspirin, either alone or in combination with β-mimetics, has been used to treat premature labor (17–19). Although adverse effects in the newborn were infrequent, maternal complications in one study included non-dose-related prolonged bleeding times and dose-related vertigo, tinnitus, headache, and hyperventilation (19).

Failure of intrauterine devices (IUD) to prevent conception has been described in two patients who consumed frequent doses of aspirin (20). The anti-inflammatory action of aspirin was proposed as the mechanism of the failure.

Low-dose aspirin (about 85 mg/day) was used to treat maternal thrombocytopenia (platelet counts $<60,000/mm^3$) in 19 patients with either intrauterine growth retardation or toxemia (21). In five women who had a definite response to the aspirin, no improvement in plasma volume or fetal welfare was demonstrated.

In women with systemic lupus erythematosus complicated with either lupus anticoagulant and/or anticardiolipin antibody (i.e., antiphospholipid antibodies), low-dose aspirin (e.g., 80 mg/day) has been used in combination with prednisone to reduce the incidence of pregnancy loss (22–25) (see reference 22 for a review of this topic). This therapy has not been associated with drug-induced fetal or neonatal complications.

Several studies have investigated the effect of low-dose aspirin (e.g., 40–150 mg/day) on the prevention of pregnancy-induced hypertension (PIH), preeclampsia, and eclampsia, and the associated fetal risks of intrauterine growth retardation and mortality (26–38) (see reference 36 for a review of this topic). Low-dose aspirin exerts its beneficial effects in these disorders by irreversible inactivation of platelet cyclo-oxygenase, resulting in the inhibition of thromboxane A_2 synthesis more so than prostacyclin production. This inhibition restores the ratio of the two substances to a more normal value. Aspirin-induced fetal and neonatal toxicity has not been observed after the chronic use of low-dose aspirin for these indications. The lack of toxicity may be partially explained by the findings of a study published in 1989 (34). In that study, 60–80 mg of aspirin/day, starting 3 weeks before delivery and continued until birth, inhibited maternal platelet cyclo-oxygenase, but not that of the newborn. These results were in agreement with other studies using 60–150 mg/day (34). Other toxicities associated with the use of full-dose aspirin near term, such as hemorrhage, premature closure of the ductus arteriosus, pulmonary hypertension, prolonged gestation, and prolonged labor, were not observed with low-dose aspirin therapy (34). Although these results are reassuring, too few studies have been reported, in the opinion of some, to allow a true estimate of the fetal risk (36). However, other recent reports have observed no serious neonatal adverse effects, including hemorrhagic complications, in their series (39, 40). In one of these studies, 33 women judged to be at risk for pregnancy-induced hypertension were randomly assigned to either an aspirin ($N = 17$) or placebo ($N = 16$) group during the 12th week of gestation in a single blind study (39). Patients in the aspirin group, treated with 60 mg/day from enrollment to delivery, had a longer duration of pregnancy (39 weeks vs. 35 weeks, $p < 0.01$) and delivered heavier infants (2922 g vs. 2264 g, $p < 0.05$). None of the aspirin-treated women developed PIH, whereas three of the placebo group did develop the complication. In a double blind study, 65 women with increased blood pressure during the rollover test administered during the 28th or 29th week of pregnancy were randomly divided into two groups: one group was treated with 100 mg/day of aspirin ($N = 34$) and the other with placebo ($N = 31$) (40). Four women (11.8%) of the aspirin-treated group developed PIH compared to 11 (35.5%) of the placebo group ($p = 0.024$).

Fetal and newborn effects, other than congenital defects, from aspirin exposure *in utero* may include increased perinatal mortality, intrauterine growth retardation, congenital salicylate intoxication, and depressed albumin-binding capacity (2, 5, 12, 41–43). For the latter effect, no increase in the incidence of jaundice was observed (2). Perinatal mortality in the Australian study was a result of stillbirths more often than neonatal deaths (5, 41). Some of the stillbirths were associated with antepartum hemorrhage and others may have been due to closure of the ductus arteriosus *in utero* (44). Closure of the ductus has been shown in animals due to aspirin inhibition of prostaglandin synthetase. In some early cases, *in utero* premature closure of the ductus arteriosus was probably due to aspirin but not suspected (45). However, a large prospective American study involving 41,337 patients, 64% of whom used aspirin sometime during gestation, failed to show that aspirin was a cause of stillbirths, neonatal deaths, or reduced birth weight (46). The difference between these findings probably relates to the chronic or intermittent use of higher doses by the patients in the Australian study (44). Excessive use of aspirin was blamed for the stillbirth of a fetus where salicylate levels in the fetal blood and liver were 25–30 mg/100 ml and 12 mg/100 ml, respectively (47). Congenital salicylate intoxication was found in two newborns exposed to high aspirin doses prior to delivery (42, 43). Although both infants survived, one infant exhibited withdrawal symptoms beginning on the 2nd neonatal day consisting of hypertonia, agitation, a shrill piercing cry, and increased reflex irritability (41). The serum salicylate level was 31 mg/100 ml. Most of the symptoms gradually subsided over 6 weeks, but some mild hypertonia may have persisted.

Aspirin given in doses of 325–650 mg during the week prior to delivery may affect the clotting ability of the newborn (48–54). In the initial study by Bleyer and Breckenridge (48), 3 of 14 newborns exposed to aspirin within 1 week of delivery had minor hemorrhagic phenomena vs. only 1 of 17 nonexposed controls. Collagen-induced platelet aggregation was absent in the aspirin group and, although of less clinical significance, factor XII activity was markedly depressed. A direct correlation was found between factor XII activity and the interval between the last dose of aspirin and birth. Neonatal purpuric rash with depressed platelet function has also been observed after maternal use of aspirin close to term (54). The use of salicylates other than aspirin may not be a problem since the acetyl moiety is apparently required to depress platelet function (55–57). In a 1982 study, 10 mothers consuming less than 1 g of aspirin within 5 days of delivery had excessive intrapartum or postpartum blood loss, resulting in hemoglobulin levels that were markedly lower than those of controls (13, 14). One mother required a transfusion. Bleeding complications seen in 9 of the 10 infants included numerous petechiae over the presenting part, hematuria, a cephalohematoma, subconjunctival hemorrhage, and bleeding from a circumcision. No life-threatening hemorrhage, effect on Apgar scores, or increased hospital stay was found, nor was bleeding observed in seven mother-infant pairs when aspirin consumption occurred 6–10 days before delivery (13, 14).

An increased incidence of intracranial hemorrhage (ICH) in premature or low-birth-weight infants may occur after maternal aspirin use near birth (58). Computed tomographic screening for ICH was conducted on 108 infants 3–7 days after delivery. All of the infants were either 34 weeks or less in gestation or 1500 g or less in birth weight. A total of 53 infants (49%) developed ICH, including 12 (71%) of the 17 aspirin-exposed newborns. This incidence was statistically significant ($p < 0.05$) when compared to the 41 (45%) non-aspirin-exposed infants who developed ICH. The conclusions of this study have been challenged and defended (59, 60). In view of the potentially serious outcome, however, full doses of aspirin should be used with extreme caution by patients in danger of premature delivery.

Aspirin readily crosses the placenta (10). When given near term, higher concentrations are found in the neonate than in the mother (61). The kinetics of salicylate elimination in the newborn have been studied (61–63).

The relationship between aspirin and congenital defects is controversial. Several studies have examined this question with findings either supporting or denying a relationship. In two large retrospective studies, mothers of 1291 malformed infants were found to have consumed aspirin during pregnancy more frequently than mothers of normal infants (64, 65). In a retrospective survey of 599 children with oral clefts, use of salicylates in the 1st trimester was almost three times more frequent in the mothers of children with this defect (66). A reviewer of these studies noted several biases, including the fact that they were retrospective, that could account for the results (46). Three other reports of aspirin teratogenicity involving a total of 10 infants have been located (67–69). In each of these cases, other drugs and factors were present.

A 1985 study found a possible association between the use of aspirin in early pregnancy and congenital heart disease (70). The risk for defects in septation of the truncus arteriosus was increased about 2-fold over nonexposed controls. In an earlier retrospective case-control comparison of the relationship between maternal drug intake and congenital heart disease, aspirin was used by 80 of 390 mothers of infants with defects vs. 203 of 1254 mothers of control infants (71). Twelve of the exposed infants had transposition of the great arteries and six had tetralogy of Fallot, but the association between the drug and these defects was weak. The study could not distinguish between the effects of the drug and the underlying condition for which the drug was used (71). A brief review of this and other investigations that have examined the relationship between aspirin and congenital heart disease was published in 1985 (72). The reviewer concluded that too few data existed to associate aspirin with cardiac defects.

A study published in 1989, however, concluded that 1st trimester use of aspirin did not increase the risk of congenital heart defects in relation to other structural anomalies (73). The interval examined encompassed the time of major cardiac development (i.e., from the 5th week after the onset of the last menstrual period to the 9th week of gestation) (73). The data, from the Slone Epidemiology Unit Birth Defects Study, involved 1381 infants with any structural cardiac defect and five subgroups with selected cardiac defects (subgroups were not mutually exclusive): aortic stenosis ($N = 43$), coarctation of the aorta ($N = 123$), hypoplastic left ventricle ($N = 98$), transposition of the great arteries ($N = 210$), and conotruncal defects ($N = 791$). A control group of 6966 infants with other malformations was used for comparison. Infants with syndromes that included cardiac defects, such as Down's syndrome or Holt-Oram syndrome, were excluded from the data, as were mothers who were uncertain about 1st trimester aspirin use or its frequency (73). After adjustment for potential confounding factors, the relative risks for the defects among aspirin users in comparison to controls were: 0.9 (95% confidence interval (CI) 0.8–1.1) for any cardiac defect, 1.2 (95% CI 0.6–2.3) for aortic stenosis, 1.0 (95% CI 0.6–1.4) for coarctation of the aorta, 0.9 (95% CI 0.6–1.4) for hypoplastic left ventricle, 0.9 (95% CI 0.6–1.2) for transposition of the great arteries, and 1.0 (95% CI 0.8–1.2) for conotruncal defects. No dose-effect relationship was observed.

The Collaborative Perinatal Project monitored 50,282 mother-child pairs, 14,864 of which used aspirin during the 1st trimester (6). For use anytime during pregnancy, 32,164 (64%) aspirin exposures were recorded. This prospective study did not find evidence of a teratogenic effect with aspirin. However, the data did not exclude the possibility that grossly excessive doses of aspirin may be teratogenic. An Australian study of 144 infants of mothers who took aspirin regularly in pregnancy also failed to find an association between salicylates and malformations (41). Based on these studies and the fact that aspirin usage in pregnancy is so common, it is not possible to determine the teratogenic risk of salicylates, if indeed it exists.

Full-dose aspirin has been reported to affect adversely the intelligence quotient (IQ) of children exposed *in utero* during the first half of pregnancy (74). In a longitudinal prospective study of the effects of prenatal alcohol exposure on child health and development conducted between 1974–1975, drug histories were obtained from 1529 women during the 5th month of pregnancy. At birth, 421 children were selected for later follow-up based on a system of prebirth criteria. Of these, 192 (45.6% had been exposed to aspirin during the first half of pregnancy. A significant and negative association was discovered between aspirin and child IQ and the children's attentional decrements when they were examined at 4 years of age. The association was not changed after adjustment for a wide variety of potentially confounding covariates. Of interest, the data indicated that girls were significantly more affected than boys (74). The physical growth parameters—height, weight, and head circumference—at 4 years of age were not significantly related to maternal use of aspirin.

In a similar study, data were collected in 19,226 pregnancies by the Collaborative Perinatal Project; aspirin exposure during the first half of pregnancy was reported by 10,159 (52.8%) (75). In contrast to the earlier report, the mean child IQs at 4 years of age in the exposed and nonexposed groups were 98.3 and 96.1, respectively ($p < 0.0001$). Adjustment for multiple confounders reduced the difference between the groups to less than one point but statistical significance remained (75). In addition, no relationship between the amount of aspirin consumed and child IQ was found. The investigators concluded that any adverse effect of *in utero* aspirin exposure on child IQ was unlikely.

In summary, the use of aspirin during pregnancy, especially of chronic or intermittent high doses, should be avoided. The drug may affect maternal and newborn hemostasis mechanisms, leading to an increased risk of hemorrhage. High doses may be related to increased perinatal mortality, intrauterine growth retardation, and teratogenic effects. Low doses, such as 80 mg/day, appear to have beneficial effects in pregnancies complicated by systemic lupus erythematosus with antiphospholipid antibodies. In pregnancies at risk for the development of pregnancy-induced hypertension and preeclampsia, and in fetuses with intrauterine growth retardation, low-dose aspirin (40–150 mg/day) may be beneficial, but more studies are required to assess accurately the risk:benefit ratio of such therapy. Near term, aspirin may prolong gestation and labor. Although aspirin has been used as a tocolytic agent, serious bleeding complications may occur in the newborn. Premature closure of the ductus arteriosus may occur in the latter part of pregnancy as a result of maternal consumption of full-dose aspirin. If an analgesic or antipyretic is needed, acetaminophen should be considered.

[*Risk Factor D if full-dose ASA used in 3rd trimester.]

Breast Feeding Summary

Aspirin and other salicylates are excreted into breast milk in low concentrations. Sodium salicylate was first demonstrated in human milk in 1935 (76). In one study of a mother taking 4 g daily, no detectable salicylate in her milk or in her infant's serum was found, but the test sensitivity was only 50 µg/ml (77). Reported milk concentrations are much lower than this level. Following single or repeated oral doses, peak milk levels occurred at around 3 hours and ranged from 1.1–10 µg/ml (78, 79). This represented a milk:plasma ratio of 0.03–0.08 at 3 hours. Since salicylates are eliminated more slowly from milk than from plasma, the ratio increased to 0.34 at 12 hours (79). Peak levels have also been reported to occur at 9 hours (80). Only one report has attributed infant toxicity to salicylates obtained in mother's milk (81). A 16-day-old female infant developed severe salicylate intoxication with a serum salicylate level of 24 mg/100 ml on the 3rd hospital day. Milk and maternal serum levels were not obtained. Although the parents denied giving the baby aspirin or other salicylates, it is unlikely, based on the above reports, that she could have received the drug from the milk in the quantities found.

Adverse effects on platelet function in the nursing infant exposed to aspirin via the milk have not been reported but are a potential risk. The American Academy of Pediatrics recommends that aspirin should be used cautiously by the mother during lactation because of potential adverse effects in the nursing infant (82).

References

1. Corby DG. Aspirin in pregnancy: maternal and fetal effects. Pediatrics 1978;62(Suppl):930–7.
2. Palmisano PA, Cassady G. Salicylate exposure in the perinate. JAMA 1969;209:556–8.
3. Forfar JO, Nelson MM. Epidemiology of drugs taken by pregnant women: drugs that may affect the fetus adversely. Clin Pharmacol Ther 1973;14:632–42.
4. Finnigan D, Burry AF, Smith IDB. Analgesic consumption in an antenatal clinic survey. Med J Aust 1974;1:761–2.
5. Collins E, Turner G. Maternal effects of regular salicylate ingestion in pregnancy. Lancet 1975;2:335–7.
6. Slone D, Heinonen OP, Kaufman DW, Siskind V, Monson RR, Shapiro S. Aspirin and congenital malformations. Lancet 1976;1:1373–5.
7. Hill RM, Craig JP, Chaney MD, Tennyson LM, McCulley LB. Utilization of over-the-counter drugs during pregnancy. Clin Obstet Gynecol 1977;20:381–94.
8. Harrison K, Thomas I, Smith I. Analgesic use during pregnancy. Med J Aust 1978;2:161.
9. Bodendorfer TW, Briggs GG, Gunning JE. Obtaining drug exposure histories during pregnancy. Am J Obstet Gynecol 1979;135:490–4.
10. Jackson AV. Toxic effects of salicylate on the foetus and mother. J Pathol Bacteriol 1948;60:587–93.
11. Lewis RN, Schulman JD. Influence of acetylsalicylic acid, an inhibitor of prostaglandin synthesis, on the duration of human gestation and labour. Lancet 1973;2:1159–61.
12. Rudolph AM. Effects of aspirin and acetaminophen in pregnancy and in the newborn. Arch Intern Med 1981;141:358–63.
13. Stuart MJ, Gross SJ, Elrad H, Graeber JE. Effects of acetylsalicylic-acid ingestion on maternal and neonatal hemostasis. N Engl J Med 1982;307:909–12.
14. Stuart MJ. Aspirin and maternal or neonatal hemostasis. N Engl J Med 1983;308:281.
15. Niebyl JR, Blake DA, Burnett LS, King TM. The influence of aspirin on the course of induced midtrimester abortion. Am J Obstet Gynecol 1976;124:607–10.

16. Castellanos JM, Aranda M, Cararach J, Cararach V. Effect of aspirin on oestriol excretion in pregnancy. Lancet 1975;1:859.
17. Babenerd VJ, Kyriakidis K. Acetylsalicylic acid in the prevention of premature delivery. Fortschr Med 1979;97:463–6.
18. Wolff F, Bolte A, Berg R. Does an additional administration of acetylsalicylic acid reduce the requirement of β-mimetics in tocolytic treatment? Geburtshilfe Frauenheilkd 1981;41:293–6.
19. Wolff F, Berg R, Bolte A. Clinical study of the labour inhibiting effects and side effects of acetylsalicylic acid (ASA). Geburtshilfe Frauenheilkd 1981;41:96–100.
20. Buhler M, Papiernik E. Successive pregnancies in women fitted with intrauterine devices who take antiinflammatory drugs. Lancet 1983;1:483.
21. Goodlin RC. Correction of pregnancy-related thrombocytopenia with aspirin without improvement in fetal outcome. Am J Obstet Gynecol 1983;146:862–4.
22. Gant NF. Lupus erythematosus, the lupus anticoagulant, and the anticardiolipid antibody. Supplement No. 6, May/June 1986, to Pritchard JA, MacDonald PC, Gant NF. Williams Obstetrics, ed 17. Norwalk:Appleton-Century-Crofts, 1985.
23. Branch DW, Scott JR, Kochenour NK, Hershgold E. Obstetric complications associated with the lupus anticoagulant. N Engl J Med 1985;313:1322–6.
24. Elder MG, DeSwiet M, Robertson A, Elder MA, Flloyd E, Hawkins DF. Low-dose aspirin in pregnancy. Lancet 1988;1:410.
25. Lockshin MD, Druzin ML, Qamar T. Prednisone does not prevent recurrent fetal death in women with antiphospholipid antibody. Am J Obstet Gynecol 1989;160:439–43.
26. Beaufils M, Uzan S, Donsimoni R, Colau JC. Prevention of pre-eclampsia by early antiplatelet therapy. Lancet 1985;1:840–2.
27. Beaufils M, Uzan S, Donsimoni R, Colau JC. Prospective controlled study of early antiplatelet therapy in prevention of preeclampsia. Adv Nephrol 1986;15:87–94.
28. Ylikorkala O, Makila U-M, Kaapa P, Viinikka L. Maternal ingestion of acetylsalicylic acid inhibits fetal and neonatal prostacyclin and thromboxane in humans. Am J Obstet Gynecol 1986;155:345–9.
29. Spitz B, Magness RR, Cox SM, Brown CEL, Rosenfeld CR, Gant NF. Low-dose aspirin. I. Effect on angiotensin II pressor responses and blood prostaglandin concentrations in pregnant women sensitive to angiotensin II. Am J Obstet Gynecol 1988;159:1035–43.
30. Wallenburg HCS, Rotmans N. Prevention of recurrent idiopathic fetal growth retardation by low-dose aspirin and dipyridamole. Am J Obstet Gynecol 1987;157:1230–5.
31. Wallenburg HCS, Rotmans N. Prophylactic low-dose aspirin and dipyridamole in pregnancy. Lancet 1988;1:939.
32. Uzan S, Beaufils M, Bazin B, Danays T. Idiopathic recurrent fetal growth retardation and aspirin-dipyridamole therapy. Am J Obstet Gynecol 1989;160:763.
33. Wallenburg HCS, Rotmans N. Idiopathic recurrent fetal growth retardation and aspirin-dipyridamole therapy. Reply. Am J Obstet Gynecol 1989;160:763–4.
34. Sibai BM, Mirro R, Chesney CM, Leffler C. Low-dose aspirin in pregnancy. Obstet Gynecol 1989;74:551–7.
35. Trudinger B, Cook CM, Thompson R, Giles W, Connelly A. Low-dose aspirin improves fetal weight in umbilical placental insufficiency. Lancet 1988;2:214–5.
36. Romero R, Lockwood C, Oyarzun E, Hobbins JC. Toxemia: new concepts in an old disease. Semin Perinatol 1988;12:302–23.
37. Lubbe WF. Low-dose aspirin in prevention of toxaemia of pregnancy. Does it have a place? Drugs 1987;34:515–8.
38. Wallenburg HCS, Dekker GA, Makovitz JW, Rotmans P. Low-dose aspirin prevents pregnancy-induced hypertension and pre-eclampsia in angiotensin-sensitive primigravidae. Lancet 1986;1:1–3.
39. Benigni A, Gregorini G, Frusca T, Chiabrando C, Ballerini S, Valcamonico A, Orisio S, Piccinelli A, Pinciroli V, Fanelli R, Gastaldi A, Remuzzi G. Effect of low-dose aspirin on fetal and maternal generation of thromboxane by platelets in women at risk for pregnancy-induced hypertension. N Engl J Med 1989;321:357–62.
40. Schiff E, Peleg E, Goldenberg M, Rosenthal T, Ruppin E, Tamarkin M, Barkai G, Ben-Baruch G, Yahal I, Blankstein J, Goldman B, Mashiach S. The use of aspirin to prevent pregnancy-induced hypertension and lower the ratio of thromboxane A_2 to prostacyclin in relatively high risk pregnancies. N Engl J Med 1989;321:351–6.

41. Turner G, Collins E. Fetal effects of regular salicylate ingestion in pregnancy. Lancet 1975;2:338–9.
42. Earle R Jr. Congenital salicylate intoxication—report of a case. N Engl J Med 1961;265:1003–4.
43. Lynd PA, Andreasen AC, Wyatt RJ. Intrauterine salicylate intoxication in a newborn. A case report. Clin Pediatr (Phila) 1976;15:912–3.
44. Shapiro S, Monson RR, Kaufman DW, Siskind V, Heinonen OP, Slone D. Perinatal mortality and birth-weight in relation to aspirin taken during pregnancy. Lancet 1976;1:1375–6.
45. Arcilla RA, Thilenius OG, Ranniger K. Congestive heart failure from suspected ductal closure *in utero*. J Pediatr 1969;75:74–8.
46. Collins E. Maternal and fetal effects of acetaminophen and salicylates in pregnancy. Obstet Gynecol 1981;58(Suppl):57S–62S.
47. Aterman K, Holzbecker M, Ellenberger HA. Salicylate levels in a stillborn infant born to a drug-addicted mother, with comments on pathology and analytical methodology. Clin Toxicol 1980;16:263–8.
48. Bleyer WA, Breckenridge RJ. Studies on the detection of adverse drug reactions in the newborn. II. The effects of prenatal aspirin on newborn hemostasis. JAMA 1970;213:2049–53.
49. Corby DG, Schulman I. The effects of antenatal drug administration on aggregation of platelets of newborn infants. J Pediatr 1971;79:307–13.
50. Casteels-Van Daele M, Eggermont E, de Gaetano G, Vermijlen J. More on the effects of antenatally administered aspirin on aggregation of platelets of neonates. J Pediatr 1972;80:685–6.
51. Haslam RR, Ekert H, Gillam GL. Hemorrhage in a neonate possible due to maternal ingestion of salicylate. J Pediatr 1974;84:556–7.
52. Ekert H, Haslam RR. Maternal ingested salicylate as a cause of neonatal hemorrhage. Reply. J Pediatr 1974;85:738.
53. Pearson H. Comparative effects of aspirin and acetaminophen on hemostasis. Pediatrics 1978;62(Suppl):926–9.
54. Haslam RR. Neonatal purpura secondary to maternal salicylism. J Pediatr 1975;86:653.
55. O'Brien JR. Effects of salicylates on human platelets. Lancet 1968;1:779–83.
56. Weiss HJ, Aledort ML, Shaul I. The effect of salicylates on the haemostatic properties of platelets in man. J Clin Invest 1968;47:2169–80.
57. Bleyer WA. Maternal ingested salicylates as a cause of neonatal hemorrhage. J Pediatr 1974;85:736–7.
58. Rumack CM, Guggenheim MA, Rumack BH, Peterson RG, Johnson ML, Braithwaite WR. Neonatal intracranial hemorrhage and maternal use of aspirin. Obstet Gynecol 1981;58(Suppl):52S–6S.
59. Soller RW, Stander H. Maternal drug exposure and perinatal intracranial hemorrhage. Obstet Gynecol 1981;58:735–7.
60. Corby DG. Editorial comment. Obstet Gynecol 1981;58:737–40.
61. Levy G, Procknal JA, Garrettson LK. Distribution of salicylate between neonatal and maternal serum at diffusion equilibrium. Clin Pharmacol Ther 1975;18:210–4.
62. Levy G, Garrettson LK. Kinetics of salicylate elimination by newborn infants of mothers who ingested aspirin before delivery. Pediatrics 1974;53:201–10.
63. Garrettson LK, Procknal JA, Levy G. Fetal acquisition and neonatal elimination of a large amount of salicylate. Study of a neonate whose mother regularly took therapeutic doses of aspirin during pregnancy. Clin Pharmacol Ther 1975;17:98–103.
64. Richards ID. Congenital malformations and environmental influences in pregnancy. Br J Prev Soc Med 1969;23:218–25.
65. Nelson MM, Forfar JO. Associations between drugs administered during pregnancy and congenital abnormalities of the fetus. Br Med J 1971;1:523–7.
66. Saxen I. Associations between oral clefts and drugs during pregnancy. Int J Epidemiol 1975;4:37–44.
67. Benawra R, Mangurten HH, Duffell DR. Cyclopia and other anomalies following maternal ingestion of salicylates. J Pediatr 1980;96:1069–71.
68. McNiel JR. The possible effect of salicylates on the developing fetus. Brief summaries of eight suggestive cases. Clin Pediatr (Phila) 1973;12:347–50.
69. Sayli BS, Asmaz A, Yemisci B. Consanguinity, aspirin, and phocomelia. Lancet 1966;1:876.
70. Zierler S, Rothman KJ. Congenital heart disease in relation to maternal use of Bendectin and other drugs in early pregnancy. N Engl J Med 1985;313:347–52.

71. Rothman KJ, Fyler DC, Goldblatt A, Kreidberg MB. Exogenous hormones and other drug expo-sures of children with congenital heart disease. Am J Epidemiol 1979;109:433–9.

72. Zierler S. Maternal drugs and congenital heart disease. Obstet Gynecol 1985;65:155–65.

73. Werler MM, Mitchell AA, Shapiro S. The relation of aspirin use during the first trimester of preg-nancy to congenital cardiac defects. N Engl J Med 1989;321:1639–42.

74. Streissguth AP, Treder RP, Barr HM, Shepard TH, Bleyer WA, Sampson PD, Martin DC. Aspirin and acetaminophen use by pregnant women and subsequent child IQ and attention decrements. Teratology 1987;35:211–9.

75. Klebanoff MA, Berendes HW. Aspirin exposure during the first 20 weeks of gestation and IQ at four years of age. Teratology 1988;37:249–55.

76. Kwit NT, Hatcher RA. Excretion of drugs in milk. Am J Dis Child 1935;49:900–4.

77. Erickson SH, Oppenheim GL. Aspirin in breast milk. J Fam Pract 1979;8:189–90.

78. Weibert RT, Bailey DN. Salicylate excretion in human breast milk (Abstract No. 7). Presented at the 1979 Seminar of the California Society of Hospital Pharmacists, Los Angeles, October 13, 1979.

79. Findlay JWA, DeAngelis RL, Kearney MF, Welch RM, Findley JM. Analgesic drugs in breast milk and plasma. Clin Pharmacol Ther 1981;29:625–33.

80. Anderson PO. Drugs and breast feeding—a review. Drug Intell Clin Pharm 1977;11:208–23.

81. Clark JH, Wilson WG. A 16-day-old breast-fed infant with metabolic acidosis caused by salicylate. Clin Pediatr (Phila) 1981;20:53–4.

82. Committee on Drugs, American Academy of Pediatrics. Transfer of drugs and other chemicals into human milk. Pediatrics 1989;84;924–36.

Name: **ATENOLOL**

Class: **Sympatholytic (β-Adrenergic Blocker)**   Risk Factor: C_M

Fetal Risk Summary

Atenolol is a cardioselective β-adrenergic blocking agent used for the treatment of hypertension. The drug readily crosses the placenta to the fetus producing steady state fetal levels that are approximately equal to those in the maternal serum (1–7). Atenolol transfer was one-third to one-fourth the transfer of the more lipid-soluble β-blockers propranolol, timolol, and labetalol in an *in vitro* experiment us-ing perfused human placentas (8). In 11 pregnant patients treated with 100 mg/day, the serum half-life (8.1 hours) and the 24-hour urinary excretion (52 mg) were similar to those in nonpregnant women (6).

Safe use of atenolol for the treatment of hypertension in the pregnant woman has been documented by several investigators (5, 9–15). No fetal malformations attributable to atenolol have been reported, but experience with the drug during the 1st trimester is lacking. Reduced birth weight and persistent β-blockade in the newborn have been observed after atenolol exposure.

In a nonrandomized study comparing atenolol with two other β-blockers for the treatment of hypertension during pregnancy, the mean birth weight of atenolol-exposed babies was markedly lower than infants exposed *in utero* to either acebutolol or pindolol (2745 g vs. 3160 g vs. 3375 g) (14, 16). A similar study comparing atenolol with labetalol found a significant difference in the birth weights of the two groups, 2750 g vs. 3280 g ($p < 0.001$) (4). No difference was found in the birth weights of atenolol- vs. placebo-exposed infants (2961 g vs. 3017 g) in a randomized, double blind investigation of 120 pregnant women with mild to mod-erate hypertension (12). The differences observed in the above studies may be related to the severity of the maternal hypertension combined with the more pronounced maternal bradycardia noted in atenolol-treated women resulting in placental insufficiency. However, in a prospective randomized study comparing 24 atenolol-treated women with 27 pindolol-treated women, no differences between the groups were found in gestational length, birth weight, Apgar scores, rates of cesarean section, or umbilical cord blood glucose levels (17). Treatment in both groups started at about 33 weeks' gestation. Intrauterine fetal deaths have been observed in women with severe hypertension treated with atenolol, but this has also occurred with other β-blockers and in hypertensive women not treated with drugs (4, 12, 18).

In eight mothers treated with atenolol or pindolol, a decrease in the basal fetal heart rate was noted only in atenolol-exposed fetuses (19). Before and during treatment, fetal heart rates in the atenolol patients were 136 and 120 beats/minute while the rates for the pindolol group were 128 and 132 beats/minute. In 60 patients treated with atenolol for pregnancy-induced hypertension, no effect was observed on fetal heart rate pattern in response to uterine contractions (20). Accelerations, variables, and late decelerations were all easily distinguishable (20).

Persistent β-blockade was observed in a newborn whose mother was treated with atenolol, 100 mg/day, for hypertension (2). At 15 hours of age, the otherwise normal infant developed bradycardia at rest and when crying, and hypotension. Serum atenolol was 0.24 μg/ml. Urinary excretion of the drug during the first 7 days ranged from 0.85–0.196 μg/ml. In another study, 39% (18 of 46) of the newborns exposed to atenolol developed bradycardia compared to only 10% (4 of 39) of placebo-exposed newborns ($p < 0.01$) (12). None of the infants required treatment for the lowered heart rate.

Doppler ultrasound was used to study maternal and fetal circulation during atenolol therapy in 14 women with pregnancy-induced hypertension at a mean gestational age of 35 weeks (range 33–38 weeks) (21). The results suggested that peripheral vascular resistance was increased on both the maternal and fetal sides of the placenta. However, the study design and techniques used have been criticized based on concerns for reproducibility, including day-to-day variability in Doppler measurements, the lack of controls in the study, and the uncertainty of the clinical significance of velocity waveform measurements (22).

Exposure to atenolol *in utero* apparently has no effect on infant growth or behavior. No differences were noted in the development at 1 year of age of offspring from mothers treated during the 3rd trimester for mild to moderate pregnancy-induced hypertension with either bed rest alone or rest combined with atenolol (23). The mean duration of therapy in the atenolol-treated patients was 5 weeks.

Newborns exposed to atenolol near delivery should be closely observed during the first 24–48 hours for signs and symptoms of β-blockade. Long-term effects of *in utero* exposure to this class of drugs have not been studied but warrant evaluation.

Breast Feeding Summary

Atenolol is excreted into breast milk (3, 6, 24–28). The drug is a weak base, and accumulation in the milk occurs with concentrations significantly greater than corresponding plasma levels (3, 24–27). Peak milk concentrations after single (50 mg) and continuous dosing (25–100 mg/day) regimens were 3.6 and 2.9 times greater than simultaneous plasma levels (26). Atenolol has been found in the serum and urine of breast-fed infants in some studies (3, 6, 24). Other studies have been unable to detect the drug in the infant serum (test limit 10 ng/ml) (25, 26).

Symptoms consistent with β-adrenergic blockade were observed in a breast-fed, 5-day-old, full-term female infant, including cyanosis, hypothermia (35.5°C rectal), and bradycardia (80 beats/minute) (28). Blood pressure was 80/40 mm Hg. Except for these findings, physical examination was normal and bacterial cultures from various sites were negative. The mother had been treated orally with atenolol, 50 mg every 12 hours, for postpartum hypertension. Breast feeding was stopped 3 days after onset of the symptoms and 6 hours later the infant's symptoms had resolved. A milk sample, collected 10 days postpartum and 1.5 hours after a 50 mg dose, contained 469 ng/ml of atenolol. Concentrations in the infant's serum, 48 and 72 hours after breast feeding, were 2010 ng/ml and 140 ng/ml, respectively. The calculated serum half-life in the infant was 6.4 hours. By extrapolation, the minimum daily dose absorbed by the infant was estimated to be 8.97 mg, approximately 9% of the mother's daily dose (28). (These calculations have been questioned and defended (29, 30).) Except for this case, adverse reactions in other infants have not been reported. However, since milk accumulation occurs with atenolol, nursing infants must be closely monitored for bradycardia and other signs and symptoms of β-blockade. Long-term effects on infants exposed to β-blockers from breast milk have not been studied but warrant evaluation. The American Academy of Pediatrics considers atenolol to be compatible with breast feeding (although the above adverse reaction report was not cited) (31).

References

1. Melander A, Niklasson B, Ingemarsson I, Liedholm H, Schersten B, Sjoberg NO. Transplacental passage of atenolol in man. Eur J Clin Pharmacol 1978;14:93–4.
2. Woods DL, Morrell DF. Atenolol: side effects in a newborn infant. Br Med J 1982;285:691–2.
3. Liedholm H. Transplacental passage and breast milk accumulation of atenolol in humans. Drugs 1983;25(Suppl 2):217–8.
4. Lardoux H, Gerard J, Blazquez G, Chouty F, Flouvat B. Hypertension in pregnancy: evaluation of two beta blockers atenolol and labetalol. Eur Heart J 1983;4(Suppl G):35–40.
5. Liedholm H. Atenolol in the treatment of hypertension of pregnancy. Drugs 1983;25(Suppl 2):206–11.
6. Thorley KJ. Pharmacokinetics of atenolol in pregnancy and lactation. Drugs 1983;25(Suppl 2):216–7.
7. Boutroy MJ. Fetal and neonatal effects of the beta-adrenoceptor blocking agents. Dev Pharmacol Ther 1987;10:224–31.
8. Schneider H, Proegler M. Placental transfer of β-adrenergic antagonists studied in an *in vitro* perfusion system of human placental tissue. Am J Obstet Gynecol 1988;159:42–7.
9. Dubois D, Petitcolas J, Temperville B, Klepper A. Beta blockers and high-risk pregnancies. Int J Biol Res Pregnancy 1980;1:141–5.
10. Thorley KJ, McAinsh J, Cruickshank JM. Atenolol in the treatment of pregnancy-induced hypertension. Br J Clin Pharmacol 1981;12:725–30.
11. Rubin PC, Butters L, Low RA, Reid JL. Atenolol in the treatment of essential hypertension during pregnancy. Br J Clin Pharmacol 1982;14:279–81.
12. Rubin PC, Butters L, Clark DM, Reynolds B, Sumner DJ, Steedman D, Low RA, Reid JL. Placebo-controlled trial of atenolol in treatment of pregnancy-associated hypertension. Lancet 1983;1:431–4.
13. Rubin PC, Butters L, Low RA, Clark DC, Reid JL. Atenolol in the management of hypertension during pregnancy. Drugs 1983;25(Suppl 2):212–4.
14. Dubois D, Peticolas J, Temperville B, Klepper A. Treatment with atenolol of hypertension in pregnancy. Drugs 1983;25(Suppl 2):215–8.
15. Frishman WH, Chesner M. Beta-adrenergic blockers in pregnancy. Am Heart J 1988;115:147–52.

16. Dubois D, Petitcolas J, Temperville B, Klepper A, Catherine P. Treatment of hypertension in pregnancy with β-adrenoceptor antagonists. Br J Clin Pharmacol 1982;13(Suppl):375S–8S.
17. Tuimala R, Hartikainen-Sorri A-L. Randomized comparison of atenolol and pindolol for treatment of hypertension in pregnancy. Curr Ther Res 1988;44:579–84.
18. Lubbe WF. More on beta-blockers in pregnancy. N Engl J Med 1982;307:753.
19. Ingemarsson I, Liedholm H, Montan S, Westgren M, Melander A. Fetal heart rate during treatment of maternal hypertension with beta-adrenergic antagonists. Acta Obstet Gynecol Scand 1984;118(Suppl):95–7.
20. Rubin PC, Butters L, Clark D, Sumner D, Belfield A, Pledger D, Low RAL, Reid JL. Obstetric aspects of the use in pregnancy-associated hypertension of the β-adrenoceptor antagonist atenolol. Am J Obstet Gynecol 1984;150:389–92.
21. Montan S, Liedholm H, Lingman G, Marsal K, Sjoberg N-O, Solum T. Fetal and uteroplacental haemodynamics during short-term atenolol treatment of hypertension in pregnancy. Br J Obstet Gynaecol 1987;94:312–7.
22. Rubin PC. Beta blockers in pregnancy. Br J Obstet Gynaecol 1987;94:292–3.
23. Reynolds B, Butters L, Evans J, Adams T, Rubin PC. First year of life after the use of atenolol in pregnancy associated hypertension. Arch Dis Child 1984;59:1061–3.
24. Liedholm H, Melander A, Bitzen PO, Helm G, Lonnerholm G, Mattiasson I, Nilsson B, Wahlin-Boll E. Accumulation of atenolol and metoprolol in human breast milk. Eur J Clin Pharmacol 1981;20:229–31.
25. Kulas J, Lunell NO, Rosing U, Steen B, Rane A. Atenolol and metoprolol. A comparison of their excretion into human breast milk. Acta Obstet Gynecol Scand 1984;118(Suppl):65–9.
26. White WB, Andreoli JW, Wong SH, Cohn RD. Atenolol in human plasma and breast milk. Obstet Gynecol 1984;63:42S–4S.
27. White WB. Management of hypertension during lactation. Hypertension 1984;6:297–300.
28. Schmimmel MS, Eidelman AJ, Wilschanski MA, Shaw D Jr, Ogilvie RJ, Koren G. Toxic effects of atenolol consumed during breast feeding. J Pediatr 1989;114:476–8.
29. Diamond JM. Toxic effects of atenolol consumed during breast feeding. J Pediatr 1989;115:336.
30. Koren G. Toxic effects of atenolol consumed during breast feeding. J Pediatr 1989;115:336–7.
31. Committee on Drugs, American Academy of Pediatrics. Transfer of drugs and other chemicals into human milk. Pediatrics 1989;84:924–36.

Name: **ATROPINE**

Class: **Parasympatholytic**　　　　　　　　　　　　　　　Risk Factor: **C**

Fetal Risk Summary

Atropine, an anticholinergic, rapidly crosses the placenta (1–3). Atropine exposure in the 1st, 2nd, and 3rd trimesters was estimated in one study to be 11.3, 6.7, and 6.3/1,000 women, respectively (4). The drug has been used to test placental function in high-risk obstetric patients by producing fetal vagal blockade and subsequent tachycardia (5). The Collaborative Perinatal Project monitored 50,282 mother-child pairs, 401 of which used atropine in the 1st trimester (6, pp. 346–353). For use anytime during pregnancy, 1,198 exposures were recorded (6, p. 439). In neither case was evidence found for an association with malformations. However, when the group of parasympatholytics were taken as a whole (2,323 exposures), a possible association with minor malformations was found (6, pp. 346–353). Atropine has been used to reduce gastric secretions prior to cesarean section without producing fetal or neonatal effects (7, 8). In a study comparing atropine and glycopyrrolate, 10 women in labor received 0.01 mg/kg of atropine intravenously (9). No statistically significant changes were noted in fetal heart rate or variability nor was there any effect on uterine acitivity.

A single case of a female infant born at 36 weeks' gestation with multiple defects, including Ebstein's anomaly, was described in a 1989 report (10). In addition to the cardiac defect, other abnormalities noted were hypertelorism, epicanthal folds, low-set posteriorly rotated ears, a cleft uvula, medially rotated hands, deafness, and blindness. The mother had taken Lomotil (diphenoxylate and atropine) for diarrhea during the 10th week of gestation. Since exposure was beyond the susceptible stages of development for these defects, the drug combination was not considered causative. However, a possible viremia in the mother as a cause of the diarrhea could not be excluded as playing a role in the infant's anomalies.

Breast Feeding Summary

The passage of atropine into breast milk is controversial (11). It has not been adequately documented if measurable amounts are excreted or, if excretion does occur, whether this may affect the nursing infant. Although neonates are particularly sensitive to anticholinergic agents, no adverse effects have been reported in nursing infants whose mothers were taking atropine and the American Academy of Pediatrics considers the agent to be compatible with breast feeding (12).

References

1. Nishimura H, Tanimura T. *Clinical Aspects of the Teratogenicity of Drugs*. New York:American Elsevier, 1976:63.
2. Kivalo I, Saarikoski S. Placental transmission of atropine at full-term pregnancy. Br J Anaesth 1977;49:1017–21.
3. Kanto J, Virtanen R, Iisalo E, Maenpaa K, Liukko P. Placental transfer and pharmacokinetics of atropine after a single maternal intravenous and intramuscular administration. Acta Anaesth Scand 1981;25:85–8.
4. Piper JM, Baum C, Kennedy DL, Price P. Maternal use of prescribed drugs associated with recognized fetal adverse drug reactions. Am J Obstet Gynecol 1988;159:1173–7.
5. Hellman LM, Fillisti LP. Analysis of the atropine test for placental transfer in gravidas with toxemia and diabetes. Am J Obstet Gynecol 1965;91:797–805.
6. Heinonen OP, Slone D, Shapiro S. *Birth Defects and Drugs in Pregnancy*. Littleton:Publishing Sciences Group, 1977.
7. Diaz DM, Diaz SF, Marx GF. Cardiovascular effects of glycopyrrolate and belladonna derivatives in obstetric patients. Bull NY Acad Med 1980;56:245–8.
8. Roper RE, Salem MG. Effects of glycopyrrolate and atropine combined with antacid on gastric acidity. Br J Anaesth 1981;53:1277–80.
9. Abboud T, Raya J, Sadri S, Grobler N, Stine L, Miller F. Fetal and maternal cardiovascular effects of atropine and glycopyrrolate. Anesth Analg 1983;62:426–30.
10. Siebert JR, Barr M Jr, Jackson JG, Benjamin DR. Ebstein's anomaly and extracardiac defects. Am J Dis Child 1989;143:570–2.
11. Stewart JJ. Gastrointestinal drugs. In Wilson JT, ed. *Drugs in Breast Milk*. Australia (Balgowlah):ADIS Press, 1981:65–71.
12. Committee on Drugs, American Academy of Pediatrics. Transfer of drugs and other chemicals into human milk. Pediatrics 1989;84:924–36.

Name: **AUROTHIOGLUCOSE**

Class: **Gold Compound**   Risk Factor: **C**

Fetal Risk Summary

See Gold Sodium Thiomalate.

Breast Feeding Summary

See Gold Sodium Thiomalate.

Name: **AZATADINE**

Class: **Antihistamine** Risk Factor: **B$_M$**

Fetal Risk Summary

No data are available. See Diphenhydramine for representative agent in this class.

Breast Feeding Summary

No data are available.

Name: **AZATHIOPRINE**

Class: **Antineoplastic/Immunosuppressant** Risk Factor: **D**

Fetal Risk Summary

Azathioprine is used primarily in patients with organ transplants or in those with inflammatory bowel disease. Prednisone is commonly combined with azathioprine in these patients. The drug readily crosses the placenta, and trace amounts of its active metabolite, 6-mercaptopurine, have been found in fetal blood (see also Mercaptopurine) (1).

Most investigators have found azathioprine to be relatively safe in pregnancy (2–20). The use of azathioprine during pregnancy in women who have received renal transplants has been reviewed (20, 21). Although teratogenic in animals, the drug has not been associated with congenital defects in humans. Sporadic anomalies have been reported but these are not believed to be related to the drug therapy (20, 21). Defects observed include pulmonary valvular stenosis (22), pre-axial polydactyly (thumb polydactyly type) (23), hypothyroidism and atrial septal defect (azathioprine therapy started in 2nd trimester) (24), hypospadias (mother also had severe diabetes mellitus) (17), plagiocephaly with neurologic damage (11), congenital heart disease (mild mitral regurgitation) (11), bilateral pes equinovarus (11), cerebral palsy (frontal hemangioma) and cerebral hemorrhage (died at 2 days of age) in twins (11), hypospadias (11), and congenital cytomegalovirus infection (11). The later infection has also been reported in another infant whose mother was taking azathioprine (8). Chromosomal aberrations were noted in three infants after *in utero* exposure to the drug, but the relationship to azathioprine and the clinical significance of the findings are questionable (11, 25).

Immunosuppression of the newborn was observed in one infant whose mother received 150 mg of azathioprine and 30 mg of prednisone daily throughout pregnancy (8). The suppression was characterized by lymphopenia, decreased survival of lymphocytes in culture, absence of immunoglobulin M, and reduced levels of immunoglobulin G. Recovery occurred at about 15 weeks of age. An infant exposed to 125 mg of azathioprine plus 12.5 mg of prednisone daily during pregnancy was born with pancytopenia and severe combined immune deficiency (26). The infant died at 28 days from complications brought on by irreversible bone marrow and lymphoid hypoplasia. To avoid neonatal leukopenia and thrombocytopenia, maternal doses of azathioprine were reduced during the 3rd trimester in a 1985 study (27). The investigators found a significant correlation between maternal leukocyte counts at 32 weeks' gestation and at delivery and cord blood leukocyte count. If the mother's count was at or below 1 standard deviation for normal pregnancy, her dose of azathioprine was halved. Before this technique was used, several newborns had leukopenia and thrombocytopenia, but no low levels were measured after institution of the new procedure.

Intrauterine growth retardation may be related to the use of azathioprine in pregnancy. Based on animal experiments and analysis of human exposures, one investigator concluded that growth retardation was associated with the drug (28). More recent reports have also supported this association (29). The incidence of small-for-gestational age infants from women who have undergone renal transplants and who are maintained on azathioprine and corticosteroids is approximately 20% (18, 20), but some centers have rates as high as 40% (29). However, the effects of the underlying disease, including hypertension, vascular disease, and renal impairment, as well as the use of multiple medications other than azathioprine, cannot be excluded as major or sole contributors to the growth retardation.

Azathioprine has been reported to interfere with the effectiveness of intrauterine contraceptive devices (IUD) (20, 30). Two renal transplant patients, maintained on azathioprine and prednisone, received a copper IUD (Cu7) and both became pregnant with the IUD in place (30). At another institution, 6 of 20 renal transplant patients have become pregnant with IUD devices *in utero* (20). Because of these failures, additional or other methods of contraception should be considered in sexually active women receiving azathioprine/prednisone.

Breast Feeding Summary

No data are available.

References

1. Sarrikoski S, Seppala M. Immunosuppression during pregnancy. Transmission of azathioprine and its metabolites from the mother to the fetus. Am J Obstet Gynecol 1973;115:1100–6.
2. Gillibrand PN. Systemic lupus erythematosus in pregnancy treated with azathioprine. Proc R Soc Med 1966;59:834.
3. Board JA, Lee HM, Draper DA, Hume DM. Pregnancy following kidney homotransplantation from a non-twin: report of a case with concurrent administration of azathioprine and prednisone. Obstet Gynecol 1967;29:318–23.
4. Kaufmann JJ, Dignam W, Goodwin WE, Martin DC, Goldman R, Maxwell MH. Successful, normal childbirth after kidney homotransplantation. JAMA 1967;200:338–41.
5. Anonymous. Eleventh annual report of human renal transplant registry. JAMA 1973;216:1197.
6. Nolan GH, Sweet RL, Laros RK, Roure CA. Renal cadaver transplantation followed by successful pregnancies. Obstet Gynecol 1974;43:732–8.
7. Sharon E, Jones J, Diamond H, Kaplan D. Pregnancy and azathioprine in systemic lupus erythematosus. Am J Obstet Gynecol 1974;118:25–7.
8. Cote CJ, Meuwissen HJ, Pickering RJ. Effects on the neonate of prednisone and azathioprine administered to the mother during pregnancy. J Pediatr 1974;85:324–8.

9. Erkman J, Blythe JG. Azathioprine therapy complicated by pregnancy. Obstet Gynecol 1972;40:708–9.
10. Price HV, Salaman JR, Laurence KM, Langmaid H. Immunosuppressive drugs and the foetus. Transplantation 1976;21:294–8.
11. The Registration Committee of the European Dialysis and Transplant Association. Successful pregnancies in women treated by dialysis and kidney transplantation. Br J Obstet Gynaecol 1980;87:839–45.
12. Golby M. Fertility after renal transplantation. Transplantation 1970;10:201–7.
13. Rabau-Friedman E, Mashiach S, Cantor E, Jacob ET. Association of hypoparathyroidism and successful pregnancy in kidney transplant recipient. Obstet Gynecol 1982;59:126–8.
14. Myers RL, Schmid R, Newton JJ. Childbirth after liver transplantation. Transplantation 1980;29:432.
15. Williams PF, Johnstone M. Normal pregnancy in renal transplant recipient with history of eclampsia and intrauterine death. Br Med J 1982;285:1535.
16. Westney LS, Callender CO, Stevens J, Bhagwanani SG, George JPA, Mims OL. Successful pregnancy with sickle cell disease and renal transplantation. Obstet Gynecol 1984;63:752–5.
17. Ogburn PL Jr, Kitzmiller JL, Hare JW, Phillippe M, Gabbe SG, Miodovnik M, Tagatz GE, Nagel TC, Williams PP, Goetz FC, Barbosa JJ, Sutherland DE. Pregnancy following renal transplantation in class T diabetes mellitus. JAMA 1986;255:911–5.
18. Marushak A, Weber T, Bock J, Birkeland SA, Hansen HE, Klebe J, Kristoffersen K, Rasmussen K, Olgaard K. Pregnancy following kidney transplantation. Acta Obstet Gynecol Scand 1986;65:557–9.
19. Key TC, Resnik R, Dittrich HC, Reisner LS. Successful pregnancy after cardiac transplantation. Am J Obstet Gynecol 1989;160:367–71.
20. Davison JM, Lindheimer MD. Pregnancy in renal transplant recipients. J Reprod Med 1982;27:613–21.
21. Kossoy LR, Herbert CM III, Wentz AC. Management of heart transplant recipients: guidelines for the obstetrician-gynecologist. Am J Obstet Gynecol 1988;159:490–9.
22. Nishimura H, Tanimura T. Clinical Aspects of the Teratogenicity of Drugs. New York:American Elsevier, 1976:106–7.
23. Williamson RA, Karp LE. Azathioprine teratogenicity: review of the literature and case report. Obstet Gynecol 1981;58:247–50.
24. Burleson RL, Sunderji SG, Aubry RH, Clark DA, Marbarger P, Cohen RS, Scruggs BF, Lagraff S. Renal allotransplantation during pregnancy. Successful outcome for mother, child, and kidney. Transplantation 1983;36:334.
25. Leb DE, Weisskopf B, Kanovitz BS. Chromosome aberrations in the child of a kidney transplant recipient. Arch Intern Med 1971;128:441–4.
26. DeWitte DB, Buick MK, Cyran SE, Maisels MJ. Neonatal pancytopenia and severe combined immunodeficiency associated with antenatal administration of azathioprine and prednisone. J Pediatr 1984;105:625–8.
27. Davison JM, Dellagrammatikas H, Parkin JM. Maternal azathioprine therapy and depressed haemopoiesis in the babies of renal allograft patients. Br J Obstet Gynaecol 1985;92:233–9.
28. Scott JR. Fetal growth retardation associated with maternal administration of immunosuppressive drugs. Am J Obstet Gynecol 1977;128:668–76.
29. Pirson Y, Van Lierde M, Ghysen J, Squifflet JP, Alexandre GPJ, van Ypersele De Strihou C. Retardation of fetal growth in patients receiving immunosuppressive therapy. N Engl J Med 1985;313:328.
30. Zerner J, Doil KL, Drewry J, Leeber DA. Intrauterine contraceptive device failures in renal transplant patients. J Reprod Med 1981;26:99–102.

b

Name: **BACAMPICILLIN**

Class: **Antibiotic**   Risk Factor: **B_M**

Fetal Risk Summary

Bacampicillin, a penicillin antibiotic, is converted to ampicillin during absorption from the gastrointestinal tract (see Ampicillin).

Breast Feeding Summary

See Ampicillin.

Name: **BACITRACIN**

Class: **Antibiotic**   Risk Factor: **C**

Fetal Risk Summary

No reports linking the use of bacitracin with congenital defects have been located. The drug is primarily used topically, although the injectable form is available. One study listed 18 patients exposed to the drug in the 1st trimester (1). The route of administration was not specified. No association with malformations was found.

Breast Feeding Summary

No data are available.

Reference

1. Heinonen OP, Slone D, Shapiro S. *Birth Defects and Drugs in Pregnancy*. Littleton:Publishing Sciences Group, 1977:297, 301.

Name: **BECLOMETHASONE**

Class: **Adrenal Hormone**   Risk Factor: **C**

Fetal Risk Summary

Beclomethasone dipropionate is given by inhalation for the chronic treatment of bronchial asthma in patients requiring corticosteroid therapy for the control of symptoms. It is also available for intranasal use and, outside of the United States, for topical application. The drug is an animal teratogen, but human reports have not associated its use during pregnancy with congenital anomalies (1–3).

In one report, beclomethasone was used during 45 pregnancies in 40 women (1). Dosage ranged between 4–16 inhalations/day (mean 9.5), with each inhalation delivering 42 μg of drug. Three of the 33 prospectively followed pregnancies ended in abortion that was not thought to be due to the maternal asthma. Forty-three living infants resulted from the remaining 42 pregnancies. Six infants had low birth weights, including two of the three premature (less than 37 weeks' gestation) newborns. There was no evidence of neonatal adrenal insufficiency. One full-term infant had cardiac malformations (double ventricular septal defect, patient ductus arteriosus, and subaortic stenosis). However, the mother's asthma was also treated with prednisone, theophylline, and epinephrine. In addition, she had schizophrenia and diabetes mellitus for which she took fluphenazine and insulin. Cardiac malformations are known to occur with diabetes mellitus (see Insulin).

Breast Feeding Summary

It is not known whether beclomethasone is excreted into breast milk. Other corticosteroids are excreted into milk in low concentrations (see Prednisone), and the manufacturer assumes that beclomethasone dipropionate is also excreted (4). One report has been located that notes three cases of maternal beclomethasone use during breast feeding (3). Effects on the nursing infants were not mentioned.

References

1. Greenberger PA, Patterson R. Beclomethasone dipropionate for severe asthma during pregnancy. Ann Intern Med 1983;98:478–80.
2. Mawhinney H, Spector SL. Optimum management of asthma in pregnancy. Drugs 1986;32:178–87.
3. Brown HM, Storey G. Treatment of allergy of the respiratory tract with beclomethasone dipropionate steroid aerosol. Postgrad Med J 1975;51(Suppl 4):59–64.
4. Product information. Vanceril Inhaler. Schering Corporation, 1990.

Name: **BELLADONNA**

Class: **Parasympatholytic**   Risk Factor: **C**

Fetal Risk Summary

Belladonna is an anticholinergic agent. The Collaborative Perinatal Project monitored 50,282 mother-child pairs, 554 of which used belladonna in the 1st trimester (1, pp. 346–353). Belladonna was found to be associated with malformations in general and with minor malformations. For use anytime during pregnancy, 1,355 exposures were recorded (1, p. 439). No association was found in this case.

Breast Feeding Summary

See Atropine.

Reference

1. Heinonen OP, Slone D, Shapiro S. *Birth Defects and Drugs in Pregnancy.* Littleton:Publishing Sciences Group, 1977.

Name: **BENDROFLUMETHIAZIDE**

Class: **Diuretic**   Risk Factor: **D***

Fetal Risk Summary

See Chlorothiazide.

[*Risk Factor C according to manufacturer — Princeton Pharmaceutical Products, 1990.]

Breast Feeding Summary

Bendroflumethiazide has been used to suppress lactation (see Chlorothiazide).

Name: **BENZTHIAZIDE**

Class: **Diuretic**   Risk Factor: **D**

Fetal Risk Summary

See Chlorothiazide.

Breast Feeding Summary

See Chlorothiazide.

Name: **BENZTROPINE**

Class: **Parasympatholytic**   Risk Factor: **C**

Fetal Risk Summary

Benztropine is an anticholinergic agent structurally related to atropine (see also Atropine). It also has antihistaminic activity. In a large prospective study, 2323 patients were exposed to this class of drugs during the 1st trimester, 4 of whom took benztropine (1). A possible association was found between the total group and minor malformations. Paralytic ileus has been observed in two newborns exposed to chlorpromazine and benztropine at term (2). In one of these infants, other anticholinergic drugs may have contributed to the effect (see Doxepin). The small left colon syndrome was characterized by decreased intestinal motility, abdominal distention, vomiting, and failure to pass meconium. The condition cleared rapidly in both infants following a Gastrografin enema.

Breast Feeding Summary

No data are available (see Atropine).

References

1. Heinonen OP, Slone D, Shapiro S. *Birth Defects and Drugs in Pregnancy*. Littleton:Publishing Sciences Group, 1977:346–53.

2. Falterman CG, Richardson CJ. Small left colon syndrome associated with maternal ingestion of psychotropic drugs. J Pediatr 1980;97:308–10.

Name: β-**CAROTENE**

Class: **Vitamin** Risk Factor: **C**

Fetal Risk Summary

β-Carotene, a natural precursor to vitamin A found in green and yellow vegetables as well as commercially available, is partially converted in the small intestine to vitamin A (1). Even with therapeutic doses of the drug, serum levels of vitamin A do not rise above normal. No reports of the therapeutic use of this vitamin in human pregnancy have been located. Studies in animals have failed to show a teratogenic effect (see also Vitamin A) (2).

Breast Feeding Summary

No data are available.

References

1. American Hospital Formulary Service. *Drug Information 1990*. Bethesda:American Society of Hospital Pharmacists, 1990:2108–9.
2. Nishimura H, Tanimura T. *Clinical Aspects of The Teratogenicity of Drugs*. New York:American Elsevier, 1978:252.

Name: **BETAMETHASONE**

Class: **Corticosteroid** Risk Factor: **C**

Fetal Risk Summary

No reports linking the use of betamethasone with congenital defects have been located. Betamethasone is often used in patients with premature labor at about 26–34 weeks' gestation to stimulate fetal lung maturation (1–15). The benefits of this therapy are:

Reduction in incidence of respiratory distress syndrome (RDS)
Decreased severity of RDS if it occurs
Decreased incidence of, and mortality from, intracranial hemorrhage
Increased survival of premature infants

Betamethasone crosses the placenta to the fetus (16). The drug is partially metabolized (47%) by the perfused placenta to its inactive 11-ketosteroid derivative but less so than other corticosteroids, although the differences are not statistically significant (17).

In patients with premature rupture of the membranes (PROM), administration of betamethasone to the mother does not always reduce the frequency of RDS or perinatal mortality (18–22). An increased risk of maternal infection has also been observed in patients with PROM treated with corticosteroids (19, 20). In a study comparing betamethasone therapy with nonsteroid management of women with PROM, neonatal sepsis was observed in 23% (5 of 22) of steroid-exposed newborns vs. only 2% (1 of 46) of the non-steroid-exposed group (21). A 1985 study also found increased neonatal sepsis in exposed newborns who were delivered more than 48 hours after PROM, 18.6% (14 of 75) vs. 7.4% (4 of 54) of nonexposed controls (22). In addition, moderate to severe respiratory morbidity was increased over that in controls, 21.3% vs. 11.1%, as well as over-all mortality, 8% vs. 1.8% (22). Other reports, however, have noted beneficial effects of betamethasone administration to patients with PROM with no increase in infectious morbidity (15, 23, 24). In women colonized with group B streptococci, the combined use of betamethasone and ampicillin improved the outcome of preterm pregnancies with PROM (25).

Betamethasone therapy is less effective in decreasing the incidence of RDS in male infants than in female infants (23, 26, 27). The reasons for this difference have not been discovered. Slower lung maturation in male fetuses has been cited as a major contributing factor to the sex differential noted in neonatal mortality (28). Therapy is also less effective in multiple pregnancies, even when doses have been doubled (27). In twins, only the first-born seems to be benefited by antenatal steroid therapy (27).

An increased incidence of hypoglycemia in newborns exposed *in utero* to betamethasone has been reported (29). Other reports have not observed this effect.

In the initial study examining the effect of betamethasone on RDS, investigators reported an increased risk of fetal death in patients with severe preeclampsia (1). They proposed that the corticosteroid had an adverse effect on placentas already damaged by vascular disease. A second study did not confirm these findings (7).

Leukocytosis was observed in an 880-g, 30-weeks'-gestation female infant whose mother received 12 mg of betamethasone 4 hours prior to delivery (30). The white blood cell count returned to normal in about 1 week. A 1984 study examined the effect of betamethasone on leukocyte counts in mothers with PROM or premature labor (31). No effect, as compared to untreated controls, was found in either group.

Respiratory crisis secondary to acute exacerbation of muscular weakness was described in a woman with myasthenia gravis treated with betamethasone and ritodrine for premature labor (32). Adrenocorticosteroids are known to aggravate myasthenia so the condition was thought to be due to betamethasone. Hypertensive crisis associated with the use of ritodrine and betamethasone has been reported (33). Systolic blood pressure was above 300 mm Hg with a diastolic pressure of 120 mm Hg. Although the hypertension was probably caused by ritodrine, it is not known whether the corticosteroid was a contributing factor.

The effect of betamethasone administration on patent ductus arteriosus (PDA) was investigated in premature infants with birth weights less than 2000 g (34). Infants of nontreated mothers had a PDA incidence of 44% vs. 6.5% for infants of treated mothers ($p < 0.01$). This reduction in the incidence of PDA after betamethasone therapy has also been observed in other studies (25). A study published in 1989 indicated that betamethasone caused transient, mild constriction of the ductus arteriosus (35). Eleven women with placenta previa with a mean gestational age of 31.7 weeks (range 27.3–37.3) were administered two 12-mg intramuscular doses of the drug, 24 hours apart, to promote fetal lung maturation. Fetal Doppler echocardiography of the ductus arteriosus was conducted just prior to the first dose then at 5 and 30 hours postdose. Two of the fetuses showed mild constriction of the ductus 4–5 hours after the first injection, but the tests were normal when performed at 30 hours. No evidence of tricuspid regurgitation was observed (35). The authors concluded that the changes were probably not clinically significant.

A 1984 article discussed the potential benefits of combining thyroid hormones with corticosteroids to produce an additive or synergistic effect on fetal lung phosphatidylcholine synthesis (36). The therapy may offer advantages over corticosteroid therapy alone, but it is presently not possible due to the lack of commercially available thyroid stimulators that cross the placenta. The thyroid hormones, T4 and T3, are poorly transported across the placenta and thus would not be effective.

Five premature infants (three males and two females), exposed *in utero* to two 8-mg intramuscular doses of betamethasone administered to the mother 48 and 24 hours prior to birth, were evaluated to determine the effect of the drug on endogenous progesterone, mineralocorticoid, and glucocorticoid activity (37). Plasma levels of the mineralocorticoids, aldosterone and 11-deoxycorticosterone, were not significantly decreased in the newborns at birth or during the next few days. Glucocorticoid activity in the newborn, as measured by levels of corticosterone, cortisol, cortisone, and 11-deoxycortisol, was significantly depressed at birth but rebounded above normal values at 2 hours of age and then returned to normal ranges shortly after this time. Progesterone and 17-hydroxyprogesterone levels in the fetuses and neonates were not affected by betamethasone.

Although human studies have usually shown a benefit, the use of corticosteroids in animals has been associated with several toxic effects (38, 39):

Reduced fetal head circumference
Reduced fetal adrenal weight
Increased fetal liver weight
Reduced fetal thymus weight
Reduced placental weight

Fortunately, none of these effects has been observed in human investigations. In children born of mothers treated with betamethasone for premature labor, studies conducted at ages 4 and 6 years have found no differences from controls in cognitive and psychosocial development (40, 41). Studies conducted on very-low-birth-weight infants (500–1500 g) at 2 years of age indicated that, compared to nonexposed controls, antenatal betamethasone therapy was associated with a significant improvement in survival, improved growth, and a decrease in early respiratory morbidity (42). Further study of the children at 5 years of age, but limited to those with birth weights of 500–999 g, found significantly improved survival but without significantly improved growth or decrease in early respiratory morbidity (43).

Breast Feeding Summary

No data are available.

References

1. Liggins GC, Howie RN. A controlled trial of antepartum glucocorticoid treatment for prevention of the respiratory distress syndrome in premature infants. Pediatrics 1972;50:515–25.
2. Gluck L. Administration of corticosteroids to induce maturation of fetal lung. Am J Dis Child 1976;130:976–8.
3. Ballard RA, Ballard PL. Use of prenatal glucocorticoid therapy to prevent respiratory distress syndrome: a supporting view. Am J Dis Child 1976;130:982–7.
4. Mead PB, Clapp JF III. The use of betamethasone and timed delivery in management of premature rupture of the membranes in the preterm pregnancy. J Reprod Med 1977;19:3–7.
5. Block MF, Kling OR, Crosby WM. Antenatal glucocorticoid therapy for the prevention of respiratory distress syndrome in the premature infant. Obstet Gynecol 1977;50:186–90.
6. Ballard RA, Ballard PL, Granberg JP, Sniderman S. Prenatal administration of betamethasone for prevention of respiratory distress syndrome. J Pediatr 1979;94:97–101.
7. Nochimson DJ, Petrie RH. Glucocorticoid therapy for the induction of pulmonary maturity in severely hypertensive gravid women. Am J Obstet Gynecol 1979;133:449–51.
8. Eggers TR, Doyle LW, Pepperell RJ. Premature labour. Med J Aust 1979;1:213–6.
9. Doran TA, Swyer P, MacMurray B, et al. Results of a double-blind controlled study on the use of betamethasone in the prevention of respiratory distress syndrome. Am J Obstet Gynecol 1980;136:313–20.
10. Schutte MF, Treffers PE, Koppe JG, Breur W. The influence of betamethasone and orciprenaline on the incidence of respiratory distress syndrome in the newborn after preterm labour. Br J Obstet Gynaecol 1980;87:127–31.
11. Dillon WP, Egan EA. Aggressive obstetric management in late second-trimester deliveries. Obstet Gynecol 1981;58:685–90.
12. Johnson DE, Munson DP, Thompson TR. Effect of antenatal administration of betamethasone on hospital costs and survival of premature infants. Pediatrics 1981;68:633–7.
13. Bishop EH. Acceleration of fetal pulmonary maturity. Obstet Gynecol 1981;58(Suppl):48S–51S.
14. Ballard PL, Ballard RA. Corticosteroids and respiratory distress syndrome: status 1979. Pediatrics 1979;63:163–5.
15. Gamsu HR, Mullinger BM, Donnai P, Dash CH. Antenatal administration of betamethasone to prevent respiratory distress syndrome in preterm infants: report of a UK multicentre trial. Br J Obstet Gynaecol 1989;96:401–10.
16. Ballard PL, Granberg P, Ballard RA. Glucocorticoid levels in maternal and cord serum after prenatal betamethasone therapy to prevent respiratory distress syndrome. J Clin Invest 1975;56:1548–54.
17. Levitz M, Jansen V, Dancis J. The transfer and metabolism of corticosteroids in the perfused human placenta. Am J Obstet Gynecol 1978;132:363–6.
18. Eggers TR, Doyle LW, Pepperell RJ. Premature rupture of the membranes. Med J Aust 1979;1:209–13.
19. Garite TJ, Freeman RK, Linzey EM, Braly PS, Dorchester WL. Prospective randomized study of corticosteroids in the management of premature rupture of the membranes and the premature gestation. Am J Obstet Gynecol 1981;141:508–15.
20. Garite TJ. Premature rupture of the membranes: the enigma of the obstetrician. Am J Obstet Gynecol 1985;151:1001–5.
21. Nelson LH, Meis PJ, Hatjis CG, Ernest JM, Dillard R, Schey HM. Premature rupture of membranes: a prospective, randomized evaluation of steroids, latent phase, and expectant management. Obstet Gynecol 1985;66:55–8.
22. Simpson GF, Harbert GM Jr. Use of β-methasone in management of preterm gestation with premature rupture of membranes. Obstet Gynecol 1985;66:168–75.
23. Kuhn RJP, Speirs AL, Pepperell RJ, Eggers TR, Doyle LW, Hutchison A. Betamethasone, albuterol, and threatened premature delivery: benefits and risks. Obstet Gynecol 1982;60:403–8.
24. Schmidt PL, Sims ME, Strassner HT, Paul RH, Mueller E, McCart D. Effect of antepartum glucocorticoid administration upon neonatal respiratory distress syndrome and perinatal infection. Am J Obstet Gynecol 1984;148:178–86.
25. Morales WJ, Angel JL, O'Brien WF, Knuppel RA. Use of ampicillin and corticosteroids in premature rupture of membranes: a randomized study. Obstet Gynecol 1989;73:721–6.

26. Ballard PL, Ballard RA, Granberg JP, et al. Fetal sex and prenatal betamethasone therapy. J Pediatr 1980;97:451–4.
27. Avery ME, Aylward G, Creasy R, Little AB, Stripp B. Update on prenatal steroid for prevention of respiratory distress: report of a conference — September 26–28, 1985. Am J Obstet Gynecol 1986;155:2–5.
28. Khoury MJ, Marks JS, McCarthy BJ, Zaro SM. Factors affecting the sex differential in neonatal mortality: the role of respiratory distress syndrome. Am J Obstet Gynecol 1985;151:777–82.
29. Papageorgiou AN, Desgranges MF, Masson M, Colle E, Shatz R, Gelfand MM. The antenatal use of betamethasone in the prevention of respiratory distress syndrome: a controlled double-blind study. Pediatrics 1979;63:73–9.
30. Bielawski D, Hiatt IM, Hegyi T. Betamethasone-induced leukaemoid reaction in pre-term infant. Lancet 1978;1:218–9.
31. Ferguson JE, Hensleigh PA, Gill P. Effects of betamethasone on white blood cells in patients with premature rupture of the membranes and preterm labor. Am J Obstet Gynecol 1984;150:439–41.
32. Catanzarite VA, McHargue AM, Sandberg EC, Dyson DC. Respiratory arrest during therapy for premature labor in a patient with myasthenia gravis. Obstet Gynecol 1984;64:819–22.
33. Gonen R, Samberg I, Sharf M. Hypertensive crisis associated with ritodrine infusion and beta-methasone administration in premature labor. Eur J Obstet Gynecol Reprod Biol 1982;13:129–32.
34. Waffarn F, Siassi B, Cabal LA, Schmidt PL. Effect of antenatal glucocorticoids on clinical closure of the ductus arteriosus. Am J Dis Child 1983;137:336–8.
35. Wasserstrum N, Huhta JC, Mari G, Sharif DS, Willis R, Neal NK. Betamethasone and the human fetal ductus arteriosus. Obstet Gynecol 1989;74:897–900.
36. Ballard PL. Combined hormonal treatment and lung maturation. Semin Perinatol 1984;8:283–92.
37. Dorr HG, Versmold HT, Sippell WG, Bidlingmaier F, Knorr D. Antenatal betamethasone therapy: effects on maternal, fetal, and neonatal mineralocorticoids, glucocorticoids, and progestins. J Pediatr 1986;108:990–3.
38. Taeusch HW Jr. Glucocorticoid prophylaxis for respiratory distress syndrome: a review of potential toxicity. J Pediatr 1975;87:617–23.
39. Johnson JWC, Mitzner W, London WT, Palmer AE, Scott R. Betamethasone and the rhesus fetus: multisystemic effects. Am J Obstet Gynecol 1979;133:677–84.
40. MacArthur BA, Howie RN, Dezoete JA, Elkins J. Cognitive and psychosocial development of 4-year-old children whose mothers were treated antenatally with betamethasone. Pediatrics 1981;68:638–43.
41. MacArthur BA, Howie RN, Dezoete JA, Elkins J. School progress and cognitive development of 6-year-old children whose mothers were treated antenatally with betamethasone. Pediatrics 1982;70:99–105.
42. Doyle LW, Kitchen WH, Ford GW, Rickards AL, Lissenden JV, Ryan MM. Effects of antenatal steroid therapy on mortality and morbidity in very low birth weight infants. J Pediatr 1986;108:287–92.
43. Doyle LW, Kitchen WH, Ford GW, Rickards AL, Kelly EA. Antenatal steroid therapy and 5-year outcome of extremely low birth weight infants. Obstet Gynecol 1989;73:743–6.

Name: **BETHANECHOL**

Class: **Parasympathomimetic (Cholinergic)**   Risk Factor: **C$_M$**

Fetal Risk Summary

The use of bethanechol in pregnancy has been reported, but too little information is available to analyze (1).

Breast Feeding Summary

Although specific data on the excretion of bethanechol into breast milk are lacking, one author cautioned that mothers receiving regular therapy with this drug should not breast feed (2). Abdominal pain and diarrhea have been reported in a nursing infant exposed to bethanechol in milk (3).

References

1. Heinonen OP, Slone D, Shapiro S. *Birth Defects and Drugs in Pregnancy*. Littleton:Publishing Sciences Group, 1977:345–56.
2. Platzker ACD, Lew CD, Stewart D. Drug "administration" via breast milk. Hosp Pract 1980;15:111–22.
3. Shore MF. Drugs can be dangerous during pregnancy and lactations. Can Pharmaceut J 1970;103:358. As cited in: Committee on Drugs, American Academy of Pediatrics. The transfer of drugs and other chemicals into human breast milk. Pediatrics 1983;72:375–83.

Name: **BIPERIDEN**

Class: **Parasympatholytic**   Risk Factor: **C$_M$**

Fetal Risk Summary

Biperiden is an anticholinergic agent used in the treatment of parkinsonism. No reports of its use in pregnancy have been located (see also Atropine).

Breast Feeding Summary

No data are available (see also Atropine).

Name: **BLEOMYCIN**

Class: **Antineoplastic**   Risk Factor: **D**

Fetal Risk Summary

No reports linking the use of bleomycin with congenital defects have been located. Chromosomal aberrations in human marrow cells have been reported, but the significance to the fetus is unknown (1). Two separate cases of non-Hodgkin's lymphoma in pregnancy were treated during the 2nd and 3rd trimesters with bleomycin and other antineoplastic agents (2, 3). Normal infants without anomalies or chromosome changes were delivered. In another case, a 21-year-old woman with a Ewing's sarcoma of the pelvis was treated with bleomycin and four other antineoplastic agents at approximately 25 weeks' gestation (4). Nine weeks later, recurrence of tumor growth necessitated delivery of the normal infant by cesarean section to allow for more definitive treatment of the tumor. The child was reported to be developing normally at 4 years of age.

A 1989 case report described the effect of maternal chemotherapy on a premature newborn delivered at approximately 27 weeks' gestation (5). The mother was treated with bleomycin (30 mg), etoposide (165 mg), and cisplatin (55 mg) (all given daily for 3 days), 1 week prior to delivery, for an unknown primary cancer with metastases to the eye and liver. The mother developed profound neutropenia just prior to delivery. On the 3rd day after delivery, the 1190-g female infant also developed a profound leukopenia with neutropenia, 10 days after *in utero* exposure to the antineoplastic agents. The condition resolved after 10 days. At 10 days of age, the infant began losing her scalp hair along with a rapid loss of lanugo (5). Etoposide was thought to be the most likely cause of the neutropenia and the alopecia (5). By 12 weeks of age, substantial hair regrowth had occurred, and at 1 year follow-up, the child was developing normally except for moderate bilateral hearing loss. The investigators could not determine if the sensorineural deafness was due to the maternal and/or neonatal gentamicin therapy, or to the maternal cisplatin chemotherapy (5).

Combination chemotherapy with bleomycin was used for teratoma of the testis in two men (6). In both cases, recovery of spermatogenesis with apparently successful fertilization occurred but the possibility of alternate paternity could not be excluded.

The long-term effects of combination chemotherapy on menstrual and reproductive function were described in a 1988 report (7). Only 7 of 40 women treated for malignant ovarian germ cell tumors received bleomycin. The results of this study are discussed in the monograph for cyclophosphamide (see Cyclophosphamide).

Occupational exposure of the mother to antineoplastic agents during pregnancy may present a risk to the fetus. A position statement from the National Study Commission on Cytotoxic Exposure and a research article involving some antineoplastic agents are presented in the monograph for cyclophosphamide (see Cyclophosphamide).

Breast Feeding Summary

No data are available.

References

1. Bornstein RS, Hungerford DA, Haller G, Engstrom PF, Yarbro JW. Cytogenic effects of bleomycin therapy in man. Cancer Res 1971;31:2004–7.
2. Ortega J. Multiple agent chemotherapy including bleomycin of non-Hodgkin's lymphoma during pregnancy. Cancer 1977;40:2829–35.
3. Falkson HC, Simson IW, Falkson G. Non-Hodgkin's lymphoma in pregnancy. Cancer 1980;45:1679–82.
4. Haerr RW, Pratt AT. Multiagent chemotherapy for sarcoma diagnosed during pregnancy. Cancer 1985;56:1028–33.
5. Raffles A, Williams J, Costeloe K, Clark P. Transplacental effects of maternal cancer chemotherapy: case report. Br J Obstet Gynaecol 1989;96:1099–1100.
6. Rubery ED. Return of fertility after curative chemotherapy for disseminated teratoma of testis. Lancet 1983;1:186.
7. Gershenson DM. Menstrual and reproductive function after treatment with combination chemotherapy for malignant ovarian germ cell tumors. J Clin Oncol 1988;6:270–5.

Name: **BRETYLIUM**

Class: **Antiarrhythmic**　　　　　　　　　　　　　　　　Risk Factor: **C**

Fetal Risk Summary

Bretylium, a quaternary ammonium compound, is an adrenergic blocker used as an antiarrhythmic agent. No information on its use in pregnancy has been located.

Hypotension has been observed in 50% of patients after bretylium (1). Although reports are lacking, reduced uterine blood flow with fetal hypoxia (bradycardia) is a potential risk.

Breast Feeding Summary

No data are available.

Reference

1. Product information. Bretylol. Du Pont Critical Care, 1988.

Name: **BROMIDES**

Class: **Anticonvulsant/Sedative**   Risk Factor: **D**

Fetal Risk Summary

The Collaborative Perinatal Project monitored 50,282 mother-child pairs, 986 of which had 1st trimester exposure to bromides (1, pp. 402–406). For use anytime during pregnancy, 2,610 exposures were recorded (1, p. 444). In neither case was evidence found to suggest a relationship to large categories of major or minor malformations. Four possible associations with individual malformations were found, but the statistical significance of these is unknown and independent confirmation is required:

Polydactyly (14 cases)
Gastrointestinal anomalies (10 cases)
Clubfoot (7 cases)
Congenital dislocation of hip (anytime use) (92 cases)

Two infants with intrauterine growth retardation have been described from a mother who chronically ingested a proprietary product containing bromides (Bromo-Seltzer) (2). Both male infants were microcephalic (one at the 2nd percentile and one less than the 2nd percentile) and one had congenital heart disease (atrial septal defect with possible pulmonary insufficiency). The woman did not use the product in three other pregnancies, two before and one after the affected children, and all three of these children were of normal height. In a similar case, a woman chronically ingested tablets containing bromides throughout gestation and eventually gave birth to a female infant who was growth retarded (all parameters below the 10th percentile) (3). Follow-up of the infant at 2.5 years of age indicated persistent developmental delay.

Neonatal bromide intoxication from transplacental accumulation has been described in four infants (4–7). In each case, the mother had either taken bromide-containing medications (three cases) or was exposed from employment in a photographic laboratory (one case). Bromide concentrations in three of the four infants were 3650, 2000, and 2420 μg/ml on day 6, 5, and 5, respectively (4–6). In the fourth case, a serum sample was not obtained until 18 days after birth and contained 150 μg/ml (7). All four infants exhibited symptoms of neonatal bromism consisting of poor suck, weak cry, diminished Moro reflex, lethargy, and hypotonia. One of the infants also had cyanosis and a large head with dysmorphic face (7). Subsequent examinations of three of the above infants revealed normal growth and development after several months (4–6). One infant, however, had mild residual hypotonia of the neck muscles persisting at 6 and 9.5 months (7).

Cord serum bromide levels were determined on 1267 newborn infants born in Rochester, New York, during the first half of 1984 (8). Mean bromide concentrations were 8.6 μg/ml (range 3.1–28.5 μg/ml), well below the serum bromide level (>720 μg/ml) that is considered toxic (8). The measured concentrations were not related to Apgar scores, neonatal condition, or congenital abnormalities. None of the mothers was taking bromide-containing drugs (most have been removed from the market), and the concentrations in cord blood were thought to have resulted from occupational exposure to photographic chemicals or from the low levels encountered in food and water.

Breast Feeding Summary

The excretion of bromides into breast milk has been known since at least 1907 (9). A 1938 report reviewed this topic and demonstrated the presence of bromides in milk in an additional 10 mothers (9). A 1935 report measured milk concentrations of 1666 μg/ml in two patients treated with 5 g daily for 1 month (10). Rash and sedation of varying degrees in several nursing infants have been reported as a result of maternal consumption of bromides during lactation (9–11). Although bromide-containing medications are no longer available in the United States, these drugs may be available in other countries. In addition, high maternal serum levels may be obtained from close, frequent exposure to chemicals used in photographic developing. Women exposed to such chemicals who are breast feeding should be alert for symptoms of sedation or drowsiness and unexplained rashes in their infants. Monitoring of bromide levels in these women may be beneficial. Breast feeding is not recommended for women receiving bromide-containing medications.

References

1. Heinonen OP, Slone D, Shapiro S. *Birth Defects and Drugs in Pregnancy*. Littleton:Publishing Sciences Group, 1977.
2. Opitz JM, Grosse RF, Haneberg B. Congenital effects of bromism? Lancet 1972;1:91–2.
3. Rossiter EJR, Rendel-Short TJ. Congenital effects of bromism? Lancet 1972;2:705.
4. Finken RL, Robertson WO. Transplacental bromism. Am J Dis Child 1963;106:224–6.
5. Mangurten HH, Ban R. Neonatal hypotonia secondary to transplacental bromism. J Pediatr 1974;85:426–8.
6. Pleasure JR, Blackburn MG. Neonatal bromide intoxication: prenatal ingestion of a large quantity of bromides with transplacental accumulation in the fetus. Pediatrics 1975;55:503–6.
7. Mangurten HH, Kaye CI. Neonatal bromism secondary to maternal exposure in a photographic laboratory. J Pediatr 1982;100:596–8.
8. Miller ME, Cosgriff JM, Roghmann KJ. Cord serum bromide concentration: variation and lack of association with pregnancy outcome. Am J Obstet Gynecol 1987;157:826–30.
9. Tyson RM, Shrader EA, Perlman HH. Drugs transmitted through breast milk. III. Bromides. J Pediatr 1938;13:91–3.
10. Kwit NT, Hatcher RA. Excretion of drugs in milk. Am J Dis Child 1935;49:900–4.
11. Van der Bogert F. Bromin poisoning through mother's milk. Am J Dis Child 1921;21:167.

Name: **BROMOCRIPTINE**

Class: **Miscellaneous**   Risk Factor: **C$_M$**

Fetal Risk Summary

Bromocriptine has been used during all stages of pregnancy. In 1982, Turkalj and co-workers (1) reviewed the results of 1410 pregnancies in 1335 women exposed to bromocriptine during gestation. The drug, used for the treatment of infertility due to hyperprolactinemia or pituitary tumors including acromegaly, was usually discontinued as soon as pregnancy was diagnosed. The mean duration of exposure after conception was 21 days. The review included all reported cases from 1973, the year bromocriptine was introduced, through 1980. Since then, 11 other studies have reported the results of treatment in 121 women with 145 pregnancies (2–12). The results of the pregnancies in the combined studies are:

Total patients/pregnancies	1456/1555
Liveborn infants	1369 (88%)
Stillborn infants	5 (0.3%)
Multiple pregnancies (30 twins/3 triplets)	33*(2.1%)
Spontaneous abortions	166 (10.7%)
Elective abortions	26 (1.7%)
Extrauterine pregnancies	12 (0.8%)
Hydatidiform moles (2 patients)	3 (0.2%)
Pregnant at time of report—outcome unknown	10

*2 women with twins were also treated with clomiphene or gonadotropin.

A total of 48 (3.5%) of the 1374 liveborn/stillborn infants had detectable anomalies at birth (1, 2). This incidence is similar to the expected rate of congenital defects found in the general population. In the review of Turkalj and co-workers, the mean duration of fetal exposure to bromocriptine was similar between children with congenital abnormalities and normal children. No distinguishable pattern of anomalies was found. Malformations detected at birth were:

Major	No.	Minor	No.
Down's syndrome	2	Bat ear/plagiocephalus	1
Hydrocephalus/multiple atresia of		Cleft palate	1
esophagus and intestine	1	Ear lobe deformity	1
Microcephalus/encephalopathy	1	Head posture constrained	1
Omphalocele/talipes	1	Hip dislocation	
Pulmonary artery atresia	1	(aplasia of cup)	9
Reduction deformities	4	Hydrocele	3
Renal agenesis	1	Hydrocele/omphalocele	1
Pierre Robin syndrome	1	Hypospadias	1
		Inguinal hernia	2
		Skull soft/open fontanella	1
		Single palmar crease	1
		Single umbilical artery	1
		Syndactyly	2
		Talipes	5
		Umbilical hernia	1
		Cutaneous hemangioma	4
		Testicular ectopia*	1
		(*spontaneous correction at age 7 months)	
Total	12	Total	36

Long-term studies on 213 children followed up to 6 years of age have shown normal mental and physical development (1, 2).

In summary, bromocriptine apparently does not pose a significant risk to the fetus. The pattern and incidence of anomalies are similar to those expected in a nonexposed population.

Breast Feeding Summary

Since bromocriptine is indicated for the prevention of physiologic lactation, breast feeding is not possible during therapy (13, 14). However, in one report, a mother taking 5 mg/day for a pituitary tumor was able to breast feed her infant successfully (3). No effects on the infant were mentioned. Because bromocriptine suppresses lactation, the American Academy of Pediatrics considers the drug to be contraindicated during breast feeding (15).

References

1. Turkalj I, Braun P, Krupp P. Surveillance of bromocriptine in pregnancy. JAMA 1982;247:1589–91.
2. Konopka P, Raymond JP, Merceron RE, Seneze J. Continuous administration of bromocriptine in the prevention of neurological complications in pregnant women with prolactinomas. Am J Obstet Gynecol 1983;146:935–8.
3. Canales ES, Garcia IC, Ruiz JE, Zarate A. Bromocriptine as prophylactic therapy in prolactinoma during pregnancy. Fertil Steril 1981;36:524–6.
4. Bergh T, Nillius SJ, Larsson SG, Wide L. Effects of bromocriptine-induced pregnancy on prolactin-secreting pituitary tumors. Acta Endocrinol 1981;98:333.
5. Yuen BH, Cannon W, Sy L, Booth J, Burch P. Regression of pituitary microadenoma during and following bromocriptine therapy: persistent defect in prolactin regulation before and throughout pregnancy. Am J Obstet Gynecol 1982;142:634–9.
6. Maeda T, Ushiroyama T, Okuda K, Fujimoto A, Ueki M, Sugimoto O. Effective bromocriptine treatment of a pituitary macroadenoma during pregnancy. Obstet Gynecol 1983;61:117–21.
7. Hammond CB, Haney AF, Land MR, van der Merwe JV, Ory SJ, Wiebe RH. The outcome of pregnancy in patients with treated and untreated prolactin-secreting pituitary tumors. Am J Obstet Gynecol 1983;147:148–57.
8. Cundy T, Grundy EN, Melville H, Sheldon J. Bromocriptine treatment of acromegaly following spontaneous conception. Fertil Steril 1984;42:134–6.
9. Randall S, Laing I, Chapman AJ, Shalet SM, Beardwell CG, Kelly WF, Davies D. Pregnancies in women with hyperprolactinaemia: obstetric and endocrinological management of 50 pregnancies in 37 women. Br J Obstet Gynaecol 1982;89:20–33.
10. Andersen AN, Starup J, Tabor A, Jensen HK, Westergaard JG. The possible prognostic value of serum prolactin increment during pregnancy in hyperprolactinaemic patients. Acta Endocrinol 1983;102:1–5.
11. van Roon E, van der Vijver JCM, Gerretsen G, Hekster REM, Wattendorff RA. Rapid regression of a suprasellar extending prolactinoma after bromocriptine treatment during pregnancy. Fertil Steril 1981;36:173–77.
12. Crosignani P, Ferrari C, Mattei AM. Visual field defects and reduced visual acuity during pregnancy in two patients with prolactinoma: rapid regression of symptoms under bromocriptine. Case reports. Br J Obstet Gynaecol 1984;91:821–3.
13. Product information. Parlodel. Sandoz Pharmaceuticals, 1985.
14. Thorbert G, Akerlund M. Inhibition of lactation by cyclofenil and bromocriptine. Br J Obstet Gynaecol 1983;90:739–42.
15. Committee on Drugs, American Academy of Pediatrics. Transfer of drugs and other chemicals into human milk. Pediatrics 1989;84;924–36.

Name: **BROMODIPHENHYDRAMINE**

Class: **Antihistamine**   Risk Factor: **C**

Fetal Risk Summary

Bromodiphenhydramine is a derivative of Diphenhydramine (see Diphenhydramine).

Breast Feeding Summary

No data are available.

Name: **BROMPHENIRAMINE**

Class: **Antihistamine**   Risk Factor: **C$_M$**

Fetal Risk Summary

The Collaborative Perinatal Project monitored 50,282 mother-child pairs, 65 of which had 1st trimester exposure to brompheniramine (1, pp. 322–325). Based on 10 malformed infants, a statistically significant association ($p < 0.01$) was found between this drug and congenital defects. This relationship was not found with other antihistamines. For use anytime during pregnancy, 412 exposures were recorded (1, p. 437). In this case, no evidence was found for an association with malformations.

The use of antihistamines in general (specific agents and dose not given) during the last 2 weeks of pregnancy has been associated with an increased risk of retrolental fibroplasia in premature infants (2). Infants weighing less than 1750 g, who had no detectable congenital anomalies and who survived for at least 24 hours after birth, were enrolled in the multicenter National Collaborative Study on Patent Ductus Arteriosus in Premature Infants conducted between 1979–1981 (2). After exclusions, 3026 infants were available for study. Exposures to antihistamines and other drugs were determined by interview and maternal record review. The incidence of retrolental fibroplasia in infants exposed to antihistamines during the last 2 weeks of gestation was 22% (19 of 86) vs. 11% (324 of 2940) not exposed during this interval. Adjustment for severity of disease did not change the estimated rate ratio.

Breast Feeding Summary

A single case report has been located describing adverse effects in a 3-month-old nursing infant of a mother consuming a long-acting preparation containing 6 mg of dexbrompheniramine and 120 mg of *d*-isoephedrine (3). The mother had begun taking the preparation on a twice-daily schedule about 1 or 2 days prior to the onset of symptoms in the infant. Symptoms consisted of irritability, excessive crying, and disturbed sleeping patterns, which resolved spontaneously within 12 hours when breast feeding was stopped. One manufacturer considers the drug to be contraindicated for nursing mothers (4). The American Academy of Pediatrics considers dexbrompheniramine usually to be compatible with breast feeding (5).

References

1. Heinonen OP, Slone D, Shapiro S. *Birth Defects and Drugs in Pregnancy.* Littleton:Publishing Sciences Group, 1977.
2. Zierler S, Purohit D. Prenatal antihistamine exposure and retrolental fibroplasia. Am J Epidemiol 1986;123:192–6.
3. Mortimer EA Jr. Drug toxicity from breast milk? Pediatrics 1977;60:780–1.
4. Product information. Dimetane. AH Robins Company, 1990.
5. Committee on Drugs, American Academy of Pediatrics. Transfer of drugs and other chemicals into human milk. Pediatrics 1989;84:924–36.

Name: **BUCLIZINE**

Class: **Antihistamine/Antiemetic**   Risk Factor: **C**

Fetal Risk Summary

Buclizine is a piperazine antihistamine that is used as an antiemetic (see also Cyclizine and Meclizine for closely related drugs). The drug is teratogenic in animals, but its effects on the human fetus have not been thoroughly studied.

The Collaborative Perinatal Project monitored 50,282 mother-child pairs, 44 of which had 1st trimester exposure to buclizine (1, pp. 323–324). No evidence was found to suggest a relationship to large categories of major or minor malformations. For use anytime during pregnancy, 62 exposures were recorded (1, p. 437). A possible association with congenital defects, based on the report of three malformed children, was found from this exposure. The manufacturer considers the drug to be contraindicated in early pregnancy (2).

An association between exposure during the last 2 weeks of pregnancy to antihistamines in general and retrolental fibroplasia in premature infants has been reported. See Brompheniramine for details.

Breast Feeding Summary

No data are available.

References

1. Heinonen OP, Slone D, Shapiro S. *Birth Defects and Drugs in Pregnancy.* Littleton:Publishing Sciences Group, 1977.
2. Product information. Bucladin. Stuart Pharmaceuticals, 1990.

Name: **BUSULFAN**

Class: **Antineoplastic**   Risk Factor: **D**

Fetal Risk Summary

Busulfan is an alkylating antineoplastic agent. The use of this drug has been reported in 38 pregnancies, 22 in the 1st trimester (1, 2). Six malformed infants have been observed (1, 3–5):

Unspecified malformations, aborted at 20 weeks

Anomalous deviation left lobe liver, bilobar spleen, pulmonary atelectasis

Pyloric stenosis

Cleft palate, microphthalmia, cytomegaly, hypoplasia of ovaries and thyroid
  gland, corneal opacity, intrauterine growth retardation (IUGR)

Myeloschisis, aborted at 6 weeks

IUGR, left hydronephrosis and hydroureter, absent right kidney and ureter,
  hepatic subcapsular calcifications

Data from one review indicated that 40% of the infants exposed to anticancer
drugs were of low birth weight (1). This finding was not related to the timing of the
exposure. Long-term studies of growth and mental development in offspring exposed to busulfan during the 2nd trimester, the period of neuroblast multiplication,
have not been conducted (6). However, a few infants have been followed for periods up to 10 years without evidence of adverse outcome (2).

Chromosomal damage has been associated with busulfan therapy, but the
clinical significance of this to the fetus is unknown (7). Irregular menses and
amenorrhea, the latter at times permanent, have been reported in women receiving busulfan (8, 9). Reversible ovarian failure with delivery of a normal infant has
also been reported after busulfan therapy (10).

Occupational exposure of the mother to antineoplastic agents during pregnancy
may present a risk to the fetus. A position statement from the National Study
Commission on Cytotoxic Exposure and a research article involving some antineoplastic agents are presented in the monograph for cyclophosphamide (see Cyclophosphamide).

Breast Feeding Summary

No data are available.

References

1. Nicholson HO. Cytotoxic drugs in pregnancy: review of reported cases. J Obstet Gynaecol Br
   Commonw 1968;75:307–12.
2. Lee RA, Johnson CE, Hanlon DG. Leukemia during pregnancy. Am J Obstet Gynecol
   1962;84:455–8.
3. Diamond I, Anderson MM, McCreadie SR. Transplacental transmission of busulfan (Myleran) in a
   mother with leukemia: production of fetal malformation and cytomegaly. Pediatrics 1960;25:85–
   90.
4. Abramovici A, Shaklai M, Pinkhas J. Myeloschisis in a six weeks embryo of a leukemic woman
   treated by busulfan. Teratology 1978;18:241–6.
5. Gililland J, Weinstein L. The effects of cancer chemotherapeutic agents on the developing fetus.
   Obstet Gynecol Surv 1983;38:6–13.
6. Dobbing J. Pregnancy and leukaemia. Lancet 1977;1:1155.
7. Gebhart E, Schwanitz G, Hartwich G. Chromosomal aberrations during busulphan therapy. Dtsch
   Med Wochenschr 1974;99:52–6.
8. Galton DAG, Till M, Wiltshaw E. Busulfan: summary of clinical results. Ann NY Acad Sci
   1958;68:967–73.
9. Schilsky RL, Lewis BJ, Sherins RJ, Young RC. Gonadal dysfunction in patients receiving chemotherapy for cancer. Ann Intern Med 1980;93:109–14.
10. Shalev O, Rahav G, Milwidsky A. Reversible busulfan-induced ovarian failure. Eur J Obstet Gyne-
    col Reprod Biol 1987;26:239–42.

Name: **BUTALBITAL**

Class: **Sedative**   Risk Factor: **C***

Fetal Risk Summary

Butalbital is a short-acting barbiturate that is contained in a number of analgesic mixtures. In a large prospective study, 112 patients were exposed to this drug during the 1st trimester (1). No association with malformations was found. Severe neonatal withdrawal was described in a male infant whose mother took 150 mg of butalbital daily during the last 2 months of pregnancy in the form of a proprietary headache mixture (Esgic—butalbital 50 mg, caffeine 40 mg, and acetaminophen 325 mg/dose) (2). The infant was also exposed to oxycodone, pentazocine, and acetaminophen during the 1st trimester, but apparently these had been discontinued prior to the start of the butalbital product. Onset of withdrawal occurred within 2 days of birth.

[*Risk Factor D if used for prolonged periods or in high doses at term.]

Breast Feeding Summary

No data are available (see also Pentobarbital).

References

1. Heinonen OP, Slone D, Shapiro S. *Birth Defects and Drugs in Pregnancy.* Littleton:Publishing Sciences Group, 1977:336–7.
2. Ostrea EM. Neonatal withdrawal from intrauterine exposure to butalbital. Am J Obstet Gynecol 1982;143:597–9.

Name: **BUTAPERAZINE**

Class: **Tranquilizer**   Risk Factor: **C**

Fetal Risk Summary

Butaperazine is a piperazine phenothiazine in the same group as prochlorperazine (see Prochlorperazine). The phenothiazines readily cross the placenta (1). No specific information on the use of butaperazine in pregnancy has been located. Although occasional reports have attempted to link various phenothiazine compounds with congenital malformations, the bulk of the evidence indicates that these drugs are safe for the mother and fetus (see also Chlorpromazine).

Breast Feeding Summary

No data are available.

Reference

1. Moya F, Thorndike V. Passage of drugs across the placenta. Am J Obstet Gynecol 1962;84:1778–98.

Name: **BUTORPHANOL**

Class: **Analgesic**   Risk Factor: **B***

Fetal Risk Summary

No reports linking the use of butorphanol with congenital defects have been located. Since it has both narcotic agonist and antagonist properties, prolonged use during gestation may result in fetal addiction with subsequent withdrawal in the newborn (see also Pentazocine).

At term, butorphanol rapidly crosses the placenta, producing cord serum levels averaging 84% of maternal concentrations (1, 2). Depressant effects on the newborn from *in utero* exposure during labor are similar to those seen with meperidine (1–3).

The use of 1 mg of butorphanol combined with 25 mg of promethazine administered intravenously to a woman in active labor was associated with a sinusoidal fetal heart rate pattern (4). Onset of the pattern occurred 6 minutes after drug injection and persisted for approximately 58 minutes. The newborn infant showed no effects from the abnormal heart pattern. A subsequent study to determine the incidence of sinusoidal fetal heart rate pattern after butorphanol administration was published in 1986 (5). Fifty-one women in labor who received butorphanol, 1 mg intravenously, were compared to a control group of 55 women who did not receive narcotic analgesia. Sinusoidal fetal heart rate pattern was observed in 75% (38 of 51) of the treated women vs. 13% (7 of 55) of controls ($p < 0.001$). The mean time of onset of the abnormal tracing was 12.74 minutes after butorphanol with a duration of 31.26 minutes. This duration was significantly longer than that observed in the nontreated controls (13.86 minutes; $p < 0.02$). Since no short-term maternal or neonatal adverse effects were observed, the investigators concluded that, in the absence of other signs, the abnormal heart rate pattern was not indicative of fetal hypoxia (5).

A study comparing neonatal neurobehavior was conducted in 135 patients during their 1st day of life (6). Maternal analgesia consisted of 1 mg of butorphanol (68 patients) or 40 mg of meperidine (67 patients). No difference between the drugs was observed.

[*Risk Factor D if used for prolonged periods or in high doses at term.]

Breast Feeding Summary

Butorphanol passes into breast milk in concentrations paralleling levels in maternal serum (2). Milk:plasma ratios after intramuscular (12 mg) or oral (8 mg) doses were 0.7 and 1.9, respectively. Using 2 mg intramuscularly or 8 mg orally four times a day would result in 4 µg excreted in the full daily milk output (1000 ml). Although it has not been studied, this amount is probably insignificant. The American Academy of Pediatrics considers butorphanol to be compatible with breast feeding (7).

References

1. Maduska AL, Hajghassemali M. A double-blind comparison of butorphanol and merperidine in labour: maternal pain relief and effect on the newborn. Can Anaesth Soc J 1978;25:398–404.
2. Pittman KA, Smyth RD, Losada M, Zighelboim I, Maduska AL, Sunshine A. Human perinatal distribution of butorphanol. Am J Obstet Gynecol 1980;138:797–800.

3. Quilligan EJ, Keegan KA, Donahue MJ. Double-blind comparison of intravenously injected butorphanol and meperidine in parturients. Int J Gynaecol Obstet 1980;18:363–7.
4. Angel JL, Knuppel RA, Lake M. Sinusoidal fetal heart rate pattern associated with intravenous butorphanol administration: a case report. Am J Obstet Gynecol 1984;149:465–7.
5. Hatjis CG, Meis PJ. Sinusoidal fetal heart rate pattern associated with butorphanol administration. Obstet Gynecol 1986;67:377–80.
6. Hodgkinson R, Huff RW, Hayashi RH, Husain FJ. Double-blind comparison of maternal analgesia and neonatal neurobehaviour following intravenous butorphanol and meperidine. J Int Med Res 1979;7:224–30.
7. Committee on Drugs, American Academy of Pediatrics. Transfer of drugs and other chemicals into human milk. Pediatrics 1989;84;924–36.

Name: **BUTRIPTYLINE**

Class: **Antidepressant**   Risk Factor: **D**

Fetal Risk Summary

No data are available (see Imipramine).

Breast Feeding Summary

No data are available (see Imipramine).

Name: **CAFFEINE**

Class: **Central Stimulant**   Risk Factor: **B**

Fetal Risk Summary

Caffeine is one of the most popular drugs in the world (1). It is frequently used in combination products containing aspirin, phenacetin, and codeine and is present in a number of commonly consumed beverages, such as coffee, teas, and colas, as well as many food items. The mean caffeine content in the usual servings of some common beverages was reported as caffeinated coffee (66–146 mg), nonherbal tea (20–46 mg), and caffeinated soft drinks (47 mg) (2), but these amounts may vary widely. (For example, see also reference 26 where it is reported that the average caffeine content in two cups of regular coffee totaled 454 mg, and the average content in a similar amount of decaffeinated coffee totaled 12 mg.)

Caffeine crosses the placenta, and fetal blood and tissue levels similar to maternal concentrations are achieved (1, 3–5). Cord blood levels of 1–1.6 µg/ml have been measured (3). Caffeine has also been found in newborns exposed to theophylline *in utero* (6).

The mutagenicity and carcinogenicity of caffeine have been evaluated in over 50 studies involving laboratory animals, human and animal cell tissue cultures, and human lymphocytes *in vivo* (1, 3). The significance of mutagenic and carcinogenic effects found in nonmammalian systems has not been established in man. The drug is an animal teratogen only when doses high enough to cause toxicity in the mother have been given (1).

The Collaborative Perinatal Project (CPP) monitored 50,282 mother-child pairs, 5,378 of which had 1st trimester exposure to caffeine (7, pp. 366–370). No evidence of a relationship to congenital defects was found. For use anytime during pregnancy, 12,696 exposures were recorded (7, pp. 493–494). In this case, slightly increased relative risks were found for musculoskeletal defects, hydronephrosis, adrenal anomalies, and hemangiomas/granulomas, but the results are uninterpretable without independent confirmation (7, pp. 493–494). A follow-up analysis by the CPP on 2,030 malformed infants and maternal use of caffeine-containing beverages did not support caffeine as a teratogen (8). Other reports have also found no association between the use of caffeine during pregnancy and congenital malformations (9–12).

Several authors have associated high caffeine consumption (six to eight cups of coffee/day) with decreased fertility, increased incidence of spontaneous abortion, and low birth weights (3, 13–17). Unfortunately, few of these studies have isolated the effects of caffeine from cigarette or alcohol use, both of which are positively associated with caffeine consumption (3). One German study has observed that high coffee use alone is associated with low birth weights (18). In an American study of more than 12,400 women, low birth weights and short gestations occurred more often among offspring of women who drank four or more cups of coffee/day and who also smoked (12). No relationship between low birth weights/ short gestation and caffeine was found after controlling for smoking, alcohol intake, and demographic characteristics. However, other investigators have questioned whether this study accurately assessed the total caffeine intake of the women (19, 20). A Canadian study retrospectively investigated 913 newborn infants for the effects of caffeine and cigarette smoking on birth weight and placental weight (21). Significant caffeine-cigarette interactions were found when daily consumption of caffeine was 300 mg or more. Compared to nonsmokers, cigarette smoking significantly lowered mean birth weight. When caffeine use was considered, daily consumption of 300 mg or more combined with smoking 15 cigarettes or more caused an additional significant reduction in weight. Head circumference and body length were not affected by any level of caffeine consumption. Placental weight, which normally increases with cigarette smoking, an effect hypothesized to be due to compensatory hypertrophy induced by chronic fetal hypoxia, was found to decrease significantly in women smoking 15 cigarettes or more/day and ingesting 300 mg or more of caffeine/day (21).

A 1986 prospective cohort study examined the relationship between caffeine intake and the incidence of late spontaneous abortion in 3135 predominantly white, educated, professional women (22). A total of 2483 (79%) of this population used caffeine during pregnancy. Caffeine consumption was calculated based on the intake of coffee (107 mg/serving), tea (34 mg/serving), colas (47 mg/serving), and drugs. Moderate to heavy consumption, defined as 151 mg or more of caffeine intake/day, occurred in 28% (879) and was associated with a 2-fold increased risk of late 1st and 2nd trimester spontaneous abortion (relative risk 1.95, $p = 0.07$). Consumption of greater than 200 mg/day did not increase this risk. In women who had a spontaneous abortion in their last pregnancy, light use of caffeine (0–150 mg/day) was associated with a 4-fold increase in late pregnancy loss (relative risk 4.18, $p = 0.04$). The data were adjusted for such factors as demographic characteristics, obstetric and medical histories, contraceptive use, smoking, and alcohol exposure. The investigators cautioned, however, that other independent epidemiologic studies were required to confirm their findings since spontaneous abortion is of multifactorial etiology (22, 23).

A 1988 publication, evaluating studies published between 1981–1986, reviewed the effects of caffeine consumption on human pregnancies in terms of congenital malformations, low birth weight, preterm birth, spontaneous abortions, and behavior in *in utero* exposed children (24). Based on this evaluation of the literature, the author concluded that moderate intake of caffeine was not related to any adverse pregnancy outcome. A second 1988 article (120 references) reviewed the effect of caffeine on pregnancy outcome in both animals and humans (25). This author also concluded that modest amounts of caffeine present no proven risk to the fetus, but that limitation of daily amounts to less than 300 mg/ day may lessen the possibility of growth retardation.

Research on the effects of caffeine consumption on human fecundability (i.e., the probability of becoming clinically pregnant in a given menstrual cycle) was reported in 1988 (26). Utilizing women they had enrolled in a study of very early pregnancy loss, the investigators chose 104 women who had not become pregnant in the first 3 months. Data were recorded daily by the women on menstrual bleeding, intercourse, and caffeine and other substance exposures. Caffeine consumption was calculated by assuming brewed coffee contained 100 mg, instant coffee 65 mg, tea 50 mg, and soft drinks 40 mg. The subjects were primarily white, college educated, and in their late twenties or early thirties. Caffeinated beverages were consumed by 93% (97 of 104) of the sample. The women were divided into lower caffeine consumers (less than 3150 mg/month, or about one cup of brewed coffee/day) and higher consumers (using more than 3150 mg/month). Based on this division, the higher consumers were consistently less likely to become pregnant than the lower consumers, with a weighted mean of fecundability ratios across 13 cycles of 0.59. (The fecundability ratio was determined in each cycle by dividing the number of women who became pregnant by the total number of woman-cycles at risk and then by dividing the fraction obtained in the higher caffeine consumption group by the fraction obtained for the lower consumption group.) The ratio was less than 1.0 in every cycle. For cycles occurring after 6 months, the ratio was 0.53, indicating a slightly stronger association between higher caffeine consumption and the inability to become pregnant (26). Statistical adjustment of the data for age, frequency of intercourse, age at menarche, cigarette smoking, vitamin and analgesic intake, alcohol and marijuana use, and the mother's weight and height did not significantly change these findings. Moreover, when caffeine consumption was further subdivided, a partial dose-response relationship was observed with a ratio of 0.26 for women consuming more than 7000 mg/month (i.e., more than 70 cups of coffee/month). Unadjusted data on infertility (defined as women who failed to achieve pregnancy after 1 year) indicated that only 6% of the lower consumption group met this definition compared to 28% of the higher consumption group, an estimated relative risk of 4.7 ($p < 0.005$) (26). Evidence was also found to suggest that the effects of caffeine on fertility were short-acting since recent consumption was far more important than previous consumption. Although the study attempted to include all related factors, the investigators did caution that they could not exclude the possibility that some unknown factor or condition might have accounted for these results and that independent confirmation was required (26, 27). Partial confirmation of this study was reported in 1989 (28). In a retrospective analysis of data collected from 1959–1967 on 6303 pregnancies, a dose-response relationship was found between caffeine consumption and difficulty in becoming pregnant. Using data adjusted for ethnicity (white, black), parity (0, 1), and smoking, the relative risk of decreased fertility for less than one cup of coffee/day was 1.00, one to three cups/day 1.20, four to six cups/day 1.88, and more than seven cups/day 1.96 (28).

Some investigators have expressed concern over the altering of catecholamine levels in the fetus by caffeine (29). Two cups of regular coffee containing a total of 454 mg of caffeine have been shown to increase maternal epinephrine levels significantly but not norepinephrine or dopamine concentrations (30). Decaffeinated coffee (12 mg of caffeine in two cups) did not affect these catecholamine levels. The clinical effect of these changes, if any, on human development is unknown.

A 1989 single blind, crossover study of eight women at 32–36 weeks of gestation investigated the effects of two cups of caffeinated (regular) or decaffeinated coffee on fetal breathing movements and heart rate (30). Administration of the test beverages, containing a total of 454 mg and 12 mg of caffeine, respectively, were separated by 1 week, and in each case, were consumed over a 15-minute period.

Fetal breathing movements increased significantly during the 3rd hour after regular coffee, rising from 144 breaths/hour to 614 breaths/hour ($p < 0.01$). Fetal heart rate fell 9% ($p < 0.05$) at 1–1.5 hours after the regular coffee and then slowly rose toward control levels at 2 and 4 hours. However, the mean number, amplitude, and duration of fetal rate accelerations did not differ statistically from the control period. Decaffeinated coffee also caused a significant increase in fetal breathing movements, rising to 505 breaths/hour during the 2nd hour, but this beverage caused only a slight, nonsignificant lowering of the fetal heart rate. In an earlier study using 200-mg tablets of caffeine, no increase in fetal breathing rates was observed (31). The differences between the two studies may have been due to the lower dose and/or the dosage form of caffeine.

In summary, although the amount of caffeine in commonly used beverages varies widely, caffeine consumption in pregnancy in modest amounts apparently does not pose a measurable risk to the fetus. When used in moderation, no association with congenital malformations, spontaneous abortions, preterm birth, and low birth weight has been proven. Use of high doses may be associated with spontaneous abortions, difficulty in becoming pregnant, and infertility. A dose-response relationship may exist for the latter two areas. However, confirmation of these findings is needed before any firm conclusions can be drawn. The consumption of high caffeine doses with cigarette smoking may increase the risk for delivery of infants with lower birth weight than that induced by smoking alone.

Breast Feeding Summary

Caffeine is excreted into breast milk (32–39). Milk:plasma ratios of 0.5 and 0.76 have been reported (33, 34). Following ingestion of coffee or tea containing known amounts of caffeine (36–335 mg), peak milk levels of 2.09–7.17 μg/ml occurred within 1 hour (35). An infant consuming 90 ml of milk every 3 hours would ingest 0.01–1.64 mg of caffeine over 24 hours after the mother drank a single cup of caffeinated beverage (35). In another study, peak milk levels after a 100-mg dose were 3.0 μg/ml at 1 hour (34). In this and an earlier study, the authors estimated a nursing infant would receive 1.5–3.1 mg of caffeine after a single cup of coffee (33, 34).

Nine breast-feeding mothers consumed a measured amount of caffeine (750 mg/day) added to decaffeinated coffee for 5 days then abstained from all caffeine ingestion for the next 4 days (38). In six women, 24-hour pooled aliquots of milk samples from each feeding were collected on days 5 and 9. In another mother, pooled aliquots were collected daily for 9 days. The average milk caffeine concentrations from these seven mothers on day 5 were 4.3 μg/ml (range <0.25–15.7 μg/ml). Caffeine was not detected (i.e., <0.25 μg/ml) in any of the seven samples on day 9. Serum levels in the infants of these seven mothers on day 5 averaged 1.4 μg/ml (range 0.8–2.8 μg/ml in five infants, nondetectable in two). On day 9, caffeine was only detectable in the sera of two infants, decreasing from 0.8 μg/ml on day 5 to 0.6 μg/ml on day 9 in one, and decreasing from 2.8 to 2.4 μg/ml in the other. The remaining two mothers collected milk samples with each feeding over the entire 9 days of the study but did not pool the samples. These mothers were breast feeding infants aged 79 and 127 days, and their mean daily milk caffeine levels on days 1–5 ranged from 4.0–28.6 μg/ml. Caffeine could not be detected in any of the milk samples after 5 days. Infant serum contained <0.25 μg/ml (mother's milk 13.4 μg/ml) and 3.2 μg/ml (mother's milk 28.6 μg/ml), respectively, on day 5, and both were <0.25 μg/ml on day 9. The wide variance in milk concentrations of caffeine was attributed to the mother's ability to metabolize caffeine (38). Based on the average level of 4.3 μg/ml, and assuming an infant consumed 150–180 ml/kg/day, the author calculated the infant would receive 0.6–0.8 mg/kg/day of caffeine (38).

In an extension of the above study, the effect of 500 mg of caffeine consumption/day on infant heart rate and sleep time was evaluated in 11 mother-infant pairs (39). Mothers consumed decaffeinated coffee daily for 5 days and then decaffeinated coffee with added caffeine for another 5-day period. Milk caffeine levels on the last day of the caffeine period ranged from 1.6–6.2 μg/ml, providing an estimated 0.3–1.0 mg/kg/day of caffeine to their infants. No significant difference in 24-hour heart rate or sleep time was observed between the two phases of the study.

The elimination half-life of caffeine is approximately 80 hours in term newborns and 97.5 hours in premature babies (36). A 1987 study investigated the metabolism of caffeine in breast-fed and formula-fed infants given oral doses of caffeine citrate (40). The serum half-lives of caffeine were greater than three times as long in the breast-fed infants as compared to the formula-fed infants (76 vs. 21 hours at 47–50 weeks postconceptional age; 54 vs. 16 hours at 51–54 weeks postconceptional age). The investigators attributed the findings to inhibition or suppression of caffeine metabolism by the hepatic cytochrome P-450 system by some element of breast milk (40).

The amounts of caffeine in breast milk after maternal ingestion of caffeinated beverages are probably too low to be clinically significant. However, accumulation may occur in infants when mothers use moderate-to-heavy amounts of caffeinated beverages. Irritability and poor sleeping patterns have been observed in nursing infants during periods of heavy maternal use of caffeine (37). The American Academy of Pediatrics considers usual amounts of caffeinated beverages to be compatible with breast feeding (41).

References

1. Soyka LF. Effects of methylxanthines on the fetus. Clin Perinatol 1979;6:37–51.
2. Bunker ML, McWilliams M. Caffeine content of common beverages. J Am Diet Assoc 1979;74:28–32.
3. Soyka LF. Caffeine ingestion during pregnancy: *in utero* exposure and possible effects. Semin Perinatol 1981;5:305–9.
4. Goldstein A, Warren R. Passage of caffeine into human gonadal and fetal tissue. Biochem Pharmacol 1962;17:166–8.
5. Parsons WD, Aranda JV, Neims AH. Elimination of transplacentally acquired caffeine in fullterm neonates. Pediatr Res 1976;10:333.
6. Brazier JL, Salle B. Conversion of theophylline to caffeine by the human fetus. Semin Perinatol 1981;5:315–20.
7. Heinonen OP, Slone D, Shapiro S. *Birth Defects and Drugs in Pregnancy*. Littleton:Publishing Sciences Group, 1977.
8. Rosenberg L, Mitchell AA, Shapiro S, Slone D. Selected birth defects in relation to caffeine-containing beverages. JAMA 1982;247:1429–32.
9. Van't Hoff W. Caffeine in pregnancy. Lancet 1982;1:1020.
10. Kurppa K, Holmberg PC, Kuosma E, Saxen L. Coffee consumption during pregnancy. N Engl J Med 1982;306:1548.
11. Curatolo PW, Robertson D. The health consequences of caffeine. Ann Intern Med 1983;98(Part 1):641–53.
12. Linn S, Schoenbaum SC, Monson RR, Rosner B, Stubblefield PG, Ryan KJ. No association between coffee consumption and adverse outcomes of pregnancy. N Engl J Med 1982;306:141–5.

13. Weathersbee PS, Olsen LK, Lodge JR. Caffeine and pregnancy. Postgrad Med 1977;62:64–9.
14. Anonymous. Caffeine and birth defects—another negative study. Pediatr Alert 1982;7:23–4.
15. Hogue CJ. Coffee in pregnancy. Lancet 1981;2:554.
16. Weathersbee PS, Lodge JR, Caffeine: its direct and indirect influence on reproduction. J Reprod Med 1977;19:55–63.
17. Lechat MF, Borlee I, Bouckaert A, Misson C. Caffeine study. Science 1980;207:1296–7.
18. Mau G, Netter P. Kaffee- und alkoholkonsum-riskofaktoren in der schwangerschaft? Geburtshilfe Frauenheilkd 1974;34:1018–22.
19. Bracken MB, Bryce-Buchanan C, Silten R, Srisuphan W. Coffee consumption during pregnancy. N Engl J Med 1982;306:1548–9.
20 Luke B. Coffee consumption during pregnancy. N Engl J Med 1982;306:1549.
21. Beaulac-Baillargeon L, Desrosiers C. Caffeine-cigarette interaction on fetal growth. Am J Obstet Gynecol 1987;157:1236–40.
22. Srisuphan W, Bracken MB. Caffeine consumption during pregnancy and association with late spontaneous abortion. Am J Obstet Gynecol 1986;154:14–20.
23. Bracken MB. Caffeine consumption during pregnancy and association with late spontaneous abortion: reply. Am J Obstet Gynecol 1986;155:1147.
24. Leviton A. Caffeine consumption and the risk of reproductive hazards. J Reprod Med 1988;33:175–8.
25. Berger A. Effects of caffeine consumption on pregnancy outcome: a review. J Reprod Med 1988;33:945–56.
26. Wilcox A, Weinberg C, Baird D. Caffeinated beverages and decreased fertility. Lancet 1988;2:1453–6.
27. Wilcox AJ. Caffeinated beverages and decreased fertility. Lancet 1989;1:840
28. Christianson RE, Oechsli FW, van den Berg BJ. Caffeinated beverages and decreased fertility. Lancet 1989;1:378.
29. Bellet S, Roman L, DeCastro O, et al. Effect of coffee ingestion on catecholamine release. Metabolism 1969;18:288–91.
30. Salvador HS, Koos BJ. Effects of regular and decaffeinated coffee on fetal breathing and heart rate. Am J Obstet Gynecol 1989;160:1043–7.
31. McGowan J, Devoe LD, Searle N, Altman R. The effects of long- and short-term maternal caffeine ingestion on human fetal breathing and body movements in term gestations. Am J Obstet Gynecol 1987;157:726–9.
32. Jobe PC. Psychoactive substances and antiepileptic drugs. In Wilson JT, ed. *Drugs in Breast Milk*. Balgowlah, Australia:ADIS Press, 1981:40.
33. Tyrala EE, Dodson WE. Caffeine secretion into breast milk. Arch Dis Child 1979;54:787–800.
34. Sargraves R, Bradley JM, Delgado MJM, Wagner D, Sharpe GL, Stavchansky S. Pharmacokinetics of caffeine in human breast milk after a single oral dose of caffeine. Drug Intell Clin Pharm 1984;18:507 (Abstr).
35. Berlin CM Jr, Denson HM, Daniel CH, Ward RM. Disposition of dietary caffeine in milk, saliva, and plasma of lactating women. Pediatrics 1984;73:59–63.
36. Berlin CM Jr. Excretion of the methylxanthines in human milk. Semin Perinatol 1981;5:389–94.
37. Hill RM, Craig JP, Chaney MD, Tennyson LM, McCulley LB. Utilization of over-the-counter drugs during pregnancy. Clin Obstet Gynecol 1977;20:381–94.
38. Ryu JE. Caffeine in human milk and in serum of breast-fed infants. Dev Pharmacol Ther 1985;8:329–37.
39. Ryu JE. Effect of maternal caffeine consumption on heart rate and sleep time of breast-fed infants. Dev Pharmacol Ther 1985;8:355–63.
40. Le Guennec J-C, Billon B. Delay in caffeine elimination in breast-fed infants. Pediatrics 1987;79:264–8.
41. Committee on Drugs, American Academy of Pediatrics. Transfer of drugs and other chemicals into human milk. Pediatrics 1989:84:924–36.

Name: **CALCIFEDIOL**

Class: **Vitamin**   Risk Factor: **A***

Fetal Risk Summary

Calcifediol is converted in the kidneys to calcitriol, one of the active forms of vitamin D. See Vitamin D.

[*Risk Factor D if used in doses above the recommended daily allowance.]

Breast Feeding Summary

See Vitamin D.

Name: **CALCITONIN**

Class: **Calcium Regulation Hormone**   Risk Factor: **B**

Fetal Risk Summary

No reports linking the use of calcitonin with congenital defects have been located. Marked increases of calcitonin concentrations in fetal serum over maternal levels have been demonstrated at term (1). The significance of this finding is unknown. The hormone does not cross the placenta (2).

Breast Feeding Summary

No data are available. Calcitonin has been shown to inhibit lactation in animals. Mothers wishing to breast feed should be informed of this potential complication (2).

References

1. Kovarik J, Woloszczuk W, Linkesch W, Pavelka R. Calcitonin in pregnancy. Lancet 1980;1:199–200.
2. Product information. Calcimar. Armour Laboratories. 1985.

Name: **CALCITRIOL**

Class: **Vitamin**   Risk Factor: **A***

Fetal Risk Summary

Calcitriol is one of three physiologically active forms of vitamin D. See Vitamin D.

[*Risk Factor D if used in doses above the recommended daily allowance.]

Breast Feeding Summary

See Vitamin D.

Name: **CAMPHOR**

Class: **Antipruritic/Local Anesthetic** Risk Factor: **C**

Fetal Risk Summary

No reports linking the use of topically applied camphor with congenital defects have been located. Camphor is toxic and potentially a fatal poison if taken orally in sufficient quantities. Four cases of fetal exposure after accidental ingestion, including a case of fetal death and neonatal respiratory failure, have been reported (1–4). The drug crosses the placenta (2).

Breast Feeding Summary

No data are available.

References

1. Figgs J, Hamilton R, Homel S, McCabe J. Camphorated oil intoxication in pregnancy. Report of a case. Obstet Gynecol 1965;25:255–8.
2. Weiss J, Catalano P. Camphorated oil intoxication during pregnancy. Pediatrics 1973;52:713–4.
3. Blackman WB, Curry HB. Camphor poisoning: report of case occurring during pregnancy. J Fla Med Assoc 1957;43:99.
4. Jacobziner H, Raybin HW. Camphor poisoning. Arch Pediatr 1962;79:28.

Name: **CAPTOPRIL**

Class: **Antihypertensive** Risk Factor: **C$_M$**

Fetal Risk Summary

Captopril, a competitive inhibitor of angiotensin I-converting enzyme, is used for the treatment of hypertension and in the management of heart failure. Data on the use of this agent in 48 human pregnancies involving 50 fetuses (two sets of twins) have been located and are reviewed in the sections below.

Captopril is embryocidal in animals and has been shown to cause an increase in stillbirths in some species (1). Because of this toxicity, a committee of the National Institutes of Health recommended in 1984 that captopril be avoided during pregnancy (2). Other than the two cases described below, where the association between captopril and the defects is unknown, malformations have not been observed when the drug was used in the 1st or other trimesters. However, stillbirths and severe renal toxicity in the newborn (i.e., anuria), at times leading to death, have been reported in human fetuses exposed to the drug.

A malformed fetus was discovered following voluntary abortion in a patient with renovascular hypertension (3). The patient had been treated during the 1st trimester with captopril, propranolol, and amiloride. The left leg ended at midthigh without distal development, and no obvious skull formation was noted above the brain tissue. However, because of the very small size of the fetus (1.5 cm), the pathologist could not be certain that the defects were not a result of the abortion (4). In a second case, a mother with a history of renal artery stenosis and malignant hypertension was treated throughout gestation with captopril, minoxidil, and propranolol (5). Three of her four previous pregnancies had ended in midgestation stillbirths. The most recent stillbirth, her fourth pregnancy, involved a 500-g male infant with low-set ears but no gross anomalies. The mother had been treated with the above regimen plus furosemide. In her second pregnancy, she had been treated only with hydrochlorothiazide and she had delivered a normal term infant. No information was available on the first and third pregnancies, both of which ended in stillbirths. In her current pregnancy, daily doses of the three drugs were 50 mg, 10 mg, and 160 mg, respectively. The infant, delivered by cesarean section at 38 weeks, had multiple abnormalities including an omphalocele (repaired on the 2nd day), pronounced hypertrichosis of the back and extremities, depressed nasal bridge, low-set ears, micrognathia, bilateral fifth finger clinodactyly, undescended testes, a circumferential midphallic constriction, a large ventriculoseptal defect, and a brain defect consisting of slightly prominent sulci, especially the basal cisterns and interhemispheric fissure. Growth retardation was not evident, but the weight (3170 g, 60th percentile), length (46 cm, 15th percentile), and head circumference (32.5 cm, 25th percentile) were disproportionate. Neurologic examinations, as well as examinations of the skeleton and kidneys, were normal. Marked hypotension (30–50 mm Hg systolic) was present, which resolved after 24 hours. Heart rate, blood glucose, and renal function were normal. The infant's hospital course was marked by failure to thrive, congestive heart failure, prolonged physiologic jaundice, and eight episodes of hyperthermia (>38.5°C without apparent cause) between 2–6 weeks of age. The hypertrichosis, which was much less prominent at 2 months of age, is a known adverse effect of minoxidil therapy in both children and adults, and the condition in this infant was thought to be due to that drug (5). The etiology of the other defects could not be determined, but a chromosome abnormality was excluded based on a normal male karyotype (46X,Y) determined after a midgestation amniocentesis.

Several case reports have described the use of captopril, usually in combination with other antihypertensive agents and often after the failure of other medications, for the treatment of resistant hypertension during pregnancy (6–12). One case involved a mother with polyarteritis nodosa treated throughout gestation with captopril, hydralazine, and furosemide (13). The pregnancy was electively terminated at approximately 31 weeks' gestation because of worsening maternal disease. A normal, non-growth-retarded infant was delivered who did well in the neonatal period. A woman, who was treated at 25 weeks' gestation developed oligohydramnios after 3 weeks of therapy (6). Cesarean section at 29 weeks' gestation produced a 1040-g infant with dehydration, marked peripheral vasodilation, severe hypotension, respiratory distress, and anuria. Epidermolysis of the trunk and extremities appeared after birth. Diagnostic studies indicated a normal bladder, but neither kidney was perfused. Angiotensin-converting enzyme activity was reported as very low. The infant died on day 8 as a result of persistent anuria. At autopsy, hemorrhagic foci were discovered in the renal cortex and medulla, but nephrogenesis was adequate for the gestational age. In a second case, a woman was treated at 27 weeks' gestation with daily doses of captopril (200 mg), labetalol (1600 mg), and furosemide (80 mg) (7). Fourteen days after treatment was begun, signs of fetal distress, attributed to the maternal hypertension, appeared and the infant was delivered by cesarean section. No adverse effects of the drug treatment were observed in the infant. A pregnant woman with nephrotic syndrome and arterial hypertension was treated throughout pregnancy with captopril and acebutolol (8). Intrauterine growth retardation (IUGR), most probably due to the severe maternal disease (although a contribution from drug therapy could not be excluded), was identified early in the 2nd trimester and became progressively worse. The growth-retarded male infant was delivered prematurely at 34 weeks by cesarean section. Captopril was found in the cord blood with levels in the mother and fetus less than 100 ng/ml, 4 hours after the last dose. Angiotensin-converting enzyme activity was below normal limits in both the mother and the newborn. Neonatal respiratory arrest occurred 15 minutes after delivery with varying degrees of hypotension persisting over the first 10 days. A patent ductus arteriosus was also present.

A woman with hypertension secondary to bilateral renal artery stenosis was treated with captopril, 150 mg/day (9). She became pregnant 6 weeks after starting captopril. Daily drug therapy during pregnancy consisted of captopril (600 mg), methyldopa (750 mg), and furosemide (80 mg). Oligohydramnios and IUGR were diagnosed at 35 weeks' gestation, at which time a cesarean section was performed to deliver the 2120-g male infant. Some of the abnormalities in the infant, such as pulmonary hypoplasia, small skull circumference (28.5 cm, <3rd percentile), hypoplastic skull bones with wide sutures, and contractures of the extremities, were probably due to the oligohydramnios and severe maternal disease (9). However, the severe hypotension (27/20 mm Hg), which slowly resolved over 5 days in spite of volume expansion and pressor agents, and the anuria were most likely due to captopril. The infant was anuric for 7 days, then oliguric with 7–10 ml/day output for the next 12 days. All diagnostic tests during the first 10 days after birth indicated apparently normal kidneys. Peritoneal dialysis was commenced on the 20th day, but the infant died at 1 month of age.

A 1985 case report described a woman with twins treated throughout pregnancy with captopril (75–100 mg/day), hydralazine (75 mg/day), metoprolol (200 mg/day), and chlorthalidone (25 mg/day; stopped after 3 months) (10). Three previous pregnancies complicated by severe hypertension had ended with one term, mentally retarded infant and two spontaneous abortions, one at 5 months and one at 7 months. Two weeks before term the dose of captopril was reduced to 37.5 mg/day. Other than their small size (weight and length of both were less than the 10th percentile), both infants were normal and had normal mental and physical growth at 10 months. In another case report, a woman who had had a renal transplant was treated throughout gestation with daily doses of captopril (75 mg), cyclosporine (200 mg), atenolol (200 mg), cimetidine (800 mg), and amoxicillin (500 mg) (11). Oligohydramnios was diagnosed at 18 weeks' gestation and IUGR with gross oligohydramnios was discovered at 26 weeks. Ultrasound scanning at 27 weeks indicated renal dysplasia. Intrauterine fetal death occurred at 29 weeks. No congenital anomalies were found at autopsy. The kidneys appeared normal, but no urine was found in the ureters or bladder. The authors attributed the renal dysgenesis to the captopril therapy (11).

A 18-year-old woman with severe chronic hypertension became pregnant while taking captopril, hydralazine, and propranolol (12). Captopril and hydralazine were discontinued on presentation at 10 weeks' gestation for unspecified reasons. Because her subsequent blood pressure control was so poor, her therapy was changed at 20 weeks' gestation to captopril (37.5 mg/day, but later increased to 75 mg/day), atenolol (100 mg/day), and nifedipine (40 mg/day). IUGR was identified by serial scanning. A healthy, 1590-g female infant was delivered by cesarean section at 30 weeks' gestation. No other additional information was provided, other than that the infant survived.

The result of a survey on the use of captopril during pregnancy was published in 1988 (14). The mothers had been treated for chronic essential or renal hypertension. The outcomes of therapy in the 37 pregnancies (38 fetuses, one set of twins) were three stillbirths, 11 premature births, four small-for-gestational-age infants, four cases of patent ductus arteriosus, and two neonatal deaths secondary to anuria. Except for the anuria, the severe maternal disease, premature delivery, and fetal/newborn hypoxia were probably the most likely causes of the adverse outcomes. Investigators at the Food and Drug Administration (FDA) summarized some of the known cases of captopril-induced neonatal anuria in a 1989 report (15). These cases have been described above (6, 8, 9). The FDA authors cautioned that if captopril was used during pregnancy, then preparations should be made for neonatal hypotension and renal failure (15).

In summary, captopril does not appear to be a human teratogen, although two case reports have described multiple defects after exposure to captopril and other drug therapy. The etiology of the defects in both cases was unknown. However, further studies are needed to determine if structural kidney defects are produced by captopril (15). (See Enalapril for a report of possible drug-induced renal anomalies.) The use of captopril during pregnancy may compromise the fetal renal system and result in severe, and at times fatal, anuria. Severe neonatal hypotension may also occur. Two reviews of fetal and newborn renal function, published in 1988, indicated that both renal perfusion and glomerular plasma flow are low during gestation and that high levels of angiotensin II may be physiologically necessary to maintain glomerular filtration at low perfusion pressures (16, 17). Captopril prevents the conversion of angiotensin I to angiotensin II and, thus, may lead to *in utero* renal failure. In cases in which the mother's disease requires captopril, the lowest possible dose should be used. Close monitoring of amniotic fluid levels and fetal well-being should be conducted during gestation followed by close observation of renal function and blood pressure in the newborn.

Breast Feeding Summary

Captopril is excreted into breast milk in low concentrations. In 12 mothers given 100 mg three times a day, average peak milk levels were 4.7 ng/ml at 3.8 hours after their last dose (18, 19). This represented an average milk:plasma ratio of 0.012. No differences were found in captopril levels in pre- and postdrug milk. No effects on the nursing infants were observed. The American Academy of Pediatrics considers captopril compatible with breast feeding (20).

References

1. Broughton Pipkin F, Turner SR, Symonds EM. Possible risk with captopril in pregnancy: some animal data. Lancet 1980;1:1256.
2. Anonymous. The 1984 report of the joint national committee on detection, evaluation, and treatment of high blood pressure. Arch Intern Med 1984;144:1045–6.
3. Duminy PC, Burger PT. Fetal abnormality associated with the use of captopril during pregnancy. S Afr Med J 1981;60:805.
4. Broude AM. Fetal abnormality associated with captopril during pregnancy. S Afr Med J 1982;61:68.
5. Kaler SG, Patrinos ME, Lambert GH, Myers TF, Karlman R, Anderson CL. Hypertrichosis and congenital anomalies associated with maternal use of minoxidil. Pediatrics 1987;79:434–6.
6. Guignard JP, Burgener F, Calame A. Persistent anuria in a neonate: a side effect of captopril? Int J Pediatr Nephrol 1981;2:133 (Abstr).

7. Millar JA, Wilson PD, Morrison N. Management of severe hypertension in pregnancy by a combined drug regimen including captopril: case report. NZ Med J 1983;96:796–8.
8. Boutroy MJ, Vert P, Hurault de Ligny B, Miton A. Captopril administration in pregnancy impairs fetal angiotensin converting enzyme activity and neonatal adaptation. Lancet 1984;2:935–6.
9. Rothberg AD, Lorenz R. Can captopril cause fetal and neonatal renal failure? Pediatr Pharmacol 1984;4:189–92.
10. Coen G, Cugini P, Gerlini G, Finistauri D, Cinotti GA. Successful treatment of long-lasting severe hypertension with captopril during a twin pregnancy. Nephron 1985;40:498–500.
11. Knott PD, Thorpe SS, Lamont CAR. Congenital renal dysgenesis possibly due to captopril. Lancet 1989;1:451.
12. Smith AM. Are ACE inhibitors safe in pregnancy? Lancet 1989;2:750–1.
13. Owen J, Hauth JC. Polyarteritis nodosa in pregnancy: a case report and brief literature review. Am J Obstet Gynecol 1989;160:606–7.
14. Kreft-Jais C, Plouin P-F, Tchobroutsky C, Boutroy J. Angiotensin-converting enzyme inhibitors during pregnancy: a survey of 22 patients given captopril and nine given enalapril. Br J Obstet Gynaecol 1988;95:420–2.
15. Rosa FW, Bosco LA, Graham CF, Milstien JB, Dreis M, Creamer J. Neonatal anuria with maternal angiotensin-converting enzyme inhibition. Obstet Gynecol 1989;74:371–4.
16. Robillard JE, Nakamura KT, Matherne GP, Jose PA. Renal hemodynamics and functional adjustments to postnatal life. Semin Perinatol 1988;12:143–50.
17. Guignard JP, Gouyon JB. Adverse effects of drugs on the immature kidney. Biol Neonate 1988;53:243–52.
18. Devlin RG, Fleiss PM. Selective resistance to the passage of captopril into human milk. Clin Pharmacol Ther 1980;27:250.
19. Devlin RG, Fleiss PM. Captopril in human blood and breast milk. J Clin Pharmacol 1981;21:110–3.
20. Committee on Drugs, American Academy of Pediatrics. Transfer of drugs and other chemicals into human milk. Pediatrics 1989;84:924–36.

Name: **CARBACHOL**

Class: **Parasympathomimetic (Cholinergic)**   Risk Factor: **C**

Fetal Risk Summary

Carbachol is used in the eye. No reports of its use in pregnancy have been located. As a quaternary ammonium compound, it is ionized at physiologic pH and transplacental passage in significant amounts would not be expected.

Breast Feeding Summary

No data are available.

Name: **CARBAMAZEPINE**

Class: **Anticonvulsant**   Risk Factor: **C$_M$**

Fetal Risk Summary

Carbamazepine, a tricyclic anticonvulsant, has been in clinical use since 1962. The drug crosses the placenta with highest concentrations found in fetal liver and kidneys (1–3). Fetal levels are approximately 50–80% of maternal serum levels (3).

Placental function in women taking carbamazepine has been evaluated (4). No effect was detected from carbamazepine as measured by serum human placental lactogen, 24-hour urinary total estriol excretion, placental weight, and birth weight.

Use of carbamazepine during the 1st trimester has been reported in over 600 pregnancies (4–19). Multiple anomalies were found in one stillborn infant where carbamazepine was the only anticonvulsant used by the mother (12). These included closely set eyes, flat nose with single nasopharynx, polydactylia, atrial septal defect, patent ductus arteriosus, absent gallbladder and thyroid, and collapsed fontanel. Individual defects observed in this and other cases include talipes, meningomyelocele, anal atresia, ambiguous genitalia, congenital heart disease, hyperterolism, hypoplasia of the nose, cleft lip, congenital hip dislocation, inguinal hernia, hypoplasia of the nails, and torticollis (5–15). Decreased head circumference, 7 mm less than controls, has been observed in infants exposed only to carbamazepine during gestation (16). The head size was still small by 18 months of age with no catch-up growth evident. In a 1982 review, Janz (20) stated that nearly all possible malformations had been observed in epileptic patients. Minor malformations, such as those seen in the fetal hydantoin syndrome (FHS) (see Phenytoin), have also been observed with carbamazepine monotherapy, causing Janz to conclude that the term FHS was misleading (20). Since carbamazepine was thought to present a lower risk to the fetus, the drug has been recommended as the treatment of choice for women who may become pregnant and who require anticonvulsant therapy for the first time (21). However, a 1989 report has indicated that carbamazepine is also probably a human teratogen (19).

Eight children were identified retrospectively after *in utero* exposure to carbamazepine either alone ($N = 4$), or in combination with other anticonvulsants (phenobarbital $N = 2$, primidone $N = 1$, phenobarbital and clonazepam $N = 1$) (19). In six mothers, daily carbamazepine doses ranged from 600–1600 mg (dosage unknown in two). The following defects were noted in the children: intrauterine growth retardation (two cases), poor neonatal performance (three cases), postnatal growth deficiency (three cases) (not determined in four), developmental delay (three cases) (not determined in four), microcephaly (three cases) (not determined in four), upslanting palpebral fissures (two cases), short nose with long philtrum (two cases), hypoplastic nails (four cases), cardiac defect (two cases). Concurrently with the above evaluations, a prospective study involving 72 women treated with carbamazepine in early pregnancy was conducted (19). Fifty-four liveborn children were evaluated from the 72 mothers with the remaining 18 excluded for various reasons (seven spontaneous abortions, five therapeutic abortions, and six lost to follow-up before delivery). A control group of 73 pregnant women was prospectively selected for comparison. Anticonvulsant drug therapy in the study group consisted of carbamazepine either alone ($N = 50$) or in combination with phenobarbital ($N = 12$), phenobarbital and valproic acid ($N = 4$), primidone ($N = 3$), valproic acid ($N = 1$), ethosuximide ($N = 1$), and primidone and ethosuximide ($N = 1$). Carbamazepine dosage varied from 200–1200 mg/day. Seizures occurred at least once during pregnancy in 59% of the women, but they did not correlate with either malformations or developmental delay in the offspring (19). Of the 54 liveborn children, 48 were examined by the study investigators. Five (10%) of these children had major anomalies consisting of lumbosacral meningomyelocele (N = 1), multiple ventricular septal defects (N = 1), indirect inguinal hernia (N = 1) (all three exposed to carbamazepine alone), and cleft uvula (N = 2) (exposed to carbamazepine and phenobarbital). Five (7%) of the control infants also had major anomalies. The incidence of children with two minor malformations was statistically similar for the study and control groups, 23% (11 of 48) vs. 13% (9 of 70), respectively. Those presenting with three or more minor anomalies, however, were more frequent in the exposed group (38%, 18 of 48) than in controls (6%, 4 of 70) (p = 0.001). The various pregnancy outcomes and abnormalities were classified by treatment group (see reference 19 for full details). Based on the combined results from the retrospective and prospective studies, the investigators concluded that carbamazepine exposure was associated with a pattern of congenital malformations whose principal features consisted of minor craniofacial defects, fingernail hypoplasia, and developmental delay (19). Because these defects were similar to those observed with the fetal hydantoin syndrome, and because both carbamazepine and phenytoin are metabolized through the arene oxide pathway, a mechanism was proposed that attributed the teratogenicity to the epoxide intermediates rather to the specific drugs themselves (19).

In later correspondence concerning the above study, the investigators cited unofficial data obtained from the Food and Drug Administration involving 1307 pregnancies in which the maternal use of carbamazepine was not confounded by the concomitant use of valproic acid (22). Eight infants with spina bifida were identified in the offspring of these mothers. The incidence of 0.6% (1 in 163) represented a 9-fold relative risk for the neural tube defect (22).

In a study designed to evaluate the effect of *in utero* exposure to anticonvulsants on intelligence, 148 Finnish children of epileptic mothers were compared to 105 controls (18). Previous studies (briefly reviewed in reference 18) had either shown intellectual impairment from this exposure or no effect. Of the 148 children of epileptic mothers, 129 were exposed to anticonvulsant therapy during the first 20 weeks of pregnancy, two were only exposed after 20 weeks, and 17 were not exposed. In those mothers treated during pregnancy, 42 received carbamazepine (monotherapy in nine cases) during the first 20 weeks, and one received the drug after 20 weeks. The children were evaluated at 5.5 years of age for both verbal and nonverbal measures of intelligence. A child was considered mentally deficient if the results of both tests were less than 71. Two of the 148 children of epileptic mothers were diagnosed as mentally deficient and two others had borderline intelligence (the mother of one of these latter children had not been treated with anticonvulsant medication). None of the controls was considered mentally deficient. One child with profound mental retardation had been exposed *in utero* to carbamazepine monotherapy, but the condition was compatible with dominant inheritance and was not thought to be due to drug exposure. Both verbal and nonverbal intelligence scores were significantly lower in the study group children than in controls. In both groups, intelligence scores were significantly lower when seven or more minor anomalies were present (p = 0.03). However, the presence of hypertelorism and digital hypoplasia, two minor anomalies considered typical of exposure to some anticonvulsants (e.g., phenytoin), was not predictive of low intelligence.

The effect of carbamazepine on maternal and fetal vitamin D metabolism was examined in a 1984 study (23). In comparison to normal controls, several significant differences were found in the level of various vitamin D compounds and in serum calcium, but the values were still within normal limits. No alterations were found in alkaline phosphatase and phosphate concentrations. The authors doubted if the observed differences were of major clinical significance.

Breast Feeding Summary

Carbamazepine is excreted into breast milk, producing milk:plasma ratios of 0.24–0.69 (1, 3, 7, 12, 24). The amount of carbamazepine measured in infant serum is low, with typical levels around 0.4 μg/ml, but levels may be as high as 0.5–1.8 μg/ml (1). Accumulation does not seem to occur. The American Academy of Pediatrics considers the drug to be compatible with breast feeding (25).

References

1. Pynnonen S, Knato J, Stilanpaa M, Erkkola R. Carbamazepine: placental transport, tissue concentrations in the foetus and newborns, and level in milk. Acta Pharmacol Toxicol 1977;41:244–53.
2. Rane A, Bertilsson L, Palmer L. Disposition of placentally transferred carbamazepine (Tegretol) in the newborn. Eur J Clin Pharmacol 1975;8:283–4.
3. Nau H, Kuhnz W, Egger HJ, Rating D, Helge H. Anticonvulsants during pregnancy and lactation: transplacental, maternal and neonatal pharmacokinetics. Clin Pharmacokinet 1982;7:508–43.
4. Hiilesmaa VK. Evaluation of placental function in women on antiepileptic drugs. J Perinat Med 1983;11:187–92.
5. Geigy Pharmaceuticals. Tegretol in epilepsy. In Monograph 319–80950, Ciba-Geigy, Ardsley, 1978:18–19.
6. McMullin GP. Teratogenic effects of anticonvulsants. Br Med J 1971;4:430.
7. Pynnonen S, Sillanpaa M. Carbamazepine and mothers milk. Lancet 1975;2:563.
8. Lander CM, Edwards VE, Endie MJ, Tyrer JH. Plasma anticonvulsant concentrations during pregnancy. Neurology 1977;27:128–31.
9. Nakane Y, Okuma T, Takahashi R, et al. Multi-institutional study on the teratogenicity and fetal toxicity to antiepileptic drugs: a report of a collaborative study group in Japan. Epilepsia 1980;21:633–80.
10. Janz D. The teratogenic risk of antiepileptic drugs. Epilepsia 1975;16:159–69.
11. Meyer JG. Teratogenic risk of anticonvulsants and the effects on pregnancy and birth. Eur Neurol 1979;10:179–90.
12. Niebly JR, Blake DA, Freeman JM, Luff RD. Carbamazepine levels in pregnancy and lactation. Obstet Gynecol 1979;53:139–40.
13. Hicks EP. Carbamazepine in two pregnancies. Clin Exp Neurol 1979;16:269–75.
14. Thomas D, Buchanan N. Teratogenic effects of anticonvulsants. J Pediatr 1981;99:163.
15. Niesen M, Froscher W. Finger- and toenail hypoplasia after carbamazepine monotherapy in late pregnancy. Neuropediatrics 1985;16:167–8.
16. Hiilesmaa VK, Teramo K, Granstrom ML, Bardy AH. Fetal head growth retardation associated with maternal antiepileptic drugs. Lancet 1981;2:165–7.
17. Hiilesmaa VK, Bardy A, Teramo K. Obstetric outcome in women with epilepsy. Am J Obstet Gynecol 1985;152:499–504.
18. Gaily E, Kantola-Sorsa E, Granstrom M-L. Intelligence of children of epileptic mothers. J Pediatr 1988;113:677–84.
19. Jones KL, Lacro RV, Johnson KA, Adams J. Pattern of malformations in the children of women treated with carbamazepine during pregnancy. N Engl J Med 1989;320:1661–6.
20. Janz D. Antiepileptic drugs and pregnancy: altered utilization patterns and teratogenesis. Epilepsia 1982;23(Suppl 1):S53–S63.
21. Paulson GW, Paulson RB. Teratogenic effects of anticonvulsants. Arch Neurol 1981;38:140–3.
22. Jones KL, Johnson KA, Adams J, Lacro RV. Teratogenic effects of carbamazepine. N Engl J Med 1989;321:1481.
23. Markestad T, Ulstein M, Strandjord RE, Aksnes L, Aarskog D. Anticonvulsant drug therapy in human pregnancy: effects on serum concentrations of vitamin D metabolites in maternal and cord blood. Am J Obstet Gynecol 1984;150:254–8.

24. Kok THHG, Taitz LS, Bennett MJ, Holt DW. Drowsiness due to clemastine transmitted in breast milk. Lancet 1982;1:914–5.
25. Committee on Drugs, American Academy of Pediatrics. Transfer of drugs and other chemicals into human milk. Pediatrics 1989;84:924–36.

Name: **CARBARSONE**

Class: **Amebicide**   Risk Factor: **D**

Fetal Risk Summary

No reports linking the use of carbarsone with congenital defects have been located. However, carbarsone contains approximately 29% arsenic, which has been associated with lesions of the central nervous system (1). In view of potential tissue accumulation and reported fetal fatalities secondary to arsenic poisonings, carbarsone is not recommended during pregnancy (1, 2).

Breast Feeding Summary

No data are available.

References

1. Arnold W. Morphologic und pathogenese der Salvarsan-schadigungen des zentralnervensystems. Virchows Arch (Pathol Anat) 1944;311:1.
2. Lugo G, Cassady G, Palmisano P. Acute maternal arsenic intoxication with neonatal death. Am J Dis Child 1969;117:328.

Name: **CARBENICILLIN**

Class: **Antibiotic**   Risk Factor: **B**

Fetal Risk Summary

Carbenicillin is a penicillin antibiotic (see also Penicillin G). The drug crosses the placenta and distributes to most fetal tissues (1, 2). Following a 4-g intramuscular dose, mean peak concentrations in cord and maternal serums at 2 hours were similar. Amniotic fluid levels averaged 7–11% of maternal peak concentrations.

No reports linking the use of carbenicillin with congenital defects have been located. The Collaborative Perinatal Project monitored 50,282 mother-child pairs, 3,546 of which had documented 1st trimester exposure to penicillin derivatives (3, pp. 297–313). For use anytime during pregnancy, 7,171 exposures were recorded (3, p. 435). In neither case was evidence found to suggest a relationship to large categories of major or minor malformations or to individual defects.

Breast Feeding Summary

No data are available (see Penicillin G).

References

1. Biro L, Ivan E, Elek E, Arr M. Data on the tissue concentration of antibiotics in man. Tissue concentrations of semi-synthetic penicillins in the fetus. Int Z Pharmakol Ther Toxikol 1970;4:321–4.
2. Elek E, Ivan E, Arr M. Passage of penicillins from mother to foetus in humans. Int J Clin Pharmacol Ther Toxicol 1972;6:223–8.
3. Heinonen OP, Slone D, Shapiro S. *Birth Defects and Drugs in Pregnancy*. Littleton:Publishing Sciences Group, 1977.

Name: **CARBIMAZOLE**

Class: **Antithyroid**   Risk Factor: **D**

Fetal Risk Summary

Carbimazole is converted *in vivo* to methimazole (1). See Methimazole.

Breast Feeding Summary

See Methimazole.

Reference

1. Haynes RC Jr, Murad F. Thyroid and antithyroid drugs. In Gilman AG, Goodman LS, Gilman A, eds. *The Pharmacological Basis of Therapeutics*, 5th ed. New York:MacMillan Publishing Co, 1980:1411.

Name: **CARBINOXAMINE**

Class: **Antihistamine**   Risk Factor: **C**

Fetal Risk Summary

No data are available. See Diphenhydramine for representative agent in this class.

Breast Feeding Summary

No data are available.

Name: **CARPHENAZINE**

Class: **Tranquilizer**   Risk Factor: **C**

Fetal Risk Summary

Carphenazine is a piperazine phenothiazine in the same group as prochlorperazine (see Prochlorperazine). Phenothiazines readily cross the placenta (1). No specific information on the use of carphenazine in pregnancy has been located. Although occasional reports have attempted to link various phenothiazine compounds with congenital malformations, the bulk of the evidence indicates that these drugs are safe for the mother and fetus (see also Chlorpromazine).

Breast Feeding Summary

No data are available.

Reference

1. Moya F, Thorndike V. Passage of drugs across the placenta. Am J Obstet Gynecol 1962;84:1778–98.

Name: **CASANTHRANOL**

Class: **Purgative**   Risk Factor: **C**

Fetal Risk Summary

Casanthranol is an anthraquinone purgative. In a large prospective study, 109 patients were exposed to this agent during pregnancy, 21 in the 1st trimester (1). No evidence of an increased risk for malformations was found (see also Cascara Sagrada).

Breast Feeding Summary

See Cascara Sagrada.

Reference

1. Heinonen OP, Slone D, Shapiro S. *Birth Defects and Drugs in Pregnancy*. Littleton:Publishing Sciences Group, 1977:384–7, 442.

Name: **CASCARA SAGRADA**

Class: **Purgative**   Risk Factor: **C**

Fetal Risk Summary

Cascara sagrada is an anthraquinone purgative. In a large prospective study, 53 mother-child pairs were exposed to cascara sagrada during the 1st trimester (1, pp. 384–387). Although the numbers are small, no evidence for an increased risk of malformations was found. For anytime use during pregnancy, 188 exposures were recorded (1, pp. 438, 442, 497). The relative risk for benign tumors was higher than expected, but the statistical significance is unknown and independent confirmation is required (1, pp. 438, 442, 497).

Breast Feeding Summary

Most reviewers acknowledge the presence of anthraquinones in breast milk and warn of the consequences for the nursing infant (2–4). A comprehensive review that describes the excretion of laxatives into human milk has been published (5). The authors state that little is actually known about the presence of these agents in breast milk. Two reports suggest an increased incidence of diarrhea in infants when nursing mothers are given cascara sagrada or senna for postpartum constipation (6, 7).

References

1. Heinonen OP, Slone D, Shapiro S. *Birth Defects and Drugs in Pregnancy*. Littleton:Publishing Sciences Group, 1977.
2. Knowles JA. Breast milk: a source of more than nutrition for the neonate. Clin Toxicol 1974;7:69–82.
3. O'Brien TE. Excretion of drugs in human milk. Am J Hosp Pharm 1974;31:844–54.
4. Edwards A. Drugs in breast milk—a review of the recent literature. Aust J Hosp Pharm 1981;11:27–39.
5. Stewart JJ. Gastrointestinal drugs. In Wilson JT, ed. *Drugs in Breast Milk*. Australia (Balgowlah):ADIS Press, 1981:65–71.
6. Tyson RM, Shrader EA, Perlman HH. Drugs transmitted through breast milk. Part I. Laxatives. J Pediatr 1937;11:824–32.
7. Greenleaf JO, Leonard HSD. Laxatives in the treatment of constipation in pregnant and breast-feeding mothers. Practitioner 1973;210:259–63.

Name: **CEFACLOR**

Class: **Antibiotic**   Risk Factor: **B$_M$**

Fetal Risk Summary

Cefaclor is a cephalosporin antibiotic. No reports on its use in pregnancy have been located.

Breast Feeding Summary

Cefaclor is excreted into breast milk in low concentrations. Following a single 500-mg oral dose, average milk levels ranged from 0.16–0.21 µg/ml over a 5-hour period (1). Only trace amounts of the antibiotic could be measured at 1 and 6 hours. Although these levels are low, three potential problems exist for the nursing infant: modification of bowel flora, direct effects on the infant, and interference with the interpretation of culture results if a fever workup is required.

Reference

1. Takase Z. Clinical and laboratory studies of cefaclor in the field of obstetrics and gynecology. Chemotherapy (Tokyo) 1979;27(Suppl):668.

Name: **CEFADROXIL**

Class: **Antibiotic**   Risk Factor: **B$_M$**

Fetal Risk Summary

Cefadroxil is a cephalosporin antibiotic. No controlled studies on its use in pregnancy have been located. At term, a 500-mg oral dose produced an average peak cord serum level of 4.6 µg/ml at 2.5 hours (about 40% of maternal serum) (1).

Amniotic fluid levels achieved a peak of 4.4 μg/ml at 10 hours. No infant data were given.

Breast Feeding Summary

Cefadroxil is excreted into breast milk in low concentrations. Following a single 500-mg oral dose, peak milk levels of about 0.6–0.7 μg/ml occurred at 5–6 hours (1). A 1-g oral dose given to six mothers produced peak milk levels averaging 1.83 μg/ml (range 1.2–2.4 μg/ml) at 6–7 hours (2). In this latter group, milk:plasma ratios at 1, 2, and 3 hours were 0.009, 0.011, and 0.019, respectively. Although these levels are low, three potential problems exist for the nursing infant: modification of bowel flora, direct effects on the infant, and interference with the interpretation of culture results if a fever workup is required. The American Academy of Pediatrics considers cefadroxil to be compatible with breast feeding (3).

References

1. Takase Z, Shirafuji H, Uchida M. Experimental and clinical studies of cefadroxil in the treatment of infections in the field of obstetrics and gynecology. Chemotherapy (Tokyo) 1980;28(Suppl 2):424–31.
2. Kafetzi D, Siafas C, Georgakopoulos P, Papdatos C. Passage of cephalosporins and amoxicillin into the breast milk. Acta Paediatr Scand 1981;70:285–8.
3. Committee on Drugs, American Academy of Pediatrics. Transfer of drugs and other chemicals into human milk. Pediatrics 1989;84:924–36.

Name: **CEFAMANDOLE**

Class: **Antibiotic**   Risk Factor: **B**_M

Fetal Risk Summary

Cefamandole is a cephalosporin antibiotic. No controlled studies on its use in pregnancy have been located. Although pregnant patients were excluded from clinical trials of cefamandole, one patient did receive the drug in the 1st trimester (J.T. Anderson, personal communication, Lilly Research Laboratories, 1981). No apparent adverse effects were noted in the newborn.

Breast Feeding Summary

Cefamandole is excreted into breast milk in low concentrations. Following a 1-g intravenous dose, average milk levels in four patients ranged from 0.46 (1 hour) to 0.19 μg/ml (6 hours) (J.T. Anderson, personal communication. Lilly Research Laboratories, 1981). The milk:plasma ratio at 1 hour was 0.02. No neonate information was given. Although these levels are low, three potential problems exist for the nursing infant: modification of bowel flora, direct effects on the infant, and interference with the interpretation of culture results if a fever workup is required.

Name: **CEFATRIZINE**

Class: **Antibiotic**   Risk Factor: **B$_M$**

Fetal Risk Summary

Cefatrizine is a cephalosporin antibiotic. No controlled studies on its use in pregnancy have been located. Transplacental passage of cefatrizine has been demonstrated in women undergoing elective therapeutic surgical abortion in the 1st and 2nd trimesters (1). None of the fetuses from prostaglandin $F_{2\alpha}$ abortions revealed evidence of cefatrizine.

Breast Feeding Summary

Most cephalosporins are excreted into breast milk in low concentrations, but data for cefatrizine are lacking. For potential problems during breast feeding, see Cephalothin.

Reference

1. Bernard B, Thielen P, Garcia-Cazares SJ, Ballard CA. Maternal-fetal pharmacology of cefatrizine in the first 20 weeks of pregnancy. Antimicrob Agents Chemother 1977;12:231–6.

Name: **CEFAZOLIN**

Class: **Antibiotic**   Risk Factor: **B$_M$**

Fetal Risk Summary

Cefazolin is a cephalosporin antibiotic. No controlled studies on its use in pregnancy have been located. Cefazolin crosses the placenta into the cord serum and amniotic fluid (1–4). In early pregnancy, distribution is limited to the body fluids and these concentrations are considerably lower than those found in the 2nd and 3rd trimesters (2). At term, 15–70 minutes after a 500-mg dose, cord serum levels range from 35–69% of maternal serum (3). The maximum concentration in amniotic fluid after 500 mg was 8 μg/ml at 2.5 hours (4). No data on the newborns were given.

Breast Feeding Summary

Cefazolin is excreted into breast milk in low concentrations. Following a 2-g intravenous dose, average milk levels ranged from 1.2–1.5 μg/ml over 4 hours (milk:plasma ratio 0.02) (5). When cefazolin was given as a 500-mg intramuscular dose, one to three times daily, the drug was not detectable (4). Although these levels are low, three potential problems exist for the nursing infant: modification of bowel flora, direct effects on the infant, and interference with the interpretation of culture results if a fever workup is required. The American Academy of Pediatrics considers cefazolin to be compatible with breast feeding (6).

References

1. Dekel A, Elian I, Gibor Y, Goldman JA. Transplacental passage of cefazolin in the first trimester of pregnancy. Eur J Obstet Gynecol Reprod Biol 1980;10:303–7.

2. Bernard B, Barton L, Abate M, Ballard CA. Maternal-fetal transfer of cefazolin in the first twenty weeks of pregnancy. J Infect Dis 1977;136:377–82.
3. Cho N, Ito T, Saito T, et al. Clinical studies on cefazolin in the field of obstetrics and gynecology. Chemotherapy (Tokyo) 1970;18:770–7.
4. von Kobyletzki D, Reither K, Gellen J, Kanyo A, Glocke M. Pharmacokinetic studies with cefazolin in obstetrics and gynecology. Infection 1974;2(Suppl):60–7.
5. Yoshioka H, Cho K, Takimato M, Maruyama S, Shimizu T. Transfer of cefazolin into human milk. J Pediatr 1979;94:151–2.
6. Committee on Drugs, American Academy of Pediatrics. Transfer of drugs and other chemicals into human milk. Pediatrics 1989;84:924–36.

Name: **CEFONICID**

Class: **Antibiotic**   Risk Factor: **B$_M$**

Fetal Risk Summary

Cefonicid is a cephalosporin antibiotic. No studies on its use in pregnancy have been located.

Breast Feeding Summary

Cefonicid is excreted into breast milk in low concentrations. Milk levels 1 hour after a 1-g intramuscular dose were equal to or less than 0.3 μg/ml, averaging 0.16 μg/ml (1). Although these concentrations are low, three potential problems exist for the nursing infant: modification of bowel flora, direct effects on the infant, and interference with the interpretation of culture results if a fever workup is required.

Reference

1. Lou MA Sr, Wu YH, Jacob LS, Pitkin DH. Penetration of cefonicid into human breast milk and various body fluids and tissues. Rev Infect Dis 1984;6(Suppl 4):S816–20.

Name: **CEFOPERAZONE**

Class: **Antibiotic**   Risk Factor: **B$_M$**

Fetal Risk Summary

Cefoperazone is a cephalosporin antibiotic. Following a 1-g intravenous (IV) or intramuscular (IM) dose, cord blood levels averaged 34.4 and 33.2%, respectively, of the maternal serum (1). Peak concentrations occurred at about 1 hour after both IV and IM doses. Amniotic fluid levels were 3–4 μg/ml within 6 hours of administration. Continuous IV dosing (1 g given two to four times every 12 hours) produced higher levels with cord blood averaging 40–48% of maternal serum and amniotic fluid levels increasing to 3.8–8.8 μg/ml. In a second study, 1 g IV produced peak cord blood concentrations averaging about 45% of maternal serum (25 μg/ml vs. 56.1 μg/ml) at 70 minutes with amniotic fluid concentrations varying between 2.8–4.8 μg/ml at 180 minutes (2). No effects on the newborns were reported in either study. In an *in vitro* experiment, placental transfer of cefoperazone was shown to occur only by simple diffusion (3).

Breast Feeding Summary

Cefoperazone is excreted into breast milk in low concentrations. An intravenous dose of 1 g produced milk levels ranging from 0.4–0.9 μg/ml (C.E. Jacobson, personal communication, Roerig, 1985). Although these concentrations are low, three potential problems exist for the nursing infant: modification of bowel flora, direct effects on the infant, and interference with the interpretation of culture results if a fever workup is required.

References

1. Matsuda S, Tanno M, Kashiwagura T, Furuya H. Placental transfer of cefoperazone (T-1551) and a clinical study of its use in obstetrics and gynecological infections. Cur Chemo Infect Dis 1979;2:167–8.
2. Shimizu K. Cefoperazone: absorption, excretion, distribution, and metabolism. Clin Ther 1980;3(Special Issue):60–79.
3. Fortunato SJ, Bawdon RE, Baum M. Placental transfer of cefoperazone and sulbactam in the isolated in vitro perfused human placenta. Am J Obstet Gynecol 1988;159:1002–6.

Name: **CEFORANIDE**

Class: **Antibiotic**   Risk Factor: **B$_M$**

Fetal Risk Summary

Ceforanide is a cephalosporin antibiotic. No data on its use in pregnancy have been located.

Breast Feeding Summary

No studies on the excretion of ceforanide into breast milk have been located. Like other cephalosporins, however, excretion should be expected, resulting in three potential problems for the nursing infant: modification of bowel flora, direct effects on the infant, and interference with the interpretation of culture results if a fever workup is required.

Name: **CEFOTAXIME**

Class: **Antibiotic**   Risk Factor: **B$_M$**

Fetal Risk Summary

Cefotaxime is a cephalosporin antibiotic. No controlled studies on its use in pregnancy have been located. During the 2nd trimester, the drug readily crosses the placenta (1). The half-life of cefotaxime in fetal serum and in amniotic fluid was 2.3 and 2.8 hours, respectively.

Breast Feeding Summary

Cefotaxime is excreted into breast milk in low concentrations. Following a 1-g intravenous dose, mean peak milk levels of 0.33 μg/ml were measured at 2–3 hours (1, 2). The half-life in milk ranged from 2.36–3.89 hours (mean 2.93). The milk:plasma ratios at 1, 2, and 3 hours were 0.027, 0.09, and 0.16, respectively. Although these levels are low, three potential problems exist for the nursing infant: modification of bowel flora, direct effects on the infant, and interference with the interpretation of culture results if a fever workup is required. The American Academy of Pediatrics considers cefotaxime to be compatible with breast feeding (3).

References

1. Kafetzis DA, Lazarides CV, Siafas CA, Georgakopoulos PA, Papadatos CJ. Transfer of cefotaxime in human milk and from mother to foetus. J Antimicrob Chemother 1980;6(Suppl A):135–41.
2. Kafetzis DA, Siafas CA, Georgakopoulos PA, Papadatos CJ. Passage of cephalosporins and amoxicillin into the breast milk. Acta Paediatr Scand 1981;70:285–8.
3. Committee on Drugs, American Academy of Pediatrics. Transfer of drugs and other chemicals into human milk. Pediatrics 1989;84:924–36.

Name: **CEFOXITIN**

Class: **Antibiotic** Risk Factor: **B**

Fetal Risk Summary

Cefoxitin is a cephalosporin antibiotic. No controlled studies of its use in pregnancy have been located, but multiple reports have described its transplacental passage (1–13). Two patients were given 1 g intravenously (IV) just prior to therapeutic abortion at 9 and 10 weeks' gestation (9). At 55 minutes, the serum level in one woman was 10.5 μg/ml while none was found in the fetal tissues. In the second patient, at 4.25 hours the maternal serum was "nil," while the fetal tissue level was 35.7 μg/ml.

At term, following intramuscular or rapid IV doses of 1 or 2 g, cord serum levels up to 22 μg/ml (11–90%) of maternal levels have been measured (6–9). Amniotic fluid concentrations peaked at 2–3 hours in the 3 to 15 μg/ml range (6, 7, 9, 10, 13). No apparent adverse effects were noted in any of the newborns.

Breast Feeding Summary

Cefoxitin is excreted into breast milk in low concentrations (5, 9, 11, 12, 14). Up to 2 μg/ml have been detected in the milk of women receiving therapeutic doses (J.J. Whalen, personal communication, Merck, Sharpe & Dohme, May 13, 1981). No data on the infants were given. Following prophylactic administration of 2–4 g of cefoxitin to 18 women during and following cesarean section, milk samples were collected a mean 25 hours (range 9–56 hours) after the last dose of antibiotic (14). Only one sample, collected 19 hours after the last dose, contained measurable concentrations of cefoxitin (0.9 μg/ml). Although these levels are low, three potential problems exist for the nursing infant: modification of bowel flora, direct effects on the infant, and interference with the interpretation of culture results if a fever workup is required. The American Academy of Pediatrics considers the drug to be compatible with breast feeding (15).

References

1. Bergone-Berezin B, Kafe H, Berthelot G, Morel O, Benard Y. Pharmacokinetic study of cefoxitin in bronchial secretions. In *Current Chemotherapy: Proceedings of the 10th International Congress of Chemotherapy*, Zurich, Switzerland, September 18–23, 1977. Washington:American Society for Microbiology, 1978.
2. Aokawa H, Minagawa M, Yamamiohi K, Sugiyama A. Studies on cefoxitin. Chemotherapy (Tokyo) 1977;(Suppl):394.
3. Matsuda S, Tanno M, Kashiwakura S, Furuya H. Basic and clinical studies on cefoxitin. Chemotherapy (Tokyo) 1977;(Suppl):396.
4. Berthelot G, Bergogne-Berezin B, Morel O, Kafe H, Benard Y. Cefoxitin: pharmacokinetic study in bronchial secretions—transplacental diffusion. Paper presented at 10th International Congress of Chemotherapy, Zurich, Switzerland, September 18–23, 1977, program abstract No. 80.
5. Mashimo K, Mihashi S, Fukaya I, Okubo B, Ohgob M, Saito A. New drug symposium IV. Cefoxitin. Chemotherapy (Tokyo) 1978;26:114–9.
6. Matsuda S, Tanno M, Kashiwakura T, Furuya H. Laboratory and clinical studies on cefoxitin in the field of obstetrics and gynecology. Chemotherapy (Tokyo) 1978;26(Suppl 1):460–7.
7. Cho N, Ubhara K, Suigizaki K, et al. Clinical studies of cefoxitin in the field of obstetrics and gynecology. Chemotherapy (Tokyo) 1978;26(Suppl 1):468–75.
8. Seiga K, Minagawa M, Yamaji K, Sugiyama Y. Study on cefoxitin. Chemotherapy (Tokyo) 1978;26(Suppl 1):491–501.
9. Takase Z, Shirafuji H, Uchida M. Clinical and laboratory studies on cefoxitin in the field of obstetrics and gynecology. Chemotherapy (Tokyo) 1978;26(Suppl 1):502–5.
10. Bergogne-Berezin B, Lambert-Zeohovsky N, Rouvillois JL. Placental transfer of cefoxitin. Paper presented at the 18th Interscience Conference on Antimicrobial Agents and Chemotherapy, Atlanta, Georgia, October 1–4, 1978, program abstract No. 314.
11. Brogden RN, Heel RC, Speight TM, Avery GS. Cefoxitin: a review of its antibacterial activity, pharmacological properties and therapeutic use. Drugs 1979;17:1–37.
12. Dubois M, Delapierre D, Demonty J, Lambotte R, Dresse A. Transplacental and mammary transfer of cefoxitin. Paper presented at 11th International Congress of Chemotherapy and 19th Interscience Conference on Antimicrobial Agents and Chemotherapy, Boston, Massachusetts, October 1–5, 1979, program abstract No. 118.
13. Bergogne-Berezin B, Morel O, Kafe H, et al. Pharmacokinetic study of cefoxitin in man: diffusion into the bronchi and transfer across the placenta. Therapie 1979;34:345–54.
14. Roex AJM, van Loenen AC, Puyenbroek JI, Arts NFT. Secretion of cefoxitin in breast milk following short-term prophylactic administration in caesarean section. Eur J Obstet Gynecol Reprod Biol 1987;25:299–302.
15. Committee on Drugs, American Academy of Pediatrics. Transfer of drugs and other chemicals into human milk. Pediatrics 1989;84:924–36.

Name: **CEFTIZOXIME**

Class: **Antibiotic**   Risk Factor: **B_M**

Fetal Risk Summary

Ceftizoxime is a cephalosporin antibiotic. Following 1- or 2-g intravenous (IV) doses administered to women at term, peak cord blood levels occurred at 1–2 hours with concentrations ranging between 12–30 μg/ml (1–5). Amniotic fluid concentrations were lower with peak levels of 10–20 μg/ml at 2–3 hours. The mean fetal:maternal ratio reported in one group of patients after a 2-g IV dose was 0. 28 (5). In a different study, maternal, fetal, and amniotic concentrations were measured in women who had received at least three doses of ceftizoxime 2 g at 8-hour intervals (6). Mean levels at delivery in the various compartments were 11.96 μg/ml, 24.54 μg/ml, and 43.45 μg/ml, respectively. Cord blood levels averaged 1.6 times higher than maternal levels with average amniotic fluid concentrations 2.9 times those in the maternal serum (6). No adverse fetal or newborn effects were noted in any of the trials.

Breast Feeding Summary

Ceftizoxime is excreted into breast milk in low concentrations (5, 7). Mean levels following single doses of 1 and 2 g were less than 0.5 μg/ml. Although these levels are low, three potential problems exist for the nursing infant: modification of bowel flora, direct effects on the infant, and interference with the interpretation of culture results if a fever workup is required.

References

1. Cho N, Fukunaga K, Kunii K. Studies on ceftizoxime (CZX) in the field of obstetrics and gynecology. Chemotherapy (Tokyo) 1980;28(Suppl 5):821–30.
2. Matsuda S, Seida A. Clinical use of ceftizoxime in obstetrics and gynecology. Chemotherapy (Tokyo) 1980;28(Suppl 5):812–20.
3. Okada E, Kawada A, Shirakawa N. Clinical studies on transplacental diffusion of ceftizoxime into fetal blood and treatment of infections in obstetrics and gynecology. Chemotherapy (Tokyo) 1980;28(Suppl 5):874–87.
4. Seiga K, Minagawa M, Egawa J, Yamaji K, Sugiyama Y. Clinical and laboratory studies on ceftizoxime (CZX) in the field of obstetrics and gynecology. Chemotherapy (Tokyo) 1980;28(Suppl 5):845–62.
5. Motomura R, Kohno M, Mori H, Yamabe T. Basic and clinical studies of ceftizoxime in obstetrics and gynecology. Chemotherapy (Tokyo) 1980;28(Suppl 5):888–99.
6. Fortunato SJ, Bawdon RE, Welt SI, Swan KF. Steady-state cord and amniotic fluid ceftizoxime levels continuously surpass maternal levels. Am J Obstet Gynecol 1988;159:570–3.
7. Gerding DN, Peterson LR. Comparative tissue and extravascular fluid concentrations of ceftizoxime. J Antimicrob Chemother 1982;10(Suppl C):105–16.

Name: **CEFTRIAXONE**

Class: **Antibiotic**   Risk Factor: **B_M**

Fetal Risk Summary

Ceftriaxone is a cephalosporin antibiotic. Peak levels in cord blood following 1- or 2-g intravenous doses occurred at 4 hours with concentrations varying between 19.6–40.6 μg/ml (1–8 hours) (1–3). Amniotic fluid levels over 24 hours ranged from 2.2–23.4 μg/ml with peak levels occurring at 6 hours (1–3). Ceftriaxone concentrations in the first voided newborn urine were highly variable, ranging from 6–92 μg/ml. Elimination half-lives from cord blood (7 hours), amniotic fluid (6.8 hours), and placenta (5.4 hours) were nearly identical to maternal serum (1, 2, 4). No adverse effects in the newborns were mentioned.

Breast Feeding Summary

Ceftriaxone is excreted into breast milk in low concentrations. Following either 1- or 2-g intravenous (IV) or intramuscular (IM) doses, peak levels of 0.5–0.7 μg/ml occurred at 5 hours, approximately 3–4% of maternal serum (1, 2). High protein binding in maternal serum probably limited transfer to the milk (1, 2). The antibiotic was still detectable in milk at 24 hours (1). Elimination half-lives after IV and IM doses were 12.8 and 17.3 hours, respectively (1). Chronic dosing would eventually produce calculated steady-state levels in 1.5–3 days in the 3–4 μg/ml range (2). Although these levels are low, three potential problems exist for the nursing infant: modification of bowel flora, direct effects on the infant, and interference with the interpretation of culture results if a fever workup is required. The American Academy of Pediatrics considers the drug to be compatible with breast feeding (5).

References

1. Kafetzis DA, Brater DC, Fanoursakis JE, Voyatzis J, Georgakopoulos P. Placental and breast-milk transfer of ceftriaxone (C). In Proceedings of the 22nd Intersci Conf on Antimicrob Ag Chemother, Miami, Florida, October 4–6, 1982:155. New York:Academic Press, 1983.
2. Kafetzis DA, Brater DC, Fanourgakis JE, Voyatzis J, Georgakopoulos P. Ceftriaxone distribution between maternal blood and fetal blood and tissues at parturition and between blood and milk postpartum. Antimicrob Agents Chemother 1983;23:870–3.
3. Cho N, Kunii K, Fukunago K, Komoriyama Y. Antimicrobial acitivity, pharmacokinetics and clinical studies of ceftriaxone in obstetrics and gynecology. In Proceedings of the 13th Inter Cong Chemother, Vienna, Austria, August 28 to September 2, 1983:100/64–66. Princeton:Excerpta Medica, 1984.
4. Graber H, Magyar T. Pharmacokinetics of ceftriaxone in pregnancy. Am J Med 1984;77:117–8.
5. Committee on Drugs, American Academy of Pediatrics. Transfer of drugs and other chemicals into human milk. Pediatrics 1989;84:924–36.

Name: **CEFUROXIME**

Class: **Antibiotic**   Risk Factor: **B**_M

Fetal Risk Summary

Cefuroxime is a cephalosporin antibiotic. No controlled studies on its use in pregnancy have been located. Cefuroxime readily crosses the placenta in late pregnancy and labor, achieving therapeutic concentrations in fetal serum and amniotic fluid (1–5). Therapeutic antibiotic levels in infants can be demonstrated up to 6 hours after birth with measurable concentrations persisting for 26 hours. The pharmacokinetics of cefuroxime in pregnancy have been reported (7). The antibiotic has been used for the treatment of pyelonephritis in pregnancy (8). Adverse effects in the newborn after *in utero* exposure have not been observed.

Breast Feeding Summary

Most cephalosporins are excreted into breast milk in low concentrations, but data for cefuroxime are lacking. For potential problems during breast feeding, see Cephalothin.

References

1. Craft I, Mullinger BM, Kennedy MRK. Placental transfer of cefuroxime. Br J Obstet Gynaecol 1981;88:141–5.
2. Bousfield P, Browning AK, Mullinger BM, Elstein M. Cefuroxime: potential use in pregnant women at term. Br J Obstet Gynaecol 1981;88:146–9.

3. Bergogne-Berezin E, Pierre J, Even P, Rouvillois JL, Dumez Y. Study of penetration of cefuroxime into bronchial secretions and of its placental transfer. Therapie 1980;35:677–84.
4. Tzingounis V, Makris N, Zolotas J, Michalas S, Aravantinos D. Cefuroxime prophylaxis in caesarean section. Pharmatherapeutica 1982;3:140–2.
5. Coppi G, Berti MA, Chehade A, Franchi I, Magro B. A study of the transplacental transfer of cefuroxime in humans. Curr Ther Res 1982;32:712–6.
6. Bousefield PF. Use of cefuroxime in pregnant women at term. Res Clin Forums 1984;6:53–8.
7. Philipson A, Stiernstedt G. Pharmacokinetics of cefuroxime in pregnancy. Am J Obstet Gynecol 1982;142:823–8.
8. Faro S, Pastorek JG II, Plauche WC, Korndorffer FA, Aldridge KE. Short-course parenteral antibiotic therapy for pyelonephritis in pregnancy. S Med J 1984;77:455–7.

Name: **CEPHALEXIN**

Class: **Antibiotic**   Risk Factor: **B$_M$**

Fetal Risk Summary

Cephalexin is a cephalosporin antibiotic. Several reports have described the administration of cephalexin to pregnant patients in various stages of gestation (1–9). None of these has linked the use of cephalexin with congenital defects or toxicity in the newborn.

Transplacental passage of cephalexin has been demonstrated only near term (1, 2). Following a 1-g oral dose, peak concentrations (μg/ml) for maternal serum, cord serum, and amniotic fluid were about 34 (1 hour), 11 (4 hours), and 13 (6 hours), respectively (2). Patients in whom labor was induced were observed to have falling concentrations of cephalexin in all samples when labor was prolonged beyond 18 hours (3). In one report, all fetal blood samples gave a negative Coombs' reaction (1).

The manufacturer has unpublished information on 46 patients treated with cephalexin during pregnancy (C.L. Lynch, personal communication, Dista Products, 1981). Two of these patients received the drug from 1–2 months prior to conception to term. No effects on the fetus attributable to the antibiotic were observed. Follow-up examination on one infant at 2 months was normal.

Breast Feeding Summary

Cephalexin is excreted into breast milk in low concentrations. A 1-g oral dose given to six mothers produced peak milk levels at 4–5 hours averaging 0.51 μg/ml (range 0.24–0.85 μg/ml) (10). Mean milk:plasma ratios at 1, 2, and 3 hours were 0.008, 0.021, and 0.14, respectively. Although these levels are low, three potential problems exist for the nursing infant: modification of bowel flora, direct effects on the infant, and interference with the interpretation of culture results if a fever workup is required.

References

1. Paterson ML, Henderson A, Lunan CB, McGurk S. Transplacental transfer of cephalexin. Clin Med 1972;79:22–4.
2. Creatsas G, Pavlatos M, Lolis D, Kaskarelis D. A study of the kinetics of cephapirin and cephalexin in pregnancy. Curr Med Res Opin 1980;7:43–6.

3. Hirsch HA. Behandlung von harnwegsinfektionen in gynakologic und geburtshilfe mit cephalexin. Int J Clin Pharmacol 1969;2(Suppl):121–3.
4. Brumfitt W, Pursell R. Double-blind trial to compare ampicillin, cephalexin, co-trimoxazole, and trimethoprim in treatment of urinary infection. Br Med J 1972;2:673–6.
5. Mizuno S, Metsuda S, Mori S. Clinical evaluation of cephalexin in obstetrics and gynaecology. In Proceedings of a Symposium on the Clinical Evaluation of Cephalexin, Royal Society of Medicine, London, June 2 and 3, 1969.
6. Guttman D. Cephalexin in urinary tract infections—preliminary results. In Proceedings of a Symposium on the Clinical Evaluation of Cephalexin, Royal Society of Medicine, London, June 2 and 3, 1969.
7. Soto RF, Fesbre F, Cordido A, et al. Ensayo con cefalexina en el tratamiento de infecciones urinarias en pacientes embarazadas. Rev Obst Gin Venezuela 1972;32:637–41.
8. Campbell-Brown M, McFadyen IR. Bacteriuria in pregnancy treated with a single dose of cephalexin. Br J Obstet Gynaecol 1983;90:1054–9.
9. Jakobi P, Neiger R, Merzbach D, Paldi E. Single-dose antimicrobial therapy in the treatment of asymptomatic bacteriuria in pregnancy. Am J Obstet Gynecol 1987;156:1148–52.
10. Kafetzis D, Siafas C, Georgakopoulos P, Papadatos CJ. Passage of cephalosporins and amoxicillin into the breast milk. Acta Paediatr Scand 1981;70:285–8.

Name: **CEPHALOTHIN**

Class: **Antibiotic**   Risk Factor: **B$_M$**

Fetal Risk Summary

Cephalothin, a cephalosporin antibiotic, has been used during all stages of gestation (1–3). No reports linking this use with congenital defects or toxicity in the newborn have been located. The drug crosses the placenta and distributes in fetal tissues (4–10). Following a 1-g dose, average peak cord serum levels were found at 1–2 hours for the intramuscular route (2.8 μg/ml—16% of maternal peak) and at 10 minutes for intravenous (IV) administration (12.5 μg/ml—41% of maternal) (4–6). In amniotic fluid, cephalothin was slowly concentrated reaching an average level of 21 μg/ml at 4–5 hours (5).

Breast Feeding Summary

Cephalothin is excreted into breast milk in low concentrations. A 1-g IV bolus dose given to six mothers produced peak milk levels at 1–2 hours averaging 0.51 μg/ml (range 0.36–0.62 μg/ml) (11). Mean milk:plasma ratios at 1, 2, and 3 hours were 0.073, 0.26, and 0.50, respectively. Although these levels are low, three potential problems exist for the nursing infant: modification of bowel flora, direct effects on the infant, and interference with the interpretation of culture results if a fever workup is required.

References

1. Cunningham FG, Morris GB, Mickal A. Acute pyelonephritis of pregnancy: a clinical review. Obstet Gynecol 1973;42:112–7.
2. Harris RE, Gilstrap LC. Prevention of recurrent pyelonephritis during pregnancy. Obstet Gynecol 1974;44:637–41.
3. Moro M, Andrews M. Prophylactic antibiotics in cesarean section. Obstet Gynecol 1974;44:688–92.
4. MacAulay MA, Charles D. Placental transfer of cephalothin. Am J Obstet Gynecol 1968;100:940–5.

5. Sheng KT, Huang NN, Promadhattavedi V. Serum concentrations of cephalothin in infants and children and placental transmission of the antibiotic. Antimicrob Agents Chemother 1964:200–6.
6. Fukada M. Studies on chemotherapy during the perinatal period with special reference to such derivatives of Cephalosporin C as cefazolin, cephaloridine and cephalothin. Jpn J Antibiot 1973;26:197–212.
7. Paterson L, Henderson A, Lunan CB, McGurk S. Transfer of cephalothin sodium to the fetus. J Obstet Gynaecol Br Commonw 1970;77:565–6.
8. Morrow S, Palmisano P, Cassady G. The placental transfer of cephalothin. J Pediatr 1968;73:262–4.
9. Stewart KS, Shafi M, Andrews J, Williams JD. Distribution of parenteral ampicillin and cephalosporins in late pregnancy. J Obstet Gynaecol Br Commonw 1973;80:902–8.
10. Corson SL, Bolognese RJ. The behavior of cephalothin in amniotic fluid. J Reprod Med 1970;4:105–8.
11. Kafetzis D, Siafas C, Georgakopoulos P, Papadatos CJ. Passage of cephalosporins and amoxicillin into the breast milk. Acta Paediatr Scand 1981;70:285–8.

Name: **CEPHAPIRIN**

Class: **Antibiotic**   Risk Factor: **B$_M$**

Fetal Risk Summary

Cephapirin is a cephalosporin antibiotic. At term, following a 1-g intramuscular dose, peak concentrations (μg/ml) for maternal serum, cord serum and amniotic fluid were about 17 (0.5 hour), 10 (4 hours), and 13 (6 hours), respectively (1). No data on the newborns were given.

Breast Feeding Summary

Cephapirin is excreted into breast milk in low concentrations. A 1-g intravenous bolus dose given to six mothers produced peak milk levels at 1–2 hours averaging 0.49 μg/ml (range 0.30–0.64 μg/ml) (2). Mean milk:plasma ratios at 1, 2, and 3 hours were 0.068, 0.250, and 0.480, respectively. Although these levels were low, three potential problems exist for the nursing infant: modification of bowel flora, direct effects on the infant, and interference with the interpretation of culture results if a fever workup is required.

References

1. Creatsas G, Pavlatos M, Lolis D, Kasharelis D. A study of the kinetics of cephapirin and cefalexin in pregnancy. Curr Med Res Opin 1980;7:43–6.
2. Kafetzis D, Siafas C, Georgakopoulos P, Papadatos CJ. Passage of cephalosporins and amoxicillin into the breast milk. Acta Paediatr Scand 1981;70:285–8.

Name: **CEPHRADINE**

Class: **Antibiotic**   Risk Factor: **B$_M$**

Fetal Risk Summary

Cephradine is a cephalosporin antibiotic. The drug rapidly crosses the placenta throughout gestation (1–4). In the 1st and 2nd trimesters, intravenous (IV) or oral doses produce amniotic fluid levels in the 1 μg/ml range or less. Between 15–30 weeks of gestation, a 1-g IV dose produces therapeutic fetal levels peaking in 40–50 minutes (1). At term, oral doses of 2 g/day for 2 days or more allowed cephradine to concentrate in the amniotic fluid, producing levels in the range of 3–15 μg/ml (2, 3). A 2-g IV dose 17 minutes prior to delivery produced high cord serum levels (29 μg/ml) but low amniotic fluid concentrations (1.1 μg/ml) (4). Serum samples taken from two of the newborns within 20 hours of birth indicated cephradine is excreted by the neonate (4). No other infant data were given in any of the studies.

Breast Feeding Summary

Cephradine is excreted into breast milk in low concentrations. After 500 mg orally every 6 hours for 48 hours, constant milk concentrations of 0.6 μg/ml were measured over 6 hours, a milk:plasma ratio of about 0.2 (2, 3). Although these levels are low, three potential problems exist for the nursing infant: modification of bowel flora, direct effects on the infant, and interference with the interpretation of culture results if a fever workup is required.

References

1. Lange IR, Rodeck C, Cosgrove R. The transfer of cephradine across the placenta. Br J Obstet Gynaecol 1984;91:551–4.
2. Mischler TW, Corson SL, Bolognese RJ, Letocha MJ, Neiss ES. Presence of cephradine in body fluids of lactating and pregnant women. Clin Pharmacol Ther 1974;15:214.
3. Mischler TW, Corson SL, Larranaga A, Bolognese RJ, Neiss ES, Vukovich RA. Cephradine and epicillin in body fluids of lactating and pregnant women. J Reprod Med 1978;21:130–6.
4. Craft I, Forster TC. Materno-fetal cephradine transfer in pregnancy. Antimicrob Agents Chemother 1978;14:924–6.

Name: **CHLORAL HYDRATE**

Class: **Sedative/Hypnotic**   Risk Factor: **C_M**

Fetal Risk Summary

No reports linking the use of chloral hydrate with congenital defects have been located. The drug has been given in labor and demonstrated in cord blood at concentrations similar to maternal levels (1). Sedative effects on the neonate have not been studied.

Breast Feeding Summary

Chloral hydrate and its active metabolite are excreted into breast milk. Peak concentrations of about 8 μg/ml were obtained about 45 minutes after a 1.3-g rectal dose (2). Only trace amounts are detectable after 10 hours.

Mild drowsiness was observed in the nursing infant of a mother taking 1300 mg of dichloralphenazone every evening (3). The mother was also consuming chlorpromazine 100 mg three times daily. Dichloralphenazone is metabolized to trichlorethanol, the same active metabolite of chloral hydrate. Milk levels of trichlorethanol were 60–80% of the maternal serum. The highest milk concentration measured was 0.27 mg/100 ml. Infant growth and development remained normal during the exposure and at follow-up 3 months after the drug was stopped. The American Academy of Pediatrics considers the drug to be compatible with breast feeding (4).

References

1. Bernstine JB, Meyer AE, Hayman HB. Maternal and fetal blood estimation following the administration of chloral hydrate during labor. J Obstet Gynecol Br Emp 1954;61:683–5.
2. Bernstine JB, Meyer AE, Bernstine RL. Maternal blood and breast milk estimation following the administration of chloral hydrate during the puerperium. J Obstet Gynecol Br Emp 1956;63:228–31.
3. Lacey JH. Dichloralphenazone and breast milk. Br Med J 1971;4:684.
4. Committee on Drugs, American Academy of Pediatrics. Transfer of drugs and other chemicals into human milk. Pediatrics 1989;84:924–36.

Name: **CHLORAMBUCIL**

Class: **Antineoplastic**　　　　　　　　　　　Risk Factor: **D$_M$**

Fetal Risk Summary

The use of chlorambucil during pregnancy has resulted in both normal and deformed infants (1–5). Two reports observed unilateral agenesis of the left kidney and ureter in male fetuses following 1st trimester exposure to chlorambucil (3, 4). Similar defects have been found in animals exposed to the drug (6). In a third case, a pregnant patient was treated with chlorambucil at the 10th week of gestation (5). A full-term infant was delivered but died 3 days later of multiple cardiovascular anomalies.

Chlorambucil is mutagenic as well as carcinogenic (7–11). These effects have not been reported in newborns following *in utero* exposure. Data from one review indicated that 40% of the infants exposed to anticancer drugs were of low birth weight (12). Long-term studies of growth and mental development in offspring exposed to chlorambucil during the 2nd trimester, the period of neuroblast multiplication, have not been conducted (13).

Amenorrhea and reversible azoospermia with high doses have been reported (14–18). Long-term follow-up of menstrual and reproductive function in women treated with various antineoplastic agents was reported in 1988 (18). Only two of the 40 women studied, however, may have been exposed to chlorambucil (see Cyclophosphamide).

Occupational exposure of the mother to antineoplastic agents during pregnancy may present a risk to the fetus. A position statement from the National Study Commission on Cytotoxic Exposure and a research article involving some antineoplastic agents are presented in the monograph for cyclophosphamide (see Cyclophosphamide).

Breast Feeding Summary

No data are available.

References

1. Sokal JE, Lessmann EM. Effects of cancer chemotherapeutic agents on the human fetus. JAMA 1960;172:1765–71.
2. Jacobs C, Donaldson SS, Rosenberg SA, Kaplan HS. Management of the pregnant patient with Hodgkin's disease. Ann Intern Med 1981;95:669–75.
3. Shotton D, Monie IW. Possible teratogenic effect of chlorambucil on a human fetus. JAMA 1963;186:74–5.
4. Steege JF, Caldwell DS. Renal agenesis after first trimester exposure to chlorambucil. South Med J 1980;73:1414–5.
5. Thompson J, Conklin KA. Anesthetic management of a pregnant patient with scleroderma. Anesthesiology 1983;59:69–71.
6. Monie IW. Chlorambucil-induced abnormalities of urogenital system of rat fetuses. Anat Rec 1961;139:145.
7. Lawler SD, Lele KP. Chromosomal damage induced by chlorambucil and chronic lymphocytic leukemia. Scand J Haematol 1972;9:603–12.
8. Westin J. Chromosome abnormalities after chlorambucil therapy of polycythemia vera. Scand J Haematol 1976;17:197–204.
9. Catovsky D, Galton DAG. Myelomonocytic leukaemia supervening on chronic lymphocytic leukaemia. Lancet 1971;1:478–9.
10. Rosner R. Acute leukemia as a delayed consequence of cancer chemotherapy. Cancer 1976;37:1033–6.
11. Reimer RR, Hover R, Fraumeni JF, Young RC. Acute leukemia after alkylating-agent therapy of ovarian cancer. N Engl J Med 1977;297:177–81.
12. Nicholson HO. Cytotoxic drugs in pregnancy: review of reported cases. J Obstet Gynaecol Br Commonw 1968;75:307–12.
13. Dobbing J. Pregnancy and leukaemia. Lancet 1977;1:1155.
14. Freckman HA, Fry HL, Mendex FL, Maurer ER. Chlorambucil-prednisolone therapy for disseminated breast carcinoma. JAMA 1964;189:111–4.
15. Richter P, Calamera JC, Morganfeld MC, Kierszenbaum AL, Lavieri JC, Mancinni RE. Effect of chlorambucil on spermatogenesis in the human malignant lymphoma. Cancer 1970;25:1026–30.
16. Morgenfeld MC, Goldberg V, Parisier H, Bugnard SC, Bur GE. Ovarian lesions due to cytostatic agents during the treatment of Hodgkin's disease. Surg Gynecol Obstet 1972;134:826–8.
17. Schilsky RL, Lewis BJ, Sherins RJ, Young RC. Gonadal dysfunction in patients receiving chemotherapy for cancer. Ann Intern Med 1980;93:109–14.
18. Gershenson DM. Menstrual and reproductive function after treatment with combination chemotherapy for malignant ovarian germ cell tumors. J Clin Oncol 1988;6:270–5.

Name: **CHLORAMPHENICOL**

Class: **Antibiotic**   Risk Factor: **C**

Fetal Risk Summary

No reports linking the use of chloramphenicol with congenital defects have been located. The drug crosses the placenta at term producing cord serum concentrations 30–106% of maternal levels (1, 2).

The Collaborative Perinatal Project monitored 50,282 mother-child pairs, 98 of which had 1st trimester exposure to chloramphenicol (3, pp. 297–301). For use anytime in pregnancy, 348 exposures were recorded (3, p. 435). In neither case was evidence found to suggest a relationship to large categories of major or minor malformations or to individual defects. A 1977 case report described a 14-day course of intravenous chloramphenicol, 2 g daily, given to a patient with typhoid fever in the 2nd trimester (4). A normal infant was delivered at term. Twenty-two patients, in various stages of gestation, were treated with chloramphenicol for acute pyelonephritis (5). No difficulties in the newborn could be associated with the antibiotic. In a controlled study, 110 patients received one to three antibiotics during the 1st trimester for a total of 589 weeks (6). Chloramphenicol was given for a total of 205 weeks. The incidence of birth defects was similar to that in controls.

Although apparently nontoxic to the fetus, chloramphenicol should be used with caution at term. Although specific details were not provided, one report claimed that cardiovascular collapse (gray syndrome) developed in babies delivered from mothers treated with chloramphenicol during the final stage of pregnancy (7). Additional reports of this severe adverse effect have not been located, although it is well known that newborns exposed directly to high doses of chloramphenicol may develop the gray syndrome (8–10). Because of this risk, some authors consider the drug to be contraindicated during pregnancy (11).

Breast Feeding Summary

Chloramphenicol is excreted into human breast milk. Two milk samples, separated by 24 hours in the same patient, were reported as 16 and 25 μg/ml, representing milk:plasma ratios of 0.51 and 0.61, respectively (12). Both active drug and inactive metabolite were measured. No effect on the infant was mentioned. No infant toxicity was mentioned in a 1964 report that found peak levels occurring in milk 1–3 hours after a single 1-g oral dose (13). In a similar study, continuous excretion of chloramphenicol into breast milk was established after the 1st day of therapy (14). Minimum and maximum milk concentrations were determined for five patients receiving 250 mg orally every 6 hours (0.54 and 2.84 μg/ml) and for five patients receiving 500 mg orally every 6 hours (1.75 and 6.10 μg/ml). No infant data were given.

The safety of maternal chloramphenicol consumption and breast feeding is unknown. The American Academy of Pediatrics classifies the antibiotic as an agent whose effect on the nursing infant is unknown but may be of concern because of the potential for idiosyncratic bone marrow suppression (15). Another publication recommended that chloramphenicol not be used in the lactating patient (16). Milk levels of this antibiotic are too low to precipitate the gray syndrome, but a theoretical risk does exist for bone marrow depression. Two other potential problems of lesser concern involve the modification of bowel flora and possible interference with the interpretation of culture results if a fever workup is required. Several adverse effects were reported in 50 breast-fed infants whose mothers were being treated with chloramphenicol including refusal of the breast, falling asleep during feeding, intestinal gas, and heavy vomiting after feeding (17).

References

1. Scott WC, Warner RF. Placental transfer of chloramphenicol (Chloromycetin). JAMA 1950;142:1331–2.
2. Ross S, Burke RG, Sites J, Rice EC, Washington JA. Placental transmission of chloramphenicol (Chloromycetin). JAMA 1950;142:1361.
3. Heinonen OP, Slone D, Shapiro S. *Birth Defects and Drugs in Pregnancy*. Littleton:Publishing Sciences Group, 1977.
4. Schiffman P, Samet CM, Fox L, Neimand KM, Rosenberg ST. Typhoid fever in pregnancy—with probable typhoid hepatitis. NY State J Med 1977;77:1778–9.

5. Cunningham FG, Morris GB, Mickal A. Acute pyelonephritis of pregnancy: a clinical review. Obstet Gynecol 1973;42:112–7.
6. Ravid R, Roaff R. On the possible teratogenicity of antibiotic drugs administered during pregnancy. In Klingberg MA, Abramovici H, Chemke J, eds. *Drugs and Fetal Development*. New York:Plenum Press, 1972:505–10.
7. Oberheuser F. Praktische erfahrungen mit medikamenten in der schwangerschaft. Therapiewoche 1971;31:2200. As reported in Manten A. Antibiotic drugs. In Dukes MNG, ed. *Meyler's Side Effects of Drugs*, Vol VIII. New York:American Elsevier, 1975:604.
8. Sutherland JM. Fatal cardiovascular collapse of infants receiving large amounts of chloramphenicol. J Dis Child 1959;97:761–7.
9. Weiss CV, Glazko AJ, Weston JK. Chloramphenicol in the newborn infant. A physiologic explanation of its toxicity when given in excessive doses. N Engl J Med 1960;262:787–94.
10. Oberheuser F. Praktische erfahrungen mit medikamenten in der schwangerschaft. Therapiewoche 1971;31:2200.
11. Schwarz RH, Crombleholme WR. Antibiotics in pregnancy. South Med J 1979;72:1315–8.
12. Smadel JE, Woodward TE, Ley HL Jr, Lewthwaite R. Chloramphenicol (Chloromycetin) in the treatment of Tsutsugamushi disease (scrub typhus). J Clin Invest 1949;28:1196–215.
13. Prochazka J, Havelka J, Hejzlar M. Excretion of chloramphenicol by human milk. Cas Lek Cesk 1964;103:378–80.
14. Prochazka J, Hejzlar M, Popov V, Viktorinova D, Prochazka J. Excretion of chloramphenicol in human milk. Chemotherapy 1968;13:204–11.
15. Committee on Drugs, American Academy of Pediatrics. Transfer of drugs and other chemicals into human milk. Pediatrics 1989;84:924–36.
16. Anonymous. Update: drugs in breast milk. Med Lett Drugs Ther 1979;21:21–4.
17. Havelka J, Frankova A. Contribution to the question of side effects of chloramphenicol therapy in newborns. Cesk Pediatr 1972;21:31–3.

Name: **CHLORCYCLIZINE**

Class: **Antihistamine**   Risk Factor: **C**

Fetal Risk Summary

No data are available. See Meclizine for representative agent in this class.

Breast Feeding Summary

No data are available.

Name: **CHLORDIAZEPOXIDE**

Class: **Sedative**   Risk Factor: **D**

Fetal Risk Summary

Chlordiazepoxide is a benzodiazepine (see also Diazepam). In a study evaluating 19,044 live births, the use of chlordiazepoxide was associated with a greater than 4-fold increase in severe congenital anomalies (1). In 172 patients exposed to the drug during the first 42 days of gestation, the following defects were observed: mental deficiency; spastic diplegia and deafness; microcephaly and retardation; duodenal atresia and Meckel's diverticulum (1). Although not statistically significant, an increased fetal death rate was also found with maternal chlordiazepoxide ingestion (1). A survey of 390 infants with congenital heart disease matched with 1,254 normal infants found a higher rate of exposure to several drugs, including chlordiazepoxide, in the offspring with defects (2). Other studies have not confirmed a relationship with increased defects or mortality (3–6).

The Collaborative Perinatal Project monitored 50,282 mother-child pairs, 257 of which were exposed in the 1st trimester to chlordiazepoxide (4, 7). No association with large classes of malformations or to individual defects was found.

Neonatal withdrawal consisting of severe tremulousness and irritability has been attributed to maternal use of chlordiazepoxide (8). The onset of withdrawal symptoms occurred on the 26th day of life. Chlordiazepoxide readily crosses the placenta at term in an approximate 1:1 ratio (9–11). The drug has been used to reduce pain during labor, but the maternal benefit was not significant (12, 13). Marked depression was observed in three infants whose mothers received chlordiazepoxide within a few hours of delivery (11). The infants were unresponsive, hypotonic, hypothermic, and fed poorly. Hypotonicity persisted for up to a week. Other studies have not seen depression (9, 10).

Breast Feeding Summary

No data are available (see Diazepam).

References

1. Milkovich L, van den Berg BJ. Effects of prenatal meprobamate and chlordiazepoxide hydrochloride on human embryonic and fetal development. N Engl J Med 1974;291:1268–71.
2. Rothman KJ, Fyler DC, Golblatt A, Kreidberg MB. Exogenous hormones and other drug exposures of children with congenital heart disease. Am J Epidemiol 1979;109:433–9.
3. Crombie DL, Pinsent RJ, Fleming DM, Rumeau-Rouguette C, Goujard J, Huel G. Fetal effects of tranquilizers in pregnancy. N Engl J Med 1975;293:198–9.
4. Hartz SC, Heinonen OP, Shapiro S, Siskind V, Slone D. Antenatal exposure to meprobamate and chlordiazepoxide in relation to malformations, mental development, and childhood mortality. N Engl J Med 1975;292:726–8.
5. Bracken MB, Holford TR. Exposure to prescribed drugs in pregnancy and association with congenital malformations. Obstet Gynecol 1981;58:336–44.
6. Committee on Drugs, American Academy of Pediatrics. Psychotropic drugs in pregnancy and lactation. Pediatrics 1982;69:241–4.
7. Heinonen OP, Slone D, Shapiro S. Birth Defects and Drugs in Pregnancy. Littleton:Publishing Sciences Group, 1977:336–7.
8. Athinarayanan P, Pierog SH, Nigam SK, Glass L. Chlordiazepoxide withdrawal in the neonate. Am J Obstet Gynecol 1976;124:212–3.
9. Decancq HG Jr, Bosco JR, Townsend EH Jr. Chlordiazepoxide in labour: its effect on the newborn infant. J Pediatr 1965;67:836–40.
10. Mark PM, Hamel J. Librium for patients in labor. Obstet Gynecol 1968;32:188–94.
11. Stirrat GM, Edington PT, Berry DJ. Transplacental passage of chlordiazepoxide. Br Med J 1974;2:729.
12. Duckman S, Spina T, Attardi M, Meyer A. Double-blind study of chlordiazepoxide in obstetrics. Obstet Gynecol 1964;24:601–5.
13. Kanto JH. Use of benzodiazepines during pregnancy, labour and lactation, with particular reference to pharmacokinetic considerations. Drugs 1982;23:354–80.

Name: **CHLOROQUINE**

Class: **Antimalarial**   Risk Factor: **C**

Fetal Risk Summary

Chloroquine is the drug of choice for the prophylaxis and treatment of sensitive malaria species during pregnancy (1–4). The drug is also indicated for the treatment of extraintestinal invasion by the protozoan parasite, *Entamoeba histolytica* (5). The drug is generally considered safe for these purposes by most authorities (1–7).

Choroquine crosses the placenta to the fetus with fetal concentrations approximating those in the mother (8). In seven mothers at term in the second stage of labor, chloroquine, 5 mg/kg administered intramuscularly, produced mean levels in maternal blood, cord venous blood, and cord arterial blood of 0.736, 0.703, and 0.663 µg/ml, respectively. The time interval from administration to sampling averaged 5.3 hours (range 2.4–10.5 hours). The calculated cord:maternal serum ratio was 0.93.

Congenital defects have been reported in three infants delivered from one mother who was treated with 250–500 mg/day of chloroquine during pregnancy for discoid lupus erythematosus (9). In addition, this woman also had two normal infants, who had not been exposed to chloroquine during gestation, and one normal infant who had been exposed. Anomalies in the three infants were Wilms' tumor at age 4 years, left-sided hemihypertrophy (one infant), and cochleovestibular paresis (two infants).

A 1985 report summarized the results of 169 infants exposed *in utero* to 300 mg of chloroquine base once weekly throughout pregnancy (10). The control group consisted of 454 nonexposed infants. Two infants (1.2%) in the study group had anomalies (tetralogy of Fallot and congenital hypothyroidism) compared to four control infants who had defects (0.9%). Based on these data, the authors concluded that chloroquine is not a major teratogen, but a small increase in birth defects could not be excluded (10).

Breast Feeding Summary

Chloroquine is excreted into human breast milk (8, 11). When chloroquine, 5 mg/kg intramuscular, was administered to six nursing mothers 17 days postpartum, mean milk and serum concentrations 2 hours later were 0.227 µg/ml (range 0.163–0.319 µg/ml) and 0.648 µg/ml (range 0.46–0.95 µg/ml), respectively. The mean milk:blood ratio was 0.358 (range 0.268–0.462). Based on an average consumption of 500 ml of milk/day, an infant would have received about 114 µg/day of chloroquine, an amount considered safe by the investigators (8). In an earlier study, three women were given a single dose of 600 mg of chloroquine 2–5 days postpartum (11). Serum and milk samples were collected up to 227 hours after administration. The milk:plasma area under the concentration-time curve ratios for chloroquine and the principal metabolite, desethylchloroquine, ranged from 1.96–4.26 and 0.54–3.89, respectively. Based on a daily milk intake of 1000 ml, the nursing infants would have ingested between 2.2–4.2% of the maternal doses over a 9-day period (11). The American Academy of Pediatrics considers the drug to be compatible with breast feeding (12).

References

1. Gilles HM, Lawson JB, Sibelas M, Voller A, Allan N. Malaria, anaemia and pregnancy. Ann Trop Med Parasitol 1969;63:245–63.
2. Diro M, Beydoun SN. Malaria in pregnancy. South Med J 1982;75:959–62.
3. Anonymous. Malaria in pregnancy. Lancet 1983;2:84–5.
4. Strang A, Lachman E, Pitsoe SB, Marszalek A, Philpott RH. Malaria in pregnancy with fatal complications: case report. Br J Obstet Gynaecol 1984;91:399–403.
5. D'Alauro F, Lee RV, Pao-In K, Khairallah M. Intestinal parasites and pregnancy. Obstet Gynecol 1985;66:639–43.
6. Ross JB, Garatsos S. Absence of chloroquine induced ototoxicity in a fetus. Arch Dermatol 1974;109:573.
7. Lewis R, Lauresen NJ, Birnbaum S. Malaria associated with pregnancy. Obstet Gynecol 1973;42:698–700.
8. Akintonwa A, Gbajumo SA, Biola Mabadeje AF. Placental and milk transfer of chloroquine in humans. Ther Drug Monit 1988;10:147–9.
9. Hart CW, Naunton RF. The ototoxicity of chloroquine phosphate. Arch Otolaryngol 1964;80:407–12.
10. Wolfe MS, Cordero JF. Safety of chloroquine in chemosuppression of malaria during pregnancy. Br Med J 1985;290:1466–7.
11. Edstein MD, Veenendaal JR, Newman K, Hyslop R. Excretion of chloroquine, dapsone and pyrimethamine in human milk. Br J Clin Pharmacol 1986;22:733–5.
12. Committee on Drugs, American Academy of Pediatrics. Transfer of drugs and other chemicals into human milk. Pediatrics 1989;84:924–36.

Name: **CHLOROTHIAZIDE**

Class: **Diuretic**   Risk Factor: **D**

Fetal Risk Summary

Chlorothiazide is a member of the thiazide group of diuretics. The information in this monograph applies to all members of the group, including the structurally related diuretics, chlorthalidone, metolazone, and quinethazone. Thiazide and related diuretics are rarely administered during the 1st trimester. In the past, when these drugs were routinely given to prevent or treat toxemia, therapy was usually begun in the 2nd or 3rd trimester and adverse effects in the fetus were rare (1–10). No increases in the incidence of congenital defects were discovered, and thiazides were considered non-teratogenic (11–14). In contrast, the Collaborative Perinatal Project monitored 50,282 mother-child pairs, 233 of which were exposed in the 1st trimester to thiazide or related diuretics (15, pp. 371–373). All of the mothers had cardiovascular disorders, which makes interpretation of the data difficult. However, an increased risk for malformations was found for chlorthalidone (20 patients) and miscellaneous thiazide diuretics (35 patients, excluding chlorothiazide and hydrochlorothiazide). For use anytime during pregnancy, 17,492 exposures were recorded and only polythiazide showed a slight increase in risk (15, p. 441).

Many investigators consider diuretics contraindicated in pregnancy, except for patients with heart disease, since they do not prevent or alter the course of toxemia and they may decrease placental perfusion (7, 16–20). A 1984 study determined that the use of diuretics for hypertension in pregnancy prevented normal plasma volume expansion and did not change perinatal outcome (21). In 4,035 patients treated for edema in the last half of the 3rd trimester (hypertensive patients were excluded), higher rates were found for induction of labor, stimulation of labor, uterine inertia, meconium staining, and perinatal mortality (19). All except perinatal mortality were statistically significant from 13,103 controls. In another study, a decrease in endocrine function of the placenta as measured by placental clearance of estradiol was found in three patients treated with hydrochlorothiazide (22).

Chlorothiazide readily crosses the placenta at term, and fetal serum levels may equal those of the mother (23). Chlorthalidone also crosses the placenta (24). Other diuretics probably cross to the fetus in similar amounts, although specific data are lacking. Thiazides are considered mildly diabetogenic since they can induce hyperglycemia (17). Several investigators have noted this effect in pregnant patients treated with thiazides (25–28). Other studies have failed to show maternal hyperglycemia (29, 30). Although apparently a low risk, newborns exposed to thiazide diuretics near term should be observed closely for symptoms of hypoglycemia resulting from maternal hyperglycemia (28).

Neonatal thrombocytopenia has been reported following the use near term of chlorothiazide, hydrochlorothiazide, and methyclothiazide (14, 25, 31–36). Other studies have not found a relationship between thiazide diuretics and platelet counts (37, 38). The positive reports involve only 11 patients, and although the numbers are small, two of the affected infants died (25, 32). The mechanism of the thrombocytopenia is unknown, but the transfer of antiplatelet antibody from the mother to the fetus has been demonstrated (36). Thiazide-induced hemolytic anemia in two newborns was described in 1964 following the use of chlorothiazide and bendroflumethiazide at term (31). Thiazide diuretics may induce severe electrolyte imbalances in the mother's serum, in amniotic fluid, and in the newborn (39–41). In one case, a stillborn fetus was attributed to electrolyte imbalance and/or maternal hypotension (39). Two hypotonic newborns were discovered to be hyponatremic, a condition believed to have resulted from maternal diuretic therapy (40). Fetal bradycardia, 65–70 beats/minute, was shown to be secondary to chlorothiazide-induced maternal hypokalemia (41). In a 1963 study, no relationship was found between neonatal jaundice and chlorothiazide (42). Maternal and fetal deaths in two cases of acute hemorrhagic pancreatitis were attributed to the use of chlorothiazide in the 2nd and 3rd trimesters (43).

In summary, 1st trimester use of thiazide and related diuretics may cause an increased risk of congenital defects based on the results of one large study. Use in later trimesters does not seem to carry this risk. In addition to malformations, other risks to the fetus or newborn include hypoglycemia, thrombocytopenia, hyponatremia, hypokalemia, and death from maternal complications. Thiazide diuretics may have a direct effect on smooth muscle and inhibit labor. Use of diuretics during pregnancy should be discouraged except in patients with heart disease.

Breast Feeding Summary

Chlorothiazide is excreted into breast milk in low concentrations (44). Following a single 500-mg oral dose, milk levels were less than 1 µg/ml at 1, 2, and 3 hours. The authors speculated that the risks of pharmacologic effects in nursing infants would be remote. However, it has been stated that thrombocytopenia can occur in the nursing infant if the mother is taking chlorothiazide (45). Documentation of this is needed (46). Chlorthalidone has a very low milk:plasma ratio of 0.05 (24).

In one mother taking 50 mg of hydrochlorothiazide (HCTZ) daily, peak milk levels of the drug occurred 5–10 hours after a dose and were about 25% of maternal blood concentrations (47). The mean milk concentration of HCTZ was about 80 ng/ml. An infant consuming 600 ml of milk/day would thus ingest about 50 μg of the drug, probably an insignificant amount (47). The diuretic could not be detected in the serum of the nursing 1-month-old infant, and measurements of serum electrolytes, blood glucose, and blood urea nitrogen were all normal.

Thiazide diuretics have been used to suppress lactation (48, 49). However, the American Academy of Pediatrics considers bendroflumethiazide, chlorthalidone, chlorothiazide, and hydrochlorothiazide to be compatible with breast feeding (50).

References

1. Finnerty FA Jr, Buchholz JH, Tuckman J. Evaluation of chlorothiazide (Diuril) in the toxemias of pregnancy. Analysis of 144 patients. JAMA 1958;166:141–4.
2. Zuspan FP, Bell JD, Barnes AC. Balance-ward and double-blind diuretic studies during pregnancy. Obstet Gynecol 1960;16:543–9.
3. Sears RT. Oral diuretics in pregnancy toxaemia. Br Med J 1960;2:148.
4. Assoli NS. Renal effects of hydrochlorothiazide in normal and toxemic pregnancy. Clin Pharmacol Ther 1960;1:48–52.
5. Tatum H, Waterman EA. The prophylactic and therapeutic use of the thiazides in pregnancy. GP 1961;24:101–5.
6. Flowers CE, Grizzle JE, Easterling WE, Bonner OB. Chlorothiazide as a prophylaxis against toxemia of pregnancy. Am J Obstet Gynecol 1962;84:919–29.
7. Weseley AC, Douglas GW. Continuous use of chlorothiazide for prevention of toxemia in pregnancy. Obstet Gynecol 1962;19:355–8.
8. Finnerty FA Jr. How to treat toxemia of pregnancy. GP 1963;27:116–21.
9. Fallis NE, Plauche WC, Mosey LM, Langford HG. Thiazide versus placebo in prophylaxis of toxemia of pregnancy in primagravid patients. Am J Obstet Gynecol 1964;88:502–4.
10. Landesman R, Aguero O, Wilson K, LaRussa R, Campbell W, Penaloza O. The prophylactic use of chlorthalidone, a sulfonamide diuretic, in pregnancy. J Obstet Gynaecol Br Commonw 1965;72:1004–10.
11. Cuadros A, Tatum H. The prophylactic and therapeutic use of bendroflumethiazide in pregnancy. Am J Obstet Gynecol 1964;89:891–7.
12. Finnerty FA Jr, Bepko FJ Jr. Lowering the perinatal mortality and the prematurity rate. The value of prophylactic thiazides in juveniles. JAMA 1966;195:429–32.
13. Kraus GW, Marchese JR, Yen SSC. Prophylactic use of hydrochlorothiazide in pregnancy. JAMA 1966;198:1150–4.
14. Gray MJ. Use and abuse of thiazides in pregnancy. Clin Obstet Gynecol 1968;11:568–78.
15. Heinonen OP, Slone D, Shapiro S. Birth Defects and Drugs in Pregnancy. Littleton:Publishing Sciences Group, 1977.
16. Watt JD, Philipp EE. Oral diuretics in pregnancy toxemia. Br Med J 1960;1:1807.
17. Pitkin RM, Kaminetzky HA, Newton M, Pritchard JA. Maternal nutrition: a selective review of clinical topics. Obstet Gynecol 1972;40:773–85.
18. Lindheimer MD, Katz AI. Sodium and diuretics in pregnancy. N Engl J Med 1973;288:891–4.
19. Christianson R, Page EW. Diuretic drugs and pregnancy. Obstet Gynecol 1976;48:647–52.
20. Lammintausta R, Erkkola R, Eronen M. Effect of chlorothiazide treatment of renin-aldosterone system during pregnancy. Acta Obstet Gynecol Scand 1978;57:389–92.
21. Sibai BM, Grossman RA, Grossman HG. Effects of diuretics on plasma volume in pregnancies with long-term hypertension. Am J Obstet Gynecol 1984;150:831–5.
22. Shoemaker ES, Grant NF, Madden JD, MacDonald PC. The effect of thiazide diuretics on placental function. Tex Med 1973;69:109–15.
23. Garnet J. Placental transfer of chlorothiazide. Obstet Gynecol 1963;21:123–5.
24. Mulley BA, Parr GD, Pau WK, Rye RM, Mould JJ, Siddle NC. Placental transfer of chlorthalidone and its elimination in maternal milk. Eur J Clin Pharmacol 1978;13:129–31.
25. Menzies DN. Controlled trial of chlorothiazide in treatment of early pre-eclampsia. Br Med J 1964;1:739–42.

26. Ladner CN, Pearson JW, Herrick CN, Harrison HE. The effect of chlorothiazide on blood glucose in the third trimester of pregnancy. Obstet Gynecol 1964;23:555–60.

27. Goldman JA, Neri A, Ovadia J, Eckerling B, DeVries A. Effect of chlorothiazide on intravenous glucose tolerance in pregnancy. Am J Obstet Gynecol 1969;105:556–60.

28. Senior B, Slone D, Shapiro S, Mitchell AA, Heinonen OP. Benzothiadiazides and neonatal hypoglycaemia. Lancet 1976;2:377.

29. Lakin N, Zeytinoglu J, Younger M, White P. Effect of chlorothiazide on insulin requirements of pregnant diabetic women. JAMA 1960;173:353–4.

30. Esbenshade JH Jr, Smith RT. Thiazides and pregnancy: a study of carbohydrate tolerance. Am J Obstet Gynecol 1965;92:270–1.

31. Harley JD, Robin H, Robertson SEJ. Thiazide-induced neonatal haemolysis? Br Med J 1964;1:696–7.

32. Rodriguez SU, Leikin SL, Hiller MC. Neonatal thrombocytopenia associated with ante-partum administration of thiazide drugs. N Engl J Med 1964;270:881–4.

33. Leikin SL. Thiazide and neonatal thrombocytopenia. N Engl J Med 1964;271:161.

34. Prescott LF. Neonatal thrombocytopenia and thiazide drugs. Br Med J 1964;1:1438.

35. Jones JE, Reed JF Jr. Renal vein thrombosis and thrombocytopenia in the newborn infant. J Pediatr 1965;67:681–2.

36. Karpatkin S, Strick N, Karpatkin MB, Siskind GW. Cumulative experience in the detection of antiplatelet antibody in 234 patients with idiopathic thrombocytopenic purpura, systemic lupus erythematosus and other clinical disorders. Am J Med 1972;52:776–85.

37. Finnerty FA Jr, Assoli NS. Thiazide and neonatal thrombocytopenia. N Engl J Med 1964;271:160–1.

38. Jerkner K, Kutti J, Victoria L. Platelet counts in mothers and their newborn infants with respect to antepartum administration of oral diuretics. Acta Med Scand 1973;194:473–5.

39. Pritchard JA, Walley PJ. Severe hypokalemia due to prolonged administration of chlorothiazide during pregnancy. Am J Obstet Gynecol 1961;81:1241–4.

40. Alstatt LB. Transplacental hyponatremia in the newborn infant. J Pediatr 1965;66:985–8.

41. Anderson GG, Hanson TM. Chronic fetal bradycardia: possible association with hypokalemia. Obstet Gynecol 1974;44:896–8.

42. Crosland D, Flowers C. Chlorothiazide and its relationship to neonatal jaundice. Obstet Gynecol 1963;22:500–4.

43. Minkowitz S, Soloway HB, Hall JE, Yermakov V. Fatal hemorrhagic pancreatitis following chlorothiazide administration in pregnancy. Obstet Gynecol 1964;24:337–42.

44. Werthmann MW Jr, Krees SV. Excretion of chlorothiazide in human breast milk. J Pediatr 1972;81:781–3.

45. Anonymous. Drugs in breast milk. Med Lett Drugs Ther 1976;16:25–7.

46. Dailey JW. Anticoagulant and cardiovascular drugs. In Wilson JT, ed. Drugs in Breast Milk. Australia (Balgowlah):ADIS Press, 1981:61–4.

47. Miller ME, Cohn RD, Burghart PH. Hydrochlorothiazide disposition in a mother and her breast-fed infant. J Pediatr 1982;101:789–91.

48. Healy M. Suppressing lactation with oral diuretics. Lancet 1961;1:1353–4.

49. Catz CS, Giacoia GP. Drugs and breast milk. Pediatr Clin North Am 1972;19:151–66.

50. Committee on Drugs, American Academy of Pediatrics. Transfer of drugs and other chemicals into human milk. Pediatrics 1989;84:924–36.

Name: CHLOROTRIANISENE

Class: **Estrogenic Hormone**   Risk Factor: X_M

Fetal Risk Summary

No data are available. Use of estrogenic hormones during pregnancy is contraindicated (see Oral Contraceptives).

Breast Feeding Summary

See Oral Contraceptives.

Name: **CHLORPHENIRAMINE**

Class: **Antihistamine/Antiemetic** Risk Factor: **B**

Fetal Risk Summary

The Collaborative Perinatal Project monitored 50,282 mother-child pairs, 1,070 of which had 1st trimester exposure to chlorpheniramine (1, pp. 322–334). For use anytime during pregnancy, 3,931 exposures were recorded (1, pp. 437, 488). In neither case was evidence found to suggest a relationship to large categories of major or minor malformations. Several possible associations with individual malformations were found, but the statistical significance of these is unknown. Independent confirmation is required to determine the actual risk.

Polydactyly in blacks (7 cases in 272 blacks)
Gastrointestinal defects (13 cases)
Eye and ear defects (7 cases)
Inguinal hernia (22 cases)
Hydrocephaly (8 cases)
Congenital dislocation of hip (16 cases)
Malformations of the female genitalia (6 cases)

In a 1971 study, significantly fewer infants with malformations were exposed to antihistamines in the 1st trimester as compared to controls (2). Chlorpheniramine was the sixth most commonly used antihistamine.

A case of infantile malignant osteopetrosis was described in a 4-month-old boy exposed *in utero* on several occasions to Contac (chlorpheniramine, phenylpropranolamine, and belladonna alkaloids) but this is a known genetic defect (3). The boy also had a continual "stuffy" nose.

An association between exposure during the last 2 weeks of pregnancy to antihistamines in general and retrolental fibroplasia in premature infants has been reported. See Brompheniramine for details.

Breast Feeding Summary

No data are available.

References

1. Heinonen OP, Slone D, Shapiro S. *Birth Defects and Drugs in Pregnancy*. Littleton:Publishing Sciences Group, 1977.
2. Nelson MM, Forfar JO. Associations between drugs administered during pregnancy and congenital abnormalities of the fetus. Br Med J 1971;1:523–7.
3. Golbus MS, Koerper MA, Hall BD. Failure to diagnose osteopetrosis *in utero*. Lancet 1976;2:1246

Name: **CHLORPROMAZINE**

Class: **Tranquilizer**   Risk Factor: **C**

Fetal Risk Summary

Chlorpromazine is a propylamino phenothiazine. The drug readily crosses the placenta (1–4). In animals, selective accumulation and retention occur in the fetal pigment epithelium (5). Although delayed ocular damage from high prolonged doses in pregnancy has not been reported in humans, concern has been expressed for this potential toxicity (5, 6).

Chlorpromazine has been used for the treatment of nausea and vomiting of pregnancy during all stages of gestation, including labor, since the mid-1950s (7–9). The drug seems to be safe and effective for this indication. Its use in labor to promote analgesia and amnesia is usually safe, but some patients, up to 18% in one series, have a marked unpredictable fall in blood pressure that could be dangerous to the mother and the fetus (10–14). Use of chlorpromazine during labor should be discouraged because of this adverse effect. One psychiatric patient, who consumed 8000 mg of chlorpromazine in the last 10 days of pregnancy, delivered a hypotonic, lethargic infant with depressed reflexes and jaundice (4). The adverse effects resolved within 3 weeks.

An extrapyramidal syndrome (EPS), which may persist for months, has been observed in some infants whose mothers received chlorpromazine near term (15–19). This reaction is characterized by tremors, increased muscle tone with spasticity, and hyperactive deep tendon reflexes. Hypotonicity has been observed in one newborn and paralytic ileus in two after exposure at term to chlorpromazine (4, 20). However, most reports describing the use of chlorpromazine in pregnancy have concluded that it does not adversely affect the fetus or newborn (21–26).

The Collaborative Perinatal Project monitored 50,282 mother-child pairs, 142 of which had 1st trimester exposure to chlorpromazine (27). For use anytime during pregnancy, 284 exposures were recorded. No evidence was found in either group to suggest a relationship to malformations or an effect on perinatal mortality rate, birth weight, or intelligence quotient scores at 4 years of age. Opposite results were found in a prospective French study that compared 315 mothers exposed to phenothiazines during the 1st trimester with 11,099 nonexposed controls (28). Malformations were observed in 11 exposed infants (3.5%) and in 178 controls (1.6%) ($p < 0.01$). In the phenothiazine group, chlorpromazine was taken by 57 women who produced four infants with malformations:

Syndactyly
Microcephaly, clubfoot/hand, muscular abdominal aplasia (also exposed to
    acetylpromazine)
Endocardial fibroelastosis, brachymesophalangy, clinodactyly (also exposed to
    pipamazine)
Microcephaly (also exposed to promethazine)

The case of microcephaly, although listed as a possible drug-induced malformation, was considered by the authors to be more likely a genetic defect since the mother had already delivered two previous children with microcephaly (28). However, even after exclusion of this case, the association between phenothiazines and malformations remained significant (28). In another report, a stillborn fetus delivered at 28 weeks with ectromelia/omphalocele was attributed to the combined use of chloropromazine and meclizine in the 1st trimester (29).

In an *in vitro* study, chlorpromazine was shown to be a potent inhibitor of sperm motility (30). A concentration of 53 μM produced a 50% reduction in motility.

In summary, although one survey found an increased incidence of defects and a report of ectromelia exists, most studies have found chlorpromazine to be safe for both mother and fetus if used occasionally in low doses. Other reviewers have also concluded that the phenothiazines are not teratogenic (24, 31). However, use near term should be avoided due to the danger of maternal hypotension and adverse effects in the newborn.

Breast Feeding Summary

Chlorpromazine is excreted into breast milk in very small concentrations. Following a 1200 mg oral dose (20 mg/kg), peak milk levels of 0.29 μg/ml were measured at 2 hours (32). This represented a milk:plasma ratio of less than 0.5. The drug could not be detected following a 600 mg oral dose. In a study of four lactating mothers consuming unspecified amounts of the neuroleptic, milk concentrations of chlorpromazine ranged from 7–98 ng/ml with maternal serum levels ranging from 16–52 ng/ml (33). In two mothers, more drug was found in the milk than in the plasma. Only two of the mothers breast fed their infants. One infant, consuming milk with a level of 7 ng/ml, showed no ill effects, but the second took milk containing 92 ng/ml and became drowsy and lethargic.

With the one exception described above, there has been a lack of reported adverse effects in breast-fed babies whose mothers were ingesting chlorpromazine (24). Based on this report, however, nursing infants exposed to the agent in milk should be observed for sedation. The American Academy of Pediatrics classifies chlorpromazine as an agent whose effect on the nursing infant is unknown but may be of concern because of the drowsiness and lethargy observed in the infant described above, and due to the galactorrhea induced in adults (34).

References

1. Franchi G, Gianni AM. Chlorpromazine distribution in maternal and fetal tissues and biological fluids. Acta Anaesthesiol (Padava) 1957;8:197–207.
2. Moya F, Thorndike V. Passage of drugs across the placenta. Am J Obstet Gyencol 1962;84:1778–98.
3. O'Donoghue SEF. Distribution of pethidine and chlorpromazine in maternal, foetal and neonatal biological fluids. Nature 1971;229:124–5.
4. Hammond JE, Toseland PA. Placental transfer of chlorpromazine. Arch Dis Child 1970;45:139–40.
5. Ullberg S, Lindquist NG, Sjostrand SE. Accumulation of chorio-retinotoxic drugs in the foetal eye. Nature 1970;227:1257–8.
6. Anonymous. Drugs and the fetal eye. Lancet 1971;1:122.
7. Karp M, Lamb VE, Benaron HBW. The use of chlorpromazine in the obstetric patient: a preliminary report. Am J Obstet Gynecol 1955;69:780–5.
8. Benaron HBW, Dorr EM, Roddick WJ, et al. Use of chlorpromazine in the obstetric patient: a preliminary report I. In the treatment of nausea and vomiting of pregnancy. Am J Obstet Gynecol 1955;69:776–9.
9. Sullivan CL. Treatment of nausea and vomiting of pregnancy with chlorpromazine. A report of 100 cases. Postgrad Med 1957;22:429–32.
10. Harer WB. Chlorpromazine in normal labor. Obstet Gynecol 1956;8:1–9.
11. Lindley JE, Rogers SF, Moyer JH. Analgesic-potentiation effect of chlorpromazine during labor; a study of 2093 patients. Obstet Gynecol 1957;10:582–6.

12. Bryans CI Jr, Mulherin CM. The use of chlorpromazine in obstetrical analgesia. Am J Obstet Gynecol 1959;77:406–11.
13. Christhilf SM Jr, Monias MB, Riley RA Jr, Sheehan JC. Chlorpromazine in obstetric analgesia. Obstet Gynecol 1960;15:625–9.
14. Rodgers CD, Wickard CP, McCaskill MR. Labor and delivery without terminal anesthesia. A report of the use of chlorpromazine. Obstet Gynecol 1961;17:92–5.
15. Hill RM, Desmond MM, Kay JL. Extrapyramidal dysfunction in an infant of a schizophrenic mother. J Pediatr 1966;69:589–95.
16. Ayd FJ Jr, ed. Phenothiazine therapy during pregnancy—effects on the newborn infant. Int Drug Ther Newslett 1968;3:39–40.
17. Tamer A, McKay R, Arias D, Worley L, Fogel BJ. Phenothiazine-induced extrapyramidal dysfunction in the neonate. J Pediatr 1969;75:479–80.
18. Levy W, Wisniewski K. Chlorpromazine causing extrapyramidal dysfunction in newborn infant of psychotic mother. NY State J Med 1974;74:684–5.
19. O'Connor M, Johnson GH, James DI. Intrauterine effect of phenothiazines. Med J Aust 1981;1:416–7.
20. Falterman CG, Richardson J. Small left colon syndrome associated with maternal ingestion of psychotropic drugs. J Pediatr 1980;97:308–10.
21. Kris EB, Carmichael DM. Chlorpromazine maintenance therapy during pregnancy and confinement. Psychiatr Q 1957;31:690–5.
22. Kris EB. Children born to mothers maintained on pharmacotherapy during pregnancy and postpartum. Recent Adv Biol Psychiatry 1962;4:180–7.
23. Sobel DE. Fetal damage due to ECT, insulin coma, chlorpromazine, or reserpine. Arch Gen Psychiatry 1960;2:606–11.
24. Ayd FJ Jr. Children born of mothers treated with chlorpromazine during pregnancy. Clin Med 1964;71:1758–63.
25. Sobel DE. Fetal damage due to ECT, insulin coma, chlorpromazine, or reserpine. Arch Gen Psychiatry 1960;2:606–11.
26. Loke KH, Salleh R. Electroconvulsive therapy for the acutely psychotic pregnant patient: a review of 3 cases. Med J Malaysia 1983;38:131–3.
27. Slone D, Siskind V, Heinonen OP, Monson RR, Kaufman DW, Shapiro S. Antenatal exposure to the pheothiazines in relation to congenital malformations, perinatal mortality rate, birth weight, and intelligence quotient score. Am J Obstet Gynecol 1977;128:486–8.
28. Rumeau-Rouquette C, Goujard J, Huel G. Possible teratogenic effect of phenothiazines in human beings. Teratology 1976;15:57–64.
29. O'Leary JL, O'Leary JA. Nonthalidomide ectromelia; report of a case. Obstet Gynecol 1964;23:17–20.
30. Levin RM, Amsterdam JD, Winokur A, Wein AJ. Effects of psychotropic drugs on human sperm motility. Fertil Steril 1981;36:503–6.
31. Ananth J. Congenital malformations with psychopharmacologic agents. Compr Psychiatry 1975;16:437–45.
32. Blacker KH, Weinstein BJ, Ellman GL. Mothers milk and chlorpromazine. Am J Psychol 1962;114:178–9.
33. Wiles DH, Orr MW, Kolakowska T. Chlorpromazine levels in plasma and milk of nursing mothers. Br J Clin Pharmacol 1978;5:272–3.
34. Committee on Drugs, American Academy of Pediatrics. Transfer of drugs and other chemicals into human milk. Pediatrics 1989;84:924–36.

Name: **CHLORPROPAMIDE**

Class: **Oral Hypoglycemic**   Risk Factor: **D***

Fetal Risk Summary

Chlorpropamide is a sulfonylurea used for the treatment of adult-onset diabetes mellitus. It is not indicated for the pregnant diabetic. When administered near term, the drug crosses the placenta and may persist in the neonatal serum for several days (1, 2). One mother, who took 500 mg/day throughout pregnancy, delivered an infant whose serum level was 15.4 mg/100 ml at 77 hours of life (1). Infants of three other mothers, who were consuming 100–250 mg/day at term, had serum levels varying between 1.8–2.8 mg/100 ml 8–35 hours after delivery (2). All four infants had prolonged symptomatic hypoglycemia secondary to hyper-insulinism lasting for 4–6 days. In other reports, totaling 69 pregnancies, chlor-propamide in doses of 100–200 mg or more/day either gave no evidence of neo-natal hypoglycemia/hyperinsulinism or no constant relationship between daily maternal dosage and neonatal complications (3, 4). However, chlorpropamide should be stopped at least 48 hours before delivery to avoid this potential compli-cation (5).

Although teratogenic in animals, an increased incidence of congenital defects, other than that expected in diabetes mellitus, has not been found with chlor-propamide (6–15). Four malformed infants have been attributed to chlor-propamide but the relationship is unclear (6, 9):

Hand/finger anomalies (6)
Stricture of lower ileum, death (6)
Preauricular sinus (6)
Microcephaly/spastic quadriplegia (9)

Maternal diabetes is known to increase the rate of malformations 2- to 4-fold, but the mechanism(s) are not understood (see also Insulin). In spite of the lack of evidence for chlorpropamide teratogenicity, the drug should not be used in preg-nancy since it will not provide good control in patients who cannot be controlled by diet alone (5).

[*Risk Factor C according to manufacturer — Pfizer, 1990.]

Breast Feeding Summary

Chlorpropamide is excreted into breast milk. Following a 500 mg oral dose, the milk concentration in a composite of two samples obtained at 5 hours was 5 μg/ml (G.G. D'Ambrosio, personal communication, Pfizer Laboratories, 1982). The ef-fects on a nursing infant from this amount of drug are unknown.

References

1. Zucker P, Simon G. Prolonged symptomatic neonatal hypoglycemia associated with maternal chlorpropamide therapy. Pediatrics 1968;42:824–5.
2. Kemball ML, McIver C, Milnar RDG, Nourse CH, Schiff D, Tiernan JR. Neonatal hypoglycaemia in infants of diabetic mothers given sulphonylurea drugs in pregnancy. Arch Dis Child 1970;45:696–701.
3. Sutherland HW, Stowers JM, Cormack JD, Bewsher PD. Evaluation of chlorpropamide in chemi-cal diabetes diagnosed during pregnancy. Br Med J 1973;3:9–13.
4. Sutherland HW, Bewsher PD, Cormack JD, et al. Effect of moderate dosage of chlorpropamide in pregnancy on fetal outcome. Arch Dis Child 1974;49:283–91.
5. Friend JR. Diabetes. Clin Obstet Gynecol 1981;8:353–82.
6. Soler NG, Walsh CH, Malins JM. Congenital malformations in infants of diabetic mothers. Q J Med 1976;45:303–13.
7. Adam PAJ, Schwartz R. Diagnosis and treatment: should oral hypoglycemic agents be used in pediatric and pregnant patients? Pediatrics 1968;42:819–23.
8. Dignan PSJ. Teratogenic risk and counseling in diabetes. Clin Obstet Gynecol 1981;24:149–59.
9. Campbell GD. Chlorpropamide and foetal damage. Br Med J 1963;1:59–60.

10. Jackson WPU, Campbell GD, Notelovitz M, Blumsohn D. Tolbutamide and chlorpropamide during pregnancy in human diabetes. Diabetes 1962;11(Suppl):98–101.
11. Jackson WPU, Campbell GD. Chlorpropamide and perinatal mortality. Br Med J 1963;2:1652.
12. Macphail I. Chlorpropamide and foetal damage. Br Med J 1963;1:192.
13. Malins JM, Cooke AM, Pyke DA, Fitzgerald MG. Sulphonylurea drugs in pregnancy. Br Med J 1964;2:187.
14. Moss JM, Connor EJ. Pregnancy complicated by diabetes. Report of 102 pregnancies including eleven treated with oral hypoglycemic drugs. Med Ann DC 1965;34;253–60.
15. Douglas CP, Richards R. Use of chlorpropamide in the treatment of diabetes in pregnancy. Diabetes 1967;16:60–1.

Name: **CHLORPROTHIXENE**

Class: **Tranquilizer**   Risk Factor: **C**

Fetal Risk Summary

Chlorprothixene is structurally and pharmacologically related to chlorpromazine and thiothixene. No specific data on its use in pregnancy have been located (see also Chlorpromazine).

Breast Feeding Summary

Chlorprothixene is excreted into breast milk (1). Serum and milk concentrations of chlorprothixene and its metabolite, chlorprothixene sulphoxide, were determined in two women consuming 200 mg/day. In one woman, plasma concentrations of the parent drug and the metabolite, 1.5–24 hours after the 200-mg dose, ranged from 13–51 nmol/L and 75–130 nmol/L, respectively. Simultaneously obtained milk levels ranged from 6–60 nmol/L and 42–96 nmol/L, respectively. The second patient had a single determination drawn 30 hours after a 200-mg dose with levels in the plasma and milk for the parent compound and metabolite of 38 and 98 (plasma) and 115 and 54 nmol/L (milk), respectively. The milk:plasma ratio for chlorprothixene varied between 1.2–2.6, while that of the metabolite varied from 0.5–0.8. The test method used was able to recover 90–100% of the drugs from the plasma but only 60–70% from the milk. No adverse effects were noted in the nursing infants. The investigators calculated that a nursing infant consuming 800 ml of milk/day would ingest no more than 15 μg of chlorprothixene/day. The American Academy of Pediatrics classifies chlorprothixene as an agent whose effect on the nursing infant is unknown but may be of concern (2).

References

1. Matheson I, Evang A, Fredricson Overo K, Syversen G. Presence of chlorprothixene and its metabolites in breast milk. Eur J Clin Pharmacol 1984;27:611–3.
2. Committee on Drugs, American Academy of Pediatrics. Transfer of drugs and other chemicals into human milk. Pediatrics 1989;84:924–36.

Name: **CHLORTETRACYCLINE**

Class: **Antibiotic** Risk Factor: **D**

Fetal Risk Summary

See Tetracycline.

Breast Feeding Summary

Chlortetracycline is excreted into breast milk. Eight patients were given 2–3 g orally/day for 3–4 days (1). Average maternal and milk concentrations were 4.1 and 1.25 µg/ml respectively, producing a milk:plasma ratio of 0.4. Infant data were not given.

Theoretically, dental staining and inhibition of bone growth could occur in breast-fed infants whose mothers were consuming chlortetracycline. However, this theoretical possibility seems remote because in infants exposed to a closely related antibiotic, tetracycline, serum levels were undetectable (less than 0.05 µg/ml) (2). The American Academy of Pediatrics considers tetracycline to be compatible with breast feeding (3). Three potential problems may exist for the nursing infant, even though there are no reports in this regard: modification of bowel flora, direct effects on the infant, and interference with the interpretation of culture results if a fever workup is required.

References

1. Guilbeau JA, Schoenbach EB, Schuab IG, Latham DV. Aureomycin in obstetrics; therapy and prophylaxis. JAMA 1950;143:520–6.
2. Posner AC, Prigot A, Konicoff NG. Further observations on the use of tetracycline hydrochloride in prophylaxis and treatment of obstetric infections. *Antibiotics Annual 1954–55,* New York:Medical Encyclopedia, 1955:594–8.
3. Committee on Drugs, American Academy of Pediatrics. Transfer of drugs and other chemicals into human milk. Pediatrics 1989;84:924–36.

Name: **CHLORTHALIDONE**

Class: **Diuretic** Risk Factor: **D**

Fetal Risk Summary

Chlorthalidone is structurally related to the thiazide diuretics. See Chlorothiazide.

Breast Feeding Summary

See Chlorothiazide.

Name: **CHLORZOXAZONE**

Class: **Muscle Relaxant**   Risk Factor: **C**

Fetal Risk Summary

No data are available.

Breast Feeding Summary

No data are available.

Name: **CHOLECALCIFEROL**

Class: **Vitamin**   Risk Factor: **A***

Fetal Risk Summary

Cholecalciferol (vitamin D_3) is converted in the liver to calcifediol, which in turn is converted in the kidneys to calcitriol, one of the active forms of vitamin D. See Vitamin D.

[*Risk Factor D if used in doses above the recommended daily allowance.]

Breast Feeding Summary

See Vitamin D.

Name: **CHOLESTYRAMINE**

Class: **Antilipemic**   Risk Factor: **C**

Fetal Risk Summary

Cholestyramine is a resin used to bind bile acids in a nonabsorbable complex. The resin has been used for the treatment of cholestasis of pregnancy (1–3). No adverse fetal effects were observed. Cholestyramine also binds fat-soluble vitamins, and long-term use could result in deficiencies of these agents in either mother or fetus (4). However, in one study, treatment with 9 g daily up to a maximum duration of 12 weeks was not associated with fetal or maternal complications (1).

Breast Feeding Summary

No data are available.

References

1. Lutz EE, Margolis AJ. Obstetric hepatosis: treatment with cholestyramine and interim response to steroids. Obstet Gynecol 1969;33:64–71.
2. Heikkinen J, Maentausta O, Ylostalo P, Janne O. Serum bile acid levels in intrahepatic cholestasis of pregnancy during treatment with phenobarbital or cholestyramine. Eur J Obstet Gynecol Reprod Biol 1982;14:153–62.

3. Shaw D, Frohlich J, Wittmann BAK, Willms M. A prospective study of 18 patients with cholestasis of pregnancy. Am J Obstet Gynecol 1982;142:621–5.
4. American Hospital Formulary Service. *Drug Information 1990*. Bethesda:American Society of Hospital Pharmacists, 1990:883–7.

Name: **CICLOPIROX**

Class: **Antifungal**   Risk Factor: **B**$_M$

Fetal Risk Summary

Ciclopirox is a synthetic anti-infective agent used topically for its antifungal properties. No reports of its use in human pregnancy have been located, nor is there evidence of teratogenic effects in animals. The manufacturer has no case reports of congenital abnormalities occurring after use of ciclopirox (C.K. Whitmore, personal communication, Hoechst-Roussel Pharmaceuticals, Inc., 1987).

Breast Feeding Summary

No data are available.

Name: **CIMETIDINE**

Class: **Antihistamine**   Risk Factor: **B**

Fetal Risk Summary

Cimetidine is an H_2-receptor antagonist that inhibits gastric acid secretion. In pregnancy, the antihistamine is primarily used for the treatment of peptic ulcer disease and for the prevention of gastric acid aspiration (Mendelson's syndrome) prior to delivery.

Cimetidine crosses the placenta to the fetus by simple diffusion (1). The drug is not metabolized by the placenta (1). At term, cimetidine crosses the placenta, resulting in a peak mean fetal:maternal ratio of 0.84 at 1.5–2 hours (2).

No reports linking the use of cimetidine with congenital defects have been located. The manufacturer has received a number of reports of women who took the drug during pregnancy, including throughout gestation (B. Dickson, personal communication, Smith Kline & French Laboratories, 1986). They are aware of three isolated incidences of congenital defects, apparently unrelated to cimetidine therapy, including congenital heart disease, mental retardation detected later in life, and clubfoot. The drug has been used throughout pregnancy in a case ending in intrauterine fetal death, but the adverse outcome was believed to be due to severe maternal disease and captopril therapy (see Captopril). Three pregnant women with gastric hemorrhage secondary to peptic ulcer disease were described in a 1982 reference (3). The women, at 16 weeks', 12 weeks', and 31 weeks' gestation, respectively, were treated for various lengths of time with cimetidine and other standard therapy and all delivered healthy newborns without congenital defects or metabolic disturbances. Transient liver impairment has been described in a newborn exposed to cimetidine at term (4). However, other reports have not confirmed this toxicity (5–22).

Cimetidine has been used at term either with or without other antacids to prevent maternal gastric acid aspiration pneumonitis (Mendelson's syndrome) (7–22). No neonatal adverse effects were noted in these studies.

Breast Feeding Summary

Cimetidine is excreted into breast milk and may accumulate in concentrations greater than that found in maternal plasma (23). Following a single 400-mg oral dose a theoretical milk:plasma ratio of 1.6 has been calculated (23). Multiple oral doses of 200 and 400 mg result in milk:plasma ratios of 4.6 to 7.44, respectively. An estimated 6 mg of cimetidine/L of milk could be ingested by the nursing infant. The clinical significance of this ingestion is unknown. Theoretically, the drug could adversely affect the nursing infant's gastric acidity, inhibit drug metabolism, and produce central nervous system stimulation, but these effects have not been reported. The American Academy of Pediatrics considers cimetidine to be compatible with breast feeding (24).

References

1. Schenker S, Dicke J, Johnson RF, Mor LL, Henderson GI. Human placental transport of cimetidine. J Clin Invest 1987;80:1428–34.
2. Howe JP, McGowan WAW, Moore J, McCaughey W, Dundee JW. The placental transfer of cimetidine. Anaesthesia 1981;36:371–5.
3. Corazza GR, Gasbarrini G, Di Nisio Q, Zulli P. Cimetidine (Tagamet) in peptic ulcer therapy during pregnancy: a report of three cases. Clin Trials J 1982;19:91–3.
4. Glade G, Saccar CL, Pereira GR. Cimetidine in pregnancy: apparent transient liver impairment in the newborn. Am J Dis Child 1980;134:87–8.
5. McGowan WAW. Safety of cimetidine treatment during pregnancy. J R Soc Med 1979;72:902–7.
6. Zulli P, DiNisio Q. Cimetidine treatment during pregnancy. Lancet 1978;2:945–6.
7. Husemeyer RP, Davenport HT. Prophylaxis for Mendelson's syndrome before elective caesarean sections. A comparison of cimetidine and magnesium trisilicate mixture regimens. Br J Obstet Gynaecol 1980;87:565–70.
8. Pickering BG,, Palahniuk RJ, Cumming M. Cimetidine premedication in elective caesarean section. Can Anaesth Soc J 1980;27:33–5.
9. Dundee JW, Moore J, Johnston JR, McCaughey W. Cimetidine and obstetric anaesthesia. Lancet 1981;2:252.
10. McCaughey W, Howe JP, Moore J, Dundee JW. Cimetidine in elective caesarean section. Effect on gastric acidity. Anaesthesia 1981;36:167–72.
11. Crawford JS. Cimetidine in elective caesarean section. Anaesthesia 1981;36:641–2.
12. McCaughey W, Howe JP, Moore J, Dundee JW. Cimetidine in elective caesarean section. Anaesthesia 1981;36:642.
13. Hodgkinson R, Glassenberg R, Joyce TH III, Coombs DW, Ostheimer GW, Gibbs CP. Safety and efficacy of cimetidine and antacid in reducing gastric acidity before elective cesarean section. Anesthesiology 1982;57:A408.
14. Ostheimer GW, Morrison JA, Lavoie C, Sepkoski C, Hoffman J, Datta S. The effect of cimetidine on mother, newborn and neonatal neurobehavior. Anesthesiology 1982;57:A405.
15. Hodgkinson R, Glassenberg R, Joyce TH III, Coombs DW, Ostheimer GW, Gibbs CP. Comparison of cimetidine (Tagamet) with antacid for safety and effectiveness in reducing gastric acidity before elective cesarean section. Anesthesiology 1983;59:86–90.
16. Qvist N, Storm K. Cimethidine pre-anesthetic: a prophylactic method against Mendelson's syndrome in cesarean section. Acta Obstet Gynecol Scand 1983;62:157–9.
17. Okasha AS, Motaweh MM, Bali A. Cimetidine-antacid combination as premedication for elective caesarean section. Can Anaesth Soc J 1983;30:593–7.
18. Frank M, Evans M, Flynn P, Aun C. Comparison of the prophylactic use of magnesium trisilicate mixture B.P.C., sodium citrate mixture or cimetidine in obstetrics. Br J Anaesth 1984;56:355–62.

19. McAuley DM, Halliday HL, Johnston JR, Moore J, Dundee JW. Cimetidine in labour: absence of adverse effect on the high-risk fetus. Br J Obstet Gynaecol 1985;92:350–5.
20. Johnston JR, McCaughey W, Moore J, Dundee JW. Cimetidine as an oral antacid before elective caesarean section. Anaesthesia 1982;37:26–32.
21. Johnston JR, McCaughey W, Moore J, Dundee JW. A field trial of cimetidine as the sole oral antacid in obstetric anaesthesia. Anaesthesia 1982;37:33–8.
22. Thorburn J, Moir DD. Antacid therapy for emergency caesarean section. Anaesthesia 1987;42:352–5.
23. Somogyi A, Gugler R. Cimetidine excretion into breast milk. Br J Clin Pharmacol 1979;7:627–9.
24. Committee on Drugs, American Academy of Pediatrics. Transfer of drugs and other chemicals into human milk. Pediatrics 1989;84:924–36.

Name: **CINNARIZINE**

Class: **Antihistamine**　　　　　　　　Risk Factor: **C**

Fetal Risk Summary

No data are available. See Meclizine for representative agent in this class.

Breast Feeding Summary

No data are available.

Name: **CINOXACIN**

Class: **Urinary Germicide**　　　　　　Risk Factor: **B$_M$**

Fetal Risk Summary

No data are available. The manufacturer recommends that it not be used in pregnancy because of cinoxacin-induced arthropathy in immature animals (1).

Breast Feeding Summary

No data are available. The manufacturer recommends that it not be used in the lactating woman (1).

Reference

1. Product information. Cinobac. Dista Products, 1990.

Name: **CISPLATIN**

Class: **Antineoplastic**　　　　　　　　Risk Factor: **D**

Fetal Risk Summary

Only two cases of cisplatin usage during pregnancy have been located (1, 2). In one case, the mother, in her 10th week of gestation, received a single intravenous dose of 50 mg/kg for carcinoma of the uterine cervix. Two weeks later, a radical hysterectomy was performed. The male fetus was morphologically normal for its developmental age. A 1989 case report described the effect of maternal chemotherapy on a premature newborn delivered at approximately 27 weeks' gestation (2). The mother had been treated with cisplatin (55 mg), bleomycin (30 mg), and etoposide (165 mg) (all given daily for 3 days), 1 week prior to delivery, for an unknown primary cancer with metastases to the eye and liver. The mother developed profound neutropenia just prior to delivery. On the 3rd day after birth, the 1190-g female infant also developed a profound leukopenia with neutropenia, 10 days after *in utero* exposure to the antineoplastic agents. The condition resolved after 10 days. At 10 days of age, the infant began losing her scalp hair along with a rapid loss of lanugo. Etoposide was thought to be the most likely cause of the neutropenia and the alopecia (2). By 12 weeks of age, substantial hair regrowth had occurred, and at 1 year follow-up, the child was developing normally except for moderate bilateral hearing loss. The investigators could not determine if the sensorineural deafness was due to the maternal and/or neonatal gentamicin therapy or to the maternal cisplatin chemotherapy (2).

The long-term effects of cisplatin and other antineoplastic agents on menstrual and reproductive function after treatment of malignant ovarian germ cell tumors have been described (3). Of the 40 women studied, cisplatin was used in six. The results of this study have been discussed in the monograph for cyclophosphamide (see Cyclophosphamide).

Reversible azoospermia occurred in a male treated for teratoma of the testis with cisplatin, vinblastine, bleomycin, surgery, and radiation (4). Fifteen months after the end of therapy, the sperm count was <50,000 sperm/μl with 70% motile and a high percentage of abnormal forms. Three months later the patient and his wife reported a pregnancy, which was terminated on their request.

Occupational exposure of the mother to antineoplastic agents during pregnancy may present a risk to the fetus. A position statement from the National Study Commission on Cytotoxic Exposure and a research article involving some antineoplastic agents are presented in the monograph for cyclophosphamide (see Cyclophosphamide).

Breast Feeding Summary

Two studies, with opposite results, have examined the excretion of cisplatin into human milk. In a 1985 study, a 31-year-old woman, 7 months postpartum with ovarian cancer, was treated with doxorubicin and cisplatin (5). Doxorubicin (90 mg) was given intravenously over 15 minutes followed by intravenous cisplatin (130 mg; 100 mg/m^2) infused over 26 hours. Blood and milk samples were collected frequently for cisplatin determination from 0.25–71.25 hours after the start of the infusion. Peak plasma concentrations of platinum reached 2.99 μg/ml, but platinum was undetectable (sensitivity 0.1 μg/ml) in the milk.

Opposite results were obtained in a 1989 study (6). A 24-year-old woman with an entodermal sinus tumor of the left ovary was treated with cisplatin, 30 mg/m^2 intravenously over 4 hours daily, for 5 consecutive days. Etoposide and bleomycin were also administered during this time. On the 3rd day of therapy, milk and serum samples were collected 30 minutes before the cisplatin dose. Cisplatin concentrations in the milk and plasma were 0.9 and 0.8 μg/ml, respectively, a milk:plasma ratio of 1.1. The infant was not allowed to breast feed. Probably because this latter report was not available prior to publication of their statement, the American Academy of Pediatrics classified cisplatin as compatible with breast feeding (7). However, based on the 1989 report, breast feeding during cisplatin therapy should be considered contraindicated.

References

1. Jacobs AJ, Marchevsky A, Gordon RE, Deppe G, Cohen CJ. Oat cell carcinoma of the uterine cervix in a pregnant woman treated with cis-diamminedichloroplatinum. Gynecol Oncol 1980;9:405–10.
2. Raffles A, Williams J, Costeloe K, Clark P. Transplacental effects of maternal cancer chemotherapy: case report. Br J Obstet Gynaecol 1989;96:1099–1100.
3. Gershenson DM. Menstrual and reproductive function after treatment with combination chemotherapy for malignant ovarian germ cell tumors. J Clin Oncol 1988;6:270–5.
4. Rubery ED. Return of fertility after curative chemotherapy for disseminated teratoma of testis. Lancet 1983;1:186.
5. Egan PC, Costanza ME, Dodion P, Egorin MJ, Bachur NR. Doxorubicin and cisplatin excretion into human milk. Cancer Treat Rep 1985;69:1387–9.
6. De Vries EGE, Van Der Zee AGJ, Uges DRA, Sleijfer DTh. Excretion of platinum into breast milk. Lancet 1989;1:497.
7. Committee on Drugs, American Academy of Pediatrics. Transfer of drugs and other chemicals into human milk. Pediatrics 1989;84:924–36.

Name: **CLEMASTINE**

Class: **Antihistamine** Risk Factor: **C**

Fetal Risk Summary

No data are available. See Diphenhydramine for representative agent in this class.

Breast Feeding Summary

Clemastine is excreted into breast milk (1). A 10-week-old girl developed drowsiness, irritability, refusal to feed, neck stiffness, and a high-pitched cry 12 hours after the mother began taking the antihistamine, 1 mg twice daily. The mother was also taking phenytoin and carbamazepine. Twenty hours after the last dose, clemastine levels in maternal plasma and milk were 20 and 5–10 ng/ml, respectively, a milk:plasma ratio of 0.25–0.5. The drug could not be detected in the infant's plasma. Symptoms in the baby resolved within 24 hours after the drug was stopped, although breast feeding was continued. Examination 3 weeks later was also normal. Due to the above case report, the American Academy of Pediatrics believes the drug should be used with caution during breast feeding (2).

References

1. Kok THHG, Taitz LS, Bennett MJ, Holt DW. Drowsiness due to clemastine transmitted in breast milk. Lancet 1982;1:914–5.
2. Committee on Drugs, American Academy of Pediatrics. Transfer of drugs and other chemicals into human milk. Pediatrics 1989;84:924–36.

Name: **CLIDINIUM**

Class: **Parasympatholytic**   Risk Factor: **C**

Fetal Risk Summary

Clidinium is an anticholinergic quaternary ammonium bromide. In a large prospective study, 2323 patients were exposed to this class of drugs during the 1st trimester, 4 of whom took clidinium (1). A possible association was found between the total group and minor malformations.

Breast Feeding Summary

No data are available (see also Atropine).

Reference

1. Heinonen OP, Slone D, Shapiro S. *Birth Defects and Drugs in Pregnancy*. Littleton:Publishing Sciences Group, 1977:346–53.

Name: **CLINDAMYCIN**

Class: **Antibiotic**   Risk Factor: **B**

Fetal Risk Summary

No reports linking the use of clindamycin with congenital defects have been located. The drug crosses the placenta, achieving maximum cord serum levels of approximately 50% of the maternal serum (1, 2). Levels in the fetus were considered therapeutic for susceptible pathogens. A study published in 1988 measured a mean cord:maternal ratio of 0.15 in three women given an unknown amount of clindamycin in labor for the treatment of chorioamnionitis (3). At the time of sampling, mean maternal blood, cord blood, and placental membrane concentrations of the antibiotic were 1.67 μg/ml, 0.26 μg/ml, and 1.86 μg/g, respectively (placenta:maternal ratio 1.11). Fetal tissue levels increase following multiple dosing with the drug concentrating in the fetal liver (1). Maternal serum levels after dosing at various stages of pregnancy were similar to those of nonpregnant patients (2, 4). Clindamycin has been used for prophylactic therapy prior to cesarean section (5).

Breast Feeding Summary

Clindamycin is excreted into breast milk. In two patients receiving 600 mg intravenously every 6 hours, milk levels varied from 2.1–3.8 μg/ml (0.2–3.5 hours after drug) (6). When the patients were changed to 300 mg orally every 6 hours, levels varied from 0.7–1.8 μg/ml (2–7 hours after drug). Maternal serum levels were not given. Two grossly bloody stools were observed in a nursing infant whose mother was receiving clindamycin and gentamicin (7). No relationship to either drug could be established. However, the condition cleared rapidly when breast feeding was stopped. Except for this one case, no other adverse effects in nursing infants have been reported. Three potential problems that may exist for the nursing infant are modification of bowel flora, direct effects on the infant, and interference with the interpretation of culture results if a fever workup is required. The American Academy of Pediatrics considers clindamycin to be compatible with breast feeding (8).

References

1. Philipson A, Sabath LD, Charles D. Transplacental passage of erythromycin and clindamycin. N Engl J Med 1973;288:1219–21.
2. Weinstein AJ, Gibbs RS, Gallagher M. Placental transfer of clindamycin and gentamicin in term pregnancy. Am J Obstet Gynecol 1976;124:688–91.
3. Gilstrap LC III, Bawdon RE, Burris J. Antibiotic concentration in maternal blood, cord blood, and placental membranes in chorioamnionitis. Obstet Gynecol 1988;72:124–5.
4. Philipson A, Sabath LD, Charles D. Erythromycin and clindamycin absorption and elimination in pregnant women. Clin Pharmacol Ther 1976;19:68–77.
5. Rehu M, Jahkola M. Prophylactic antibiotics in caesarean section: effect of a short preoperative course of benzyl penicillin or clindamycin plus gentamicin on postoperative infectious morbidity. Ann Clin Res 1980;12:45–8.
6. Smith JA, Morgan JR, Rachlis AR, Papsin FR. Clindamycin in human breast milk. Can Med Assoc J 1975;112:806.
7. Mann CF. Clindamycin and breast-feeding. Pediatrics 1980;66:1030–1.
8. Committee on Drugs, American Academy of Pediatrics. Transfer of drugs and other chemicals into human milk. Pediatrics 1989;84:924–36.

Name: **CLOFIBRATE**

Class: **Antilipemic Agent**   Risk Factor: **C**

Fetal Risk Summary

No reports linking the use of clofibrate with congenital defects have been located. There is pharmacologic evidence that clofibrate crosses the rat placenta and reaches measurable levels, but data in humans are lacking (1). The drug is metabolized by glucuronide conjugation. Because this system is immature in the newborn, accumulation may occur. Consequently, the use of clofibrate near term is not recommended.

Breast Feeding Summary

No data are available. Animal studies suggest that the drug is excreted into milk (1).

Reference

1. Chhabra S, Kurup CKR. Maternal transport of chlorophenoxyisobutyrate at the foetal and neonatal stages of development. Biochem Pharmacol 1978;27:2063–5.

Name: **CLOMIPHENE**

Class: **Fertility Agent (Nonhormonal)**   Risk Factor: X_M

Fetal Risk Summary

Clomiphene is used to induce ovulation and is contraindicated after conception has occurred. Several case reports of neural tube defects have been reported after ovulation stimulation with clomiphene (1–5). However, an association between the drug and these defects has not been established (6–10). In one review, the percentage of congenital anomalies after clomiphene use was no greater than in the normal population (6). Similarly, another study involving 1034 pregnancies after clomiphene-induced ovulation found no association with the incidence or type of malformation (11). Congenital malformations reported in patients who received clomiphene prior to conception include (5, 6, 12–25):

Hydatidiform mole	Retinal aplasia
Syndactyly	Clubfoot
Pigmentation defects	Microcephaly
Congenital heart defects	Cleft lip/palate
Down's syndrome	Ovarian dysplasia
Hypospadias	Polydactyly
Hemangioma	Anencephaly

A single case of hepatoblastoma in a 15-month-old female was thought to be due to the use of clomiphene and follicle-stimulating/luteinizing hormone prior to conception (26).

Inadvertent use of clomiphene early in the 1st trimester has been reported in two patients (18, 24). A ruptured lumbosacral meningomyelocele was observed in one infant exposed during the 4th week of gestation (18). There was no evidence of neurologic defect in the lower limbs or of hydrocephalus. The second infant was delivered with esophageal atresia with fistula, congenital heart defects, hypospadias, and absent left kidney (24). The mother also took methyldopa throughout pregnancy for mild hypertension.

Patients requiring the use of clomiphene should be cautioned that each new course of the drug should be started only after pregnancy has been excluded.

Breast Feeding Summary

No data are available.

References

1. Barrett C, Hakim C. Anencephaly, ovulation stimulation, subfertility, and illegitimacy. Lancet 1973;2:916–7.
2. Dyson JL, Kohler HG, Anencephaly and ovulation stimulation. Lancet 1973;1:1256–7.
3. Field B, Kerr C. Ovulation stimulation and defects of neural tube closure. Lancet 1974;2:1511.
4. Sandler B. Anencephaly and ovulation stimulation. Lancet 1973;2:379.
5. Biale Y, Leventhal H, Altaras M, Ben-Aderet N. Anencephaly and clomiphene-induced pregnancy. Acta Obstet Gynecol Scand 1978;57:483–4.
6. Asch RH, Greenblatt RB. Update on the safety and efficacy of clomiphene citrate as a therapeutic agent. J Reprod Med 1976;17:175–180.
7. Harlap S. Ovulation induction and congenital malformations. Lancet 1976;2:961.
8. James WH, Clomiphene, anencephaly, and spina bifida. Lancet 1977;1:603.
9. Ahlgren M, Kallen B, Rannevik G. Outcome of pregnancy after clomiphene therapy. Acta Obstet Gynecol Scand 1976;55:371–5.
10. Elwood JM. Clomiphene and anencephalic births. Lancet 1974;1:31.
11. Kurachi K, Aono T, Minagawa J, Miyake A. Congenital malformations of newborn infants after clomiphene-induced ovulation. Fertil Steril 1983;40:187–9.
12. Miles PA, Taylor HB, Hill WC. Hydatidiform mole in a clomiphene related pregnancy: a case report. Obstet Gynecol 1971;37:358–9.
13. Schneiderman CI, Waxman B. Clomid therapy and subsequent hydatidiform mole formation: a case report. Obstet Gynecol 1972;39:787–8.

14. Wajntraub G, Kamar R, Pardo Y. Hydatidiform mole after treatment with clomiphene. Fertil Steril 1974;25:904–5.
15. Berman P. Congenital abnormalities associated with maternal clomiphene ingestion. Lancet 1975;2:878.
16. Drew AL. Letter to the editor. Dev Med Child Neurol 1974;16:276.
17. Hack M, Brish M, Serr DM, Insler V, Salomy M, Lunenfeld B. Outcome of pregnancy after induced ovulation. Follow-up of pregnancies and children born after clomiphene therapy. JAMA 1972;220:1329–33.
18. Ylikorkala O. Congenital anomalies and clomiphene. Lancet 1975;2:1262–3.
19. Laing IA, Steer CR, Dudgeon J, Brown JK. Clomiphene and congenital retinopathy. Lancet 1981;2:1107–8.
20. Ford WDA, Little KET. Fetal ovarian dysplasia possibly associated with clomiphene. Lancet 1981;2:1107.
21. Kistner RW. Induction of ovulation with clomiphene citrate. Obstet Gynecol Surv 1965;20:873–99.
22. Goldfarb AF, Morales A, Rakoff AE, Protos P. Critical review of 160 clomiphene-related pregnancies. Obstet Gynecol 1968;31:342–5.
23. Oakely GP, Flynt IW. Increased prevalence of Down's syndrome (mongolism) among the offspring of women treated with ovulation-inducing agents. Teratology 1972;5:264.
24. Singhi M, Singhi S. Possible relationship between clomiphene and neural tube defects. J Pediatr 1978;93:152.
25. Mor-Joseph S, Anteby SO, Granat M, Brzezinsky A, Evron S. Recurrent molar pregnancies associated with clomiphene citrate and human gonadotropins. Am J Obstet Gynecol 1985;151:1085–6.
26. Melamed I, Bujanover Y, Hammer J, Spirer Z. Hepatoblastoma in an infant born to a mother after hormonal treatment for sterility. N Engl J Med 1982;307:820.

Name: **CLOMIPRAMINE**

Class: **Antidepressant**   Risk Factor: **D**

Fetal Risk Summary

The use of clomipramine throughout pregnancy to treat maternal depression has been described in three women (1, 2). All three newborns developed toxic morbidity shortly after birth. Clinical symptoms included lethargy, hypotonia, cyanosis, jitteriness, irregular respirations with respiratory acidosis, and hypothermia. The hypothermia persisted for 4 days (1). In one infant serum levels of clomipramine on the 1st and 3rd days were <20 ng/ml but levels at these times of the active metabolite, chlordesipramine, were 116 and 96 ng/ml, respectively (1). The toxicity observed in these cases may have been due to the anticholinergic properties of the drug. The infants were successfully treated with phenobarbital and subsequently developed normally.

Convulsions in two newborns exposed *in utero* to clomipramine have been reported (3). Both mothers had combined clomipramine and desmethyl-clomipramine concentrations higher than the suggested therapeutic range. In one of the cases, the convulsions were controlled by administering clomipramine to the newborn infant. The first infant was exposed during the last 7 weeks of gestation. At birth, his serum levels of clomipramine and the metabolite, desmethyl-clomipramine, were estimated to be 190 and 160 ng/ml, respectively. Seizures occurred at 8 hours after birth and then persisted intermittently until he was 53 hours of age despite treatment with phenobarbital and paraldehyde. Hypertonicity, jitteriness, and ankle clonus continued until the 11th day of life, and anticonvulsant therapy was stopped 3 days later. The mother of the second infant was treated throughout gestation with clomipramine and flurazepam. The infant was delivered at 33 weeks' gestation and began convulsing at 7 hours of age. Seizures in the form of myoclonic jerks continued in spite of phenobarbital. Intravenous clomipramine was started at 24 hours with an initial dose of 0.4 mg over 2 hours. Convulsions stopped completely for 11 hours. Upon their recurrence, a dose of 0.5 mg over 2 hours was given, followed by a continuous tapering infusion until age 12 days when oral therapy was started (doses not given). No additional convulsions were observed, but the infant remained jittery. All therapy was stopped at age 17 days. Follow-up of these infants was not reported.

Breast Feeding Summary

No data are available (see Imipramine).

References

1. Ben Muza A, Smith CS. Neonatal effects of maternal clomipramine therapy. Arch Dis Child 1979;54:405.
2. Ostergaard GZ, Pedersen SE. Neonatal effects of maternal clomipramine treatment. Pediatrics 1982;69:233–4.
3. Cowe L, Lloyd DJ, Dawling S. Neonatal convulsions caused by withdrawal from maternal clomipramine. Br Med J 1982;284:1837–8.

Name: **CLOMOCYCLINE**

Class: **Antibiotic**   Risk Factor: **D**

Fetal Risk Summary

See Tetracycline.

Breast Feeding Summary

See Tetracycline.

Name: **CLONAZEPAM**

Class: **Anticonvulsant**   Risk Factor: **C**

Fetal Risk Summary

Clonazepam is a benzodiazepine anticonvulsant that is chemically and structurally similar to diazepam (1). The drug is used either alone or in combination with other anticonvulsants. In a small series of patients (N = 150) matched with nonepileptic controls, anticonvulsant therapy, including five women using clonazepam, had no effect on the incidence of pregnancy-induced hypertension, albuminuria, premature contractions, premature labor, bleeding in pregnancy, duration of labor, blood loss at delivery, cesarean sections, and vacuum extractions (2).

Toxicity in the newborn, apparently related to clonazepam, has been reported. A 36 weeks' gestational age infant, exposed throughout pregnancy to an unspecified amount of clonazepam, developed apnea, cyanosis, lethargy, and hypotonia at 6 hours of age (3). There was no evidence of congenital defects in the 2750-g newborn. Cord and maternal serum levels of clonazepam were 19 and 32 ng/ml, respectively, a ratio of 0.59. Both levels were within the therapeutic range (5–70 ng/ml) (3). At 18 hours of age, the clonazepam level in the infant's serum measured 4.4 ng/ml. Five episodes of prolonged apnea (16–43 seconds/occurrence) were measured by pneumogram over the next 12 hours. Hypotonia and lethargy resolved within 5 days, but overt clinical apnea persisted for 10 days. Follow-up pneumograms demonstrated apnea spells until 10 weeks of age, but the presence of the drug in breast milk may have contributed to the condition (see Breast Feeding Summary). The authors concluded that apnea due to prematurity was not a significant factor. Neurologic development was normal at 5 months.

Breast Feeding Summary

Clonazepam is excreted into breast milk. In a woman treated with an unspecified amount of the anticonvulsant, milk concentrations remained constant between 11 and 13 ng/ml (3). The milk:maternal serum ratio was approximately 0.33. After 7 days of nursing, the infant, described above, had a serum concentration of 2.9 ng/ml. A major portion of this probably resulted from *in utero* exposure because the elimination half-life of clonazepam in neonates is thought to be prolonged (3). No evidence of drug accumulation after breast feeding was found. Persistent apnea spells, lasting until 10 weeks of age, were observed, but it was not known whether breast feeding contributed to the condition. Based on this case, the authors recommended that infants exposed *in utero* or during breast feeding to clonazepam should have serum levels of the drug determined and be closely monitored for central nervous system depression or apnea (3).

References

1. Reith H, Schafer H. Antiepileptic drugs during pregnancy and the lactation period. Pharmacokinetic data. Dtsch Med Wochenschr 1979;104:818–23.
2. Hiilesmaa VK, Bardy A, Teramo K. Obstetric outcome in women with epilepsy. Am J Obstet Gynecol 1985;152:499–504.
3. Fisher JB, Edgren BE, Mammel MC, Coleman JM. Neonatal apnea associated with maternal clonazepam therapy: a case report. Obstet Gynecol 1985;66(Suppl):34S–5S.

Name: **CLONIDINE**

Class: **Antihypertensive**   Risk Factor: **C**

Fetal Risk Summary

No reports linking the use of clonidine with congenital defects have been located. The drug has been used during all trimesters, but experience during the 1st trimester is very limited. Adverse fetal effects attributable to clonidine have not been observed (1–8).

The pharmacokinetics of clonidine during pregnancy have been reported (9). The mean maternal and cord serum concentrations in 10 women were 0.46 and

0.41 ng/ml, respectively, corresponding to a cord:maternal ratio 0.89. The mean amniotic fluid concentration was 1.50 ng/ml. The mean maternal dose was 330 μg/day. Results of neurologic examinations and limited blood chemistry tests in the exposed infants were similar to those in untreated controls. No neonatal hypotension was observed.

Breast Feeding Summary

Clonidine is secreted into breast milk (8, 9). Following a 150-μg oral dose, milk concentrations of 1.5 ng/ml may be achieved (milk:plasma ratio 1.5) (P.A. Bowers, personal communication, Boehringer Ingelheim, Ltd., 1981). In a study of nine nursing women taking mean daily doses of 391.7 μg (postpartum days 1–5), 309.4 μg (postpartum days 10–14), and 241.7 μg (postpartum days 45–60), milk concentrations were approximately twice those in maternal serum (9). Mean milk levels were close to 2 ng/ml or higher during the three sampling periods. Hypotension was not observed in the nursing infants, although clonidine was found in the serum of the infants (mean levels less than maternal). The long-term significance of this exposure is not known.

References

1. Turnbull AC, Ahmed S. Catapres in the treatment of hypertension in pregnancy, a preliminary study. In *Catapres in Hypertension*. Symposium of the Royal College of Surgeons. London, 1970:237–45.
2. Johnston CI, Aickin DR. The control of high blood pressure during labour with clonidine. Med J Aust 1971;2:132.
3. Raftos J, Bauer GE, Lewis RG, Stokes GS, Mitchell AS, Young AA, Maclachlan I. Clonidine in the treatment of severe hypertension. Med J Aust 1973;1:786–93.
4. Horvath JS, Phippard A, Korda A, Henderson-Smart DJ, Child A, Tiller DJ. Clonidine hydrochloride — a safe and effective antihypertensive agent in pregnancy. Obstet Gynecol 1985;66:634–8.
5. Horvath JS, Korda A, Child A, Henderson-Smart D, Phippard A, Duggin GC, Hall BM, Tiller DJ. Hypertension in pregnancy: a study of 142 women presenting before 32 weeks' gestation. Med J Aust 1985;143:19–21.
6. NG Wingtin L, Frelon JH, Beaute Y, Pellerin M, Guillaumin JP. Clonidine et traitement de l'hypertension arterielle de la femme enceinte. Cah Anesthesiol 1986;34:389–93.
7. Ng-Wing Tin L, Frelon JH, Beaute Y, Pellerin M, Guillaumin JP, Bazin C. Clonidine et traitement de l'hypertension arterielle de la femme enceinte. Rev Franc Gynecol Obstet 1986;81:563–6.
8. Ng Wing-Tin L, Frelon JH, Hardy F, Bazin C. Clonidine et traitement des urgences hypertensives de la femme enceinte. Rev Franc Gynecol Obstet 1987;82:519–22.
9. Hartikainen-Sorri A-L, Heikkinen JE, Koivisto M. Pharmacokinetics of clonidine during pregnancy and nursing. Obstet Gynecol 1987;69:598–600.

Name: **CLOTRIMAZOLE**

Class: **Antifungal Antibiotic**   Risk Factor: **B**

Fetal Risk Summary

No reports linking the use of clotrimazole with congenital defects have been located. The topical use of the drug in pregnancy has been studied (1–4). No adverse effects attributable to clotrimazole were observed. In a retrospective analysis of 104,339 women who had delivered in Michigan hospitals during 1980–1983, suspected birth defect diagnoses occurred in 6,564 (5). First trimester vaginitis treatment with clotrimazole occurred in 74 of the 6,564 deliveries linked to birth defect diagnoses and in 1,012 of the 97,775 cases not linked to such diagnoses. The estimated relative risk of birth defects when clotrimazole was used was 1.09 (95% confidence limits 0.9–1.4). Although an increased relative risk was not found, this study could not exclude the possibility of an association with a specific birth defect (5).

Breast Feeding Summary

No data are available.

References

1. Tan CG, Good CS, Milne LJR, Loudon JDO. A comparative trial of six day therapy with clotrimazole and nystatin in pregnant patients with vaginal candidiasis. Postgrad Med 1974;50(Suppl 1):102–5.
2. Frerich W, Gad A. The frequency of Candida infections in pregnancy and their treatment with clotrimazole. Curr Med Res Opin 1977;4:640–4.
3. Haram K, Digranes A. Vulvovaginal candidiasis in pregnancy treated with clotrimazole. Acta Obstet Gynecol Scand 1978;57:453–5.
4. Svendsen E, Lie S, Gunderson TH, Lyngstad-Vik I, Skuland J. Comparative evaluation of miconazole, clotrimazole and nystatin in the treatment of candidal vulvo-vaginitis. Curr Ther Res 1978;23:666–72.
5. Rosa FW, Baum C, Shaw M. Pregnancy outcomes after first-trimester vaginitis drug therapy. Obstet Gynecol 1987;69:751–5.

Name: **CLOXACILLIN**

Class: **Antibiotic** Risk Factor: **B$_M$**

Fetal Risk Summary

Cloxacillin is a penicillin antibiotic (see also Penicillin G). No reports linking its use with congenital defects have been located. The Collaborative Perinatal Project monitored 50,282 mother-child pairs, 3,546 of which had 1st trimester exposure to penicillin derivatives (1, pp. 297–313). For use anytime during pregnancy, 7,171 exposures were recorded (1, p. 435). In neither case was evidence found to suggest a relationship to large categories of major or minor malformations or to individual defects.

Breast Feeding Summary

No data are available (see Penicillin G).

Reference

1. Heinonen OP, Slone D, Shapiro S. *Birth Defects and Drugs in Pregnancy*. Littleton:Publishing Sciences Group, 1977.

Name: **COCAINE**
Class: **Sympathomimetic**   Risk Factor: **C***

Fetal Risk Summary

Cocaine, a naturally occurring alkaloid, is legally available in the United States as a topical anesthetic, but its illegal use as a central nervous system stimulant far exceeds any medicinal market for the drug. Cocaine is a sympathomimetic, producing hypertension and vasoconstriction as a result of its direct cardiovascular activity. The increasing popularity of cocaine is due to its potent ability to produce euphoria, an effect that is counterbalanced by the strong addictive properties of the drug (1). As of 1985, an estimated 30 million Americans had used cocaine and 5 million were believed to be using it regularly (1). Although the exact figures are unknown, current usage probably exceeds these estimates. Preliminary results of a study conducted between July 1984 and June 1987 in the Boston area indicated that 117 (17%) of 679 urban women used cocaine at least once during pregnancy as determined by prenatal and postpartum interviews and urine assays for cocaine metabolites (2). Final results from this study, now involving a total of 1226 mothers, found that 216 (18%) used cocaine during pregnancy, but that only 165 (76%) of these women would have been detected by history alone (3). Fifty-one women who had denied use of cocaine had positive urine assays for cocaine metabolites. Other investigators have reported similar findings (4). Of 138 women who had positive urine screens for cocaine at delivery, only 59 (43%) would have been identified by drug history alone. In this same study, the increasing prevalence of maternal cocaine abuse was demonstrated (4). Over a 24-month period (September 1986–August 1988), the incidence of positive urine screens for cocaine in women at delivery rose steadily, starting at 4% in the first 6-month quarter and increasing to 12% in the final quarter. The total number of women (1776) was approximately equally divided among the four quarters.

Illicitly obtained cocaine varies greatly in purity, and it is commonly adulterated with such substances as lactose, mannitol, lidocaine, and procaine (5). Cocaine is detoxified by liver and plasma cholinesterases (1, 5). Activity of the latter enzyme system is much lower in the fetus and in infants and is decreased in pregnant women, resulting in slower metabolism and elimination of the drug (1, 5). Moreover, most studies have found a correlation between cocaine use and the use of other abuse drugs such as heroin, methadone, methamphetamine, marijuana, tobacco, and alcohol. Compared to drug-free women, this correlation was highly significant ($p < 0.0001$), and, further, users were significantly more likely to be heavy abusers of these substances ($p < 0.0001$) (2).

Research on the effects of maternal and fetal cocaine exposure has focused on several different areas and reflects the wide-ranging concerns for fetal safety this drug has produced:

  Placental transfer of cocaine
  Pregnancy complications
    Placental receptor function
    Duration of gestation
    Premature labor and delivery
    Spontaneous abortions

Premature rupture of membranes
Placenta previa
Pregnancy-induced hypertension
Abruptio placentae
Rupture of ectopic pregnancy
Maternal mortality
Fetal complications
 Growth retardation
 Fetal distress
  Meconium staining
  Bradycardia/tachycardia
  Apgar scores
 Cerebrovascular accidents
 Congenital anomalies
Neonatal neurobehavior

Although the placental transfer of cocaine has not been quantified in humans, cocaine metabolites are frequently found in the urine of *in utero*-exposed newborns. Since cocaine has high water and lipid solubility, low molecular weight (approximately 340), and low ionization at physiologic pH, it should freely cross to the fetus (5). In pregnant sheep given intravenous cocaine, 0.5 mg/kg, to produce plasma levels similar to those observed in humans, fetal plasma levels at 5 minutes were 46.8 ng/ml compared to simultaneous maternal levels of 405 ng/ml (fetus 12% of mother) (6). At 30 minutes, the levels for fetal and maternal plasma had decreased to 11.8 and 83 ng/ml, respectively (fetus 14% of mother). Uterine blood flow was decreased in a dose-dependent manner by 36% after the above dose (6). Decreases in uterine blood flow of similar magnitude have also been observed in other studies with pregnant sheep (7, 8). In one report, the reduction was accompanied by fetal hypoxemia, hypertension, and tachycardia, which were more severe then when cocaine was administered directly to the fetus (8).

In a study examining the effects of prenatal cocaine exposure on human placental tissue, significant decreases, as compared to nonexposed controls, were found for the total number of β-adrenergic receptor-binding sites (202 vs. 313 fmol/mg, $p < 0.01$), μ-opiate receptor-binding sites (77 vs. 105 fmol/mg, $p < 0.05$), and δ-opiate receptor-binding sites (77 vs. 119 fmol/mg, $p < 0.01$) (9). These effects were interpreted as a true down-regulation of the receptor population and may be associated with increased levels of adrenergic compounds (9, 10). The authors speculated that if a similar down-regulation of the fetal adrenergic receptor-binding sites also occurred, it could result in disruption of synaptic development of the fetal nervous system. However, the clinical significance of these findings has not yet been determined (9).

The effect of maternal cocaine use on the duration of gestation has been included in several research papers (3, 4, 11–25). When compared with non-drug-using controls, *in utero* cocaine exposure invariably resulted in significantly shortened mean gestational periods ranging up to 2 weeks. A statistically significant mean shorter (1.9 weeks) gestational period was also observed when cocaine-polydrug users (20% used heroin) were compared with noncocaine-polydrug users (26% used heroin) (13). Two other studies, comparing cocaine/amphetamine (18) or cocaine/methadone (17) consumption with noncocaine heroin/methadone-abusing women, found nonsignificantly shorter gestational lengths, 37.9 vs. 38.3 weeks and 37.2 vs. 38.1 weeks, respectively. A third study classified some of their subjects into two subgroups: cocaine only ($N = 24$) and cocaine plus polyabuse drugs ($N = 46$) (20). No statistical differences were measured for gestational age at delivery (36.6 vs. 37.4 weeks) or for the incidence of preterm (<37 weeks) delivery (25.0% vs. 23.9%). When included as part of the research format, the incidence of premature labor and delivery was significantly increased in comparison to that in drug-free women (4, 11, 18–25). When comparisons were made with noncocaine opiate abusers, the incidences were higher but not significant. One investigation also found that cocaine use significantly increased the incidence of precipitous labor (11). Although objective data were not provided, a 1985 report mentioned that several cocaine-exposed women had noted uterine contractions and increased fetal activity within minutes of using cocaine (26). This same group reported in 1989 that infants who had been exposed to cocaine throughout pregnancy ($N = 52$) (average maternal dose/use $= 0.5$ g) had a significantly shorter mean gestational age than infants of drug-free women ($N = 40$), 38.0 weeks vs. 39.8 weeks ($p < 0.001$), respectively (24). The gestational period of those who used cocaine only during the 1st trimester was a mean 38.9 weeks, which was not significantly different from that of either of the other two groups. The incidence of preterm delivery (defined as <38 weeks) in the three groups was 17% (4 of 23; 1st trimester use only), 31% (16 of 52; cocaine use throughout pregnancy), and 3% (1 of 40; drug-free controls) (24). Only the difference between the latter two groups was statistically significant ($p < 0.003$). In another 1989 study, bivariate comparisons of 114 cocaine users (as determined by positive urine assays) with 1010 nonusers (as determined by interview and negative urine assays) indicated the difference in gestational length to be statistically significant (38.8 weeks vs. 39.3 weeks, $p < 0.05$) (3). However, multivariate analyses to control the effect of other substances and maternal characteristics known to affect pregnancy outcome adversely resulted in a loss of significance, thus demonstrating that, in this population, cocaine exposure alone did not affect the duration of gestation (3).

A 1985 report found an increased rate of spontaneous abortions in previous pregnancies of women using cocaine either alone or with narcotics compared to women using only narcotics and women not abusing drugs (26). These data were based on patient recall so the authors were unable to determine if a causal relationship existed. In a subsequent report on this patient population, the incidence of previous abortions (not differentiated between elective and spontaneous) was significantly greater in women who predominantly used cocaine either alone or with opiates when compared to those who used only opiates or to non-drug-using controls (25). A statistically significant ($p < 0.05$) higher incidence of one or more spontaneous abortions was found in 117 users (30%) compared to 562 nonusers (21%) (2). Other studies, examining cocaine consumption in current pregnancies, found no correlation between the drug and spontaneous abortions (5, 15–17, 22).

Premature rupture of the membranes (PROM) was observed in 2% of 46 women using cocaine and/or methamphetamine vs. 10% of 49 women using narcotics vs. 4.4% of 45 drug-free controls (differences not significant) (18). Similarly, no difference in PROM rates were noted between two groups of women admitted in labor without previous prenatal care (cocaine group $N = 124$, noncocaine group $N = 218$) (23). However, a 1989 report found a statistically significant increase in the incidence of PROM in women with a positive urine screen for cocaine (29 of 138, 21%) in comparison to non-cocaine-using controls (3 of 88, 3%) ($p < 0.0005$) (4). Although not statistically significant, the risk of PROM was higher in women who predominantly used cocaine either alone (10%, 6 of 63) or with opiates (14%, 4 of 28) than in drug-free controls (2%, 3 of 123) (26). The incidence of placenta previa was also not increased by cocaine use in this study (22). In contrast, 33% of 50 "crack" (alkaloidal cocaine that is smoked) users had PROM compared to 18% of non-drug-using controls ($p = 0.05$) (21). Drug abuse patterns in both groups were determined by interview, which may have introduced classification error into the results, but the authors reasoned that any error would have underestimated the actual effect of the cocaine exposure (21).

Two studies have measured the incidence of pregnancy-induced hypertension in their patients (22, 23). In one, the rate of this complication in cocaine-exposed and nonexposed women was too low to report (22). In the second, 25% (13 of 53) of cocaine-exposed women vs. 4% (4 of 100) of nonexposed controls had the disorder ($p < 0.05$) (23). Such other factors as maternal age, race, use of multiple abuse drugs, small numbers, and self-reported cocaine exposure may have accounted for this difference.

Two cases of abruptio placentae after intravenous and intranasal cocaine use were reported in 1983 (27). Since this initial observation, a number of similar cases of this complication have been described (1, 4, 5, 11, 14, 18, 19, 21, 24–26, 28–30), although some investigators either did not observe any cases (31) or the number of cases in the studied patients was too low to report (22). The findings of one study indicated that abruptio placentae-induced stillbirths in cocaine users ($N = 50$), multiple drug users (some of whom used cocaine) ($N = 110$), and drug-free controls ($N = 340$) were 8%, 4.5%, and 0.8%, respectively (5). The difference between the cocaine-only group and the controls was significant ($p < 0.001$). The four mothers in the cocaine group suffered placental abruption after intravenous and intranasal administration (one each) and smoking (two cases). Two of the five mothers in the multiple drug use group suffered the complication after injection of a "speed ball" (heroin plus cocaine) (5). Thus, 6 of the 12 cases were associated with cocaine use. Onset of labor with abruptio placentae was observed in 4 of 23 women after the use of intravenous cocaine (25). Additional information was provided by these investigators in a series of papers extending into 1989 (11, 14, 20, 24, 25). The latest data indicated that in women who had used cocaine during pregnancy ($N = 75$, 23 of whom used cocaine only during the 1st trimester), 10 (13.3%) had suffered abruptio placentae compared to none of the 40 drug-free controls ($p < 0.05$) (24). Retroplacental hemorrhages, including placental abruption, were significantly increased in a cocaine and/or methamphetamine group (13% of 46) in comparison to either opiate users (2% of 49) or drug-free controls (2.2% of 45) ($p < 0.05$) (18). Two cases of abruptio placentae were observed in 55 women using "crack" (none in 55 drug-free controls) (21) and one case in a woman using cocaine in 102 consecutive deliveries at a Texas hospital (28). Three additional cases of sonographically diagnosed abruption probably related to cocaine use were described in a 1988 report (29). While the exact mechanism of cocaine-induced abruptio placentae is still unknown, the pharmacologic effects of the drug offer a reasonable explanation. Cocaine prevents norepinephrine reuptake at nerve terminals, producing peripheral and placental vasoconstriction, reflex tachycardia with acute hypertension, and uterine contractions. The net effect of these actions in some cases may be abruptio placentae (1, 5, 11, 18, 24, 26, 27, 32).

Two cases of rupture of ectopic pregnancies were reported in 1989 (33). In both incidences, the women described severe abdominal pain immediately after consuming cocaine (smoking in one, nasally in the other). While the authors of this report could not totally exclude spontaneous rupture of the tubal pregnancies, they concluded that the short time interval between cocaine ingestion and the onset of symptoms made the association appear likely (33).

Fatalities following adult cocaine use have been reported frequently, but only two cases have been located that involve pregnant women (34, 35). A 24-year-old woman, who smoked "crack" daily, presented at 34 weeks' gestation with acute onset of severe headache and photophobia (34). Her symptoms were determined to be due to subarachnoid hemorrhage resulting from a ruptured aneurysm. Following surgery to relieve intracranial pressure and an unsuccessful attempt to isolate the aneurysm, the patient gave birth to a normal 2400-g male infant. Her condition subsequently worsened on postpartum day 21 and she expired 4 days later from recurrent intracranial hemorrhage. The second case involved a 21-year-old in her approximate 16th week of pregnancy (35). She was admitted to the hospital in a comatose condition after about 1.5 g of cocaine had been placed in her vagina. She was maintained on life support systems and eventually delivered, by cesarean section, a female infant at 33 weeks' gestation with severe brain abnormalities. The infant died at 10 days of age, and the mother expired approximately 4 months later.

Fetal complications reported after exposure to cocaine include growth retardation, fetal distress, cerebrovascular accidents, and congenital anomalies. A large number of studies have examined the effect of *in utero* cocaine exposure on fetal growth parameters (birth weight, length, and head circumference) (2–5, 11–26, 36–39). The majority of these found, after correcting for confounding variables, that cocaine exposure, when compared to non-drug-abuse populations, was associated with reduced fetal growth. This reduction was comparable, in most cases, to that observed in fetuses exposed to opiates, such as heroin or methadone. A survey of 117 users compared to 562 nonusers discovered that 14% of the former had given birth to a low-birth-weight infant vs. 8% of the nonexposed women ($p < 0.05$) (2). In one investigation, when maternal drug use included both cocaine (or amphetamines) and narcotics, the infants ($N = 9$) had a significant reduction in birth weight, length, and head circumference compared to either stimulant or narcotic use alone (18). In an earlier report, no significant differences were observed in fetal growth parameters between groups of women consuming cocaine ($N = 12$), cocaine plus methadone ($N = 11$), methadone ($N = 15$), and noncocaine/nonmethadone controls ($N = 15$) (26). However, in a subsequent publication from these researchers, women who used cocaine throughout gestation (as opposed to those who only used it during the 1st trimester) were significantly more likely than drug-free controls to deliver low-birth-weight infants; 25% (13 of 52) vs. 5% (2 of 40) ($p < 0.003$), respectively (24). Fetal growth parameters (birth weight, length, and head circumference) were also significantly ($p < 0.001$) depressed compared to those of controls if the woman used cocaine throughout pregnancy (24). Exposure during the 1st trimester only resulted in reduced growth but the difference was not significant. Some investigators have suggested that the decrease in fetal growth in two studies may have been due to poor nutrition or to alcohol intake (40, 41). In both instances, however, women abusing alcohol either had been excluded or their exclusion would not have changed the findings (42, 43). In one study that found no statistical difference in birth weights between infants of cocaine users and noncocaine users, only 10 cocaine-exposed newborns were involved (28). The cocaine group had been identified from obstetric records of 102 consecutively delivered women. However, the sample size is very small and the character of cocaine use (e.g., dose, frequency, etc.) could not always be determined. In addition, recent research has shown that self-reporting of cocaine use probably underestimates actual usage (3, 4).

A single case of oligohydramnios at 17 weeks' gestation with increased serum α-fetoprotein levels (125 µg/L and 168 µg/L) has been described, but any relationship between these events and the mother's history of cocaine abuse is unknown (44). Intrauterine growth retardation was diagnosed at 26 weeks' gestation followed shortly thereafter by fetal death *in utero*. Analysis of fetal whole blood showed a cocaine level of 1 µg/ml, within the range associated with fatalities in adults (44).

In a prospective 1989 study involving 1226 mothers, 18% used cocaine as determined by interview or urine assay (3). After controlling for potentially confounding variables and other substance abuse, infants of women with positive urine assay for cocaine, compared to infants of nonusers, had lower birth weights (93 g less, $p = 0.07$), lengths (0.7 cm less, $p = 0.01$), and head circumferences (0.43 cm less, $p = 0.01$). The effect of cocaine on birth weight was even greater if prepregnancy weight and pregnancy weight gain were not considered. The mean reduction in infant birth weight was now 137 g vs. 93 g when these factors were considered ($p < 0.01$). In those cases where the history of cocaine use was positive but the urine assay was negative, no significant differences were found by multivariate analyses. The authors concluded that cocaine impaired fetal growth but that urine assays (or another biologic marker) were important to show the association (3).

Multiple ultrasound examinations (two to four) were used to evaluate fetal growth in a series of 43 women with primary addiction to cocaine (45). An additional 24 women were studied, but their ultrasound examinations were incomplete in one aspect or another and they were not included in the analysis. Careful attention was given to establishing gestational age. Complete ultrasonic parameters included biparietal diameter, femur length, and head and abdominal circumferences. The number of addicted infants with birth weight, head circumference, and femur length at the equal to or <50th, equal to or <25th, and equal to or <10th percentile ranks did not differ significantly from expected standard growth charts. However, the number of examinations yielding values for biparietal diameter and abdominal circumference at the equal to or <50th and equal to or <25th percentile ranks was significantly more than expected ($p = 0.001$). Since biparietal diameter and head circumference are not independent parameters, each being an indicator of fetal head size, the authors speculated that the most logical explanation for their findings was late-onset dolichocephalia (45). Based on these findings, the study concluded that maternal cocaine use had adversely affected fetal growth. If only birth weight had been used as a criterion, this effect may have been missed (45).

Several studies have included measurements of fetal distress in their research findings (11, 15–21, 23, 26, 31, 37, 39). In some reports, perinatal distress was significantly ($p < 0.05$) increased in cocaine abusers over women using heroin/ methadone (11, 12) and drug-free controls (19). Perinatal distress was also noted more frequently in other studies comparing cocaine users to drug-free controls (10% vs. 5.7% and 11.1% vs. 3.7%, respectively), but the differences were not significant (20, 21). Compared to nondrug users, higher rates of fetal tachycardia (2% vs. 0%) and bradycardia (17% vs. 6%) have been observed, but, again, the differences were not significant (18). One-minute Apgar scores were lower after *in utero* cocaine exposure in several studies (4, 15–17, 20, 23, 37), but only statistically significant in some (15–17, 23), and no different in another (25). In contrast, only two studies, one a series of three reports on the same group of patients, found a significant lowering of the 5-minute Apgar score (15–17, 25). Other studies observed no difference in this value (4, 20, 23, 26, 31, 37, 39). Significantly more ($p < 0.05$) meconium-stained infants were observed in studies comparing cocaine users to methadone-maintained women (25% vs. 8.2%) (10) and to noncocaine/other drug-exposed subjects (25% vs. 4%) (23). Three other studies observed nonsignificant increased rates of meconium staining or passage (22% vs. 17%, 29% vs. 23%, and 73% vs. 58%) (18, 20, 25), and a fourth reported a lower incidence (22% vs. 27%), compared to non-drug-using controls (21).

Eight reports have described perinatal or newborn cerebrovascular accidents and resulting brain damage in infants exposed *in utero* to cocaine (11, 14, 18, 46–50). The first report of this condition was published in 1986 (46). A mother, who had used an unknown amount of cocaine intranasally during the first 5 weeks of pregnancy and approximately 5 g during the 3 days before delivery, gave birth to a full-term, 3660-g male infant. The last dose of approximately 1 g had been consumed 15 hours before delivery. Fetal monitoring during the 12 hours before delivery showed tachycardia (180–200 beats/minute) and multiple variable decelerations. At birth, the infant was limp, he had a heart rate of 80 beats/minute, and thick meconium staining (without aspiration) was noted. Apnea, cyanosis, multiple focal seizures, intermittent tachycardia (up to 180 beats/minute), hypertension (up to 140 mm Hg by palpation), abnormalities in tone (both increased and decreased depending on the body part), and miotic pupils were noted beginning at 16 hours of age. Noncontrast computed tomography scan at 24 hours of age showed an acute infarction in the distribution of the left middle cerebral artery. Repeat scans showed a persistent left-sided infarct with increased gyral density (age 7 days) and a persistent area of focal encephalomalacia at the site of the infarction (age 2.5 months). One other infant with perinatal cerebral infarction associated with maternal cocaine use in the 48–72 hours prior to delivery has been mentioned by these investigators (11, 14, 24). A separate report described a mother who had used cocaine and multiple other abuse drugs during gestation who delivered a female infant (gestational age not specified) with bilateral cerebrovascular accident and resulting porencephaly (47). The infant expired at 2.5 months of age. In another study of 55 infants exposed to cocaine (with or without opiates), one infant with perinatal asphyxia had a cerebral infarction (18). A severely depressed male infant delivered at 38 weeks' gestation had an electroencephalogram and cranial ultrasound suggestive of hemorrhagic infarction (48). Follow-up during the neonatal period indicated mild to moderate neurodevelopmental abnormalities. Brain lesions were described in 39% (11 of 28) of infants with a positive urine assay for cocaine and in 33% (5 of 15) of newborns with a positive assay for methamphetamine (49). The brain injuries, which were not differentiated by drug type, were hemorrhagic infarction in the deep brain (six cases; three around the internal capsule/basal ganglion), cystic lesions in the deep brain (four cases), large posterior fossa hemorrhage (three cases), absent septum pellucidum with atrophy (one case), diffuse atrophy (one case), and brain edema (one case) (49). In a control group of 20 term infants with severe asphyxia, only one had a similar brain lesion. A second report also described brain lesions in infants exposed *in utero* to cocaine (50). The 11 infants all had major central nervous system (CNS) anomalies, and 10 of the infants also had craniofacial defects (described later). The CNS defects were hydranencephaly (one case), porencephaly (two cases), hypoplastic corpus callosum with unilateral parietal lobe cleft and heterotopias (one case), intraparenchymal hemorrhage (five cases), unilateral three-vessel hemispheric infarction (one case), and encephalomalacia (one case). In addition, three infants had arthrogryposis multiplex congenita of central origin (50). Four of the infants died, and the other seven had serious neurodevelopmental disabilities (50).

Echoencephalography (ECHO) was performed within 3 days of birth on 74 term (>37 weeks) infants who had tested positive for cocaine or methamphetamine, but who otherwise had uncomplicated perinatal courses (51). The infants had no other known risk factors for cerebral injury. The 74 newborns were classified into three groups: 32 (43%) cocaine exposed, 24 (32%) methamphetamine exposed, and 18 (24%) exposed to cocaine plus heroin or methadone, or both. Two comparison groups were formed: a group of 87 term, drug-free infants studied by ECHO because of clinical concerns for hypoxic-ischemic encephalopathy, and a normal group of 19 drug-free term newborns. Both groups of comparison infants were also studied by ECHO within 3 days of birth. Only one structural anomaly, consisting of an absent septum pellucidum, was observed in the infants examined. The affected newborn, exposed to methamphetamine, was also found to have bilateral optic nerve atrophy and diffuse attenuation of the white matter. Twenty-six (35.1%) of the drug-exposed infants had cranial abnormalities detected by ultrasonography, which was similar to the 27.6% (24 of 87) incidence in the ill comparison group ($p = 0.7$). The normal controls had an incidence of 5.3% (1 of 19) ($p < 0.01$ in comparison to both of the other groups). The lesions observed in the drug-exposed infants were intraventricular hemorrhage, echodensities known to be associated with necrosis, and cavitary lesions. Lesions were concentrated in the basal ganglion, frontal lobes, and posterior fossa (51). Cerebral infarction was found in two cocaine-exposed infants. The ECHO abnormalities were not predicted by standard neonatal clinical assessment and were believed to be consistent with those observed in adult abusers of cocaine and amphetamines (51).

Maternal cocaine abuse has been associated with numerous other congenital malformations. In a series of publications extending from 1985–1989, a group of investigators described the onset of ileal atresia (with bowel infarction in one) within the first 24 hours after birth in two infants and genitourinary tract malformations in nine infants (11, 13, 20, 24, 26). The abnormalities in the nine infants were prune belly syndrome with urethral obstruction, bilateral cryptorchidism (one also had absent digits 3 and 4 on the left hand and a second-degree hypospadias) (two males), female pseudohermaphroditism (one case) (defects included hydronephrosis, ambiguous genitalia with absent uterus and ovaries, anal atresia, absent digits 3 and 4 on the left hand, and clubfoot), secondary hypospadias (two cases), hydronephrosis (three cases), and unilateral hydronephrosis with renal infarction of the opposite kidney (one case). Data from the metropolitan Atlanta Birth Defects Case-Control study, involving 4929 liveborn and stillborn infants with major defects compared to 3029 randomly selected controls, showed a statistically significant association between cocaine use and urinary tract malformations (adjusted odds ratio 4.81, 95% confidence interval 1.15–20.14) (52, 53). The adjusted risk for anomalies of the genitalia was 2.27 (not statistically significant). Cocaine exposure for this analysis was based on self-reported use any time from 1 month before conception through the first 3 months of pregnancy (52, 53).

The rates of major congenital malformations in a study involving 50 cocaine-only users, 110 cocaine plus polydrug users, and 340 drug-free controls were 10% (five cases), 4.5% (five cases), and 2% (seven cases), respectively (4). The groups were classified by history and infant urine assays, and chronic alcohol abusers were excluded. The difference between the first and last groups was significant ($p < 0.01$). The incidence of minor abnormalities (e.g., hypertelorism, epicanthal folds, and micrognathia) was similar among the groups (5). Congenital heart defects were observed in all three groups as follows: transposition of the great arteries (one case), hypoplastic right heart syndrome (one case) (both cocaine-only), ventricular septal defects (three cases) (cocaine plus polydrug), ventricular septal defect (one case), patent ductus arteriosus (one case), pulmonary stenosis (one case) (three controls). Skull defects were observed in three infants in the cocaine-only group: exencephaly (stillborn), interparietal encephalocele, and parietal bone defects without herniation of meninges or cerebral tissue. One infant in the cocaine plus polydrug group had microcephalia. Significantly more major and minor malformations were seen in a group of cocaine-exposed infants ($N = 53$) (five major/four minor) than in a matched nonexposed sample ($N = 100$) (two major/four minor) ($p < 0.05$) (23). Congenital heart defects occurred in four of the cocaine-exposed infants: atrial septal defect (one case), ventricular septal defects (two cases), and cardiomegaly (one case). None of the infants born from controls had heart defects ($p < 0.01$). The authors noted, however, that their findings were weakened by the self-reported nature of the drug histories (23).

A 1989 report of 138 women at delivery with positive urine cocaine tests found 10 (7%) infants with congenital anomalies: ventricular septal defect (two), atrial septal defect (one), complete heart block (one), inguinal hernia (two), esophageal atresia (one), hypospadias (one), cleft lip and palate with trisomy 13 (one), and polydactyly (one) (4). Only two (2%) of 88 non-cocaine-using controls had congenital defects, but the difference between the two groups was not significant. When the cocaine group was divided into cocaine only (114 women) and cocaine plus other abuse drugs (24 women), five infants in each group were found to have a malformation. The difference between these subgroups was highly significant ($p < 0.005$).

Necrotizing enterocolitis has been described in two infants after *in utero* cocaine exposure (48). One of the infants was also exposed to heroin and methamphetamine. The proposed mechanism for the injuries was cocaine-induced ischemia of the fetal bowel followed by invasion of anaerobic bacteria (48). In another report, three newborns (two may have been described immediately above) presented with intestinal defects: one each with midcolonic atresia, ileal atresia, and widespread infarction of the bowel distal to the duodenum (54). Five other infants plus one of those with intestinal disruption had congenital limb reduction defects: unilateral terminal transverse defect (three), Poland sequence (i.e., unilateral defect of pectoralis muscle and syndactyly of hand (55)) and bilateral upper limb anomalies including ulnar ray deficiencies (one), bilateral radial ray defects (two) (54). The defects were thought to be due to cocaine-induced vascular disruption or hypoperfusion (54).

Facial defects seen in 10 of 11 infants exposed either to cocaine alone (6 of 11) or to cocaine plus other abuse drugs (5 of 11) included blepharophimosis (two), ptosis and facial diplegia (one), unilateral oro-orbital cleft (one), Pierre Robin anomaly (one), cleft palate (one), cleft lip and palate (one), skin tags (two), and cutis aplasia (one) (50). All of the infants had major brain abnormalities, which have been described above.

Ocular defects consisting of persistent hyperplastic primary vitreous in one eye and changes similar to those observed in retinopathy of prematurity in the other eye were described in a case report of an infant exposed throughout gestation to cocaine and multiple other abuse drugs (56). The association of the two defects was thought to be coincidental and not likely due to cocaine (56). Thirteen newborns with cocaine toxicity (each infant with multiple symptoms and positive urine assay) had a complete ophthalmic examination; six were discovered to have marked dilation and tortuosity of the iris vasculature (57). The five infants who were most severely affected were followed for at least 3 months and all showed a gradual resolution of the defects without apparent visual impairment. The transient iris vasculature defects have also been found in infants of diabetic mothers (both gestational and insulin-dependent) (58) and in non-cocaine-exposed controls (57, 59). However, the vascular changes have not yet been observed in infants of mothers abusing methadone, heroin, amphetamines, marijuana, or a combination of these drugs (specific data on the number of infants examined in these categories were not given) (58).

Two mothers who had used cocaine during the 1st trimester produced infants with unusual abnormalities (60, 61). Both mothers used other abuse drugs, heroin in one case and marijuana and methaqualone in the other. The anomalies observed were chromosome aneuploidy 45,X, bilaterally absent fifth toes, and features consistent with Turner's syndrome in one (60); multiple defects including hypothalamic hamartoblastoma in one (61). Hydrocephaly was noted in one infant (from a group of 10) exposed *in utero* to cocaine, marijuana, and amphetamines (28). No major anomalies were seen in eight infants exposed to cocaine (all had positive urine assays for cocaine) and other abuse drugs, but two infants had minor defects consisting of a sacral exostosis and capillary hemangioma in one, and a capillary hemangioma in the other (37). In the latter case, the mother claimed to have used cocaine only during the month preceding delivery. Cocaine was not considered a causative agent in any of these cases (28, 37, 60, 61).

In contrast to the above reports, no congenital abnormalities were observed in series of cocaine-exposed women totaling 55 (21), 39 (31), 56 (39), and 38 (62) subjects. A prospective 1989 study mentioned previously found cocaine metabolites in the urine assays from 114 (9.3%) of 1226 women (3). After controlling for the effects of other substances and maternal characteristics known to affect pregnancy outcome adversely, no significant association was found between cocaine and one or more minor anomalies, a constellation of three minor anomalies, or one major anomaly (3). An association with the latter two, however, was suggested by the data ($p = 0.10$) (3). Although animal data cannot be directly extrapolated to humans, administration of cocaine to pregnant rats and mice did not increase the incidence of congenital abnormalities (63).

Newborn infants who have been exposed *in utero* to cocaine may have significant neurobehavior impairment in the neonatal period. An increased degree of irritability, tremulousness, and muscular rigidity has been observed by a number of researchers (4, 11, 15–19, 21, 23, 26, 62, 64). Gastrointestinal symptoms (vomiting, diarrhea) have also been observed (4, 21). The onset of these symptoms usually occurs 1–2 days after birth with peak severity of symptoms occurring on days 2 and 3 (19, 21, 62, 64). Seizures, which may have been related to withdrawal, have been observed (14, 23). The overall incidence of severe withdrawal symptoms, however, is apparently not increased over that expected in opiate-addicted newborns (15–17). In one report that identified 138 infants whose mothers tested positive for cocaine, 24 (17%) of the mothers also tested positive for other abuse substances, usually opiates (4). The incidence of withdrawal in the cocaine-only group infants was 25% (28 of 114) vs. 54% (13 of 24) of the multiple abuse drug group ($p < 0.005$).

The Neonatal Behavior Assessment Scale (NBAS) has been employed in several studies to quantify the observed symptoms (11, 24, 26, 64). In a blinded study comparing infants of methadone-maintained women to those of cocaine-exposed women, the latter group had a significantly increased degree of irritability, tremulousness, and state lability ($p < 0.03$) (11). Expansion of this study to include drug-free controls and cluster analysis of the NBAS revealed that the cocaine group had significant impairment in state organization compared to either the opiate group infants or controls (24, 26). The NBAS was used to evaluate 16 term newborn infants with cocaine-positive urine assays (65). All demonstrated no to very poor visual attention and tracking, abnormal state regulation, and mild to moderate hypertonicity with decreased spontaneous movement (65). Flash evoked visual potentials were abnormal in 11 of 12 infants studied, and the disturbances remained in six infants studied at 4–6 months (65).

Ultrasound was used in a study published in 1989 to evaluate the behavior of 20 fetuses exposed to cocaine as a predictor of neonatal outcome (66). All fetuses were exposed to cocaine during the 1st trimester; four during the 1st trimester only, seven during the 1st and 2nd trimesters, and nine throughout gestation. The investigators were able to document that fetal state organization was predictive of newborn neurobehavioral well-being and state organization. In this study, the most frequent indicators of neurobehavioral well-being were excessive tremulousness of the extremities, unexplained tachypnea, or both (66). Abnormal state organization was shown by hyperresponsiveness and difficulty in arousal (66).

Electroencephalographic (EEG) abnormalities indicative of cerebral irritation have been documented in cocaine-exposed neonates (31, 64, 65). Normalization of the EEG abnormalities may require up to 12 months (31, 64).

Increased perinatal mortality was observed in a study published in 1989, although in comparison to controls, the higher incidence was not significant (4). Seven (5%) of 140 infants (138 mothers, two sets of twins) whose mothers tested positive for cocaine at delivery died compared to none of 88 infants whose mothers did not test positive for cocaine at delivery (50 vs. 0/1000, respectively). The seven cases included three intrauterine fetal deaths and four neonatal deaths.

An increased risk of sudden infant death syndrome (SIDS) has been suggested by three studies (11, 17, 67). Two infants, from a group of 50 exposed *in utero* to cocaine and methadone, died of SIDS, one at 1 month of age and the other at 3 months (17). It could not be determined if a relationship existed between the deaths and maternal cocaine use (17). In one study, 10 of 66 infants (15%) exposed to cocaine *in utero* died of SIDS over a 9–180-day interval (mean 46 days) following birth (11). This incidence was estimated to be approximately 30 times that observed in the general population and almost 4 times that seen in the infants of opiate-abusing women (11). Based on this experience, a prospective study was commenced and the results were reported in 1989 (67). Thirty-two infants of cocaine-using mothers were compared to 18 infants of heroin/methadone-addicted mothers. Eight of the mothers in the cocaine group also used heroin/methadone. The mothers of both groups received similar prenatal care, and they used similar amounts of alcohol, cigarettes, and marijuana. Infants in both groups were delivered at a gestational age of 38 weeks or more, and mean birth weight, length, and head circumference were identical. Cardiorespiratory recordings (pneumograms), conducted in most cases at 8–14 days of age, were abnormal in 13 infants, 12 cocaine exposed and 1 opiate exposed ($p < 0.05$). Five of the cocaine-exposed infants had an episode of life-threatening apnea of infancy requiring home resuscitation before the pneumograms could be performed. The 13 infants were treated with theophylline until age 6 months, or longer if the pneumogram had not yet normalized. No cases of SIDS were observed in any of the 50 infants. In an earlier study, pneumograms were used to quantify abnormal sleeping ventilatory patterns in infants of substance-abusing mothers (68). Of three cocaine-exposed infants, one had an abnormal pneumogram. Apnea and/or abnormal pneumograms were observed in 20 (14%) of 138 infants whose mothers tested positive for cocaine at delivery (4). None of the 88 control infants whose mothers tested negative for cocaine at delivery had apnea or abnormal pneumograms ($p < 0.0005$). In a large study examining the relationship between SIDS and cocaine exposure, one infant of 175 exposed to cocaine died from SIDS compared to four infants of 821 who were not exposed (36). The risks per 1000 in the two groups were similar, 5.6 and 4.9, respectively, corresponding to a relative risk for SIDS among infants of cocaine-abusing women of 1.17 (95% confidence interval 0.13, 10.43) (36). Based on these data, the study concluded that the increased rates reported previously probably reflected other risk factors that were independently associated with SIDS (36). However, since the study relied on self-reported cocaine use and urine screens (only detects recent exposure), some of the women may have been misclassified as nonusers (69). Analysis of the hair, where the drug accumulates for months, has been advocated as a technique to assure accurate assessment of past exposure (69).

Increased neonatal hospitalization in infants whose mothers tested positive for cocaine at delivery has been reported (4). In 137 infants (138 mothers, two sets of twins, three fetal deaths excluded), the mean days hospitalized was 19.2 compared to 5.1 for 88 infants of mothers who tested negative for cocaine at delivery ($p < 0.0001$). Moreover, the incidence of neonatal hospitalization for longer than 3 and 10 days were both significantly greater for the cocaine group (80% vs. 24%, respectively, $p < 0.00001$; and 35% vs. 10%, respectively, $p < 0.0005$). The implications of these findings on the limited resources available to hospitals are, obviously, very important.

In summary, the widespread abuse of cocaine has resulted in major toxicity in the mother, the fetus, and the newborn. The use of cocaine is often significantly correlated with the heavy use of other abuse drugs. Many of the studies reviewed here were unable completely to separate this usage in their patient populations or were unable to verify self-reported usage of cocaine, thus resulting in the possible misclassification of patients into the various groups. Whether the reported consequences of maternal cocaine exposure are due to these biases, to cocaine itself, to other drugs acting independently or in conjunction with cocaine, to poor lifestyles, or to other maternal characteristics is not presently clear. It is clear, however, that women who use cocaine during pregnancy are at significant risk for shorter gestations, premature delivery, spontaneous abortions, abruptio placentae, and death. The drug decreases uterine blood flow and induces uterine contractions. An increased risk may exist for premature rupture of the membranes but apparently not for placenta previa. The unborn children of these women may be growth retarded or severely distressed, and they are at risk for increased mortality. *In utero* cerebrovascular accidents with profound morbidity and mortality may occur. Congenital abnormalities involving the genitourinary tract, heart, limbs, and face may occur, and cocaine abuse should be considered teratogenic. Bowel atresias have also been observed in newborn infants, which may be due to intrauterine bowel infarctions. The exact mechanism of cocaine-induced malformations is presently uncertain, but it may be related to the placental vasoconstriction and fetal hypoxia produced by the drug with the resulting intermittent vascular disruptions and ischemia actually causing the fetal damage. Interactions with other drugs, however, may play a role. In addition to the above toxicities, the newborn child exposed to cocaine during gestation is at risk for severe neurobehavior and neurophysiologic abnormalities that may persist for months. An increased incidence of sudden infant death syndrome in the first few months after birth may also be a consequence of maternal cocaine abuse in conjunction with other factors. Long-term studies of cocaine-exposed children need to be completed before a true assessment of the damage caused by this drug can be determined.

[*Risk Factor X if nonmedicinal use.]

Breast Feeding Summary

Milk:plasma ratios of cocaine in human breast milk have not been determined. In one case, the urine of a normal, breast-fed, 6-week-old boy was positive for a cocaine metabolite (70). The mother was using an unspecified amount of cocaine. In another patient, a milk sample 12 hours after the last dose of approximately 0.5 g taken intranasally over 4 hours contained measurable levels (specific data not given) of cocaine and the metabolite, benzoylecgonine, that persisted until 36 hours after the dose (71). The 14-day-old infant was breast fed five times over the 4-hour period during which the mother ingested the cocaine. Approximately 3 hours after the first dose, the child became markedly irritable with onset of vomiting and diarrhea. Other symptoms observed upon examination were tremulousness, increased startle response, hyperactive Moro reaction, increased, symmetrical deep tendon reflexes with bilateral ankle clonus, and marked lability of mood (71). The irritability and tremulousness steadily improved over the next 48 hours. Large amounts of cocaine and the metabolite were found in the infant's urine 12 hours after the mother's last dose, which persisted until 60 hours postdose. On discharge (time not specified), the physical and neurologic examinations were normal. Additional follow-up of the infant was not reported.

In an unusual case report, a mother applied cocaine powder to her nipples to relieve soreness shortly before breast feeding her 11-day-old infant (72). Although a breast shield was used, the unsheathed nipple protruded to allow feeding. Three hours after feeding, the infant was found gasping, choking, and blue. Seizures, which occurred with other symptoms of acute cocaine ingestion, stopped 2 hours after admission to the hospital. The mother's milk was negative for cocaine and metabolites but the infant's urine was positive. Physical and neurologic examinations were normal on discharge 5 days later and again at 6 months. Computed tomography (CT) scan during hospitalization showed a small area of lucency in the left frontal lobe and an EEG at this time was abnormal. A repeat CT scan and EEG were normal at age 2 months.

Based on the toxicity exhibited in the infant after exposure via the milk, maternal cocaine use during breast feeding should be strongly discouraged and considered contraindicated. Obviously, mothers should also be warned against using the drug topically for nipple soreness. The American Academy of Pediatrics considers cocaine to be contraindicated during breast feeding (73).

References

1. Cregler LL, Mark H. Special report: medical complications of cocaine abuse. N Engl J Med 1986;315:1495–500.
2. Frank DA, Zuckerman BS, Amaro H, Aboagye K, Bauchner H, Cabral H, Fried L, Hingson R, Kayne H, Levenson SM, Parker S, Reece H, Vinci R. Cocaine use during pregnancy: prevalence and correlates. Pediatrics 1988;82:888–95.
3. Zuckerman B, Frank DA, Hingson R, Amaro H, Levenson SM, Kayne H, Parker S, Vinci R, Aboagye K, Fried LE, Cabral H, Timperi R, Bauchner H. Effects of maternal marijuana and cocaine use on fetal growth. N Engl J Med 1989;320:762–8.
4. Neerhof MG, MacGregor SN, Retzky SS, Sullivan TP. Cocaine abuse during pregnancy: peripartum prevalence and perinatal outcome. Am J Obstet Gynecol 1989;161:633–8.
5. Bingol N, Fuchs M, Diaz V, Stone RK, Gromisch DS. Teratogenicity of cocaine in humans. J Pediatr 1987;110:93–6.
6. Moore TR, Sorg J, Miller L, Key TC, Resnik R. Hemodynamic effects of intravenous cocaine on the pregnant ewe and fetus. Am J Obstet Gynecol 1986;155:883–8.
7. Foutz SE, Kotelko DM, Shnider SM, Thigpen JW, Rosen MA, Brookshire GL, Koike M, Levinson G, Elias-Baker B. Placental transfer and effects of cocaine on uterine blood flow and the fetus. Anesthesiology 1983;59:A422.
8. Woods JR Jr, Plessinger MA, Clark KE. Effect of cocaine on uterine blood flow and fetal oxygenation. JAMA 1987;257:957–61.
9. Wang CH, Schnoll SH. Prenatal cocaine use associated with down regulation of receptors in human placenta. Neurotoxicol Teratol 1987;9:301–4.
10. Wang CH, Schnoll SH. Prenatatal cocaine use associated with down regulation of receptors in human placenta. Natl Inst Drug Abuse Res Monogr Ser 1987;76:277.
11. Chasnoff IJ, Burns KA, Burns WJ. Cocaine use in pregnancy: perinatal morbidity and mortality. Neurotoxicol Teratol 1987;9:291–3.
12. Chasnoff IJ. Cocaine- and methadone-exposed infants: a comparison. Natl Inst Drug Abuse Res Monogr Ser 1987;76:278.
13. Chasnoff IJ, Chisum GM, Kaplan WE. Maternal cocaine use and genitourinary tract malformations. Teratology 1988;37:201–4.
14. Chasnoff I, MacGregor S. Maternal cocaine use and neonatal morbidity. Pediatr Res 1987;21:356A.
15. Ryan L, Ehrlich S, Finnegan L. Outcome of infants born to cocaine using drug dependent women. Pediatr Res 1986;20:209A.
16. Ryan L, Ehrlich S, Finnegan LP. Cocaine abuse in pregnancy: effects on the fetus and newborn. Natl Inst Drug Abuse Res Monogr Ser 1987;76:280.

17. Ryan L, Ehrlich S, Finnegan L. Cocaine abuse in pregnancy: effects on the fetus and newborn. Neurotoxicol Teratol 1987;9:295–9.
18. Oro AS, Dixon SD. Perinatal cocaine and methamphetamine exposure: maternal and neonatal correlates. J Pediatr 1987;111:571–8.
19. Dixon SD, Oro A. Cocaine and amphetamine exposure in neonates: perinatal consequences. Pediatr Res 1987;21:359A.
20. MacGregor SN, Keith LG, Chasnoff IJ, Rosner MA, Chisum GM, Shaw P, Minogue JP. Cocaine use during pregnancy: adverse perinatal outcome. Am J Obstet Gynecol 1987;157:686–90.
21. Cherukuri R, Minkoff H, Feldman J, Parekh A, Glass L. A cohort study of alkaloidal cocaine ("crack") in pregnancy. Obstet Gynecol 1988;72:147–51.
22. Chouteau M, Namerow PB, Leppert P. The effect of cocaine abuse on birth weight and gestational age. Obstet Gynecol 1988;72:351–4.
23. Little BB, Snell LM, Klein VR, Gilstrap LC III. Cocaine abuse during pregnancy: maternal and fetal implications. Obstet Gynecol 1989;73:157–60.
24. Chasnoff IJ, Griffith DR, MacGregor S, Dirkes K, Burns KA. Temporal patterns of cocaine use in pregnancy: perinatal outcome. JAMA 1989;261:1741–4.
25. Keith LG, MacGregor S, Friedell S, Rosner M, Chasnoff IJ, Sciarra JJ. Substance abuse in pregnant women: recent experience at the Perinatal Center for Chemical Dependence of Northwestern Memorial Hospital. Obstet Gynecol 1989;73:715–20.
26. Chasnoff IJ, Burns WJ, Schnoll SH, Burns KA. Cocaine use in pregnancy. N Engl J Med 1985;313:666–9.
27. Acker D, Sachs BP, Tracey KJ, Wise WE. Abruptio placentae associated with cocaine use. Am J Obstet Gynecol 1983;146:220–1.
28. Little BB, Snell LM, Palmore MK, Gilstrap LC III. Cocaine use in pregnant women in a large public hospital. Am J Perinatol 1988;5:206–7.
29. Townsend RR, Laing FC, Jeffrey RB Jr. Placental abruption associated with cocaine abuse. AJR 1988;150:1339–40.
30. Collins E, Hardwick RJ, Jeffery H. Perinatal cocaine intoxication. Med J Aust 1989;150:331–4.
31. Doberczak TM, Shanzer S, Senie RT, Kandall SR. Neonatal neurologic and electroencephalographic effects of intrauterine cocaine exposure. J Pediatr 1988;113:354–8.
32. Finnegan L. The dilemma of cocaine exposure in the perinatal period. Natl Inst Drug Abuse Res Monogr Ser 1988;81:379.
33. Thatcher SS, Corfman R, Grosso J, Silverman DG, DeCherney AH. Cocaine use and acute rupture of ectopic pregnancies. Obstet Gynecol 1989;74:478–9.
34. Henderson CE, Torbey M. Rupture of intracranial aneurysm associated with cocaine use during pregnancy. Am J Perinatol 1988;5:142–3.
35. Greenland VC, Delke I, Minkoff HL. Vaginally administered cocaine overdose in a pregnant woman. Obstet Gynecol 1989;74:476–7.
36. Bauchner H, Zuckerman B, McClain M, Frank D, Fried LE, Kayne H. Risk of sudden infant death syndrome among infants with in utero exposure to cocaine. J Pediatr 1988;113:831–4.
37. Madden JD, Payne TF, Miller S. Maternal cocaine abuse and effect on the newborn. Pediatrics 1986;77:209–11.
38. Fulroth R, Phillips B, Durand DJ. Perinatal outcome of infants exposed to cocaine and/or heroin in utero. Am J Dis Child 1989;143:905–10.
39. Hadeed AJ, Siegel SR. Maternal cocaine use during pregnancy: effect on the newborn infant. Pediatrics 1989;84:205–10.
40. Bauchner H, Zuckerman B, Amaro H, Frank DA, Parker S. Teratogenicity of cocaine. J Pediatr 1987;111:160–1.
41. Donvito MT. Cocaine use during pregnancy: adverse perinatal outcome. Am J Obstet Gynecol 1988;159:785–6.
42. Bingol N, Fuchs M, Diaz V, Stone RK, Gromisch DS. Teratogenicity of cocaine. Reply. J Pediatr 1987;111:161.
43. MacGregor SN. Cocaine use during pregnancy: adverse perinatal outcome. Reply. Am J Obstet Gynecol 1988;159:786.
44. Critchley HOD, Woods SM, Barson AJ, Richardson T, Lieberman BA. Fetal death in utero and cocaine abuse: case report. Br J Obstet Gynaecol 1988;95:195–6.
45. Mitchell M, Sabbagha RE, Keith L, MacGregor S, Mota JM, Minoque J. Ultrasonic growth parameters in fetuses of mothers with primary addiction to cocaine. Am J Obstet Gynecol 1988;159:1104–9.

46. Chasnoff IJ, Bussey ME, Savich R, Stack CM. Perinatal cerebral infarction and maternal cocaine use. J Pediatr 1986;108:456–9.
47. Tenorio GM, Nazvi M, Bickers GH, Hubbird RH. Intrauterine stroke and maternal polydrug abuse. Clin Pediatr 1988;27:565–7.
48. Telsey AM, Merrit TA, Dixon SD. Cocaine exposure in a term neonate: necrotizing enterocolitis as a complication. Clin Pediatr 1988;27:547–50.
49. Dixon SD, Bejar R. Brain lesions in cocaine and methamphetamine exposed neonates. Pediatr Res 1988;23:405A.
50. Kobori JA, Ferriero DM, Golabi M. CNS and craniofacial anomalies in infants born to cocaine abusing mothers. Clin Res 1989;37:196A.
51. Dixon SD, Bejar R. Echoencephalographic findings in neonates associated with maternal cocaine and methamphetamine use: incidence and clinical correlates. J Pediatr 1989;115:770–8.
52. Chavez GF, Mulinare J, Cordero JF. Maternal cocaine use and the risk for genitourinary tract defects: an epidemiologic approach. Am J Hum Genet 1988;43 (Suppl):A43.
53. Chavez GF, Mulinare J, Cordero JF. Maternal cocaine use during early pregnancy as a risk factor for congenital urogenital anomalies. JAMA 1989;262:795–8.
54. Hoyme HE, Jones KL, Dixon SD, Jewett T, Hanson JW, Robinson LK, Msall ME, Allanson J. Maternal cocaine use and fetal vascular disruption. Am J Hum Genet 1988;43 (Suppl):A56.
55. Smith DW, Jones KL. Recognizable Patterns of Human Malformations, ed 3. Philadelphia:WB Saunders, 1982:224.
56. Teske MP, Trese MT. Retinopathy of prematurity-like fundus and persistent hyperplastic primary vitreous associated with maternal cocaine use. Am J Ophthalmol 1987;103:719–20.
57. Isenberg SJ, Spierer A, Inkelis SH. Ocular signs of cocaine intoxication in neonates. Am J Ophthalmol 1987;103:211–4.
58. Ricci B, Molle F. Ocular signs of cocaine intoxication in neonates. Am J Ophthalmol 1987;104:550–1.
59. Isenberg SJ, Inkelis SH, Spierer A. Ocular signs of cocaine intoxication in neonates. Reply. Am J Ophthalmol 1987;104:551.
60. Kushnick T, Robinson M, Tsao C. 45,X chromosome abnormality in the offspring of a narcotic addict. Am J Dis Child 1972;124:772–3.
61. Huff DS, Fernandes M. Two cases of congenital hypothalamic hamartoblastoma, polydactyly, and other congenital anomalies (Pallister-Hall syndrome). N Engl J Med 1982;306:430–1.
62. LeBlanc PE, Parekh AJ, Naso B, Glass L. Effects of intrauterine exposure to alkaloidal cocaine ("crack"). Am J Dis Child 1987;141:937–8.
63. Fantel AG, MacPhail BJ. The teratogenicity of cocaine. Teratology 1982;26:17–9.
64. Doberczak TM, Shanzer S, Kandall SR. Neonatal effects of cocaine abuse in pregnancy. Pediatr Res 1987;21:359A.
65. Dixon SD, Coen RW, Crutchfield S. Visual dysfunction in cocaine-exposed infants. Pediatr Res 1987;21:359A.
66. Hume RF Jr, O'Donnell KJ, Staner CL, Killam AP, Gingras JL. In utero cocaine exposure: observations of fetal behavioral state may predict neonatal outcome. Am J Obstet Gynecol 1989;161:685–90.
67. Chasnoff IJ, Hunt CE, Kletter R, Kaplan D. Prenatal cocaine exposure is associated with respiratory pattern abnormalities. Am J Dis Child 1989;143:583–7.
68. Davidson Ward SL, Schuetz S, Krishna V, Bean X, Wingert W, Wachsman L, Keens TG. Abnormal sleeping ventilatory pattern in infants of substance-abusing mothers. Am J Dis Child 1986;140:1015–20.
69. Graham K, Koren G. Maternal cocaine use and risk of sudden infant death. J Pediatr 1989;115:333.
70. Shannon M, Lacouture PG, Roa J, Woolf A. Cocaine exposure among children seen at a pediatric hospital. Pediatrics 1989;83:337–42.
71. Chasnoff IJ, Lewis DE, Squires L. Cocaine intoxication in a breast-fed infant. Pediatrics 1987;80:836–8.
72. Chaney NE, Franke J, Wadlington WB. Cocaine convulsions in a breast-feeding baby. J Pediatr 1988;112:134–5.
73. Committee on Drugs, American Academy of Pediatrics. Transfer of drugs and other chemicals into human milk. Pediatrics 1989;84;924–36.

Name: **CODEINE**

Class: **Narcotic Analgesic/Antitussive**   Risk Factor: **C***

Fetal Risk Summary

The Collaborative Perinatal Project monitored 50,282 mother-child pairs, 563 of which had 1st trimester exposure to codeine (1, pp. 287–295). No evidence was found to suggest a relationship to large categories of major or minor malformations. Associations were found with six individual defects (1, pp. 287–295, 471). Only the association with respiratory malformation is statistically significant. The significance of the other associations is unknown. However, independent confirmation is required for all associations found in this study.

Respiratory (8 cases)
Genitourinary (other than hypospadias) (7 cases)
Down's syndrome (1 case)
Tumors (4 cases)
Umbilical hernia (3 cases)
Inguinal hernia (12 cases)

For use anytime during pregnancy, 2522 exposures were recorded (1, p. 434). With the same qualifications, possible associations with four individual defects were found (1, p. 484):

Hydrocephaly (7 cases)
Pyloric stenosis (8 cases)
Umbilical hernia (7 cases)
Inguinal hernia (51 cases)

In an investigation of 1427 malformed newborns compared to 3001 controls, 1st trimester use of narcotic analgesics (codeine most common) was associated with inguinal hernias, cardiac and circulatory system defects, cleft lip and palate, dislocated hip and other musculoskeletal defects (2). Second trimester use was associated with alimentary tract defects. In a large retrospective Finnish study, the use of opiates (mainly codeine) during the 1st trimester was associated with an increased risk of cleft lip and palate (3, 4). Finally, a survey of 390 infants with congenital heart disease matched with 1254 normal infants found a higher rate of exposure to several drugs, including codeine, in the offspring with defects (5). Although all four of these studies contain several possible biases that could have affected the results, the data serve as a possible warning that indiscriminate use of codeine may present a risk to the fetus.

Use of codeine during labor produces neonatal respiratory depression to the same degree as other narcotic analgesics (6). The first known case of neonatal codeine addiction was described in 1965 (7). The mother had taken analgesic tablets containing 360–480 mg of codeine/day for 8 weeks prior to delivery.

A second report described neonatal codeine withdrawal in two infants of nonaddicted mothers (8). The mother of one infant began consuming a codeine cough medication 3 weeks prior to delivery. Approximately 2 weeks before delivery, analgesic tablets with codeine were taken at a frequency of up to six tablets/day (48 mg of codeine/day). The second mother was treated with a codeine cough medication consuming 90–120 mg of codeine/day for the last 10 days of pregnancy. Apgar scores of both infants were 8–10 at 1 and 5 minutes. Typical symptoms of narcotic withdrawal were noted in the infants shortly after birth but not in the mothers.

[*Risk Factor D if used for prolonged periods or in high doses at term.]

Breast Feeding Summary

Codeine passes into breast milk in very small amounts that are probably insignificant (9–11). The American Academy of Pediatrics considers codeine to be compatible with breast feeding (12).

References

1. Heinonen OP, Slone D, Shapiro S. *Birth Defects and Drugs in Pregnancy*. Littleton:Publishing Sciences Group, 1977.
2. Bracken MB, Holford TR. Exposure to prescribed drugs in pregnancy and association with congenital malformations. Obstet Gynecol 1981;58:336–44.
3. Saxen I. Associations between oral clefts and drugs taken during pregnancy. Int J Epidemiol 1975;4;37–44.
4. Saxen I. Epidemiology of cleft lip and palate: an attempt to rule out chance correlations. Br J Prev Soc Med 1975;29:103–10.
5. Rothman KJ, Fyler DC, Goldblatt A, Kreidberg MB. Exogeneous hormones and other drug exposures of children with congenital heart disease. Am J Epidemiol 1979;109:433–9.
6. Bonica JJ. *Principles and Practice of Obstetric Analgesia and Anesthesia*. Philadelphia:FA Davis, 1967:245.
7. Van Leeuwen G, Guthrie R, Stange F. Narcotic withdrawal reaction in a newborn infant due to codeine. Pediatrics 1965;36;635–6.
8. Mangurten HH, Benawra R. Neonatal codeine withdrawal in infants of nonaddicted mothers. Pediatrics 1980;65:159–60.
9. Kwit NT, Hatcher RA. Excretion of drugs in milk. Am J Dis Child 1935;49:900–4.
10. Horning MG, Stillwell WG, Nowlin J, Lertratanangkoon K, Stillwell RN, Hill RM. Identification and quantification of drugs and drug metabolites in human breast milk using GC-MS-COM methods. Mod Probl Paediatr 1975;15:73–9.
11. Anonymous. Drugs in breast milk. Med Lett Drugs Ther 1974;16:25–7.
12. Committee on Drugs, American Academy of Pediatrics. Transfer of drugs and other chemicals into human milk. Pediatrics 1989;84:924–36.

Name: **COLCHICINE**

Class: **Metaphase Inhibitor**   Risk Factor: **C$_M$**

Fetal Risk Summary

The original reports of colchicine cytogenetic effects have not been confirmed with recent studies (1, 2). Human lymphocytic cultures of cells have shown chromosomal damage when exposed to colchicine. No relationship between teratogenic effects and this damage has been established. Use of colchicine by the father prior to conception has been associated with teratogenicity (atypical Down's syndrome) (1). Other investigators were unable to find teratogenic or cytogenetic effects in 19 male and 19 female subjects (3). Colchicine may or may not cause azoospermia (4, 5). Until colchicine safety is established, the drug should be avoided during the reproductive years.

Breast Feeding Summary

No data are available.

References

1. Cestari AN, Vieira Filho JP, Yonenaga Y. A case of human reproductive abnormalities possibly induced by colchicine treatment. Rev Bras Biol 1965;25:253–6.
2. Serreira NR, Buoniconti A. Trisomy after colchicine therapy. Lancet 1968;2:1304.
3. Cohen MM, Levy M, Eliakim M. A cytogenetic evaluation of long-term colchicine therapy in the treatment of familial Mediterranean fever (FMF). Am J Med Sci 1977;274:147–52.
4. Merlin HE. Azoospermia caused by colchicine—a case report. Fertil Steril 1972;23:180–1.
5. Bremer WJ, Paulsen CA. Colchicine and testicular function in man. N Engl J Med 1976;294:1384–5.

Name: **COLISTIMETHATE**

Class: **Antibiotic**   Risk Factor: **B**

Fetal Risk Summary

No reports linking the use of colistimethate with congenital defects have been located. The drug crosses the placenta at term (1).

Breast Feeding Summary

Colistimethate is excreted into breast milk. The milk:plasma ratio is 0.17–0.18 (2). While this level is low, three potenital problems exist for the nursing infant: modification of bowel flora, direct effects on the infant, and interference with the interpretation of culture results if a fever workup is required.

References

1. MacAulay MA, Charles D. Placental transmission of colistimethate. Clin Pharmacol Ther 1967;8:578–86.
2. Wilson JT. Milk/plasma ratios and contraindicated drugs. In Wilson JT, ed. Drugs in Breast Milk. Balgowlah, Australia:ADIS Press, 1981:78–9.

Name: **CORTICOTROPIN/COSYNTROPIN**

Class: **Corticosteroid Stimulating Hormone**   Risk Factor: **C**

Fetal Risk Summary

Studies reporting the use of corticotropin in pregnancy have not demonstrated adverse fetal effects (1–4). However, corticosteroids have been suspected of causing malformations (see Cortisone). Since corticotropin stimulates the release of endogenous corticosteroids, this relationship should be considered when prescribing the drug to women in their reproductive years.

Breast Feeding Summary

No data are available.

References

1. Johnstone FD, Campbell S. Adrenal response in pregnancy to long-acting tetracosactrin. J Obstet Gynaecol Br Commonw 1974;81:363–7.
2. Simmer HH, Tulchinsky D, Gold EM, et al. On the regulation of estrogen production by cortisol and ACTH in human pregnancy at term. Am J Obstet Gynecol 1974;119:283–96.
3. Aral K, Kuwabara Y, Okinaga S. The effect of adrenocorticotropic hormone and dexamethasone, administered to the fetus *in utero*, upon maternal and fetal estrogens. Am J Obstet Gynecol 1972;113:316–22.
4. Potert AJ. Pregnancy and adrenalcortical hormones. Br Med J 1962;2:967–72.

Name: **CORTISONE**

Class: **Corticosteroid** Risk Factor: **D**

Fetal Risk Summary

Since cortisone is often used during pregnancy, reports of congenital defects are reflective of a much greater utilization of cortisone and not necessarily of a more potent teratogen than other glucocorticoids (see Prednisolone, Betamethasone, Dexamethasone, Corticotropin). The Collaborative Perinatal Project monitored 50,282 mother-child pairs, 34 of which had 1st trimester exposure to cortisone (1). No evidence of a relationship to congenital malformations was found. In 35 other reported cases of 1st trimester exposure, congenital defects were observed in nine infants (2–7): cataracts, cyclopia, interventricular septal defect, gastroschisis, hydrocephalus, cleft lip, coarctation of the aorta, clubfoot, and undescended testicles. Concern has been expressed that neonatal adrenal hyperplasia or insufficiency may result from maternal corticosteroid administration (8; R.K. Freeman, unpublished data, 1982).

Breast Feeding Summary

No data are available.

References

1. Heinonen OP, Slone D, Shapiro S. *Birth Defects and Drugs in Pregnancy*. Littleton:Publishing Sciences Group, 1977:389, 391.
2. Kraus AM. Congenital cataract and maternal steroid ingestion. J Pediatr Ophthalmol 1975;12:107.
3. Khudr G, Olding L. Cyclopia. Am J Dis Child 1973;125:102.
4. deVilliers DM. Kortisoon swangerskap en die ongebore kind. S Afr Med J 1967;41:781–2.
5. Malaps P. Foetal malformation and cortisone therapy. Br Med J 1965;1:795.
6. Harris JWS, Poss IP. Cortisone therapy in early pregnancy. Relation to cleft palate. Lancet 1956;1:1045–7.
7. Wells CN. Treatment of hyperemesis gravidarium with cortisone. I. Fetal results. Am J Obstet Gynecol 1953;66:598–601.
8. Sidhu RK, Hawkins DF. Corticosteroids. Clin Obstet Gynecol 1981;8:383–404.

Name: **COUMARIN DERIVATIVES**

Class: **Anticoagulant**   Risk Factor: **D**

Fetal Risk Summary

The use of coumarin derivatives during pregnancy may result in significant problems for the fetus and newborn. Since the first case of fetal coumarin embryopathy was described by DiSaia in 1966 (1), a large volume of literature has accumulated. Hall and co-workers (2) reviewed this subject in 1980 (167 references). In the 3 years following this review, a number of other reports have appeared (3–12). The principal problems confronting the fetus and newborn are:

Embryopathy (fetal warfarin syndrome)
Central nervous system defects
Spontaneous abortion
Stillbirth
Prematurity
Hemorrhage

First trimester use of coumarin derivatives may result in the fetal warfarin syndrome (FWS) (1–4). The common characteristics of the FWS are nasal hypoplasia due to failure of development of the nasal septum and stippled epiphyses. The bridge of the nose is depressed, resulting in a flattened, upturned appearance. Neonatal respiratory distress occurs frequently due to upper airway obstruction. Other features that may be present are:

Birth weight less than 10th percentile for gestational age
Eye defects (blindness, optic atrophy, microphthalmia) when drug also used in
   2nd and 3rd trimesters
Hypoplasia of the extremities (ranging from severe rhizomelic dwarfing to dys-
   trophic nails and shortened fingers)
Developmental retardation
Seizures
Scoliosis
Deafness/hearing loss
Congenital heart disease
Death

The critical period of exposure, based on Hall and co-workers (2), seems to be the 6th-9th weeks of gestation. All of the known cases of FWS were exposed during at least a portion of these weeks. Exposure after the 1st trimester carries the risk of central nervous system defects. No constant grouping of abnormalities was observed, nor was there an apparent correlation between time of exposure and the defects, except that all fetuses were exposed in the 2nd and/or 3rd trimesters. After elimination of those cases that were probably due to late fetal or neonatal hemorrhage, the central nervous system defects in 13 infants were thought to represent deformations that occurred as a result of abnormal growth arising from an earlier fetal hemorrhage and subsequent scarring (2). Two patterns were recognized:

Dorsal midline dysplasia characterized by agenesis of corpus callosum, Dandy-Walker malformations, and midline cerebellar atrophy; encephaloceles may be present

Ventral midline dysplasia characterized by optic atrophy (eye anomalies)

Other features of central nervous system damage in the 13 infants were:

Mental retardation (13 of 13)
Blindness (7 of 13)
Spasticity (4 of 13)
Seizures (3 of 13)
Deafness (1 of 13)
Scoliosis (1 of 13)
Growth failure (1 of 13)
Death (3 of 13)

Long-term effects in the children with central nervous system defects were more significant and debilitating than those from the fetal warfarin syndrome (2).

Fetal outcomes for the 463 cases of *in utero* exposure to coumarin derivatives reported through 1983 are summarized below (2–12):

1ST TRIMESTER EXPOSURE (263):
    Normal infants — 167 (63%)
    Spontaneous abortions — 41 (16%)
    Stillborn/neonatal death — 17 (6%)
    FWS — 27 (10%)
    CNS/other defects — 11 (4%)
2ND/3RD TRIMESTER EXPOSURE (208):
    Normal infants — 175 (84%)
    Spontaneous abortions — 4 (2%)
    Stillborn/neonatal death — 19 (9%)
    CNS/other defects — 10 (5%)
TOTAL INFANTS EXPOSED (471):
    Normal infants — 342 (73%)
    Spontaneous abortions — 45 (10%)
    Stillborn/neonatal death — 36 (8%)
    FWS/CNS/other defects — 48 (10%)

Hemorrhage was observed in 11 (3%) of the normal newborns (premature and term). Two of the patients in the 2nd/3rd trimester group were treated with the coumarin derivatives phenprocoumon and nicoumalone. Both infants were normal.

Congenital abnormalities that did not fit the pattern of the FWS or central nervous system defects were reported in 10 infants (2, 9). These were thought to be incidental malformations that were probably not related to the use of coumarin derivatives (see also three other cases, in which the relationship to coumarin derivatives is unknown, described in the text below, references 16, 20 and 22).

Asplenia, two-chambered heart, agenesis of pulmonary artery
Anencephaly, spina bifida, congenital absence of clavicles
Congenital heart disease, death
Fetal distress, focal motor seizures
Bilateral polydactyly
Congenital corneal leukoma
Nonspecified multiple defects
Asplenia, congenital heart disease, incomplete rotation of gut, short broad pha-
    langes, hypoplastic nails
Single kidney, toe defects, other anomalies, death
Cleft palate

A 1984 study examined 22 children, with a mean age of 4.0 years, who were exposed *in utero* to warfarin (13). Physical and mental development of the children was comparable to that of matched controls.

Since publication of the above data, a number of additional reports and studies have appeared describing the outcomes of pregnancies treated at various times with coumarin derivatives (14–22). The largest series involved 156 women with cardiac valve prostheses who had 223 pregnancies (14). Over a period of 19 years, the women were grouped based on evolving treatment regimens: group I — 68 pregnancies treated with acenocoumarol until the diagnosis of pregnancy was made, and then treated with dipyridamole and/or aspirin; group II — 128 pregnancies treated with acenocoumarol throughout gestation; group III — 12 pregnancies treated with acenocoumarol, except when heparin was substituted from pregnancy diagnosis to the 13th week of gestation, and again from the 38th week until delivery; and group IV — 15 pregnancies in women with biologic prostheses who were not treated with anticoagulant therapy. The fetal outcomes in the four groups were: spontaneous abortions 10.3% vs. 28.1% vs. 0% vs. 0% ($p <$ 0.0005); stillbirths 7.4% vs. 7.1% vs. 0% vs. 6.7%; and neonatal deaths 0% vs. 2.3% vs. 0% vs. 0%. (See reference for maternal outcomes in the various groups.) Of the 38 children examined in group II, 3 (7.9%) had features of the FWS.

In a subsequent report from these investigators, the outcomes of 72 pregnancies followed prospectively were described in 1986 (15). The pregnancies were categorized into three groups according to the anticoagulant therapy: group I — 23 pregnancies treated with acenocoumarol except for heparin from the 6th–12th weeks of gestation; group II — 12 pregnancies treated the same as group I except that heparin treatment was started after the 7th week; and group III — 37 pregnancies treated with acenocoumarol throughout gestation (pregnancies in this group were not detected until after the 1st trimester). In most patients, heparin was substituted for the coumarin derivative after the 38th week of gestation. The fetal outcomes in the three groups were: spontaneous abortions 8.7% vs. 25% vs. 16.2%; and stillbirths 0% vs. 8.3% vs. 0%. Not all of the infants born to the mothers were examined, but of those that were, the FWS was observed in 0% of group I (0 of 19), 25.0% of group II (2 of 8), and 29.6% of group III (8 of 27). Thus, 10 (28.6%) of the 35 infants examined who were exposed at least during the first 7 weeks of gestation had warfarin embryopathy.

A 1983 report described 14 pregnancies in 13 women with a prosthetic heart valve who were treated throughout pregnancy with warfarin (16). Two patients had spontaneous abortions, two delivered premature stillborn infants (one infant had anencephaly), and two newborns died during the neonatal period. The total fetal/neonatal mortality in this series was 43%. Other defects noted were corneal changes in two, bradydactyly and dysplastic nails in two, and nasal hypoplasia in one.

In 18 pregnancies of 16 women with an artificial heart valve, heparin was substituted for warfarin when pregnancy was diagnosed (between 6–8 weeks after the last menstrual period) and continued until the 13th week of gestation (17). Nine of the 18 pregnancies aborted, but none of the nine liveborn infants had congenital anomalies or other complications.

Five reports have described single cases of exposure to warfarin during pregnancy (18–22). A woman with Marfan's syndrome had replacement of her aortic arch and valve combined with coronary artery bypass performed during the 1st week of her pregnancy (1–8 days after conception) (18). She was treated with warfarin throughout gestation. A normal female infant was delivered by elective cesarean section at 34 weeks' gestation. Warfarin was used to treat a deep vein thrombosis during the 3rd trimester in a 34-year-old woman because of heparin-induced maternal thrombocytopenia (19). A normal infant was delivered at term. In another case involving a woman with a deep vein thrombosis that had occurred before the present pregnancy, warfarin therapy was continued through the first 14 weeks of gestation (20). At term, a 3660-g infant was delivered who did not breathe and who died after 35 minutes. At autopsy, an almost total agenesis of the left diaphragm and hypoplasia of both lungs were noted. The relationship between warfarin and the defect is unknown.

The use of warfarin to treat a deep vein thrombosis associated with circulating lupus anticoagulant during pregnancy has been described (21). Therapy was started after the 9th week of gestation. Because of severe pregnancy-induced hypertension, an 1830-g female infant was delivered by cesarean section at 31 weeks. No information was provided about the condition of the infant.

A woman with a mitral valve replacement 8 months prior to pregnancy was treated continuously with warfarin until 6 weeks after her last menstrual period (22). Warfarin was then stopped and except for cigarette smoking, no other drugs were taken during the pregnancy. A growth-retarded (2340 g, 3rd percentile; 50 cm length, 50th percentile; 35 cm head circumference, 50th percentile) female infant was delivered at term. Congenital abnormalities noted in the infant were triangular face with broad forehead, micrognathia, microglossia, hypoplastic finger- and toenails, and hypoplasia of the distal phalanges. No epiphyseal stippling was seen on a skeletal survey. A normal female karyotype, 46,XX was found on chromosome analysis. Psychomotor development was normal at 1 year of age but physical growth remained retarded (3rd percentile). The authors concluded that the pattern of defects represented the earliest teratogenic effects of warfarin, but they could not exclude a chance association with the drug.

In summary, the use of coumarin derivatives during the 1st trimester carries with it a significant risk to the fetus. For all cases, only about 70% of pregnancies are expected to result in a normal infant. Exposure in the 6th-9th weeks of gestation may produce a pattern of defects termed the fetal warfarin syndrome with an incidence up to 25% or greater in some series. Infants exposed before and after this period have had other congenital anomalies, but the relationship between warfarin and these defects is unknown. Infrequent central nervous system defects, which have greater clinical significance to the infant than the defects of the fetal warfarin syndrome, may be deformations related to hemorrhage and scarring with subsequent impaired growth of brain tissue. Spontaneous abortions, still-births, and neonatal deaths may also occur. If the mother's condition requires anticoagulation, the use of heparin from the start of the 6th gestational week through the end of the 12th gestational week, and again at term, may lessen the risk to the fetus of adverse outcome.

Breast Feeding Summary

Excretion of coumarin derivatives into breast milk is dependent on the agent used. Three reports on warfarin have been located totaling 28 lactating women (23–25). Doses ranged between 2–12 mg/day in 13 patients with serum levels varying from 1.6–8.5 μmol/L (23). Warfarin was not detected in the milk of these patients. Maternal dosages or levels were not provided in the other reports (24, 25). No warfarin was detected in the serum of any of the 28 breast-fed infants. Also, no effects on the bleeding time were found in the 18 infants in whom the test was performed (23–25).

Exposure to ethyl biscoumacetate in milk resulted in bleeding in 5 of 42 exposed infants in one report (26). The maternal dosage was not given. An unidentified metabolite was found in the milk that may have led to the high complication rate. A 1959 study measured ethyl biscoumacetate levels in 38 milk specimens obtained from four women taking 600–1200 mg/day (27). The drug was detected in only 13 samples with levels varying from 0.09–1.69 μg/ml. No correlation could be found between the milk concentrations and the dosage or time of administration. A total of 22 infants were breast fed from these and other mothers receiving ethyl biscoumacetate. No adverse effects were observed in the infants, but coagulation tests were not conducted.

Over 1600 postpartum women were treated with dicumarol to prevent thromboembolic complications in a 1950 study (28). Doses were titrated to adjust the prothrombin clotting time to 40–50% of normal. No adverse effects or any change in prothrombin times were noted in any of the nursing infants.

Phenindione use in a lactating woman resulted in a massive scrotal hematoma and wound oozing in a 1½-month-old breast-fed infant shortly after a herniotomy was performed (29). The mother was taking 50 mg every morning and alternating 50 mg/25 mg every night for suspected pulmonary embolism that developed post-partum. Milk levels varying from 1–5 μg/ml have been reported after 50- or 75-mg single doses of phenindione (30). When the dose was 25 mg, only 18 of 68 samples contained detectable amounts of the anticoagulant.

In summary, maternal warfarin consumption apparently does not pose a significant risk to normal, full-term, breast-fed infants. Other oral anticoagulants should be avoided by the lactating woman. The American Academy of Pediatrics considers phenindione (which is not used in the United States) to be contraindicated during breast feeding because of the risk of hemorrhage in the infant (31). Both warfarin and dicumarol (bishydroxycoumarin) are classified by the Academy to be compatible with breast feeding (31).

References

1. DiSaia PJ. Pregnancy and delivery of a patient with a Starr-Edwards mitral valve prosthesis. Obstet Gynecol 1966;28:469–71.
2. Hall JG, Pauli RM, Wilson KM. Maternal and fetal sequelae of anticoagulation during pregnancy. Am J Med 1980;68:122–40.

3. Baillie M, Allen ED, Elkington AR. The congenital warfarin syndrome: a case report. Br J Ophthalmol 1980;64:633–5.
4. Harrod MJE, Sherrod PS. Warfarin embryopathy in siblings. Obstet Gynecol 1981;57:673–6.
5. Russo R, Bortolotti U, Schivazappa L, Girolami A. Warfarin treatment during pregnancy: a clinical note. Haemostasis 1979;8:96–8.
6. Biale Y, Cantor A, Lewenthal H, Gueron M. The course of pregnancy in patients with artificial heart valves treated with dipyridamole. Int J Gynaecol Obstet 1980;18:128–32.
7. Moe N. Anticoagulant therapy in the prevention of placental infarction and perinatal death. Obstet Gynecol 1982;59:481–3.
8. Kaplan LC, Anderson GG, Ring BA. Congenital hydrocephalus and Dandy-Walker malformation associated with warfarin use during pregnancy. Birth Defects 1982;18:79–83.
9. Chen WWC, Chan CS, Lee PK, Wang RYC, Wong VCW. Pregnancy in patients with prosthetic heart valves: an experience with 45 pregnancies. Q J Med 1982;51:358–65.
10. Vellenga E, Van Imhoff GW, Aarnoudse JG. Effective prophylaxis with oral anticoagulants and low-dose heparin during pregnancy in an antithrombin III deficient woman. Lancet 1983;2:224.
11. Michiels JJ, Stibbe J, Vellenga E, Van Vliet HHDM. Prophylaxis of thrombosis in antithrombin III-deficient women during pregnancy and delivery. Eur J Obstet Gynecol Reprod Biol 1984;18:149–53.
12. Oakley C. Pregnancy in patients with prosthetic heart valves. Br Med J 1983;286:1680–3.
13. Chong MKB, Harvey D, De Swiet M. Follow-up study of children whose mothers were treated with warfarin during pregnancy. Br J Obstet Gynaecol 1984;91:1070–3.
14. Salazar E, Zajarias A, Gutierrez N, Iturbe I. The problem of cardiac valve prostheses, anticoagulants, and pregnancy. Circulation 1984;70(Suppl 1):I169–I77.
15. Iturbe-Alessio I, Fonseca MDC, Mutchinik O, Santos MA, Zajarias A, Salazar E. Risks of anticoagulant therapy in pregnant women with artificial heart valves. N Engl J Med 1986;315:1390–3.
16. Sheikhzadeh A, Ghabusi P, Hakim S, Wendler G, Sarram M, Tarbiat S. Congestive heart failure in valvular heart disease in pregnancies with and without valvular prostheses and anticoagulant therapy. Clin Cardiol 1983;6:465–70.
17. Lee P-K, Wang RYC, Chow JSF, Cheung K-L, Wong VCW, Chan T-K. Combined use of warfarin and adjusted subcutaneous heparin during pregnancy in patients with an artificial heart valve. J Am Coll Cardiol 1986;8:221–4.
18. Cola LM, Lavin JP Jr. Pregnancy complicated by Marfan's syndrome with aortic arch dissection, subsequent aortic arch replacement and triple coronary artery bypass grafts. J Reprod Med 1985;30:685–8.
19. Copplestone A, Oscier DG. Heparin-induced thrombocytopenia in pregnancy. Br J Haematol 1987;65:248.
20. Normann EK, Stray-Pedersen B. Warfarin-induced fetal diaphragmatic hernia: case report. Br J Obstet Gynaecol 1989;96:729–30.
21. Campbell JM, Tate G, Scott JS. The use of warfarin in pregnancy complicated by circulating lupus anticoagulant; a technique for monitoring. Eur J Obstet Gynecol Reprod Biol 1988;29:27–32.
22. Ruthnum P, Tolmie JL. Atypical malformations in an infant exposed to warfarin during the first trimester of pregnancy. Teratology 1987;36:299–301.
23. L'E Orme M, Lewis PJ, De Swiet M, Serlin MJ, Sibeon R, Baty JD, Breckenridge AM. May mothers given warfarin breast-feed their infants? Br Med J 1977;1:1564–5.
24. De Swiet M, Lewis PJ. Excretion of anticoagulants in human milk. N Engl J Med 1977;297:1471.
25. McKenna R, Cole ER, Vasan U. Is warfarin sodium contraindicated in the lactating mother? J Pediatr 1983;103:325–7.
26. Gostof, Momolka, Zilenka. Les substances derivees du tromexane dans le lait maternel et leurs actions paradoxales sur la prothrombine. Schweiz Med Wochenschr 1952;30:764–5. As cited in Daily JW. Anticoagulant and cardiovascular drugs. In Wilson JT, ed. *Drugs in Breast Milk*. Australia:ADIS Press, 1981:63.
27. Illingworth RS, Finch E. Ethyl biscoumacetate (Tromexan) in human milk. J Obstet Gynaecol Br Commonw 1959;66:487–8.
28. Brambel CE, Hunter RE. Effect of dicumarol on the nursing infant. Am J Obstet Gynecol 1950;59:1153–9.
29. Eckstein HB, Jack B. Breast-feeding and anticoagulant therapy. Lancet 1970;1:672–3.
30. Goguel M, Noel G, Gillet JY. Therapeutique anticoagulante et allaitement: etude du passage de la phenyl-2-dioxo,1,3 indane dans le lait maternel. Rev Fr Gynecol Obstet 1970;65:409–12. As cited in Anderson PO. Drugs and breast feeding — a review. Drug Intell Clin Pharm 1977;11:208–23.

31. Committee on Drugs, American Academy of Pediatrics. Transfer of drugs and other chemicals into human milk. Pediatrics 1989;84;924–36.

Name: **CROMOLYN SODIUM**

Class: **Miscellaneous**   Risk Factor: **B$_M$**

Fetal Risk Summary

Cromolyn sodium is used by inhalation for the treatment of bronchial asthma. The drug is generally considered safe for use during pregnancy (1–6). Although small amounts are absorbed systemically from the lungs, it is not known whether the drug crosses the placenta to the fetus (6).

Congenital malformations were noted in four (1.35%) newborns in a 1982 study of 296 women treated throughout gestation with cromolyn sodium (7). This incidence is less than the expected rate of 2–3% in a nonexposed population. The defects observed were patent ductus arteriosus, clubfoot, nonfused septum, and harelip alone. The author concluded that there was no association between the defects and cromolyn sodium (7).

As of 1983, the manufacturer had reports of 185 women treated during all or parts of pregnancy, but the small number probably reflects underreporting of the actual usage (personal communication, Fisons Corporation, 1983). From these cases, 10 infants had been born with congenital defects, at least three of which appeared to be genetic in origin. Multiple drug exposure was common. In none of the 10 cases was there evidence to link the defects with cromolyn sodium.

Breast Feeding Summary

No data are available.

References

1. Dykes MHM. Evaluation of an antiasthmatic agent cromolyn sodium (Aarane, Intal). JAMA 1974;227:1061–2.
2. Greenberger P, Patterson R. Safety of therapy for allergic symptoms during pregnancy. Ann Intern Med 1978;89:234–7.
3. Weinstein AM, Dubin BD, Podleski WK, Spector SL, Farr RS. Asthma and pregnancy. JAMA 1979;241:1161–5.
4. Pratt WR. Allergic diseases in pregnancy and breast feeding. Ann Allergy 1981;47:355–60.
5. Mawhinney H, Spector SL. Optimum management of asthma in pregnancy. Drugs 1986;32:178–87.
6. Niebyl JR. *Drug Use in Pregnancy*. Philadelphia:Lea & Febiger, 1982:53.
7. Wilson J. Use of sodium cromoglycate during pregnancy: results on 296 asthmatic women. Acta Therap 1982;8(Suppl):45–51.

Name: **CYCLACILLIN**

Class: **Antibiotic** Risk Factor: **B$_M$**

Fetal Risk Summary

Cyclacillin is a penicillin antibiotic (see also Penicillin G). No reports linking its use with congenital defects have been located. The Collaborative Perinatal Project monitored 50,282 mother-child pairs, 3,546 of which had 1st trimester exposure to penicillin derivatives (1, pp. 297–313). For use anytime during pregnancy, 7,171 exposures were recorded (1, p. 435). In neither case was evidence found to suggest a relationship to large categories of major or minor malformations or to individual defects.

Breast Feeding Summary

No data are available (see Penicillin G).

Reference

1. Heinonen OP, Slone D, Shapiro S. *Birth Defects and Drugs in Pregnancy*. Littleton:Publishing Sciences Group, 1977.

Name: **CYCLAMATE**

Class: **Sweetener** Risk Factor: **C**

Fetal Risk Summary

Controlled studies on the effects of cyclamate on the fetus have not been found. The drug crosses the placenta to produce fetal blood levels of about 25% of maternal serum (1). Cyclamate has been suspected of having cytogenetic effects in human lymphocytes (2). One group of investigators attempted to associate these effects with an increased incidence of malformations and behavioral problems, but a causal relationship could not be established (3).

Breast Feeding Summary

No data are available.

References

1. Pitkin RM, Reynolds WA, Filer LJ. Placental transmission and fetal distribution of cyclamate in early human pregnancy. Am J Obstet Gynecol 1970;108:1043–50.
2. Bauchinger M. Cytogenetic effect of cyclamate on human peripheral lymphocytes in vivo. Dtsch Med Wochenschr 1970;95:2220–3.
3. Stone D, Matalka E, Pulaski B. Do artificial sweeteners ingested in pregnancy affect the offspring? Nature 1971;231:53.

Name: **CYCLANDELATE**

Class: **Vasodilator**   Risk Factor: **C**

Fetal Risk Summary

No data are available.

Breast Feeding Summary

No data are available.

Name: **CYCLAZOCINE**

Class: **Narcotic Antagonist**   Risk Factor: **D**

Fetal Risk Summary

Cyclazocine is not available in the United States. In addition to its ability to re-verse narcotic overdose, it has been used in the treatment of narcotic dependence (1). Its actions are similar to those of nalorphine (see also Nalorphine).

Breast Feeding Summary

No data are available.

Reference

1. Wade A, ed. *Martindale. The Extra Pharmacopoeia,* ed 27. London:Pharmaceutical Press, 1977:985.

Name: **CYCLIZINE**

Class: **Antihistamine/Antiemetic**   Risk Factor: **B**

Fetal Risk Summary

Cyclizine is a piperazine antihistamine that is used as an antiemetic (see also Buclizine and Meclizine for closely related drugs). The drug is teratogenic in animals but apparently not in humans. In 111 patients given cyclizine during the 1st trimester, no increased malformation rate was observed (1). Similarly, the Collaborative Perinatal Project found no association between 1st trimester cyclizine use and congenital defects, although the number of exposed patients ($N = 15$) was small compared to the total sample (2). The Food and Drug Administration's OTC Laxative Panel acting on this data concluded that cyclizine is not teratogenic (3). In 1974, investigators searching for an association between antihistamines and oral clefts found no relationship between this defect and the cyclizine group (4). Finally, a retrospective study in 1971 found significantly fewer infants with malformations were exposed to antihistamines/antiemetics in the 1st trimester as compared to controls (5). Cyclizine was the fifth most commonly used antiemetic.

An association between exposure during the last 2 weeks of pregnancy to antihistamines in general and retrolental fibroplasia in premature infants has been reported. See Brompheniramine for details.

Breast Feeding Summary

No data are available.

References

1. Milkovich L, Van den Berg BJ. An evaluation of the teratogenicity of certain antinauseant drugs. Am J Obstet Gynecol 1976;125:244–8.
2. Heinonen OP, Slone D, Shapiro S. *Birth Defects and Drugs in Pregnancy*. Littleton:Publishing Sciences Group, 1977:323.
3. Anonymous. Meclizine;cyclizine not teratogenic. Pink Sheets. FDC Rep 1974:T&G–2.
4. Saxen I. Cleft palate and maternal diphenhydramine intake. Lancet 1974;1:407–8.
5. Nelson MM, Forfar JO. Associations between drugs administered during pregnancy and congenital abnormalities of the fetus. Br Med J 1971;1:523–7.

Name: **CYCLOPENTHIAZIDE**

Class: **Diuretic**   Risk Factor: **D**

Fetal Risk Summary

See Chlorothiazide.

Breast Feeding Summary

See Chlorothiazide.

Name: **CYCLOPHOSPHAMIDE**

Class: **Antineoplastic**   Risk Factor: **D**

Fetal Risk Summary

Cyclophosphamide is an alkylating antineoplastic agent. Both normal and malformed newborns have been reported following the use in pregnancy of cyclophosphamide (1–23). Eight malformed infants have resulted from 1st trimester exposure (1–6). Radiation therapy was given to most of the mothers, and at least one patient was treated with other antineoplastics (1, 2, 4). Defects observed in four of the infants are shown in the list below, and a fifth infant is described in the text that follows:

Flattened nasal bridge, palate defect, skin tag, four toes each foot, hypoplastic middle phalanx fifth finger, bilateral inguinal hernia sacs (1)
Toes missing, single coronary artery (2)
Hemangioma, umbilical hernia (3)
Imperforate anus, rectovaginal fistula, growth retarded (4)

A newborn exposed *in utero* to cyclophosphamide during the 1st trimester presented with multiple anomalies (6). The mother, who was being treated for a severe exacerbation of systemic lupus erythematosus, received two intravenous doses of 200 mg each between 15 and 46 days' gestation. Except for prednisone, 20 mg daily, no other medication was given during the pregnancy. The 3150-g female infant was delivered at 39 weeks' gestational age with multiple abnormalities, including dysmorphic facies, multiple eye defects including bilateral blepharophimosis with left microphthalmos, abnormally shaped, low-set ears, cleft palate, bilaterally absent thumbs, and dystrophic nails. Borderline microcephaly, hypotonia, and possible developmental delay were observed at 10 months of age.

A case report of a 16-year-old woman with ovarian endodermal sinus tumor presenting in two pregnancies was published in 1979 (17). Conservative surgery, suction curettage to terminate a pregnancy estimated to be at 8–10 weeks' gestation, and chemotherapy with cyclophosphamide, dactinomycin, and vincristine (VAC) produced a complete clinical response for 12 months. The patient then refused further therapy and presented a second time, 6 months later, with tumor recurrence and a pregnancy estimated at 18–20 weeks' gestation. She again refused chemotherapy, but her disease progressed to the point where she allowed VAC chemotherapy to be reinstated 4 weeks later. At 33 weeks' gestation, 2 weeks after her last dose of chemotherapy, she spontaneously delivered a normal 2213-g female infant. The infant was developing normally when last seen at 8 months of age. In a similar case, a woman, treated with surgery and chemotherapy in her 15th week of pregnancy for an ovarian endodermal sinus tumor, delivered a normal 2850-g male infant at 37 weeks' gestation (18). Chemotherapy, begun during the 16th gestational week, included six courses of VAC chemotherapy. The last course was administered 5 days prior to delivery. No information was provided on the subsequent growth and development of the infant.

Pancytopenia occurred in a 1000-g male infant exposed to cyclophosphamide and five other antineoplastic agents in the 3rd trimester (12). In a similar case, maternal treatment for leukemia was begun at 12.5 weeks' gestation and eventually included cyclophosphamide, five other antineoplastic agents, and whole brain radiation (22). A normally developed, premature female infant was delivered at 31 weeks, who subsequently developed transient severe bone marrow hypoplasia in the neonatal period. The myelosuppression was probably due to mercaptopurine therapy.

Data from one review indicated that 40% of the patients exposed to anticancer drugs during pregnancy delivered low-birth-weight infants (24). This finding was not related to the timing of exposure. Use of cyclophosphamide in the 2nd and 3rd trimesters does not seem to place the fetus at risk for congenital defects. Except in a few individual cases, long-term studies of growth and mental development in offspring exposed to cyclophosphamide during the 2nd trimester, the period of neuroblast multiplication, have not been conducted (25).

Cyclophosphamide is one of the most common causes of chemotherapy-induced menstrual difficulties and azoospermia (26–34). Permanent secondary amenorrhea with evidence of primary ovarian damage has been observed after long-term (20 months) use of cyclophosphamide (34). In contrast, successful pregnancies have been reported following high-dose therapy (28, 29, 35–39). Moreover, azoospermia appears to be reversible when the drug is stopped (30–33, 40).

One report associated paternal use of cyclophosphamide and three other antineoplastics prior to conception with congenital anomalies in an infant (41). Defects in the infant included syndactyly of the first and second digits of the right foot and Fallot's tetralogy. In a group of men treated over a minimum of 3.5 years with multiple chemotherapy for acute lymphocytic leukemia, one man fathered a normal child while a second fathered two children, one with multiple anomalies (42). Any relationship between these outcomes and paternal use of cyclophosphamide is doubtful because of the lack of experimental evidence and confirming reports.

Cyclophosphamide-induced chromosomal abnormalities are also of doubtful clinical significance, but have been described in some patients after use of the drug. A study published in 1974 reported chromosome abnormalities in patients treated with cyclophosphamide for rheumatoid arthritis and scleroderma (43). In contrast, chromosome studies were normal in a mother and infant treated during the 2nd and 3rd trimesters in another report (14). In another case, a 34-year-old woman with acute lymphoblastic leukemia was treated with multiple antineoplastic agents from 22 weeks' gestation until delivery of a healthy female infant 18 weeks later (19). Cyclophosphamide was administered three times between the 26th and 30th weeks of gestation. Chromosome analysis of the newborn revealed a normal karyotype (46,XX) but with gaps and a ring chromosome. The clinical significance of these findings is unknown, but since these abnormalities may persist for several years, the potential existed for an increased risk of cancer as well as for a risk of genetic damage in the next generation (19).

The long-term effects of cyclophosphamide on female and male reproductive function have been recently reported (44, 45). In a 1988 publication, 40 women who had been treated with combination chemotherapy for malignant ovarian germ cell tumors (median age of diagnosis 15 years, range 6–29) were evaluated approximately 10 years later (median age 25.5 years, range 14–40) (44). Cyclophosphamide had been used in 33 (83%) of the women. Menstrual function in these women after chemotherapy was as follows: premenarchal ($N = 1$), regular menses ($N = 27$), irregular menses ($N = 5$), oligomenorrhea ($N = 2$), amenorrhea ($N = 4$), and premature menopause ($N = 1$). Of the 12 women with menstrual difficulties, only three were considered serious or persistent. Evaluation of the reproductive status after chemotherapy revealed that 24 had not attempted to become pregnant, nine had problem-free conceptions, three had initial infertility followed by conceptions, and four had chronic infertility. Of the 12 women who had conceived on one or more occasions, one had an elective abortion at 10 weeks' gestation, and 11 had delivered 22 healthy infants, although one had amelogenesis imperfecta.

A study published in 1985 examined 30 men to determine the effect of cyclophosphamide on male hormone levels and spermatogenesis (45). The men had been treated at a mean age of 9.4 years for a mean duration of 280 days. The mean age of the men at the time of the study was 22 years with a mean interval from end of treatment to evaluation of 12.8 years. Four of the men were azoospermic, 9 were oligospermic, and 17 were normospermic. Compared to normal controls, however, the 17 men classified as normospermic had lower ejaculate volumes (3.1 vs. 3.3 ml), lower sperm density (54.5×10^6 vs. 79×10^6/ml), decreased sperm motility (42% vs. 61%, $p < 0.05$), and less normal sperm forms (61% vs. 70%, $p < 0.05$). Concentrations of testosterone, dehydroepiandrosterone sulfate, and prolactin were not significantly different between patients and controls. One oligospermic man (sperm density 12×10^6/ml) had fathered a child.

The effect of occupational exposure to antineoplastic agents on pregnancy outcome was examined in a 1985 case-control study involving 124 nurses in 17 Finnish hospitals compared to 321 matched controls (46). The cases involved nurses working in 1979–1980 in hospitals that used at least 100 g of cyclophosphamide (the most commonly administered antineoplastic agent in Finland) per year or at least 200 g of all antineoplastic drugs per year. The average total antineoplastic drug use for all hospitals was 1898 g, but a lower total use, 887 g, occurred for intravenous drugs (47). Moreover, the nurses had to be 40 years of age or younger in 1980 and had to work in patient areas where antineoplastic agents were mixed and administered (46). The agents were prepared without the use of vertical-airflow biologic-safety hoods or protective clothing (47). Exposure to these agents during the 1st trimester was significantly associated with early fetal loss (odds ratio 2.30, 95% confidence interval (CI) 1.20–4.39) ($p = 0.01$) (46). Cyclophosphamide, one of four individual antineoplastic agents to which at least 10 women had been exposed, had an odds ratio for fetal loss of 2.66 (95% CI 1.25–5.71). Other significant associations were found for doxorubicin (odds ratio 3.96, CI 1.31–11.97) and vincristine (odds ratio 2.46, CI 1.13–5.37). The association between fluorouracil and fetal loss (odds ratio 1.70, CI 0.55–5.21) was not significant. Based on the results of their study and data from previous studies, the investigators concluded that nursing personnel should exercise caution in handling these agents (46).

Although there is no current consensus on the danger posed to pregnant women from the handling of antineoplastic agents (e.g., the above study generated several letters that questioned the observed association (48–51)), pharmacy and nursing personnel should take precautions to avoid exposure to these potent agents. The National Study Commission on Cytotoxic Exposure published a position statement on this topic in January 1987 (52). Due to the importance of this issue, the statement is quoted in its entirety below:

"The Handling of Cytotoxic Agents by Women Who Are Pregnant,
Attempting to Conceive, or Breast Feeding"

"There are substantial data regarding the mutagenic, teratogenic and abortiofacient properties of certain cytotoxic agents both in animals and humans who have received therapeutic doses of these agents. Additionally the scientific literature suggests a possible association of occupational exposure to certain cytotoxic agents during the first trimester of pregnancy with fetal loss or malformation. These data suggest the need for caution when women who are pregnant or attempting to conceive, handle cytotoxic agents. Incidentally, there is no evidence relating male exposure to cytotoxic agents with adverse fetal outcome.

There are no studies which address the possible risk associated with the occupational exposure to cytotoxic agents and the passage of these agents into breast milk. Nevertheless, it is prudent that women who are breast feeding should exercise caution in handling cytotoxic agents.

If all procedures for safe handling, such as those recommended by the Commission are complied with, the potential for exposure will be minimized.

Personnel should be provided with information to make an individual decision. This information should be provided in written form and it is advisable that a statement of understanding be signed.

It is essential to refer to individual state right-to-know laws to insure compliance."

Breast Feeding Summary

Cyclophosphamide is excreted into breast milk (53). Although the concentrations were not specified, the drug was found in milk up to 6 hours after a single 500-mg intravenous dose. The mother was not nursing. A brief 1977 correspondence from investigators in New Guinea described neutropenia in a breast-fed infant whose mother received weekly injections of 800 mg of cyclophosphamide, 2 mg of vincristine, and 30-mg daily oral doses of prednisolone for 6 weeks (54). Absolute neutropenia was present 9 days after breast feeding had been stopped, which persisted for at least 12 days (54). Serial determinations of the infant's white cell and neutrophil counts were begun 2 days after the last exposure to breast milk. The lowest measured absolute lymphocyte count was 4750/µl. Except for the neutropenia and a brief episode of diarrhea, no other adverse effects were observed in the infant.

A 1979 report involved a case of an 18-year-old woman with Burkitt lymphoma diagnosed in the 26th week of gestation (55). She was treated with a 7-day course of cyclophosphamide, 10 mg/kg intravenously, as a single daily dose (total dose 3.5 g). Six weeks after the last chemotherapy dose, she delivered a normal, 2160-g male infant. Analysis of the newborn's blood counts was not conducted. The tumor recurred in the postpartum period and treatment with cyclophosphamide, 6 mg/kg/day intravenously, was started 20 days after delivery. Although she was advised not to nurse her infant, she continued to do so until her sudden death after the third dose of cyclophosphamide. Blood counts were conducted on both the mother and the infant during therapy. Immediately prior to the first dose, the infant's leukocyte and platelet counts were 4,800/mm^3 (abnormally low for age) and 270,000/mm^3, respectively. After the third maternal dose, the infant's counts were 3,200/mm^3 and 47,000/mm^3, respectively. Both counts were interpreted by the investigator as signs of cyclophosphamide-induced toxicity. It was concluded that breast feeding should be stopped during therapy with the agent (55).

The American Academy of Pediatrics considers cyclophosphamide to be contraindicated during breast feeding because of the reported case of neutropenia and because of the potential adverse effects relating to immune suppression, growth, and carcinogenesis (56).

References

1. Greenberg LH, Tanaka KR. Congenital anomalies probably induced by cyclophosphamide. JAMA 1964;188:423–6.
2. Toledo TM, Harper RC, Moser RH. Fetal effects during cyclophosphamide and irradiation therapy. Ann Intern Med 1971;74:87–91.
3. Coates A. Cyclophosphamide in pregnancy. Aust NZ J Obstet Gynaecol 1970;10:33–4.
4. Murray CL, Reichert JA, Anderson J, Twiggs LB. Multimodal cancer therapy for breast cancer in the first trimester of pregnancy. JAMA 1984;252:2607–8.
5. Sweet DL, Kinzie J. Consequences of radiotherapy and antineoplastic therapy for the fetus. J Reprod Med 1976;17:241–6.
6. Kirshon B, Wasserstrum N, Willis R, Herman GE, McCabe ERB. Teratogenic effects of first-trimester cyclophosphamide therapy. Obstet Gynecol 1988;72:462–4.

7. Lasher MJ, Geller W. Cyclophosphamide and vinblastine sulfate in Hodgkin's disease during pregnancy. JAMA 1966;195:486–8.
8. Lergier JE, Jimenez E, Maldonado N, Veray F. Normal pregnancy in multiple myeloma treated with cyclophosphamide. Cancer 1974;34:1018–22.
9. Garcia V, San Miguel J, Borrasca AL. Doxorubicin in the first trimester of pregnancy. Ann Intern Med 1981;94:547.
10. Lowenthal RM, Funnell CF, Hope DM, Stewart IG, Humphrey DC. Normal infant after combination chemotherapy including teniposide for Burkitt's lymphoma in pregnancy. Med Pediatr Oncol 1982;10:165–9.
11. Daly H, McCann SR, Hanratty TD, Temperley IJ. Successful pregnancy during combination chemotherapy for Hodgkin's disease. Acta Haematol (Basel) 1980;64:154–6.
12. Pizzuto J, Aviles A, Noriega L, Niz J, Morales M, Romero F. Treatment of acute leukemia during pregnancy: presentation of nine cases. Cancer Treat Rep 1980;64:679–83.
13. Sears HF, Reid J. Granulocytic sarcoma: local presentation of a systemic disease. Cancer 1976;37:1808–13.
14. Falkson HC, Simson IW, Falkson G. Non-Hodgkin's lymphoma in pregnancy. Cancer 1980;45:1679–82.
15. Webb GA. The use of hyperalimentation and chemotherapy in pregnancy: a case report. Am J Obstet Gynecol 1980;137:263–6.
16. Gililland J, Weinstein L. The effects of cancer chemotherapeutic agents on the developing fetus. Obstet Gynecol Surv 1983;38:6–13.
17. Weed JC Jr, Roh RA, Mendenhall HW. Recurrent endodermal sinus tumor during pregnancy. Obstet Gynecol 1979;54:653–6.
18. Kim DS, Park MI. Maternal and fetal survival following surgery and chemotherapy of endodermal sinus tumor of the ovary during pregnancy: a case report. Obstet Gynecol 1989;73:503–7.
19. Schleuning M, Clemm C. Chromosomal aberrations in a newborn whose mother received cytotoxic treatment during pregnancy. N Engl J Med 1987;317:1666–7.
20. Haerr RW, Pratt AT. Multiagent chemotherapy for sarcoma diagnosed during pregnancy. Cancer 1985;56:1028–33.
21. Turchi JJ, Villasis C. Anthracyclines in the treatment of malignancy in pregnancy. Cancer 1988;61:435–40.
22. Okun DB, Groncy PK, Sieger L, Tanaka KR. Acute leukemia in pregnancy: transient neonatal myelosuppression after combination chemotherapy in the mother. Med Pediatr Oncol 1979;7:315–9.
23. Ortega J. Multiple agent chemotherapy including bleomycin of non-Hodgkin's lymphoma during pregnancy. Cancer 1977;40:2829–35.
24. Nicholson HO. Cytotoxic drugs in pregnancy: review of reported cases. J Obstet Gynaecol Br Commonw 1968;75:307–12.
25. Dobbing J. Pregnancy and leukaemia. Lancet 1977;1:1155.
26. Schilsky RL, Lewis BJ, Sherins RJ, Young RC. Gonadal dysfunction in patients receiving chemotherapy for cancer. Ann Intern Med 1980;93:109–14.
27. Stewart BH. Drugs that cause and cure male infertility. Drug Ther 1975;5:42–8.
28. Schwartz PE, Vidone RA. Pregnancy following combination chemotherapy for a mixed germ cell tumor of the ovary. Gynecol Oncol 1981;12:373–8.
29. Bacon C, Kernahan J. Successful pregnancy in acute leukaemia. Lancet 1975;2:515.
30. Qureshji MA, Pennington JH, Goldsmith HJ, Cox PE. Cyclophosphamide therapy and sterility. Lancet 1972;2:1290–1.
31. George CRP, Evans RA. Cyclophosphamide and infertility. Lancet 1972;1:840–1.
32. Sherins RJ, DeVita VT Jr. Effect of drug treatment for lymphoma on male reproductive capacity. Ann Intern Med 1973;79:216–20.
33. Lendon M, Palmer MK, Hann IM, Shalet SM, Jones PHM. Testicular histology after combination chemotherapy in childhood for acute lymphoblastic leukaemia. Lancet 1978;2:439–41.
34. Uldall PR, Feest TG, Morley AR, Tomlinson BE, Kerr DNS. Cyclophosphamide therapy in adults with minimal-change nephrotic syndrome. Lancet 1972;2:1250–3.
35. Card RT, Holmes IH, Sugarman RG, Storb R, Thomas D. Successful pregnancy after high dose chemotherapy and marrow transplantation for treatment of aplastic anemia. Exp Hematol 1980;8:57–60.

36. Deeg HJ, Kennedy MS, Sanders JE, Thomas ED, Storb R. Successful pregnancy after marrow transplantation for severe aplastic anemia and immunosuppression with cyclosporine. JAMA 1983;250:647.

37. Javaheri G, Lifchez A, Valle J. Pregnancy following removal of and long-term chemotherapy for ovarian malignant teratoma. Obstet Gynecol 1983;61:8S–9S.

38. Rustin GJS, Booth M, Dent J, Salt S, Rustin F, Bagshawe KD. Pregnancy after cytotoxic chemotherapy for gestational trophoblastic tumours. Br Med J 1984;288:103–6.

39. Lee RB, Kelly J, Elg SA, Benson WL. Pregnancy following conservative surgery and adjunctive chemotherapy for stage III immature teratoma of the ovary. Obstet Gynecol 1989;73:853–5.

40. Hinkes E, Plotkin D. Reversible drug-induced sterility in a patient with acute leukemia. JAMA 1973;223:1490–1.

41. Russell JA, Powles RL, Oliver RTD. Conception and congenital abnormalities after chemotherapy of acute myelogenous leukaemia in two men. Br Med J 1976;1:1508.

42. Evenson DP, Arlin Z, Welt S, Claps ML, Melamed MR. Male reproductive capacity may recover following drug treatment with the L-10 protocol for acute lymphocytic leukemia. Cancer 1984;53:30–6.

43. Tolchin SF, Winkelstein A, Rodnan GP, Pan SF, Nankin HR. Chromosome abnormalities from cyclophosphamide therapy in rheumatoid arthritis and progressive systemic sclerosis (scleroderma). Arthritis Rheum 1974;17:375–82.

44. Gershenson DM. Menstrual and reproductive function after treatment with combination chemotherapy for malignant ovarian germ cell tumors. J Clin Oncol 1988;6:270–5.

45. Watson AR, Rance CP, Bain J. Long term effects of cyclophosphamide on testicular function. Br Med J 1985;291:1457–60.

46. Selevan SG, Lindbohm M-L, Hornung RW, Hemminki K. A study of occupational exposure to antineoplastic drugs and fetal loss in nurses. N Engl J Med 1985;313:1173–8.

47. Selevan SG, Hornung RW. Antineoplastic drugs and spontaneous abortion in nurses. N Engl J Med 1986;314:1050–1.

48. Kalter H. Antineoplastic drugs and spontaneous abortion in nurses. N Engl J Med 1986;314:1048–9.

49. Mulvihill JJ, Stewart KR. Antineoplastic drugs and spontaneous abortion in nurses. N Engl J Med 1986;314:1049.

50. Chabner BA. Antineoplastic drugs and spontaneous abortion in nurses. N Engl J Med 1986;314:1049–50.

51. Zellmer WA. Antineoplastic drugs and spontaneous abortion in nurses. N Engl J Med 1986;314:1050.

52. Jeffrey LP, Chairman, National Study Commission on Cytotoxic Exposure. Position statement. The handling of cytotoxic agents by women who are pregnant, attempting to conceive, or breast feeding. January 12, 1987.

53. Wiernik PH, Duncan JH. Cyclophosphamide in human milk. Lancet 1971;1:912.

54. Amato D, Niblett JS. Neutropenia from cyclophosphamide in breast milk. Med J Aust 1977;1:383–4.

55. Durodola JI. Administration of cyclophosphamide during late pregnancy and early lactation: a case report. J Natl Med Assoc 1979;71:165–6.

56. Committee on Drugs, American Academy of Pediatrics. Transfer of drugs and other chemicals into human milk. Pediatrics 1989;84;924–36.

Name: **CYCLOSERINE**

Class: **Antituberculosis Agent**   Risk Factor: **C**

Fetal Risk Summary

Cycloserine is a broad-spectrum antibiotic used primarily for active pulmonary and extrapulmonary tuberculosis. The Collaborative Perinatal Project (CPP) monitored 50,282 mother-child pairs, 3 of which had 1st trimester exposure to cycloserine (1). No evidence of adverse fetal effects was suggested by the CPP data.

The American Thoracic Society recommends avoidance of cycloserine during pregnancy, if possible, due to the lack of information on the fetal effects of the drug (2).

Breast Feeding Summary

No data are available.

References

1. Heinonen OP, Slone D, Shapiro S. *Birth Defects and Drugs in Pregnancy*. Littleton:Publishing Sciences Group, 1977:297.
2. American Thoracic Society. Medical Section of the American Lung Association: Treatment of tuberculosis and tuberculosis infection in adults and children. Am Rev Respir Dis 1986;134:355–63.

Name: **CYCLOSPORINE**

Class: **Miscellaneous**   Risk Factor: **C$_M$**

Fetal Risk Summary

Cyclosporine (cyclosporin A), an antibiotic produced by certain fungi, is used as an immunosuppressive agent to prevent rejection of kidney, liver, or heart allografts.

Cyclosporine readily crosses the placenta to the fetus (1–5). In a 1983 study, the cord blood:maternal plasma ratio at delivery was 0.63 (1). In a second study, cord blood and amniotic fluid levels 8 hours after a dose of 325 mg were 57 ng/ml and 234 ng/ml, respectively (2). Concentrations in the newborn fell to 14 ng/ml at 14 hours and were undetectable (<4 ng/ml) at 7 days. Cord blood:maternal plasma ratios in twins delivered at 35 weeks' gestation were 0.35 and 0.57, respectively (3). A similar ratio of 0.40 was reported in a case delivered at 31 weeks' gestation (4).

Several case reports describing the use of cyclosporine throughout gestation have been published (1–12). Maternal doses ranged between 260–550 mg/day (1–3, 6, 8, 9, 12). Cases usually involved maternal renal transplantation (1–3, 5–11), but one report described a successful pregnancy in a woman after heart transplantation (4), one involved a combined transplant of a kidney and paratropic segmental pancreas in a diabetic woman (9), and one involved a patient with a liver transplant (12). In addition, a report has described a successful pregnancy in a woman with aplastic anemia who was treated with bone marrow transplantation (13). In this case, however, cyclosporine therapy had been stopped prior to conception. Guidelines for counseling heart transplant patients who wish to become pregnant have been published (14).

As of October, 1987, the manufacturer had knowledge of 34 pregnancies involving cyclosporine (A. Poploski and D.A. Colasante, personal communication, Sandoz Pharmaceuticals Corporation, 1987) (14). Some of these cases are described above. These pregnancies resulted in six abortions (one after early detection of anencephaly, three elective, and two spontaneous abortions, one at 20 weeks' gestation), one pregnancy still ongoing, and 27 live births. One of the newborns died at age 3 days. Autopsy revealed a complete absence of the corpus callosum. Other problems observed in individual newborns exposed *in utero* to cyclosporine were: thrombocytopenia (thought to be due to hydralazine taken by the mother for hypertension) (6), a hydrocele that resolved spontaneously (8), asphyxia and intracerebral bleeding in an extremely premature infant (A. Poploski and D.A. Colasante, personal communication, 1987), physiologic jaundice (A. Poploski and D.A. Colasante, personal communication), leukopenia (3) (A. Poploski and D.A. Colasante, personal communication, 1987), hypoglycemia and mild disseminated intravascular coagulation that resolved spontaneously (A. Poploski and D.A. Colasante, personal communication, 1987), and bilateral cataracts (A. Poploski and D.A. Colasante, personal communication, 1987). A 1989 case report described an infant with hypoplasia of the right leg and foot after *in utero* exposure to cyclosporine (10). The right leg was 2 cm shorter than the left. Hypoplasia of the muscles and subcutaneous tissue of the right leg was also present. The authors proposed a possible mechanism for the defect, which involved cyclosporine inhibition of lymphocytic interleukin-2 release and subsequent interference with the differentiation of osteoclasts (10).

Many of the liveborn infants were growth retarded (2, 6, 8–12). Birth weights of full-term newborns ranged from 2160–3200 g (11, 12) (A. Poploski and D.A. Colasante, personal communication, 1987). A 1985 review article observed that growth retardation was common in the offspring of renal transplant patients, occurring in 8–45% of reported pregnancies (15). Although the specific cause of the diminished growth could not be determined, the most likely processes involved were considered to be maternal hypertension, renal function, and immunosuppressive drugs (15).

Follow-up of children exposed *in utero* to cyclosporine has been conducted in a few cases (3, 9) (A. Poploski and D.A. Colasante, personal communication, 1987). In 15 of 27 surviving neonates, early postnatal development was normal except for one infant with slight growth retardation (3, 9) (A. Poploski and D.A. Colasante, personal communication, 1987). Postnatal development of 10 children followed from 1–13 months revealed normal physical and mental development (3, 9) (A. Poploski and D.A. Colasante, personal communication, 1987). No abnormal renal or liver function has been reported in the exposed newborns.

In summary, based on relatively small numbers, the use of cyclosporine during pregnancy apparently does not pose a major risk to the fetus. Cyclosporine is not an animal teratogen (16), and the limited experience in women indicates that it is unlikely to be a human teratogen. No pattern of defects has emerged in the few newborns with anomalies. Skeletal defects, other then the single case of osseous malformation, have not been observed. The disease process itself, for which cyclosporine is indicated, makes these pregnancies high risk and subject to numerous potential problems, of which the most common is growth retardation. This latter problem is probably related to the mother's disease rather than to her drug therapy, but a contribution from cyclosporine and corticosteroids cannot be excluded. Long-term follow-up studies are warranted, however, to detect latent effects including those in subsequent generations.

Breast Feeding Summary

Cyclosporine is excreted into human breast milk, but no reports of its use during breast feeding have been located (1, 2, 4, 5). In a patient taking 450 mg of cyclosporine/day, milk levels on postpartum days 2, 3, and 4 were 101 ng/ml, 109 ng/ml, and 263 ng/ml, respectively (1). No details were given about the relationship of maternal doses with these levels. In another patient, milk concentrations 22 hours after a dose of 325 mg were 16 ng/ml while maternal blood levels were 52 ng/ml, a milk:plasma ratio of 0.31 (2). A milk:plasma ratio of 0.40 was reported in one study (4) and a ratio of approximately 0.17 was measured in another (5). Breast feeding was not allowed in any of these studies and has been actively discouraged by most sources because of concerns for potential toxicity in the nursing infant (11, 12, 14, 16) (A. Poploski and D.A. Colasante, personal communication, 1987). The American Academy of Pediatrics considers cyclosporine to be contraindicated during breast feeding due to the potential for immune suppression and neutropenia, an unknown effect on growth, and a possible association with carcinogenesis (17).

References

1. Lewis GJ, Lamont CAR, Lee HA, Slapak M. Successful pregnancy in a renal transplant recipient taking cyclosporin A. Br Med J 1983;286:603.
2. Flechner SM, Katz AR, Rogers AJ, Van Buren C, Kahan BD. The presence of cyclosporine in body tissues and fluids during pregnancy. Am J Kidney Dis 1985;5:60–3.
3. Burrows DA, O'Neil TJ, Sorrells TL. Successful twin pregnancy after renal transplant maintained on cyclosporine A immunosuppression. Obstet Gynecol 1988;72:459–61.
4. Lowenstein BR, Vain NW, Perrone SV, Wright DR, Boullon FJ, Favaloro RG. Successful pregnancy and vaginal delivery after heart transplantation. Am J Obstet Gynecol 1988;158:589–90.
5. Ziegenhagen DJ, Grombach G, Dieckmann M, Zehnter E, Wienand P, Baldamus CA. Pregnancy under cyclosporine administration after renal transplantation. Dtsch Med Wochenschr 1988;113:260–3.
6. Klintmalm G, Althoff P, Appleby G, Segerbrandt E. Renal function in a newborn baby delivered of a renal transplant patient taking cyclosporine. Transplantation 1984;38:198–9.
7. Grischke E, Kaufmann M, Dreikorn K, Linderkamp O, Kubli F. Successful pregnancy after kidney transplantation and cyclosporin A. Geburtshilfe Frauenheilkd 1986;46:176–9.
8. Pikrell MD, Sawers R, Michael J. Pregnancy after renal transplantation: severe intrauterine growth retardation during treatment with cyclosporin A. Br Med J 1988;296:825.
9. Calne RY, Brons IGM, Williams PF, Evans DB, Robinson RE, Dossa M. Successful pregnancy after paratopic segmental pancreas and kidney transplantation. Br Med J 1988;296:1709.
10. Pujals JM, Figueras G, Puig JM, Lloveras J, Aubia J, Masramon J. Osseous malformation in baby born to woman on cyclosporin. Lancet 1989;1:667.
11. Al-Khader AA, Absy M, Al-Hasani MK, Joyce B, Sabbagh T. Successful pregnancy in renal transplant recipients treated with cyclosporine. Transplantation 1988;45:987–8.
12. Sims CJ, Porter KB, Knuppel RA. Successful pregnancy after a liver transplant. Am J Obstet Gynecol 1989;161:532–3.
13. Deeg HJ, Kennedy MS, Sanders JE, Thomas ED, Storb R. Successful pregnancy after marrow transplantation for severe aplastic anemia and immunosuppression with cyclosporine. JAMA 1983;250:647.
14. Kossoy LR, Herbert CM III, Wentz AC. Management of heart transplant recipients: guidelines for the obstetrician-gynecologist. Am J Obstet Gynecol 1988;159:490–9.
15. Lau RJ, Scott JR. Pregnancy following renal transplantation. Clin Obstet Gynecol 1985;28:339–50.
16. Product information. Sandimmune. Sandoz Pharmaceutical Corporation, 1990.
17. Committee on Drugs, American Academy of Pediatrics. Transfer of drugs and other chemicals into human milk. Pediatrics 1989;84;924–36.

Name: **CYCLOTHIAZIDE**

Class: **Diuretic**   Risk Factor: **D**

Fetal Risk Summary

See Chlorothiazide.

Breast Feeding Summary

See Chlorothiazide.

Name: **CYCRIMINE**

Class: **Parasympatholytic**   Risk Factor: **C**

Fetal Risk Summary

Cycrimine is an anticholinergic agent used in the treatment of parkinsonism. No reports of its use in pregnancy have been located (see also Atropine).

Breast Feeding Summary

No data are available (see also Atropine).

Name: **CYPROHEPTADINE**

Class: **Antihistamine/Antiserotonin**   Risk Factor: **B$_M$**

Fetal Risk Summary

Cyproheptadine has been used as a serotonin antagonist to prevent habitual abortion in patients with increased serotonin production (1, 2). No congenital defects were observed when the drug was used for this purpose. Two patients, who were being treated with cyproheptadine for Cushing's syndrome, conceived while taking the drug (3, 4). Therapy was stopped at 3 months in one patient but continued throughout gestation in the second. Apparently healthy infants were delivered prematurely (33–34 weeks and 36 weeks) from both mothers. The 33–34 week gestational infant, exposed throughout pregnancy to the drug, developed fatal gastroenteritis at 4 months of age (3). In a separate case, a woman with Cushing's was successfully treated with cyproheptadine; 2 years after stopping the drug, she conceived and eventually delivered a healthy male infant (5).

Breast Feeding Summary

No data are available. The manufacturer considers cyproheptadine to be contraindicated in nursing mothers (6).

References

1. Sadovsky E, Pfeifer Y, Polishuk WZ, Sulman FG. A trial of cyproheptadine in habitual abortion. Isr J Med Sci 1972;8:623–5.
2. Sadovsky E. Prevention of hypothalamic habitual abortion by Periactin. Harefuah 1970;78:332–3. As reported in JAMA 1970;212:1253.
3. Kasperlik-Zaluska A, Migdalska B, Hartwig W, Wilczynska J, Marianowski L, Stopinska-Gluszak U, Lozinska D. Two pregnancies in a woman with Cushing's syndrome treated with cyproheptadine. Br J Obstet Gynaecol 1980;87:1171–3.
4. Khir ASM, How J, Bewsher PD. Successful pregnancy after cyproheptadine treatment for Cushing's disease. Eur J Obstet Gynecol Reprod Biol 1982;13:343–7.
5. Griffith DN, Ross EJ. Pregnancy after cyproheptadine treatment for Cushing's disease. N Engl J Med 1981;305:893–4.
6. Product information. Periactin. Merck Sharpe & Dohme, 1990.

Name: **CYTARABINE**

Class: **Antineoplastic**   Risk Factor: D_M

Fetal Risk Summary

Normal infants have resulted following *in utero* exposure to cytarabine during all stages of gestation (1–26). Follow-up of seven infants exposed *in utero* during the 2nd trimester to cytarabine revealed normal infants at 4–60 months (19, 21–25). Two cases of intrauterine fetal death have been located after cytarabine combination treatment (19, 22). In one case, maternal treatment for 5 weeks starting at the 15th week of gestation ended in intrauterine death at 20 weeks' gestation of a fetus without abnormalities or leukemic infiltration (19). The second case also involved a woman treated from the 15th week who developed severe pregnancy-induced hypertension at 29 weeks' gestation (22). An apparently normal fetus died 1 week later, most likely as a consequence of the preeclampsia.

Use during the 1st and 2nd trimesters has been associated with congenital and chromosomal abnormalities (20, 27–29). One leukemic patient treated during the 2nd trimester elected to have an abortion at 24 weeks' gestation (20). The fetus had trisomy for group C autosomes without mosaicism. A second pregnancy in the same patient with identical therapy ended normally. In another case, a 34-year-old woman with acute lymphoblastic leukemia was treated with multiple antineoplastic agents from 22 weeks' gestation until delivery of a healthy female infant 18 weeks later (27). Cytarabine was administered only during the 27th week of gestation. Chromosome analysis of the newborn revealed a normal karyotype (46,XX) but with gaps and a ring chromosome. The clinical significance of these findings is unknown, but because these abnormalities may persist for several years, the potential existed for an increased risk of cancer as well as for a risk of genetic damage in the next generation (27). Two women, one treated during the 1st trimester and the other treated throughout pregnancy, delivered infants with multiple anomalies:

Bilateral microtia and atresia of external auditory canals, right hand lobster claw with three digits, bilateral lower limb defects (28)

Two medial digits of both feet missing, distal phalanges of both thumbs missing
with hypoplastic remnant of right thumb (29)

Congenital anomalies have also been observed after paternal use of cytarabine
plus other antineoplastics prior to conception (30). The investigators suggested
that the antineoplastic agents may have damaged the sperm without producing
infertility in the two fathers. The relationship between use of the chemotherapy in
these men and the defects observed is doubtful due to the lack of experimental
evidence and confirming reports. The results of these pregnancies were: Fallot's
tetralogy, syndactyly of first and second digits of right foot, and a stillborn
anencephalic. Cytarabine may produce reversible azoospermia (31, 32). However, male fertility has been demonstrated during maintenance therapy with
cytarabine (33).

Pancytopenia was observed in a 1000-g male infant exposed to cytarabine and
five other antineoplastic agents during the 3rd trimester (11).

Data from one review indicated that 40% of the mothers exposed to antineoplastic drugs during pregnancy delivered low-birth-weight infants (34). This finding was not related to the timing of exposure. Except for the few cases noted
above, long-term studies of growth and mental development in offspring exposed
to cytarabine during the 2nd trimester, the period of neuroblast multiplication,
have not been conducted (35).

Occupational exposure of the mother to antineoplastic agents during pregnancy
may present a risk to the fetus. A position statement from the National Study
Commission on Cytotoxic Exposure and a research article involving some antineoplastic agents are presented in the monograph for cyclophosphamide (see Cyclophosphamide).

Breast Feeding Summary

No data are available.

References

1. Pawliger DF, McLean FW, Noyes WD. Normal fetus after cytosine arabinoside therapy. Ann Intern Med 1971;74:1012.
2. Au-Yong R, Collins P, Young JA. Acute myeloblastic leukemia during pregnancy. Br Med J
   1972;4:493–4.
3. Raich PC, Curet LB. Treatment of acute leukemia during pregnancy. Cancer 1975;36:861–2.
4. Gokal R, Durrant J, Baum JD, Bennett MJ. Successful pregnancy in acute monocytic leukaemia.
   Br J Cancer 1976;34:299–302.
5. Sears HF, Reid J. Granulocytic sarcoma: local presentation of a systemic disease. Cancer
   1976;37:1808–13.
6. Durie BGM, Giles HR. Successful treatment of acute leukemia during pregnancy. Arch Intern Med
   1977;137:90–1.
7. Lilleyman JS, Hill AS, Anderton KJ. Consequences of acute myelogenous leukemia in early pregnancy. Cancer 1977;40:1300–3.
8. Moreno H, Castleberry RP, McCann WP. Cytosine arabinoside and 6-thioguanine in the treatment
   of childhood acute myeloblastic leukemia. Cancer 1977;40:998–1004.
9. Newcomb M, Balducci L, Thigpen JT, Morrison FS. Acute leukemia in pregnancy: successful delivery after cytarabine and doxorubicin. JAMA 1978;239:2691–2.
10. Manoharan A, Leyden MJ. Acute non-lymphocytic leukaemia in the third trimester of pregnancy.
    Aust NZ J Med 1979;9:71–4.
11. Pizzuto J, Aviles A, Noriega L, Niz J, Morales M, Romero F. Treatment of acute leukemia during
    pregnancy: presentation of nine cases. Cancer Treat Rep 1980;64:679–83.

12. Colbert N, Najman A, Gorin NC, Blum F, Treisser A, Lasfargues G, Cloup M, Barrat H, Duhamel G. Acute leukaemia during pregnancy: favourable course of pregnancy in two patients treated with cytosine arabinoside and anthracyclines. Nouv Presse Med 1980;9:175–8.
13. Tobias JS, Bloom HJG. Doxorubicin in pregnancy. Lancet 1980;1:776.
14. Taylor G, Blom J. Acute leukemia during pregnancy. South Med J 1980;73:1314–5.
15. Dara P, Slater LM, Armentrout SA. Successful pregnancy during chemotherapy for acute leukemia. Cancer 1981;47:845–6.
16. Plows CW. Acute myelomonocytic leukemia in pregnancy: report of a case. Am J Obstet Gynecol 1982;143:41–3.
17. De Souza JJL, Bezwoda WR, Jetham D, Sonnendecker EWW. Acute leukaemia in pregnancy: a case report and discussion on modern management. S Afr Med J 1982;62:295–6.
18. Feliu J, Juarez S, Ordonez A, Garcia-Paredes ML, Gonzalez-Baron M, Montero JM. Acute leukemia and pregnancy. Cancer 1988;61:580–4.
19. Volkenandt M, Buchner T, Hiddemann W, Van De Loo J. Acute leukaemia during pregnancy. Lancet 1987;2:1521–2.
20. Maurer LH, Forcier RJ, McIntyre OR, Benirschke K. Fetal group C trisomy after cytosine arabinoside and thioguanine. Ann Intern Med 1971;75:809–10.
21. Lowenthal RM, Marsden KA, Newman NM, Baikie MJ, Campbell SN. Normal infant after treatment of acute myeloid leukaemia in pregnancy with daunorubicin. Aust NZ J Med 1978;8:431–2.
22. O'Donnell R, Costigan C, O'Donnell LG. Two cases of acute leukaemia in pregnancy. Acta Haematol 1979;61:298–300.
23. Doney KC, Kraemer KG, Shepard TH. Combination chemotherapy for acute myelocytic leukemia during pregnancy: three case reports. Cancer Treat Rep 1979;63:369–71.
24. Cantini E, Yanes B. Acute myelogenous leukemia in pregnancy. South Med J 1984;77:1050–2.
25. Alegre A, Chunchurreta R, Rodrigueq-Alarcon J, Cruz E, Prada M. Successful pregnancy in acute promyelocytic leukemia. Cancer 1982;49:152–3.
26. Hamer JW, Beard MEJ, Duff GB. Pregnancy complicated by acute myeloid leukaemia. NZ Med J 1979;89:212–3.
27. Schleuning M, Clemm C. Chromosomal aberrations in a newborn whose mother received cytotoxic treatment during pregnancy. N Engl J Med 1987;317:1666–7.
28. Wagner VM, Hill JS, Weaver D, Baehner RL. Congenital abnormalities in baby born to cytarabine treated mother. Lancet 1980;2:98–9.
29. Schafer AI. Teratogenic effects of antileukemic chemotherapy. Arch Intern Med 1981;141:514–5.
30. Russell JA, Powles RL, Oliver RTD. Conception and congenital abnormalities after chemotherapy of acute myelogenous leukaemia in two men. Br Med J 1976;1:1508.
31. Lendon M, Palmer MK, Hann IM, Shalet SM, Jones PHM. Testicular histology after combination chemotherapy in childhood for acute lymphoblastic leukaemia. Lancet 1978;2:439–41.
32. Lilleyman JS. Male fertility after successful chemotherapy for lymphoblastic leukaemia. Lancet 1979;2:1125.
33. Matthews JH, Wood JK. Male fertility during chemotherapy for acute leukemia. N Engl J Med 1980;303:1235.
34. Nicholson HO. Cytotoxic drugs in pregnancy: review of reported cases. J Obstet Gynaecol Br Commonw 1968;75:307–12.
35. Dobbing J. Pregnancy and leukaemia. Lancet 1977;1:1155.

d

Name: **DACARBAZINE**

Class: **Antineoplastic**   Risk Factor: **C$_M$**

Fetal Risk Summary

No data are available. See also Cyclophosphamide for occupational exposure to antineoplastic agents during pregnancy.

Breast Feeding Summary

No data are available.

Name: **DACTINOMYCIN**

Class: **Antineoplastic**   Risk Factor: **C$_M$**

Fetal Risk Summary

Dactinomycin is an antimitotic antineoplastic agent. Normal pregnancies have followed the use of this drug prior to conception (1–8). Women, however, were less likely to have a live birth following treatment with this drug than with other antineoplastics (5).

Reports on the use of dactinomycin in six pregnancies have been located (9–13). In these cases, dactinomycin was administered during the 2nd and 3rd trimesters and apparently normal infants were delivered. The infant from one of the pregnancies was continuing to do well 4 years after birth (11). Two of the other pregnancies (12, 13) are discussed in more detail in the monograph for cyclophosphamide (see Cyclophosphamide).

Data from one review indicated that 40% of the infants exposed to anticancer drugs were of low birth weight (9). This finding was not related to the timing of exposure. Long-term studies of growth and mental development in offspring exposed to dactinomycin during the 2nd trimester, the period of neuroblast multiplication, have not been conducted (14).

The long-term effects of combination chemotherapy on menstrual and reproductive function have been described in a 1988 report (15). Thirty-two of the 40 women treated for malignant ovarian germ cell tumors received dactinomycin. The results of this study are discussed in the monograph for cyclophosphamide (see Cyclophosphamide).

Occupational exposure of the mother to antineoplastic agents during pregnancy may present a risk to the fetus. A position statement from the National Study Commission on Cytotoxic Exposure and a research article involving some antineoplastic agents are presented in the monograph for cyclophosphamide (see Cyclophosphamide).

Breast Feeding Summary

No data are available.

References

1. Ross GT. Congenital anomalies among children born of mothers receiving chemotherapy for gestational trophoblastic neoplasms. Cancer 1976;37:1043–7.
2. Walden PAM, Bagshawe KD. Pregnancies after chemotherapy for gestational trophoblastic tumours. Lancet 1979;2:1241.
3. Schwartz PE, Vidone RA. Pregnancy following combination chemotherapy for a mixed germ cell tumor of the ovary. Gynecol Oncol 1981;12:373–8.
4. Pastorfide GB, Goldstein DP. Pregnancy after hydatidiform mole. Obstet Gynecol 1973;42:67–70.
5. Rustin GJS, Booth M, Dent J, Salt S, Rustin F, Bagshawe KD. Pregnancy after cytotoxic chemotherapy for gestational trophoblastic tumours. Br Med J 1984;288:103–6.
6. Evenson DP, Arlin Z, Welt S, Claps ML, Melamed MR. Male reproductive capacity may recover following drug treatment with the L-10 protocol for acute lymphocytic leukemia. Cancer 1984;53:30–6.
7. Sivanesaratnam V, Sen DK. Normal pregnancy after successful treatment of choriocarcinoma with cerebral metastases: a case report. J Reprod Med 1988;33:402–3.
8. Lee RB, Kelly J, Elg SA, Benson WL. Pregnancy following conservative surgery and adjunctive chemotherapy for stage III immature teratoma of the ovary. Obstet Gynecol 1989;73:853–5.
9. Nicholson HO. Cytotoxic drugs in pregnancy: review of reported cases. J Obstet Gynaecol Br Commonw 1968;75:307–12.
10. Gililland J, Weinstein L. The effects of cancer chemotherapeutic agents on the developing fetus. Obstet Gynecol Surv 1983;38:6–13.
11. Haerr RW, Pratt AT. Multiagent chemotherapy for sarcoma diagnosed during pregnancy. Cancer 1985;56:1028–33.
12. Weed JC Jr, Roh RA, Mendenhall HW. Recurrent endodermal sinus tumor during pregnancy. Obstet Gynecol 1979;54:653–6.
13. Kim DS, Park MI. Maternal and fetal survival following surgery and chemotherapy of endodermal sinus tumor of the ovary during pregnancy: a case report. Obstet Gynecol 1989;73:503–7.
14. Dobbing J. Pregnancy and leukaemia. Lancet 1977;1:1155.
15. Gershenson DM. Menstrual and reproductive function after treatment with combination chemotherapy for malignant ovarian germ cell tumors. J Clin Oncol 1988;6:270–5.

Name: **DANTHRON**

Class: **Purgative**   Risk Factor: **C**

Fetal Risk Summary

Danthron is an anthraquinone purgative. See Cascara Sagrada.

Breast Feeding Summary

No data are available. See Cascara Sagrada.

Name: **DAUNORUBICIN**

Class: **Antineoplastic**   Risk Factor: **D$_M$**

Fetal Risk Summary

The use of daunorubicin during pregnancy has been reported in 29 patients, four during the 1st trimester (1–18). No congenital defects were observed in the 22 (one set of twins) liveborns, but one of these infants was anemic and hypoglycemic and had multiple serum electrolyte abnormalities (7). Severe, transient, drug-induced bone marrow hypoplasia occurred in one newborn after *in utero* exposure to daunorubicin and five other antineoplastic agents (17). The myelosuppression was probably secondary to mercaptopurine. The infant made an uneventful recovery. Results of the remaining pregnancies were three elective abortions (one with enlarged spleen), three intrauterine deaths (one probably due to severe pregnancy-induced hypertension), one stillborn with diffuse myocardial necrosis, and one maternal death (7, 8, 14, 16). Eleven of the infants (including one set of twins) were followed for periods ranging from 6 months to 9 years and all showed normal growth and development (8–10, 13, 14, 16–18).

Data from one review indicated that 40% of the infants exposed to anticancer drugs were of low birth weight (19). This finding was not related to timing of the exposure. Except for the infants noted above, long-term studies of growth and mental development in offspring exposed to daunorubicin during the 2nd trimester, the period of neuroblast multiplication, have not been conducted (20).

In one report, the use of daunorubicin and other antineoplastic drugs in two males was thought to be associated with congenital defects in their offspring (21). The defects observed were Fallot's tetralogy and syndactyly of the first and second digits of the right foot, and a stillborn anencephalic. Although the authors speculated that the drugs damaged the germ cells without producing infertility, and thus were responsible for the defects, any relationship with paternal use of daunorubicin is doubtful due to the lack of experimental evidence and other confirming reports. In a third male, fertilization occurred during treatment with daunorubicin and resulted in the birth of a healthy infant (22). Successful pregnancies have also been reported in two women after treatment with daunorubicin (23).

Chromosome aberrations were observed in the fetus of a 34-year-old woman with acute lymphoblastic leukemia who was treated with multiple antineoplastic agents (11). Daunorubicin was administered for approximately 3 weeks beginning at 22 weeks' gestation. A healthy female infant was delivered 18 weeks after the start of therapy. Chromosome analysis of the newborn revealed a normal karyotype (46,XX) but with gaps and a ring chromosome. The clinical significance of these findings is unknown, but since these abnormalities may persist for several years, the potential existed for an increased risk of cancer as well as for a risk of genetic damage in the next generation (11).

Occupational exposure of the mother to antineoplastic agents during pregnancy may present a risk to the fetus. A position statement from the National Study Commission on Cytotoxic Exposure and a research article involving some antineoplastic agents are presented in the monograph for cyclophosphamide (see Cyclophosphamide).

Breast Feeding Summary

No data are available.

References

1. Sears HF, Reid J. Granulocytic sarcoma: local presentation of a systemic disease. Cancer 1976;37:1808–13.
2. Lilleyman JS, Hill AS, Anderton KJ. Consequences of acute myelogenous leukemia in early pregnancy. Cancer 1977;40:1300–3.
3. Colbert N, Najman A, Gorin NC, et al. Acute leukaemia during pregnancy: favourable course of pregnancy in two patients treated with cytosine arabinoside and anthracyclines. Nouv Presse Med 1980;9:175–8.
4. Tobias JS, Bloom HJG. Doxorubicin in pregnancy. Lancet 1980;1:776.
5. Sanz MA, Rafecas FJ. Successful pregnancy during chemotherapy for acute promyelocytic leukemia. N Engl J Med 1982;306:939.
6. Alegre A, Chunchurreta R, Rodriguez-Alarcon J, Cruz E, Prada M. Successful pregnancy in acute promyelocytic leukemia. Cancer 1982;49:152–3.
7. Gililland J, Weinstein L. The effects of cancer chemotherapeutic agents on the developing fetus. Obstet Gynecol Surv 1983;38:6–13.
8. Feliu J, Juarez S, Ordonez A, Garcia-Paredes ML, Gonzalez-Baron M, Montero JM. Acute leukaemia and pregnancy. Cancer 1988;61:580–4.
9. Volkenandt M, Buchner T, Hiddemann W, Van De Loo J. Acute leukaemia during pregnancy. Lancet 1987;2:1521–2.
10. Turchi JJ, Villasis C. Anthracyclines in the treatment of malignancy in pregnancy. Cancer 1988;61:435–40.
11. Schleuning M, Clemm C. Chromosomal aberrations in a newborn whose mother received cytotoxic treatment during pregnancy. N Engl J Med 1987;317:1666–7.
12. Gokal R, Durrant J, Baum JD, Bennett MJ. Successful pregnancy in acute monocytic leukaemia. Br J Cancer 1976;34:299–302.
13. Lowenthal RM, Marsden KA, Newman NM, Baikie MJ, Campbell SN. Normal infant after treatment of acute myeloid leukaemia in pregnancy with daunorubicin. Aust NZ J Med 1978;8:431–2.
14. O'Donnell R, Costigan C, O'Connell LG. Two cases of acute leukaemia in pregnancy. Acta Haematol 1979;61:298–300.
15. Hamer JW, Beard MEJ, Duff GB. Pregnancy complicated by acute myeloid leukaemia. NZ Med J 1979;89:212–3.
16. Doney KC, Kraemer KG, Shepard TH. Combination chemotherapy for acute myelocytic leukemia during pregnancy: three case reports. Cancer Treat Rep 1979;63:369–71.
17. Okun DB, Groncy PK, Sieger L, Tanaka KR. Acute leukemia in pregnancy: transient neonatal myelosuppression after combination chemotherapy in the mother. Med Pediatr Oncol 1979;7:315–9.
18. Cantini E, Yanes B. Acute myelogenous leukemia in pregnancy. South Med J 1984;77:1050–2.
19. Nicholson HO. Cytotoxic drugs in pregnancy: review of reported cases. J Obstet Gynaecol Br Commonw 1968;75:307–12.
20. Dobbing J. Pregnancy and leukaemia. Lancet 1977;1:1155.
21. Russell JA, Powles RL, Oliver RTD. Conception and congenital abnormalities after chemotherapy of acute myelogenous leukaemia in two men. Br Med J 1976;1:1508.
22. Matthews JH, Wood JK. Male fertility during chemotherapy for acute leukemia. N Engl J Med 1980;303:1235.
23. Estiu M. Successful pregnancy in leukaemia. Lancet 1977;1:433.

Name: **DECAMETHONIUM**

Class: **Muscle Relaxant**   Risk Factor: **C**

Fetal Risk Summary

Decamethonium is no longer manufactured in the United States. No reports linking the use of decamethonium with congenital defects have been located. The drug has been used at term for maternal analgesia (1).

Breast Feeding Summary

No data are available.

Reference

1. Moya F, Thorndyke V. Passage of drugs across the placenta. Am J Obstet Gynecol 1962;84:1778–98.

Name: **DEFEROXAMINE**

Class: **Heavy Metal Antagonist**   Risk Factor: **C$_M$**

Fetal Risk Summary

Deferoxamine is used for the treatment of acute iron intoxication and chronic iron overload. Some animal studies have shown skeletal anomalies at doses close to those used in humans (1). The use of this drug in pregnancy has been described in three pregnant women, two with acute iron overdose and one with transfusion-dependent thalassemia (2–4). Brief mention of three other pregnant patients treated with deferoxamine for acute overdose appeared in an earlier report, but no details were given except that all of the infants were normal (5). The authors have knowledge of a seventh patient treated in the 3rd trimester for overdose with normal outcome (S.M. Lovett, unpublished data, 1985).

In the thalassemia patient, deferoxamine was given by continuous subcutaneous infusion pump, 2 g every 12 hours, for the first 16 weeks of pregnancy (2). A cesarean section was performed at 33 weeks' gestation for vaginal bleeding and premature rupture of the membranes, with delivery of a normal preterm male infant. The neonatal period was complicated by hypoglycemia and prolonged jaundice lasting 6 weeks, but neither problem was thought to be related to deferoxamine.

The iron overdose cases occurred at 15 and 34 weeks, respectively (3, 4). Both women were treated with intramuscular deferoxamine, and one also received the drug nasogastrically. Spontaneous labor with rupture of the membranes occurred 8 hours after iron ingestion in the 34–week gestation patient, resulting in the vaginal delivery 6 hours later of a normal male infant (3). The cord blood iron level was 121 μg/100 ml (normal 106–227 μg/100 ml) but fell to 21 μg/100 ml at 12 hours. The infant's clinical course was normal except for low iron levels requiring iron supplementation. The authors suggested that the low neonatal iron levels were due to chelation of iron by transplacentally transferred deferoxamine. In the other case, a normal term male infant was delivered without evidence of injury from deferoxamine (4).

Breast Feeding Summary

No data are available.

References

1. Product information. Desferal. CIBA Pharmaceutical Co., 1990.
2. Thomas RM, Skalicka AE. Successful pregnancy in transfusion-dependent thalassaemia. Arch Dis Child 1980;55:572–4.
3. Rayburn WF, Donn SM, Wulf ME. Iron overdose during pregnancy: successful therapy with deferoxamine. Am J Obstet Gynecol 1983;147:717–8.
4. Blanc P, Hryhorczuk D, Danel I. Deferoxamine treatment of acute iron intoxication in pregnancy. Obstet Gynecol 1984;64:12S-4S.
5. Strom RL, Schiller P, Seeds AE, Ten Bensel R. Fatal iron poisoning in a pregnant female: case report. Minn Med 1976;59:483–9.

Name: **DEMECARIUM**

Class: **Parasympathomimetic (Cholinergic)**   Risk Factor: **C**

Fetal Risk Summary

Demecarium is used in the eye. No reports of its use in pregnancy have been located. As a quaternary ammonium compound, it is ionized at physiologic pH and transplacental passage in significant amounts would not be expected (see also Neostigmine).

Breast Feeding Summary

No data are available.

Name: **DEMECLOCYCLINE**

Class: **Antibiotic**   Risk Factor: **D**

Fetal Risk Summary

See Tetracycline.

Breast Feeding Summary

See Tetracycline.

Name: **DESIPRAMINE**

Class: **Antidepressant**   Risk Factor: **C**

Fetal Risk Summary

Desipramine is an active metabolite of imipramine (see also Imipramine). No reports linking the use of desipramine with congenital defects have been located. Neonatal withdrawal symptoms, including cyanosis, tachycardia, diaphoresis, and weight loss, were observed after desipramine was taken throughout pregnancy (1).

In an *in vitro* study, desipramine was shown to be a potent inhibitor of sperm motility (2). A concentration of 27 μM produced a 50% reduction in motility.

Breast Feeding Summary

Desipramine is excreted into breast milk (3–5). No reports of adverse effects have been located. In one patient, milk:plasma ratios of 0.4–0.9 were measured with milk levels ranging between 17–35 μg/ml (3). A 35-year-old mother in her 9th postpartum week took 300 mg of desipramine daily at bedtime for depression (5). One week later, simultaneous milk and serum samples were collected about 9 hours after a dose. Concentrations of desipramine in the milk and serum were 316 and 257 ng/ml (ratio 1.2), respectively, while levels of the metabolite, 2–hydroxydesipramine, were 381 and 234 ng/ml (ratio 1.6), respectively. The measurements were repeated 1 week later, 10.33 hours after the dose, and milk levels of the parent drug and metabolite were 328 and 327 ng/ml. No drug was detected in the infant's serum nor were any clinical signs of toxicity observed in the infant after 3 weeks of maternal treatment. The American Academy of Pediatrics classifies desipramine as an agent whose effect on the nursing infant is unknown but may be of concern (6).

References

1. Webster PA. Withdrawal symptoms in neonates associated with maternal antidepressant therapy. Lancet 1973;2:318–9.
2. Levin RM, Amsterdam JD, Winokur A, Wein AJ. Effects of psychotropic drugs on human sperm motility. Fertil Steril 1981;36:503–6.
3. Sovner R, Orsulak PJ. Excretion of imipramine and desipramine in human breast milk. Am J Psychiatry 1979;136:451–2.
4. Erickson SH, Smith GH, Heidrich F. Tricyclics and breast feeding. Am J Psychiatry 1979;136:1483.
5. Stancer HC, Reed KL. Desipramine and 2–hydroxydesipramine in human breast milk and the nursing infant's serum. Am J Psychiatry 1986;143:1597–1600.
6. Committee on Drugs, American Academy of Pediatrics. Transfer of drugs and other chemicals into human milk. Pediatrics 1989;84:924–36.

Name: **DESLANOSIDE**

Class: **Cardiac Glycoside**   Risk Factor: **C**

Fetal Risk Summary

See Digitalis.

Breast Feeding Summary

See Digitalis.

Name: **DESMOPRESSIN**

Class: **Pituitary Hormone, Synthetic**   Risk Factor: **B$_M$**

Fetal Risk Summary

Desmopressin is a synthetic polypeptide structurally related to vasopressin. See Vasopressin.

Breast Feeding Summary

See Vasopressin.

Name: **DEXAMETHASONE**

Class: **Corticosteroid**   Risk Factor: **C**

Fetal Risk Summary

No reports linking the use of dexamethasone with congenital defects have been located. Other corticosteroids have been suspected of causing malformations (see Cortisone). Maternal free estriol and cortisol are significantly depressed after dexamethasone therapy, but the effects of these changes on the fetus have not been studied (1–3).

Dexamethasone has been used in patients with premature labor at about 26–34 weeks' gestation to stimulate fetal lung maturation (4–14). Although this therapy is supported by many clinicians, its use is still controversial since the beneficial effects of steroids are greatest in singleton pregnancies with female fetuses (15–18). These benefits are:

Reduction in incidence of respiratory distress syndrome (RDS)
Decreased severity of RDS if it occurs
Decreased incidence of and mortality from intracranial hemorrhage
Increased survival of premature infants

Toxicity in the fetus and newborn following the use of dexamethasone is rare.

In studies of women with premature rupture of the membranes (PROM), administration of corticosteroids does not always reduce the frequency of RDS or perinatal mortality (19–21). In addition, an increased risk of maternal infection has been observed in patients with PROM treated with corticosteroids (20, 21). A recent report, however, found no difference in the incidence of maternal complications between treated and nontreated patients (22).

Dexamethasone crosses the placenta to the fetus (23, 24). The drug is partially metabolized (54%) by the perfused placenta to its inactive 11–ketosteroid derivative, more so than betamethasone, but the difference is not statistically significant (24).

Leukocytosis has been observed in infants exposed antenatally to dexamthasone (25, 26). The white blood cell counts returned to normal in about a week.

The use of corticosteroids, including dexamethasone, for the treatment of asthma during pregnancy has not been related to a significantly increased risk of maternal or fetal complications (27). A slight increase in the number of premature births was found, but it could not be determined whether this was an effect of the corticosteroids. An earlier study also recorded a shortening of gestation with chronic corticosteroid use (28).

In Rh-sensitized women, the use of dexamethasone may have prevented intrauterine fetal deterioration and the need for fetal transfusion (29). Five women, in the 2nd and 3rd trimesters, were treated with 24 mg of the steroid weekly for 2–7 weeks resulting, in each case, in a live newborn.

Dexamethasone, 4 mg/day for 15 days, was administered to a woman late in the 3rd trimester for the treatment of autoimmune thrombocytopenic purpura (30). Therapy was given in an unsuccessful attempt to prevent fetal/neonatal thrombocytopenia due to the placental transfer of antiplatelet antibody. Platelet counts in the newborn were 38,000–49,000/mm^3, but the infant made an uneventful recovery.

The use of dexamethasone for the pharmacologic suppression of the fetal adrenal gland has been described in two women with 21-hydroxylase deficiency (31, 32). This deficiency results in the overproduction of adrenal androgens and the virilization of female fetuses. Dexamethasone, in divided doses of 1 mg/day, was administered from early in the 1st trimester (5th week and 10th week) to term. Normal female infants resulted from both pregnancies.

Although human studies have usually shown a benefit, the use of corticosteroids in animals has been associated with several toxic effects (33, 34):

Reduced fetal head circumference
Reduced fetal adrenal weight
Increased fetal liver weight
Reduced fetal thymus weight
Reduced placental weight

Fortunately, none of these effects have been observed in human investigations. Long-term follow-up evaluations of children exposed *in utero* to dexamethasone have shown no adverse effects from this exposure (35, 36).

Breast Feeding Summary

No data are available.

References

1. Reck G, Nowostawski, Bredwoldt M. Plasma levels of free estriol and cortisol under ACTH and dexamethasone during late pregnancy. Acta Endocrinol 1977;84:86–7.
2. Kauppilla A. ACTH levels in maternal, fetal and neonatal plasma after short term prenatal dexamethasone therapy. Br J Obstet Gynaecol 1977;84:128–34.
3. Warren JC, Cheatum SG. Maternal urinary estrogen excretion: effect of adrenal suppression. J Clin Endocrinol 1967;27:436–8.

4. Caspi I, Schreyer P, Weinraub Z, Reif R, Levi I, Mundel G. Changes in amniotic fluid lecithin-sphingomyelin ratio following maternal dexamethasone administration. Am J Obstet Gynecol 1975;122:327–31.

5. Spellacy WN, Buhi WC, Riggall FC, Holsinger KL. Human amniotic fluid lecithin/sphingomyelin ratio changes with estrogen or glucocorticoid treatment. Am J Obstet Gynecol 1973;115:216–8.

6. Caspi E, Schreyer P, Weinraub Z, Reif R, Levi I, Mundel G. Prevention of the respiratory distress syndrome in premature infants by antepartum glucocorticoid therapy. Br J Obstet Gynaecol 1976;83:187–93.

7. Ballard RA, Ballard PL. Use of prenatal glucocorticoid therapy to prevent respiratory distress syndrome. Am J Dis Child 1976;130:982–7.

8. Thornfeldt RE, Franklin RW, Pickering NA, Thornfeldt CR, Amell G. The effect of glucocorticoids on the maturation of premature lung membranes: preventing the respiratory distress syndrome by glucocorticoids. Am J Obstet Gynecol 1978;131:143–8.

9. Ballard PL, Ballard RA. Corticosteroids and respiratory distress syndrome: status 1979. Pediatrics 1979;63:163–5.

10. Taeusch HW Jr, Frigoletto F, Kitzmiller J, et al. Risk of respiratory distress syndrome after prenatal dexamethasone treatment. Pediatrics 1979;63:64–72.

11. Caspi E, Schreyer P, Weinraub Z, Lifshitz Y, Goldberg M. Dexamethasone for prevention of respiratory distress syndrome: multiple perinatal factors. Obstet Gynecol 1981;57:41–7.

12. Bishop EH. Acceleration of fetal pulmonary maturity. Obstet Gynecol 1981;58(Suppl):48S-51S.

13. Farrell PM, Engle MJ, Zachman RD, Curet LB, Morrison JC, Rao AV, Poole WK. Amniotic fluid phospholipids after maternal administration of dexamethasone. Am J Obstet Gynecol 1983;145:484–90.

14. Ruvinsky ED, Douvas SG, Roberts WE, Martin JN Jr, Palmer SM, Rhodes PG, Morrison JC. Maternal administration of dexamethasone in severe pregnancy-induced hypertension. Am J Obstet Gynecol 1984;149:722–6.

15. Avery ME. The argument for prenatal administration of dexamethasone to prevent respiratory distress syndrome. J Pediatr 1984;104:240.

16. Sepkowitz S. Prenatal corticosteroid therapy to prevent respiratory distress syndrome. J Pediatr 1984;105:338–9.

17. Avery ME. Reply. J Pediatr 1984;105:339.

18. Levy DL. Maternal administration of dexamethasone to prevent RDS. J Pediatr 1984;105:339.

19. Eggers TR, Doyle LW, Pepperell RJ. Premature rupture of the membranes. Med J Aust 1979;1:209–13.

20. Garite TJ, Freeman RK, Linzey EM, Braly PS, Dorchester WL. Prospective randomized study of corticosteroids in the management of premature rupture of the membranes and the premature gestation. Am J Obstet Gynecol 1981;141:508–15.

21. Garite TJ. Premature rupture of the membranes: the enigma of the obstetrician. Am J Obstet Gynecol 1985;151:1001–5.

22. Curet LB, Morrison JC, Rao AV. Antenatal therapy with corticosteroids and postpartum complications. Am J Obstet Gynecol 1985;152:83–4.

23. Osathanondh R, Tulchinsky D, Kamali H, Fencl MdeM, Taeusch HW Jr. Dexamethasone levels in treated pregnant women and newborn infants. J Pediatr 1977;90:617–20.

24. Levitz M, Jansen V, Dancis J. The transfer and metabolism of corticosteroids in the perfused human placenta. Am J Obstet Gynecol 1978;132:363–6.

25. Otero L, Conlon C, Reynolds P, Duval-Arnould B, Golden SM. Neonatal leukocytosis associated with prenatal administration of dexamethasone. Pediatrics 1981;68:778–80.

26. Anday EK, Harris MC. Leukemoid reaction associated with antenatal dexamethasone administration. J Pediatr 1982;101:614–6.

27. Schatz M, Patterson R, Zeitz S, O'Rourke J, Melam H. Corticosteroid therapy for the pregnant asthmatic patient. JAMA 1975;233:804–7.

28. Jenssen H, Wright PB. The effect of dexamethasone therapy in prolonged pregnancy. Acta Obstet Gynecol Scand 1977;56:467–73.

29. Navot D, Rozen E, Sadovsky E. Effect of dexamethasone on amniotic fluid absorbance in Rh-sensitized pregnancy. Br J Obstet Gynaecol 1982;89:456–8.

30. Yin CS, Scott JR. Unsuccessful treatment of fetal immunologic thrombocytopenia with dexamethasone. Am J Obstet Gynecol 1985;152:316–7.

31. David M, Forest MG. Prenatal treatment of congenital adrenal hyperplasia resulting from 21-hydroxylase deficiency. J Pediatr 1984;105:799–803.

32. Evans MI, Chrousos GP, Mann DW, Larsen JW Jr, Green I, McCluskey J, Loriaux L, Fletcher JC, Koons G, Overpeck J, Schulman JD. Pharmacologic suppression of the fetal adrenal gland *in utero*. JAMA 1985;253:1015–20.
33. Taeusch HW Jr. Glucocorticoid prophylaxis for respiratory distress syndrome: a review of potential toxicity. J Pediatr 1975;87:617–23.
34. Johnson JWC, Mitzner W, London WT, Palmer AE, Scott R. Betamethasone and the rhesus fetus: multisystemic effects. Am J Obstet Gynecol 1979;133:677–84.
35. Wong YC, Beardsmore CS, Silverman M. Antenatal dexamethasone and subsequent lung growth. Arch Dis Child 1982;57:536–8.
36. Collaborative Group on Antenatal Steroid Therapy. Effects of antenatal dexamethasone administration in the infant: long-term follow-up. J Pediatr 1984;104:259–67.

Name: **DEXBROMPHENIRAMINE**

Class: **Antihistamine**   Risk Factor: **C**

Fetal Risk Summary

Dexbrompheniramine is the *dextro*-isomer of brompheniramine (see Brompheniramine). No reports linking its use with congenital defects have been located.

Breast Feeding Summary

See Brompheniramine.

Name: **DEXCHLORPHENIRAMINE**

Class: **Antihistamine**   Risk Factor: **B$_M$**

Fetal Risk Summary

Dexchlorpheniramine is the *dextro*-isomer of chlorpheniramine (see also Chlorpheniramine). No reports linking its use with congenital defects have been located. One study recorded 14 exposures in the 1st trimester without evidence for an association with malformations (1). Animal studies for chlorpheniramine have not shown a teratogenic effect (2).

An association between exposure during the last 2 weeks of pregnancy to antihistamines in general and retrolental fibroplasia in premature infants has been reported. See Brompheniramine for details.

Breast Feeding Summary

No data are available.

References

1. Heinonen OP, Slone D, Shapiro S. *Birth Defects and Drugs in Pregnancy*. Littleton:Publishing Sciences Group, 1977:323.
2. Product information. Polaramine. Schering Corporation, 1990.

Name: **DEXTROAMPHETAMINE**

Class: **Central Stimulant**   Risk Factor: C_M

Fetal Risk Summary

See Amphetamine.

Breast Feeding Summary

See Amphetamine.

Name: **DEXTROTHYROXINE**

Class: **Antilipemic**   Risk Factor: **C**

Fetal Risk Summary

Dextrothyroxine is the *dextro*-isomer of levothyroxine (see also Levothyroxine). Although formerly used to treat hypothyroidism, the drug is now used exclusively for the therapy of hyperlipidemia. In a study of placental passage of dextrothyroxine, approximately 9% of a radiolabeled dose given 2–8 hours before delivery was found in the cord blood (1). Except for this one report, no mention of its use in human pregnancy has been located.

Breast Feeding Summary

No data are available.

Reference

1. Kearns JE, Hutson W. Tagged isomers and analogues of thyroxine (their transmission across the human placenta and other studies). J Nucl Med 1963;4:453–61.

Name: **DIATRIZOATE**

Class: **Diagnostic**   Risk Factor: **D**

Fetal Risk Summary

The use of diatrizoate for amniography has been described in several studies (1–10). Except for inadvertent injection of the contrast media into the fetus during amniocentesis, the use of diatrizoate was not thought to result in fetal harm. More recent studies have examined the effect of the drug on fetal thyroid function.

All of the various preparations of diatrizoate contain a high concentration of organically bound iodine. Twenty-eight pregnant women received intra-amniotic injections (50 ml) of diatrizoate for diagnostic indications (11). When compared to nontreated controls, no effect was observed on cord blood levothyroxine (T4) and liothyronine resin uptake values regardless of the time interval between injection and delivery. The authors concluded that the iodine remained organically bound until it was eliminated in 2–4 days from the amniotic fluid.

In another report, seven patients within 13 days or less of term were injected intra-amniotically with a mixture of ethiodized oil (12 ml) and diatrizoate (30 ml) (12). Thyrotropin (TSH) levels were determined in the cord blood of five newborns and in the serum of all seven infants on the 5th day of life. TSH was markedly elevated in three of five cord samples and six of seven neonatal samples. Three of the infants had signs and symptoms of hypothyroidism:

Elevated TSH/normal T4; apathy and jaundice clearing immediately with thyroid therapy (one infant)
Elevated TSH/decreased T4 (one infant)
Elevated TSH/decreased T4 with goiter (one infant)

In contrast to the initial report, the severity of thyroid suppression seemed greater the longer the time interval between injection and delivery. The explanation offered for these different results was the utilization of the more sensitive TSH serum test and the use of only water-soluble contrast media in the first study.

In summary, diatrizoate may suppress the fetal thyroid when administered by intra-amniotic injection. Appropriate measures should be taken to diagnose and treat neonatal hypothyroidism if amniography with diatrizoate is performed.

Breast Feeding Summary

No data are available. See also Potassium Iodide.

References

1. McLain CR Jr. Amniography studies of the gastrointestinal motility of the human fetus. Am J Obstet Gynecol 1963;86:1079–87.
2. McLain CR Jr. Amniography, a versatile diagnostic procedure in obstetrics. Obstet Gynecol 1964;23:45–50.
3. McLain CR Jr. Amniography for diagnosis and management of fetal death in utero. Obstet Gynecol 1965;26:233–6.
4. Ferris EJ, Shapiro JH, Spira J. Roentgenologic aspects of intrauterine transfusion. JAMA 1966;196:127–8.
5. Wiltchik SG, Schwarz RH, Emich JP Jr. Amniography for placental localization. Obstet Gynecol 1966;28:641–5.
6. Misenhimer HR. Fetal hemorrhage associated with amniocentesis. Am J Obstet Gynecol 1966;94:1133–5.
7. Blumberg ML, Wohl GT, Wiltchik S, Schwarz R, Emich JP. Placental localization by amniography. AJR 1967;100:688–97.
8. Berner HW Jr. Amniography, an accurate way to localize the placenta. Obstet Gynecol 1967;29:200–6.
9. Creasman WT, Lawrence RA, Thiede HA. Fetal complications of amniocentesis. JAMA 1968;204:949–52.
10. Bottorff MK, Fish SA. Amniography. S Med J 1971;64:1203–6.
11. Morrison JC, Boyd M, Friedman BI, et al. The effects of Renografin-60 on the fetal thyroid. Obstet Gynecol 1973;42:99–103.
12. Rodesch F, Camus M, Ermans AM, Dodion J, Delange F. Adverse effect of amniofetography on fetal thyroid function. Am J Obstet Gynecol 1976;126:723–6.

Name: **DIAZEPAM**

Class: **Sedative**   Risk Factor: **D**

Fetal Risk Summary

Diazepam and its metabolite, n-demethyldiazepam, freely cross the placenta and accumulate in the fetal circulation with newborn levels about one to three times greater than maternal serum levels (1–10). Equilibrium between mother and fetus occurs in 5–10 minutes after intravenous administration (10). The maternal and fetal serum binding capacity for diazepam is reduced in pregnancy and is not correlated with albumin (11, 12). The plasma half-life in newborns is significantly increased due to a decreased clearance of the drug. Because the transplacental passage is rapid, timing of the intravenous administration with uterine contractions will greatly reduce the amount of drug transferred to the fetus (6).

In a case of gross overdose, a mother who took 580 mg of diazepam as a single dose on about the 43rd day of gestation delivered an infant with cleft lip/palate, craniofacial asymmetry, ocular hypertelorism, and bilateral perauricular tags (13). The authors concluded that the drug ingestion was responsible for the defects. An association between diazepam and an increased risk of cleft lip and/or palate was suggested by several studies (14–17). The findings indicated that 1st or 2nd trimester use of diazepam, and selected other drugs, is significantly greater among mothers of children born with oral clefts. However, a review of these studies, published in 1976, concluded that a causal relationship between diazepam and oral clefts had not yet been established, but even if it had, the actual risk was only 0.2% for cleft palate and only 0.4% for cleft lip with or without cleft palate (18). In addition, large retrospective studies showing no association between diazepam and cleft lip/palate have been published (19–22). The results of one of these studies has been criticized and defended (23, 24). Although no association was found with cleft lip/palate, a statistically significant association was discovered between diazepam and inguinal hernia (24). This same association, along with others, was found in another investigation (25).

In 1427 malformed newborns compared to 3001 controls, 1st trimester use of tranquilizers (diazepam most common) was associated with inguinal hernia, cardiac defects, and pyloric stenosis (25). Second trimester exposure was associated with hemangiomas and cardiac and circulatory defects. The combination of cigarette smoking and tranquilizer use increased the risk of delivering a malformed infant by 3.7–fold as compared to those who smoked but did not use tranquilizers (25). A survey of 390 infants with congenital heart disease matched with 1254 normal infants found a higher rate of exposure to several drugs, including diazepam, in the offspring with defects (26). Other congenital anomalies reported in infants exposed to diazepam include absence of both thumbs (two cases), spina bifida (one case), and absence of left forearm and syndactyly (one case) (27–29). Any relationship between diazepam and these defects is unknown.

A 1989 report described dysmorphic features, growth retardation, and central nervous system defects in eight infants exposed either to diazepam, 30 mg/day or more, or oxazepam, 75 mg/day or more throughout gestation (30). Three of the mothers denied use of drugs during pregnancy, but diazepam and its metabolite were demonstrated in their plasma in early pregnancy. The mothers did not use alcohol or street drugs, had regular prenatal care, and had no record of criminality or prostitution. The mean birth weight of the infants was 1.2 standard deviations below the Swedish average, only one having a weight above the mean, and one was small for gestational age. Six of the newborns had low Apgar scores primarily due to apnea, five needed resuscitation, all were hypotonic at birth, and all had neonatal drug withdrawal with episodes of opisthotonos and convulsions. Seven of the eight infants had feeding difficulties caused by a lack of rooting and sucking reflexes. Craniofacial defects observed in the infants (number of infants with defect shown in parenthesis) were short nose with low nasal bridge (six), uptilted nose (six), slanted eyes (eight), epicanthic folds (eight), telecanthus (two), long eyelashes (three), highly arched palate (four), cleft hard palate and bifid uvula (two), low-set/abnormal ears (four), webbed neck (three), flat upper lip (five), full lips (four), hypoplastic mandible (five), and microcephaly (two). Other defects present were small, wide-spaced nipples (two), renal defect (one), inguinal hernia (two), and cryptorchidism (two). An infant with severe psychomotor retardation died of possible sudden infant death syndrome at 11 weeks of age. Microscopic examination of the brain demonstrated slight cortical dysplasia and an increased number of single-cell neuronal heterotopias in the white matter. Six other children had varying degrees of mental retardation, some had severely disturbed visual perception, all had gross motor disability, and hyperactivity and attention deficits were common. Extensive special examinations were conducted to identify other possible etiologies, but the only common factor in the eight cases was maternal consumption of benzodiazepines (30). Based on the apparent lack of other causes, the investigators concluded that the clinical characteristics observed in the infants probably represented a teratogenic syndrome due to benzodiazepines.

Several investigators have observed that the use of diazepam during labor is not harmful to the mother or her infant (31–38). A dose response is likely as the frequency of newborn complications rises when doses exceed 30–40 mg or when diazepam is taken for extended periods, allowing accumulation to occur (39–45). Two major syndromes of neonatal complications have been observed:

Floppy infant syndrome:
    Hypotonia
    Lethargy
    Sucking difficulties
Withdrawal syndrome:
    Intrauterine growth retardation
    Tremors
    Irritability
    Hypertonicity
    Diarrhea/vomiting
    Vigorous sucking

Under miscellaneous effects, diazepam may alter thermogenesis, cause loss of beat-to-beat variability in the fetal heart rate, and decrease fetal movements (30, 46–51).

Breast Feeding Summary

Diazepam and its metabolite, n-demethyldiazepam, enter breast milk (52–57). Lethargy and loss of weight have been reported (55). Milk:plasma ratios varied between 0.2–2.7 (54).

A mother who took 6–10 mg daily throughout pregnancy delivered a full-term, normally developed male infant (57). The infant was breast fed and the mother continued to take her diazepam. Sedation was noted in the infant if nursing occurred less than 8 hours after taking a dose. Paired samples of maternal serum and breast milk were obtained on five occasions between 1–4 months after delivery. Milk concentrations of diazepam and desmethyldiazepam varied between 7.5–87 ng/ml and 19.2–77 ng/ml, respectively. The milk:serum ratios for diazepam varied between 0.14–0.21 in four samples, but was 1.0 on one sample. The ratio for demethyldiazepam varied from 0.10–0.18 on four samples, and was 0.53 on the sample with the high diazepam ratio. A serum level was drawn from the infant on one occasion, revealing levels of diazepam and the metabolite of 0.7 and 46 ng/ml, respectively.

Diazepam may accumulate in breast-fed infants, and its use in lactating women is not recommended. The American Academy of Pediatrics considers the effects of diazepam on the nursing infant to be unknown, but they may be of concern (58).

References

1. Erkkola R, Kanto J, Sellman R. Diazepam in early human pregnancy. Acta Obstet Gynecol Scand 1974;53:135–8.
2. Kanto J, Erkkola R, Sellman R. Accumulation of diazepam and n-demethyldiazepam in the fetal blood during labor. Ann Clin Res 1973;5:375–9.
3. Idanpaan-Heikkila JE, Jouppila PI, Puolakka JO, Vorne MS. Placental transfer and fetal metabolism of diazepam in early human pregnancy. Am J Obstet Gynecol 1971;109:1011–6.
4. Mandelli M, Morselli PL, Nordio S, Pardi G, Principi N. Sereni F, Tognoni G. Placental transfer of diazepam and its disposition in the newborn. Clin Pharmacol Ther 1975;17:564–72.
5. Gamble JAS, Moore J, Lamke H, Howard PJ. A study of plasma diazepam levels in mother and infant. Br J Obstet Gynaecol 1977;84:588–91.
6. Haram K, Bakke DM, Johannessen KH, Lund T. Transplacental passage of diazepam during labor: influence of uterine contractions. Clin Pharmacol Ther 1978;24:590–9.
7. Bakke OM, Haram K, Lygre T, Wallem G. Comparison of the placental transfer of thiopental and diazepam in caesarean section. Eur J Clin Pharmacol 1981;21:221–7.
8. Haram K, Bakke OM. Diazepam as an induction agent for caesarean section: a clinical and pharmacokinetic study of fetal drug exposure. Br J Obstet Gynaecol 1980;87:506–12.
9. Kanto JH. Use of benzodiazepines during pregnancy, labour and lactation, with particular reference to pharmacokinetic considerations. Drugs 1982;23:354–80.
10. Bakke OM, Haram K. Time-course of transplacental passage of diazepam: influence of injection-delivery interval on neonatal drug concentrations. Clin Pharmacokinet 1982;7:353–62.
11. Lee JN, Chen SS, Richens A, Menabawey M, Chard T. Serum protein binding of diazepam in maternal and foetal serum during pregnancy. Br J Clin Pharmacol 1982;14:551–4.
12. Ridd MJ, Brown KF, Nation RL, Collier CB. Differential transplacental binding of diazepam: causes and implications. Eur J Clin Pharmacol 1983;24:595–601.
13. Rivas F, Hernandez A, Cantu JM. Acentric craniofacial cleft in a newborn female prenatally exposed to a high dose of diazepam. Teratology 1984;30:179–80.
14. Safra JM, Oakley GP Jr. Association between cleft lip with or without cleft palate and prenatal exposure to diazepam. Lancet 1975;2:478–80.
15. Saxen I. Epidemiology of cleft lip and palate: an attempt to rule out chance correlations. Br J Prev Soc Med 1975;29:103–10.
16. Saxen I. Associations between oral clefts and drugs taken during pregnancy. Int J Epidemiol 1975;4:37–44.

17. Saxen I, Saxen L. Association between maternal intake of diazepam and oral clefts. Lancet 1975;2:498.
18. Safra MJ, Oakley GP Jr. Valium: an oral cleft teratogen? Cleft Palate J 1976;13:198–200.
19. Czeizel A. Diazepam, phenytoin, and etiology of cleft lip and/or cleft palate. Lancet 1976;1:810.
20. Rosenberg L, Mitchell AA, Parsells JL, Pashayan H, Louik C, Shapiro S. Lack of relation of oral clefts to diazepam use during pregnancy. N Engl J Med 1983;309:1282–5.
21. Shiono PH, Mills JL. Oral clefts and diazepam use during pregnancy. N Engl J Med 1984;311:919–20.
22. Lakos P, Czeizel E. A teratological evaluation of anticonvulsant drugs. Acta Paediatr Acad Sci Hung 1977;18:145–53.
23. Entman SS, Vaughn WK. Lack of relation of oral clefts to diazepam use in pregnancy. N Engl J Med 1984;310:1121–2.
24. Rosenberg L, Mitchell AA. Lack of relation of oral clefts to diazepam use in pregnancy. N Engl J Med 1984;310:1122.
25. Bracken MB, Holford TR. Exposure to prescribed drugs in pregnancy and association with congenital malformations. Obstet Gynecol 1981;58:336–44.
26. Rothman KJ, Fyler DC, Goldblatt A, Kreidberg MB. Exogenous hormones and other drug exposures of children with congenital heart disease. Am J Epidemiol 1979;109:433–9.
27. Istvan EJ. Drug-associated congenital abnormalities. Can Med Assoc J 1970;103:1394.
28. Ringrose CAD. The hazard of neurotrophic drugs in the fertile years. Can Med Assoc J 1972;106:1058.
29. Fourth Annual Report of the New Zealand Committee on Adverse Drug Reactions. NZ Med J 1969;70:118–22.
30. Laegreid L, Olegard R, Walstrom J, Conradi N. Teratogenic effects of benzodiazepine use during pregnancy. J Pediatr 1989;114:126–31.
31. Greenblatt DJ, Shader RI. Effect of benzodiazepines in neonates. N Engl J Med 1975;292:649.
32. Modif M, Brinkman CR, Assali NS. Effects of diazepam on uteroplacental and fetal hemodynamics and metabolism. Obstet Gynecol 1973;41:364–8.
33. Toaff ME, Hezroni J, Toaff R. Effect of diazepam on uterine activity during labor. Isr J Med Sci 1977;13:1007–9.
34. Shannon RW, Fraser GP, Aitken RG, Harper JR. Diazepam in preeclamptic toxaemia with special reference to its effect on the newborn infant. Br J Clin Pract 1972;26:271–5.
35. Yeh SY, Paul RIT, Cordero L, Hon EH. A study of diazepam during labor. Obstet Gynecol 1974;43:363–73.
36. Kasturilal, Shetti RN. Role of diazepam in the management of eclampsia. Curr Ther Res 1975;18:627–30.
37. Eliot BW, Hill JG, Cole AP, Hailey DM. Continuous pethidine/diazepam infusion during labor and its effects on the newborn. Br J Obstet Gynaecol 1975;82:126–31.
38. Lean TH, Retnam SS, Sivasamboo R. Use of benzodiazepines in the management of eclampsia. J Obstet Gynaecol Br Commonw 1968;75:856–62.
39. Scanlon JW. Effect of benzodiazepines in neonates. N Engl J Med 1975;292:649.
40. Gillberg C. "Floppy infant syndrome" and maternal diazepam. Lancet 1977;2:244.
41. Haram K. "Floppy infant syndrome" and maternal diazepam. Lancet 1977;2:612–3.
42. Speight AN. Floppy-infant syndrome and maternal diazepam and/or nitrazepam. Lancet 1977;1:878.
43. Rementeria JL, Bhatt K. Withdrawal symptoms in neonates from intrauterine exposure to diazepam. J Pediatr 1977;90:123–6.
44. Thearle MJ, Dunn PM. Exchange transfusions for diazepam intoxication at birth followed by jejunal stenosis. Proc R Soc Med 1973;66:13–4.
45. Backes CR, Cordero L. Withdrawal symptoms in the neonate from presumptive intrauterine exposure to diazepam: report of case. J Am Osteopath Assoc 1980;79:584–5.
46. Cree JE, Meyer J, Hailey DM. Diazepam in labour: its metabolism and effect on the clinical condition and thermogenesis of the newborn. Br Med J 1973;4:251–5.
47. McAllister CB. Placental transfer and neonatal effects of diazepam when administered to women just before delivery. Br J Anaesth 1980;52:423–7.
48. Owen JR, Irani SF, Blair AW. Effect of diazepam administered to mothers during labour on temperature regulation of neonate. Arch Dis Child 1972;47:107–10.
49. Scher J, Hailey DM, Beard RW. The effects of diazepam on the fetus. J Obstet Gynaecol Br Commonw 1972;79:635–8.

50. van Geijn HP, Jongsma HW, Doesburg WH, Lemmens WA, deHaan J, Eskes TK. The effect of diazepam administration during pregnancy or labor on the heart rate variability of the newborn infant. Eur J Obstet Gynaecol Reprod Biol 1980;10:187–201.
51. Birger M, Homberg R, Insler V. Clinical evaluation of fetal movements. Int J Gynaecol Obstet 1980;18:377–82.
52. van Geijn HP, Kenemans P, Vise T, Vanderkleijn E, Eskes TK. Pharamcokinetics of diazepam and occurrence in breast milk. In Proceedings of the Sixth International Congress of Pharmacology, Helsinki 1975:514.
53. Hill RM, Nowlin J, Lertratanangkoon K, Stillwell WG, Stillwell RN, Horning MG. The identification and quantification of drugs in human breast milk. Clin Res 1974;22:77A.
54. Cole AP, Hailey DM. Diazepam and active metabolite in breast milk and their transfer to the neonate. Arch Dis Child 1975;50:741–2.
55. Patrick MJ, Tilstone WJ, Reavey P. Diazepam and breast-feeding. Lancet 1972;1:542–3.
56. Catz CS. Diazepam in breast milk. Drug Ther 1973;3:72–3.
57. Wesson DR, Camber S, Harkey M, Smith DE. Diazepam and desmethyldiazepam in breast milk. J Psychoactive Drugs 1985;17:55–6.
58. Committee on Drugs, American Academy of Pediatrics. Transfer of drugs and other chemicals into human milk. Pediatrics 1989;84;924–36.

Name: **DIAZOXIDE**

Class: **Antihypertensive**   Risk Factor: **C$_M$**

Fetal Risk Summary

Diazoxide readily crosses the placenta and reaches fetal plasma concentrations similar to maternal levels (1). The drug has been used for the treatment of severe hypertension associated with pregnancy (1–12). Some investigators have cautioned against the use of diazoxide in pregnancy (13, 14). In one study, the decrease in maternal blood pressure was sufficient to produce a state of clinical shock and endanger placental perfusion (13). Transient fetal bradycardia has been reported in other studies following a rapid, marked decrease in maternal blood pressure (7, 15). Fatal maternal hypotension has been reported in one patient after diazoxide therapy (16). Some investigators have recommended the infusion technique for administering diazoxide rather than rapid boluses to prevent maternal and fetal complications (17). However, small bolus doses at frequent intervals (30 mg every 1–2 minutes) have been used successfully to treat maternal hypertension without producing fetal toxicity (18).

Diazoxide is a potent relaxant of uterine smooth muscle and may inhibit uterine contractions if given during labor (2, 3, 5–7, 19–21). The degree and duration of uterine inhibition are dose dependent (20). Augmentation of labor with oxytocin may be required in patients receiving diazoxide.

Hyperglycemia in the newborn (glucose 500–700 mg/dl) secondary to intravenous diazoxide therapy in a mother just prior to delivery has been observed to persist for up to 3 days (22). In some series, all of the mothers and newborns had hyperglycemia without ketoacidosis (13). The glucose levels returned to near normal within 24 hours.

The use of oral diazoxide for the last 19–69 days of pregnancy has been associated with alopecia, hypertrichosis lanuginosa, and decreased ossification of the wrist (1). However, long-term oral therapy has not caused similar problems in other newborns exposed *in utero* (4).

Since other antihypertensive drugs are available for severe maternal hypertension and the long-term effects on the infant have not been evaluated, diazoxide should be used with caution, if at all, during pregnancy. If diazoxide is needed after other therapies have failed, small doses are recommended.

Breast Feeding Summary

No data are available.

References

1. Milner RDG, Chouksey SK. Effects of fetal exposure to diazoxide in man. Arch Dis Child 1972;47:537–43.
2. Finnerty FA JR, Kakaviatos N, Tuckman J, Magill J. Clinical evaluation of diazoxide: a new treatment for acute hypertension. Circulation 1963;28:203–8.
3. Finnerty FA Jr. Advantages and disadvantages of furosemide in the edematous states of pregnancy. Am J Obstet Gynecol 1969;105:1022–7.
4. Pohl JEF, Thurston H, Davis D, Morgan MY. Successful use of oral diazoxide in the treatment of severe toxaemia of pregnancy. Br Med J 1972;2:568–70.
5. Pennington JC, Picker RH. Diazoxide and the treatment of the acute hypertensive emergency in obstetrics. Med J Aust 1972;2:1051–4.
6. Koch-Weser J. Diazoxide. N Engl J Med 1976;294:1271–4.
7. Morris JA, Arce JJ, Hamilton CJ, Davidson EC, Maidman JE, Clark JH, Bloom RS. The management of severe preeclampsia and eclampsia with intravenous diazoxide. Obstet Gynecol 1977;49:675–80.
8. Keith TA III. Hypertension crisis: recognition and management. JAMA 1977;237:1570–7.
9. MacLean AB, Doig JR, Aickin DR. Hypovolaemia, pre-eclampsia and diuretics. Br J Obstet Gynaecol 1978;85:597–601.
10. Barr PA, Gallery ED. Effect of diazoxide on the antepartum cardiotocograph in severe pregnancy-associated hypertension. Aust NZ J Obstet Gynaecol 1981;21:11–5.
11. MacLean AB, Doig JR, Chatfield WR, Aickin DR. Small-dose diazoxide administration in pregnancy. Aust NZ J Obstet Gynaecol 1981;21:7–10.
12. During VR. Clinical experience obtained from use of diazoxide (Hypertonalum) for treatment of acute intrapartum hypertensive crisis. Zentralbl Gynakol 1982;104:89–93.
13. Neuman J, Weiss B, Rabello Y, Cabal L, Freeman RK. Diazoxide for the acute control of severe hypertension complicating pregnancy: a pilot study. Obstet Gynecol 1979;53(Suppl):50S-5S.
14. Perkins RP. Treatment of toxemia of pregnancy. JAMA 1977;238:2143–4.
15. Michael CA. Intravenous diazoxide in the treatment of severe preeclamptic toxaemia and eclampsia. Aust NZ J Obstet Gynaecol 1973;13:143–6.
16. Henrich WL, Cronin R, Miller PD, Anderson RJ. Hypotensive sequelae of diazoxide and hydralazine therapy. JAMA 1977;237:264–5.
17. Thien T, Koene RAP, Schijf C, Pieters GFFM, Eskes TKAB, Wijdeveld PGAB. Infusion of diazoxide in severe hypertension during pregnancy. Eur J Obstet Gynaecol Reprod Biol 1980;10:367–74.
18. Dudley DKL. Minibolus diazoxide in the management of severe hypertension in pregnancy. Am J Obstet Gynecol 1985;151:196–200.
19. Barden TP, Keenan WJ. Effects of diazoxide in human labor and the fetus-neonate. Obstet Gynecol 1971;37:631–2 (Abstract).
20. Landesman R, Adeodato de Souza FJ, Countinho EM, Wilson KH, Bomfim de Sousa FM. The inhibitory effect of diazoxide in normal term labor. Am J Obstet Gynecol 1969;103:430–3.
21. Paulissian R. Diazoxide. Int Anesthesiol Clin 1978;16:201–36.
22. Milsap RL, Auld PAM. Neonatal hyperglycemia following maternal diazoxide administration. JAMA 1980;243:144–5.

Name: **DIBENZEPIN**

Class: **Antidepressant**   Risk Factor: **D**

Fetal Risk Summary

No data are available. See Imipramine.

Breast Feeding Summary

No data are available. See Imipramine.

Name: **DICLOXACILLIN**

Class: **Antibiotic**   Risk Factor: **B$_M$**

Fetal Risk Summary

Dicloxacillin is a penicillin antibiotic (see also Penicillin G). The drug crosses the placenta into the fetal circulation and amniotic fluid. Levels are low compared to other penicillins due to the high degree of maternal protein binding (1, 2). Following a 500-mg intravenous dose, the fetal peak serum level of 3.4 µg/ml occurred at 2 hours (8% of maternal peak) (2). A peak of 1.8 µg/ml was obtained at 6 hours in the amniotic fluid.

No reports linking the use of dicloxacillin with congenital defects have been located. The Collaborative Perinatal Project monitored 50,282 mother-child pairs, 3,546 of which had 1st trimester exposure to penicillin derivatives (3, pp. 297–313). For use anytime in pregnancy, 7,171 exposures were recorded (3, p. 435). In neither case was evidence found to suggest a relationship to large categories of major or minor malformations or to individual defects.

Breast Feeding Summary

No data are available (see Penicillin G).

References

1. MacAulay M, Berg S, Charles D. Placental transfer of dicloxacillin at term. Am J Obstet Gynecol 1968;102:1162–8.
2. Depp R, Kind A, Kirby W, Johnson W. Transplacental passage of methicillin and dicloxacillin into the fetus and amniotic fluid. Am J Obstet Gynecol 1970;107:1054–7.
3. Heinonen OP, Slone D, Shapiro S. *Birth Defects and Drugs in Pregnancy*. Littleton:Publishing Sciences Group, 1977.

Name: **DICUMAROL**

Class: **Anticoagulant**   Risk Factor: **D**

Fetal Risk Summary

See Coumarin Derivatives.

Breast Feeding Summary

See Coumarin Derivatives.

Name: **DICYCLOMINE**

Class: **Parasympatholytic**   Risk Factor: **B**

Fetal Risk Summary

See Doxylamine.

Breast Feeding Summary

See Doxylamine.

Name: **DIENESTROL**

Class: **Estrogenic Hormone**   Risk Factor: **X**

Fetal Risk Summary

Dienestrol is used topically. Estrogens are readily absorbed, and intravaginal use can lead to significant concentrations of estrogen in the blood (1, 2). The Collaborative Perinatal Project monitored 614 mother-child pairs with 1st trimester exposure to estrogenic agents, including 36 with exposure to dienestrol (3, pp. 389, 391). An increase in the expected frequency of cardiovascular defects, eye and ear anomalies, and Down's syndrome was found for estrogens as a group but not for dienestrol (3, pp. 389, 391, 395). Use of estrogenic hormones during pregnancy is contraindicated.

Breast Feeding Summary

No reports of adverse effects of dienestrol on the nursing infant have been located. It is possible that decreased milk volume and decreased nitrogen and protein content could occur (see Mestranol and Ethinyl Estradiol).

References

1. Gilman AG, Goodman LS, Gilman A. *The Pharmacological Basis of Therapeutics*. New York:MacMillan, 1980:1428.
2. Rigg LA, Hermann H, Yen SSC. Absorption of estrogens from vaginal creams. N Engl J Med 1978;298:195–7.
3. Heinonen OP, Slone D, Shapiro S. *Birth Defects and Drugs in Pregnancy*. Littleton:Publishing Sciences Group, 1977.

Name: **DIETHYLPROPION**

Class: **Central Stimulant/Anorectant**   Risk Factor: **B**

Fetal Risk Summary

No reports linking the use of diethylpropion with congenital defects have been located. The drug has been studied as an appetite suppressant in 28 pregnant patients and, although adverse effects were common in the women, no problems were observed in their offspring (1). A retrospective survey of 1232 patients exposed to diethylpropion during pregnancy found no difference in the incidence of defects (0.9%) when compared to a matched control group (1.1%) (2). Animal studies have not revealed a teratogenic potential (3).

Breast Feeding Summary

No data are available.

References

1. Silverman M, Okun R. The use of an appetitie suppressant (diethylpropion hydrochloride) during pregnancy. Curr Ther Res 1971;13:648–53.
2. Bunde CA, Leyland HM. A controlled retrospective survey in evaluation of teratogenicity. J New Drugs 1965;5:193–8.
3. Schardein JL. *Drugs as Teratogens*. Cleveland:CRC Press, 1976:73–5.

Name: **DIETHYLSTILBESTROL**

Class: **Estrogenic Hormone**   Risk Factor: **X_M**

Fetal Risk Summary

Between 1940–1971, an estimated 6 million mothers and their fetuses were exposed to diethylstilbestrol (DES) to prevent reproductive problems such as miscarriage, premature delivery, intrauterine fetal death, and toxemia (1–4). Controlled studies have since proven that DES was not successful in preventing these disorders (5, 6). This use has resulted, however, in significant complications of the reproductive system in both female and male offspring (1–12). Two large groups have been established to monitor these complications: the Registry for Research on Hormonal Transplacental Carcinogenesis and the Diethylstilbestrol Adenosis (DESAD) Project (4). The published findings and recommendations of the DESAD project through 1980 plus a number of other studies including the Registry were reviewed in a 1981 National Institutes of Health booklet available from the National Cancer Institute (4). This information was also reprinted in a 1983 journal article (13). The complications identified in female and male children exposed *in utero* to DES are:

Female
   Lower müllerian tract
      Vaginal adenosis
      Vaginal and cervical clear cell adenocarcinoma
      Cervical/vaginal fornix defects (10)

Cockscomb (hood, transverse ridge of cervix)
Collar (rim, hood, transverse ridge of cervix)
Pseudopolyp
Hypoplastic cervix (immature cervix)
Altered fornix of vagina
Vaginal defects (exclusive of fornix) (10)
Incomplete transverse septum
Incomplete longitudinal septum
Upper müllerian tract
Uterine structural defects
Fallopian tube structural defects
Male
Reproductive dysfunction
Altered semen analysis
Infertility

The Registry was established in 1971 to study the epidemiologic, clinical, and pathologic aspects of clear cell adenocarcinoma of the vagina and cervix in DES-exposed women (2). Over 400 cases of clear cell adenocarcinoma have been reported to the registry. Additional reports continue to appear in the literature (14). The risk of carcinoma is apparently higher when DES treatment was given before the 12th week of gestation and is estimated to be 0.14–1.4/1000 for women under the age of 25 years (2, 4).

A recent report described the first known case of adenosquamous carcinoma of the cervix in an exposed patient (15). In a second case, a 12-year-old exposed girl developed a fatal malignant teratoma of the ovary (16). The relationship between these tumors and DES is unknown.

The frequency of dysplasia and carcinoma in situ (CIS) of the cervix and vagina in 3980 DESAD Project patients was significantly increased over controls with an approximate 2- to 4-fold increase in risk (11). These results were different from earlier studies of these same women which had indicated no increased risk for dysplasia/CIS (17, 18). Robboy and co-workers speculated that the increased incidence now observed was related to the greater amount of squamous metaplasia found in DES-exposed women (11). Scanning electron microscopy of the cervicovaginal transformation zone has indicated that maturation of epithelium is slowed or arrested at the stage of immature squamous epithelium in some DES-exposed women (19). This process may produce greater susceptibility to such factors as herpes and papillomavirus obtained through early coitus with multiple partners and result in the observed increased rates of dysplasia/CIS (11). Of interest in this regard, a 1983 article reported detectable papillomavirus antigen in the cervical-vaginal biopsies of 16 (43%) of 37 DES-exposed women (20).

The incidence of cervical or vaginal structural changes has been reported to occur in up to 85% of exposed women, although most studies place the incidence in the 22–58% range (2, 3, 5, 7, 12, 21–24). The structural changes are outlined above. The DESAD Project reported an incidence of approximately 25% in 1655 women (10). Selection bias was eliminated by analyzing only those patients identified by record review. Patients referred by physicians and self-referrals had much higher rates of defects, about 49% and 43%, respectively. Almost all of the defects were confined to the cervical-vaginal fornix area, with only 14 patients having vaginal changes exclusive of the fornix and nearly all of these being incomplete transverse septums (10).

Reports linking the use of DES with major congenital anomalies have not been located. The Collaborative Perinatal Project monitored 614 mother-child pairs with 1st trimester exposure to estrogens, including 164 with exposure to DES (25, pp. 389, 391). Evidence for an increase in the expected frequency for cardiovascular defects, eye and ear anomalies, and Down's syndrome was found for estrogens as a group, but not for DES (25, pp. 389, 391, 395). Re-evaluation of these data in terms of timing of exposure, vaginal bleeding in early pregnancy, and previous maternal obstetric history, however, failed to support an association between estrogens and cardiac malformations (26). An earlier study also failed to find any relationship with nongenital malformations (27).

Alterations in the body of the uterus have led to concern regarding increased pregnancy wastage and premature births (8, 22, 28–31). Increased rates of spontaneous abortions, premature births and ectopic pregnancies are well established by these latter reports, although the relationship to the abnormal changes of the cervix and/or vagina is still unclear (8). Serial observations of vaginal epithelial changes indicate that the frequency of such changes decreases with age (4, 17, 24).

Spontaneous rupture of a term uterus has been described in a 25-year-old primigravid with DES-type changes in her vagina, cervix and uterus (32). Other reports of this type have not been located.

In a 1984 study, DES exposure had no effect on the age at menarche, first coitus, pregnancy or live birth, nor on a woman's ability to conceive (33). One group of investigators found that although anomalies in the upper genital tract increased the risk for poor pregnancy outcome, they could not relate specific changes to specific types of outcomes (34).

Hirsutism and irregular menses were found in 72% and 50%, respectively, of 32 DES-exposed women (35). The degree of hirsutism was age related, with the mean ages of severely and mildly hirsute women being 28.8 and 24.7 years, respectively. Based on various hormone level measurements, the authors concluded that *in utero* DES exposure may result in hypothalamic-pituitary-ovarian dysfunction (35). However, other studies in much larger exposed populations have not observed disturbances of menstruation or excessive hair growth (36).

Data on DES-exposed women who had undergone major gynecologic surgical procedures, excluding cesarean section, were reported in a 1982 study (37). Of 309 exposed women, 33 (11%) had a total of 43 procedures. The authors suggested that DES exposure resulted in an increased incidence of adnexal disease involving adhesions, benign ovarian cysts, and ectopic pregnancies (37). Surgical manipulation of the cervix (cryocautery or conization) in DES-exposed patients results in a high incidence of cervical stenosis and possible development of endometriosis (38, 39). Both studies concluded, however, that the causes of infertility in these patients were comparable to those in a non-DES-exposed population.

Adverse effects in male offspring attributable to *in utero* DES exposure have been reported (1, 5, 40–46). Abnormalities thought to occur at greater frequencies include:

Epididymal cysts
Hypotrophic testis
Microphallus
Variococele
Capsular induration
Altered semen (decreased count, concentration, motility, and morphology)

An increase in problems with passing urine and urogenital tract infections has also been observed (40).

DES exposure has been proposed as a possible cause of infertility in male off-spring (1). However, in a controlled *in vitro* study, no association was found between exposure to DES and reduced sperm penetration of zona-free hamster eggs (46). In addition, a study of 828 exposed males found no increase over controls for risk of genitourinary abnormalities, infertility, or testicular cancer (47). Based on their data, the authors proposed that previous studies showing a positive relationship may have had selection biases, differences in DES use, or both.

Testicular tumors have been reported in three DES-exposed patients (6, 48). In one case, a teratoma was discovered in a 23-year-old male (6). Two patients, 27 and 28 years of age, were included in the second report (48). Both had left-sided anaplastic seminomas, and one had epididymal cysts. A male sibling of one of the patients, also DES exposed, had severe oligospermia, and two exposed sisters had vaginal adenosis and vaginal adenocarcinoma.

Changes in the psychosexual performance of young boys have been attributed to *in utero* exposure to DES and progesterone (49, 50). The mothers received estrogen/progestogen regimens for diabetes. A trend to less heterosexual experience and fewer masculine interests than controls was shown. A 2-fold increase in psychiatric disease, especially depression and anxiety, has been observed in both male and female exposed offspring (6).

Breast Feeding Summary

No data are available. Decreased milk volume and nitrogen-protein content may occur if diethylstilbestrol is used during lactation (see Mestranol and Ethinyl Estradiol).

References

1. Stenchever MA, Williamson RA, Leonard J, Karp LE, Ley B, Shy K, Smith D. Possible relationship between *in utero* diethylstilbestrol exposure and male fertility. Am J Obstet Gynecol 1981;140:186–93.
2. Herbst AL. Diethylstilbestrol and other sex hormones during pregnancy. Obstet Gynecol 1981;58(Suppl):35s–40s.
3. Nordquist SAB, Medhat IA, Ng AB. Teratogenic effects of intrauterine exposure to DES in female offspring. Compr Ther 1979;5:69–74.
4. Robboy SJ, Noller KL, Kaufman RH, Barnes AB, Townsend D, Gundersen JH, Nash S. Information for Physicians. Prenatal diethylstilbestrol (DES) exposure: recommendations of the Diethylstilbestrol-Adenosis (DESAD) Project for the identification and management of exposed individuals. NIH Publication No. 81–2049, 1981.
5. Stillman RJ. In utero exposure to diethylstilbestrol: adverse effects on the reproductive tract and reproductive performance in male and female offspring. Am J Obstet Gynecol 1982;142:905–21
6. Vessey MP, Fairweather DVI, Norman-Smith B, Buckley J. A randomized double-blind controlled trial of the value of stilboestrol therapy in pregnancy: long-term follow-up of mothers and their offspring. Br J Obstet Gynaecol 1983;90:1007–17.

7. Prins RP, Morrow P, Townsend DE, Disaia PJ. Vaginal embryogenesis, estrogens, and adenosis. Obstet Gynecol 1976;48:246–50.

8. Sandberg EC, Riffle NL, Higdon JV, Getman CE. Pregnancy outcome in women exposed to diethylstilbestrol *in utero*. Am J Obstet Gynecol 1981;140:194–205.

9. Noller KL, Townsend DE, Kaufman RH, Barnes AB, Robboy SJ, Fish CR, Jefferies JA, Bergstralh EJ, O'Brien PC, McGorray SP, Scully R. Maturation of vaginal and cervical epithelium in women exposed *in utero* to diethylstilbestrol (DESAD Project). Am J Obstet Gynecol 1983;146:279–85.

10. Jefferies JA, Robboy SJ, O'Brien PC, Bergstralh EJ, Labarthe DR, Barnes AB, Noller KL, Hatab PA, Kaufman RH, Townsend DE. Structural anomalies of the cervix and vagina in women enrolled in the Diethylstilbestrol Adenosis (DESAD) Project. Am J Obstet Gynecol 1984;148:59–66.

11. Robboy SJ, Noller KL, O'Brien P, Kaufman RH, Townsend D, Barnes AB, Gundersen J, Lawrence WD, Bergstrahl E, McGorray S, Tilley BC, Anton J, Chazen G. Increased incidence of cervical and vaginal dysplasia in 3,980 diethylstilbestrol-exposed young women. Experience of the National Collaborative Diethylstilbestrol Adenosis Project. JAMA 1984;252:2979–83.

12. Chanen W, Pagano R. Diethylstilboestrol (DES) exposure *in utero*. Med J Aust 1984;141:491–3.

13. NCI DES Summary. Prenatal diethylstilbestrol (DES) exposure. Clin Pediatr 1983;22:139–43.

14. Kaufman RH, Korhonen MO, Strama T, Adam E, Kaplan A. Development of clear cell adenocarcinoma in DES-exposed offspring under observation. Obstet Gynecol 1982;59(Suppl):68S–72S.

15. Vandrie DM, Puri S, Upton RT, Demeester LJ. Adenosquamous carcinoma of the cervix in a woman exposed to diethylstilbestrol *in utero*. Obstet Gynecol 1983;61(Suppl):84S–7S.

16. Lazarus KH. Maternal diethylstilboestrol and ovarian malignancy in offspring. Lancet 1984;1:53.

17. O'Brien PC, Noller KL, Robboy SJ, Barnes AB, Kaufman RH, Tilley BC, Townsend DE. Vaginal epithelial changes in young women enrolled in the National Cooperative Diethylstilbestrol Adenosis (DESAD) Project. Obstet Gynecol 1979;53:300–8.

18. Robboy SJ, Kaufman RH, Prat J, Welch WR, Gaffey T, Scully RE, Richart R, Fenoglio CM, Virata R, Tilley BC. Pathologic findings in young women enrolled in the National Cooperative Diethylstilbestrol Adenosis (DESAD) Project. Obstet Gynecol 1979;53:309–17.

19. McDonnell JM, Emens JM, Jordan JA. The congenital cervicovaginal transformation zone in young women exposed to diethylstilboestrol in utero. Br J Obstet Gynaecol 1984;91:574–9.

20. Fu YS, Lancaster WD, Richart RM, Reagan JW, Crum CP, Levine RU. Cervical papillomavirus infection in diethylstilbestrol-exposed progeny. Obstet Gynecol 1983;61:59–62.

21. Ben-Baruch G, Menczer J, Mashiach S, Serr DM. Uterine anomalies in diethylstilbestrol-exposed women with fertility disorders. Acta Obstet Gynecol Scand 1981;60:395–7.

22. Pillsbury SG. Jr. Reproductive significance of changes in the endometrial cavity associated with exposure *in utero* in diethylstilbestrol. Am J Obstet Gynecol 1980;137:178–82.

23. Professional and Public Relations Committee of the Diethylstilbestrol and Adenosis Project of the Division of Cancer Control and Rehabilitation. Exposure *in utero* to diethylstilbestrol and related synthetic hormones. Association with vaginal and cervical cancers and other abnormalities. JAMA 1976;236:1107–9.

24. Burke L, Antonioli D, Friedman EA. Evolution of diethylstilbestrol-associated genital tract lesions. Obstet Gynecol 1981;57:79–84.

25. Heinonen OP, Slone D, Shapiro S. *Birth Defects and Drugs in Pregnancy.* Littleton:Publishing Sciences Group, 1977.

26. Wiseman RA, Dodds-Smith IC. Cardiovascular birth defects and antenatal exposure to female sex hormones: a reevaluation of some base data. Teratology 1984;30:359–70.

27. Wilson JG, Brent RL. Are female sex hormones teratogenic? Am J Obstet Gynecol 1981;141:567–80.

28. Herbst AL, Hubby MM, Blough RR, Azizi F. A comparison of pregnancy experience in DES-exposed daughters. J Reprod Med 1980;24:62–9.

29. Barnes AB, Colton T, Gundersen J, Noller KL, Tilley BC, Strama T, Townsend DE, Hatab P, O'Brien PC. Fertility and outcome of pregnancy in women exposed *in utero* to diethylstilbestrol. N Engl J Med 1980;302:609–13.

30. Veridiano NP, Dilke I, Rogers J, Tancer ML. Reproductive performance of DES-exposed female progeny. Obstet Gynecol 1981;58:58–61.

31. Mangan CE, Borow L, Burnett-Rubin MM, Egan V, Giuntoli RL, Mikuta JJ. Pregnancy outcome in 98 women exposed to diethylstilbestrol *in utero*, their mothers, and unexposed siblings. Obstet Gynecol 1982; 59:315–9.

32. Williamson HO, Sowell GA, Smith HE. Spontaneous rupture of gravid uterus in a patient with diethylstilbestrol-type changes. Am J Obstet Gynecol 1984;150:158–60.

33. Barnes AB. Menstrual history and fecundity of women exposed and unexposed *in utero* to diethyl-stilbestrol. J Reprod Med 1984;29:651–5.
34. Kaufman RH, Noller K, Adam E, Irwin J, Gray M, Jefferies JA, Hilton J. Upper genital tract abnor-malities and pregnancy outcome in diethylstilbestrol-exposed progeny. Am J Obstet Gynecol 1984;148:973–84.
35. Peress MR, Tsai CC, Mathur RS, Williamson HO. Hirsutism and menstrual patterns in women exposed to diethylstilbestrol *in utero*. Am J Obstet Gynecol 1982;144:135–40.
36. Verkauf BS. Discussion. Am J Obstet Gynecol 1982;144:139–40.
37. Schmidt G, Fowler WC Jr. Gynecologic operative experience in women exposed to DES *in utero*. South Med J 1982;75:260–3.
38. Haney AF, Hammond MG. Infertility in women exposed to diethylstilbestrol *in utero*. J Reprod Med 1983;28:851–6.
39. Stillman RJ, Miller LC. Diethylstilbestrol exposure *in utero* and endometriosis in infertile females. Fertil Steril 1984;41:369–72.
40. Henderson BE, Benton B, Cosgrove M, Baptista J, Aldrich J, Townsend D, Hart W, Mack TM. Urogenital tract abnormalities in sons of women treated with diethylstilbestrol. Pediatrics 1976;58:505–7.
41. Gill WB, Schumacher GFB, Bibbo M. Pathological semen and anatomical abnormalities of the genital tract in human male subjects exposed to diethylstilbestrol in utero. J Urol 1977;117:477–80.
42. Gill WB, Schumacher GFB, Bibbo M, Strous FH, Schoenberh HW. Association of diethylstilbestrol exposure in utero with cryptorchidism, testicular hypoplasia and semen abnormalities. J Urol 1979;122:36–9.
43. Gill WB, Schumacher GFB, Bibbo M. Structural and functional abnormalities in the sex organs of male offspring of mothers treated with diethylstilbestrol (DES). J Reprod Med 1976;16:147–53.
44. Driscoll SG, Taylor SM. Effects of prenatal maternal estrogen on the male urogenital system. Obstet Gynecol 1980;56:537–42.
45. Bibbo M, Gill WB, Azizi F, Blough R, Fang VS, Rosenfield RL, Schaumacher GFB, Sleeper K, Sonek MG, Wied GL. Follow-up study of male and female offspring of DES-exposed mothers. Obstet Gynecol 1977;49:1–8.
46. Shy KK, Stenchever MA, Karp LE, Berger RE, Williamson RA, Leonard J. Genital tract examina-tions and zona-free hamster egg penetration tests from men exposed *in utero* to diethylstilbestrol. Fertil Steril 1984;42:772–8.
47. Leary FJ, Resseguie LJ, Kurland LT, O'Brien PC, Emslander RF, Noller KL. Males exposed *in utero* to diethylstilbestrol. JAMA 1984;252:2984–9.
48. Conley GR, Sant GR, Ucci AA, Mitcheson HD. Seminoma and epididymal cysts in a young man with known diethylstilbestrol exposure *in utero*. JAMA 1983;249:1325–6.
49. Yalom ID, Green R, Fisk N. Prenatal exposure to female hormones. Effect on psychosexual de-velopment in boys. Arch Gen Psychiatry 1973;28:554–61.
50. Burke L, Apfel RJ, Fischer S, Shaw J. Observations on the psychological impact of diethylstilbes-trol exposure and suggestions on management. J Reprod Med 1980;24:99–102.

Name: **DIGITALIS**

Class: **Cardiac Glycoside** Risk Factor: **C**

Fetal Risk Summary

No reports linking digitalis or the various digitalis glycosides with congenital defects have been located. Animal studies have failed to show a teratogenic effect (1). Rapid passage to the fetus has been observed after digoxin and digitoxin (2–9). One group of investigators found that the amount of digitoxin recovered from the fetus was de-pendent on the length of gestation (2). In the late 1st trimester, only 0.05–0.10% of the injected dose was recovered from three fetuses. Digitoxin metabolites accounted for 0.18–0.33%. At 34 weeks of gestation, digitoxin recovery was 0.85% and metabolite recovery was 3.49% from one fetus. Average cord concentrations of digoxin in three reports were 50%, 81%, and 83% of the maternal serum (3, 4, 9). Highest fetal concentrations of digoxin in the second half of pregnancy were found in the heart (5). The fetal heart has only a limited binding capacity for digoxin in the first half of pregnancy (5). In animals, amniotic fluid acts as a reservoir for digoxin, but no data are available in humans after prolonged treatment (5). The pharmacokinetics of digoxin in pregnant women have been reported (10, 11).

Digoxin has been used for both maternal and fetal indications (e.g., congestive heart failure and supraventricular tachycardia) during all stages of gestation without causing fetal harm (12–25). Direct administration of digoxin to the fetus by periodic intramuscular injections has been used to treat supraventricular tachycardia when indirect therapy via the mother failed to control the arrhythmia (26).

Fetal toxicity resulting in neonatal death has been reported after maternal overdose (27). The mother, in her 8th month of pregnancy, took an estimated 8.9 mg of digitoxin as a single dose. Delivery occurred 4 days later. The baby demonstrated digitalis cardiac effects until death at age 3 days from prolonged intrauterine anoxia.

In a series of 22 multiparous patients maintained on digitalis, spontaneous labor occurred more than 1 week earlier than in 64 matched controls (28). The first stage of labor in the treated patients averaged 4.3 hours vs. 8 hours in the control group. In contrast, others found no effect on duration of pregnancy or labor in 122 patients with heart disease (29).

Breast Feeding Summary

Digoxin is excreted into breast milk. Data for other cardiac glycosides have not been located. Digoxin milk:plasma ratios have varied from 0.6–0.9 (4, 7, 30, 31). Although these amounts seem high, they represent very small amounts of digoxin due to significant maternal protein binding. No adverse effects in the nursing infant have been reported. The American Academy of Pediatrics considers digoxin to be compatible with breast feeding (32).

References

1. Shepard TH. *Catalog of Teratogenic Agents*, ed. 3. Baltimore:Johns Hopkins University Press, 1980:116–7.
2. Okita GT, Plotz EF, Davis ME. Placental transfer of radioactive digitoxin in pregnant women and its fetal distribution. Circ Res 1956;4:376–80.
3. Rogers MC, Willserson JT, Goldblatt A, Smith TW. Serum digoxin concentrations in the human fetus, neonate and infant. N Engl J Med 1972;287:1010–3.
4. Chan V, Tse TF, Wong V. Transfer of digoxin across the placenta and into breast milk. Br J Obstet Gynaecol 1978;85:605–9.
5. Saarikoski S. Placental transfer and fetal uptake of ^{3}H-digoxin in humans. Br J Obstet Gynaecol 1976;83:879–84.
6. Allonen H, Kanto J, Lisalo E. The foeto-maternal distribution of digoxin in early human pregnancy. Acta Pharmacol Toxicol 1976;39:477–80.
7. Finley JP, Waxman MB, Wong PY, Lickrish GM. Digoxin excretion in human milk. J Pediatr 1979;94:339–40.
8. Soyka LF. Digoxin: placental transfer, effects on the fetus, and therapeutic use in the newborn. Clin Perinatol 1975;2:23–35.
9. Padeletti L, Porciani MC, Scimone G. Placental transfer of digoxin (beta-methyl-digoxin) in man. Int J Clin Pharmacol Biopharm 1979;17:82–3.
10. Marzo A, Lo Cicero G, Brina A, Zuliani G, Ghirardi P, Pardi G. Preliminary data on the pharmacokinetics of digoxin in pregnancy. Boll Soc Ital Biol Sper 1980;56:219–23.

11. Luxford AME, Kellaway GSM. Pharmacokinetics of digoxin in pregnancy. Eur J Clin Pharmacol 1983;25:117–21.
12. Lingman G, Ohrlander S, Ohlin P. Intrauterine digoxin treatment of fetal paroxysmal tachycardia: case report. Br J Obstet Gynaecol 1980;87:340–2.
13. Kerenyi TD, Gleicher N, Meller J, Brown E, Steinfeld L, Chitkara U, Raucher H. Transplacental cardioversion of intrauterine supraventricular tachycardia with digitalis. Lancet 1980;2:393–4.
14. Harrigan JT, Kangos JJ, Sikka A, Spisso KR, Natarajan N, Rosenfeld D, Leiman S, Korn D. Successful treatment of fetal congestive heart failure secondary to tachycardia. N Engl J Med 1981;304:1527–9.
15. Diro M, Beydoun SN, Jaramillo B, O'Sullivan MJ, Kieval J. Successful pregnancy in a woman with a left ventricular cardiac aneurysm: a case report. J Reprod Med 1983;28:559–63.
16. Heaton FC, Vaughan R. Intrauterine supraventricular tachycardia: cardioversion with maternal digoxin. Obstet Gynecol 1982;60:749–52.
17. Simpson PC, Trudinger BJ, Walker A, Baird PJ. The intrauterine treatment of fetal cardiac failure in a twin pregnancy with an acardiac, acephalic monster. Am J Obstet Gynecol 1983;147:842–4.
18. Spinnato JA, Shaver DC, Flinn GS, Sibai BM, Watson DL, Marin-Garcia J. Fetal supraventricular tachycardia: in utero therapy with digoxin and quinidine. Obstet Gynecol 1984;64:730–5.
19. Bortolotti U, Milano A, Mazzucco A, Valfre C, Russo R, Valente M, Schivazappa L, Thiene G, Gallucci V. Pregnancy in patients with a porcine valve bioprosthesis. Am J Cardiol 1982;50:1051–4.
20. Rotmensch HH, Rotmensch S, Elkayam U. Management of cardiac arrhythmias during pregnancy: current concepts. Drugs 1987;33:623–33.
21. Tamari I, Eldar M, Rabinowitz B, Neufeld HN. Medical treatment of cardiovascular disorders during pregnancy. Am Heart J 1982;104:1357–63.
22. Dumesic DA, Silverman NH, Tobias S, Golbus MS. Transplacental cardioversion of fetal supraventricular tachycardia with procainamide. N Engl J Med 1982;307:1128–31.
23. Gleicher N, Elkayam U. Cardiac problems in pregnancy. II. Fetal aspects: advances in intrauterine diagnosis and therapy. JAMA 1984;252:78–80.
24. Golichowski AM, Caldwell R, Hartsough A, Peleg D. Pharmacologic cardioversion of intrauterine supraventricular tachycardia. A case report. J Reprod Med 1985;30:139–44.
25. Reece EA, Romero R, Santulli T, Kleinman CS, Hobbins JC. In utero diagnosis and management of fetal tachypnea. A case report. J Reprod Med 1985;30:221–4.
26. Weiner CP, Thompson MIB. Direct treatment of fetal supraventricular tachycardia after failed transplacental therapy. Am J Obstet Gynecol 1988;158:570–3.
27. Sherman JL Jr, Locke RV. Transplacental neonatal digitalis intoxication. Am J Cardiol 1960;6:834–7.
28. Weaver JB, Pearson JF. Influence of digitalis on time of onset and duration of labour in women with cardiac disease. Br Med J 1973;3:519–20.
29. Ho PC, Chen TY, Wong V. The effect of maternal cardiac disease and digoxin administration on labour, fetal weight and maturity at birth. Aust NZ J Obstet Gynaecol 1980;20:24–7.
30. Levy M, Granit L, Laufer N. Excretion of drugs in human milk. N Engl J Med 1977;297:789.
31. Loughnan PM. Digoxin excretion in human breast milk. J Pediatr 1978;92:1019–20.
32. Committee on Drugs, American Academy of Pediatrics. Transfer of drugs and other chemicals into human milk. Pediatrics 1989;84:924–36.

Name: **DIGITOXIN**

Class: **Cardiac Glycoside**

Risk Factor: **C$_M$**

Fetal Risk Summary

See Digitalis.

Breast Feeding Summary

See Digitalis.

Name: **DIGOXIN**

Class: **Cardiac Glycoside**   Risk Factor: **C_M**

Fetal Risk Summary

See Digitalis.

Breast Feeding Summary

See Digitalis.

Name: **DIHYDROCODEINE BITARTRATE**

Class: **Narcotic Analgesic**   Risk Factor: **B***

Fetal Risk Summary

No reports linking the use of dihydrocodeine with congenital defects have been located. Usage in pregnancy is primarily confined to labor. Respiratory depression in the newborn has been reported to be less than with meperidine, but depression is probably similar when equianalgesic doses are compared (1–3).

[*Risk Factor D if used for prolonged periods or in high doses at term.]

Breast Feeding Summary

No data are available.

References

1. Ruch WA, Ruch RM. A preliminary report on dihydrocodeine-scopolamine in obstetrics. Am J Obstet Gynecol 1957;74:1125–7.
2. Myers JD. A preliminary clinical evaluation of dihydrocodeine bitartrate in normal parturition. Am J Obstet Gynecol 1958;75:1096–100.
3. Bonica JJ. *Principles and Practice of Obstetric Analgesia and Anesthesia.* Philadelphia:FA Davis, 1967:245.

Name: **DIHYDROTACHYSTEROL**

Class: **Vitamin**   Risk Factor: **A***

Fetal Risk Summary

Dihydrotachysterol is a synthetic analogue of vitamin D. It is converted in the liver to 25-hydroxydihydrotachysterol, an active metabolite. See Vitamin D.

[*Risk Factor D if used in doses above the recommended daily allowance.]

Breast Feeding Summary

See Vitamin D.

Name: **DIMENHYDRINATE**

Class: **Antiemetic**   Risk Factor: **B_M**

Fetal Risk Summary

Dimenhydrinate is the clorotheophylline salt of the antihistamine diphenhydramine. A prospective study in 1963 compared dimenhydrinate usage in three groups of patients: 266 with malformed infants and two groups of 266 each without malformed infants (1). No difference in usage of the drug was found between the three groups. The Collaborative Perinatal Project monitored 50,282 mother-child pairs, 319 of which had 1st trimester exposure to dimenhydrinate (2, pp. 367–370). For use anytime in pregnancy, 697 exposures were recorded (2, p. 440). In neither case was evidence found to suggest a relationship to large categories of major or minor malformations. Two possible associations with individual malformations were found, but their statistical significance is unknown. The defects noted were cardiovascular defects (five cases), and inguinal hernia (eight cases). Independent confirmation is required to determine the actual risk for these anomalies from dimenhydrinate (2, p. 440).

A number of reports have described the oxytocic effect of intravenous dimenhydrinate (3–13). When used either alone or with oxytocin, most studies found a smoother, shorter labor. However, in one study of 30 patients who received a 100-mg dose over 3.5 minutes, some (at least two, but exact number not specified) also showed evidence of uterine hyperstimulation and fetal distress (e.g., bradycardia and loss of beat-to-beat variability) (13). Due to these effects, dimenhydrinate should not be used for this purpose.

Dimenhydrinate has been used for the treatment of hyperemesis gravidarum (14). In 64 women presenting with the condition prior to 13 weeks' gestation, all were treated with dimenhydrinate followed by various other antiemetics. Three of the newborns had integumentary abnormalities consisting of one case of webbed toes with an extra finger, and two cases of skin tags (one preauricular and one sacral). The defects were not thought to be related to the drug therapy (14).

An association between exposure during the last 2 weeks of pregnancy to antihistamines in general and retrolental fibroplasia in premature infants has been reported. See Brompheniramine for details.

Breast Feeding Summary

No data are available.

References

1. Mellin GW, Katzenstein M. Meclozine and fetal abnormalities. Lancet 1963;1:222–3.
2. Heinonen OP, Slone D, Shapiro S. *Birth Defects and Drugs in Pregnancy*. Littleton:Publishing Sciences Group, 1977.
3. Watt LO. Oxytocic effects of dimenhydrinate in obstetrics. Can Med Assoc J 1961;84:533–4.
4. Rotter CW, Whitaker JL, Yared J. The use of intravenous Dramamine to shorten the time of labor and potentiate analgesia. Am J Obstet Gynecol 1958:75:1101–4.
5. Scott RS, Wallace KH, Badley DN, Watson BH. Use of dimenhydrinate in labor. Am J Obstet Gynecol 1962;83:25–8.
6. Humphreys DW. Safe relief of pain during labor with dimenhydrinate. Clin Med (Winnetka) 1962;69:1165–8.
7. Cooper K. Failure of dimenhydrinate to shorten labor. Am J Obstet Gynecol 1963;86:1041–3.

8. Harkins JL, Van Praagh IG, Irwin NT. A clinical evaluation of intravenous dimenhydrinate in labor. Can Med Assoc J 1964;91:164–6.
9. Scott RS. The use of intravenous dimenhydrinate in labor. New Physician 1964;13:302–7.
10. Klieger JA, Massart JJ. Clinical and laboratory survey into the oxytocic effects of dimenhydrinate in labor. Am J Obstet Gynecol 1965;92:1–10.
11. Hay TB, Wood C. The effect of dimenhydrinate on uterine contractions. Aust NZ J Obstet Gynaecol 1967;1:81–9.
12. Shephard B, Cruz A, Spellacy W. The acute effects of Dramamine on uterine contractability during labor. J Reprod Med 1976;16:27–8.
13. Hara GS, Carter RP, Krantz KE. Dramamine in labor: potential boon or a possible bomb? J Kans Med Soc 1980;81:134–6,155.
14. Gross S, Librach C, Cecutti A. Maternal weight loss associated with hyperemesis gravidarum: a predictor of fetal outcome. Am J Obstet Gynecol 1989;160:906–9.

Name: **DIMETHINDENE**

Class: **Antihistamine**   Risk Factor: **C**

Fetal Risk Summary

No data are available. See Chlorpheniramine for representative agent in this class.

Breast Feeding Summary

No data are available.

Name: **DIMETHOTHIAZINE**

Class: **Antihistamine**   Risk Factor: **C**

Fetal Risk Summary

No data are available. See Promethazine for representative agent in this class.

Breast Feeding Summary

No data are available.

Name: **DIOXYLINE**

Class: **Vasodilator**   Risk Factor: **C**

Fetal Risk Summary

No data are available.

Breast Feeding Summary

No data are available.

Name: **DIPHEMANIL**

Class: **Parasympatholytic**   Risk Factor: **C**

Fetal Risk Summary

Diphemanil is an anticholinergic quaternary ammonium methylsulfate. No reports of its use in pregnancy have been located (see also Atropine).

Breast Feeding Summary

No data are available (see also Atropine).

Name: **DIPHENADIONE**

Class: **Anticoagulant**   Risk Factor: **D**

Fetal Risk Summary

See Coumarin Derivatives.

Breast Feeding Summary

See Coumarin Derivatives.

Name: **DIPHENHYDRAMINE**

Class: **Antihistamine**   Risk Factor: **C**

Fetal Risk Summary

The Collaborative Perinatal Project monitored 50,282 mother-child pairs, 595 of which had 1st trimester exposure to diphenhydramine (1, pp. 323–337). For use anytime during pregnancy, 2,948 exposures were recorded (1, p. 437). In neither case was evidence found to suggest a relationship to large categories of major or minor malformations. Several possible associations with individual malformations were found, but the statistical significance of these is unknown and independent confirmation is required to determine the actual risk (1, pp. 323–337, 437, 475).

Genitourinary (other than hypospadias) (5 cases)
Hypospadias (3 cases)
Eye and ear defects (3 cases)
Syndromes (other than Down's syndrome) (3 cases)
Inguinal hernia (13 cases)
Clubfoot (5 cases)
Any ventricular septal defect (open or closing) (5 cases)
Malformations of diaphragm (3 cases)

Cleft palate and diphenhydramine usage in the 1st trimester were statistically associated in a 1974 study (2). A group of 599 children with oral clefts were compared to 590 controls without clefts. *In utero* exposures to diphenhydramine in the groups were 20 and 6, respectively, a significant difference. However, in a 1971 report significantly fewer infants with malformations were exposed to antihistamines in the 1st trimester as compared to controls (3). Diphenhydramine was the second most commonly used antihistamine. In addition, a 1985 study reported 1st trimester use of diphenhydramine in 270 women from a total group of 6509 (4). No association between the use of the drug and congenital abnormalities was found.

Diphenhydramine withdrawal was reported in a newborn infant whose mother had taken 150 mg/day during pregnancy (5). Generalized tremulousness and diarrhea began on the 5th day of life. Treatment with phenobarbital resulted in the gradual disappearance of the symptoms.

A stillborn, full-term, 1000-g female infant was exposed during gestation to high doses of diphenhydramine, theophylline, ephedrine, and phenobarbital, all used for maternal asthma (6). Except for a ventricular septal defect, no other macroscopic internal or external anomalies were observed. However, complete triploidy was found in lymphocyte cultures, which is unusual because very few such infants survive until term (6). No relationship between the chromosome abnormality or the congenital defect and the drug therapy can be inferred from this case.

A potential drug interaction between diphenhydramine and temazepam resulting in the stillbirth of a term female infant has been reported (7). The mother had taken diphenhydramine 50 mg for mild itching of the skin and approximately 1.5 hours later, took 30 mg of temazepam for sleep. Three hours later she awoke with violent intrauterine fetal movements, which lasted several minutes and then abruptly stopped. The stillborn infant was delivered approximately 4 hours later. Autopsy revealed no gross or microscopic anomalies. In an experiment with pregnant rabbits, neither of the drugs alone caused fetal mortality but when combined, 51 (81%) of 63 fetuses were stillborn or died shortly after birth (7). No definite mechanism could be established for the suggested interaction.

A 1980 report described the oxytocic properties of diphenydramine when used in labor (8). Fifty women were given 50 mg intravenously over 3.5 minutes in a study designed to compare its effect with dimenhydrinate (see also Dimenhydrinate). The effects on the uterus were similar to those of dimenhydrinate but not as pronounced. Although no uterine hyperstimulation or fetal distress was observed, the drug should not be used for this purpose due to these potential complications.

An association between exposure during the last 2 weeks of pregnancy to antihistamines in general and retrolental fibroplasia in premature infants has been reported. See Brompheniramine for details.

Breast Feeding Summary

Diphenhydramine is excreted into human breast milk, but levels have not been reported (9). Although the levels are not thought to be sufficiently high after therapeutic doses to affect the infant, the manufacturer considers the drug contraindicated in nursing mothers. The reason given for this is the increased sensitivity of newborn or premature infants to antihistamines.

References

1. Heinonen OP, Sloan D, Shapiro S. *Birth Defects and Drugs in Pregnancy.* Littleton:Publishing Sciences Group, 1977.
2. Saxen I. Cleft palate and maternal diphenhydramine intake. Lancet 1974;1:407–8.
3. Nelson MM, Forfar JO. Associations between drugs administered during pregnancy and congenital abnormalities of the fetus. Br Med J 1971;1:523–7.
4. Aselton P, Jick H, Milunsky A, Hunter JR, Stergachis A. First-trimester drug use and congenital disorders. Obstet Gynecol 1985;65:451–5.
5. Parkin DE. Probable Benadryl withdrawal manifestations in a newborn infant. J Pediatr 1974;85:580.
6. Halbrecht I, Komlos L, Shabtay F, Solomon M, Bock JA. Triploidy 69,XXX in a stillborn girl. Clin Genet 1973;4:210–2.
7. Kargas GA, Kargas SA, Bruyere HJ Jr, Gilbert EF, Opitz JM. Perinatal mortality due to interaction of diphenhydramine and temazepam. N Engl J Med 1985;313:1417.
8. Hara GS, Carter RP, Krantz KE. Dramamine in labor: potential boon or a possible bomb? J Kans Med Soc 1980;81:134–6,155.
9. O'Brien TE. Excretion of drugs in human milk. Am J Hosp Pharm 1974;31:844–54.

Name: **DIPHENOXYLATE**

Class: **Antidiarrheal**   Risk Factor: **C$_M$**

Fetal Risk Summary

Diphenoxylate is a narcotic related to meperidine. It is available only in combination with atropine (to discourage overdosage) for the treatment of diarrhea. In one study, no malformed infants were observed after 1st trimester exposure in seven patients (1).

A single case of a female infant born at 36 weeks' gestation with multiple defects, including Ebstein's anomaly, was described in a 1989 report (2). In addition to the cardiac defect, other abnormalities noted were hypertelorism, epicanthal folds, low-set posteriorly rotated ears, a cleft uvula, medially rotated hands, deafness, and blindness. The mother had taken Lomotil (diphenoxylate and atropine) for diarrhea during the 10th week of gestation. Since exposure was beyond the susceptible stages of development for these defects, the drug combination was not considered causative. However, a possible viremia in the mother as a cause of the diarrhea and the defects could not be excluded.

Breast Feeding Summary

The manufacturer reports that diphenoxylate is probably excreted into breast milk, and the effects of that drug and atropine may be evident in the nursing infant (3). One source recommends that the drug should not be used in lactating mothers (4). However, the American Academy of Pediatrics considers atropine (diphenoxylate was not listed) to be compatible with breast feeding (5).

References

1. Heinonen OP, Slone D, Shapiro S. *Birth Defects and Drugs in Pregnancy.* Littleton:Publishing Sciences Group, 1977:287.
2. Siebert JR, Barr M Jr, Jackson JC, Benjamin DR. Ebstein's anomaly and extracardiac defects. Am J Dis Child 1989;143:570–2.
3. Product information. Lomotil. Searle and Company, 1990.

4. Stewart JJ. Gastrointestinal drugs. In Wilson JT, ed. *Drugs in Breast Milk.* Balgowlah, Australia:ADIS Press, 1981:71.
5. Committee on Drugs, American Academy of Pediatrics. Transfer of drugs and other chemicals into human milk. Pediatrics 1989;84:924–36.

Name: **DIPYRIDAMOLE**

Class: **Vasodilator**   Risk Factor: **C**

Fetal Risk Summary

No reports linking the use of dipyridamole with congenital defects have been located. The drug has been used in pregnancy as a vasodilator and to prevent thrombus formation in patients with prosthetic heart valves (1–8). A single intravenous 30-mg dose of dipyridamole was shown to increase uterine perfusion in the 3rd trimester in 10 patients (9). In one pregnancy, a malformed infant was delivered, but the mother was also taking coumadin (1). The multiple defects in the infant were consistent with the fetal warfarin syndrome (see Coumadin Derivatives).

In a randomized, nonblinded study to prevent preeclampsia, 52 high-risk patients treated from the 13th week of gestation through delivery with daily doses of 300 mg of dipyridamole plus 150 mg of aspirin were compared to 50 high-risk controls (10). Four treated patients were excluded from analysis (spontaneous abortions before 16 weeks) vs. five controls (two lost to follow-up plus three spontaneous abortions). Hypertension occurred in 41 patients—19 treated and 22 controls. The outcome of pregnancy was significantly better in treated patients in three areas: preeclampsia (none vs. 6, $p < 0.01$), fetal and neonatal loss (none vs. 5, $p < 0.02$), and severe intrauterine growth retardation (none vs. 4, $p < 0.05$). No fetal malformations were observed in either group. Other reports and reviews have documented the benefits of this therapy, namely a reduction in the incidence of stillbirth, placental infarction, and intrauterine growth retardation (11–17).

Breast Feeding Summary

Dipyridamole is excreted into breast milk but in levels too low to measure with current techniques (P.A. Bowers, personal communication, 1981). The manufacturer knows of no problems in breast-fed infants whose mothers were taking this drug (P.A. Bowers, personal communication, 1981).

References

1. Tejani N. Anticoagulant therapy with cardiac valve prosthesis during pregnancy. Obstet Gynecol 1973;42:785–93.
2. Del Bosque MR. Dipiridamol and anticoagulants in the management of pregnant women with cardiac valvular prosthesis. Ginecol Obstet Mex 1973;33:191–8.
3. Littler WA, Bonnar J, Redman CWG, Beilin LJ, Lee GD. Reduced pulmonary arterial compliance in hypertensive patients. Lancet 1973;1:1274–8.
4. Biale Y, Lewenthal H, Gueron M, Beu-Aderath N. Caesarean section in patient with mitral-valve prosthesis. Lancet 1977;1:907.
5. Taguchi K. Pregnancy in patients with a prosthetic heart valve. Surg Gynecol Obstet 1977;145:206–8.

6. Ahmad R, Rajah SM, Mearns AJ, Deverall PB. Dipyridamole in successful management of pregnant women with prosthetic heart valve. Lancet 1976;2:1414–5.
7. Biale Y, Cantor A, Lewenthal H, Gueron M. The course of pregnancy in patients with artificial heart valves treated with dipyridamole. Int J Gynaecol Obstet 1980;18:128–32.
8. Salazar E, Zajarias A, Gutierrez N, Iturbe I. The problem of cardiac valve prostheses, anticoagulants, and pregnancy. Circulation 1984;70(Suppl 1):I169–I177.
9. Lauchkner W, Schwarz R, Retzke U. Cardiovascular action of dipyridamole in advanced pregnancy. Zentralbl Gynaekol 1981;103:220–7.
10. Beaufils M, Uzan S, Donsimoni R, Colau JC. Prevention of pre-eclampsia by early antiplatelet therapy. Lancet 1985;1:840–2.
11. Beaufils M, Uzan S, Donsimoni R, Colau JC. Prospective controlled study of early antiplatelet therapy in prevention of preeclampsia. Adv Nephrol 1986;15:87–94.
12. Wallenburg HCS, Rotmans N. Prevention of recurrent idiopathic fetal growth retardation by low-dose aspirin and dipyridamole. Am J Obstet Gynecol 1987;157:1230–5.
13. Uzan S, Beaufils M, Bazin B, Danays T. Idiopathic recurrent fetal growth retardation and aspirin-dipyridamole therapy. Am J Obstet Gynecol 1989;160:763.
14. Wallenburg HCS, Rotmans N. Idiopathic recurrent fetal growth retardation and aspirin-dipyridamole therapy. Reply. Am J Obstet Gynecol 1989;160:763–4.
15. Wallenburg HCS, Rotmans N. Prophylactic low-dose aspirin and dipyridamole in pregnancy. Lancet 1988;1:939.
16. Capetta P, Airoldi ML, Tasca A, Bertulessi C, Rossi E, Polvani F. Prevention of pre-eclampsia and placental insufficiency. Lancet 1986;1:919.
17. Romero R, Lockwood C, Oyarzun E, Hobbins JC. Toxemia: new concepts in an old disease. Semin Perinatol 1988;12:302–23.

Name: **DISOPYRAMIDE**

Class: **Antiarrhythmic**   Risk Factor: **C**

Fetal Risk Summary

No reports linking the use of disopyramide with congenital defects in humans or animals have been located. At term, a cord blood level of 0.9 µg/ml (39% of maternal serum) was measured 6 hours after a maternal 200-mg dose (1). A 27-year-old woman took disopyramide throughout a full-term gestation, 1350 mg/day for the last 16 days, and delivered a healthy, 2920-g female infant (2). Concentrations of disopyramide and the metabolite, N-monodesalkyl disopyramide, in the cord and maternal serum were 0.7 and 0.9 µg/ml, and 2.7 and 2.1 µg/ml, respectively. The cord:maternal ratios for the parent drug and metabolite were 0.26 and 0.43, respectively (2).

Disopyramide has been used throughout other pregnancies without evidence of congenital abnormalities or growth retardation (1, 3, 4) (M.S. Anerson, personal communication, G.D. Searle and Company, 1981). Early onset of labor has been reported in one patient (5). The mother, in her 32nd week of gestation, was given 300 mg orally, followed by 100 or 150 mg every 6 hours for posterior mitral leaflet prolapse. Uterine contractions, without vaginal bleeding or cervical changes, and abdominal pain occurred 1–2 hours after each dose. When disopyramide was stopped, symptoms subsided over the next 4 hours. Oxytocin induction 1 week later resulted in the delivery of a healthy infant. In another patient, use of 200 mg twice daily during the 18th and 19th weeks of pregnancy was not associated with uterine contractions or other observable adverse effects in the mother or fetus (6).

Most reviews of antiarrhythmic drug therapy consider the drug probably safe during pregnancy (3, 7), but one does not recommend it for routine therapy (8).

Breast Feeding Summary

Disopyramide is excreted into breast milk (2, 4, 9, 10). In a woman taking 200 mg three times daily, samples obtained on the 5th–8th days of treatment revealed a mean milk:plasma ratio of 0.9 for disopyramide and 5.6 for the active metabolite (9). Neither drug was detected in the infant's plasma. In a second case, a mother was taking 450 mg of disopyramide every 8 hours 2 weeks postpartum (2). Milk and serum samples were obtained at 0, 2, 4, and 8 hours after the dose following an overnight fast. Milk concentrations of disopyramide and its metabolite, N-monodesalkyl disopyramide, ranged from 2.6–4.4 μg/ml and from 9.6–12.3 μg/ml, respectively. In both cases, the lowest levels occurred at the 8-hour sampling time. The mean milk:plasma ratios for the two were 1.06 and 6.24, respectively. Disopyramide was not detected in the infant's serum (test sensitivity 0.45 μg/ml), but both disopyramide and the metabolite were found in the infant's urine, 3.3 and 3.7 μg/ml, respectively. A brief 1985 report described a woman taking 100 mg five times a day throughout pregnancy who delivered a normal female infant (4). On the 2nd postpartum day and 2 hours after a dose, paired milk and serum sample were obtained. The concentrations of disopyramide in the aqueous phase of the milk and the serum were 4.0 and 10.3 μM/L, respectively, a milk:serum ratio of 0.4. The same ratio was obtained 2 weeks later with samples drawn 3 hours after a dose and levels of 5.0 and 11.5 μM/L, respectively. No disopyramide was found in the infant's serum (limit of test accuracy 1.5 μM/L) during the second sampling. A woman taking 200 mg twice daily had milk and serum samples drawn before and 3.5 hours after a dose (10). The concentrations in the serum were 3.7 and 5.5 μM/L, and those in the milk were 1.7 and 2.9 μM/L, respectively. The milk:serum ratios were 0.46 before and 0.53 after the dose. No adverse effects were noted in the nursing infants in any of the above cases. The American Academy of Pediatrics considers disopyramide to be compatible with breast feeding (11).

References

1. Shaxted EJ, Milton PJ. Disopyramide in pregnancy: a case report. Curr Med Res Opin 1979;6:70–2.
2. Ellsworth AJ, Horn JR, Raisys VA, Miyagawa LA, Bell JL. Disopyramide and N-monodesalkyl disopyramide in serum and breast milk. Drug Intell Clin Pharm 1989;23:56–7.
3. Rotmensch HH, Elkayam U, Frishman W. Antiarrhythmic drug therapy during pregnancy. Ann Intern Med 1983;98:487–97.
4. MacKintosh D, Buchanan N. Excretion of disopyramide in human breast milk. Br J Clin Pharmacol 1985;19:856–7.
5. Leonard RF, Braun TE, Levy AM. Initiation of uterine contractions by disopyramide during pregnancy. N Engl J Med 1978;299:84–5.
6. Stokes IM, Evans J, Stone M. Myocardial infarction and cardiac arrest in the second trimester followed by assisted vaginal delivery under epidural analgesia at 38 weeks gestation. Case report. Br J Obstet Gynaecol 1984;91:197–8.
7. Tamari I, Eldar M, Rabinowitz B, Neufeld HN. Medical treatment of cardiovascular disorders during pregnancy. Am Heart J 1982;104:1357–63.
8. Rotmensch HH, Rotmensch S, Elkayam U. Management of cardiac arrhythmias during pregnancy: current concepts. Drugs 1987;33:623–33.
9. Barnett DB, Hudson SA, McBurney A. Disopyramide and its N-monodesalkyl metabolite in breast milk. Br J Clin Pharmacol 1982;14:310–2.

10. Hoppu K, Neuvonen PJ, Korte T. Disopyramide and breast feeding. Br J Clin Pharmacol 1986;21:553.
11. Committee on Drugs, American Academy of Pediatrics. Transfer of drugs and other chemicals into human milk. Pediatrics 1989;84:924–36.

Name: **DISULFIRAM**

Class: **Unclassified**   Risk Factor: **C**

Fetal Risk Summary

Disulfiram is used to prevent alcohol consumption in patients with a history of alcohol abuse. The use of disulfiram in pregnancy has been described in seven pregnancies (1, 2). Four of the eight fetuses exposed (one set of twins) had congenital defects, and a spontaneous abortion occurred in a fifth fetus. The malformations observed were:

Clubfoot (two cases) (1)
Multiple anomalies with VACTERL syndrome
(radial aplasia, vertebral fusion, tracheo-esophageal fistula) (one case) (2)
Phocomelia of lower extremities (one case) (2)

In the two of the infants, exposure occurred in the 1st trimester and the use of other teratogens, including alcohol, was excluded (2). Although controversial, heavy alcohol intake prior to conception has been suspected of producing the fetal alcohol syndrome (FAS) (3–5). However, the anomalies described in the four infants exposed to disulfiram do not fit the pattern seen with the FAS.

In animals, disulfiram is embryotoxic, possibly due to copper chelation, but it is not teratogenic (6). Because of this, and the lack of any pattern to the defects observed in humans, further study is required before the relationship between disulfiram and human congenital malformations is known.

Breast Feeding Summary

No data are available.

References

1. Favre-Tissot M, Delatour P. Psychopharmacologie et teratogenese a propos du sulfirame: essai experimental. Annales Medico-psychogiques 1965;1:735–40. As cited in Shepard TH. *Catalog of Teratogenic Agents*, ed. 3. Baltimore:Johns Hopkins University Press, 1980:127.
2. Nora AH, Nora JJ, Blu J. Limb-reduction anomalies in infants born to disulfiram-treated alcoholic mothers. Lancet 1977;2:664.
3. Scheiner AP, Donovan CM, Bartoshesky LE. Fetal alcohol syndrome in child whose parents had stopped drinking. Lancet 1979;1:1077–8.
4. Scheiner AP. Fetal alcohol syndrome in a child whose parents had stopped drinking. Lancet 1979;2:858.
5. Smith DW, Graham JM Jr. Fetal alcohol syndrome in child whose parents had stopped drinking. Lancet 1979;2:527.
6. Shepard TH. Catalog of Teratogenic Agents, ed. 6. Baltimore:The Johns Hopkins University Press, 1989:239–40.

Name: **DOBUTAMINE**

Class: **Sympathomimetic (Adrenergic)**   Risk Factor: **C**

Fetal Risk Summary

Dobutamine is structurally related to dopamine. It has not been studied in human pregnancy (see also Dopamine). Short-term use in one patient with a myocardial infarction at 18 weeks' gestation was not associated with any known adverse effects (1).

Breast Feeding Summary

No data are available.

Reference

1. Stokes IM, Evans J, Stone M. Myocardial infarction and cardiac arrest in the second trimester followed by assisted vaginal delivery under epidural analgesia at 38 weeks gestation. Case report. Br J Obstet Gynaecol 1984;91:197–8.

Name: **DOCUSATE CALCIUM**

Class: **Laxative**   Risk Factor: **C**

Fetal Risk Summary

See Docusate Sodium.

Breast Feeding Summary

No data are available.

Name: **DOCUSATE POTASSIUM**

Class: **Laxative**   Risk Factor: **C**

Fetal Risk Summary

See Docusate Sodium.

Breast Feeding Summary

No data are available.

Name: **DOCUSATE SODIUM**

Class: **Laxative**   Risk Factor: **C**

Fetal Risk Summary

No reports linking the use of docusate sodium (DSS) with congenital defects have been located. DSS is a common ingredient in many laxative preparations available to the public. In a large prospective study, 116 patients were exposed to this drug during pregnancy (1). No evidence for an association with malformations was found. Similarly, no evidence of fetal toxicity was noted in 35 women treated with a combination of docusate sodium and dihydroxyanthraquinone (2).

Chronic use of 150–250 mg or more/day of docusate sodium throughout pregnancy was suspected of causing hypomagnesemia in a mother and her newborn (3). At 12 hours of age, the neonate exhibited jitteriness, which resolved spontaneously. Neonatal serum magnesium levels ranged from 0.9–1.1 mg/100 ml between 22–48 hours of age with a maternal level of 1.2 mg/100 ml on the 3rd postpartum day. All other laboratory parameters were normal.

Breast Feeding Summary

A combination of docusate sodium and dihydroxyanthraquinone (Normax) was given to 35 postpartum women in a 1973 study (2). One infant developed diarrhea, but the relationship between the symptom and the laxative is unknown.

References

1. Heinonen OP, Slone D, Shapiro S. *Birth Defects and Drugs in Pregnancy*. Littleton:Publishing Sciences Group, 1977:442.
2. Greenhalf JO, Leonard HSD. Laxatives in the treatment of constipation in pregnant and breast-feeding mothers. Practitioner 1973;210:259–63.
3. Schindler AM. Isolated neonatal hypomagnesaemia associated with maternal overuse of stool softener. Lancet 1984;2:822.

Name: **DOPAMINE**

Class: **Sympathomimetic (Adrenergic)**   Risk Factor: **C**

Fetal Risk Summary

Experience with dopamine in human pregnancy is limited. Since dopamine is indicated only for life-threatening situations, chronic use would not be expected. Animal studies have shown both increases and decreases in uterine blood flow (1, 2). In a study in pregnant baboons, dopamine infusion increased uterine vascular resistance and thus impaired uteroplacental perfusion (1). Because of this effect, the investigators concluded that the drug should not be used in patients with severe preeclampsia or eclampsia (1). However, although human studies on uterine perfusion have not been conducted, the use in women with severe toxemia has not been associated with fetal harm. The drug has been used to prevent renal failure in nine oligoanuric eclamptic patients by re-establishing diuresis (3). In another study of six women with severe preeclampsia and oliguria, low-dose dopamine (1–5 µg/kg/min) infusion produced a significant rise in urine and cardiac output (4). No significant changes in blood pressure, central venous pressure, or pulmonary capillary wedge pressure occurred. Dopamine has also been used to treat hypotension in 26 patients undergoing cesarean section (2). No adverse effects attributable to dopamine were observed in the fetuses or newborns of the mothers in these studies.

Breast Feeding Summary

No data are available.

References

1. Fishburne JI Jr, Dormer KJ, Payne GG, Gill PS, Ashrafzadeh AR, Rossavik IK. Effects of amrinone and dopamine on uterine blood flow and vascular responses in the gravid baboon. Am J Obstet Gynecol 1988;158:829–37.
2. Clark RB, Brunner JA III. Dopamine for the treatment of spinal hypotension during cesarean section. Anesthesiology 1980;53:514–7.
3. Gerstner G, Grunberger W. Dopamine treatment for prevention of renal failure in patients with severe eclampsia. Clin Exp Obstet Gynecol 1980;7:219–22.
4. Kirshon B, Lee W, Mauer MB, Cotton DB. Effects of low-dose dopamine therapy in the oliguric patient with preeclampsia. Am J Obstet Gynecol 1988;159:604–7.

Name: **DOTHIEPIN**

Class: **Antidepressant**   Risk Factor: **D**

Fetal Risk Summary

No data are available. See Imipramine.

Breast Feeding Summary

Dothiepin is excreted into human breast milk (1). In a single patient treated with dothiepin, 25 mg three times a day for 3 months, milk and maternal serum concentrations 3 hours after the second dose of the day were 11 and 33 ng/ml (ratio 0.33). A second woman, treated intermittently over a 6-day period with a total dose of 300 mg, had a milk level of 10 ng/ml (1). Effects of this exposure in the nursing infants were not mentioned. The American Academy of Pediatrics classifies dothiepin as an agent whose effect on the nursing infant is unknown but may be of concern (2).

References

1. Rees JA, Glass RC, Sporne GA. Serum and breast milk concentrations of dothiepen. Practitioner 1976;217:686.
2. Committee on Drugs, American Academy of Pediatrics. Transfer of drugs and other chemicals into human milk. Pediatrics 1989;84:924–36.

Name: **DOXEPIN**

Class: **Antidepressant**   Risk Factor: **C**

Fetal Risk Summary

No reports linking the use of doxepin with congenital defects have been located (see also Imipramine). Paralytic ileus has been observed in an infant exposed to doxepin at term (1). The condition was thought to be due primarily to chlorpromazine, but the authors speculated that the anticholinergic effects of doxepin worked synergistically with the phenothiazine.

Breast Feeding Summary

Doxepin and its active metabolite, N-desmethyldoxepin, are excreted into breast milk (2, 3). Two case histories on the use of this agent during lactation have been published.

A 36-year-old woman was treated with doxepin, 10 mg daily, for approximately 5 weeks starting 2 weeks after the birth of her daughter (2). The dose was increased to 25 mg three times daily 4 days before the wholly breast-fed 8-week-old infant was found pale, limp, and near respiratory arrest. Although drowsiness and shallow respirations continued on admission to the hospital, the baby made a rapid recovery and was normal in 24 hours. A peak milk concentration of doxepin, 29 ng/ml, occurred 4–5 hours after a dose, while two levels obtained just prior to a dose (12 hours after the last dose in each case) were 7 and 10 ng/ml, respectively. Milk concentrations of the metabolite ranged from "not detectable" (lower limit of detection 7 ng/ml) to 11 ng/ml. The averages of nine determinations for doxepin and the metabolite in the milk were 18 and 9 ng/ml, respectively. Maternal serum doxepin and N-desmethyldoxepin levels ranged from trace to 21 ng/ml (average 15 ng/ml) and 33–66 ng/ml (average 57 ng/ml), respectively. The milk:serum ratio for doxepin on two determinations was 0.9, while ratios for the metabolite were 0.12 and 0.17. Doxepin was almost undetectable (estimated to be 3 ng/ml) in the infant's serum, but the levels of the metabolite on two occasions were 58 and 66 ng/ml, demonstrating marked accumulation in the infant's serum. The initial infant urine sample contained 39 ng/ml of the metabolite.

The second case involved a 26-year-old woman, 30 days postpartum, who was treated with doxepin (150 mg every night) for a major depressive disorder (3). Blood samples were obtained a mean 18 hours after a dose on days 7, 14, 22, 28, 36, 43, 50, and 99 days of treatment. On the same days that blood specimens were drawn, milk samples were collected at the start of feeding (17.2 hours after the last dose) and at the end of feeding (17.7 hours after the last dose). Plasma concentrations of doxepin varied between 35–68 ng/ml, with a mean value of 46 ng/ml. Levels for the metabolite, N-desmethyldoxepin, ranged from 65–131 ng/ml, with a mean of 90 ng/ml. Mean pre- and postfeed milk:plasma ratios for doxepin were 1.08 (range 0.51–1.44) and 1.66 (range 0.79–2.39), respectively, and for the metabolite, 1.02 (range 0.54–1.45) and 1.53 (range 0.85–2.35), respectively. A plasma sample drawn from the infant on day 43 showed no detectable doxepin (sensitivity 5 ng/ml) and 15 ng/ml of the metabolite. No adverse effects of the exposure to doxepin were observed in the infant.

Although adverse effects were only observed in one of the two cases cited above, the effects were serious and potentially lethal to the nursing infant. Based on that report, doxepin should be taken with caution, if at all, by the breast-feeding woman. The American Academy of Pediatrics classifies doxepin as an agent whose effect on the nursing infant is unknown but may be of concern (4).

References

1. Falterman CG, Richardson CJ. Small left colon syndrome associated with maternal ingestion of psychotropic drugs. J Pediatr 1980;97:308–10.
2. Matheson I, Pande H, Alertsen AR. Respiratory depression caused by N-desmethyldoxepin in breast milk. Lancet 1985;2:1124.
3. Kemp J, Ilett KF, Booth J, Hackett LP. Excretion of doxepin and N-desmethyldoxepin in human milk. Br J Clin Pharmacol 1985;20:497–9.
4. Committee on Drugs, American Academy of Pediatrics. Transfer of drugs and other chemicals into human milk. Pediatrics 1989;84:924–36.

Name: **DOXORUBICIN**

Class: **Antineoplastic**   Risk Factor: **D**

Fetal Risk Summary

Several reports have described the use of doxorubicin in pregnancy, including three during the 1st trimester (1–16). One of the fetuses exposed during the 1st trimester to doxorubicin, cyclophosphamide, and unshielded radiation was borne with an imperforate anus and rectovaginal fistula (14). At about 3 months of age, the infant was small with a head circumference of 46 cm (<5th percentile) but was doing well after two corrective surgeries (14). A 1983 report described the use of doxorubicin and other antineoplastic agents in two pregnancies, one of which ended in fetal death 36 hours after treatment had begun (17). Other than maceration, no other fetal abnormalities were observed. The investigators could not determine the exact cause of the outcome but concluded that the chemotherapy was probably not responsible. The only other complication observed in exposed infants was transient polycythemia and hyperbilirubinemia in one subject. Infants who have been evaluated have shown normal growth and development.

Three studies have investigated the placental passage of doxorubicin (1, 17, 18). In one, the drug was not detected in the amniotic fluid at 20 weeks of gestation, which suggested that the drug was not transferred in measurable amounts to the fetus (1). Placental transfer was demonstrated in a 17-week-old aborted fetus, however, using high-performance liquid chromatography (HPLC) (15). High concentrations were found in fetal liver, kidney, and lung. The drug was not detected in amniotic fluid (<1.66 ng/ml), brain, intestine, or gastrocnemius muscle. A third study examined the placental passage of doxorubicin in two pregnancies, one resulting in the birth of a healthy infant at 34 weeks' gestation and one ending with a stillborn fetus at 31 weeks' gestation (17). Using HPLC, doxorubicin was demonstrated in the first case, 48 hours after a 45 mg/m² dose (total cumulative dose, 214 mg/m²), on both sides of the placenta and in the umbilical cord but not in cord blood plasma. In the stillborn, doxorubicin was not detected in any fetal tissue, 36 hours after a single dose of 45 mg/m². However, a substance was detected in all fetal tissues analyzed that the investigators concluded may have represented an unknown doxorubicin metabolite.

Long-term studies of growth and mental development of offspring exposed to doxorubicin and other antineoplastic agents in the 2nd trimester, the period of neuroblast multiplication, have not been conducted (18).

Doxorubicin may cause reversible testicular dysfunction (20, 21). Similarly, normal pregnancies have occurred in women treated before conception with doxorubicin (22). In 436 long-term survivors treated with chemotherapy for gestational trophoblastic tumors between 1958–1978, 33 (8%) received doxorubicin as part of their treatment regimens (22). Of the 33 women, five (15%) had at least one live birth (data given in parentheses refer to mean/maximum doxorubicin dose in milligrams) (100/100), two (6%) had no live births (150/200), one (3%) failed to conceive (100/100), and 25 (76%) did not try to conceive (140/400). Additional details, including congenital anomalies observed, are described in the monograph for methotrexate (see Methotrexate).

The long-term effects of combination chemotherapy on menstrual and reproductive function have been described in a 1988 report (23). Only one of the 40 women treated for malignant ovarian germ cell tumors received doxorubicin. The results of this study are discussed in the monograph for cyclophosphamide (see Cyclophosphamide).

Occupational exposure of the mother to antineoplastic agents during pregnancy may present a risk to the fetus. A position statement from the National Study Commission on Cytotoxic Exposure and a research article involving some antineoplastic agents, including doxorubicin, are presented in the monograph for cyclophosphamide (see Cyclophosphamide).

Breast Feeding Summary

Doxorubicin is excreted into human milk (24). A 31-year-old woman, 7 months postpartum, was given doxorubicin (70 mg/m^2), infused over 15 minutes, for the treatment of ovarian cancer (24). Both doxorubicin and the metabolite, doxorubicinol, were detected in the plasma and the milk. Peak concentrations of the two substances in the plasma occurred at the first sampling time (0.5 hour) and were 805 and 82 ng/ml, respectively. In the milk, the peak concentrations occurred at 24 hours with levels of 128 and 111 ng/ml, respectively. The "area under concentration time curves" (AUC) of the parent compound and metabolite in the plasma were 8.3 and 1.7 μM $\times$ hours, respectively, while the AUCs in the milk were 9.9 and 16.5 μM $\times$ hours, respectively. The highest milk:plasma ratio, 4.43, was measured at 24 hours. Although milk concentrations often exceeded those in the plasma, the total amount of active drug available in the milk was only 0.24 μg/ml (24). However, although these amounts may be considered negligible, the American Academy of Pediatrics considers doxorubicin to be contraindicated during breast feeding because of concerns for possible immune suppression, carcinogenesis, neutropenia, and unknown effects on growth (25).

References

1. Roboz J, Gleicher N, Wu K, Kerenyi T, Holland J. Does doxorubicin cross the placenta? Lancet 1979;2:1382–3.
2. Khursid M, Saleem M. Acute leukaemia in pregnancy. Lancet 1978;2:534–5.
3. Newcomb M, Balducci L, Thigpen JT, Morrison FS. Acute leukemia in pregnancy: successful delivery after cytarabine and doxorubicin. JAMA 1978;239:2691–2.
4. Hassenstein E, Riedel H. Zur teratogenitat von Adriamycin ein fallbericht. Geburtshilfe Frauenheilkd 1978;38:131–3.

5. Cervantes F, Rozman C. Adriamycina y embarazo. Sangre (Barc) 1980;25:627.
6. Pizzuto J, Aviles A, Noriega L, Niz J, Morales M, Romero F. Treatment of acute leukemia during pregnancy: presentation of nine cases. Cancer Treat Rep 1980;64:679–83.
7. Tobias JS, Bloom HJG. Doxorubicin in pregnancy. Lancet 1980;1:776.
8. Garcia V, San Miguel J, Borrasca AL. Doxorubicin in the first trimester of pregnancy. Ann Intern Med 1981;94:547.
9. Garcia V, San Miguel IJ, Borrasca AL. Adriamycin and pregnancy. Sangre (Barc) 1981;26:129.
10. Dara P, Slater LM, Armentrout SA. Successful pregnancy during chemotherapy for acute leukemia. Cancer 1981;47:845–6.
11. Lowenthal RM, Funnell CF, Hope DM, Stewart IG, Humphrey DC. Normal infant after combination chemotherapy including teniposide for Burkitt's lymphoma in pregnancy. Med Pediatr Oncol 1982;10:165–9.
12. Webb GA. The use of hyperalimentation and chemotherapy in pregnancy: a case report. Am J Obstet Gynecol 1980;137:263–6.
13. Gililland J, Weinstein L. The effects of cancer chemotherapeutic agents on the developing fetus. Obstet Gynecol Surv 1983;38:6–13.
14. Murray CL, Reichert JA, Anderson J, Twiggs LB. Multimodal cancer therapy for breast cancer in the first trimester of pregnancy. A case report. JAMA 1984;252:2607–8.
15. Haerr RW, Pratt AT. Multiagent chemotherapy for sarcoma diagnosed during pregnancy. Cancer 1985;56:1028–33.
16. Turchi JJ, Villasis C. Anthracyclines in the treatment of malignancy in pregnancy. Cancer 1988;61:435–40.
17. Karp GI, Von Oeyen P, Valone F, Khetarpal VK, Israel M, Mayer RJ, Frigoletto FD, Garnick MB. Doxorubicin in pregnancy: possible transplacental passage. Cancer Treat Rep 1983;67:773–7.
18. D'Incalci M, Broggini M, Buscaglia M, Pardi G. Transplacental passage of doxorubicin. Lancet 1983;1:75.
19. Dobbing J. Pregnancy and leukaemia. Lancet 1977;1:1155.
20. Lendon M, Palmer MK, Hann IM, Shalet SM, Jones PHM. Testicular histology after combination chemotherapy in childhood for acute lymphoblastic leukaemia. Lancet 1978;2:439–41.
21. Schilsky RL, Lewis BJ, Sherins RJ, Young RC. Gonadal dysfunction in patients receiving chemotherapy for cancer. Ann Intern Med 1980;93:109–14.
22. Rustin GJS, Booth M, Dent J, Salt S, Rustin F, Bagshawe KD. Pregnancy after cytotoxic chemotherapy for gestational trophoblastic tumours. Br Med J 1984;288:103–6.
23. Gershenson DM. Menstrual and reproductive function after treatment with combination chemotherapy for malignant ovarian germ cell tumors. J Clin Oncol 1988;6:270–5.
24. Egan PC, Costanza ME, Dodion P, Egorin MJ, Bachur NR. Doxorubicin and cisplatin excretion into human milk. Cancer Treat Rep 1985;69:1387–9.
25. Committee on Drugs, American Academy of Pediatrics. Transfer of drugs and other chemicals into human milk. Pediatrics 1989;84:924–36.

Name: **DOXYCYCLINE**

Class: **Antibiotic**   Risk Factor: **D**

Fetal Risk Summary

See Tetracycline.

Breast Feeding Summary

Doxycycline is excreted into breast milk. Oral doxycycline, 200 mg followed after 24 hours by 100 mg, was given to 15 nursing mothers (1). Milk:plasma ratios determined at 3 and 24 hours after the second dose were 0.3 and 0.4, respectively. Mean milk concentrations were 0.77 and 0.38 µg/ml.

Theoretically, dental staining and inhibition of bone growth could occur in breast-fed infants whose mothers were consuming doxycycline. However, this theoretical possibility seems remote, because in infants exposed to a closely related antibiotic, tetracycline, serum levels were undetectable (less than 0.05 μg/ml) (2). The American Academy of Pediatrics considers tetracycline compatible with breast feeding (3). Three potential problems may exist for the nursing infant even though there are no reports in this regard: modification of bowel flora, direct effects on the infant, and interference with the interpretation of culture results if a fever workup is required.

References

1. Morganti G, Ceccarelli G, Ciaffi EG. Comparative concentrations of a tetracycline antibiotic in serum and maternal milk. Antibiotica 1968;6:216–23.
2. Posner AC, Prigot A, Konicoff NG. Further observations on the use of tetracycline hydrochloride in prophylaxis and treatment of obstetric infections. *Antibiotics Annual 1954–55.* New York:Medical Encyclopedia, 1955:594–8.
3. Committee on Drugs, American Academy of Pediatrics. Transfer of drugs and other chemicals into human milk. Pediatrics 1989;84:924–36.

Name: **DOXYLAMINE**

Class: **Antiemetic**   Risk Factor: **B**

Fetal Risk Summary

The combination of doxylamine, pyridoxine, and dicyclomine (Bendectin, others) was originally marketed in 1956. The drug was reformulated in 1976 (USA and Canada) to eliminate dicyclomine because that component was not found to contribute to its effectiveness as an antiemetic. Over 33 million women have taken this product during pregnancy, making it one of the most heavily prescribed drugs for this condition. The manufacturer ceased producing the drug combination in 1983 because of litigation over its alleged association with congenital limb defects. Although no longer available as a fixed combination, the individual components are still marketed by various manufacturers.

Over 160 cases of congenital defects have been reported in the literature or to the Food and Drug Administration (FDA) as either "Bendectin-induced" or associated with use of the drug in the 1st trimester (1–6). Defects observed included skeletal, limb, and cardiac anomalies as well as cleft lip or palate. A possible association between doxylamine-pyridoxine and diaphragmatic hernia was reported in 1983 and assumed to reflect earlier findings of a large prospective study (6). Authors of the latter study, however, cautioned that their results were uninterpretable, even when apparently strong associations existed, without independent confirmation (7, 8). In a large case-control study, infants exposed *in utero* to the combination had a slightly greater relative risk (1.40) for congenital defects (9). The risk was more than doubled (2.91) if the mother also smoked. An increased risk for heart value anomalies (2.99) was also found. A significant association was discovered in this study between Bendectin and pyloric stenosis (4.33 to 5.24), representing about a 4-fold increase in risk for this anomaly. Similarly, the Boston Collaborative Drug Surveillance Programs reported preliminary findings to the

FDA indicating a 2.7-fold increase in risk (10). A 1983 case-control study, however, found no association between Bendectin use and the anomaly (11). In evaluating these three reports, the FDA considered them the best available information on the topic but concluded that no definite causal relationship had been shown between Bendectin and pyloric stenosis (10). In addition, the FDA commented that even if there was evidence for an association between the drug and the defect, it did not necessarily constitute evidence of a causal relationship since the nausea and vomiting itself, or the underlying disease causing the condition, could be responsible for the increased risk (10). A 1985 study, which appeared after the above FDA evaluation, found a possible association with pyloric stenosis but could not eliminate the possibility that it was due to other factors (12). A minimal relationship was found between congenital heart disease and doxylamine (Bendectin) use in early pregnancy in another 1985 report comparing 298 cases with 738 controls (13). The authors went to great efforts to assure that their drug histories were accurate. Their findings provided evidence that if an association did exist at all, it was very small.

The evidence indicating that doxylamine-pyridoxine is safe in pregnancy is impressive. A number of large studies, many reviewed in a 1983 article (14), have discovered no relationship between the drug and birth weight, length, head circumference, gestational age, congenital malformations, or other adverse fetal outcome (14–30). A 1985 study also found no association with defects other than pyloric stenosis (12). One study was unable to observe chromosomal abnormalities associated with the drug combination, whereas a second study found that use of the drugs was not related to the Poland anomaly (unilateral absence of the pectoralis major muscle with or without ipsilateral hand defect) (31, 32).

Although the literature supports the relative safety of this product, when compared to the normal background of malformations, it is not possible to state that it was completely without risk to the fetus. As some have indicated, it is not completely possible to prove a negative in the field of teratology (14, 33).

Breast Feeding Summary

No data are available (see also Pyridoxine).

References

1. Korcok M. The Bendectin debate. Can Med Assoc J 1980;123:922–8.
2. Soverchia G, Perri PF. Two cases of malformations of a limb in infants of mothers treated with an antiemetic in a very early phase of pregnancy. Pediatr Med Chir 1981;3:97–9.
3. Donaldson GL, Bury RG. Multiple congenital abnormalities in a newborn boy associated with maternal use of fluphenazine enanthate and other drugs during pregnancy. Acta Paediatr Scand 1982;71:335–8.
4. Grodofsky MP, Wilmott RW. Possible association of use of Bendectin during early pregnancy and congenital lung hypoplasia. N Engl J Med 1984;311:732.
5. Fisher JE, Nelson SJ, Allen JE, Holsman RS. Congenital cystic adenomatoid malformation of the lung. A unique variant. Am J Dis Child 1982;136:1071–4.
6. Bracken MB, Berg A. Bendectin (Debendox) and congenital diaphragmatic hernia. Lancet 1983;1:586.
7. Heinonen OP, Slone D, Shapiro S. Birth Defects and Drugs in Pregnancy. Littleton:Publishing Sciences Group, 1977:474–5.
8. Ohga K, Yamanaka R, Kinumaki H, Awa S, Kobayashi N. Bendectin (Debendox) and congenital diaphragmatic hernia. Lancet 1983;1:930.
9. Eskenazi B, Bracken MB. Bendectin (Debendox) as a risk factor for pyloric stenosis. Am J Obstet Gynecol 1982;144:919–24.

10. Bendectin and pyloric stenosis. FDA Drug Bull 1983;13:14–5.
11. Mitchell AA, Schwingl PJ, Rosenberg L, Louik C, Shapiro S. Birth defects in relation to Bendectin use in pregnancy. II. Pyloric stenosis. Am J Obstet Gynecol 1983;147:737–42.
12. Aselton P, Jick H, Milunsky A, Hunter JR, Stergachis A. First-trimester drug use and congenital disorders. Obstet Gynecol 1985;65:451–5.
13. Zierler S, Rothman KJ. Congenital heart disease in relation to maternal use of Bendectin and other drugs in early pregnancy. N Engl J Med 1985;313:347–52.
14. Holmes LB. Teratogen update: Bendectin. Teratology 1983;27:277–81.
15. Milkovich L, van den Berg BJ. An evaluation of the teratogenicity of certain antinauseant drugs. Am J Obstet Gynecol 1976;125:244–8.
16. Shapiro S, Heinonen OP, Siskind V, Kaufman DW, Monson RR, Slone D. Antenatal exposure to doxylamine succinate and dicyclomine hydrochloride (Bendectin) in relation to congenital malformations, perinatal mortality rate, birth weight, intelligence quotient score. Am J Obstet Gynecol 1977;128:480–5.
17. Rothman KJ, Flyer DC, Goldblatt A, Kreidberg MB. Exogenous hormones and other drug exposures of children with congenital heart disease. Am J Epidemiol 1979;109:433–9.
18. Bunde CA, Bowles DM. A technique for controlled survey of case records. Curr Ther Res 1963;5:245–8.
19. Gibson GT, Collen DP, McMichael AJ, Hartshorne JM. Congenital anomalies in relation to the use of doxylamine/dicyclomine and other antenatal factors. An ongoing prospective study. Med J Aust 1981;1:410–4.
20. Correy JF, Newman NM. Debendox and limb reduction deformities. Med J Aust 1981;1:417–8.
21. Clarke M, Clayton DG. Safety of Debendox. Lancet 1981;2:659–60.
22. Harron DWG, Griffiths K, Shanks RG. Debendox and congenital malformations in Northern Ireland. Br Med J 1980;4:1379–81.
23. Smithells RW, Sheppard S. Teratogenicity testing in humans: a method demonstrating safety of Bendectin. Teratology 1978;17:31–5.
24. Morelock S, Hingson R, Kayne H, et al. Bendectin and fetal development: a study at Boston City Hospital. Am J Obstet Gynecol 1982;142:209–13.
25. Cordero JF, Oakley GP, Greenberg F, James LM. Is Bendectin a teratogen? JAMA 1981;245:2307–10.
26. Mitchell AA, Rosenberg L, Shapiro S, Slone D. Birth defects related to Bendectin use in pregnancy: I. Oral clefts and cardiac defects. JAMA 1981;245:2311–4.
27. Fleming DM, Knox JDE, Crombie DL. Debendox in early pregnancy and fetal malformation. Br Med J 1981;283:99–101.
28. Greenberg G, Inman WHW, Weatherall JAC, Adelstein AM, Haskey JC. Maternal drug histories and congenital abnormalities. Br Med J 1977;2:853–6.
29. Aselton PJ, Jick H. Additional follow-up of congenital limb disorders in relation to Bendectin use. JAMA 1983;250:33–4.
30. McCredie J, Kricker A, Elliott J, Forrest J. The innocent bystander: doxylamine/dicyclomine/pyridoxine and congenital limb defects. Med J Aust 1984;140:525–7.
31. Hughes DT, Cavanagh N. Chromosomal studies on children with phocomelia, exposed to Debendox during early pregnancy. Lancet 1983;2:399.
32. David TJ. Debendox does not cause the Poland anomaly. Arch Dis Child 1982;57:479–80.
33. Brent RR. Editorial. The Bendectin saga: another American tragedy. Teratology 1983;27:283–6.

Name: **DROPERIDOL**

Class: **Tranquilizer**   Risk Factor: **C_M**

Fetal Risk Summary

Droperidol is a butyrophenone derivative structurally related to haloperidol (see also Haloperidol). The drug has been used to promote analgesia for cesarean section patients without affecting the respiration of the newborn (1, 2). The placental transfer of droperidol is slow (2). The drug was used during labor as a sedative in a study comparing 48 women treated with droperidol with 52 women receiving promethazine (3). These investigators noted eight other reports where the drug was used in a similar manner. No serious maternal or fetal adverse effects were observed. Droperidol has also been used for the treatment of hyperemesis gravidarum (4). The authors have administered the drug as a continuous intravenous infusion for hyperemesis during all trimesters without apparent fetal harm (G.G. Briggs and R.K. Freeman, unpublished data, 1990).

Breast Feeding Summary

No data are available.

References

1. Smith AM, McNeil WT. Awareness during anesthesia. Br Med J 1969;1:572–3.
2. Zhdanov GG, Ponomarev GM. The concentration of droperidol in the venous blood of the parturients and in the blood of the umbilical cord of neonates. Anesteziol Reanimatol 1980;4:14–6.
3. Pettit GP, Smith GA, McIlroy WL. Droperidol in obstetrics: a double-blind study. Milit Med 1976;141:316–7.
4. Martynshin MYA, Arkhengel'skii AE. Experience in treating early toxicoses of pregnancy with metoclopramide. Akush Ginekol 1981;57:44–5.

Name: **DYPHYLLINE**

Class: **Spasmolytic/Vasodilator**   Risk Factor: **C$_M$**

Fetal Risk Summary

No data are available. See also Theophylline.

Breast Feeding Summary

Dyphylline is excreted into breast milk. In 20 normal lactating women a single 5 mg/kg intramuscular dose produced an average milk:plasma ratio of 2.08 (1). The milk and serum elimination rates were equivalent. Although the drug accumulates in milk, the American Academy of Pediatrics considers dyphylline compatible with breast feeding (2).

References

1. Jarboe CH, Cook LN, Malesic I, Fleischaker J. Dyphylline elimination kinetics in lactating women: blood to milk transfer. J Clin Pharmacol 1981;21:405–10.
2. Committee on Drugs, American Academy of Pediatrics. Transfer of drugs and other chemicals into human milk. Pediatrics 1989;84:924–36.

Name: **ECHOTHIOPHATE**

Class: **Parasympathomimetic (Cholinergic)**   Risk Factor: **C**

Fetal Risk Summary

Echothiophate is used in the eye. No reports of its use in pregnancy have been located. As a quaternary ammonium compound, it is ionized at physiologic pH and transplacental passage in significant amounts would not be expected (see also Neostigmine).

Breast Feeding Summary

No data are available.

Name: **EDROPHONIUM**

Class: **Parasympathomimetic (Cholinergic)**   Risk Factor: **C**

Fetal Risk Summary

Edrophonium is a quaternary ammonium chloride with anticholinesterase activity used in the diagnosis of myasthenia gravis. The drug has been used in pregnancy without producing fetal malformations (1–7). Because it is ionized at physiologic pH, edrophonium would not be expected to cross the placenta in significant amounts. Caution has been advised against the use in pregnancy of intravenous anticholinesterases because they may cause premature labor (1, 3). This effect on the pregnant uterus increases near term. Intramuscular neostigmine should be used in place of intravenous edrophonium if diagnosis of myasthenia gravis is required in a pregnant patient (3). In one report, however, intravenous edrophonium was given to a woman in the 2nd trimester in an unsuccessful attempt to treat tachycardia secondary to Wolff-Parkinson-White syndrome (6). No effect on the uterus was mentioned and she continued with an uneventful full-term pregnancy.

Transient muscular weakness has been observed in about 20% of newborns of mothers with myasthenia gravis (8). The neonatal myasthenia is due to transplacental passage of anti-acetylcholine receptor immunoglobulin G antibodies (8).

Breast Feeding Summary

Because it is ionized at physiologic pH, edrophonium would not be expected to be excreted into breast milk (9).

References

1. Foldes FF, McNall PG. Myasthenia gravis: a guide for anesthesiologists. Anesthesiology 1962;23:837–72.
2. Plauche WG. Myasthenia gravis in pregnancy. Am J Obstet Gynecol 1964;88:404–9.
3. McNall PG, Jafarnia MR. Management of myasthenia gravis in the obstetrical patient. Am J Obstet Gynecol 1965;92:518–25.
4. Hay DM. Myasthenia gravis in pregnancy. J Obstet Gynaecol Br Commonw 1969;76:323–9.
5. Heinonen OP, Slone D, Shapiro S. *Birth Defects and Drugs in Pregnancy*. Littleton:Publishing Sciences Group, 1977:345–56.
6. Gleicher N, Meller J, Sandler RZ, Sullum S. Wolff-Parkinson-White syndrome in pregnancy. Obstet Gynecol 1981;58:748–52.
7. Blackhall MI, Buckley GA, Roberts DV, Roberts JB, Thomas BH, Wilson A. Drug-induced neonatal myasthenia. J Obstet Gynaecol Br Commonw 1969;76:157–62.
8. Plauche WC. Myasthenia gravis in pregnancy: an update. Am J Obstet Gynecol 1979;135:691–7.
9. Wilson JT. Pharmacokinetics of drug excretion. In Wilson JT, ed. *Drugs in Breast Milk*. Australia (Balgowlah):ADIS Press, 1981:17.

Name: **ENALAPRIL**

Class: **Antihypertensive**   Risk Factor: C_M

Fetal Risk Summary

Enalapril, a competitive inhibitor of angiotensin I-converting enzyme, is used for the treatment of hypertension (see also Captopril). Data on the use of enalapril in 20 pregnancies have been located (1–7).

In an European survey on the use on angiotensin-converting enzyme inhibitors in pregnancy, the results in nine mother-child pairs were briefly reviewed (1). Indications for use of the drug were seven cases of essential hypertension, one case of lupus-induced hypertension, and one case of renal hypertension (glomerulopathy). Two spontaneous abortions occurred: one at 7 weeks in a 44-year-old woman, and one at 11 weeks in a 41-year-old diabetic patient. Enalapril, 20 mg/day, had been used from conception until abortion in the first case and from conception until 6 weeks' gestation in the second. In both cases, factors other than the drug therapy were probably responsible for the pregnancy losses. In a third case, enalapril (30 mg/day) was started at 24 weeks; the patient, with severe glomerulopathy, delivered a stillborn infant 2 weeks later. It is not known whether enalapril therapy was associated with the adverse outcome. The remaining six women were being treated at the time of conception with 10 mg/day (two) or 20 mg/day (four) for essential hypertension or lupus-induced hypertension. Therapy was discontinued by 7 weeks' gestation in four pregnancies, at 28 weeks in one, and was continued throughout gestation (40 weeks) in one. Two infants were small for gestational age; one had been exposed only during the first 4 weeks, and one was exposed throughout (40 weeks). No anomalies were mentioned, nor were any other problems in the exposed liveborn infants. The growth retardation was probably due to the severe maternal disease (1).

A 1988 case report described a woman with pregnancy-induced hypertension who was treated with methyldopa and verapamil for 6 weeks with poor control of her blood pressure (2). At 32 weeks' gestation, methyldopa was discontinued and enalapril (20 mg/day) was combined with verapamil (360 mg/day), resulting in good control. An elective cesarean section was performed after 17 days of combination therapy. Oligohydramnios was noted, as was meconium staining. The 2100-g female infant was anuric during the first 2 days, although tests indicated normal kidneys without obstruction. A renal biopsy showed hyperplasia of the juxtaglomerular apparatus. She began producing urine on the 3rd day (2 ml over 24 hours), 12 hours after the onset of peritoneal dialysis. She remained oliguric when dialysis was stopped at age 10 days, producing only 30 ml of urine over 24 hours. By the 19th postnatal day, her urine output had reached 125 ml/24 hours. The plasma enalaprilat concentration was 28 ng/ml before dialysis and then fell to undetectable (<0.16 ng/ml) levels after dialysis. Angiotensin-converting enzyme levels (normal 95 $+/-$ 29 nmol/ml minute) were <1 (days 2 and 3), 2.1 (day 5), 15.6 (day 8), 127 (day 31), and >130 (day 90). Angiotensin II concentrations (normal 182 $+/-$ 89 fmol/ml) were still suppressed (39.8) on day 31; plasma renin activity, active renin, and total renin were all markedly elevated until day 90. By this time, renal function had returned to normal. Clinical follow-up at 1 year of age was normal.

A renal transplant patient was treated with enalapril, azathioprine, atenolol, and prednisolone (doses not given) throughout pregnancy (3). Ultrasound at 32 weeks' gestation indicated oligohydramnios and asymmetrical growth retardation. A cesarean section delivered a 1280-g (10th percentile) male infant with a head circumference of 25.7 cm (3rd percentile). Severe hypotension (mean 25 mm Hg), present at birth, was resistant to volume expansion and pressor agents. The newborn was anuric for 72 hours, then oliguric, passing only 2.5 ml over the next 36 hours. Ultrasonography revealed a normal-sized kidney and a normal urinary tract. Peritoneal dialysis was commenced on day 8, but the infant died 2 days later. Defects secondary to oligohydramnios were squashed facies, contractures of the extremities, and pulmonary hypoplasia. Ossification of the occipital skull was absent, but the etiology of this defect was unknown. A chromosome abnormality was excluded based on a normal male karyotype (46X,Y). The renal failure was most likely due to enalapril.

A 24-year-old woman with malignant hypertension and familial hypophosphatemic rickets was treated from before conception with enalapril (10 mg/day), furosemide (40 mg/day), calciferol (1.25 mg/day), and slow phosphate (1200 mg/day) (4). Blood pressure was normal at 15 weeks' gestation as was fetal growth. However, oligohydramnios developed 2 weeks later, and by 20 weeks' gestation, virtually no fluid was present. Fetal growth retardation was also evident at this time. Enalapril and furosemide therapy were slowly replaced by labetalol over the next week and a steady improvement in amniotic fluid volume was noted by 24 weeks. Volume was normal at 27 weeks' gestation, but shortly thereafter, abruptio placentae occurred, requiring an emergency cesarean section. A 720-g (below 3rd percentile) male infant was delivered who died on day 6. A postmortem examination indicated a normal urogenital tract.

An 18-year-old woman with severe chronic hypertension had four pregnancies over an approximately 4-year period, all while taking angiotensin-converting enzyme inhibitors and other antihypertensives (5). During her first pregnancy, she had been maintained on captopril and she delivered a premature, growth-retarded, but otherwise healthy female infant who survived. In the postpartum period, captopril was discontinued and enalapril (10 mg/day) was started while continuing atenolol (100 mg/day) and nifedipine (40 mg/day). She next presented in the 13th week of her second pregnancy with unchanged antihypertensive therapy. Fetal death occurred at 18 weeks' gestation. The 340-g male fetus was macerated but otherwise normal. Her third and fourth pregnancies, again with basically unchanged antihypertensive therapy except for the addition of aspirin (75 mg/day) at the 10th week, resulted in the delivery of an 1170-g female and a 1540-g male, both at 29 weeks.

Investigators at the Food and Drug Administration (FDA) reviewed five cases of enalapril-induced neonatal renal failure, one of which had been published previously in a 1989 report (6). The remaining four unpublished cases involved two mothers with hypertension of unspecified cause, one with chronic hypertension and glomerulonephritis, and one with hypertension after a kidney transplant. Enalapril doses ranged from 10–45 mg/day. Two of the mothers were treated throughout gestation, one was treated from 27–34 weeks' gestation, and one was treated during the last 3 weeks only. All of the infants required dialysis for anuria. Renal function eventually recovered in two infants, it was still abnormal 1 month after birth in one, and tubular acidosis occurred in the fourth infant 60 days after delivery. Hypotension was reported in three of the four newborns. The FDA authors cautioned that if enalapril was used during pregnancy, then preparations should be made for neonatal hypotension and renal failure (6).

A 1990 case report may indicate that structural kidney defects may be a consequence of enalapril therapy (7). A 22-year-old mother, with systemic lupus erythematosus and severe chronic hypertension, was treated throughout gestation with enalapril (20 mg/day), propranolol (40 mg/day), and hydrochlorothiazide (50 mg/day). Blood pressure was well controlled on this regimen, and no evidence of active lupus occurred during pregnancy. Normal amniotic fluid volume was documented at 16 weeks' gestation followed by severe oligohydramnios as 27 weeks. Although normal fetal growth was observed, the male infant was delivered at 34 weeks' gestation by emergency cesarean section because thick meconium was found on amniocentesis. No meconium was found below the vocal cords. The profound neonatal hypotension induced by enalapril required aggressive treatment with fluids and pressor agents. The newborn had the characteristic features of the oligohydramnios sequence. Both kidneys were morphologically normal by renal ultrasonogram, but no urine output was observed, and no urine was found in the bladder. The infant died at about 25 hours of age. Pulmonary hypoplasia, a condition secondary to oligohydramnios, was found at autopsy. Except for their large size, approximately 1.5 times the expected weight, the kidneys were grossly normal with normal vessels and ureters, and a contracted bladder. Microscopic examination revealed a number of kidney abnormalities: irregular corticomedullary junctions; glomerular maldevelopment with a decreased number of lobulations in many of the glomeruli, and some congested glomeruli; a reduced number of tubules in the upper portion of the medulla with increased mesenchymal tissue; and tubular distension in the cortex and medulla (7). The investigators could not determine if the renal defects were due to reduced renal blood flow secondary to enalapril, a direct teratogenic effect of the drug, or an effect of the specific drug combination. However, no renal anomalies have been reported after use of the other two drugs (see Hydrochlorothiazide and Propranolol), and similar renal defects have not been reported as a complication of maternal lupus (7).

The limited experience with enalapril in early gestation does not allow an assessment of its teratogenic potential. However, the case report cited describing major renal malformations should be carefully considered before this drug is used in early gestation. Further studies are needed to determine if structural kidney anomalies are induced by enalapril (6). The severe hypotension present at birth and the renal failure observed were due to enalapril (see also Captopril). The use of angiotensin I-converting enzyme inhibitors during pregnancy may compromise the fetal renal system. Two reviews of fetal and newborn renal function, published in 1988, indicated that both renal perfusion and glomerular plasma flow are low during gestation and that high levels of angiotensin II may be physiologically necessary to maintain glomerular filtration at low perfusion pressures (8, 9). Enalapril prevents the conversion of angiotensin I to angiotensin II and, thus, may lead to *in utero* renal failure. In those cases where the mother's disease requires enalapril, close monitoring of amniotic fluid levels and fetal well-being are required. If oligohydramnios ensues, changing to other antihypertensive agents may reverse the condition based on one case history, but it is not known if this will result in improved fetal outcome. Newborn renal function and blood pressure should be closely monitored after *in utero* exposure to enalapril.

Breast Feeding Summary

No data are available (see also Captopril).

References

1. Kreft-Jais C, Plouin P-F, Tchobroutsky C, Boutroy M-J. Angiotensin-converting enzyme inhibitors during pregnancy: a survey of 22 patients given captopril and nine given enalapril. Br J Obstet Gynaecol 1988;95:420–2.
2. Schubiger G, Flury G, Nussberger J. Enalapril for pregnancy-induced hypertension: acute renal failure in a neonate. Ann Intern Med 1988;108:215–6.
3. Mehta N, Modi N. ACE inhibitors in pregnancy. Lancet 1989;2:96.
4. Broughton Pipkin F, Baker PN, Symonds EM. ACE inhibitors in pregnancy. Lancet 1989;2:96–7.
5. Smith AM. Are ACE inhibitors safe in pregnancy? Lancet 1989;2:750–1.
6. Rosa FW, Bosco LA, Graham CF, Milstien JB, Dreis M, Creamer J. Neonatal anuria with maternal angiotensin-converting enzyme inhibition. Obstet Gynecol 1989;74:371–4.
7. Cunniff C, Jones KL, Phillipson J, Benirschke K, Short S, Wujek J. Oligohydramnios sequence and renal tubular malformation associated with maternal enalapril use. Am J Obstet Gynecol 1990;162:187–9.
8. Robillard JE, Nakamura KT, Matherne GP, Jose PA. Renal hemodynamics and functional adjustments to postnatal life. Semin Perinatol 1988;12:143–50.
9. Guignard J-P, Gouyon J-B. Adverse effects of drugs on the immature kidney. Biol Neonate 1988;53:243–52.

Name: **ENCAINIDE**

Class: **Antiarrhythmic**   Risk Factor: **B$_M$**

Fetal Risk Summary

Encainide is a cardiac agent used for the treatment of ventricular arrhythmias. Neither animal nor human teratogenicity has been observed, but human experience is very limited.

The parent compound and its two active metabolites (more potent than encainide on a per milligram basis), o-demethyl encainide and 3-methoxy-o-demethyl encainide, cross the placenta to the fetus (B.D. Quart, personal communication, Bristol-Myers Company, 1988). Concentrations of encainide and its metabolites in fetal plasma have ranged from 30–300% of simultaneously collected maternal serum levels (B.D. Quart, personal communication, 1988). Excessive accumulation of the drug or its metabolites in the fetal plasma apparently does not occur. Amniotic fluid levels of the three compounds in one case were 2–3 times greater than in fetal plasma (B.D. Quart, personal communication, 1988).

Encainide has been successfully used to treat a fetal cardiac arrhythmia *in utero*, but a high maternal dose, 50 mg four times a day, was required to control the abnormality (B.D. Quart, personal communication, 1988). The gestational age of the fetus was not given nor was the length of therapy. In this case, encainide could not be found in fetal plasma, and concentrations of the two metabolites were less than 100 ng/ml. Very high concentrations of the metabolites were measured in the newborn's first several urine samples.

Breast Feeding Summary

Encainide and its active metabolites are excreted in breast milk. In one patient taking 50 mg four times a day, milk levels of encainide and one metabolite, o-demethyl encainide, were 200–400 ng/ml and 100–200 ng/ml, respectively (B.D. Quart, personal communication, 1988). These levels were comparable to maternal peak plasma levels. A third metabolite, 3-methoxy-o-demethyl encainide, evidently was not produced by the mother because it was not found in her plasma or milk. However, based on animal experiments, it is also expected to cross into the milk if present in the maternal plasma (B.D. Quart, personal communication, 1988).

Name: **EPHEDRINE**

Class: **Sympathomimetic (Adrenergic)**   Risk Factor: **C**

Fetal Risk Summary

Ephedrine is a sympathomimetic used widely for bronchial asthma, allergic disorders, hypotension, and the alleviation of symptoms caused by upper respiratory infections. It is a common component of proprietary mixtures containing antihistamines, bronchodilators, and other ingredients. Thus it is difficult to separate the effects of ephedrine on the fetus from other drugs, disease states and viruses. Ephedrine-like drugs are teratogenic in some animal species, but human teratogenicity has not been suspected (1, 2). The Collaborative Perinatal Project monitored 50,282 mother-child pairs, 373 of which had 1st trimester exposure to ephedrine (3, pp. 345–356). For use anytime during pregnancy, 873 exposures were recorded (3, p. 439). No evidence for a relationship to large categories of major or minor malformations or to individual defects was found. However, an association in the 1st trimester was found between the sympathomimetic class of drugs as a whole and minor malformations (not life-threatening or major cosmetic defects), inguinal hernia, and clubfoot (3, pp. 345–356).

Ephedrine is routinely used to treat or prevent maternal hypotension following spinal anesthesia (4–7). Significant increases in fetal heart rate and beat-to-beat variability may occur, but these effects may have been the result of normal reflexes following hypotension-associated bradycardias. A recent study, however, has demonstrated the placental passage of ephedrine with fetal levels at delivery approximately 70% of the maternal concentration (8). The presence of ephedrine in the fetal circulation is probably a major cause of the fetal heart rate changes.

Breast Feeding Summary

A single case report has been located describing adverse effects in a 3-month-old nursing infant of a mother consuming a long-acting preparation containing 120 mg of d-isoephedrine and 6 mg of dexbrompheniramine (9). The mother had begun taking the preparation on a twice daily schedule 1 or 2 days prior to onset of the infant's symptoms. The infant exhibited irritability, excessive crying, and disturbed sleeping patterns that resolved spontaneously within 12 hours when breast feeding was stopped.

References

1. Nishimura H, Tanimura T. *Clinical Aspects of the Teratogenity of Drugs*. Amsterdam:Excerpta Medica, 1976:231.
2. Shepard TH. *Catalog of Teratogenic Agents*, ed. 3. Baltimore:Johns Hopkins University Press, 1980:134–5.
3. Heinonen OP, Slone D, Shapiro S. *Birth Defects and Drugs in Pregnancy*. Littleton:Publishing Sciences Group, 1977.
4. Wright RG, Shnider SM, Levinson G, Rolbin SH, Parer JT. The effect of maternal administration of ephedrine on fetal heart rate and variability. Obstet Gynecol 1981;57:734–8.
5. Antoine C, Young BK. Fetal lactic acidosis with epidural anesthesia. Am J Obstet Gynecol 1982;142:55–9.
6. Datta S, Alper MH, Ostheimer GW, Weiss JB. Method of ephedrine administration and nausea and hypotension during spinal anesthesia for cesarean section. Anesthesiology 1982;56:68–70.
7. Antoine C, Young BK. Fetal lactic acidosis with epidural anesthesia. Am J Obstet Gynecol 1982;142:55–9.
8. Hughes SC, Ward MG, Levinson G, Shnider SM, Wright RG, Gruenke LD, Craig JC. Placental transfer of ephedrine does not affect neonatal outcome. Anesthesiology 1985;63:217–9.
9. Mortimer EA Jr. Drug toxicity from breast milk? Pediatrics 1977;60:780–1.

Name: **EPINEPHRINE**

Class: **Sympathomimetic (Adrenergic)** Risk Factor: **C**

Fetal Risk Summary

Epinephrine is a sympathomimetic that is widely used for conditions such as shock, glaucoma, allergic reactions, bronchial asthma, and nasal congestion. Because it occurs naturally in all humans, it is difficult to separate the effects of its administration from effects on the fetus induced by endogenous epinephrine, other drugs, disease states, and viruses. The drug readily crosses the placenta (1). Epinephrine is teratogenic in some animal species, but human teratogenicity has not been suspected (2, 3). The Collaborative Perinatal Project monitored 50,282 mother-child pairs, 189 of which had 1st trimester exposure to epinephrine (4, pp. 345–356). For use anytime during pregnancy, 508 exposures were recorded (4, p. 439). A statistically significant association was found between 1st trimester use of epinephrine and major and minor malformations. An association was also found with inguinal hernia after both 1st trimester and anytime use (4, pp. 477, 492). Although not specified, these data may reflect the potentially severe maternal status for which epinephrine administration is indicated.

Theoretically, epinephrine's α-adrenergic properties might lead to a decreased in uterine blood flow. A large intravenous dose of epinephrine, 1.5 ml of a 1:1000 solution over 1 hour to reverse severe hypotension secondary to an allergic reaction, may have contributed to intrauterine anoxic insult to a 28-week-old fetus (5). Decreased fetal movements occurred after treatment and the infant, delivered at 34 weeks' gestation, had evidence of intracranial hemorrhage at birth and died 4 days later. Thus, in situations such as maternal hypotension where a pressor agent is required, use of ephedrine may be a better choice.

Breast Feeding Summary

No data are available.

References

1. Morgan CD, Sandler M, Panigel M. Placental transfer of catecholamines in vitro and in vivo. Am J Obstet Gynecol 1972;112:1068–75.
2. Nishimura H, Tanimura T. *Clinical Aspects of the Teratogenicity of Drugs.* Amsterdam:Excerpta Medica, 1976:231.
3. Shepard TH. *Catalog of Teratogenic Agents*, ed. 3. Baltimore:Johns Hopkins University Press, 1980:134–5.
4. Heinonen OP, Slone D, Shapiro S. *Birth Defects and Drugs in Pregnancy.* Littleton:Publishing Sciences Group, 1977.
5. Entman SS, Moise KJ. Anaphylaxis in pregnancy. S Med J 1984;77:402.

Name: **ERGOCALCIFEROL**

Class: **Vitamin**   Risk Factor: **A***

Fetal Risk Summary

Ergocalciferol (vitamin D_2) is converted in the liver to 25-hydroxyergocalciferol, which in turn is converted in the kidneys to 1,25-dihydroxyergocalciferol, one of the active forms of vitamin D. See Vitamin D.

[*Risk Factor D if used in doses above the recommended daily allowance.]

Breast Feeding Summary

See Vitamin D.

Name: **ERYTHRITYL TETRANITRATE**

Class: **Vasodilator**

Risk Factor: **C$_M$**

Fetal Risk Summary

See Nitroglycerin or Amyl Nitrite.

Breast Feeding Summary

No data are available.

Name: **ERYTHROMYCIN**

Class: **Antibiotic**

Risk Factor: **B**

Fetal Risk Summary

No reports linking the use of erythromycin with congenital defects have been located. The drug crosses the placenta but in concentrations too low to treat most pathogens (1–3). Fetal tissue levels increase after multiple doses (3). However, a case has been described in which erythromycin was used successfully to treat maternal syphilis but failed to treat the fetus adequately (4). During pregnancy, erythromycin serum concentrations vary greatly as compared to those in normal men and nonpregnant women, which might account for the low levels observed in the fetus (5).

The estolate salt of erythromycin has been observed to induce hepatotoxicity in pregnant patients (6). Approximately 10% of 161 women treated with the estolate form in the 2nd trimester had abnormally elevated levels of serum glutamic-oxaloacetic transaminase, which returned to normal after therapy was discontinued.

The use of erythromycin in the 1st trimester was reported in a mother who delivered an infant with left absence-of-tibia syndrome (7). The mother was also exposed to other drugs, which makes a relationship to the antibiotic unlikely.

The Collaborative Perinatal Project monitored 50,282 mother-child pairs, 79 of which had 1st trimester exposure to erythromycin (8, pp. 297–313). For use anytime during pregnancy, 230 exposures were recorded (8, p. 435). No evidence was found to suggest a relationship to large categories of major and minor malformations or to individual defects. Erythromycin, like many other antibiotics, lowers urine estriol concentrations (see also Ampicillin for mechanism and significance) (9). The antibiotic has been used during the 3rd trimester to reduce maternal and infant colonization with group B β-hemolytic streptococcus (10, 11). Erythromycin has also been used during pregnancy for the treatment of genital mycoplasmas (12, 13). A reduction in the rates of pregnancy loss and low-birth-weight infants was seen in patients with mycoplasma infection after treatment with erythromycin.

Breast Feeding Summary

Erythromycin is excreted into breast milk (14). Following oral doses of 400 mg every 8 hours, milk levels ranged from 0.4–1.6 µg/ml. Oral doses of 2 g/day produced milk concentrations of 1.6–3.2 μg/ml. The milk:plasma ratio in both groups was 0.5. No reports of adverse effects in infants exposed to erythromycin in breast milk have been located. However, three potential problems exist for the nursing infant: modification of bowel flora, direct effects on the infant, and interference with the interpretation of culture results if a fever workup is required. The American Academy of Pediatrics considers the antibiotic to be compatible with breast feeding (15).

References

1. Heilman FR, Herrell WE, Wellman WE, Geraci JE. Some laboratory and clinical observations on a new antibiotic, erythromycin (Ilotycin). Proc Staff Meet Mayo Clin 1952;27:285–304.
2. Kiefer L, Rubin A, McCoy JB, Foltz EL. The placental transfer of erythromycin. Am J Obstet Gynecol 1955;69:174–7.
3. Philipson A, Sabath LD, Charles D. Transplacental passage of erythromycin and clindamycin. N Engl J Med 1973;288:1219–20.
4. Fenton LJ, Light LJ. Congenital syphilis after maternal treatment with erythromycin. Obstet Gynecol 1976;47:492–4.
5. Philipson A, Sabath LD, Charles D. Erythromycin and clindamycin absorption and elimination in pregnant women. Clin Pharmacoal Ther 1976;19:68–77.
6. McCormack WM, George H, Donner A, Kodgis LF, Albert S, Lowe EW, Kass EH. Hepatotoxicity of erythromycin estolate during pregnancy. Antimicrob Agents Chemother 1977;12:630–5.
7. Jaffe P, Liberman MM, McFadyen I, Valman HB. Incidence of congenital limb-reduction deformities. Lancet 1975;1:526–7.
8. Heinonen OP, Slone D, Shapiro S. *Birth Defects and Drugs in Pregnancy*. Littleton:Publishing Sciences Group, 1977.
9. Gallagher JC, Ismail MA, Aladjem S. Reduced urinary estriol levels with erythromycin therapy. Obstet Gynecol 1980;56:381–2.
10. Merenstein GB, Todd WA, Brown G, Yost CC, Luzier T. Group B B-hemolytic streptococcus: randomized controlled treatment study at term. Obstet Gynecol 1980;55:315–8.
11. Easmon CSF, Hastings MJG, Deeley J, Bloxham B, Rivers RPA, Marwood R. The effect of intrapartum chemoprophylaxis on the vertical transmission of group B streptococci. Br J Obstet Gynaecol 1983;90:633–5.
12. Quinn PA, Shewchuk AB, Shuber J, Lie KI, Ryan E, Chipman ML, Nocilla DM. Efficacy of antibiotic therapy in preventing spontaneous pregnancy loss among couples colonized with genital mycoplasmas. Am J Obstet Gynecol 1983;145:239–44.
13. Kass EH, McCormack WM. Genital mycoplasma infection and perinatal morbidity. N Engl J Med 1984;311:258.
14. Knowles JA. Drugs in milk. Pediatr Currents 1972;21:28–32.
15. Committee on Drugs, American Academy of Pediatrics. Transfer of drugs and other chemicals into human milk. Pediatrics 1989;84:924–36.

Name: **ESMOLOL**

Class: **Sympatholytic**   Risk Factor: **C$_M$**

Fetal Risk Summary

Esmolol is a short-acting cardioselective β-adrenergic blocking agent that is structurally related to atenolol and metoprolol (1). The drug is used for the rapid, temporary treatment of supraventricular tachyarrhythmias (e.g., atrial flutter and/or fibrillation, sinus tachycardia) and for hypertension occurring during surgery. No reports of the use of esmolol in human pregnancy have been located. In pregnant sheep, the mean fetal:maternal serum ratio at the end of an infusion of esmolol was 0.08 (2). The drug was not detectable in the fetus 10 minutes after the end of the infusion. However, the hemodynamic effects, in terms of decreases in mean arterial pressure and heart rate, in the fetal sheep were similar to those in the mothers. The drug is not an animal teratogen (1). Because hypotension may occur with its use — up to 50% of patients in some trials — the potential for decreased uterine blood flow and resulting fetal hypoxia should be considered.

Breast Feeding Summary

No data are available.

References

1. Product information, Brevibloc. Dupont Critical Care, 1989.
2. Ostman PL, Chestnut DH, Robillard JE, Weiner CP, Hdez MJ. Transplacental passage and hemodynamic effects of esmolol in the gravid ewe. Anesthesiology 1988;69:738–41.

Name: **ESTRADIOL**

Class: **Estrogenic Hormone**   Risk Factor: **X**

Fetal Risk Summary

Estradiol and its salts (cypionate, valerate) are used for treatment of menopausal symptoms, female hypogonadism, and primary ovarian failure. The Collaborative Perinatal Project monitored 614 mother-child pairs with 1st trimester exposure to estrogenic agents (including 48 with exposure to estradiol) (1, pp. 389, 391). An increase in the expected frequency of cardiovascular defects, eye and ear anomalies, and Down's syndrome was found for estrogens as a group but not for estradiol (1, pp. 389, 391, 395). Re-evaluation of these data in terms of timing of exposure, vaginal bleeding in early pregnancy, and previous maternal obstetric history, however, failed to support an association between estrogens and cardiac malformations (2). An earlier study also failed to find any relationship with nongenital malformations (3).

Developmental changes in the psychosexual performance of boys has been attributed to *in utero* exposure to estradiol and progesterone (4). The mothers received an estrogen/progestogen regimen for their diabetes. Hormone-exposed males demonstrated a trend to have less heterosexual experience and fewer masculine interests than controls. Estradiol has been administered to women in labor in an attempt to potentiate the cervical ripening effects of prostaglandins (5). No detectable effect was observed. Use of estrogenic hormones during pregnancy is contraindicated.

Breast Feeding Summary

Estradiol is used to suppress postpartum breast engorgement in patients who do not desire to breast feed. Following the administration of vaginal suppositories containing 50 or 100 mg of estradiol to six lactating women who wished to stop breast feeding, less than 10% of the dose appeared in breast milk (6). The American Academy of Pediatrics considers estradiol to be compatible with breast feeding (7).

References

1. Heinonen OP, Slone D, Shapiro S. *Birth Defects and Drugs in Pregnancy*. Littleton:Publishing Sciences Group, 1977.
2. Wiseman RA, Dodds-Smith IC. Cardiovascular birth defects and antenatal exposure to female sex hormones: a reevaluation of some base data. Teratology 1984;30:359–70.
3. Wilson JG, Brent RL. Are female sex hormones teratogenic? Am J Obstet Gynecol 1981;141:567–80.
4. Yalom ID, Green R, Fisk N. Prenatal exposure to female hormones. Effect of psychosexual development in boys. Arch Gen Psychiatry 1973;28:554–61.
5. Luther ER, Roux J, Popat R, Gardner A, Gray J, Soubiran E, Korcaz Y. The effect of estrogen priming on induction of labor with prostaglandins. Am J Obstet Gynecol 1980;137:351–7.
6. Nilsson S, Nygren KG, Johansson EDB. Transfer of estradiol to human milk. Am J Obstet Gynecol 1978;132:653–7.
7. Committee on Drugs, American Academy of Pediatrics. Transfer of drugs and other chemicals into human milk. Pediatrics 1989;84:924–36.

Name: **ESTROGENS, CONJUGATED**

Class: **Estrogenic Hormone**   Risk Factor: X_M

Fetal Risk Summary

Conjugated estrogens are a mixture of estrogenic substances (primarily estrone). The Collaborative Perinatal Project monitored 13 mother-child pairs who were exposed to conjugated estrogens during the 1st trimester (1, pp. 389, 391). An increased risk for malformations was found, although identification of the malformations was not provided. Estrogenic agents as a group were monitored in 614 mother-child pairs. An increase in the expected frequency of cardiovascular defects, eye and ear anomalies, and Down's syndrome was reported (1, p. 395). Reevaluation of these data in terms of timing of exposure, vaginal bleeding in early pregnancy, and previous maternal obstetric history, however, failed to support an association between estrogens and cardiac malformations (2). An earlier study also failed to find any relationship with nongenital malformations (3). No adverse effects were observed in one infant exposed during the 1st trimester to conjugated estrogens (4). However, in a second infant exposed during the 4th–7th weeks of gestation, multiple anomalies were found: cleft palate, wormian bones, heart defect, dislocated hips, absent tibiae, polydactyly, and abnormal dermal pattern (5).

Conjugated estrogens have been used to induce ovulation in anovulatory women (6). They have also been used as partially successful contraceptives when given within 72 hours of unprotected, midcycle coitus (7). No fetal adverse effects were mentioned in either of these reports.

Breast Feeding Summary

No reports of adverse effects from conjugated estrogens in the nursing infant have been located. It is possible that decreased milk volume and decreased nitrogen and protein content could occur (see Mestranol, Ethinyl Estradiol).

References

1. Heinonen OP, Slone D, Shapiro S. *Birth Defects and Drugs in Pregnancy*. Littleton:Publishing Sciences Group, 1977.
2. Wiseman RA, Dodds-Smith IC. Cardiovascular birth defects and antenatal exposure to female sex hormones: a reevaluation of some base data. Teratology 1984;30:359–70.
3. Wilson JG, Brent RL. Are female sex hormones teratogenic? Am J Obstet Gynecol 1981;141:567–80.
4. Hagler S, Schultz A, Hankin H, Kunstadter RH. Fetal effects of steroid therapy during pregnancy. Am J Dis Child 1963;106:586–90.
5. Ho CK, Kaufman RL, McAlister WH. Congenital malformations. Am J Dis Child 1975;129:714–6.
6. Price R. Pregnancies using conjugated oestrogen therapy. Med J Aust 1980;2:341–2.
7. Dixon GW, Schlesselman JJ, Ory HW, Blye RP. Ethinyl estradiol and conjugated estrogens as postcoital contraceptives. JAMA 1980;244:1336–9.

Name: **ESTRONE**

Class: **Estrogenic Hormone**   Risk Factor: **X**

Fetal Risk Summary

See Estrogens, Conjugated.

Breast Feeding Summary

See Estrogens, Conjugated.

Name: **ETHACRYNIC ACID**

Class: **Diuretic**   Risk Factor: **D**

Fetal Risk Summary

Ethacrynic acid is a potent diuretic. It has been used for toxemia, pulmonary edema, and diabetes insipidus during pregnancy (1–10). Although it is not an animal teratogen, and limited 1st trimester human experience has not shown an increased incidence of malformations, ethacrynic acid is not recommended for use in pregnant women (11, 12). Diuretics do not prevent or alter the course of toxemia, and they may decrease placental perfusion (see also Chlorothiazide) (13–15). Ototoxicity has been observed in a mother and her newborn following the use of ethacrynic acid and kanamycin during the 3rd trimester (16).

Breast Feeding Summary

No data are available (see also Chlorothiazide). The manufacturer considers ethacrynic acid contraindicated in nursing mothers (11).

References

1. Delgado Urdapilleta J, Dominguez Robles H, Villalobos Roman M, Perez Diaz A. Ethacrynic acid in the treatment of toxemia of pregnancy. Ginecol Obstet Mex 1968;23:271–80.

2. Felman D, Theoleyre J, Dupoizat H. Investigation of ethacrynic acid in the treatment of excessive gain in weight and pregnancy arterial hypertension. Lyon Med 1967;217:1421–8.
3. Sands RX, Vita F. Ethacrynic acid (a new diuretic), pregnancy, and excessive fluid retention. Am J Obstet Gynecol 1968;101:603–9.
4. Kittaka S, Aizawa M, Tokue I, Shimizu M. Clinical results in Edecril tablet in the treatment of toxemia of late pregnancy. Obstet Gynecol (Jpn) 1968;36:934–7.
5. Mahon R, Dubecq JP, Baudet E, Coqueran J. Use of Edecrin in obstetrics. Bull Fed Soc Gynecol Obstet Lang Fr 1968;20:440–2.
6. Imaizumi S, Suzuoki Y, Torri M, et al. Clinical trial of ethacrynic acid (Edecril) for toxemia of pregnancy. Jpn J Med Consult New Remedies 1969;6:2364–8.
7. Young BK, Haft JI. Treatment of pulmonary edema with ethacrynic acid during labor. Am J Obstet Gynecol 1970;107:330–1.
8. Harrison KA, Ajabor LN, Lawson JB. Ethacrynic acid and packed-blood-cell transfusion in treatment of severe anaemia in pregnancy. Lancet 1971;1:11–4.
9. Fort AT, Morrison JC, Fisk SA. Iatrogenic hypokalemia of pregnancy by furosemide and ethacrynic acid: two case reports. J Reprod Med 1971;6:21–2.
10. Pico I, Greenblatt RB. Endocrinopathies and infertility. IV. Diabetes insipidus and pregnancy. Fertil Steril 1969;20:384–92.
11. Product information. Edecrin. Merck Sharpe & Dohme, 1985.
12. Wilson AL, Matzke GR. The treatment of hypertension in pregnancy. Drug Intell Clin Pharm 1981;15:21–6.
13. Pitkin RM, Kaminetzky HA, Newton M, Pritchard JA. Maternal nutrition: a selective review of clinical topics. Obstet Gynecol 1972;40:773–85.
14. Lindheimer MD, Katz AI. Sodium and diuretics in pregnancy. N Engl J Med 1973;288:891–4.
15. Christianson R, Page EW. Diuretic drugs and pregnancy. Obstet Gynecol 1976;48:647–52.
16. Jones HC. Intrauterine ototoxicity: a case report and review of literature. J Natl Med Assoc 1973;65:201–3.

Name: **ETHAMBUTOL**

Class: **Antituberculosis Agent**   Risk Factor: **B**

Fetal Risk Summary

No reports linking the use of ethambutol with congenital defects have been located. The drug crosses the placenta to the fetus (1, 2). In a woman delivered at 38 weeks' gestation, ethambutol concentrations in the cord and maternal blood 30 hours after an 800-mg (15 mg/kg) dose were 4.1 and 5.5 ng/ml, respectively, a cord:maternal serum ratio of 0.75 (1). The amniotic fluid ethambutol level was 9.5 ng/ml (1). These levels were within the range (1–5 ng/ml) required to inhibit the growth of *Mycobacterium tuberculosis* (1).

The literature supports the safety of ethambutol in combination with isoniazid and rifampicin during pregnancy (3–7). One investigator studied 38 patients (42 pregnancies) receiving antitubercular therapy (3). The minor abnormalities noted were within the expected frequency of occurrence. Another researcher observed six aborted fetuses at 5–12 weeks of age (4). Embryonic optic systems were specifically examined and were found to be normal. Most reviewers consider ethambutol, along with isoniazid and rifampin, to be the safest antituberculosis therapy (8, 9). However, long-term follow-up examinations for ocular damage have not been reported, causing concern among some clinicians (10).

Breast Feeding Summary

Ethambutol is excreted into human milk (11). Milk concentrations in two women, based on unpublished data, were 1.4 μg/ml (after an oral dose of 15 mg/kg) and 4.60 μg/ml (dosage not given), respectively. Corresponding maternal serum levels were 1.5 μg/ml and 4.62 μg/ml, respectively, indicating milk:serum ratios of approximately 1:1. The American Academy of Pediatrics considers ethambutol to be compatible with breast feeding (12).

References

1. Shneerson JM, Francis RS. Ethambutol in pregnancy—foetal exposure. Tubercle 1979;60:167–9.
2. Holdiness MR. Transplacental pharmacokinetics of the antituberculosis drugs. Clin Pharmacokinet 1987;13:125–9.
3. Bobrowitz ID. Ethambutol in pregnancy. Chest 1974;66:20–4.
4. Lewit T, Nebel L, Terracina S, Karman S. Ethambutol in pregnancy: observations on embryogenesis. Chest 1974;66:25–6.
5. Snider DE, Layde PM, Johnson MW, Lyle MA. Treatment of tuberculosis during pregnancy. Am Rev Respir Dis 1980;122:65–79.
6. Brock PG, Roach M. Antituberculous drugs in pregnancy. Lancet 1981;1:43.
7. Kingdom JCP, Kennedy DH. Tuberculous meningitis in pregnancy. Br J Obstet Gynaecol 1989;96:233–5.
8. American Thoracic Society. Treatment of tuberculosis and tuberculosis infection in adults and children. Am Rev Respir Dis 1986;134:355–63.
9. Medchill MT, Gillum M. Diagnosis and management of tuberculosis during pregnancy. Obstet Gynecol Surv 1989;44:81–4.
10. Wall MA. Treatment of tuberculosis during pregnancy. Am Rev Respir Dis 1980;122:989.
11. Snider DE Jr, Powell KE. Should women taking antituberculosis drugs breast-feed? Arch Intern Med 1984;144:589–90.
12. Committee on Drugs, American Academy of Pediatrics. Transfer of drugs and other chemicals into human milk. Pediatrics 1989;84:924–36.

Name: **ETHANOL**

Class: **Sedative** Risk Factor: **D***

Fetal Risk Summary

The teratogenic effects of ethanol (alcohol) have been recognized since antiquity, but this knowledge gradually fell into disfavor and was actually dismissed as superstition in the 1940s (1). Approximately three decades later, the characteristic pattern of anomalies that came to be known as the fetal alcohol syndrome (FAS) were rediscovered, first in France and then in the United States (2–5). By 1981, over 800 clinical and research papers on the FAS had been published (6).

Mild FAS (low birth weight) has been induced by the daily consumption of as little as two drinks (1 ounce of absolute alcohol or about 30 ml) in early pregnancy, but the complete syndrome is usually seen when maternal consumption is four to five drinks (60–75 ml of absolute alcohol) per day or more. The Council on Scientific Affairs of the American Medical Association, and the American Council on Science and Health have each published reports on the consequences of maternal alcohol ingestion during pregnancy (7, 8). The incidence of the FAS, depending upon the population studied, is estimated to be between 1/300 and 1/2000 live births with 30–40% of the offspring of alcoholic mothers expected to show the complete syndrome (7). The true incidence may be even higher because the diagnosis of FAS can be delayed for many years (9) (e.g., see reference 25 below). In addition, the incidence of alcohol abuse seems to be rising. A 1989 report found that alcohol abuse during 1987 in 1032 pregnant women was 1.4% compared to 0.7% of 5602 pregnant women during 1977–1980 (10). The difference in frequency was significant ($p < 0.05$).

Heavy alcohol intake by the father prior to conception has been suspected of producing the FAS (11, 12), although this association has been challenged (13). The report by the AMA Council states that growth retardation and some adverse aspects of fetal development may be due to paternal influence but conclusive evidence for the complete FAS is lacking (7).

Evidence supporting an association between "regular drinking" by the father in the month before conception and the infant's birth weight was published in two reports, both by the same authors (14, 15). "Regular drinking" was defined as "an average of at least 30 ml of ethanol daily or of 75 ml or more on a single occasion at least once a month" (14). "Occasional drinking" was defined as anything less than this. The mean birth weight, 3465 g, of 174 infants of "regular drinking" fathers was 181 g less than the mean birth weight, 3646 g, of 203 infants of "occasional drinking" fathers, a significant difference ($p < 0.001$). Using regression analysis, a 137-g decrease in birth weight was predicted (15). Statistical significance was also present when the data were categorized by sex (males 3561 g vs. 3733 g ($p < 0.05$), females 3364 g vs. 3538 g ($p < 0.05$)), percentage of infants less than 3000 g (15% vs. 9% ($p < 0.05$)), and percentage of infants at or greater than 4000 g (12% vs. 23% ($p < 0.01$)). Infant characteristics unrelated to the father's drinking were length, head circumference, gestational age, and Apgar scores (15). Consideration of the mother's drinking, smoking, and marijuana use did not change the statistical significance of the data. Nor could the differences be attributed to any of 20 reproductive and socioeconomic variables that were examined, including paternal smoking and marijuana use. No increases in structural defects were detected in the infants of the "regular drinking" fathers, but the sample size may have been too small to detect such an increase (14). In contrast to these data, other researchers have been unable to find an association between paternal drinking and infant birth weight (16). Thus, additional research is required, especially because the biologic mechanisms for the proposed association have not been determined (15).

The mechanism of ethanol's teratogenic effect is unknown but may be related to acetaldehyde, a metabolic byproduct of ethanol (7). One researcher reported higher blood levels of acetaldehyde in mothers of children with FAS than in alcoholics who delivered normal children (17). However, the analysis techniques used in that study have been questioned, and the high concentrations may have been due to artifactual formation of acetaldehyde (18). At the cellular level, alcohol or one of its metabolites may disrupt protein synthesis, resulting in cellular growth retardation with serious consequences for fetal brain development (19). Other proposed mechanisms that may contribute, as reviewed by Shepard (20), include poor protein intake, vitamin B deficiency, lead contamination of alcohol, and genetic predisposition. Of interest, metronidazole, a commonly used anti-infective agent, has been shown to markedly potentiate the fetotoxicity and teratogenicity of alcohol in mice (21). Human studies of this possible interaction have not been reported.

The complete FAS consists of abnormalities in three areas with a fourth area often involved: (a) craniofacial dysmorphology, (b) prenatal and antenatal growth deficiencies, (c) central nervous system dysfunction, and (d) various other abnormalities (7, 8). Problems occurring in the latter area include cardiac and renogenital defects, and hemangiomas in about one-half of the cases (3–5, 22). Cardiac malformations were described in 43 patients (57%) in a series of 76 children with the FAS evaluated for 0–6 years (age: birth to 18 years) (23). Functional murmurs (12 cases, 16%) and ventricular septal defects (VSD) (20 patients, 26%) accounted for the majority of anomalies. Other cardiac lesions present, in descending order of frequency, were: double outlet right ventricle and pulmonary atresia, dextrocardia (with VSD), patent ductus arteriosus with secondary pulmonary hypertension, and cor pulmonale. Liver abnormalities have also been reported (24, 25). Behavioral problems, including minimal brain dysfunction, are long-term effects of the FAS (1).

Ten-year follow-up of the original 11 children who were first diagnosed as having the FAS was reported in 1985 (25). Of the 11 children, two were dead, one was lost to follow-up, four had borderline intelligence with continued growth deficiency and were dysmorphic, and four had severe intelligence deficiency as well as growth deficiency and dysmorphic appearance. Moreover, the degree of growth deficiency and intellectual impairment was directly related to the degree of craniofacial abnormalities (25). In the eight children examined, height, weight, and head circumference were deficient, especially the latter two parameters. The authors concluded that the slow head growth after birth may explain why, in some cases, the FAS is not diagnosed until 9–12 months of age (25). Cardiac malformations originally observed in the infants, atrial septal defect (one), patent ductus arteriosus (one), and ventricular septal defect (six), had either resolved spontaneously or were no longer clinically significant. Three new features of the FAS were observed: dental malalignments, malocclusions, and eustachian tube dysfunction (associated with maxillary hypoplasia and leading to chronic serous otitis media) (25).

Fetal Alcohol Syndrome (2–9, 11–13, 22–38)
  Craniofacial
    Eyes: short palpebral fissures, ptosis, strabismus, epicanthal folds, myopia, microphthalmia, blepharophimosis
    Ears: poorly formed concha, posterior rotation, eustachian tube dysfunction
    Nose: short, upturned hypoplastic philtrum
    Mouth: prominent lateral palatine ridges, thinned upper vermilion, retrognathia in infancy, micrognathia or relative prognathia in adolescence, cleft lip or palate, small teeth with faulty enamel, Class III malocclusion, poor dental alignment
    Maxilla: hypoplastic
  Central nervous system
    Dysfunction demonstrated by mild to moderate retardation, microcephaly, poor coordination, hypotonia, irritability in infancy and hyperactivity in childhood
  Growth
    Prenatal (affecting body length more than weight) and postnatal deficiency (length, weight, and head circumference)

Cardiac
  Murmurs, atrial septal defect, ventricular septal defect, great vessel anom-
    alies, tetralogy of Fallot
Renogenital
  Labial hypoplasia, hypospadias, renal defects
Cutaneous
  Hemangiomas, hirsutism in infancy
Skeletal
  Abnormal palmar creases, pectus excavatum, restriction of joint move-
    ment, nail hypoplasia, radioulnar synostosis, pectus carinatum, bifid
    xiphoid, Klippel-Feil anomaly, scoliosis
Muscular
  Hernias of diaphragm, umbilicus or groin, diastasis recti

A study published in 1987 found that craniofacial abnormalities were closely
related to alcohol consumption in a dose-response manner (39). Although a distinct threshold was not defined, the data indicated that the consumption of more
than six drinks (90 ml of ethanol) per day was clearly related to structural defects,
with the critical period for alcohol-induced teratogenicity around the time of conception (39). A 1989 study that examined 595 live singleton births found a significant correlation between alcohol use in the first 2 months of pregnancy and intrauterine growth retardation and structural abnormalities (40). Analysis of alcohol
use during the other periods of pregnancy did not show a significant association
with these outcomes.

A prospective study conducted between 1974–1977 at the Kaiser-Permanente
health maintenance organization in Northern California was conducted to determine if light to moderate drinking during pregnancy was associated with congenital abnormalities (41). A total of 32,870 women met all of the criteria for enrollment
in the study. Of the total study population, 15,460 (47%) used alcohol during pregnancy, 17,114 (52%) denied use, and 296 (1%) provided incomplete information
on their drinking. Of those drinking, 14,502 (94%) averaged less than one drink/
day, 793 (5%) drank one to two drinks/day, 127 (0.8%) consumed three to five
drinks/day, and 38 (0.2%) drank six or more drinks/day. The total (major and minor) malformation rates were similar between nondrinkers and light (less than one
drink/day) or moderate (one to two drinks/day) drinkers; 78.1/1000, 77.3/1000,
and 83.2/1000, respectively. A significant trend ($p = 0.034$) was found with increasing alcohol use and congenital malformations of the sex organs (e.g., absence or hypertrophy of the labia, clitoris, and vagina; defects of the ovaries, fallopian tubes, and uterus; hypoplastic or absent penis or scrotum; intersex and
unspecified genital anomalies) (41). Rates per 1000 for defects of the sex organs
in nondrinkers and the four drinking groups were 2.8, 2.6, 6.3, 7.9, and 26.3, respectively. Genitourinary malformations (i.e., cryptorchidism, hypospadias, and
epispadias) also followed an increasing trend with rates per 1000 women of 27.2,
27.5, 31.5, 47.2, and 78.9 (p value for trend = 0.04), respectively. At the levels of
alcohol consumption observed in the study, no increase in the other malformations commonly associated with the FAS was found with increasing alcohol use.

A strong association between moderate drinking (>30 ml of absolute alcohol
twice per week) and 2nd trimester (15–27 weeks) spontaneous abortions has
been found (27, 28). Alcohol consumption at this level may increase the risk of

miscarriage by 2–4-fold, apparently by acting as an acute fetal toxin. Consumption of smaller amounts of alcohol, such as one drink (approximately 15 ml of absolute alcohol) per week, was not associated with an increased risk of miscarriage in a 1989 report (42).

Ethanol was once used to treat premature uterine contractions. In a retrospective analysis of women treated for premature labor between 1968–1973, 239 singleton pregnancies were identified (43). In 136, the women had received oral and/or intravenous (IV) ethanol, in addition to bed rest and oral β-mimetics. The remaining 103 women had been treated only with bed rest and oral β-mimetics. The alcohol group received an average of 38 g of ethanol/day for 2–34 days. In addition, 73 of these women continued to use oral alcohol at home as needed to arrest uterine contractions. Treatment with ethanol was begun at 12 weeks' gestation or less in 82 (60.3%) of the treated women. The mean birth weights of the alcohol-exposed and nonexposed infants were similar, 3385 g vs. 3283 g, respectively. No significant differences were found between the groups in the number of infants who were small for gestational age (weight or length <10th percentile), birth length, fetal and neonatal deaths, and infants with anomalies. No relationship was found between ethanol dose and birth weight, length, or neonatal outcome. None of the exposed infants had features of the typical fetal alcohol syndrome. Psychomotor development (age to sit, walk, speak few-word sentences, and read) and growth velocity were similar between the two groups. One of the infants whose mother had been treated with intravenous alcohol was growth retarded from birth to 14 years of age. Eight (6.1%) of 131 alcohol-exposed infants were considered to have problems in school (hyperactivity, carelessness, etc) compared to two (2.0%) of 99 controls, but the difference was not significant. Other complications observed were aphasia and impaired hearing in two of the treated group and a third infant with blindness in the right eye (this infant was delivered at 27 weeks' gestation and the condition was thought to be due to oxygen therapy). The authors concluded that the alcohol treatment for threatened 1st or 2nd trimester abortions did not cause fetal damage (43). However, an earlier study concluded that adverse effects occurred after even short-term exposure (44). This conclusion was reached in an evaluation of 25 children 4–7 years of age whose mothers had been treated with alcohol infusions to prevent preterm labor (44). In comparison with matched controls, seven children born during or within 15 hours of termination of the infusion had significant pathology in developmental and personality evaluations.

Two reports have described neural tube defects in six infants exposed to heavy amounts of alcohol during early gestation (45, 46). Lumbosacral meningomyelocele was observed in five of the newborns and anencephaly in one. One of the infants also had a dislocated hip and clubfeet (45).

A possible association between maternal drinking and clubfoot was proposed in a short 1985 report (47). Three of 43 infants, delivered from maternal alcoholics, had fetal talipes equinovarus (clubfoot), an incidence significantly greater than expected ($p < 0.00001$).

Gastroschisis has been observed in dizygotic twins delivered from a mother who consumed 150–180 ml of absolute ethanol/day during the first 10 weeks of gestation (48). Although an association could not be proven, the authors speculated that the defects resulted from the heavy alcohol ingestion.

A 1982 report described four offspring of alcoholic mothers with clinical and laboratory features of combined FAS and DiGeorge syndrome (49). Several characteristics of the two syndromes are similar, including craniofacial, cardiac, central nervous system, renal, and immune defects (49). Features not shared are hypoparathyroidism (part of DiGeorge syndrome) and skeletal anomalies (part of FAS). A possible causative relationship was suggested between maternal alcoholism and the DiGeorge syndrome.

An unusual chromosome anomaly was discovered in a 2-year-old girl whose mother drank heavily during early gestation (50). The infant's karotype revealed an isochromosome for the long arm of number 9: 46,XX, $-9, +i(9q)$. The infant had several characteristics of the FAS, including growth retardation. The relationship between the chromosome defect and alcohol is unknown.

Prospective analysis of 31,604 pregnancies found that the percentage of newborns below the 10th percentile of weight for gestational age increased sharply as maternal alcohol intake increased (51). In comparison to nondrinkers, mean birth weight was reduced 14 g in those drinking less than one drink/day and 165 g in those drinking three to five drinks/day. The risk for growth retardation was markedly increased by the ingestion of one to two drinks each day. Other investigators discovered that women drinking more than 100 g of absolute alcohol/week at the time of conception had an increased risk of delivering a growth-retarded infant (52). The risk was twice that of women ingesting less than 50 g/week. Of special significance, the risk for growth retardation was not reduced if drinking was reduced later in pregnancy. However, a 1983 report found that if heavy drinkers reduced their consumption in midpregnancy, growth impairment was also reduced, although an increased incidence of congenital defects was still evident (53). Significantly smaller head circumferences have been measured in offspring of mothers who drank more than an average of 20 ml of alcohol/day compared to nondrinkers (54). In this same study, the incidence of major congenital anomalies in drinkers and nondrinkers was 1.2% vs none (54). These authors concluded that there was no safe level of alcohol consumption in pregnancy.

Alcohol ingestion has been shown to abolish fetal breathing (55). Eleven women, at 37–40 weeks' gestation, were given 0.25 g/kg of ethanol. Within 30 minutes, fetal breathing movements were almost abolished and remained so for 3 hours. No effect on gross fetal body movements or fetal heart rate was observed. However, a 1986 report described four women admitted to a hospital because of marked alcohol intoxication (56). In each case, fetal heart rate tracings revealed no or poor variability and no reactivity to fetal movements or external stimuli. Because of suspected fetal distress, an emergency cesarean section was performed in one patient, but no signs of hypoxia were present in the healthy infant. In the remaining three women, normalization of the fetal heart rate patterns occurred within 11–14 hours when the mothers became sober.

A study of the relationship between maternal alcohol ingestion and the risk of respiratory distress syndrome (RDS) in their infants was published in 1987 (57). Of the 531 infants in the study, 134 were delivered at a gestational age of 28–36 weeks. The 134 mothers of these preterm infants were classified by the amount of alcohol they consumed per occasion into abstainers ($N = 58$) (none), occasional ($N = 21$) (less than 15 ml), social ($N = 15$) (15–30 ml), binge ($N = 12$) (greater than 75 ml), and alcoholic ($N = 28$). The incidence of RDS in the infants from the five groups was 44.8%, 38.1%, 26.7%, 16.7%, and 21.4%, respectively. The difference between abstainers and those frankly alcoholic was significant ($p < 0.05$). Moreover, assuming equal intervals of alcohol intake among the five groups, the decrease in incidence of RDS with increasing alcohol intake was significant ($p <$

0.02). Adjustment of the data for smoking, gestational age, birth weight, Apgar score, and sex of the infant did not change the findings. The authors concluded that chronic alcohol ingestion may have enhanced fetal lung maturation (57).

Neonatal alcohol withdrawal has been demonstrated in offspring of mothers ingesting a mean of 21 ounces (630 ml) of alcohol/week during pregnancy (58). In comparison to infants exposed to an equivalent amount of ethanol only during early gestation or to infants whose mothers never drank, the heavily exposed infants had significantly more withdrawal symptoms. No differences were found between the infants exposed only during early gestation and those never exposed. Electroencephalogram (EEG) testing of infants at 4–6 weeks of age indicated that the irritability and tremors may be due to a specific effect of ethanol on the fetal brain and not to withdrawal or prematurity (59). Persistent EEG hypersynchrony was observed in those infants delivered from mothers who drank more than 60 ml of alcohol/day during pregnancy. The EEG findings were found in the absence of dysmorphology and as a result, the authors suggested that this symptom should be added to the definition of the FAS (59).

Combined fetal alcohol and hydantoin syndromes have been described in several reports (60–63). The infants exhibited numerous similar features from exposure to alcohol and phenytoin. The possibility that the agents are also carcinogenic *in utero* has been suggested by the finding of ganglioneuroblastoma in a 35-month-old boy and Hodgkin's disease in a 45-month-old girl, both with the combined syndromes (see also Phenytoin) (61–63). Adrenal carcinoma in a 13-year-old girl with FAS has also been reported (64). These findings may be fortuitous, but long-term follow-up of children with the FAS is needed.

An unusual cause of FAS was described in 1981 (65). A woman consumed, throughout pregnancy, 480–840 ml/day of an over-the-counter cough preparation. Since the cough syrup contained 9.5% alcohol, the woman was ingesting 45.6–79.8 ml of ethanol/day. The infant had the typical facial features of the FAS, plus an umbilical hernia and hypoplastic labia. Irritability, tremors, and hypertonicity were also evident.

In summary, ethanol is a teratogen and its use during pregnancy, especially during the first 2 months after conception, is associated with significant risk to the fetus and newborn. Heavy maternal use is related to a spectrum of defects collectively termed the fetal alcohol syndrome. Even moderate use may be related to spontaneous abortions and to developmental and behavioral dysfunction in the infant. A safe level of maternal alcohol consumption has not been established (7, 8, 66). Based on practical considerations, the American Council on Science and Health recommends that pregnant women limit their alcohol consumption to no more than two drinks daily (1 ounce or 30 ml of absolute alcohol) (8). However, the safest course for women who are pregnant, or who are planning to become pregnant, is abstinence (7, 66).

[*Risk Factor X if used in large amounts or for prolonged periods.]

Breast Feeding Summary

Although alcohol passes freely into breast milk, reaching concentrations approximating maternal serum levels, the effect on the infant has been considered insignificant except in rare cases or at very high concentrations (67). Recent research on the effects of chronic exposure of the nursing infant to alcohol in breast milk, however, should cause a reassessment of this position.

Chronic exposure to alcohol in breast milk was found to have an adverse effect on psychomotor development of breast-feeding infants in a 1989 report (68). In this study, "breast-fed" was defined as a breast-feeding child who received no more than 473 ml (16 ounces) of its nourishment in the form of supplemental feedings/day. Statistical methods were used to control for alcohol exposure during gestation. Of the 400 infants studied, 153 were breast fed by mothers who were classified as "heavier" drinkers (i.e., an average daily consumption of one ounce of ethanol or about two drinks, or binge drinkers who consumed 2.5 ounces or more of ethanol on a single occasion). The population sampled was primarily white, well-educated, middle-class women who belonged to a health maintenance organization. The investigators measured the mental and psychomotor development of the infants at 1 year of age using the Bayley Scales of Infant Development. Mental development was unrelated to maternal drinking during breast feeding. In contrast, psychomotor development was adversely affected in a dose-response relation (p for linear trend, 0.006). The mean Psychomotor Development Index (PDI) of infants of mothers who had at least one drink daily was 98, compared to 103 for infants of mothers consuming less alcohol ($p < 0.01$). The decrease in PDI was even greater if only those women not supplementing breast feeding were considered. Regression analysis predicted that the PDI of totally breast-fed infants of mothers who consumed an average of two drinks daily would decrease by 7.5 points. These associations persisted even after more than 100 potentially confounding variables, including maternal tobacco, marijuana, and heavy caffeine exposures, were controlled for during pregnancy and the first 3 months after delivery. The authors cautioned that their findings were only suggestive and should not be extrapolated to other patient populations because of the relative homogeneity of their sample (68). Although the conclusions of this study have been criticized and defended (69, 70), judgment on the risks to the nursing infant from alcohol in milk must be withheld until additional research has been completed.

The toxic metabolite of ethanol, acetaldehyde, apparently does not pass into milk even though considerable levels can be measured in the mother's blood (71). One report calculated the amount of alcohol received in a single feeding from a mother with a blood concentration of 100 mg/dl (equivalent to a heavy, habitual drinker) as 164 mg, an insignificant amount (72). Maternal blood alcohol levels have to reach 300 mg/dl before mild sedation might be seen in the baby. However, a 1937 report described a case of alcohol poisoning in an 8-day-old breast-fed infant whose mother drank an entire bottle (750 ml) of port wine (73). Symptoms in the child included deep sleep, no response to painful stimuli, abnormal reflexes, and weakly reactive pupils. Alcohol was detected in the infant's blood. The child made an apparently uneventful recovery.

Potentiation of severe hypoprothrombic bleeding, a pseudo-Cushing syndrome, and an effect on the milk-ejecting reflex have been reported in nursing infants of alcoholic mothers (74–76). The American Academy of Pediatrics considers maternal ethanol use to be compatible with breast feeding, although it is recognized that adverse effects may occur (77).

References

1. Shaywitz BA. Fetal alcohol syndrome: an ancient problem rediscovered. Drug Ther 1978;8:95–108.
2. Lemoine P, Harroussean H, Borteyrn JP. Les enfants de parents alcooliques: anomalies observees. A propos de 127 cas. Quest Med 1968;25:477–82.
3. Ulleland CN. The offspring of alcoholic mothers. Ann NY Acad Sci 1972;197:167–9.

4. Jones KL, Smith DW, Ulleland CN, Streissguth AP. Pattern of malformation in offspring of chronic alcoholic mothers. Lancet 1973;1:1267–71.

5. Jones KL, Smith DW. Recognition of the fetal alcohol syndrome in early infancy. Lancet 1973;2:999–1001.

6. Abel EL. *Fetal Alcohol Syndrome, Vol 1: An Annotated and Comprehensive Bibliography*. Boca Raton, Fl:CRC Press, 1981. As cited in Alcohol and the fetus — is zero the only option? Lancet 1983;1:682–3.

7. Council on Scientific Affairs, American Medical Association. Fetal effects of maternal alcohol use. JAMA 1983;249:2517–21.

8. Alcohol use during pregnancy. A report by the American Council on Science and Health. As reprinted in Nutrition Today 1982;17:29–32.

9. Lipson AH, Walsh DA, Webster WS. Fetal alcohol syndrome. A great paediatric imitator. Med J Aust 1983;1:266–9.

10. Little BB, Snell LM, Gilstrap LC III, Gant NF, Rosenfeld CR. Alcohol abuse during pregnancy: changes in frequency in a large urban hospital. Obstet Gynecol 1989;74:547–50.

11. Scheiner AP, Donovan CM, Burtoshesky LE. Fetal alcohol syndrome in child whose parents had stopped drinking. Lancet 1979;1:1077–8.

12. Scheiner AP. Fetal alcohol syndrome in a child whose parents had stopped drinking. Lancet 1979;2:858.

13. Smith DW, Graham JM Jr. Fetal alcohol syndrome in child whose parents had stopped drinking. Lancet 1979;2:527.

14. Little RE, Sing CF. Association of father's drinking and infant's birth weight. N Engl J Med 1986;314:1644–5.

15. Little RE, Sing CF. Father's drinking and infant birth weight; report of an association. Teratology 1987;36:59–65.

16. Rubin DH, Leventhal JM, Krasilnikoff PA, Weile B, Berget A. Fathers' drinking (and smoking) and infants' birth weight. N Engl J Med 1986;315:1551.

17. Veghelyi PV. Fetal abnormality and maternal ethanol metabolism. Lancet 1983;2:53–4.

18. Ryle PR, Thomson AD. Acetaldehyde and the fetal alcohol syndrome. Lancet 1983;2:219–20.

19. Kennedy LA. The pathogenesis of brain abnormalities in the fetal alcohol syndrome: an integrating hypothesis. Teratology 1984;29:363–8.

20. Shepard TH. *Catalog of Teratogenic Agents*. 6th ed. Baltimore:The Johns Hopkins University Press, 1989:54.

21. Damjanov I. Metronidazole and alcohol in pregnancy. JAMA 1986;256:472.

22. FDA Drug Bulletin, *Fetal Alcohol Syndrome*, vol. 7. National Institute on Alcohol Abuse and Alcoholism, 1977:4.

23. Sandor GGS, Smith DF, MacLeod PM. Cardiac malformations in the fetal alcohol syndrome. J Pediatr 1981;98:771–3.

24. Habbick BF, Casey R, Zaleski WA, Murphy F. Liver abnormalities in three patients with fetal alcohol syndrome. Lancet 1979;1:580–1.

25. Streissguth AP, Clarren SK, Jones KL. Natural history of the fetal alcohol syndrome: a 10-year follow-up of eleven patients. Lancet 1985;2:85–91.

26. Khan A, Bader JL, Hoy GR, Sinks LF. Hepatoblastoma in child with fetal alcohol syndrome. Lancet 1979;1:1403–4.

27. Harlap S, Shiono PH. Alcohol, smoking and incidence of spontaneous abortions in the first and second trimester. Lancet 1980;2:173–6.

28. Kline J, Shrout P, Stein Z, Susser M, Warburton D. Drinking during pregnancy and spontaneous abortion. Lancet 1980;2:176–80.

29. Hanson JW, Jones KL, Smith DW. Fetal alcohol syndrome experience with 41 patients. JAMA 1976;235:1458–60.

30. Goetzman BW, Kagan J, Blankenship WJ. Expansion of the fetal alcohol syndrome. Clin Res 1975;23:100A.

31. DeBeukelaer MM, Randall CL, Stroud DR. Renal anomalies in the fetal alcohol syndrome. J Pediatr 1977;91:759–60.

32. Qazi Q, Masakawa A, Milman D, McGann B, Chua A, Haller J. Renal anomalies in fetal alcohol syndrome. Pediatrics 1979;63:886–9.

33. Steeg CN, Woolf P. Cardiovascular malformations in the fetal alcohol syndrome. Am Heart J 1979;98:636–7.

34. Halliday HL, Reid MM, McClure G. Results of heavy drinking in pregnancy. Br J Obstet Gynaecol 1982;89:892–5.

35. Beattie JO, Day RE, Cockburn F, Garg RA. Alcohol and the fetus in the west of Scotland. Br Med J 1983;287:17–20.

36. Tsukahara M, Kajii T. Severe skeletal dysplasias following intrauterine exposure to ethanol. Teratology 1988;37:79–80.

37. Charness ME, Simon RP, Greenberg DA. Ethanol and the nervous system. N Engl J Med 1989;321:442–54.

38. Golden NL, Sokol RJ, Kuhnert BR, Bottoms S. Maternal alcohol use and infant development. Pediatrics 1982;70:931–4.

39. Ernhart CB, Sokol RJ, Martier S, Moron P, Nadler D, Ager JW, Wolf A. Alcohol teratogenicity in the human: a detailed assessment of specificity, critical period, and threshold. Am J Obstet Gynecol 1987;156:33–9.

40. Day NL, Jasperse D, Richardson G, Robles N, Sambamoorthi U, Taylor P, Scher M, Stoffer D, Cornelius M. Prenatal exposure to alcohol: effect on infant growth and morphologic characteristics. Pediatrics 1989;84:536–41.

41. Mills JL, Graubard BI. Is moderate drinking during pregnancy associated with an increased risk for malformations? Pediatrics 1987;80:309–14.

42. Halmesmaki E, Valimaki M, Roine R, Ylikahri R, Ylikorkala O. Maternal and paternal alcohol consumption and miscarriage. Br J Obstet Gynaecol 1989;96:188–91.

43. Halmesmaki E, Ylikorkala O. A retrospective study on the safety of prenatal ethanol treatment. Obstet Gynecol 1988;72:545–9.

44. Sisenwin FE, Tejani NA, Boxer HS, DiGiuseppe R. Effects of maternal ethanol infusion during pregnancy on the growth and development of children at four to seven years of age. Am J Obstet Gynecol 1983;147:52–6.

45. Friedman JM. Can maternal alcohol ingestion cause neural tube defects? J Pediatr 1982;101:232–4.

46. Castro-Gago M, Rodriguez-Cervilla J, Ugarte J, Novo I, Pombo M. Maternal alcohol ingestion and neural tube defects. J Pediatr 1984;104:796–7.

47. Halmesmaki E, Raivio K, Ylikorkala O. A possible association between maternal drinking and fetal clubfoot. N Engl J Med 1985;312:790.

48. Sarda P, Bard H. Gastroschisis in a case of dizygotic twins: the possible role of maternal alcohol consumption. Pediatrics 1984;74:94–6.

49. Ammann AJ, Wara DW, Cowan MJ, Barrett DJ, Stiehm ER. The DiGeorge syndrome and the fetal alcohol syndrome. Am J Dis Child 1982;136:906–8.

50. Gardner LI, Mitter N, Coplan J, Kalinowski DP, Sanders KJ. Isochromosome 9q in an infant exposed to ethanol prenatally. N Engl J Med 1985;312:1521.

51. Mills JL, Graubard BI, Harley EE, Rhoads GG, Berendes HW. Maternal alcohol consumption and birth weight. How much drinking during pregnancy is safe? JAMA 1984;252:1875–9.

52. Wright JT, Waterson EJ, Barrison IG, Toplis PJ, Lewis IG, Gordon MG, MacRae KD, Morris NF, Murray-Lyon IM. Alcohol consumption, pregnancy, and low birthweight. Lancet 1983;1:663–5.

53. Rosett HL, Weiner L, Lee A, Zuckerman B, Dooling E, Oppenheimer E. Patterns of alcohol consumption and fetal development. Obstet Gynecol 1983;61:539–46.

54. Davis PJM, Partridge JW, Storrs CN. Alcohol consumption in pregnancy. How much is safe? Arch Dis Child 1982;57:940–3.

55. McLeod W, Brien J, Loomis C, Carmichael L, Probert C, Patrick J. Effect of maternal ethanol ingestion on fetal breathing movements, gross body movements, and heart rate at 37 to 40 weeks' gestational age. Am J Obstet Gynecol 1983;145:251–7.

56. Halmesmaki E, Ylikorkala O. The effect of maternal ethanol intoxication on fetal cardiotocography: a report of four cases. Br J Obstet Gynaecol 1986;93:203–5.

57. Ioffe S, Chernick V. Maternal alcohol ingestion and the incidence of respiratory distress syndrome. Am J Obstet Gynecol 1987;156:1231–5.

58. Coles CD, Smith IE, Fernhoff PM, Falek A. Neonatal ethanol withdrawal: characteristics in clinically normal, nondysmorphic neonates. J Pediatr 1984;105:445–51.

59. Ioffe S, Childiaeva R, Chernick V. Prolonged effects of maternal alcohol ingestion on the neonatal electroencephalogram. Pediatrics 1984;74:330–5.

60. Wilker R, Nathenson G. Combined fetal alcohol and hydantoin syndromes. Clin Pediatr 1982;21:331–4.

61. Seeler RA, Israel JN, Royal JE, Kaye CI, Rao S, Abulaban M. Ganglioneuroblastoma and fetal hydantoin-alcohol syndromes. Pediatrics 1979;63:524–7.
62. Ramilo J, Harris VJ. Neuroblastoma in a child with the hydantoin and fetal alcohol syndrome. The radiographic features. Br J Radiol 1979;52:993–5.
63. Bostrom B, Nesbit ME Jr. Hodgkin disease in a child with fetal alcohol-hydantoin syndrome. J Pediatr 1983;103:760–2.
64. Hornstein L, Crowe C, Gruppo R. Adrenal carcinoma in child with history of fetal alcohol syndrome. Lancet 1977;2:1292–3.
65. Chasnoff IJ, Diggs G, Schnoll SH. Fetal alcohol effects and maternal cough syrup abuse. Am J Dis Child 1981;135:968.
66. Anonymous. Alcohol and the fetus - is zero the only option? Lancet 1983;1:682–3.
67. Anonymous. Update: drugs in breast milk. Med Lett Drugs Ther 1979;21:21.
68. Little RE, Anderson KW, Ervin CH, Worthington-Roberts B, Clarren SK. Maternal alcohol use during breast-feeding and infant mental and motor development at one year. N Engl J Med 1989;321:425–30.
69. Lindmark B. Maternal use of alcohol and breast-fed infants. N Engl J Med 1990;322:338–9.
70. Little RE. Maternal use of alcohol and breast-fed infants. N Engl J Med 1990;322:339.
71. Kesaniemi YA. Ethanol and acetaldehyde in the milk and peripheral blood of lactating women after ethanol administration. J Obstet Gynaecol Br Commonw 1974;81:84–6.
72. Wilson JT, Brown RD, Cherek DR, Dailey JW, Hilman B, Jobe PC, Manno BR, Manno JE, Redetzki HM, Stewart JJ. Drug excretion in human breast milk. Principles, pharmacokinetics and projected consequences. Clin Pharmacol 1980;5:1–66.
73. Bisdom CJW. Alcohol and nicotine poisoning in nurslings. Maandschrift voor Kindergeneeskunde, Leyden 1937;6:332. As cited in JAMA 1937;109:178.
74. Hoh TK. Severe hypoprothrombinaemic bleeding in the breast-fed young infant. Singapore Med J 1969;10:43–9.
75. Binkiewicz A, Robinson MJ, Senior B. Pseudo-Cushing syndrome caused by alcohol in breast milk. J Pediatr 1978;93:965.
76. Cobo E. Effect of different doses of ethanol on the milk-ejecting reflex in lactating women. Am J Obstet Gynecol 1973;115:817–21.
77. Committee on Drugs, American Academy of Pediatrics. Transfer of drugs and other chemicals into human milk. Pediatrics 1989;84:924–36.

Name: **ETHCHLORVYNOL**

Class: **Hypnotic**   Risk Factor: **C$_M$**

Fetal Risk Summary

No reports linking the use of ethchlorvynol with congenital defects have been located. The Collaborative Perinatal Project reported 68 patients with 1st trimester exposure to miscellaneous tranquilizers and nonbarbiturate sedatives, 12 of which had been exposed to ethchlorvynol (1). For the group as a whole, six infants with malformations occurred, but details on individual exposures were not given. Animal data indicate that rapid equilibrium occurs between maternal and fetal blood with maximum fetal blood levels measured within 2 hours of maternal ingestion (2). The authors concluded that following maternal ingestion of a toxic or lethal dose, delivery should be accomplished before equilibrium occurs. Neonatal withdrawal symptoms, consisting of mild hypotonia, poor suck, absent rooting, poor grasp, and delayed-onset jitteriness, have been reported (B.H. Rumack, P.A. Walravens, personal communication, Dept. of Pediatrics, Univ. of Colorado Medical Center, 1981). The mother had been taking 500 mg daily during the 3rd trimester.

Breast Feeding Summary

No data are available.

References

1. Heinonen OP, Slone D, Shapiro S. *Birth Defects and Drugs in Pregnancy*. Littleton:Publishing Sciences Group, 1977:336–7.
2. Hume AS, Williams JM, Douglas BH. Disposition of ethchlorvynol in maternal blood, fetal blood, amniotic fluid, and chorionic fluid. J Reprod Med 1971;6:54–6.

Name: **ETHINAMATE**

Class: **Hypnotic**   Risk Factor: **C$_M$**

Fetal Risk Summary

Ethinamate is a hypnotic used for insomnia. Animal reproduction studies have not been conducted with this drug. The Collaborative Perinatal Project monitored 50,282 mother-child pairs, 68 of which had 1st trimester exposure to miscellaneous tranquilizers and nonbarbiturate sedatives (1). Three of these exposures were to ethinamate. From the total group of 68, six infants with malformations occurred but details on individual exposures were not given.

Breast Feeding Summary

No data are available.

Reference

1. Heinonen OP, Slone D, Shapiro S. *Birth Defects and Drugs in Pregnancy*. Littleton:Publishing Sciences Group, 1977:336.

Name: **ETHINYL ESTRADIOL**

Class: **Estrogenic Hormone**   Risk Factor: **X**

Fetal Risk Summary

Ethinyl estradiol is used frequently in combination with progestins for oral contraception (see Oral Contraceptives). The Collaborative Perinatal Project monitored 89 mother-child pairs who were exposed to ethinyl estradiol during the 1st trimester (1, pp. 389, 391). An increased risk for malformations was found, although identification of the malformations was not provided. Estrogenic agents as a group were monitored in 614 mother-child pairs. An increase in the expected frequency of cardiovascular defects, eye and ear anomalies, and Down's syndrome was reported (1, p. 395). Reevaluation of these data in terms of timing of exposure, vaginal bleeding in early pregnancy, and previous maternal obstetric history, however, failed to support an association between estrogens and cardiac malformations (2). An earlier study also failed to find any relationship with nongenital malformations (3). In a smaller study, 12 mothers were exposed to ethinyl estradiol during the 1st trimester (4). No fetal abnormalities were observed. Ethinyl estradiol has also been used as a contraceptive when given within 72 hours of unprotected midcycle coitus (5). Use of estrogenic hormones during pregnancy is contraindicated.

Breast Feeding Summary

Estrogens are frequently used for suppression of postpartum lactation (6, 7). Very small amounts are excreted in milk (7). When used in oral contraceptives, ethinyl estradiol has been associated with decreased milk production and decreased composition of nitrogen and protein content in human milk (8). Although the magnitude of these changes is low, the differences in milk production and composition may be of nutritional importance to nursing infants of malnourished mothers. If breast feeding is desired, the lowest dose of oral contraceptives should be chosen. Monitoring of infant weight gain and the possible need for nutritional supplementation should be considered (see Oral Contraceptives).

References

1. Heinonen OP, Slone D, Shapiro S. *Birth Defects and Drugs in Pregnancy*. Littleton:Publishing Sciences Group, 1977.
2. Wiseman RA, Dodds-Smith IC. Cardiovascular birth defects and antenatal exposure to female sex hormones: a reevaluation of some base data. Teratology 1984;30:359–70.
3. Wilson JG, Brent RL. Are female sex hormones teratogenic? Am J Obstet Gynecol 1981;141:567–80.
4. Hagler S, Schultz A, Hankin H, Kunstadler RH. Fetal effects of steroid therapy during pregnancy. Am J Dis Child 1963;106:586–90.
5. Dixon GW, Schlesselman JJ, Ory HW, Blye RP. Ethinyl estradiol and conjugated estrogens as postcoital contraceptives. JAMA 1980;244:1336–9.
6. Gilman AG, Goodman LS, Gilman A, eds. *The Pharmacological Basis of Therapeutics*, ed 6. New York:MacMillan Publishing Co, 1980:1431.
7. Klinger G, Claussen C, Schroder S. Excretion of ethinyloestradiol sulfonate in the human milk. Zentralbl Gynaekol 1981;103:91–5.
8. Lonnerdal B, Forsum E, Hambraeus L. Effect of oral contraceptives on composition and volume of breast milk. Am J Clin Nutr 1980;33:816–24.

Name: **ETHIODIZED OIL**

Class: **Diagnostic**   Risk Factor: **D**

Fetal Risk Summary

Ethiodized oil contains a high concentration of organically bound iodine. Use of this agent close to term has been associated with neonatal hypothyroidism (see Diatrizoate).

Breast Feeding Summary

See Potassium Iodide.

Name: **ETHISTERONE**

Class: **Progestogenic Hormone**   Risk Factor: **D**

Fetal Risk Summary

The Food and Drug Administration mandated deletion of pregnancy-related indications for all progestins because of a possible association with congenital anomalies. No reports linking the use of ethisterone alone with congenital defects have been located. The Collaborative Perinatal Project monitored 866 mother-child pairs with 1st trimester exposure to progestational agents (including two with exposure to ethisterone) (1, pp. 389, 391). An increase in the expected frequency of cardiovascular defects and hypospadias was observed for the progestational agents as a group, but not for ethisterone as a single agent (1, p. 394). In a subsequent report from the Collaborative Study, a single case of tricuspid atresia and ventricular septal defect was identified with 3rd trimester exposure to ethisterone and ethinyl estradiol (2). Reevaluation of these data in terms of timing of exposure, vaginal bleeding in early pregnancy, and previous maternal obstetric history, however, failed to support an association between female sex hormones and cardiac malformations (3). An earlier study also failed to find any relationship with nongenital malformations (4). (See also Hydroxyprogesterone and Medroxyprogesterone)

Breast Feeding Summary

See Oral Contraceptives.

References

1. Heinonen OP, Slone D, Shapiro S. *Birth Defects and Drugs in Pregnancy*. Littleton:Publishing Sciences Group, 1977.
2. Heinonen OP, Slone D, Monson RR, Hook EB, Shapiro S. Cardiovascular birth defects and antenatal exposure to female sex hormones. N Engl J Med 1977;296:67–70.
3. Wiseman RA, Dodds-Smith IC. Cardiovascular birth defects and antenatal exposure to female sex hormones: a reevaluation of some base data. Teratology 1984;30:359–70.
4. Wilson JG, Brent RL. Are female sex hormones teratogenic? Am J Obstet Gynecol 1981;141:567–80.

Name: **ETHOHEPTAZINE**

Class: **Analgesic**   Risk Factor: **C**

Fetal Risk Summary

The Collaborative Perinatal Project monitored 50,282 mother-child pairs, 60 of which had 1st trimester exposure to ethoheptazine (1, pp. 287–295). For use anytime during pregnancy, 300 exposures were recorded (1, p. 434). Although the numbers were small, a possible relationship may exist between this drug and major or minor malformations. Further, a possible association with individual defects was observed (1, p. 485). The statistical significance of these associations is unknown, and independent confirmation is required.

Congenital dislocation of the hip (three cases)

Umbilical hernia (three cases)
Inguinal hernia (eight cases)

Breast Feeding Summary

No data are available.

Reference

1. Heinonen OP, Slone D, Shapiro S. *Birth Defects and Drugs in Pregnancy*. Littleton:Publishing Sciences Group, 1977.

Name: **ETHOPROPAZINE**

Class: **Parasympatholytic (Anticholinergic)**   Risk Factor: **C**

Fetal Risk Summary

Ethopropazine is a phenothiazine compound with anticholinergic activity that is used in the treatment of parkinsonism (see also Atropine and Promethazine). No reports of its use in pregnancy have been located.

Breast Feeding Summary

No data are available (see also Atropine and Promethazine).

Name: **ETHOSUXIMIDE**

Class: **Anticonvulsant**   Risk Factor: **C**

Fetal Risk Summary

Ethosuximide is a succinimide anticonvulsant used in the treatment of petit mal epilepsy. The use of ethosuximide has been reported in 163 pregnancies (1–11). Due to the lack of specific information on the observed malformations, multiple drug therapies, and differences in study methodology, conclusions linking the use of ethosuximide with congenital defects are difficult. Spontaneous hemorrhage in the neonate following *in utero* exposure to ethosuximide has been reported (see also Phenytoin and Phenobarbital) (6). Abnormalities identified with ethosuximide use in 10 pregnancies include:

Patent ductus arteriosus (eight cases)
Cleft lip and/or palate (seven cases)
Mongoloid facies, short neck, altered palmar crease and an accessory nipple (one case)
Hydrocephalus (one case)

Ethosuximide has a much lower teratogenic potential than the oxazolidinedione class of anticonvulsants (see also Trimethadione and Paramethadione) (11, 12).

The succinimide anticonvulsants should be considered the anticonvulsants of choice for the treatment of petit mal epilepsy during the 1st trimester.

Breast Feeding Summary

Ethosuximide freely enters the breast milk in concentrations similar to the maternal serum (13–15). Two reports measured similar milk:plasma ratios of 1.0 and 0.78 (13, 14). No adverse effects on the nursing infant have been reported. The American Academy of Pediatrics considers ethosuximide to be compatible with breast feeding (16).

References

1. Speidel BD, Meadow SR. Maternal epilepsy and abnormalities of the fetus and newborn. Lancet 1972;2:839–43.
2. Fedrick J. Epilepsy and pregnancy: a report from the Oxford Record Linkage Study. Br Med J 1973;2:442–8.
3. Lowe CR. Congenital malformations among infants born to epileptic women. Lancet 1973; 1:9–10.
4. Starreveld-Zimmerman AAE, van der Kolk WJ, Meinardi H, Elshve J. Are anticonvulsants teratogenic? Lancet 1973;2:48–9.
5. Kuenssberg EV, Knox JDE. Teratogenic effect of anticonvulsants. Lancet 1973;2:198.
6. Speidel BD, Meadow SR. Epilepsy, anticonvulsants and congenital malformations. Drugs 1974;8:354–65.
7. Janz D. The teratogenic risk of antiepileptic drugs. Epilepsia 1975;16:159–69.
8. Nakane Y, Okuma T, Takahashi R, et al. Multi-institutional study on the teratogenicity and fetal toxicity of antiepileptic drugs: a report of a collaborative study group in Japan. Epilepsia 1980;21:663–80.
9. Heinonen OP, Slone D, Shapiro S. Birth Defects and Drugs in Pregnancy. Littleton:Publishing Sciences Group, 1977:358–9.
10. Dansky L, Andermann E, Andermann F. Major congenital malformations on the offspring of epileptic patients: genetic and environment risk factors. In Epilepsy, Pregnancy and the Child. Proceedings of a workshop held in Berlin, September 1980. New York:Raven Press, 1981.
11. Fabro S, Brown NA. Teratogenic potential of anticonvulsants. N Engl J Med 1979;300:1280–1.
12. The National Institute of Health. Anticonvulsants found to have teratogenic potential. JAMA 1981;241:36.
13. Koup JR, Rose JQ, Cohen ME. Ethosuximide pharmacokinetics in pregnant patient and her newborn. Epilepsia 1978;19:535.
14. Kaneko S, Sato T, Suzuki K. The levels of anticonvulsants in breast milk. Br J Clin Pharmacol 1979;7:624–6.
15. Horning MG, Stillwell WG, Nowlin J, Lertratanangkoon K, Stillwill RN, Hill RM. Identification and quantification of drugs and drug metabolites in human breast milk using GC-MS-COM methods. Mod Probl Paediatr 1975;15:73–9.
16. Committee on Drugs, American Academy of Pediatrics. The transfer of drugs and other chemicals into human breast milk. Pediatrics 1983;72:375–83.

Name: ETHOTOIN

Class: **Anticonvulsant**   Risk Factor: **D**

Fetal Risk Summary

Ethotoin is a low-potency hydantoin anticonvulsant (1). The fetal hydantoin syndrome has been associated with the use of the more potent phenytoin (see Phenytoin). Only six reports describing the use of ethotoin during the 1st trimester have been located (2–4). Congenital malformations observed in two of these cases included cleft lip/palate and patent ductus arteriosus (3, 4). No cause and effect relationship was established. Although the toxicity of ethotoin appears to be lower than the more potent phenytoin, the occurrence of congenital defects in two fetuses exposed to ethotoin suggests that a teratogenic potential may exist.

Breast Feeding Summary

No data are available.

References

1. Schmidt RP, Wilder BJ. Epilepsy. In *Contemporary Neurology Services*, vol. 2. Philadelphia:FA Davis Co, 1968:154.
2. Heinonen OP, Slone D, Shapiro S. *Birth Defects and Drugs in Pregnancy*. Littleton:Publishing Sciences Group, 1977:358–9.
3. Zablen M, Brand N. Cleft lip and palate with the anticonvulsant ethantoin. N Engl J Med 1978;298:285.
4. Nakane Y, Okuma T, Takahashi R, et al. Multi-institutional study on the teratogenicity and fetal toxicity of antiepileptic drugs: a report of a collaborative study group in Japan. Epilepsia 1980;21:663–80.

Name: **ETHYL BISCOUMACETATE**

Class: **Anticoagulant**   Risk Factor: **D**

Fetal Risk Summary

See Coumarin Derivatives.

Breast Feeding Summary

See Coumarin Derivatives.

Name: **ETHYNODIOL**

Class: **Progestogenic Hormone**   Risk Factor: **D**

Fetal Risk Summary

Ethynodiol is used primarily in oral contraceptive products (see Oral Contraceptives).

Breast Feeding Summary

See Oral Contraceptives.

Name: **ETRETINATE**

Class: **Vitamin**   Risk Factor: **X_M**

Fetal Risk Summary

Etretinate, an orally active synthetic retinoid and vitamin A derivative, is used for the treatment of severe recalcitrant psoriasis. It is contraindicated in pregnant women and in those likely to become pregnant. Following oral administration, etretinate is stored in subcutaneous fat and is slowly released over a prolonged interval (1, 2). In some patients after chronic therapy, detectable serum drug levels may occur up to 2.9 years after treatment has been stopped (2, 3). Due to this variable excretion pattern, the exact length of time that pregnancy must be avoided after discontinuing treatment is unknown (2, 3).

Like other retinoids (see also Isotretinoin and Vitamin A), etretinate is a potent animal teratogen (4). Data accumulated since release of this drug now indicate that it must be considered a human teratogen as well (1–3, 5, 6).

As of June, 1986, a total of 51 pregnancies had occurred during treatment with etretinate (1, 7, 8). Of these pregnancies, 23 were still ongoing at the time of the reports and were unable to be evaluated (1). In the remaining 28 cases, 17 resulted in normal infants and three were normal fetuses after induced abortion. Skeletal anomalies were evident in eight cases: three liveborns, one stillbirth at 5 months, and four induced abortions. In addition, marked cerebral abnormalities, including meningomyeloceles, were observed in the stillborn and in three of the aborted fetuses.

A 1988 correspondence listed 22 documented etretinate exposures during pregnancy in West Germany as of September, 1988 (9). The outcomes of these pregnancies were six induced abortions (no anomalies observed), four spontaneous abortions (no anomalies observed), six normal infants, and six infants with malformations (9).

Fifty-three pregnancies are known to have occurred following discontinuance of etretinate therapy (1, 10). Of the 38 evaluable cases, two malformed infants were observed. In one case, a 22-year-old woman, treated intermittently over 5 years, became pregnant 4 months after etretinate therapy had been stopped (1, 11, 12). Serum concentrations of etretinate and the metabolite, etretin, were 7 ng/ml and 8 ng/ml, respectively, during the 8th week of gestation (6 months after the last dose). Following induced abortion at 10 weeks' gestation, the fetus was found to have unilateral skeletal defects of the lower limb consisting of a rudimentary left leg with one toe, missing tibia and fibula, and a hypoplastic femur (11, 12). Evaluation of the face, skull, and brain was not possible. The defect was attributed to etretinate.

The second case also involved a 22-year-old woman who conceived 51 weeks after her last dose of etretinate (10). Other than the use of metoclopramide at 8 weeks' gestation for nausea and vomiting, no other drug history was mentioned. A growth-retarded (2850 g; 46 cm long, 3rd percentile) female infant was delivered by cesarean section at 38 weeks' gestation. Multiple congenital anomalies were noted involving the central nervous system, head, face, and heart, which included tetralogy of Fallot, microcephaly, hair whorls, small mandible, asymmetrical nares, protruding ears with malformed antihelices, absent lobules, and enlarged, keyhole-shaped entrances to the external ear canals, strabismus, left peripheral facial nerve paresis, and poor head control. Etretinate was detected in the mother's serum 3.5 months after delivery, but the concentration was below the test's lower limit of accuracy (2 ng/ml). No etretinate was detected in the infant's serum. Etretinate was considered responsible for the defects based partially on the presence of the drug in the mother's serum, and the fact that the pattern of malformation was identical to that observed with isotretinoin, another synthetic retinoid. The author also concluded that women treated with etretinate should avoid conception indefinitely (10).

Some of the defects noted in the above infant are also components of the CHARGE (coloboma, heart defects, choanal atresia, retardation, genital [males only], and ear anomalies) association (13), but in a response, the author of the case immediately above noted that such a relationship does not exclude etretinate as the etiology of the defects (14). Others have questioned whether an indefinite recommendation to avoid pregnancy is practical or necessary (15, 16). In West Germany, 2 years of conception avoidance are recommended followed by determination of serum levels of etretinate and its metabolites (16). In six women treated with etretinate from 4–78 months, plasma concentrations of the drug were detected after 12 months in three patients (4, 8, and 8 ng/ml each) and after 18 months in one patient (10 ng/ml) (16). Two women had no measurable etretinate 12 and 14 months after stopping therapy. The metabolites, acitretin and cis-acitretin, were detectable in two women (at 8 and 18 months) and five women (at 8–18 months), respectively.

The range of malformations, as listed by the manufacturer, includes meningomyelocele, meningoencephalocele, multiple synostoses, facial dysmorphia, syndactylies, absence of terminal phalanges, malformations of hip, ankle and forearm, low-set ears, high palate, decreased cranial volume, and alterations of the skull and cervical vertebrae (2).

Pronounced jaundice with elevations of the transaminase enzymes, glutamic-oxaloacetic transaminase and glutamic-pyruvic transaminase, was observed in an otherwise normal male newborn following *in utero* exposure to etretinate (17). The cause of the liver pathology was unknown. No other abnormalities were observed, and the infant was normal at 5 months of age.

One source has suggested that male patients treated with etretinate should avoid fathering children during treatment; if this does occur, ultrasound of the fetus is indicated (18). Although there is no evidence that etretinate adversely affects sperm, and even if it did, that this could result in birth defects, the authors defended their comment as practicing "defensive" medicine (19, 20).

Breast Feeding Summary

It is not known if etretinate is excreted into human milk (2). The closely related retinoid, vitamin A, is excreted (see Vitamin A) and the presence of etretinate in breast milk should be expected. The manufacturer considers use of the drug during lactation to be contraindicated due to the potential for adverse effects (2).

References

1. Orfanos CE, Ehlert R, Gollnick H. The retinoids: a review of their clinical pharmacology and therapeutic use. Drugs 1987;34:459–503.
2. Roche scientific summary. The clinical evaluation of Tegison. Roche Laboratories, Division of Hoffmann-La Roche, Inc, 1986.
3. Anonymous. Etretinate approved. FDA Drug Bull 1986;16:16–7.
4. Kamm JJ. Toxicology, carcinogenicity, and teratogenicity of some orally administered retinoids. J Am Acad Dermatol 1982;6:652–9.
5. Anonymous. Etretinate (Tegison) for skin disease. Drug Ther Bull 1983;21:9–11.
6. Anonymous. Etretinate for psoriasis. Med Lett Drugs Ther 1987;29:9–10.
7. Happle R, Traupe H, Bounameaux Y, Fisch T. Teratogenicity of etretinate in humans. Dtsch Med Wochenschr 1984;109:1476–80.

8. Rosa FW, Wilk AL, Kelsey FO. Teratogen update: vitamin A congeners. Teratology 1986;33:355–64.
9. Hopf G, Mathias B. Teratogenicity of isotretinoin and etretinate. Lancet 1988;2:1143.
10. Lammer EJ. Embryopathy in infant conceived one year after termination of maternal etretinate. Lancet 1988;2:1080–1.
11. Grote W, Harms D, Janig U, Kietzmann H, Ravens U, Schwarze I. Malformation of fetus conceived 4 months after termination of maternal etretinate treatment. Lancet 1985;1:1276.
12. Kietzmann H, Schwarze I, Grote W, Ravens U, Janig U, Harms D. Fetal malformation after maternal etretinate treatment of Darier's disease. Dtsch Med Wochenschr 1986;111:60–2.
13. Blake KD, Wyse RKH. Embryopathy in infant conceived one year after termination of maternal etretinate: a reappraisal. Lancet 1988;2:1254.
14. Lammer E. Etretinate and pregnancy. Lancet 1989;1:109.
15. Greaves MW. Embryopathy in infant conceived one year after termination of maternal etretinate: a reappraisal. Lancet 1988;2:1254.
16. Rinck G, Gollnick H, Orfanos CE. Duration of contraception after etretinate. Lancet 1989;1:845–6.
17. Jager K, Schiller F, Stech P. Congenital ichthyosiforme erythroderma, pregnancy under aromatic retinoid treatment. Hautarzt 1985;36:150–3.
18. Ellis CN, Voorhees JJ. Etretinate therapy. J Am Acad Dermatol 1987;16:267–91.
19. Katz R. Etretinate and paternity. J Am Acad Dermatol 1987;17:509.
20. Ellis CN, Voorhees JJ. Etretinate and paternity. Reply. J Am Acad Dermatol 1987;17:509.

Name: **EVANS BLUE**

Class: **Dye**   Risk Factor: **C**

Fetal Risk Summary

No reports linking the use of Evans blue with congenital defects have been located. The dye is teratogenic in some animal species (1). Evans blue has been injected intra-amniotically for diagnosis of ruptured membranes without apparent effect on the fetus except for temporary staining of the skin (2, 3). The use of Evans blue during pregnancy for plasma volume determinations is routine (4–7). No problems in the fetus or newborn have been attributed to this use.

Breast Feeding Summary

No data are available.

References

1. Wilson JG. Teratogenic activity of several azo dyes chemically related to trypan blue. Anat Rec 1955;123:313–34.
2. Atley RD, Sutherst JR. Premature rupture of the fetal membranes confirmed by intraamniotic injection of dye (Evans blue T-1824). Am J Obstet Gynecol 1970;108:993–4.
3. Morrison L, Wiseman HJ. Intra-amniotic injection of Evans blue dye. Am J Obstet Gynecol 1972;113:1147.
4. Quinlivan WLG, Brock JA, Sullivan H. Blood volume changes and blood loss associated with labor. I. Correlation of changes in blood volume measured by I^{131}-albumin and Evans blue dye, with measured blood loss. Am J Obstet Gynecol 1970;106:843–9.
5. Sibai BM, Abdella TN, Anderson GD, Dilts PV Jr. Plasma volume findings in pregnant women with mild hypertension: therapeutic considerations. Am J Obstet Gynecol 1983;145:539–44.
6. Goodlin RC, Anderson JC, Gallagher TF. Relationship between amniotic fluid volume and maternal plasma volume expansion. Am J Obstet Gynecol 1983;146:505–11.
7. Hays PM, Cruikshank DP, Dunn LJ. Plasma volume determination in normal and preeclamptic pregnancies. Am J Obstet Gynecol 1985;151:958–66.

Name: **FENFLURAMINE**

Class: **Central Stimulant/Anorectant**   Risk Factor: **C**$_M$

Fetal Risk Summary

No data are available (see Diethylpropion, Dextroamphetamine).

Breast Feeding Summary

No data are available.

Name: **FENOPROFEN**

Class: **Nonsteroidal Anti-inflammatory**   Risk Factor: **B***

Fetal Risk Summary

No reports linking the use of fenoprofen with congenital defects have been located. The drug was used during labor in one study (1). No data were given except that the drug could not be detected in cord blood or amniotic fluid. If the drug did reach the fetus, fenoprofen, a prostaglandin synthetase inhibitor, could theoretically cause constriction of the ductus arteriosus *in utero* (2). Persistent pulmonary hypertension of the newborn should also be considered (2). Drugs in this class have been shown to inhibit labor and prolong pregnancy (3).

[*Risk Factor D if used in the 3rd trimester or near delivery.]

Breast Feeding Summary

Fenoprofen passes into breast milk in very small quantities. The milk:plasma ratio in nursing mothers given 600 mg every 6 hours for 4 days was approximately 0.017 (1). The clinical significance of this amount is unknown.

References

1. Rubin A, Chernish SM, Crabtree R, et al. A profile of the physiological disposition and gastrointestinal effects of fenoprofen in man. Curr Med Res Opin 1974;2:529–44.
2. Levin DL. Effects of inhibition of prostaglandin synthesis on fetal development, oxygenation, and the fetal circulation. Semin Perinatol 1980;4:35–44.
3. Fuchs F. Prevention of prematurity. Am J Obstet Gynecol 1976;126:809–20.

Name: **FENOTEROL**

Class: **Sympathomimetic (Adrenergic)**   Risk Factor: **B**

Fetal Risk Summary

No reports linking the use of fenoterol with congenital defects have been located. Fenoterol, a β-sympathomimetic, has been used to prevent premature labor (1, 2). The effects in the mother, fetus, and newborn are similar to those produced by the parent compound (see Metaproterenol). Fenoterol has been shown to inhibit prostaglandin-induced uterine activity at term (3).

Fenoterol was administered to 11 patients 30 minutes prior to cesarean section under general anesthesia at an infusion rate of 3 μg/minute (4). No adverse effects were seen in the mother, fetus or newborn after this short exposure. Infusion in hypertensive pregnant patients caused a greater drop in diastolic blood pressure than did the same dose in normotensive pregnant women (5). Other cardiovascular parameters in the mothers and fetuses were comparable between the two groups.

Breast Feeding Summary

No data are available.

References

1. Lipshitz J, Baillie P, Davey DA. A comparison of the uterine beta-2-adrenoreceptor selectivity of fenoterol, hexoprenaline, ritodrine and salbutamol. S Afr Med J 1976;50:1969–72.
2. Lipshitz J. The uterine and cardiovascular effects of oral fenoterol hydrochloride. Br J Obstet Gynaecol 1977;84:737–9.
3. Lipshitz J, Lipshitz EM. Uterine and cardiovascular effects of fenoterol and hexoprenaline in prostaglandin $F_{2\alpha}$-induced labor in humans. Obstet Gynecol 1984;63:396–400.
4. Jouppila R, Kauppila A, Tuimala R, Pakarinen A, Moilanen K. Maternal, fetal and neonatal effects of beta-adrenergic stimulation in connection with cesarean section. Acta Obstet Gynecol Scand 1980;59:489–93.
5. Oddoy UA, Joschko K. Effects of fenoterol on blood pressure, heart rate, and cardiotocogram of hypertensive and normotensive women in advanced pregnancy. Zentralbl Gynakol 1982;104:415–21.

Name: **FENTANYL**

Class: **Narcotic Analgesic**   Risk Factor: **B***

Fetal Risk Summary

No reports linking the use of fentanyl with congenital defects have been located. In a study comparing women in labor who received 50 μg or 100 μg of fentanyl intravenously every hour as needed ($N = 137$) (mean dose 140 μg ± 42 μg, range 50–600 μg) to those not requiring analgesia (epidural or narcotic) ($N = 112$), no statistical differences were found in newborn outcome in terms of the incidence of depressed respirations, Apgar scores, and the need for naloxone (1). In blinded measurements taken at 2–4 hours and at 24 hours, no differences were observed between the two groups of infants in respiratory rate, heart rate, blood pressure, adaptive capacity, neurologic evaluation, and overall assessment. The last dose of fentanyl was given a mean 112 minutes before delivery. Cord blood levels of the narcotic were always significantly lower than maternal serum levels (cord:maternal ratios approximately 0.5 but exact data not given) ($p < 0.03$). Doses used were considered equianalgesic to 5–10 mg of morphine or 37.5–75 mg of meperidine (1).

Respiratory depression has been observed in one infant whose mother received epidural fentanyl during labor (2). Fentanyl may produce loss of fetal heart rate variability without causing fetal hypoxia (1, 3). The narcotic has been combined with bupivacaine for spinal anesthesia during labor (4, 5).

In 15 women undergoing elective cesarean section, fentanyl 1 μg/kg given intravenously within 10 minutes of delivery produced an average cord blood:maternal blood ratio over 10 minutes of 0.31 (range 0.06–0.43 ng/ml) (6). No respiratory depression was observed, and all neurobehavioral scores were normal at 4 and 24 hours.

[*Risk Factor D if used for prolonged periods or in high doses at term.]

Breast Feeding Summary

No data are available.

References

1. Rayburn W, Rathke A, Leuschen MP, Chleborad J, Weidner W. Fentanyl citrate analgesia during labor. Am J Obstet Gynecol 1989;161:202–6.
2. Carrie LES, O'Sullivan GM, Seegobin R. Epidural fentanyl in labour. Anaesthesia 1981;36:965–9.
3. Johnson ES, Colley PS. Effects of nitrous oxide and fentanyl anesthesia on fetal heart-rate variability intra- and postoperatively. Anesthesiology 1980;52:429–30.
4. Justins DM, Francis D, Houlton PG, Reynolds F. A controlled trial of extradural fentanyl in labour. Br J Anaesth 1982;54:409–13.
5. Milon D, Bentue-Ferrer D, Noury D, Reymann JM, Sauvage J, Allain H, Saint-Marc C, van den Driessche J. Peridural anesthesia for cesarean section employing a bupivacaine-fentanyl combination. Ann Fr Anesth Reanim 1983;2:273–9.
6. Eisele JH, Wright R, Rogge P. Newborn and maternal fentanyl levels at cesarean section. Anesth Anal 1982;61:179–80 (Abstr).

Name: **FLECAINIDE**

Class: **Antiarrhythmic** Risk Factor: **C$_M$**

Fetal Risk Summary

Flecainide is an antiarrhythmic agent that is structurally related to encainide and procainamide. The drug is teratogenic in some animal species (1). Two reports of human use have been located, but it appears that a single incidence of exposure to the drug has been separately described by different groups of authors (2, 3). Intravenous flecainide was given to a pregnant woman at 30 weeks' gestation for persistent fetal supraventricular tachycardia resistent to digoxin (2, 3). The fetal heart rate pattern quickly converted to a sinus rhythm and the mother was maintained on oral flecainide, 100 mg three times daily, until delivery was induced at 38 weeks' gestation. The 3450-g female infant had no cardiac problems during the 10 days of observation. Flecainide concentrations in the cord blood and maternal serum at delivery 5 hours after the last dose were 533 and 833 ng/ml, respectively (ratio 0.63) (2).

Breast Feeding Summary

No data are available.

References

1. Product information, Tambocor. Riker Laboratories, 1990.
2. Wren C, Hunter S. Maternal administration of flecainide to terminate and suppress fetal tachycardia. Br Med J 1988;296:249.
3. Macphail S, Walkinshaw SA. Fetal supraventricular tachycardia: detection by routine auscultation and successful in-utero management: case report. Br J Obstet Gynaecol 1988;95:1073–6.

Name: **FLUCYTOSINE**

Class: **Antifungal**   Risk Factor: **C**

Fetal Risk Summary

Flucytosine is embryotoxic and teratogenic in some species of animals, but its use in human pregnancy has not been studied. Following oral administration, about 4% of the drug is metabolized to 5-fluorouracil, an antineoplastic agent (1). Fluorouracil is suspected of producing congenital defects in humans (see Fluorouracil). Three case reports of pregnant patients treated in the 2nd and 3rd trimesters with flucytosine have been located (2–4). No defects were observed in the newborns.

Breast Feeding Summary

No data are available.

References

1. Diasio RB, Lakings DE, Bennett JE. Evidence for conversion of 5-fluorocytosine to 5-fluorouracil in humans: possible factor in 5-fluorocytosine clinical toxicity. Antimicrob Agents Chemother 1978;14:903–8.
2. Philpot CR, Lo D. Cryptococcal meningitis in pregnancy. Med J Aust 1972;2:1005–7.
3. Schonebeck J, Segerbrand E. Candida albicans septicaemia during first half of pregnancy successfully treated with 5-fluorocytosine. Br Med J 1973;4:337–8.
4. Curole DN. Cryptococcal meningitis in pregnancy. J Reprod Med 1981;26:317–9.

Name: **FLUNITRAZEPAM**

Class: **Hypnotic**   Risk Factor: **D**

Fetal Risk Summary

Flunitrazepam is a benzodiazepine (see also Diazepam). No reports linking the use of flunitrazepam with congenital defects have been located, but other drugs in this group have been suspected of causing fetal malformations (see also Diazepam or Chlordiazepoxide). In contrast to other benzodiazepines, flunitrazepam crosses the placenta slowly (1, 2). About 12 hours after a 1-mg oral dose, cord:maternal blood ratios in early and late pregnancy were about 0.5 and 0.22, respectively. Amniotic fluid:maternal serum ratios were in the 0.02–0.07 range in both cases. Accumulation in the fetus may occur after repeated doses (1).

Breast Feeding Summary

Flunitrazepam is excreted into breast milk. Following a single 2-mg oral dose in five patients, mean milk:plasma ratios at 11, 15, 27, and 39 hours were 0.61, 0.68, 0.9, and 0.75, respectively (1, 2). The effects of these levels on the nursing infant are unknown but they are probably insignificant.

References

1. Kanto J, Aaltonen L, Kangas L, Erkkola R, Pitkanen Y. Placental transfer and breast milk levels of flunitrazepam. Curr Ther Res 1979;26:539–46.
2. Kanto JH. Use of benzodiazepines during pregnancy, labour and lactation, with special reference to pharmacokinetic considerations. Drugs 1982;23:354–80.

Name: **FLUOROURACIL**

Class: **Antineoplastic**   Risk Factor: **D**

Fetal Risk Summary

Experience with fluorouracil during pregnancy is limited. There are no reports of fetal effects after topical use of the drug. Following systemic therapy in the 1st trimester (also exposed to 5 rad of irradiation), multiple defects were observed in an aborted fetus: radial aplasia; absent thumbs and three fingers; hypoplasia of lungs, aorta, thymus, and bile duct; aplasia of esophagus, duodenum, and ureters; single umbilical artery; absent appendix; imperforate anus; and a cloaca (1).

A 33-year-old woman with metastatic breast cancer was treated with a modified radical mastectomy during her 3rd month of pregnancy followed by oophorectomy at 13 weeks' gestation (2). Chemotherapy, consisting of 5-fluorouracil, cyclophosphamide, and doxorubicin, was started at approximately 11 weeks' gestation and continued for six 3-week cyclic courses. Methotrexate was substituted for doxorubicin at this time and the new three-drug regimen was continued until delivery by cesarean section at 35 weeks of a 2260-g female infant. No abnormalities were noted at birth, and continued follow-up at 24 months of age revealed normal growth and development. Toxicity consisting of cyanosis and jerking extremities has been reported in a newborn exposed to fluorouracil in the 3rd trimester (3).

Amenorrhea has been observed in women treated with fluorouracil for breast cancer, but this was probably due to concurrent administration of melphalan (see also Melphalan) (4, 5). The long-term effects of combination chemotherapy on menstrual and reproductive function have been described in two 1988 reports (6, 7). In one report, only two of the 40 women treated for malignant ovarian germ cell tumors received fluorouracil (6). The results of this study are discussed in the monograph for cyclophosphamide (see Cyclophosphamide). The other report described the reproductive results of 265 women who had been treated from 1959–1980 for gestational trophoblastic disease (7). Single agent chemotherapy was administered to 91 women, including 54 cases in which 5-fluorouracil was the only agent used; sequential (single agent) and combination therapy were administered to 67 and 107 women, respectively. Of the total group, 241 were exposed to pregnancy and 205 (85%) of these women conceived, with a total of 355 pregnancies. The time interval between recovery and pregnancy was 1 year or less (8.5%), 1–2 years (32.1%), 2–4 years (32.4%), 4–6 years (15.5%), 6–8 years (7.3%), 8–10 years (1.4%), and more than 10 years (2.8%). A total of 303 (four sets of twins) liveborn infants resulted from the 355 pregnancies, three of whom had congenital malformations: anencephaly, hydrocephalus, and congenital heart disease (one in each case). No gross developmental abnormalities were observed in the dead fetuses. Cytogenetic studies were conducted on the peripheral lymphocytes of 94 children, and no significant chromosomal abnormalities were noted. Moreover, follow-up of the children, more than 80% of the group older than 5 years of age (the oldest was 25 years), revealed normal development. The reproductive histories and pregnancy outcomes of the treated women were comparable to those of the normal population (7).

Occupational exposure of the mother to antineoplastic agents during pregnancy may present a risk to the fetus. A position statement from the National Study Commission on Cytotoxic Exposure and a research article involving some antineoplastic agents are presented in the monograph for cyclophosphamide (see Cyclophosphamide).

Breast Feeding Summary

No data are available.

References

1. Stephens JD, Golbus MS, Miller TR, Wilber RR, Epstein CJ. Multiple congenital anomalies in a fetus exposed to 5-fluorouracil during the first trimester. Am J Obstet Gynecol 1980; 137:747–9.
2. Turchi JJ, Villasis C. Anthracyclines in the treatment of malignancy in pregnancy. Cancer 1988;61:435–440.
3. Stadler HE, Knowles J. Fluorouracil in pregnancy: effect on the neonate. JAMA 1971; 217:214–5.
4. Fisher B, Sherman B, Rockette H, Redmond C, Margolese K, Fisher ER. L-Phenylalanine (L-PAM) in the management of premenopausal patients with primary breast cancer. Cancer 1979;44:847–57.
5. Schilsky RL, Lewis BJ, Sherins RJ, Young RC. Gonadal dysfunction in patients receiving chemotherapy for cancer. Ann Intern Med 1980;93:109–14.
6. Gershenson DM. Menstrual and reproductive function after treatment with combination chemotherapy for malignant ovarian germ cell tumors. J Clin Oncol 1988;6:270–5.
7. Song H, Wu P, Wang Y, Yang X, Dong S. Pregnancy outcomes after successful chemotherapy for choriocarcinoma and invasive mole: long-term follow-up. Am J Obstet Gynecol 1988;158:538–45.

Name: **FLUPENTHIXOL**

Class: **Tranquilizer**   Risk Factor: **C**

Fetal Risk Summary

Flupenthixol crosses the placenta with cord blood levels averaging 24% of maternal serum levels (1). Amniotic fluid concentrations are similar to those in cord blood. Flupenthixol 1 mg daily was used throughout the 2nd and 3rd trimesters in one patient with borderline psychotic depression (2). None of the infants in the above studies was apparently affected by the exposure to flupenthixol.

Breast Feeding Summary

Flupenthixol is excreted into breast milk (1, 2). In one study, concentrations were about 30% higher than those in maternal serum (1). In a second study, a mother received 1 mg daily throughout the 2nd and 3rd trimesters (2). The dose was increased to 4 mg daily on the 1st postpartum day, then tapered to 2 mg daily over the next 7 weeks. The mother was also receiving nortriptyline. While receiving the 4-mg daily dose, milk concentrations, measured 2–4.5 hours after a dose on postpartum days 6 (four samples) and 20 (two samples), ranged from 2.0–6.8 ng/ml, with a mean of 3.2 ng/ml. The milk:serum ratios for these samples ranged from 0.50–1.62, with a mean of 0.85. No effects of the drug exposure were observed in the nursing infant, who had normal motor development over the first 4 months (2). The significance of chronic exposure of the nursing infant to this drug is unknown, but concern was expressed about the effects of long-term exposure on the infant's neurobehavioral mechanisms (2).

References

1. Kirk L, Jorgensen A. Concentrations of cis(z)-flupenthixol in maternal serum, amniotic fluid, umbilical cord serum, and milk. Psychopharmacology (Berlin) 1980;72:107–8.
2. Matheson I, Skjaeraasen J. Milk concentrations of flupenthixol, nortriptyline and zuclopenthixol and between-breast differences in two patients. Eur J Clin Pharmacol 1988;35:217–20.

Name: **FLUPHENAZINE**

Class: **Tranquilizer**   Risk Factor: **C**

Fetal Risk Summary

Fluphenazine is a piperazine phenothiazine in the same group as prochlorperazine. Phenothiazines readily cross the placenta (1). Extrapyramidal symptoms in the newborn have been attributed to *in utero* exposure to fluphenazine (see also Chlorpromazine) (2). An infant with multiple anomalies was born to a mother treated with fluphenazine enanthate injections throughout pregnancy (3). The mother also took Debendox (see Doxylamine) during the 1st trimester. Anomalies included: ocular hypertelorism with telecanthus, cleft lip and palate, imperforate anus, hypospadias of penoscrotal type, jerky, roving eye movements, episodic rapid nystagmoid movements, rectourethral fistula, and poor ossification of frontal skull bone. Other reports have indicated that the phenothiazines are relatively safe during pregnancy (see also Prochlorperazine).

Breast Feeding Summary

No data are available. See also Prochlorperazine.

References

1. Moya F, Thorndike V. Passage of drugs across the placenta. Am J Obstet Gynecol 1962;84:1778–98.
2. Cleary MF. Fluphenazine decanoate during pregnancy. Am J Psychiatry 1977;134:815–6.
3. Donaldson GL, Bury RG. Multiple congenital abnormalities in a newborn boy associated with maternal use of fluphenazine enanthate and other drugs during pregnancy. Acta Paediatr Scand 1982;71:335–8.

Name: **FOLIC ACID**

Class: **Vitamin**   Risk Factor: **A***

Fetal Risk Summary

Folic acid, a water-soluble B complex vitamin, is essential for nucleoprotein synthesis and the maintenance of normal erythropoiesis (1). The American recommended daily allowance for folic acid in pregnancy is 0.8 mg (2). However, a recommended dietary intake of 0.5 mg/day has been proposed that would meet the needs of women with poor folate stores, those with essentially no other dietary folate, and those with multiple pregnancies (3).

Rapid transfer of folic acid to the fetus occurs in pregnancy (4–6). One investigation indicated that the placenta stores folic acid and transfer occurs only after placental tissue vitamin receptors are saturated (7). Results compatible with this hypothesis were found in a 1975 study using radiolabeled folate in women undergoing 2nd trimester abortions (8).

Folic acid deficiency is common during pregnancy (9–12). If not supplemented, maternal serum and red blood cell (RBC) folate values decline during pregnancy (9, 13–17). Even with vitamin supplements, however, maternal folate hypovitaminemia may result (9). This depletion is thought to result from preferential uptake of folic acid by the fetal circulation such that at birth, newborn levels are significantly higher than maternal levels (9, 16–19). At term, mean serum folate in 174 mothers was 5.6 ng/ml (range 1.5–7.6) and in their newborns 18 ng/ml (range 5.5–66.0) (9). In an earlier study, similar serum values were measured with RBC folate decreasing from 157 ng/ml at 15 weeks' gestation to 118 ng/ml at 38 weeks (13). Folic acid supplementation prevented the decrease in both serum and RBC folate. Although supplementation is common during pregnancy in some countries, not all authorities believe this is necessary for the entire population (20, 21). The main controversy between some is whether all women should receive supplements because of the cost involved in identifying those at risk (20) or if supplements should be given only to those in whom a clear indication has been established (21).

The most common complication of maternal folic acid deficiency is megaloblastic anemia (10, 22–31). Pancytopenia secondary to folate deficiency has also

been reported during pregnancy (32). The three main factors involved in the pathogenesis of megaloblastic anemia of pregnancy are depletion of maternal folic
acid stores by the fetus, inadequate maternal intake of the vitamin, and faulty
absorption (28). Multiple pregnancy, hemorrhage, and hemolytic anemia hasten
the decline of maternal levels (14, 28). A 1969 study used 1-mg daily supplements
to uniformly produce a satisfactory hematologic response in these conditions (30).

The effects on the mother and fetus resulting from folate deficiency are controversial. These effects can be summarized as:

Fetal anomalies
Placental abruption
Pregnancy-induced hypertension (PIH, toxemia, preeclampsia)
Abortions
Placenta previa
Low birth weight
Premature delivery

Folic acid deficiency is a well-known experimental animal teratogen (33). In
humans, the relationship between fetal defects and folate deficiency is less
clear. Several reports have claimed an increase in congenital malformations associated with low levels of this vitamin (10, 25–27, 34–37). Other investigators
have stated that maternal deficiency does not result in fetal anomalies (23, 24,
38–44). One study found the folate status of mothers giving birth to severely
malformed fetuses to be no different from that of the general obstetric population and much better than that of mothers with overt megaloblastic anemia (38).
Similar results were found in other series (42–44). In one of these, 10 mg/day of
folic acid were given to one patient from about the 6th week through term (42).
The mother, who had given birth to previous children with neural tube defects
(NTDs), gave birth to a child with spina bifida and craniolacunae. A subsequent
pregnancy in this woman, without supplementation, resulted in a healthy infant.
A 1985 publication of a study conducted in Dublin found no difference in serum
folate or vitamin B_{12} levels in mothers whose pregnancies ended with an NTD
infant/fetus when compared to 395 normal controls (45). The serum samples
were obtained during a routine screening program for rubella antibody conducted in three Dublin hospitals. After testing, the samples were frozen and
then later used for this study. A total of 116 cases of NTDs were identified during the study period, but serum was available for only 32 of the cases: 16 with
anencephalus, 15 with spina bifida, and one encephalocele. In half of the cases,
serum was obtained between 9–13 weeks' gestation. The mean serum folate
concentrations in the cases and controls were both 3.4 ng/ml, while levels of B_{12}
were 297 and 277 pg/ml, respectively.

A 1987 publication found significantly lower red cell folate levels in pregnancies
ending with a NTD (46). This Scottish study measured vitamin levels in 20 women
under the age of 35 years who had a history of two or more NTD pregnancies. A
control group of 20 women with no pregnancies ending in NTD, but matched for
age, obstetric history, and social class, was used for comparison. No significant
differences between the two groups were found in assays for plasma or serum
vitamin A, thiamine, riboflavin, pyridoxine, vitamin B_{12}, folate, vitamin C, vitamin E,
total protein, albumin, transferrin, copper, magnesium, zinc, and white cell vitamin

C. Red cell folate, however, was significantly lower in the case mothers than in controls, 178 vs. 268 ng/ml ($p = 0.005$), respectively, although both were within the normal range (106–614 ng/ml). Moreover, a linear relationship was found between red cell folate and the number of NTD pregnancies. Women who had three or four such pregnancies also had the lowest concentrations of red cell folate (46). The dietary intake of folic acid was lower in the case mothers than in controls, but the difference was not statistically significant. Since the lower red cell folate levels could not be attributed entirely to dietary intake of folic acid, the authors theorized that one factor predisposing to the occurrence of NTD may be an inherited disorder of folate metabolism (46).

The data of other investigators have suggested a relationship between folic acid deficiency and NTD (See also Vitamins, Multiple; especially study by Milunsky and co-workers, 1989). In a randomized double blind trial to prevent recurrences of NTD, 44 women took 4 mg/day of folic acid from before conception through early pregnancy (34). There were no recurrences in this group. A placebo group of 51 women plus 16 noncompliant patients from the treated group had four and two recurrences, respectively. The difference between the supplemented and nonsupplemented patients was significant ($p = 0.04$). Other researchers reported significantly lower RBC folate levels in mothers of infants with NTD than in mothers of normal infants, but not all of the affected group had low serum folate (47). In a subsequent report by these investigators, very low vitamin B_{12} concentrations were found, suggesting that the primary deficiency may have been due to this latter vitamin with resulting depletion of RBC and tissue folate (48). A large retrospective study found a protective effect with folate administration during pregnancy, leading to a possible conclusion that deficiency of this vitamin could be teratogenic (37).

Evidence was published in 1989 that dietary intake of folic acid is related to the occurrence of NTDs (49). In this Australian population-based case-control study, 77 mothers whose pregnancies involved an isolated NTD were compared to 77 mothers of infants with other defects (control group 1) and 154 mothers of normal infants (control group 2). Free folate intake was classified into four levels (in micrograms/day): 8.0–79.8, 79.9–115.4, 115.5–180.5, and 180.6–1678.0. After adjustment for potential confounding variables, a statistically significant trend for protection against an NTD outcome was observed with increasing free folate intake in comparison to both control groups: $p = 0.02$ for control group 1, and $p < 0.001$ for control group 2. The odds ratios (95% confidence intervals) for the highest intake compared to the control groups were 0.31 (0.10–0.97) and 0.16 (0.06–0.49), respectively. When total folate intake was examined, the trends were less: $p = 0.10$ for control group 1 and $p = 0.03$ for control group 2. In an accompanying editorial comment, criticism of the above study focused on the authors' estimation of dietary folate intake (50). The commentary cited evidence that nutrition tables are unreliable for the estimation of folate content, and that the only conclusion the study could claim was that dietary factors, but not necessarily folate, had a role in the etiology of NTD.

The strongest evidence for an association between folic acid and fetal defects comes from examining patients treated with drugs that are either folic acid antagonists or induce folic acid deficiency, although agreement with the latter is not universal (41, 51, 52). The folic acid antagonists, aminopterin and methotrexate, are known teratogens (see Aminopterin and Methotrexate). A very high incidence of defects resulted when aminopterin was used as an unsuccessful abortifacient in the 1st trimester. These antineoplastic agents may cause fetal injury by blocking the conversion of folic acid to tetrahydrofolic acid in both the fetus and the mother.

In contrast, certain anticonvulsants, such as phenytoin and phenobarbital, induce maternal folic acid deficiency, possibly by impairing gastrointestinal absorption or increasing hepatic metabolism of the vitamin (41, 51, 52). Whether these agents also induce folic acid deficiency in the fetus is less certain, because the fetus seems to be efficient in drawing on available maternal stores of folic acid. Low maternal folate levels, however, have been proposed as a mechanism for the increased incidence of defects observed in infants exposed *in utero* to anticonvulsants. In a 1984 article, investigators reported research on the relationship between folic acid, anticonvulsants, and fetal defects (51). In the retrospective part of this study, a group of 24 women who were treated with phenytoin and other anticonvulsants produced 66 infants, of whom 10 (15%) had major anomalies. Two of the mothers with affected infants had markedly low RBC folate concentrations. A second group of 22 epileptic women was then given supplements of daily folic acid, 2.5–5.0 mg, starting before conception in 26 pregnancies and within the first 40 days in six. This group produced 33 newborns (32 pregnancies—1 set of twins) with no defects, a significant difference from the group not receiving supplementation. Negative associations between anticonvulsant-induced folate deficiency and birth defects have also been reported (41, 52). Investigators studied a group of epileptic women taking anticonvulsants and observed only two defects (2.9%) in pregnancies producing a live baby, a rate similar to that expected in a healthy population (41). Although folate levels were not measured in this retrospective survey, maternal folate deficiency was predicted by the authors, based on their current research with folic acid in patients taking anticonvulsants. Another group of researchers observed 20 infants (15%) with defects from 133 women taking anticonvulsants (52). No neural tube defects were found, but this defect is rare in Finland and an increase in the anomaly could have been missed (52). All of the women were given supplements of 0.1–1.0 mg (average 0.5 mg) of folate/day from the 6th–16th weeks of gestation until delivery. Folate levels were usually within the normal range (normals considered to be: serum >1.8 ng/ml, RBC >203 ng/ml).

Maternal folic acid status may be associated with placental abruption (26, 27, 29, 36, 53). In a review and analysis of 506 consecutive cases of abruptio placentae, defective folate metabolism was found as a predisposing factor in 97.5%. The authors theorized that folic acid deficiency early in pregnancy caused irreversible damage to the fetus, chorion, and decidua, leading to abruption, abortion, premature delivery, low birth weight, and fetal malformations. Other studies have discovered that 60% of their patients with abruption were folate deficient, but their numbers were too small for statistical analysis (54). In other series, no correlation was found between low levels of folic acid and this complication (17, 40, 55).

A relationship between folate deficiency and PIH is doubtful. In a study of women with megaloblastic anemia, 14% had PIH compared to the predicted incidence of 6% for that population (23). In another report, although 22 of 36 PIH patients had folate deficiency, the authors were unable to conclude that a positive association existed (36, 54). Other investigators have also failed to find a relationship between low levels of the vitamin and PIH (24, 28). In one of these studies, the incidence of PIH in megaloblastic anemia was 12.2% compared to 14.0% in normoblastic anemia (28). A second group of investigators studied folate levels in 101 preeclamptic and 17 eclamptic women and compared them to 52 normal controls and 29 women with overt megaloblastic anemia (56). No correlation was found between levels of folic acid and the complications.

Several papers have associated folic acid deficiency with abortion (26, 27, 36, 53, 57–59). The etiology of some abortions, as proposed by some, is faulty folate metabolism in early pregnancy, producing irreversible injury to the fetus and placenta (53). Others have been unable to detect any significant relationship between serum and RBC folate levels and abortion (13, 39, 60). In a series of 66 patients with early spontaneous abortions, the incidence of folate deficiency was the same as in those with uncomplicated pregnancies (60). These researchers did find a relationship between low folic acid levels and placenta previa. However, others found no evidence of an association between folate deficiency and either abortion or antepartum hemorrhage (13).

The relationship between prematurity, low birth weight, and folic acid levels has been investigated. In one study, significantly lower folate levels were measured in the blood of low-birth-weight neonates as compared to normal-weight infants (19). The incidences of both premature delivery and birth weight under 2500 g were increased in folate-deficient mothers in a 1960 report (23). These patients all had severe megaloblastic anemia and a poor standard of nutrition. In a later study of 510 infants from folate-deficient mothers, 276 (56%) weighed 2500 g or less compared to a predicted incidence of 8.6% (53). A study of women with uterine bleeding during pregnancy found a significant association between serum folate and low birth weight (58). Similarly, another study reported a significant relationship between folate levels at the end of the 2nd trimester and newborn birth weight (61). In contrast, others have found no association between folic acid deficiency and prematurity (28, 40, 62, 63) or between serum folate and birth weight (13, 40, 64, 65).

Two reports have alluded to problems with high folic acid levels in the mother during pregnancy (66, 67). An isolated case report described an anencephalic fetus whose mother was under psychiatric care (66). She had been treated with very high doses of folic acid and vitamins B_1, B_6, and C. The relationship between the vitamins and the defect is questionable. A 1984 study examined the effect of folic acid, zinc, and other nutrients on pregnancy outcome (67). Total complications of pregnancy (infection, bleeding, fetal distress, prematurity or death, PIH, and tissue fragility) were associated with high serum folate and low serum zinc levels. The explanation offered for these surprising findings was that folate inhibits intestinal absorption of zinc, which, they proposed, was responsible for the complications. This study also found an association between low folate and abortion.

In summary, folic acid deficiency during pregnancy is a common problem in undernourished women and in women not receiving supplements. The relationship between folic acid levels and various maternal or fetal complications appears to be complex. Evidence has accumulated that interference with folic acid metabolism by some drugs early in pregnancy will result in congenital anomalies. Evidence has also accumulated that non-drug-induced maternal folic acid deficiency, or abnormal folate metabolism, may be related to the occurrence of NTD (see also Vitamins, Multiple). The timing of folic acid deficiency (i.e., very early 1st trimester vs. later 1st trimester) is important, especially for the prevention of NTD. For other complications, it is probable that a number of factors, of which folic acid may be one, contribute to poor pregnancy outcome. Consequently, to assure good maternal and fetal health, supplementation of the pregnant woman with the folic acid RDA or sufficient amounts to maintain normal maternal folate levels is recommended.

[*Risk Factor C if used in doses above the RDA.]

Breast Feeding Summary

Folic acid is actively excreted in human breast milk (68–77). Accumulation of folate in milk takes precedence over maternal folate needs (68). Levels of folic acid are relatively low in colostrum but as lactation proceeds, concentrations of the vitamin rise (69–71). Folate levels in newborns and breast-fed infants are consistently higher than those in mothers and normal adults (72, 73). In Japanese mothers, mean breast milk folate concentrations were 141.4 ng/ml, resulting in a total intake by the infant of 14–25 µg/kg/day (73). Much lower mean levels were measured in pooled human milk in an English study examining preterm (26 mothers—29–34 weeks) and term (35 mothers—39 weeks or longer) patients (70). Preterm milk rose from 10.6 ng/ml (colostrum) to 30.5 ng/ml (16–196 days), whereas term milk increased over the same period from 17.6–42.3 ng/ml.

Supplementation with folic acid is apparently not needed in mothers with good nutritional habits (71–75). Folic acid deficiency and megaloblastic anemia did not develop in women not receiving supplements even when lactation exceeded I year (71, 72). In another study, maternal serum and red blood cell folate levels increased significantly after 1 mg of folic acid/day for 4 weeks, but milk folate levels remained unchanged (73). Investigators gave well-nourished lactating women a multivitamin preparation containing 0.8 mg of folic acid (74). At 6 months postpartum, milk concentrations of folate did not differ significantly from those of controls not receiving supplements. Other investigators measured more than adequate blood folate levels in American breast-fed infants during the 1st year of life (75). The mean milk concentration of folate consumed by these infants was 85 ng/ml.

In patients with poor nutrition, lactation may lead to severe maternal folic acid deficiency and megaloblastic anemia (68). For these patients, there is evidence that low folate levels, as part of the total nutritional status of the mother, are related to the length of the lactation period (71). Lactating mothers with megaloblastic anemia, in one study, were treated with 5 mg/day of folic acid for 3 days (69). Breast milk folate rose from 7–9 ng/ml to 15–40 ng/ml 1 day after treatment began. The elevated levels were maintained for 3 weeks without further treatment. Nine low socioeconomic status women were treated with multivitamins containing 0.8 mg of folic acid and compared with seven untreated controls (76). Breast milk folate was significantly higher in the treated women. In another study of lactating women with low nutritional status, supplementation with folic acid, 0.2–10.0 mg/day, resulted in mean milk concentrations of 2.3–5.6 ng/ml (77). Milk concentrations were directly proportional to dietary intake.

Folic acid concentrations were determined in preterm and term milk in a study to determine the effect of storage time and temperature (78). Storage of milk in a freezer resulted in progressive decreases over 3 months such that the RDA of folate for infants could not be provided from milk stored for this length of time. Storage in a refrigerator for 24 hours did not affect folate levels.

The American RDA for folic acid during lactation is 0.5 mg (2). If the lactating woman's diet adequately supplies this amount, maternal supplementation with folic acid is not needed. Maternal supplementation with the RDA for folic acid is recommended for those patients with inadequate nutritional intake. The American Academy of Pediatrics considers maternal consumption of folic acid to be compatible with breast feeding (79).

References

1. American Hospital Formulary Service. *Drug Information 1990*. Bethesda:American Society of Hospital Pharmacists, 1990:2111–2.
2. *Recommended Dietary Allowances*, 9th ed. Washington:National Academy of Sciences, 1980.
3. Herbert V. Recommended dietary intakes (RDI) of folate in humans. Am J Clin Nutr 1987;45:661–70.
4. Frank O, Walbroehl G, Thomson A, Kaminetzky H, Kubes Z, Baker H. Placental transfer: fetal retention of some vitamins. Am J Clin Nutr 1970;23:662–3.
5. Kaminetzky HA, Baker H, Frank O, Langer A. The effects of intravenously administered water-soluble vitamins during labor in normovitaminemic and hypovitaminemic gravidas on maternal and neonatal blood vitamin levels at delivery. Am J Obstet Gynecol 1974;120:697–703.
6. Hill EP, Longo LD. Dynamics of maternal-fetal nutrient transfer. Fed Proc 1980;39:239–44.
7. Baker H, Frank O, Deangelis B, Feingold S, Kaminetzky HA. Role of placenta in maternal-fetal vitamin transfer in humans. Am J Obstet Gynecol 1981;141:792–6.
8. Landon MJ, Eyre DH, Hytten FE. Transfer of folate to the fetus. Br J Obstet Gynaecol 1975;82:12–9.
9. Baker H, Frank O, Thomason AD, Langer A, Munves ED, De Angelis B, Kaminetzky HA. Vitamin profile of 174 mothers and newborns at parturition. Am J Clin Nutr 1975;28:59–65.
10. Kaminetzky HA, Baker H. Micronutrients in pregnancy. Clin Obstet Gynecol 1977;20:263–80.
11. Dostalova L. Correlation of the vitamin status between mother and newborn during delivery. Dev Pharmacol Ther 1982;4 (Suppl 1):45–57.
12. Bruinse HW, Berg HVD, Haspels AA. Maternal serum folacin levels during and after normal pregnancy. Eur J Obstet Gynecol Reprod Biol 1985;20:153–8.
13. Chanarin I, Rothman D, Ward A, Perry J. Folate status and requirement in pregnancy. Br Med J 1968;2:390–4.
14. Ball EW, Giles C. Folic acid and vitamin B_{12} levels in pregnancy and their relation to megaloblastic anemia. J Clin Pathol 1964;17:165–74.
15. Ek J, Magnus EM. Plasma and red blood cell folate during normal pregnancies. Acta Obstet Gynecol Scand 1981;60:247–51.
16. Baker H, Ziffer H, Pasher I, Sobotka H. A Comparison of maternal and foetal folic acid and vitamin B_{12} at parturition. Br Med J 1958;1:978–9.
17. Avery B, Ledger WJ. Folic acid metabolism in well-nourished pregnant women. Obstet Gynecol 1970;35:616–24.
18. Ek J. Plasma and red cell folate values in newborn infants and their mothers in relation to gestational age. J Pediatr 1980;97:288–92.
19. Baker H, Thind IS, Frank O, DeAngelis B, Caterini H, Lquria DB. Vitamin levels in low-birth-weight newborn infants and their mothers. Am J Obstet Gynecol 1977;129:521–4.
20. Horn E. Iron and folate supplements during pregnancy: supplementing everyone treats those at risk and is cost effective. Br Med J 1988;297:1325,1327.
21. Hibbard BM. Iron and folate supplements during pregnancy: supplementation is valuable only in selected patients. Br Med J 1988;297:1324,1326.
22. Chanarin I, MacGibbon BM, O'Sullivan WJ, Mollin DL. Folic-acid deficiency in pregnancy: the pathogenesis of megaloblastic anaemia of pregnancy. Lancet 1959;2:634–9.
23. Gatenby PBB, Lillie EW. Clinical analysis of 100 cases of severe megaloblastic anaemia of pregnancy. Br Med J 1960;2:1111–4.
24. Pritchard JA, Mason RA, Wright MR. Megaloblastic anemia during pregnancy and the puerperium. Am J Obstet Gynecol 1962;83:1004–20.

25. Fraser JL, Watt HJ. Megaloblastic anemia in pregnancy and the puerperium. Am J Obstet Gynecol 1964;89:532–4.

26. Hibbard BM. The role of folic acid in pregnancy: with particular reference to anaemia, abruption and abortion. J Obstet Gynaecol Br Commonw 1964;71:529–42.

27. Hibbard BM, Hibbard ED, Jeffcoate TNA. Folic acid and reproduction. Acta Obstet Gynecol Scand 1965;44:375–400.

28. Giles C. An account of 335 cases of megaloblastic anaemia of pregnancy and the puerperium. J Clin Pathol 1966;19:1–11.

29. Streiff RR, Little AB. Folic acid deficiency in pregnancy. N Engl J Med 1967;276:776–9.

30. Pritchard JA, Scott DE, Whalley PJ. Folic acid requirements in pregnancy-induced megaloblastic anemia. JAMA 1969;208:1163–7.

31. Rothman D. Folic acid in pregnancy. Am J Obstet Gynecol 1970;108:149–75.

32. Solano FX Jr, Councell RB. Folate deficiency presenting as pancytopenia in pregnancy. Am J Obstet Gynecol 1986;154:1117–8.

33. Shepard TH. Catalog of Teratogenic Agents, 3rd ed. Baltimore:Johns Hopkins University Press, 1980:153–4.

34. Laurence KM, James N, Miller MH, Tennant GB, Campbell H. Double-blind randomised controlled trial of folate treatment before conception to prevent recurrence of neural-tube defects. Br Med J 1981;282:1509–11.

35. Hibbard ED, Smithells RW. Folic acid metabolism and human embryopathy. Lancet 1965;1:1254.

36. Stone ML. Effects on the fetus of folic acid deficiency in pregnancy. Clin Obstet Gynecol 1968;11:1143–53.

37. Nelson MM, Forfar JO. Associations between drugs administered during pregnancy and congenital abnormalities of the fetus. Br Med J 1971;1:523–7.

38. Scott DE, Whalley PJ, Pritchard JA. Maternal folate deficiency and pregnancy wastage. II. Fetal malformation. Obstet Gynecol 1970;36:26–8.

39. Pritchard JA, Scott DE, Whalley PJ, Haling RF Jr. Infants of mothers with megaloblastic anemia due to folate deficiency. JAMA 1970;211:1982–4.

40. Kitay DZ, Hogan WJ, Eberle B, Mynt T. Neutrophil hypersegmentation and folic acid deficiency in pregnancy. Am J Obstet Gynecol 1969;104:1163–73.

41. Pritchard JA, Scott DE, Whalley PJ. Maternal folate deficiency and pregnancy wastage. IV. Effects of folic acid supplements, anticonvulsants, and oral contraceptives. Am J Obstet Gynecol 1971;109:341–6.

42. Emery AEH, Timson J, Watson-Williams, EJ. Pathogenesis of spina bifida. Lancet 1969;2:909–10.

43. Hall MH. Folates and the fetus. Lancet 1977;1:648–9.

44. Emery AEH. Folates and fetal central-nervous-system malformations. Lancet 1977;1:703.

45. Molloy AM, Kirke P, Hillary I, Weir DG, Scott JM. Maternal serum folate and vitamin B_{12} concentrations in pregnancies associated with neural tube defects. Arch Dis Child 1985;60:660–5.

46. Yates JRW, Ferguson-Smith MA, Shenkin A, Guzman-Rodriguez R, White M, Clark BJ. Is disordered folate metabolism the basis for the genetic predisposition to neural tube defects? Clin Genet 1987;31:279–87.

47. Smithells RW, Sheppard S, Schorah CJ. Vitamin deficiencies and neural tube defects. Arch Dis Child 1976;51:944–50.

48. Schorah CJ, Smithells RW, Scott J. Vitamin B_{12} and anencephaly. Lancet 1980;1:880.

49. Bower C, Stanley FJ. Dietary folate as a risk factor for neural-tube defects: evidence from a case-control study in Western Australia. Med J Aust 1989;150:613–9.

50. Mann J. Dietary folate and neural-tube defects. Med J Aust 1989;150:609.

51. Biale Y, Lewenthal H. Effect of folic acid supplementation on congenital malformations due to anticonvulsive drugs. Eur J Obstet Gynecol Reprod Biol 1984;18:211–6.

52. Hiilesmaa VK, Teramo K, Granstrom M-L, Bardy AH. Serum folate concentrations during pregnancy in women with epilepsy: relation to antiepileptic drug concentrations, number of seizures, and fetal outcome. Br Med J 1983;287:577–9.

53. Hibbard BM, Jeffcoate TNA. Abruptio placentae. Obstet Gynecol 1966;27:155–67.

54. Stone ML, Luhby AL, Feldman R, Gordon M, Cooperman JM. Folic acid metabolism in pregnancy. Am J Obstet Gynecol 1967;99:638–48.

55. Whalley PJ, Scott DE, Pritchard JA. Maternal folate deficiency and pregnancy wastage. I. Placental abruption. Am J Obstet Gynecol 1969;105:670–8.

56. Whalley PJ, Scott DE, Pritchard JA. Maternal folate deficiency and pregnancy wastage. III. Pregnancy-induced hypertension. Obstet Gynecol 1970;36:29–31.
57. Martin JD, Davis RE. Serum folic acid activity and vaginal bleeding in early pregnancy. J Obstet Gynaecol Br Commonw 1964;71:400–3.
58. Martin RH, Harper TA, Kelso W. Serum-folic-acid in recurrent abortions. Lancet 1965;1:670–2.
59. Martin JD, Davis RE, Stenhouse N. Serum folate and vitamin B12 levels in pregnancy with particular reference to uterine bleeding and bacteriuria. J Obstet Gynaecol Br Commonw 1967;74:697–701.
60. Streiff RR, Little B. Folic acid deficiency as a cause of uterine hemorrhage in pregnancy. J Clin Invest 1965;44:1102.
61. Whiteside MG, Ungar B, Cowling DC. Iron, folic acid and vitamin B_{12} levels in normal pregnancy, and their influence on birth-weight and the duration of pregnancy. Med J Aust 1968;1:338–42.
62. Husain OAN, Rothman D, Ellis L. Folic acid deficiency in pregnancy. J Obstet Gynaecol Br Commonw 1963;70:821–7.
63. Abramowicz M, Kass EH. Pathogenesis and prognosis of prematurity (continued). N Engl J Med 1966;275:938–43.
64. Scott KE, Usher R. Fetal malnutrition: its incidence, causes, and effects. Am J Obstet Gynecol 1966;94:951–63.
65. Varadi S, Abbott D, Elwis A. Correlation of peripheral white cell and bone marrow changes with folate levels in pregnancy and their clinical significance. J Clin Pathol 1966;19:33–6.
66. Averback P. Anencephaly associated with megavitamin therapy. Can Med Assoc J 1976;114:995.
67. Mukherjee MD, Sandstead HH, Ratnaparkhi MV, Johnson LK, Milne DB, Stelling HP. Maternal zinc, iron, folic acid, and protein nutriture and outcome of human pregnancy. Am J Clin Nutr 1984;40:496–507.
68. Metz J. Folate deficiency conditioned by lactation. Am J Clin Nutr 1970;23:843–7.
69. Cooperman JM, Dweck HS, Newman LJ, Garbarino C, Lopez R. The folate in human milk. Am J Clin Nutr 1982;36:576–80.
70. Ford JE, Zechalko A, Murphy J, Brooke OG. Comparison of the B vitamin composition of milk from mothers of preterm and term babies. Arch Dis Child 1983;58:367–72.
71. Ek J. Plasma, red cell, and breast milk folacin concentrations in lactating women. Am J Clin Nutr 1983;38:929–35.
72. Ek J, Magnus EM. Plasma and red blood cell folate in breastfed infants. Acta Paediatr Scand 1979;68:239–43.
73. Tamura T, Yoshimura Y, Arakawa T. Human milk folate and folate status in lactating mothers and their infants. Am J Clin Nutr 1980;33:193–7.
74. Thomas MR, Sneed SM, Wei C, Nail PA, Wilson M, Sprinkle EE III. The effects of vitamin C, vitamin B_6, vitamin B_{12}, folic acid, riboflavin, and thiamine on the breast milk and maternal status of well-nourished women at 6 months postpartum. Am J Clin Nutr 1980;33:2151–6.
75. Smith AM, Picciano MF, Deering RH. Folate intake and blood concentrations of term infants. Am J Clin Nutr 1985;41:590–8.
76. Sneed SM, Zane C, Thomas MR. The effects of ascorbic acid, vitamin B_6, vitamin B_{12}, and folic acid supplementation on the breast milk and maternal nutritional status of low socioeconomic lactating women. Am J Clin Nutr 1981;34:1338–46.
77. Deodhar AD, Rajalakshmi R, Ramakrishnan CV. Studies on human lactation. Part III. Effect of dietary vitamin supplementation on vitamin contents of breast milk. Acta Paediatr (Stockholm) 1964;53:42–8.
78. Bank MR, Kirksey A, West K, Giacoia G. Effect of storage time and temperature on folacin and vitamin C levels in term and preterm human milk. Am J Clin Nutr 1985;41:235–42.
79. Committee on Drugs, American Academy of Pediatrics. Transfer of drugs and other chemicals into human milk. Pediatrics 1989;84:924–36.

Name: **FURAZOLIDONE**

Class: **Anti-infective**   Risk Factor: **C**

Fetal Risk Summary

No reports linking the use of furazolidone with congenital defects have been located. The Collaborative Perinatal Project monitored 50,282 mother-child pairs, 132 of which had 1st trimester exposure to furazolidone (1). No association with malformations was found. Theoretically, furazolidone could produce hemolytic anemia in a glucose-6-phosphate-dehydrogenase-deficient newborn if given at term. Placental passage of the drug has not been reported.

Breast Feeding Summary

No data are available.

Reference

1. Heinonen OP, Slone D, Shapiro S. *Birth Defects and Drugs in Pregnancy.* Littleton:Publishing Sciences Group, 1977:299–302.

Name: **FUROSEMIDE**

Class: **Diuretic**   Risk Factor: **C$_M$**

Fetal Risk Summary

Furosemide is a potent diuretic. Cardiovascular disorders, such as pulmonary edema, severe hypertension, or congestive heart failure, are probably the only valid indications for this drug in pregnancy. Furosemide crosses the placenta (1). Following oral doses of 25–40 mg, peak concentrations in cord serum of 330 ng/ml were recorded at 9 hours. Maternal and cord levels were equal at 8 hours. Increased fetal urine production after maternal furosemide therapy has been observed (2, 3). Administration of furosemide to the mother has been used to assess fetal kidney function by provoking urine production which is then visualized by ultrasonic techniques (4, 5). Diuresis was found more often in newborns exposed to furosemide shortly before birth than in controls (6). Urinary sodium and potassium levels in the treated newborns were significantly greater than in the nonexposed controls.

Furosemide is rarely given during the 1st trimester. After the 1st trimester, furosemide has been used for edema, hypertension, and toxemia of pregnancy without causing fetal or newborn adverse effects (7–29). Many investigators now consider diuretics contraindicated in pregnancy, except for patients with cardiovascular disorders, since they do not prevent or alter the course of toxemia and they may decrease placental perfusion (30–33). A 1984 study determined that the use of diuretics for hypertension in pregnancy prevented normal plasma volume expansion and did not change perinatal outcome (34).

Administration of the drug during pregnancy does not significantly alter amniotic fluid volume (28). Serum uric acid levels, which are increased in toxemia, are further elevated by furosemide (35). No association was found in a 1973 study between furosemide and low platelet counts in the neonate (36). Unlike the thiazide diuretics, neonatal thrombocytopenia has not been reported for furosemide.

Breast Feeding Summary

Furosemide is excreted into breast milk (37). No reports of adverse effects in nursing infants have been found. Thiazide diuretics have been used to suppress lactation (see Chlorothiazide).

References

1. Beermann B, Groschinsky-Grind M, Fahraeus L, Lindstroem B. Placental transfer of furosemide. Clin Pharmacol Ther 1978;24:560–2.
2. Wladimiroff JW. Effect of furosemide on fetal urine production. Br J Obstet Gynaecol 1975;82:221–4.
3. Stein WW, Halberstadt E, Gerner R, Roemer E. Effect of furosemide on fetal kidney function. Arch Gynekol 1977;224:114–5.
4. Barrett RJ, Rayburn WF, Barr M Jr. Furosemide (Lasix) challenge test in assessing bilateral fetal hydronephrosis. Am J Obstet Gynecol 1983;147:846–7.
5. Harman CR. Maternal furosemide may not provoke urine production in the compromised fetus. Am J Obstet Gynecol 1984;150:322–3.
6. Pecorari D, Ragni N, Autera C. Administration of furosemide to women during confinement, and its action on newborn infants. Acta Biomed (Italy) 1969;40:2–11.
7. Pulle C. Diuretic therapy in monosymptomatic edema of pregnancy. Minerva Med 1965;56:1622–3.
8. DeCecco L. Furosemide in the treatment of edema in pregnancy. Minerva Med 1965;56:1586–91.
9. Bocci A, Pupita F, Revelli E, Bartoli E, Molaschi M, Massobrio A. The water-salt metabolism in obstetrics and gynecology. Minerva Ginecol 1965;17:103–10.
10. Sideri L. Furosemide in the treatment of oedema in gynaecology and obstetrics. Clin Ter 1966;39:339–46.
11. Wu CC, Lee TT, Kao SC. Evaluation of new diuretic (furosemide) on pregnant women. A pilot study. J Obstet Gynecol Republ China 1966;5:318–20.
12. Loch EG. Treatment of gestosis with diuretics. Med Klin 1966;61:1512–5.
13. Buchheit H, Nicolai KH. Influence of furosemide (Lasix) on gestational edemas. Med Klin 1966;61:1515–8.
14. Tanaka T. Studies on the clinical effect of Lasix in edema of pregnancy and toxemia of pregnancy. Sanka To Fujinka 1966;41:914–20.
15. Merger R, Cohen J, Sadut R. Study of the therapeutic effects of furosemide in obstetrics. Rev Fr Gynecol 1967;62:259–65.
16. Nascimento R, Fernandes R, Cunha A. Furosemide as an accessory in the therapy of the toxemia of pregnancy. Hospital (Portugal) 1967;71:137–40.
17. Finnerty FA Jr. Advantages and disadvantages of furosemide in the edematous states of pregnancy. Am J Obstet Gynecol 1969;105:1022–7.
18. Das Gupta S. Furosemide in blood transfusion for severe anemia in pregnancy. J Obstet Gynaecol India 1970;20:521–5.
19. Kawathekar P, Anusuya SR, Sriniwas P, Lagali S. Diazepam (Calmpose) in eclampsia: a preliminary report of 16 cases. Curr Ther Res 1973;15:845–55.
20. Pianetti F. Our results in the treatment of parturient patients with oedema during the five years 1966–1970. Atti Accad Med Lomb 1973;27:137–40.
21. Azcarte Sanchez S, Quesada Rocha T, Rosas Arced J. Evaluation of a plan of treatment in eclampsia (first report). Ginecol Obstet Mex 1973;34:171–86.
22. Bravo Sandoval J. Management of pre-eclampsia-eclampsia in the third gyneco-obstetrical hospital. Cir Cirjjands 1973;41:487–94.
23. Franck H, Gruhl M. Therapeutic experience with nortensin in the treament of toxemia of pregnancy. Munch Med Wochenschr 1974;116:521–4.
24. Cornu P, Laffay J, Ertel M, Lemiere J. Resuscitation in eclampsia. Rev Prat 1975;25:809–30.
25. Finnerty FA Jr. Management of hypertension in toxemia of pregnancy. Hosp Med 1975;11:52–65.
26. Saldana-Garcia RH. Eclampsia: maternal and fetal mortality. Comparative study of 80 cases. In VIII World Congress of Gynecology and Obstetrics. Int Cong Ser 1976;396:58–9.

27. Palot M, Jakob L, Decaux J, Brundis JP, Quereux C, Wahl P. Arterial hypertensions of labor and the postpartum period. Rev Fr Gynecol Obstet 1979;74:173–6.

28. Votta RA, Parada OH, Windgrad RH, Alvarez OH, Tomassinni TL, Patori AA. Furosemide action on the creatinine concentration of amniotic fluid. Am J Obstet Gynecol 1975;123:621–4.

29. Clark AD, Sevitt LH, Hawkins DF. Use of furosemide in severe toxaemia of pregnancy. Lancet 1972;1:35–6.

30. Pitkin RM, Kaminetzky HA, Newton M, Pritchard JA. Maternal nutrition: a selective review of clinical topics. Obstet Gynecol 1972;40:773–85.

31. Lindheimer MD, Katz AI. Sodium and diuretics in pregnancy. N Engl J Med 1973;288:891–4.

32. Christianson R, Page EW. Diuretic drugs and pregnancy. Obstet Gynecol 1976;48:647–52.

33. Gant NF, Madden JD, Shteri PK, MacDonald PC. The metabolic clearance rate of dehydroisoandrosterone sulfate. IV. Acute effects of induced hypertension, hypotension, and natriuresis in normal and hypertensive pregnancies. Am J Obstet Gynecol 1976;124:143–8.

34. Sibai BM, Grossman RA, Grossman HG. Effects of diuretics on plasma volume in pregnancies with long-term hypertension. Am J Obstet Gynecol 1984;150:831–5.

35. Carswell W, Semple PF. The effect of furosemide on uric acid levels in maternal blood, fetal blood and amniotic fluid. J Obstet Gynaecol Br Commonw 1974;81:472–4.

36. Jerkner K, Kutti J, Victorin L. Platelet counts in mothers and their newborn infants with respect to antepartum administration of oral diuretics. Acta Med Scand 1973;194:473–5.

37. Product information. Lasix. Hoechst-Roussel Pharmaceuticals, 1990.

Name: **GENTAMICIN**

Class: **Antibiotic**   Risk Factor: **C**

Fetal Risk Summary

Gentamicin is an aminoglycoside antibiotic. The drug rapidly crosses the placenta into the fetal circulation and amniotic fluid (1–8). Following 40–80-mg intramuscular (IM) doses given to patients in labor, peak cord serum levels averaging 34–44% of maternal levels were obtained at 1–2 hours (1, 4, 8). No toxicity attributable to gentamicin was seen in any of the newborns. Patients undergoing 1st and 2nd trimester abortions were given 1 mg/kg IM (5). Gentamicin could not be detected in their cord serum before 2 hours. Amniotic fluid levels were undetectable at this dosage up to 9 hours postinjection. Doubling the dose to 2 mg/kg allowed detectable levels in the fluid in one of two samples 5 hours postinjection.

Intra-amniotic instillations of gentamicin were given to 11 patients with premature rupture of the membranes (9). Ten patients received 25 mg every 12 hours and one received 25 mg every 8 hours, for a total of 1–19 doses per patient. Maternal gentamicin serum levels ranged from 0.063–6 µg/ml (all but one were less than 0.6 µg/ml and that one was believed to be due to error). Cord serum levels varied from 0.063–2 µg/ml (all but two were less than 0.6 µg/ml). No harmful effects were seen in the newborns after prolonged exposure to high local concentrations of gentamicin.

No reports linking the use of gentamicin to congenital defects have been located. Ototoxicity, which is known to occur after gentamicin therapy, has not been reported as an effect of *in utero* exposure. However, eighth cranial nerve toxicity in the fetus is well known following exposure to other aminoglycosides (see Kanamycin and Streptomycin) and may potentially occur with gentamicin. Gentamicin and vancomycin, both of which can cause ototoxicity and nephrotoxicity, have been used together during pregnancy without apparent harm to the fetus or newborn (see Vancomycin).

Potentiation of $MgSO_4$-induced neuromuscular weakness has been reported in a neonate exposed during the last 32 hours of pregnancy to 24 g of $MgSO_4$ (10). The depressed infant was treated with gentamicin for sepsis at 12 hours of age. After the second dose, the infant's condition worsened with rapid onset of respiratory arrest. Emergency treatment was successful, and no lasting effects of the toxic interaction were noted.

Breast Feeding Summary

Data on the excretion of gentamicin into breast milk are lacking. In one case report, a nursing infant developed two grossly bloody stools while his mother was receiving gentamicin and clindamycin (10). The condition cleared rapidly when breast feeding was discontinued. Clindamycin is known to be excreted into breast milk, as are other aminoglycosides (see Amikacin, Kanamycin, Streptomycin, and Tobramycin).

References

1. Percetto G, Baratta A, Menozzi M. Observations on the use of gentamicin in gynecology and obstetrics. Minerva Ginecol 1969;21:1–10.
2. von Kobyletzki D. Experimental studies on the transplacental passage of gentamicin. Presented at Fifth International Congress on Chemotherapy, Vienna, 1967.
3. von Koblyetzki D, Wahlig H, Gebhardt F. Pharmacokinetics of gentamicin during delivery. Antimicrobial Anticancer Chemotherapy—Proceedings of the Sixth International Congress on Chemotherapy, Tokyo, 1969;1:650–2.
4. Yoshioka H, Monma T, Matsuda S. Placental transfer of gentamicin. J Pediatr 1972;80:121–3.
5. Garcia S, Ballard C, Martin C, Ivler D, Mathies A, Bernard B. Perinatal pharmacology of gentamicin. Clin Res 1972;20:252.
6. Daubenfeld O, Modde H, Hirsch H. Transfer of gentamicin to the foetus and the amniotic fluid during a steady state in the mother. Arch Gynecol 1974;217:233–40.
7. Kauffman R, Morris J, Azarnoff D. Placental transfer and fetal urinary excetion of gentamicin during constant rate maternal infusion. Pediatr Res 1975;9:104–7.
8. Weistein A, Gibbs R, Gallagher M. Placental transfer of clindamycin and gentamicin in term pregnancy. Am J Obstet Gynecol 1976;124:688–91.
9. Freeman D, Matsen J, Arnold N. Amniotic fluid and maternal and cord serum levels of gentamicin after intra-amniotic instillation in patients with premature rupture of the membranes. Am J Obstet Gynecol 1972;113:1138–41.
10. L'Hommedieu CS, Nicholas D, Armes DA, Jones P, Nelson T, Pickering LK. Potentiation of magnesium sulfate-induced neuromuscular weakness by gentamicin, tobramycin, and amikacin. J Pediatr 1983;102:629–31.
11. Mann CF. Clindamycin and breast-feeding. Pediatrics 1980;66:1030–1.

Name: **GENTIAN VIOLET**

Class: **Disinfectant/Anthelmintic**   Risk Factor: **C**

Fetal Risk Summary

The Collaborative Perinatal Project monitored 50,282 mother-child pairs, 40 of which had 1st trimester exposure to gentian violet (1). Evidence was found to suggest a relationship to malformations based on defects in 4 patients. Independent confirmation is required to determine the actual risk.

Breast Feeding Summary

No data are available.

Reference

1. Heinonen OP, Slone D, Shapiro S. *Birth Defects and Drugs in Pregnancy*. Littleton:Publishing Sciences Group 1977:302.

Name: **GITALIN**

Class: **Cardiac Glycoside**   Risk Factor: **C**

Fetal Risk Summary

See Digitalis.

Breast Feeding Summary

See Digitalis.

Name: **GLYCERIN**

Class: **Diuretic**   Risk Factor: **C**

Fetal Risk Summary

No data are available.

Breast Feeding Summary

No data are available.

Name: **GLYCOPYRROLATE**

Class: **Parasympatholytic (Anticholinergic)**   Risk Factor: **B$_M$**

Fetal Risk Summary

Glycopyrrolate is an anticholinergic agent. In a large prospective study, 2323 patients were exposed to this class of drugs during the 1st trimester, only 4 of whom took glycopyrrolate (1). A possible association was found between the total group and minor malformations. Glycopyrrolate has been used prior to cesarean section to decrease gastric secretions (2–5). Maternal heart rate, but not blood pressure, was increased. Uterine activity increased as expected for normal labor. Fetal heart rate and variability were not changed significantly, confirming the limited placental transfer of this quaternary ammonium compound. No effects in the newborns were observed.

Breast Feeding Summary

No data are available (see also Atropine).

References

1. Heinonen OP, Slone D, Shapiro S. *Birth Defects and Drugs in Pregnancy*. Littleton:Publishing Sciences Group, 1977:346–53.
2. Diaz DM, Diaz SF, Marx GF. Cardiovascular effects of glycopyrrolate and belladonna derivatives in obstetric patients. Bull NY Acad Med 1980;56:245–8.
3. Abboud TK, Read J, Miller F, Chen T, Valle R, Henriksen EH. Use of glycopyrrolate in the parturient: effect on the maternal and fetal heart and uterine activity. Obstet Gynecol 1981;57:224–7.

4. Roper RE, Salem MG. Effects of glycopyrrolate and atropine combined with antacid on gastric acidity. Br J Anaesth 1981;53:1277–80.
5. Abboud T, Raya J, Sadri S, Grobler N, Stine L, Miller F. Fetal and maternal cardiovascular effects of atropine and glycopyrrolate. Anesth Analg 1983;62:426–30.

Name: **GOLD SODIUM THIOMALATE**

Class: **Gold Compound**   Risk Factor: **C**

Fetal Risk Summary

Gold compounds have been used for the treatment of maternal rheumatoid arthritis and other conditions in a small number of pregnancies (1–6). One review noted that several pregnant patients had been treated with gold salts without harmful effects observed in the newborns (1). In a Japanese report, 119 patients were treated during the 1st trimester with gold, 26 of whom received the drug throughout pregnancy (2). Two anomalies were observed in the newborns—a dislocated hip in one infant and a flattened acetabulum in another—but the association with the therapy is unknown. A German case history involved a woman who received her last injection of gold for chronic polyarthritis in the 3rd week of pregnancy (3). A growth-retarded, 1750-g female infant was delivered at 40 weeks' gestation. Other than the low birth weight, no other abnormalities were noted in the infant, whose development during the next 2 years was normal. In another case, a woman had been treated with gold sodium thiomalate (sodium aurothiomalate) for 2 years immediately prior to pregnancy, receiving her last dose when several weeks pregnant (4). No adverse effects in the newborn were mentioned.

Gold compounds cross the placenta. A patient who had received a total dose of 570 mg of gold sodium thiomalate from before conception through the 20th week of gestation elected to terminate her pregnancy (5). No obvious fetal abnormalities were observed, but gold deposits were found in the fetal liver and kidneys. A second patient received monthly 100-mg injections of gold throughout pregnancy (6). The last dose, given 3 days prior to delivery, produced a cord serum concentration of 2.25 μg/ml, 57% of the simultaneous maternal serum level. No anomalies were observed in the infant.

Although gold compounds apparently do not pose a major risk to the fetus, the clinical experience is limited and long-term follow-up studies of exposed fetuses have not been reported.

Breast Feeding Summary

Gold is excreted in milk (4, 7–9). A woman received a total aurothioglucose dose of 135 mg in the postpartum period (7). Gold levels in two milk samples collected a week apart were 8.64 μg/ml and 9.97 μg/ml. The validity of these figures has been challenged on a mathematical basis, so the exact amount excreted is open to question (8). In addition, the timing of the samples in relation to the dose was not given. Of interest, however, was the demonstration of gold levels in the infant's red blood cells (0.354 μg/ml) and serum (0.712 μg/ml) obtained on the same date as the second milk sample. The author speculated that this unexpected oral absorption may have been the cause of various unexplained adverse reactions noted in nursing infants of mothers receiving gold injections, such as rashes, nephritis, hepatitis, and hematologic abnormalities (7).

Another report described a lactating woman who was treated with 50 mg of gold sodium thiomalate weekly for 7 weeks after an initial 20-mg dose (total dose 370 mg) (9). Milk and infant urine samples collected 66 hours after the last dose yielded gold levels of 22 ng/ml and 0.4 ng/ml, respectively. Repeat samples collected 7 days after an additional 25-mg dose produced milk and urine levels of 40 ng/ml and <0.4 ng/ml, respectively. Three months after cessation of therapy, transient facial edema was observed in the nursing infant, but it was not known if this was related to the maternal gold administration.

In a 1986 report, two women were given intramuscular injections of gold sodium thiomalate (4). One patient received 20 mg on day 1 followed by 50 mg on day 3. Milk concentrations rose from a low of 17 ng/ml (1.4% of simultaneous maternal serum) 10 hours after the first dose to a peak of 153 ng/ml (approximately 4.6% of maternal serum) 22 hours after the second dose. The second patient received three doses of the gold salt consisting of 10 mg on day 1, 20 mg on day 8, and 20 mg on day 12. The peak milk concentration, 185 ng/ml (10.4% of maternal serum), occurred 3 hours after the third dose. The levels of gold in the milk of both patients increased steadily over the sampling periods. The investigators estimated that the nursing infant would receive about 20% of the maternal dose (4).

In summary, three studies have described the excretion of gold into breast milk with milk concentrations, in two of the studies, similar in magnitude. Gold absorption by the nursing infant has been documented. Although adverse effects have been suggested, a direct cause and effect relationship has not been proven. At least one set of investigators cautioned that, due to the prolonged maternal elimination time after gold administration and the potential for toxicity in the infant, nursing should be avoided (4). However, the American Academy of Pediatrics considers gold salts to be compatible with breast feeding (10).

References

1. Freyberg RH, Ziff M, Baum J. Gold therapy for rheumatoid arthritis. In Hollander JL, McCarty DJ Jr, eds. Arthritis and Allied Conditions, 8th ed. Philadelphia:Lea & Febiger, 1972:479.
2. Miyamoto T, Miyaji S, Horiuchi Y, Hara M, Ishihara K. Gold therapy in bronchial asthma—special emphasis upon blood level of gold and its teratogenicity. J Jpn Soc Intern Med 1974; 63:1190–7.
3. Fuchs U, Lippert TH. Gold therapy and pregnancy. Dtsch Med Wochenschr 1986;111:31–4.
4. Ostensen M, Skavdal K, Myklebust G, Tomassen Y, Aarbakke J. Excretion of gold into human breast milk. Eur J Clin Pharmacol 1986;31:251–2.
5. Rocker I, Henderson WJ. Transfer of gold from mother to fetus. Lancet 1976;2:1246.
6. Cohen DL, Orzel J, Taylor A. Infants of mothers receiving gold therapy. Arthritis Rheum 1981;24:104–5.
7. Blau SP. Metabolism of gold during lactation. Arthritis Rheum 1973;16:777–8.
8. Gottlieb NL. Suggested errata. Arthritis Rheum 1974;17:1057.
9. Bell RAF, Dale IM. Gold secretion in maternal milk. Arthritis Rheum 1976;19:1374.
10. Committee on Drugs, American Academy of Pediatrics. Transfer of drugs and other chemicals into human milk. Pediatrics 1989;84:924–36.

Name: **GRISEOFULVIN**

Class: **Antifungal**   Risk Factor: **C**

Fetal Risk Summary

Griseofulvin is embryotoxic and teratogenic in some species of animals, but its use in human pregnancy is limited. Because of the animal toxicity, at least one publication suggested that it not be given during pregnancy (1). Placental transfer of griseofulvin has been demonstrated at term (2).

A possible interaction between oral contraceptives and griseofulvin has been reported in 22 women (3). Transient intermenstrual bleeding in 15, amenorrhea in 5, and unintended pregnancies in 2 were described.

In a report from investigators at the US Food and Drug Administration, two sets of conjoined twins were observed in a sample of more than 20,000 birth defect cases with 1st trimester drug exposure (4). The first case involved female twins conjoined at the head and chest (craniothoracopagus syncephalus), while the second involved male dicephalic twins joined in the thorax and lumbar areas with a single seven-chamber heart. In both cases the mothers had taken griseofulvin during early pregnancy. Fission with twinning is normally completed by the 20th day after ovulation, and thus, the cause of conjoined twinning would have to be present prior to this time (4). In both cases, maternal griseofulvin use was the only drug exposure (of those drugs under surveillance by the FDA). Because the incidence of conjoined twins is rare (approximately 1 in 50,000 births) and thoracopagus is even less common (1 in 250,000), the authors concluded that the cases provided evidence for an association with griseofulvin (4). The FDA investigators also examined other data on 1st trimester griseofulvin exposure involving 55,736 deliveries from one geographical area between 1980–1983 (4). Of these cases, griseofulvin was taken during the first 3 months by 37 mothers, two of whom delivered infants with birth defects—one with a congenital heart defect and one with an unknown defect. The incidence of 5.4% (2 of 37) was approximately the incidence in the total sample. However, in 4264 women with spontaneous or threatened abortion diagnoses, seven had been prescribed the drug during the preceding 3 months, a relative risk of 2.5 (95% confidence limits 1.01–6.1) (4).

Prompted by the above report, investigators in two other countries reported data from their respective congenital anomaly registries (5, 6). One of these, from Hungary, found 39 sets of conjoined twins in a sample of more than 100,000 cases of congenital anomalies observed between 1970–1986 (griseofulvin was marketed in Hungary in 1970) (5). None of the mothers of the 39 conjoined twins took griseofulvin. The prevalence of conjoined twins in Hungary is approximately 1 in 60,000 births (5). The investigators also reported data from their case-control surveillance system for the period 1980–1984 (5). Of 6786 congenital anomaly cases, two were exposed to griseofulvin—one infant with a heart defect was exposed during the 2nd and 3rd months, and one infant with pyloric stenosis was exposed during the 1st month. Three exposures occurred in the 10,962 matched controls, all in the late 2nd and 3rd trimesters. The second report involved data from the International Clearinghouse for Birth Defects Monitoring Systems (6). None of the 47 sets of conjoined twins in over 3 million births had been exposed to griseofulvin. Thus, neither of these reports was able to support the FDA report of an association between griseofulvin and the rare defect. However, since the use of an antifungal agent is seldom essential during pregnancy, griseofulvin should be avoided during this time (4).

Breast Feeding Summary

No data are available.

References

1. Anonymous. Griseofulvin: a new formulation and some old concerns. Med Lett Drugs Ther 1976;18:17.
2. Rubin A, Dvornik D. Placental transfer of griseofulvin. Am J Obstet Gynecol 1965;92:882–3.
3. van Dijke CPH, Weber JCP. Interaction between oral contraceptives and griseofulvin. Br Med J 1984;288:1125–6.
4. Rosa FW, Hernandez C, Carlo WA. Griseofulvin teratology, including two thoracopagus conjoined twins. Lancet 1987;1:171.
5. Metneki J, Czeizel A. Griseofulvin teratology. Lancet 1987;1:1042.
6. Knudsen LB. No association between griseofulvin and conjoined twinning. Lancet 1987;2:1097.

Name: **GUAIFENESIN**

Class: **Expectorant**   Risk Factor: **C**

Fetal Risk Summary

The Collaborative Perinatal Project monitored 197 mother-child pairs with 1st trimester exposure to guaifenesin (1, p. 478). An increase in the expected frequency of inguinal hernias was found. For use anytime during pregnancy, 1336 exposures were recorded (1, p. 442). In this latter case, no evidence for an association with malformations was found. In another large study in which 241 women were exposed to the drug during pregnancy, no strong association was found between guaifenesin and congenital defects (2).

A 1981 report described a woman who consumed, throughout pregnancy, 480–840 ml/day of a cough syrup (3). The potential maximum daily doses based on 840 ml of syrup were 16.8 g of guaifenesin, 5.0 g of pseudoephedrine, 1.68 g of dextromethorphan, and 79.8 ml of ethanol. The infant had features of the fetal alcohol syndrome (see Ethanol) and displayed irritability, tremors, and hypertonicity. It is not known if guaifenesin or the other drugs, other than ethanol, were associated with the adverse effects observed in the infant.

Breast Feeding Summary

No data are available.

References

1. Heinonen OP, Slone D, Shapiro S. *Birth Defects and Drugs in Pregnancy*. Littleton:Publishing Sciences Group, 1977.
2. Aselton P, Jick H, Milunsky A, Hunter JR, Stergachis A. First-trimester drug use and congenital disorders. Obstet Gynecol 1985;65:451–5.
3. Chasnoff IJ, Diggs G, Schnoll SH. Fetal alcohol effects and maternal cough syrup abuse. Am J Dis Child 1981;135:968.

Name: **HALOPERIDOL**

Class: **Tranquilizer**   Risk Factor: **C**

Fetal Risk Summary

Two reports describing limb reduction malformations after 1st trimester use of haloperidol have been located (1, 2). In one of these cases, high doses (15 mg/day) were used (2). Other investigations have not found these defects (3–7). Defects observed in the two infants were:

Ectrophocomelia (1)
Multiple upper and lower limb defects,
    aortic valve defect, death (2)

In 98 of 100 patients treated with haloperidol for hyperemesis gravidarum in the 1st trimester, no effects were produced on birth weight, duration of pregnancy, sex ratio, or fetal or neonatal mortality, and no malformations were found in abortuses, stillborn, or liveborn infants (3). Two of the patients were lost to follow-up. In 31 infants with severe reduction deformities born over a 4-year period, none of the mothers remembered taking haloperidol (4). Haloperidol has been used for the control of chorea gravidarum and manic-depressive illness during the 2nd and 3rd trimesters (8, 9). During labor, the drug has been administered to the mother without causing neonatal depression or other effects in the newborn (5).

Breast Feeding Summary

Haloperidol is excreted into breast milk. In one patient receiving an average of 29.2 mg/day, a milk level of 5 ng/ml was detected (10). When the dose was decreased to 12 mg, a level of 2 ng/ml was measured. In a second patient taking 10 mg daily, milk levels up to 23.5 ng/ml were found (11). A milk:plasma ratio of 0.6–0.7 was calculated. No adverse effects were noted in the nursing infant. The American Academy of Pediatrics classifies haloperidol as an agent whose effect on the nursing infant is unknown but may be of concern (12).

References

1. Dieulangard P, Coignet J, Vidal JC. Sur un cas d'ectro-phocomelie peut-etre d'origine medicamenteuse. Bull Fed Gynecol Obstet 1966;18:85–7.
2. Kopelman AE, McCullar FW, Heggeness L. Limb malformations following maternal use of haloperidol. JAMA 1975;231:62–4.
3. Van Waes A, Van de Velde E. Safety evaluation of haloperidol in the treatment of hyperemesis gravidarum. J Clin Pharmacol 1969;9:224–7.
4. Hanson JW, Oakley GP. Haloperidol and limb deformity. JAMA 1975;231:26.
5. Ayd FJ Jr. Haloperidol: fifteen years of clinical experience. Dis Nerv Syst 1972;33:459–69.
6. Magnier P. On hyperemesis gravidarum; a therapeutical study of R 1625. Gynecol Prat 1964;15:17–23.

7. Loke KH, Salleh R. Electroconvulsive therapy for the acutely psychotic pregnant patient: a review of 3 cases. Med J Malaysia 1983;38:131–3.
8. Donaldson JO. Control of chorea gravidarum with haloperidol. Obstet Gynecol 1982;59:381–2.
9. Nurnberg HG. Treatment of mania in the last six months of pregnancy. Hosp Community Psychiatry 1980;31:122–6.
10. Stewart RB, Karas B, Springer PK. Haloperidol excretion in human milk. Am J Psychiatry 1980;137:849–50.
11. Whalley LJ, Blain PG, Prime JK. Haloperidol secreted in breast milk. Br Med J 1981;282:1746–7.
12. Committee on Drugs, American Academy of Pediatrics. Transfer of drugs and other chemicals into human milk. Pediatrics 1989;84:924–36.

Name: **HEPARIN**

Class: **Anticoagulant**   Risk Factor: **C**

Fetal Risk Summary

No reports linking the use of heparin during gestation with congenital defects have been located. Other problems, at times lethal to the fetus or neonate, may be related to heparin or to the severe maternal disease necessitating anticoagulant therapy. Hall and co-workers (1) reviewed the use of heparin and other anticoagulants during pregnancy (167 references) (see also Coumarin Derivatives). They concluded from the published cases in which heparin was used without other anticoagulants that significant risks existed for the mother and fetus and that heparin was not a clearly superior form of anticoagulation during pregnancy. Nageotte and co-workers (2) analyzed the same data to arrive at a different conclusion.

	Hall	Nageotte
Total number of cases	135	120
Term liveborn—no complications	86	86
Premature—survived without complications	19	19
Liveborn—complications (not specified)	1	1
Premature—expired		
Heparin therapy appropriate*	10	5
Heparin therapy not appropriate*		4[a]
Severe maternal disease making successful		
outcome of pregnancy unlikely		1[b]
Spontaneous abortions		
Unknown cause	2	1
Maternal death due to pulmonary embolism		1
Stillbirths		
Heparin therapy appropriate*	17	8
Heparin therapy not appropriate*		7[c]
Heparin and coumadin used		2

*Appropriateness as determined by current standards
[a]Hypertension of pregnancy (4)
[b]Tricuspid atresia (1)
[c]Hypertension of pregnancy (6); proliferative glomerulonephritis (1)

By eliminating the 15 cases in which maternal disease or other drugs were the most likely cause of the fetal problem, the analysis of Nageotte and co-workers results in a 13% (15 of 120) unfavorable outcome vs. the 22% (30 of 135) of Hall and associates. This new value appears to be significantly better than the 31%

(133 of 426) abnormal outcome reported for coumarin derivatives (see Coumarin Derivatives). Furthermore, in contrast to coumarin derivatives where a definite drug-induced pattern of malformations has been observed (fetal warfarin syndrome), heparin has not been related to congenital defects nor does it cross the placenta (3–5). Consequently, the mechanism of heparin's adverse effect on the fetus, if it exists, must be indirect. Hall and co-workers theorized that fetal effects may be due to calcium (or other cation) chelation resulting in the deficiency of that ion(s) in the fetus. A more likely explanation, in light of the report of the Nageotte group, is severe maternal disease that could be relatively independent of heparin. Thus, heparin appears to have major advantages over oral anticoagulants as the treatment of choice during pregnancy (6–13).

A retrospective study, published in 1989, lends support to the argument that heparin therapy is safe for the mother and fetus (14). A total of 77 women were treated with heparin during 100 pregnancies. In 98 pregnancies, therapy was administered for the prevention or treatment of venous thromboembolism, and in two, treatment was because of prosthetic heart valves. In comparison to normal pregnancies, no difference was seen in the case mothers in terms of prematurity, spontaneous abortions, stillbirths, neonatal deaths, or congenital malformations (6). Two bleeding episodes occurred, but there were no symptomatic thrombolic events.

Long-term heparin therapy during pregnancy has been associated with maternal osteopenia (15–19). Both low-dose (10,000 units/day) and high-dose heparin have been implicated, but the latter is more often related to this complication. One study found bone demineralization to be dose related, with more severe changes occurring after long-term therapy (>25 weeks) and in patients who had also received heparin in a previous pregnancy (18). The significant decrease in 1,25-dihydroxyvitamin D levels measured in heparin-treated pregnant patients may be related to the pathogenesis of this adverse effect (16, 17). Similar problems have not been reported in newborns.

Breast Feeding Summary

Heparin is not excreted into breast milk due to its high molecular weight (15,000) (20).

References

1. Hall JG, Pauli RM, Wilson KM. Maternal and fetal sequelae of anticoagulation during pregnancy. Am J Med 1980;68:122–40.
2. Nageotte MP, Freeman RK, Garite TJ, Block RA. Anticoagulation in pregnancy. Am J Obstet Gynecol 1981;141:472.
3. Flessa HC, Kapstrom AB, Glueck HI, Will JJ, Miller MA, Brinker B. Placental transport of heparin. Am J Obstet Gynecol 1965;93:570–3.
4. Russo R, Bortolotti U, Schivazappa L, Girolami A. Warfarin treatment during pregnancy: a clinical note. Haemostasis 1979;8:96–8.
5. Moe N. Anticoagulant-therapy in the prevention of placental infarction and perinatal death. Obstet Gynecol 1982;59:481–3.
6. Hellgren M, Nygards EB. Long-term therapy with subcutaneous heparin during pregnancy. Gynecol Obstet Invest 1982;13:76. As cited in Obstet Gynecol Surv 1982;37:615–6.
7. Cohen AW, Gabbe SG, Mennuti MT. Adjusted-dose heparin therapy by continuous intravenous infusion for recurrent pulmonary embolism during pregnancy. Am J Obstet Gynecol 1983;146:463–4.
8. Howell R, Fidler J, Letsky E. The risks of antenatal subcutaneous heparin prophylaxis: a controlled trial. Br J Obstet Gynaecol 1983;90:1124–8.

9. Vellenga E, van Imhoff GW, Aarnoudse JG. Effective prophylaxis with oral anticoagulants and low-dose heparin during pregnancy in an antithrombin III deficient woman. Lancet 1983;2:224.
10. Bergqvist A, Bergqvist D, Hallbook T. Deep vein thrombosis during pregnancy. Acta Obstet Gynecol Scand 1983;62:443–8.
11. Michiels JJ, Stibbe J, Vellenga E, van Vliet HHDM. Prophylaxis of thrombosis in antithrombin III-deficient women during pregnancy and delivery. Eur J Obstet Gynecol Reprod Biol 1984;18:149–53.
12. Nelson DM, Stempel LE, Fabri PJ, Talbert M. Hickman catheter use in a pregnant patient requiring therapeutic heparin anticoagulation. Am J Obstet Gynecol 1984;149:461–2.
13. Romero R, Duffy TP, Berkowitz RL, Chang E, Hobbins JC. Prolongation of a preterm pregnancy complicated by death of a single twin in utero and disseminated intravascular coagulation: effects of treatment with heparin. N Engl J Med 1984;310:772–4.
14. Ginsberg JS, Kowalchuk G, Hirsh J, Brill-Edwards P, Burrows R. Heparin therapy during pregnancy: risks to the fetus and mother. Arch Intern Med 1989;149:2233–6.
15. Wise PH, Hall AJ. Heparin-induced osteopenia in pregnancy. Br Med J 1980;281:110–1.
16. Aarskog D, Aksnes L, Lehmann V. Low 1,25-dihydroxyvitamin D in heparin-induced osteopenia. Lancet 1980;2:650–1.
17. Aarskog D, Aksnes L, Markestad T, Ulstein M, Sagen N. Heparin-induced inhibition of 1,25-dihydroxyvitamin D formation. Am J Obstet Gynecol 1984;148:1141–2.
18. De Swiet M, Dorrington Ward P, Fidler J, Horsman A, Katz D, Letsky E, Peacock M, Wise PH. Prolonged heparin therapy in pregnancy causes bone demineralization. Br J Obstet Gynaecol 1983;90:1129–34.
19. Griffiths HT, Liu DTY. Severe heparin osteoporosis in pregnancy. Postgrad Med J 1984;60:424–5.
20. O'Reilly RA. Anticoagulant, antithrombotic, and thrombolytic drugs. In Gilman AG, Goodman LS, Gilman A, eds. The Pharmacological Basis of Therapeutics, ed. 6. New York:MacMillan, 1980:1350.

Name: **HEROIN**

Class: **Narcotic Analgesic**   Risk Factor: **B***

Fetal Risk Summary

In the United States, heroin exposure during pregnancy is confined to illicit use as opposed to other countries, such as Great Britain, where the drug is commercially available. The documented fetal toxicity of heroin derives from the illicit use and resulting maternal-fetal addiction. In the form available to the addict, heroin is adulterated with various substances (such as lactose, glucose, mannitol, starch, quinine, amphetamines, strychnine, procaine, or lidocaine) or contaminated with bacteria, viruses or fungi (1, 2). Maternal use of other drugs, abuse and nonabuse, is likely. It is, therefore, difficult to separate entirely the effects of heroin on the fetus from the possible effects of other chemical agents, multiple diseases with addiction, and life style.

Heroin rapidly crosses the placenta, entering fetal tissues within 1 hour of administration. Withdrawal of the drug from the mother causes the fetus to undergo simultaneous withdrawal. Intrauterine death may occur from meconium aspiration (3, 4).

Assessment of fetal maturity and status is often difficult due to uncertain dates and an accelerated appearance of mature lecithin:sphingomyelin ratios (5).

Until recently, the incidence of congenital anomalies was not thought to be increased (6–8). Current data, however, suggest that a significant increase in major anomalies can occur (9). In a group of 830 heroin-addicted mothers, the incidence of infants with congenital abnormalities was significantly greater than in a group of 400 controls (9). Higher rates of jaundice, respiratory distress syndrome, and low Apgar scores were also found. Malformations reported with heroin are multiple and varied with no discernible patterns of defects (6–13). In addition, all of the mothers in the studies reporting malformed infants were consuming numerous other drugs, including drugs of abuse.

Characteristics of the infant delivered from a heroin-addicted mother may be (14):

Accelerated liver maturity with a lower incidence of jaundice (8, 15)
Lower incidence of hyaline membrane disease after 32 weeks' gestation (5, 16)
Normal Apgar scores (6)

(*Note*: The findings of Ostrea and Chavez (9) are in disagreement with the above statements.)

Low birth weight; up to 50% weigh less than 2500 g
Small size for gestational age
Narcotic withdrawal in about 85% (58–91%): symptoms apparent usually within the first 48 hours with some delaying up to 6 days; incidence is directly related to daily dose and length of maternal addiction; hyperactivity, respiratory distress, fever, diarrhea, mucus secretion, sweating, convulsions, yawning and face scratching (7, 8)
Meconium staining of amniotic fluid
Elevated serum magnesium levels when withdrawal signs are present (up to twice normal)
Increased perinatal mortality; rates up to 37% in some series (13)

Random chromosome damage was significantly higher when Apgar scores were 6 or less (12, 17). However, only one case has appeared relating chromosome abnormalities to congenital anomalies (12). The clinical significance of this is doubtful. The lower incidence of hyaline membrane disease may be due to elevated prolactin blood levels in fetuses of addicted mothers (18).

Long-term effects on growth and behavior have been reported (19). As compared to controls, children aged 3–6 years delivered from addicted mothers were found to have lower weights, lower heights, and impaired behavior, perceptual, and organizational abilities.

[*Risk factor D if used for prolonged periods or in high doses at term.]

Breast Feeding Summary

Heroin crosses into breast milk in sufficient quantities to cause addiction in the infant (20). A milk:plasma ratio has not been reported. Previous investigators have considered nursing as one method for treating the addicted newborn (21). The American Academy of Pediatrics classifies heroin abuse as a contraindication to breast feeding (22).

References

1. Anonymous. Diagnosis and management of reactions to drug abuse. Med Lett Drugs Ther 1980;22:74.
2. Thomas L. Notes of a biology-watcher. N Engl J Med 1972;286:531–3.

3. Chappel JN. Treatment of morphine-type dependence. JAMA 1972;221:1516.
4. Rementeria JL, Nunag NN. Narcotic withdrawal in pregnancy: stillbirth incidence with a case re-port. Am J Obstet Gynecol 1973;116:1152–6.
5. Gluck L, Kulovich MV. Lecithin/sphingomyelin ratios in amniotic fluid in normal and abnormal pregnancy. Am J Obstet Gynecol 1973;115:539–46.
6. Reddy AM, Harper RG, Stern G. Observations on heroin and methadone withdrawal in the new-born. Pediatrics 1971;48:353–8.
7. Stone ML, Salerno LJ, Green M, Zelson C. Narcotic addiction in pregnancy. Am J Obstet Gynecol 1971;109:716–23.
8. Zelson C, Rubio E, Wasserman E. Neonatal narcotic addiction: 10 year observation. Pediatrics 1971;48:178–89.
9. Ostrea EM, Chavez CJ. Perinatal problems (excluding neonatal withdrawal) in maternal drug ad-diction: a study of 830 cases. J Pediatr 1979;94:292–5.
10. Perlmutter JF. Drug addiction in pregnant women. Am J Obstet Gynecol 1967;99:569–72.
11. Krause SO, Murray PM, Holmes JB, Burch RE. Heroin addiction among pregnant women and their newborn babies. Am J Obstet Gynecol 1958;75:754–8.
12. Kushnick T, Robinson M, Tsao C. 45,X chromosome abnormality in the offspring of a narcotic addict. Am J Dis Child 1972;124:772–3.
13. Naeye RL, Blanc W, Leblanc W, Khatamee MA. Fetal complications of maternal heroin addiction: abnormal growth, infections and episodes of stress. J Pediatr 1973;83:1055–61.
14. Perlmutter JF. Heroin addiction and pregnancy. Obstet Gynecol Surv 1974;29:439–46.
15. Nathenson G, Cohen MI, Liff IF, McNamara H. The effect of maternal heroin addiction on neona-tal jaundice. J Pediatr 1972;81:899–903.
16. Glass L, Rajegowda BK, Evans HE. Absence of respiratory distress syndrome in premature in-fants of heroin-addicted mothers. Lancet 1971;2:685–6.
17. Amarose AP, Norusis MJ. Cytogenetics of methadone-managed and heroin-addicted pregnant women and their newborn infants. Am J Obstet Gynecol 1976;124:635–40.
18. Parekh A, Mukherjee TK, Jhaveri R, Rosenfeld W, Glass L. Intrauterine exposure to narcotics and cord blood prolactin concentrations. Obstet Gynecol 1981;57:447–9.
19. Wilson GS, McCreary R, Kean J, Baxter JC. The development of preschool children of heroin-addicted mothers: a controlled study. Pediatrics 1979;63:135–41.
20. Lichlenstein PM. Infant drug addiction. NY Med J 1915;102:905. As reported by Cobrinik RW, et al, in Pediatrics 1959;24:288–304.
21. Cobrinik RW, Hood RT Jr, Chusid E. The effect of maternal narcotic addiction on the newborn infant. Pediatrics 1959;24:288–304.
22. Committee on Drugs, American Academy of Pediatrics. Transfer of drugs and other chemicals into human milk. Pediatrics 1989;84:924–36.

Name: **HETACILLIN**

Class: **Antibiotic**   Risk Factor: **B**

Fetal Risk Summary

Hetacillin, a penicillin antibiotic, breaks down in aqueous solution to ampicillin and acetone (see Ampicillin).

Breast Feeding Summary

See Ampicillin.

Name: **HEXAMETHONIUM**

Class: **Antihypertensive**   Risk Factor: **C**

Fetal Risk Summary

No reports linking the use of hexamethonium with congenital defects have been located. Hexamethonium crosses the placenta and accumulates in the amniotic fluid. The drug has been used in the treatment of preeclampsia and essential hypertension. Its use in these conditions is no longer recommended. Three cases of paralytic ileus and one case of delayed passage of meconium have been reported (1, 2).

Breast Feeding Summary

No data are available.

References

1. Morris N. Hexamethonium in the treatment of pre-eclampsia and essential hypertension during pregnancy. Lancet 1953;1:322–4.
2. Hallum JL, Hatchuel WLF. Congenital paralytic ileus in a premature baby as a complication of hexamethonium bromide therapy for toxemia of pregnancy. Arch Dis Child 1954;29:354–6.

Name: **HEXOCYCLIUM**

Class: **Parasympatholytic (Anticholinergic)**   Risk Factor: **C**

Fetal Risk Summary

Hexocyclium is an anticholinergic agent. No reports of its use in pregnancy have been located (see also Atropine).

Breast Feeding Summary

No data are available (see also Atropine).

Name: **HOMATROPINE**

Class: **Parasympatholytic (Anticholinergic)**   Risk Factor: **C**

Fetal Risk Summary

Homatropine is an anticholinergic agent. The Collaborative Perinatal Project monitored 50,282 mother-child pairs, 26 of which used homatropine in the 1st trimester (1, pp. 346–353). For use anytime during pregnancy, 86 exposures were recorded (1, p. 439). Only for anytime use was a possible association with congenital defects discovered. In addition, when the group of parasympatholytics was taken as a whole (2323 exposures), a possible association with minor malformations was found (1, pp. 346–353).

Breast Feeding Summary

See Atropine.

Reference

1. Heinonen OP, Slone D, Shapiro S. *Birth Defects and Drugs in Pregnancy*. Littleton:Publishing Sciences Group, 1977.

Name: **HORMONAL PREGNANCY TEST TABLETS**

Class: **Estrogenic/Progestogenic Hormones**   Risk Factor: **X**

Fetal Risk Summary

See Oral Contraceptives.

Breast Feeding Summary

See Oral Contraceptives.

Name: **HYDRALAZINE**

Class: **Antihypertensive**   Risk Factor: C_M

Fetal Risk Summary

No reports linking the use of hydralazine with congenital defects have been located. In England, hydralazine is the most commonly used antihypertensive agent in pregnant women (1). Neonatal thrombocytopenia and bleeding secondary to maternal ingested hydralazine have been reported in three infants (2). In each case, the mother had consumed the drug daily throughout the 3rd trimester. This complication has also been reported in series examining severe maternal hypertension and may be related to the disease rather than to the drug (3, 4).

Hydralazine readily crosses the placenta to the fetus (5). Serum concentrations in the fetus are equal to or greater than those in the mother.

The Collaborative Perinatal Project monitored 50,282 mother-child pairs, eight of which had 1st trimester exposure to hydralazine (6, p. 372). For use anytime during pregnancy, 136 cases were recorded (6, p. 441). No defects were observed with 1st trimester use. There were eight infants born with defects who were exposed in the 2nd or 3rd trimesters. This incidence (5.8%) is greater than the expected frequency of occurrence, but the severe maternal disease necessitating the use of hydralazine is probably responsible. Patients with preeclampsia are at risk for a marked increase in fetal mortality (7–10).

A number of studies involving the use of hydralazine either alone or in combination with other antihypertensives have found the drug to be relatively safe for the fetus (4, 7–17). Fatal maternal hypotension has been reported in one patient after combined therapy with hydralazine and diazoxide (18). Two reports published in

1989 associated adverse effects in the fetus and newborn with maternal hydralazine therapy (19, 20).

In a woman with chronic hypertension maintained on methyldopa, an increase in blood pressure at about 35 weeks' gestation prompted the addition of hydralazine, 25 mg twice daily, to the treatment regimen (19). Fetal premature atrial contractions were diagnosed 1 week later, but tachyarrhythmias, which can be initiated by premature atrial contractions, were not observed (19). Hospitalization with bed rest allowed the patient's blood pressure to decline enough to discontinue hydralazine therapy. Within 24 hours of stopping hydralazine, the fetal arrhythmia resolved. The infant was delivered at 38 weeks and cardiac evaluation after discharge at 3 days indicated a regular heart rate. A syndrome resembling lupus erythematosus was diagnosed in a 29-year-old woman treated with intravenous hydralazine during the 28th week of pregnancy (20). The patient received 425 mg over a 6-day period for the treatment of hypertension. Intravenous methyldopa was administered on the 6th day of therapy. Labor was induced for fetal distress and a 780-g growth-retarded male infant was delivered vaginally. The infant expired at 36 hours of age secondary to cardiac tamponade induced by 7 ml of clear sterile transudate in the pericardial space. Lupus-like symptoms consisting of macular rash, arthralgia, and bilateral pleural effusion developed in the mother on the 5th day of hydralazine therapy and gradually resolved after discontinuance of the drug and delivery. The findings of pericardial effusion and cardiac tamponade in the infant were also thought to represent clinical evidence of a lupus-like syndrome (20). The symptoms in both the mother and fetus were attributed to hydralazine sensitivity resulting in the induction of a lupus-like syndrome.

Breast Feeding Summary

Hydralazine is excreted into breast milk (5). In one patient treated with 50 mg three times daily, the milk:plasma ratio 2 hours after a dose was 1.4. This value is in close agreement with the predicted ratio calculated from the pK_a (21). The available dose of hydralazine in 75 ml of milk was estimated to be 13 μg (5). No adverse effects were noted in the nursing infant from this small concentration. The American Academy of Pediatrics considers hydralazine to be compatible with breast feeding (22).

References

1. de Swiet M. Antihypertensive drugs in pregnancy. Br Med J 1985;291:365–6.
2. Widerlov E, Karlman I. Storsater J. Hydralazine-induced neonatal thrombocytopenia. N Engl J Med 1980;303:1235.
3. Brazy JE, Grimm JK, Little VA. Neonatal manifestations of severe maternal hypertension occurring before the thirty-sixth week of pregnancy. J Pediatr 1982;100:265–71.
4. Sibai BM, Anderson GD. Pregnancy outcome of intensive therapy in severe hypertension in first trimester. Obstet Gynecol 1986;67:517–22.
5. Liedholm H, Wahlin-Boll E, Ingemarsson I, Melander A. Transplacental passage and breast milk concentrations of hydralazine. Eur J Clin Pharmacol 1982;21:417–9.
6. Heinonen OP, Slone D, Shapiro S. Birth Defects and Drugs in Pregnancy. Littleton:Publishing Sciences Group, 1977.
7. Bott-Kanner G, Schweitzer A, Schoenfeld A, Joel-Cohen J, Rosenfeld JB. Treatment with propranolol and hydralazine throughout pregnancy in a hypertensive patient. Isr J Med Sci 1978;14:466–8.
8. Pritchard JA, Pritchard SA. Standardized treatment of 154 consecutive cases of eclampsia. Am J Obstet Gynecol 1975;123:543–52.
9. Chapman ER, Strozier WE, Magee RA. The clinical use of Apresoline in the toxemias of pregnancy. Am J Obstet Gynecol 1954;68:1109–17.

10. Johnson GT, Thompson RB. A clinical trial of intravenous Apresoline in the management of toxemia of late pregnancy. J Obstet Gynecol 1958;65:360–6.
11. Kuzniar J, Skret A, Piela A, Szmigiel Z, Zaczek T. Hemodynamic effects of intravenous hydralazine in pregnant women with severe hypertension. Obstet Gynecol 1985;66:453–8.
12. Hogstedt S, Lindeberg S, Axelsson O, Lindmark G, Rane A, Sandstrom B, Lindberg BS. A prospective controlled trial of metoprolol-hydralazine treatment in hypertension during pregnancy. Acta Obstet Scand 1985;64:505–10.
13. Gallery EDM, Ross MR, Gyory AZ. Antihypertensive treatment in pregnancy: analysis of different responses to oxprenolol and methyldopa. Br Med J 1985;291:563–6.
14. Horvath JS, Korda A, Child A, Henderson-Smart D, Phippard A, Duggin GG, Hall BM, Tiller DJ. Hypertension in pregnancy: a study of 142 women presenting before 32 weeks' gestation. Med J Aust 1985;143:19–21.
15. Rosenfeld J, Bott-Kanner G, Boner G, Nissenkorn A, Friedman S, Ovadia J, Merlob P, Reisner S, Paran E, Zmora E, Biale Y, Insler V. Treatment of hypertension during pregnancy with hydralazine monotherapy or with combined therapy with hydralazine and pindolol. Eur J Obstet Gynecol Reprod Biol 1986;22:197–204.
16. Mabie WC, Gonzalez AR, Sibai BM, Amon E. A comparative trial of labetalol and hydralazine in the acute management of severe hypertension complicating pregnancy. Obstet Gynecol 1987;70:328–33.
17. Owen J, Hauth JC. Polyarteritis nodosa in pregnancy: a case report and brief literature review. Am J Obstet Gynecol 1989;160:606–7.
18. Henrich WL, Cronin R, Miller PD, Anderson RJ. Hypotensive sequelae of diazoxide and hydralazine therapy. JAMA 1977;237:264–5.
19. Lodeiro JG, Feinstein SJ, Lodeiro SB. Fetal premature atrial contractions associated with hydralazine. Am J Obstet Gynecol 1989;160:105–7.
20. Yemini M, Shoham(Schwartz) Z, Dgani R, Lancet M, Mogilner BM, Nissim F, Bar-Khayim Y. Lupus-like syndrome in a mother and newborn following administration of hydralazine: a case report. Eur J Obstet Gynecol Reprod Biol 1989;30:193–7.
21. Daily JW. Anticoagulant and cardiovascular drugs. In Wilson JT, ed. Drugs in Breast Milk. Balgowlah, Australia:ADIS Press, 1981:61–4.
22. Committee on Drugs, American Academy of Pediatrics. Transfer of drugs and other chemicals into human milk. Pediatrics 1989;84:924–36.

Name: **HYDRIODIC ACID**

Class: **Expectorant**   Risk Factor: **D**

Fetal Risk Summary

The active ingredient of hydriodic acid is iodide (see Potassium Iodide).

Breast Feeding Summary

See Potassium Iodide.

Name: **HYDROCHLOROTHIAZIDE**

Class: **Diuretic**   Risk Factor: **D**

Fetal Risk Summary

See Chlorothiazide.

Breast Feeding Summary

See Chlorothiazide.

Name: **HYDROCODONE**

Class: **Narcotic Analgesic/Antitussive** Risk Factor: **B***

Fetal Risk Summary

No reports linking the use of hydrocodone with congenital defects have been located. Due to its narcotic properties, withdrawal could theoretically occur in infants exposed *in utero* to prolonged maternal ingestion of hydrocodone.

[*Risk Factor D if used for prolonged periods or in high doses at term.]

Breast Feeding Summary

No data are available.

Name: **HYDROFLUMETHIAZIDE**

Class: **Diuretic** Risk Factor: **D**

Fetal Risk Summary

See Chlorothiazide.

Breast Feeding Summary

See Chlorothiazide.

Name: **HYDROMORPHONE**

Class: **Narcotic Analgesic** Risk Factor: **B***

Fetal Risk Summary

No reports linking the use of hydromorphone with congenital defects have been located. Withdrawal could occur in infants exposed *in utero* to prolonged maternal ingestion of hydromorphone. Use of the drug in pregnancy is primarily confined to labor. Respiratory depression in the neonate similar to that produced by meperidine or morphine should be expected (1).

[*Risk Factor D if used for prolonged periods or in high doses at term.]

Breast Feeding Summary

No data are available.

Reference

1. Bonica J. *Principles and Practice of Obstetric Analgesia and Anesthesia.* Philadelphia:FA Davis, 1967:251.

Name: **HYDROXYPROGESTERONE**

Class: **Progestogenic Hormone**   Risk Factor: **D**

Fetal Risk Summary

The Food and Drug Administration mandated deletion of pregnancy-related indications from all progestins because of a possible association with congenital anomalies. Ambiguous genitalia of both male and female fetuses have been reported with hydroxyprogesterone (see also Norethindrone, Norethynodrel) (1–3). The Collaborative Perinatal Project monitored 866 mother-child pairs with 1st trimester exposure to progestational agents (including 162 with exposure to hydroxyprogesterone) (4, pp. 389, 391). An increase in the expected frequency of cardiovascular defects and hypospadias was observed for both estrogens and progestogens (4, p. 394; 5). Reevaluation of these data in terms of timing of exposure, vaginal bleeding in early pregnancy, and previous maternal obstetric history, however, failed to support an association between female sex hormones and cardiac malformations (6).

Dillion (7, 8) reported six infants with malformations exposed to hydroxyprogesterone during various stages of gestation. The congenital defects included spina bifida, anencephalus, hydrocephalus, Fallot's tetralogy, common truncus arteriosus, cataract, and ventricular septal defect. Complete absence of both thumbs and dislocated head of the right radius in a child have been associated with hydroxyprogesterone (8). Use of diazepam in early pregnancy and the lack of similar reports make an association doubtful.

A 1985 study described 2754 offspring born to mothers who had vaginal bleeding during the 1st trimester (9). Of the total group, 1608 of the newborns were delivered from mothers treated during the 1st trimester with either oral medroxyprogesterone (20–30 mg/day), 17-hydroxyprogesterone (500 mg/week by injection), or a combination of the two. Medroxyprogesterone was used exclusively in 1274 (79.2%) of the study group. The control group consisted of 1146 infants delivered from mothers who bled during the 1st trimester but who were not treated. There were no differences between the study and control groups in the overall rate of malformations (120 vs. 123.9/1000, respectively) or in the rate of major malformations (63.4 vs. 71.5/1000, respectively). Another 1985 study compared 988 infants, exposed *in utero* to various progesterones, to a matched cohort of 1976 unexposed controls (10). No association between the use of progestins, primarily progesterone and 17-hydroxyprogesterone, and fetal malformations was discovered.

Developmental changes in the psychosexual performance of boys has been attributed to *in utero* exposure to hydroxyprogesterone (11). The mothers received an estrogen/progestogen regimen for their diabetes. Hormone-exposed males demonstrated a trend to have less heterosexual experience and fewer masculine interests than controls.

The use of high-dose hydroxprogesterone during the 2nd and 3rd trimesters has been advocated for the prevention of premature labor (12, 13). However, the use of the steroid was not effective in twin pregnancies (14). Fetal adverse effects were not observed.

Breast Feeding Summary

No data are available.

References

1. Dayan E, Rosa FW. Fetal ambiguous genitalia associated with sex hormone use early in pregnancy. ADR Highlights 1981:1–14. Food and Drug Administration, Division of Drug Experience.
2. Wilkins L. Masculinization of female fetus due to use of orally given progestins. JAMA 1960;172;1028–32.
3. Wilkins L, Jones HW, Holman GH, Stempfel RS Jr. Masculinization of the female fetus associated with administration of oral and intramuscular progestins during gestation: non-adrenal female pseudohermaphrodism. J Clin Endocrinol Metab 1958;68:559–85
4. Heinonen OP, Slone D, Shapiro S. Birth Defects and Drugs in Pregnancy. Littleton:Publishing Sciences Group, 1977.
5. Heinonen OP, Slone D, Monson RR, Hook EB, Shapiro S. Cardiovascular birth defects and antenatal exposure to female sex hormones. N Engl J Med 1977;296:67–70.
6. Wiseman RA, Dodds-Smith IC. Cardiovascular birth defects and antenatal exposure to female sex hormones: a reevaluation of some base data. Teratology 1984;30:359–70.
7. Dillion S. Congenital malformations and hormones in pregnancy. Br Med J 1976;2:1446.
8. Dillon S. Progestogen therapy in early pregnancy and associated congenital defects. Practitioner 1970;205:80–4.
9. Katz Z, Lancet M, Skornik J, Chemke J, Mogilner BM, Klinberg M. Teratogenicity of progestogens given during the first trimester of pregnancy. Obstet Gynecol 1985;65:775–80.
10. Resseguie LJ, Hick JF, Bruen JA, Noller KL, O'Fallon WM, Kurland LT. Congenital malformations among offspring exposed in utero to progestins, Olmsted County, Minnesota, 1936–1974. Fertil Steril 1985;43:514–9.
11. Yalom ID, Green R, Fisk N. Prenatal exposure to female hormones. Effect on psychosexual development in boys. Arch Gen Psychiatry 1973;28:554–61.
12. Johnson JWC, Austin KL, Jones GS, Davis GH, King TM. Efficacy of 17-hydroxyprogesterone caproate in the prevention of premature labor. N Engl J Med 1975;293:675–80.
13. Johnson JWC, Lee PA, Zachary AS, Calhoun S, Migeon CJ. High-risk prematurity-progestin treatment and steroid studies. Obstet Gynecol 1979;54:412–8.
14. Hartikainen-Sorri AL, Kauppila A, Tuimala R. Inefficacy of 17-hydroxyprogesterone caproate in the prevention of prematurity in twin pregnancy. Obstet Gynecol 1980;56:692–5.

Name: **HYDROXYUREA**

Class: **Antineoplastic**   Risk Factor: **D**

Fetal Risk Summary

Hydroxyurea, an antineoplastic agent, is teratogenic in animals, but human pregnancy experience is very limited. Two women, both with acute myelocytic leukemia, were treated with five-drug chemotherapy regimens at 17' and 27 weeks' gestation, respectively (1). In both cases, hydroxyurea (8 mg) was given as an initial, single intravenous dose. One woman underwent an elective abortion of a grossly normal fetus 4 weeks after the start of chemotherapy. The second patient delivered a premature infant at 31 weeks, again 4 weeks after the start of therapy. Follow-up at 13.5 months revealed normal growth and development.

The outcomes of pregnancies exposed to chemotherapy prior to conception were described in a 1984 report (2). In 436 long-term survivors treated with chemotherapy for gestational trophoblastic neoplasms between 1958–1978, 69 (16%) received hydroxyurea as part of their treatment regimens (2). Of the 69 women, 14 (20%) had at least one live birth (numbers in parentheses refer to mean/maximum hydroxyurea dose in grams) (3.6/8.0), three (4%) had no live births (6.3/16.0), three (4%) failed to conceive (3.0/6.0), and 49 (71%) did not try to conceive (9.4/47.0). Additional details, including congenital anomalies observed, are described in the monograph for methotrexate (see Methotrexate).

Occupational exposure of the mother to antineoplastic agents during pregnancy may present a risk to the fetus. A position statement from the National Study Commission on Cytotoxic Exposure and a research article involving some antineoplastic agents are presented in the monograph for cyclophosphamide (see Cyclophosphamide).

Breast Feeding Summary

Hydroxyurea is excreted into human milk. A 29-year-old breast-feeding woman with recently diagnosed chronic myelogenous leukemia was treated with oral hydroxyurea, 500 mg orally three times daily (3). Breast feeding was halted prior to initiation of the chemotherapy. Milk samples were collected 2 hours after the last dose for 7 days. Due to technical difficulties with the analysis, milk concentrations of hydroxyurea could only be determined on days 1, 3, and 4. The mean level of hydroxyurea was 6.1 µg/ml (range 3.8–8.4 µg/ml). Serum concentrations were not measured. Although these concentrations are low, the potential for adverse effects in the infant indicates that nursing should be considered contraindicated during hydroxyurea therapy.

References

1. Doney KC, Kraemer KG, Shepard TH. Combination chemotherapy for acute myelocytic leukemia during pregnancy: three case reports. Cancer Treat Rep 1979;63:369–71.
2. Rustin GJS, Booth M, Dent J, Salt S, Rustin F, Bagshawe KD. Pregnancy after cytotoxic chemotherapy for gestational trophoblastic tumours. Br Med J 1984;288:103–6.
3. Sylvester RK, Lobell M, Teresi ME, Brundage D, Dubowy R. Excretion of hydroxyurea into milk. Cancer 1987;60:2177–8.

Name: **HYDROXYZINE**

Class: **Tranquilizer**   Risk Factor: **C**

Fetal Risk Summary

Hydroxyzine belongs to the same class of compounds as buclizine, cyclizine, and meclizine. Although an animal teratogen in high doses, human teratogenicity has not been proven. In 100 patients treated in the 1st trimester with oral hydroxyzine (50 mg daily) for nausea and vomiting, no significant difference from nontreated controls was found in fetal wastage or anomalies (1). The Collaborative Perinatal Project monitored 50,282 mother-child pairs, 50 of which had 1st trimester exposure to hydroxyzine (2, pp. 335–337, 341). For use anytime during pregnancy, 187 exposures were recorded (2, p. 438). Based on five malformed children, a possible relationship was found between 1st trimester use and congenital defects, but the numbers were too small to determine statistical significance. The manufacturer considers the drug to be contraindicated in early pregnancy (3). During labor, hydroxyzine has been shown to be safe and effective for the relief of anxiety (4). No effect on the progress of labor or on neonatal Apgar scores was observed.

Breast Feeding Summary

No data are available.

References

1. Erez S, Schifrin BS, Dirim O. Double-blind evaluation of hydroxyzine as an antiemetic in pregnancy. J Reprod Med 1971;7:57–9.
2. Heinonen OP, Slone D, Shapiro S. *Birth Defects and Drugs in Pregnancy*. Littleton:Publishing Sciences Group, 1977.
3. Product information. Vistaril. Pfizer Laboratories, 1990.
4. Zsigmond EK, Patterson RL. Double-blind evaluation of hydroxyzine hydrochloride in obstetric anesthesia. Anesth Analg (Cleve) 1967;46:275.

Name: *l*-HYOSCYAMINE

Class: **Parasympatholytic (Anticholinergic)**   Risk Factor: **C**

Fetal Risk Summary

l-Hyoscyamine is an anticholinergic agent. No reports of its use in pregnancy have been located (see also Belladonna or Atropine).

Breast Feeding Summary

See Atropine.

Name: **HYPERALIMENTATION, PARENTERAL**

Class: **Nutrient**   Risk Factor: **C**

Fetal Risk Summary

Parenteral hyperalimentation (TPN) is the administration of an intravenous solution designed to provide complete nutritional support for a patient unable to maintain adequate nutritional intake. The solution is normally composed of dextrose (5–35%), amino acids (3.5–5%), vitamins, electrolytes, and trace elements. Lipids (intravenous fat emulsions) are often given with TPN to supply essential fatty acids and calories (see Lipids). A number of studies describing the use of TPN in pregnant women have been published (1–23). A report of four additional cases with a review of the literature appeared in 1986 (24). Maternal indications for TPN have been varied, with duration of therapy ranging from a few days to the entire pregnancy. Eleven patients were treated during the 1st trimester (1–5). No fetal complications attributable to TPN, including newborn hypoglycemia, have been identified in any of the reports. Intrauterine growth retardation occurred in five infants and one of these died, but the retarded growth and neonatal death were most likely due to the underlying maternal disease (2–4, 6–9, 22). In a group of eight women treated with TPN for severe hyperemesis gravidarum and who delivered live babies, the ratio of birth weight to standard mean weight for gestational age was greater than 1.0 in each case (5).

Obstetric complications included the worsening of one mother's renal hypertension after TPN was initiated, but the relationship between the effect and the therapy is not known (8). In a second case, resistance to oxytocin-induced labor was observed, but, again, the relationship to TPN is not clear (9).

Maternal and fetal death secondary to cardiac tamponade during central hyperalimentation has been reported (25). A 22-year-old woman in the 3rd trimester of pregnancy was treated with TPN for severe hyperemesis gravidarum. Seven days after commencing central TPN therapy, the patient experienced acute sharp retrosternal pain and dyspnea (25). Cardiac tamponade was subsequently diagnosed, but the mother and the fetus expired before the condition could be corrected. Percutaneous pericardiocentesis yielded 70 ml of fluid that was a mixture of the TPN and lipid solutions that the patient had been receiving.

In summary, the use of total parenteral hyperalimentation does not seem to pose a risk to the fetus or newborn provided that normal procedures, as with nonpregnant patients, are followed to prevent maternal complications.

Breast Feeding Summary

No problems should be expected in nursing infants whose mothers are receiving total parenteral hyperalimentation.

References

1. Hew LR, Deitel M. Total parenteral nutrition in gynecology and obstetrics. Obstet Gynecol 1980;55:464–8.
2. Tresadern JC, Falconer GF, Turnberg LA, Irving MH. Successful completed pregnancy in a patient maintained on home parenteral nutrition. Br Med J 1983;286:602–3.
3. Tresadern JC, Falconer GF, Turnberg LA, Irving MH. Maintenance of pregnancy in a home parenteral nutrition patient. JPEN 1984;8:199–202.
4. Breen KJ, McDonald IA, Panelli D, Ihle B. Planned pregnancy in a patient who was receiving home parenteral nutrition. Med J Aust 1987;146:215–7.
5. Levine MG, Esser D. Total parenteral nutrition for the treatment of severe hyperemesis gravidarum: maternal nutritional effects and fetal outcome. Obstet Gynecol 1988;72:102–7.
6. Gineston JL, Capron JP, Delcenserie R, Delamarre J, Blot M, Boulanger JC. Prolonged total parenteral nutrition in a pregnant woman with acute pancreatitis. J Clin Gastroenterol 1984;6:249–52.
7. Lakoff KM, Feldman JD. Anorexia nervosa associated with pregnancy. Obstet Gynecol 1972;39:699–701.
8. Lavin JP Jr, Gimmon Z, Miodovnik M, von Meyenfeldt M, Fischer JE. Total parenteral nutrition in a pregnant insulin-requiring diabetic. Obstet Gynecol 1982;59:660–4.
9. Weinberg RB, Sitrin MD, Adkins GM, Lin CC. Treatment of hyperlipidemic pancreatitis in pregnancy with total parenteral nutrition. Gastroenterology 1982;83:1300–5.
10. Di Costanzo J, Martin J, Cano N, Mas JC, Noirclerc M. Total parenteral nutrition with fat emulsions during pregnancy — nutritional requirements: a case report. JPEN 1982;6:534–8.
11. Young KR. Acute pancreatitis in pregnancy: two case reports. Obstet Gynecol 1982;60:653–7.
12. Rivera-Alsina ME, Saldana LR, Stringer CA. Fetal growth sustained by parenteral nutrition in pregnancy. Obstet Gynecol 1984;64:138–41.

13. Seifer DB, Silberman H, Catanzarite VA, Conteas CN, Wood R, Ueland K. Total parenteral nutrition in obstetrics. JAMA 1985;253:2073–5.
14. Benny PS, Legge M, Aickin DR. The biochemical effects of maternal hyperalimentation during pregnancy. NZ Med J 1978;88:283–5.
15. Cox KL, Byrne WJ, Ament ME. Home total parenteral nutrition during pregnancy: a case report. JPEN 1981;5:246–9.
16. Gamberdella FR. Pancreatic carcinoma in pregnancy: a case report. Am J Obstet Gynecol 1984;149:15–7.
17. Loludice TA, Chandrakaar C. Pregnancy and jejunoileal bypass: treatment complications with total parenteral nutrition. South Med J 1980;73:256–8.
18. Main ANH, Shenkin A, Black WP, Russell RI. Intravenous feeding to sustain pregnancy in patient with Crohn's disease. Br Med J 1981;283:1221–2.
19. Webb GA. The use of hyperalimentation and chemotherapy in pregnancy: a case report. Am J Obstet Gynecol 1980;137:263–6.
20. Stowell JC, Bottsford JE Jr, Rubel HR. Pancreatitis with pseudocyst and cholelithiasis in third trimester of pregnancy: management with total parenteral nutrition. South Med J 1984;77:502–4.
21. Martin R, Trubow M, Bistrian BR, Benotti P, Blackburn GL. Hyperalimentation during pregnancy: a case report. JPEN 1985;9:212–5.
22. Herbert WNP, Seeds JW, Bowes WA, Sweeney CA. Fetal growth response to total parenteral nutrition in pregnancy: a case report. J Reprod Med 1986;31:263–6.
23. Hatjis CG, Meis PJ. Total parenteral nutrition in pregnancy. Obstet Gynecol 1985;66:585–9.
24. Lee RV, Rodgers BD, Young C, Eddy E, Cardinal J. Total parenteral nutrition during pregnancy. Obstet Gynecol 1986;68:563–71.
25. Greenspoon JS, Masaki DI, Kurz CR. Cardiac tamponade in pregnancy during central hyperalimentation. Obstet Gynecol 1989;73:465–6.

Name: **IBUPROFEN**

Class: **Nonsteroidal Anti-inflammatory**   Risk Factor: **B***

Fetal Risk Summary

No published reports linking the use of ibuprofen with congenital defects have been located. The manufacturer has received information by a voluntary reporting system on the use of ibuprofen in 50 pregnancies (1). Seven of these cases were reported retrospectively and 43 prospectively. The results of the retrospective cases included one fetal death (cause of death unknown, no abnormalities observed) after 3rd trimester exposure, and one spontaneous abortion without abnormality. Five infants with defects were observed including an anencephalic infant exposed during the 1st trimester to ibuprofen and Bendectin (doxylamine succinate and pyridoxine hydrochloride), petit mal seizures progressing to grand mal convulsions, cerebral palsy (also exposed to other drugs), a hearsay report of microophthalmia with nasal cleft and mildly rotated palate, and tooth staining (1) (M.M. Westland, personal communication, The Upjohn Company, 1981). A cause and effect relationship between the drug and these defects is doubtful.

Prospectively, 23 of the exposed pregnancies ended in normal outcomes, one infant was stillborn, and one ended in spontaneous abortion, both without apparent abnormality (1). Seven of the pregnancies were electively terminated, three had unknown outcomes, and eight of the pregnancies were still progressing at the time of the report.

The use of ibuprofen as a tocolytic agent has been associated with reduced amniotic fluid volume (2). Fourteen (82.3%) of 17 women treated with a nonsteroidal anti-inflammatory agent had decreased amniotic fluid volume. Of the 17 women, ibuprofen, 1200–2400 mg/day, was used alone in three pregnancies and was combined with ritodrine in one. The other 13 women were treated with indomethacin (see also Indomethacin). One woman who was treated with ibuprofen for 44 days had a return to a normal amniotic fluid volume after the drug was stopped (time for reversal not specified).

Theoretically, ibuprofen, a prostaglandin synthetase inhibitor, could cause constriction of the ductus arteriosus *in utero* (3). Persistent pulmonary hypertension of the newborn should also be considered (3). However, no reports of early closure of the ductus arteriosus have been located and none have been reported to the manufacturer (1). Drugs in this class have been shown to inhibit labor and prolong pregnancy (4).

[*Risk Factor D if used in the 3rd trimeter.]

Breast Feeding Summary

Ibuprofen does not enter human milk in significant quantities. In 12 patients taking 400 mg every 6 hours for 24 hours, an assay capable of detecting 1 μg/ml failed to demonstrate ibuprofen in the milk (5, 6). In another case report, a woman was treated with 400 mg twice daily for 3 weeks (7). Milk levels shortly before and up to 8 hours after drug administration were all less than 0.5 μg/ml. The American Academy of Pediatrics considers ibuprofen to be compatible with breast feeding (8).

References

1. Barry WS, Meinzinger MM, Howse CR. Ibuprofen overdose and exposure in utero: results from a postmarketing voluntary reporting system. Am J Med 1984;77(1A):35–9.
2. Hickok DE, Hollenbach KA, Reilley SF, Nyberg DA. The association between decreased amniotic fluid volume and treatment with nonsteroidal anti-inflammatory agents for preterm labor. Am J Obstet Gynecol 1989;160:1525–31.
3. Levin DL. Effects of inhibition of prostaglandin synthesis on fetal development, oxygenation, and the fetal circulation. Semin Perinatol 1980;4:35–44.
4. Fuchs F. Prevention of prematurity. Am J Obstet Gynecol 1976;126:809–20.
5. Townsend RJ, Benedetti T, Erickson S, Gillespie WR, Albert KS. A study to evaluate the passage of ibuprofen into breast milk. Drug Intell Clin Pharm 1982;16:482–3 (Abstract).
6. Townsend RJ, Benedetti TJ, Erickson S, Cengiz C, Gillespie WR, Gschwend J, Albert KS. Excretion of ibuprofen into breast milk. Am J Obstet Gynecol 1984;149:184–6.
7. Weibert RT, Townsend RJ, Kaiser DG, Naylor AJ. Lack of ibuprofen secretion into human milk. Clin Pharm 1982;1:457–8.
8. Committee on Drugs, American Academy of Pediatrics. Transfer of drugs and other chemicals into human milk. Pediatrics 1989;84:924–36.

Name: **IDOXURIDINE**

Class: **Antiviral**   Risk Factor: **C**

Fetal Risk Summary

Idoxuridine has not been studied in human pregnancy. The drug is teratogenic in some species of animals after injection and ophthalmic use (1, 2).

Breast Feeding Summary

No data are available.

References

1. Nishimura H, Tanimura T. *Clinical Aspects of the Teratogenicity of Drugs*. Amsterdam:Excerpta Medica, 1976:148,258–9.
2. Itoi M, Gefter JW, Kaneko N, Ishii Y, Ramer RM, Gasset AR. Teratogenicities of ophthalmic drugs. I. Antiviral ophthalmic drugs. Arch Ophthalmol 1975;93:46–51.

Name: **IMIPRAMINE**

Class: **Antidepressant**   Risk Factor: **D**

Fetal Risk Summary

Bilateral amelia was reported in one child whose mother had ingested imipramine during pregnancy (1). An analysis of 546,505 births, 161 with 1st trimester exposure to imipramine, however, failed to find an association with limb reduction defects (2–14). Reported malformations other than limb reduction include (3–5):

Defective abdominal muscles (one case)
Diaphragmatic hernia (two cases)
Exencephaly, cleft palate, adrenal hypoplasia (one case)
Cleft palate (two cases)
Renal cystic degeneration (one case)

These reports indicate that imipramine is not a major cause of congenital limb deformities.

Neonatal withdrawal symptoms have been reported with the use of imipramine during pregnancy (15–17). Symptoms observed in the infants during the 1st month after birth were colic, cyanosis, rapid breathing, and irritability (15–17). Urinary retention in the neonate has been associated with maternal use of nortriptyline (chemically related to imipramine) (18).

Breast Feeding Summary

Imipramine and its metabolite, desipramine, enter breast milk in low concentrations (19, 20). A milk:plasma ratio of 1 has been suggested (19). Assuming a therapeutic serum level of 200 ng/ml, an infant consuming 1000 ml of breast milk would ingest a daily dose of about 0.2 mg. The clinical significance of this amount is not known. The American Academy of Pediatrics classifies imipramine as an agent whose effect on the nursing infant is unknown but may be of concern (21).

References

1. McBride WG. Limb deformities associated with iminodibenzyl hydrochloride. Med J Aust 1972;1:492.
2. Heinonen OP, Slone D, Shapiro S. *Birth Defects and Drugs in Pregnancy*. Littleton:Publishing Sciences Group, 1977:336–7.
3. Kuenssberg EV, Knox JDE. Imipramine in pregnancy. Br Med J 1972;2:29.
4. Barson AJ. Malformed infant. Br Med J 1972; 2:45.
5. Idanpaan-Heikkila J, Saxen L. Possible teratogenicity of imipramine/chloropyramine. Lancet 1973;2:282–3.
6. Crombie DL, Pinsent R, Fleming D. Imipramine in pregnancy. Br Med J 1972; 1:745.
7. Sim M. Imipramine and pregnancy. Br Med J 1972; 2:45.
8. Scanlon FJ. Use of antidepressant drugs during the first trimester. Med J Aust 1969;2:1077.
9. Rachelefsky GS, Flynt JW, Eggin AJ, Wilson MG. Possible teratogenicity of tricyclic antidepressants. Lancet 1972;1:838.
10. Banister P, Dafoe C, Smith ESO, Miller J. Possible teratogenicity of tricyclic antidepressants. Lancet 1972; 1:838–9.
11. Jacobs D. Imipramine (Tofranil). S Afr Med J 1972;46:1023.
12. Australian Drug Evaluation Committee. Tricyclic antidepressant and limb reduction deformities. Med J Aust 1973;1:766–9.
13. Morrow AW. Imipramine and congenital abnormalities. NZ Med J 1972;75:228–9.
14. Wilson JG. Present status of drugs as teratogens in man. Teratology 1973;7:3–15.

15. Hill RM. Will this drug harm the unborn infant? South Med J 1977;67:1476–80.
16. Eggermont E. Withdrawal symptoms in neonate associated with maternal imipramine therapy. Lancet 1973;2:680.
17. Shrand H. Agoraphobia and imipramine withdrawal? Pediatrics 1982;70:825.
18. Shearer WT, Schreiner RL, Marshall RE. Urinary retention in a neonate secondary to maternal ingestion of nortriptyline. J Pediatr 1972;81:570–2.
19. Sovner R, Orsulak PJ. Excretion of imipramine and desipramine in human breast milk. Am J Psychiatry 1979;136:451–2.
20. Erickson SH, Smith GH, Heidrich F. Tricyclics and breast feeding. Am J Psychiatry 1979;136:1483.
21. Committee on Drugs, American Academy of Pediatrics. Transfer of drugs and other chemicals into human milk. Pediatrics 1989;84:924–36.

Name: **IMMUNE GLOBULIN, HEPATITIS B**

Class: **Serum**   Risk Factor: **B**

Fetal Risk Summary

Hepatitis B immune globulin is used to provide passive immunity following exposure to hepatitis B. When hepatitis B occurs during pregnancy, an increased rate of abortion and prematurity may be observed (1). No risk to the fetus from the immune globulin has been reported (1, 2). The American College of Obstetricians and Gynecologists Technical Bulletin No. 64 recommends use of hepatitis B immune globulin in pregnancy for postexposure prophylaxis (1).

Breast Feeding Summary

No data are available.

References

1. American College of Obstetricians and Gynecologists. *ACOG Technical Bulletin*, Number 64, May 1982.
2. Amstey MS. Vaccination in pregnancy. Clin Obstet Gynaecol 1983;10:13–22.

Name: **IMMUNE GLOBULIN, RABIES**

Class: **Serum**   Risk Factor: **B**

Fetal Risk Summary

Rabies immune globulin is used to provide passive immunity following exposure to rabies combined with active immunization with rabies vaccine (1). Since rabies is nearly 100% fatal if contracted, both the immune globulin and the vaccine should be given for postexposure prophylaxis (1). No risk to the fetus from the immune globulin has been reported (see also Vaccine, Rabies Human) (1, 2).

Breast Feeding Summary

No data are available.

References

1. American College of Obstetricians and Gynecologists. *ACOG Technical Bulletin*, Number 64, May 1982.
2. Amstey MS. Vaccination in pregnancy. Clin Obstet Gynaecol 1983;10:13–22.

Name: **IMMUNE GLOBULIN, TETANUS**

Class: **Serum**   Risk Factor: **B**

Fetal Risk Summary

Tetanus immune globulin is used to provide passive immunity following exposure to tetanus combined with active immunization with tetanus toxoid (1). Tetanus produces severe morbidity and mortality in both the mother and newborn. No risk to the fetus from the immune globulin has been reported (1, 2).

Breast Feeding Summary

No data are available.

References

1. American College of Obstetricians and Gynecologists. *ACOG Technical Bulletin*, Number 64, May 1982.
2. Amstey MS. Vaccination in pregnancy. Clin Obstet Gynaecol 1983;10:13–22.

Name: **INDIGO CARMINE**

Class: **Dye**   Risk Factor: **B**

Fetal Risk Summary

Indigo carmine is used as a diagnostic dye. No reports linking its use with congenital defects have been located. Intra-amniotic injection has been conducted without apparent effect on the fetus (1, 2). Due to its known toxicities after intravenous administration, however, the dye should not be considered totally safe (3).

Breast Feeding Summary

No data are available.

References

1. Elias S, Gerbie AB, Simpson JL, Nadler HL, Sabbagha RE, Shkolnik A. Genetic amniocentesis in twin gestations. Am J Obstet Gynecol 1980;138:169–74.
2. Horger EO III, Moody LO. Use of indigo carmine for twin amniocentesis and its effect on bilirubin analysis. Am J Obstet Gynecol 1984;150:858–60.
3. Fribourg S. Safety of intraamniotic injection of indigo carmine. Am J Obstet Gynecol 1981;140:350–1.

Name: **INDOMETHACIN**

Class: **Nonsteroidal Anti-inflammatory Analgesic**   Risk Factor: **B***

Fetal Risk Summary

Indomethacin is a nonsteroidal anti-inflammatory agent that is occasionally used in the treatment of premature labor (1–27). The drug acts as a prostaglandin synthetase inhibitor and is apparently effective as a tocolytic agent, including in those cases resistant to β-mimetics. Niebyl (26) reviewed this topic in 1981. Daily doses ranged from 100–200 mg usually by the oral route, but rectal administration was often used. In most cases, indomethacin, either alone or in combination with other tocolytics, was successful in postponing delivery until fetal lung maturation had occurred.

In a 1986 report, 46 infants exposed *in utero* to indomethacin for maternal tocolysis were compared with two control groups: (*a*) 43 infants exposed to other tocolytics and (*b*) 46 infants whose mothers were not treated with tocolytics (27). Indomethacin-treated women received one or two courses of 150 mg orally over 24 hours, all before 34 weeks' gestation. No significant differences were observed between the groups in Apgar scores, birth weight, or gestational age at birth. Similarly, no differences were found in the number of neonatal complications such as hypocalcemia, hypoglycemia, respiratory distress syndrome, need for continuous positive airway pressure, pneumothorax, patent ductus arteriosus, sepsis, exchange transfusion for hyperbilirubinemia, congenital anomalies, or mortality.

A 1989 study compared indomethacin, 100-mg rectal suppository followed by 25 mg orally every 4 hours for 48 hours, with intravenous ritodrine in 106 women in preterm labor with intact membranes who were at a gestational age of 32 weeks or less (28). Fifty-two women received indomethacin and 54 received ritodrine. Thirteen (24%) of the ritodrine group developed adverse drug reactions severe enough to require discontinuance of the drug and a change to magnesium sulfate: cardiac arrhythmia (one), chest pain (two), tachycardia (three), and hypotension (seven). None of the indomethacin-treated women developed drug intolerance ($p < 0.01$). The outcomes of the pregnancies were similar, regardless of whether delivery occurred close to the time of therapy or not. Of those delivered within 48 hours of initiation of therapy, the mean glucose level in the ritodrine-exposed newborns ($N = 9$) was significantly higher than the level in those exposed to indomethacin ($N = 8$), 198 mg/dl vs. 80 mg/dl ($p < 0.05$), respectively. No cases of premature closure of the ductus arteriosus or pulmonary hypertension were observed. A reduction in amniotic fluid volume was noted in three (5.6%) of the ritodrine group and in six (11.5%) of those treated with indomethacin. On a cost basis, tocolysis with indomethacin was 17 times less costly than tocolysis with ritodrine (28).

Complications associated with the use of indomethacin during pregnancy may include premature closure of the ductus arteriosus, resulting in primary pulmonary hypertension of the newborn and in severe cases, neonatal death (1–5, 29–36). These effects are due to the shunting of the right ventricular outflow into the pulmonary vessels when the fetal ductus arteriosus closes, which causes pulmonary arterial hypertrophy (36). Persistent fetal circulation occurs after birth due to the pulmonary hypertension forcing blood to be shunted through the foramen ovale, bypassing the lungs (36).

Using fetal echocardiography, Moise and co-workers described the above effects in a study of 13 women (14 fetuses, 1 set of twins) between the gestational ages of 26.5–31.0 weeks (36). The patients were treated with 100–150 mg of indomethacin orally per day. Fetal ductal constriction occurred in 7 of 14 fetuses 9.5–25.5 hours after the first dose and was not correlated with either gestational age or maternal indomethacin serum levels. In two other cases not included in the present series, ductal constriction did not occur until several weeks after the start of therapy. Tricuspid regurgitation was observed in three of the fetuses with ductal constriction. This defect was due to the constriction-induced elevated pressure in the right ventricular outflow tract producing mild endocardial ischemia with papillary muscle dysfunction (36). All cases of constriction, including two of the three with tricuspid regurgitation, resolved within 24 hours after indomethacin was discontinued. The third tricuspid case returned to normal 40 hours after resolution of the ductal constriction. No cases of persistent fetal circulation were observed in the 11 newborns studied. Some disagreement has been published, however, concerning the methods used in the above study and whether the results actually reflected fetal ductal constriction (37). In response, the authors of the original paper defended their techniques based on both animal and human experimental findings (38).

In contrast to the studies above, a 1987 report described a patient with premature labor who was treated for 29 days between 27–32 weeks' gestation with a total indomethacin dose of 6.2 g (39). The woman delivered a female infant who had patent ductus arteriosus that persisted for 4 weeks. A macerated twin fetus, delivered at the same time as the surviving infant, was thought to have expired prior to the initiation of treatment.

Administration of indomethacin to the mother results in reduced fetal urine output. Severe oligohydramnios, meconium staining, constriction of the ductus arteriosus, and death were reported in the offspring of three women treated for preterm labor at 32–33 weeks' gestation (40). Indomethacin doses were 100 mg (one case) and 400 mg (two cases) during the first 24 hours followed by 100 mg/day for 2–5 days. Two of the fetuses were stillborn, and the third died within 3 hours of birth. A second report described a woman with preterm labor at 24 weeks' gestation who was treated with intravenous ritodrine and indomethacin, 300 mg/day, for 8 weeks (41). A reduction in the amount of amniotic fluid was noted at 28 weeks' gestation (after 4 weeks of therapy), and severe oligohydramnios was present 4 weeks later. Filling of the fetal bladder could not be visualized at this time. The infant, who expired 47 hours after birth, had the characteristic facies of the Potter syndrome (i.e., oligohydramnios sequence), but autopsy revealed a normal urinary tract with normal kidneys. Both cardiac ventricles were hypertrophic and the normal lungs showed no evidence of pulmonary hypertension.

In a 1987 study involving eight patients with polyhydramnios and premature uterine contractions, indomethacin, administered by oral tablets or vaginal suppositories in a dose of 2.2–3.0 mg/kg/day, resolved the condition in each case (42). Four of the patients had diabetes mellitus. The gestational age of the patients at the start of treatment ranged between 21.5–34 weeks. The duration of therapy, which was stopped between 34.5–38 weeks' gestation, ranged from 2–11 weeks. The average gestational age at birth was 38.6 weeks (none was premature) with average Apgar scores of 5 and 10 at 1 and 5 minutes, respectively. All infants were normal at birth and at follow-up for 2–6 months. In addition to the reduced urine output, indomethacin was thought to have minimized the amount of fluid produced by the amnion and chorion (42). In a single case report, a 33-year-old woman with a low serum α-fetoprotein level at 16 weeks' gestation and symptomatic polyhydramnios and preterm labor at 26 weeks' gestation was treated with indomethacin, 25 mg orally every 4 hours, after therapeutic decompression had removed 3000 ml of amniotic fluid (43). During the 9 weeks of therapy, periodic fetal echocardiography was conducted to ensure that the fetal ductus arteriosus remained patent. Fetal urine output declined significantly (<50%) as determined by ultrasound examinations during therapy. Therapy was stopped at 35 weeks' gestation, and a 2280-g female infant was delivered vaginally a week later. Chromosome analysis of the amniotic fluid at 26 weeks and of the infant after birth revealed 46 chromosomes with an additional marker or ring chromosome. No structural defects were noted in the infant, who was developing normally at 3 months of age.

In two women treated for premature labor, indomethacin-induced oligohydramnios was observed 1 week and 3.5 weeks after starting therapy (44). Treatment was continued for 3 weeks in one patient and for 8 weeks in the other, with therapy discontinued at 31 weeks' and 32 weeks' gestation, respectively. Within a week of stopping indomethacin, amniotic fluid volume had returned to normal in both patients. Ultrasonography revealed that both fetuses had regular filling of their bladders. The newborns, delivered 3–4 weeks after indomethacin treatment was halted, had normal urine output. Neither premature closure of the ductus arteriosus nor pulmonary hypertension was observed. Another case of reversible indomethacin-induced oligohydramnios was reported in 1989 (45). The woman was treated from 20–28 weeks' gestation with indomethacin, 100–200 mg/day, plus various other tocolytic agents for premature labor. Ten days after indomethacin therapy was stopped, the volume of amniotic fluid was normal. She was eventually delivered of a 2905-g female infant at 36 weeks' gestation. Development was normal at 1 year of age.

The effects of tocolytic therapy on amniotic fluid volume were the subject of a 1989 study (46). Of 27 women meeting the criteria for the study, 13 were treated either with indomethacin alone ($N = 9$) or indomethacin combined with ritodrine ($N = 2$), terbutaline ($N = 1$), or magnesium sulfate ($N = 1$). Indomethacin dosage varied from 100–200 mg/day with a mean duration of treatment of 15.3 days (range 5–44 days). Four other patients were treated with ibuprofen, another nonsteroidal anti-inflammatory agent. Fourteen of the 17 patients (82.3%) either had a decrease in amniotic fluid volume to low normal levels or had oligohydramnios compared to none of the 10 women treated only with terbutaline, ritodrine, or magnesium sulfate ($p < 0.001$). The mean time required to reaccumulate amniotic fluid in seven women after stopping nonsteroidal anti-inflammatory therapy was 4.4 days. In one other woman who had an ultrasound examination after therapy was discontinued, amniotic fluid volume remained in the low normal range.

A study published in 1988 described the treatment with indomethacin, 100–150 mg/day, for premature labor in eight women at 27–32 weeks' gestation (47). Fetal urine output fell from a mean pretreatment value of 11.2 ml/hour to 2.2 ml/hour at 5 hours, then stabilized at 1.8 ml/hour at 12 and 24 hours. Mean output 24 hours after stopping indomethacin was 13.5 ml/hour. No correlation was found between maternal indomethacin serum levels and hourly fetal urine output. Three of the four fetuses treated with indomethacin every 4 hours had ductal constriction at 24 hours that apparently resolved after therapy was halted. All newborns had normal renal function in the neonatal period.

A probable drug interaction between indomethacin and β-blockers resulting in severe maternal hypertension was reported in two women in 1989 (48). One woman, with a history of labile hypertension of 6 years' duration, was admitted at 30 weeks' gestation for control of her blood pressure. She was treated with propranolol 80 mg/day with good response. Indomethacin was started because of premature uterine contractions occurring at 32 weeks' gestation. An initial 200-mg rectal dose was followed by 25 mg orally/day. On the 4th day of therapy, the patient suffered a marked change in blood pressure, which rose from 135/85 mm Hg to 240/140 mm Hg, with cardiotocographic signs of fetal distress. A cesarean section was performed, but the severely growth-retarded newborn died 72 hours later. The second patient developed signs and symptoms of preeclampsia at 31 weeks' gestation. She was treated with pindolol 15 mg/day with good blood pressure response. Two weeks later, indomethacin was started, as in the first case, for preterm labor. On the 5th day of therapy, blood pressure rose to 230/130 mm Hg. Signs of fetal distress were evident and a cesarean section was performed. The low-weight infant survived. The mechanism of this interaction is unknown, but one source has reviewed several cases of this interaction with the observation that indomethacin may inhibit the effects of β-blockers, as well as antihypertensives in general (49).

Severe complications after *in utero* exposure to indomethacin have been reported in three preterm infants (50). The three mothers had been treated with indomethacin, 200–300 mg/day, for 4 weeks, 3 days, and 2 days, respectively, immediately prior to delivery. Complications in the newborns included edema or hydrops, oliguric renal failure (<0.5 ml/kg/hour) lasting for 1–2 days, gastrointestinal bleeding occurring on the 4th and 6th days (two infants), subcutaneous bruising, intraventricular hemorrhage (one infant), absent platelet aggregation (two infants; not determined in the third infant), and perforation of the terminal ileum. The authors attributed the problems to maternal indomethacin therapy because of (a) the absence of predisposing factors, and the lack of diagnostic evidence, for necrotizing enterocolitis, and (b) the close similarity and sequential pattern of the signs and symptoms in the three newborns.

A single case of phocomelia with agenesis of the penis has been described, but the relationship between indomethacin and this defect is unknown (51). Finally, inhibition of platelet aggregation may have contributed to postpartum hemorrhage in 3 of 16 women given a 100-mg indomethacin suppository during term labor (12).

In summary, the use of indomethacin as a tocolytic agent during the latter half of pregnancy may cause constriction of the fetal ductus arteriosus, with or without tricuspid regurgitation. Premature closure of the ductus arteriosus can result in primary pulmonary hypertension of the newborn that, in severe cases, may be fatal. Reduced fetal urine output should be expected when indomethacin is administered to the mother. This may be therapeutic in cases of polyhydramnios, but the complications of this therapy may be severe. Oliguric renal failure, hemorrhage, and intestinal perforation have been reported in premature infants exposed immediately prior to delivery. Use of indomethacin with antihypertensive agents, particularly the β-blockers, may cause severe maternal hypertension with resulting fetal distress. Short courses of indomethacin, such as 24–48 hours with allowance of at least 24 hours or more between the last dose and delivery, should prevent complications of this therapy in the newborn. Use of the smallest effective dose is essential, although maternal serum levels of indomethacin that are effective for tocolysis have not yet been defined (36). Restriction of indomethacin tocolysis to pregnancies of less than 34–35 weeks' gestation, when therapy for premature labor is most appropriate, will also lessen the incidence of complications (26). Other uses of indomethacin, such as for analgesia or inflammation, have not been studied in pregnancy but should be approached with caution due to the effects described above.

[*Risk Factor D if used for longer than 48 hours or after 34 weeks' gestation.]

Breast Feeding Summary

Indomethacin is excreted in human breast milk, but a milk:plasma ratio has not been reported. It is known that milk levels are similar to maternal plasma levels (52). There is one case report of possible indomethacin-induced seizures in a breast-fed infant, although the causal link between the two events has been questioned (52, 53). The mother was taking 200 mg/day (3 mg/kg/day). The American Academy of Pediatrics noted the above possible adverse reaction, but considers indomethacin to be compatible with breast feeding (54).

References

1. Atad J, David A, Moise J, Abramovici H. Classification of threatened premature labor related to treatment with a prostaglandin inhibitor: indomethacin. Biol Neonate 1980;37:291–6.
2. Gonzalez CHL, Jimenez PG, Pezzotti y R MA, Favela EL. Hipertension pulmonar persistente en el recien nacido por uso prenatal de inhibidores de las prostaglandinas (indometacina). Informe de un caso. Ginec Obstet Mex 1980;48:103–10.
3. Sureau C, Piovani P. Clinical study of indomethacin for prevention of prematurity. Eur J Obstet Gynecol Reprod Biol 1983;46:400–2.
4. Van Kets H, Thiery M, Derom R, Van Egmond H, Baele G. Perinatal hazards of chronic antenatal tocolysis with indomethacin. Prostaglandins 1979;18:893–907.
5. Van Kets H, Thiery M, Derom R, Van Egmond H, Baele G. Prostaglandin synthase inhibitors in preterm labor. Lancet 1980;2:693.
6. Blake DA, Niebyl JR, White RD, Kumor KM, Dubin NH, Robinson JC, Egner PG. Treatment of premature labor with indomethacin. Adv Prostaglandin Thromboxane Res 1980;8:1465–7.
7. Grella P, Zanor P. Premature labor and indomethacin. Prostaglandins 1978;16:1007–17.
8. Karim SMM. On the use of blockers of prostaglandin synthesis in the control of labor. Adv Prostaglandin Thromboxane Res 1978;4:301–6.
9. Katz Z, Lancet M, Yemini M, Mogilner BM, Feigl A, Ben Hur H. Treatment of premature labor contractions with combined ritodrine and indomethacine. Int J Gynaecol Obstet 1983;21:337–42.
10. Niebyl JR, Blake DA, White RD, Kumor KM, Dubin NH, Robinson JC, Egner PG. The inhibition of premature labor with indomethacin. Am J Obstet Gynecol 1980;136:1014–9.
11. Peteja J. Indometacyna w zapobieganiu porodom przedwczesnym. Ginekol Pol 1980;51:347–53.
12. Reiss U, Atad J, Rubinstein I, Zuckerman H. The effect of indomethacin in labour at term. Int J Gynaecol Obstet 1976;14:369–74.
13. Souka AR, Osman N, Sibaie F, Einen MA. Therapeutic value of indomethacin in threatened abortion. Prostaglandins 1980;19:457–60.
14. Spearing G. Alcohol, indomethacin, and salbutamol. Obstet Gynecol 1979;53:171–4.
15. Chimura T. The treatment of threatened premature labor by drugs. Acta Obstet Gynaecol Jpn 1980;32:1620–4.
16. Suzanne F, Fresne JJ, Portal B, Baudon J. Essai therapeutique de l'indometacine dans les menaces d'accouchement premature: a propos de 30 observations. Therapie 1980;35:751–60.
17. Tinga DJ, Aranoudse JG. Post-partum pulmonary oedema associated with preventive therapy for premature labor. Lancet 1979;1:1026.
18. Dudley DKL, Hardie MJ. Fetal and neonatal effects of indomethacin used as a tocolytic agent. Am J Obstet Gynecol 1985;151:181–4.

19. Gamissans O, Canas E, Cararach V, Ribas J, Puerto B, Edo A. A study of indomethacin com- bined with ritodrine in threatened preterm labor. Eur J Obstet Gynecol Reprod Biol 1978;8:123–8.
20. Wiqvist N, Lundstrom V, Green K. Premature labor and indomethacin. Prostaglandins 1975;10:515–26.
21. Wiqvist N, Kjellmer I, Thiringer K, Ivarsson E, Karlsson K. Treatment of premature labor by pros- taglandin synthetase inhibitors. Acta Biol Med Germ 1978;37:923–30.
22. Zuckerman H, Reiss U, Rubinstein I. Inhibition of human premature labor by indomethacin. Obstet Gynecol 1974;44:787–92.
23. Zuckerman H, Reiss U, Atad J, Lampert I, Ben Ezra S, Sklan D. The effect of indomethacin on plasma levels of prostaglandin $F_{2\alpha}$ in women in labour. Br J Obstet Gynaecol 1977;84:339–43.
24. Zuckerman H, Shalev E, Gilad G, Katzuni E. Further study of the inhibition of premature labor by indomethacin. Part I. J Perinat Med 1984;12:19–23.
25. Zuckerman H, Shalev E, Gilad G, Katzuni E. Further study of the inhibition of premature labor by indomethacin. Part II. Double-blind study. J Perinat Med 1984;12:25–9.
26. Niebyl JR. Prostaglandin synthetase inhibitors. Semin Perinatol 1981;5:274–87.
27. Niebyl JR, Witter FR. Neonatal outcome after indomethacin treatment for preterm labor. Am J Obstet Gynecol 1986;155:747–9.
28. Morales WJ, Smith SG, Angel JL, O'Brien WF, Knuppel RA. Efficacy and safety of indomethacin versus ritodrine in the management of preterm labor: a randomized study. Obstet Gynecol 1989;74:567–72.
29. Levin DL. Effects of inhibition of prostaglandin synthesis on fetal development, oxygenation, and the fetal circulation. Semin Perinatol 1980;4:35–44.
30. Csaba IF, Sulyok E, Ertl T. Relationship of maternal treatment with indomethacin to persistence of fetal circulation syndrome. J Pediatr 1978;92:484.
31. Levin DL, Fixler DE, Morriss FC, Tyson J. Morphologic analysis of the pulmonary vascular bed in infants exposed in utero to prostaglandin synthetase inhibitors. J Pediatr 1978;92:478–83.
32. Rubaltelli FF, Chiozza ML, Zanardo V, Cantarutti F. Effect on neonate of maternal treatment with indomethacin. J Pediatr 1979;94:161.
33. Manchester D, Margolis HS, Sheldon RE. Possible association between maternal indomethacin therapy and primary pulmonary hypertension of the newborn. Am J Obstet Gynecol 1976;126:467–9.
34. Goudie BM, Dossetor JFB. Effect on the fetus of indomethacin given to suppress labour. Lancet 1979;2:1187–8.
35. Mogilner BM, Ashkenazy M, Borenstein R, Lancet M. Hydrops fetalis caused by maternal in- domethacin treatment. Acta Obstet Gynecol Scand 1982;61:183–5.
36. Moise KJ Jr, Huhta JC, Sharif DS, Ou CN, Kirshon B, Wasserstrum N, Cano L. Indomethacin in the treatment of premature labor: effects on the fetal ductus arteriosus. N Engl J Med 1988;319:327–31.
37. Ovadia M. Effects of indomethacin on the fetus. N Engl J Med 1988;319:1484.
38. Moise KJ Jr, Huhta JC, Mari G. Effects of indomethacin on the fetus. N Engl J Med 1988;319:1485.
39. Atad J, Lissak A, Rofe A, Abramovici H. Patent ductus arteriosus after prolonged treatment with indomethacin during pregnancy: case report. Int J Gynaecol Obstet 1987;25:73–6.
40. Itskovitz J, Abramovici H, Brandes JM. Oligohydramnion, meconium and perinatal death concur- rent with indomethacin treatment in human pregnancy. J Reprod Med 1980;24:137–40.
41. Veersema D, de Jong PA, van Wijck JAM. Indomethacin and the fetal renal nonfuction syndrome. Eur J Obstet Gynecol Reprod Biol 1983;16:113–21.
42. Cabrol D, Landesman R, Muller J, Uzan M, Sureau C, Saxena BB. Treatment of polyhydramnios with prostaglandin synthetase inhibitor (indomethacin). Am J Obstet Gynecol 1987;157:422–6.
43. Kirshon B, Cotton DB. Polyhydramnios associated with a ring chromosome and low maternal serum α-fetoprotein levels managed with indomethacin. Am J Obstet Gynecol 1988;158:1063–4.
44. De Wit W, Van Mourik I, Wiesenhaan PF. Prolonged maternal indomethacin therapy associated with oligohydramnios: case reports. Br J Obstet Gynecol 1988;95:303–5.
45. Goldenberg RL, Davis RO, Baker RC. Indomethacin-induced oligohydramnios. Am J Obstet Gy- necol 1989;160:1196–7.
46. Hickok DE, Hollenbach KA, Reilley SF, Nyberg DA. The association between decreased amniotic fluid volume and treatment with nonsteroidal anti-inflammatory agents for preterm labor. Am J Obstet Gynecol 1989;160:1525–31.

47. Kirshon B, Moise KJ Jr, Wasserstrum N, Ou CN, Huhta JC. Influence of short-term indomethacin therapy on fetal urine output. Obstet Gynecol 1988;72:51–3.

48. Schoenfeld A, Freedman S, Hod M, Ovadia Y. Antagonism of antihypertensive drug therapy in pregnancy by indomethacin? Am J Obstet Gynecol 1989;161:1204–5.

49. Hansen PD. Drug Interactions, 5th ed. Philadelphia:Lea & Febiger, 1985:36.

50. Vanhaesebrouck P, Thiery M, Leroy JG, Govaert P, de Praeter C, Coppens M, Cuvelier C, Dhont M. Oligohydramnios, renal insufficiency, and ileal perforation in preterm infants after intrauterine exposure to indomethacin. J Pediatr 1988;113:738–43.

51. Di Battista C, Landizi L, Tamborino G. Focomelia ed agenesia del pene in neonato. Minerva Pediatr 1975;27:675. As cited in Dukes MNG, ed. Side Effects of Drugs Annual 1. Amsterdam:Excerpta Medica, 1977:89.

52. Eeg-Olofsson O, Malmros I, Elwin CE, Steen B. Convulsions in a breast-fed infant after maternal indomethacin. Lancet 1978;2:215.

53. Fairhead FW. Convulsions in a breast-fed infant after maternal indomethacin. Lancet 1978;2:576.

54. Committee on Drugs, American Academy of Pediatrics. Transfer of drugs and other chemicals into human milk. Pediatrics 1989;84;924–36.

Name: **INSULIN**

Class: **Antidiabetic**   Risk Factor: **B**

Fetal Risk Summary

Insulin, a naturally occurring hormone, is the drug of choice for the control of diabetes mellitus in pregnancy. Infants of diabetic mothers are at risk for an increased incidence of congenital anomalies, up to 2–4 times that of normal controls (1–4). The rate of malformations seems to be related to the severity of the maternal disease. The exact mechanisms causing this increase are unknown. Human insulin does not cross the placenta, at least when administered in the 2nd trimester (5). Studies prior to this time have not been conducted. This distinction is of interest since most major malformations observed in infants of diabetic mothers were induced sometime prior to the 7th week of gestation (1). Several mechanisms have been offered as a cause of the malformations, including exogenous insulin itself and insulin-induced hypoglycemia. However, a recent study using hemoglobin A_{1c}, a normal minor hemoglobin whose levels are indicative of diabetic control, found a significantly higher percentage of major congenital anomalies in the offspring of mothers with elevated levels of this hemoglobin (3). The authors concluded that poorly controlled diabetes (i.e., hyperglycemia) was associated with an increased risk of defects. Congenital malformations are now the most common cause of perinatal death in infants of diabetic mothers (1, 2). Not only is the frequency of major defects increased, but also the frequency of multiple malformations (affecting more than one organ system) (1). Malformations observed in infants of diabetic mothers usually involve one or more of five systems (1):

Most common
    Skeletal: vertebrae and limbs
    Cardiovascular: transposition of great vessels; ventricular septal defects; coarctation of the aorta
    Central nervous system: neural tube defects

Less common
  Genitourinary: varied
  Gastrointestinal: tracheoesophageal fistula; bowel atresias; imperforate anus; narrowed colon

Infants of diabetic mothers may have significant perinatal morbidity, even when the mothers have been under close diabetic control (6). Perinatal morbidity in one series affected 65% (169/260) of the infants and included hypoglycemia, hyperbilirubinemia, hypocalcemia, and polycythemia (6).

Breast Feeding Summary

Insulin is a naturally occurring constituent of the blood. It does not pass into breast milk.

References

1. Dignan PSJ. Teratogenic risk and counseling in diabetes. Clin Obstet Gynecol 1981;24:149–59.
2. Friend JR. Diabetes. Clin Obstet Gynaecol 1981;8:353–82.
3. Miller E, Hare JW, Cloherty JP, et al. Elevated maternal hemoglobin A_{1c} in early pregnancy and major congenital anomalies in infants of diabetic mothers. N Engl J Med 1981;304:1331–4.
4. Soler NG, Walsh CH, Malins JM. Congenital malformations in infants of diabetic mothers. Q J Med 1976;45:303–13.
5. Adam PAJ, Teramo K, Raiha N, Gitlin D, Schwartz R. Human fetal insulin metabolism early in gestation. Diabetes 1969;18:409–16.
6. Gabbe SG, Mestman JH, Freeman RK, et al. Management and outcome of pregnancy in diabetes mellitus, classes B to R. Am J Obstet Gynecol 1977;129:723–32.

Name: **IOCETAMIC ACID**

Class: **Diagnostic**   Risk Factor: **D**

Fetal Risk Summary

Iocetamic acid contains a high concentration of organically bound iodine. See Diatrizoate for possible effects on the fetus and neonate.

Breast Feeding Summary

See Potassium Iodide.

Name: **IODAMIDE**

Class: **Diagnostic**   Risk Factor: **D**

Fetal Risk Summary

The various preparations of iodamide contain a high concentration of organically bound iodine. See Diatrizoate for possible effects on the fetus and newborn.

Breast Feeding Summary

See Potassium Iodide.

Name: **IODINATED GLYCEROL**

Class: **Expectorant**   Risk Factor: X_M

Fetal Risk Summary

Iodinated glycerol is a stable complex containing 50% organically bound iodine (see Potassium Iodide).

Breast Feeding Summary

See Potassium Iodide.

Name: **IODINE**

Class: **Anti-infective**   Risk Factor: **D**

Fetal Risk Summary

See Potassium Iodide.

Breast Feeding Summary

See Potassium Iodide.

Name: **IODIPAMIDE**

Class: **Diagnostic**   Risk Factor: **D**

Fetal Risk Summary

The various preparations of iodipamide contain a high concentration of organically bound iodine. See Diatrizoate for possible effects on the fetus and newborn.

Breast Feeding Summary

See Potassium Iodide.

Name: **IODOQUINOL**

Class: **Amebicide**   Risk Factor: **C**

Fetal Risk Summary

Iodoquinol (di-iodohydroxyquinoline; diiodohydroxyquin) has been used in pregnancy apparently without causing fetal harm. Two case reports described the use of iodoquinol in pregnancy for the treatment of a rare skin disease. The first case involved a woman with chronic acrodermatitis enteropathica who was treated with the amebicide in the 2nd and 3rd trimesters of her first pregnancy (1). She delivered a typical achondroplastic dwarf who died in 30 minutes. The second case also involved a woman with the same disorder who took iodoquinol throughout gestation (2). Dosage during the 1st trimester, 1.3 g/day, was systematically increased during pregnancy in an attempt to control the cutaneous lesions, eventually reaching 6.5 g/day during the last 4 weeks. A normal male infant was delivered at term. Physical examinations of the infant, including ophthalmic examinations, were normal at birth and at 6 weeks' follow-up.

The Collaborative Perinatal Project monitored 50,282 mother-child pairs, 169 of which had 1st trimester exposure to iodoquinol (3, pp. 299, 302). Ten of the infants were born with a congenital malformation, corresponding to a hospital standardized relative risk (SRR) of 0.88. Based on three infants, an SRR of 6.6 for congenital dislocation of the hip was calculated, but this association is uninterpretable without confirming evidence (3, pp. 467, 473). For use anytime during pregnancy, 172 exposures were recorded (3, pp. 434, 435). With the same caution as noted above, an SRR of 1.68 (95% confidence interval 0.62–3.58) was estimated based on malformations in six infants. The SRR for congenital dislocation of the hip after use anytime during pregnancy was 6.5 (3, p. 486).

Breast Feeding Summary

No data are available.

References

1. Vedder JS, Griem S. Acrodermatitis enteropathica (Danbolt-Closs) in five siblings: efficacy of di-odoquin in its management. J Pediatr 1956;48:212–9.
2. Verburg DJ, Burd LI, Hoxtell EO, Merrill LK. Acrodermatitis enteropathica and pregnancy. Obstet Gynecol 1974;44:233–7.
3. Heinonen OP, Slone D, Shapiro S. *Birth Defects and Drugs in Pregnancy*. Littleton:Publishing Sciences Group, 1977.

Name: **IODOTHYRIN**

Class: **Thyroid**   Risk Factor: **A**

Fetal Risk Summary

Iodothyrin is a combination product containing thyroid, iodized calcium, and peptone. See Thyroid.

Breast Feeding Summary

See Levothyroxine and Liothyronine.

Name: **IODOXAMATE**

Class: **Diagnostic**   Risk Factor: **D**

Fetal Risk Summary

The various preparations of iodoxamate contain a high concentration of organically bound iodine. See Diatrizoate for possible effects on the fetus and newborn.

Breast Feeding Summary

See Potassium Iodide.

Name: **IOPANOIC ACID**

Class: **Diagnostic**   Risk Factor: **D**

Fetal Risk Summary

Iopanoic acid contains a high concentration of organically bound iodine. See Diatrizoate for possible effects on the fetus and newborn.

Breast Feeding Summary

Iopanoic acid is excreted in breast milk. Cholecystography was performed in 11 lactating patients with iopanoic acid (1). The mean amount of iodine administered to five patients was 2.77 g (range 1.98–3.96 g) and the mean amount excreted in breast milk during the next 19–29 hours was 20.8 mg (0.08%) (range 6.72–29.9 mg). The nursing infants showed no reaction to the contrast media.

Reference

1. Holmdahl KH. Cholecystography during lactation. Acta Radiol 1956;45: 305–7.

Name: **IOTHALAMATE**

Class: **Diagnostic**   Risk Factor: **D**

Fetal Risk Summary

Iothalamate has been used for diagnostic procedures during pregnancy. Amniography was performed in one patient to diagnose monoamniotic twinning shortly before an elective cesarean section (1). No effect on the two newborns was mentioned. In a second study, 17 women were given either iothalamate or metrizoate for ascending phlebography during various stages of pregnancy (2). Two patients, one exposed in the 1st trimester and one in the 2nd trimester, were diagnosed as having deep vein thrombosis and were treated with heparin. The baby from the 2nd trimester patient was normal, but the other newborn had hyperbilirubinemia and undescended testis. The relationship between the diagnostic agents (or other drugs) and the defects is not known.

Use of other organically bound iodine preparations near term has resulted in hypothyroidism in some newborns (see Diatrizoate). Thus, appropriate measures should be taken to treat neonatal hypothyroidism if diagnostic tests with iothalamate are required close to delivery.

Breast Feeding Summary

See Potassium Iodide.

References

1. Dunnihoo DR, Harris RE. The diagnosis of monoamniotic twinning by amniography. Am J Obstet Gynecol 1966;96:894–5.
2. Kierkegaard A. Incidence and diagnosis of deep vein thrombosis associated with pregnancy. Acta Obstet Gynecol Scand 1983;62:239–43.

Name: **IPODATE**

Class: **Diagnostic**   Risk Factor: **D**

Fetal Risk Summary

Ipodate contains a high concentration of organically bound iodine. See Diatrizoate for possible effects on the fetus and newborn.

Breast Feeding Summary

See Potassium Iodide.

Name: **IPRINDOLE**

Class: **Antidepressant**   Risk Factor: **D**

Fetal Risk Summary

No data are available (see Imipramine).

Breast Feeding Summary

No data are available (see Imipramine).

Name: **IPRONIAZID**

Class: **Antidepressant**   Risk Factor: **C**

Fetal Risk Summary

No data are available (see Phenelzine).

Breast Feeding Summary

No data are available (see Phenelzine).

Name: **ISOCARBOXAZID**

Class: **Antidepressant**   Risk Factor: **C**

Fetal Risk Summary

Isocarboxazid is a monoamine oxidase inhibitor. The Collaborative Perinatal Project monitored 21 mother-child pairs exposed to these drugs during the 1st trimester, 1 which was exposed to isocarboxazid (1). An increased risk of malformations was found. Details of the single case with exposure to isocarboxazid were not given.

Breast Feeding Summary

No data are available.

Reference

1. Heinonen OP, Slone D, Shapiro S. *Birth Defects and Drugs in Pregnancy*. Littleton:Publishing Sciences Group, 1977:336–7.

Name: **ISOETHARINE**

Class: **Sympathomimetic (Adrenergic)**   Risk Factor: **C**

Fetal Risk Summary

No reports linking the use of isoetharine with congenital defects have been located. Isoetharine-like drugs are teratogenic in some animal species, but human teratogenicity has not been suspected (1, 2). Recent data may require a reappraisal of this opinion. The Collaborative Perinatal Project monitored 50,282 mother-child pairs, 3,082 of which had 1st trimester exposure to sympathomimetic drugs (3, pp. 345–356). For use anytime during pregnancy, 9,719 exposures were recorded (3, p. 439). An association in the 1st trimester was found between the sympathomimetic class of drugs as a whole and minor malformations (not life-threatening or major cosmetic defects), inguinal hernia, and clubfoot (3, pp. 345–356). Sympathomimetics are often administered in combination with other drugs to alleviate the symptoms of upper respiratory infections. Thus, the fetal effects of sympathomimetics, other drugs, and viruses cannot be totally separated. However, indiscriminate use of this class of drugs, especially in the 1st trimester, is not without risk.

Breast Feeding Summary

No data are available.

References

1. Nishimura H, Tanimura T. *Clinical Aspects of the Teratogenicity of Drugs*. Amsterdam:Excerpta Medica, 1976:231.
2. Shepard TH. *Catalog of Teratogenic Agents*, ed. 3. Baltimore:Johns Hopkins University Press, 1980:134–5.
3. Heinonen OP, Slone D, Shapiro S. *Birth Defects and Drugs in Pregnancy*. Littleton:Publishing Sciences Group, 1977.

Name: **ISOFLUROPHATE**

Class: **Parasympathomimetic (Cholinergic)**   Risk Factor: **C**

Fetal Risk Summary

Isoflurophate is used in the eye. No reports of its use in pregnancy have been located. As a quaternary ammonium compound, it is ionized at physiologic pH and transplacental passage in significant amounts would not be expected (see also Neostigmine).

Breast Feeding Summary

No data are available.

Name: **ISONIAZID**

Class: **Antituberculosis Agent**   Risk Factor: **C**

Fetal Risk Summary

An official statement of the American Thoracic Society, published in 1986, recommends isoniazid as part of the treatment regimen for women who have tuberculosis during pregnancy (1). Other reviewers also consider isoniazid as part of the treatment of choice for tuberculosis occurring during pregnancy (2).

Isoniazid crosses the placenta to the fetus (3–5). In a 1955 study, 19 women in labor were given a single 100-mg dose of isoniazid 0.25–4.25 hours before delivery (3). The mean maternal serum concentration at birth was 0.32 μg/ml compared to a cord blood level of 0.22 μg/ml. The mean cord:maternal ratio was 0.73, but in seven of the patients, cord blood concentrations exceeded those in the maternal plasma. Another study examined the placental transfer of isoniazid in two women who had been treated with 300 mg/day during the 3rd trimester (4). One hour prior to delivery, the women were given a single 300-mg intramuscular dose. Mean cord blood and maternal serum concentrations were 4 and 6.5 μg/ml, respectively, a ratio of 0.62. These studies and the elimination kinetics of intrauterine acquired isoniazid in the newborn were reviewed in 1987 (5).

Reports discussing fetal effects of isoniazid (INH) during pregnancy reflect multiple drug therapies. Early reports identified retarded psychomotor activity, psychic retardation, convulsions, myoclonia, myelomeningocele with spina bifida and talipes, and hypospadias as possible effects related to isoniazid therapy during pregnancy (6, 7). The Collaborative Perinatal Project monitored 85 patients who received isoniazid during the 1st trimester (8, pp. 299, 313). They observed 10 malformations, an incidence almost twice the expected rate, but they cautioned that their findings required independent confirmation. For use anytime during pregnancy, 146 mother-child pairs were exposed to isoniazid, with malformations that may have been produced after the 1st trimester observed in 4 infants (8, p. 435). This was close to the expected frequency. Adverse outcomes in the fetus and newborn after intrauterine exposure to isoniazid have not been confirmed by other studies (9–14). Retrospective analysis of over 4900 pregnancies in which isoniazid was administered demonstrated rates of malformations similar to those in control populations (0.7%–2.3%). A 1980 review also found no association between isoniazid and fetal anomalies (15).

A case report of a malignant mesothelioma in a 9-year-old child who was exposed to isoniazid *in utero* was published in 1980 (16). The authors suggested a possible carcinogenic effect of isoniazid because of the rarity of malignant mesotheliomas during the first decade and supportive animal data. However, an earlier study followed 660 children up to 16 years of age and found no association with carcinogenic effects (17).

An association between isoniazid and hemorrhagic disease of the newborn has been suspected in two infants (18). The mothers were also treated with rifampin and ethambutol and in a third case, only with these latter two drugs. Although other reports of this potentially serious reaction have not been found, prophylactic vitamin K is recommended at birth (see Phytonadione).

In summary, isoniazid does not appear to be a human teratogen. The American Thoracic Society recommends use of the drug for tuberculosis occurring during pregnancy because, "Untreated tuberculosis represents a far greater hazard to a pregnant woman and her fetus than does treatment of the disease" (1).

Breast Feeding Summary

No reports of isoniazid-induced effects in the nursing infant have been located, but the potential for interference with nucleic acid function and for hepatotoxicity may exist (19, 20). Both isoniazid and its metabolite, acetylisoniazid, are excreted in breast milk (20–22). A woman was given a single oral dose of 300 mg after complete weaning of her infant (20). Both isoniazid and the metabolite were present in her milk within 1 hour with peak levels of isoniazid (16.6 μg/ml) occurring at 3 hours and those of the metabolite (3.76 μg/ml) at 5 hours. At 5 and 12 hours after the dose, isoniazid levels in the milk were twice the levels in simultaneously obtained plasma. Levels of acetylisoniazid were similar in plasma and milk at 5 and 12 hours. The elimination half-life for milk isoniazid was calculated to be 5.9 hours, whereas that of the metabolite was 13.5 hours. Both were detectable in milk 24 hours after the dose. The 24-hour excretion of isoniazid was estimated to be 7 mg. Two other studies also reported substantial excretion of isoniazid into human milk (21, 22). A milk:plasma ratio of 1.0 was reported in one of these studies (21). In another, milk levels 3 hours after a maternal 5 mg/kg dose were 6 µg/ml (22). Doubling the maternal dose doubled the milk concentration.

Based on the above information, at least one review concluded that women can safely breast feed their infants while taking isoniazid if, among other precautions, the infant is periodically examined for signs and symptoms of peripheral neuritis or hepatitis (19). Moreover, the American Academy of Pediatrics considers isoniazid to be compatible with breast feeding (23).

References

1. American Thoracic Society. Treatment of tuberculosis and tuberculosis infection in adults and children. Am Rev Respir Dis 1986;134:355–63.
2. Medchill MT, Gillum M. Diagnosis and management of tuberculosis during pregnancy. Obstet Gynecol Surv 1989;44:81–4.
3. Bromberg YM, Salzberger M, Bruderman I. Placental transmission of isonicotinic acid hydrazide. Gynaecologia 1955;140:141–4.
4. Miceli JN, Olson WA, Cohen SN. Elimination kinetics of isoniazid in the newborn infant. Dev Pharmacol Ther 1981;2:235–9.
5. Holdiness MR. Transplacental pharmacokinetics of the antituberculosis drugs. Clin Pharmacokinet 1987;13:125–9.
6. Weinstein L, Dalton AC. Host determinants of response to antimicrobial agents. N Engl J Med 1968;279:524–31.
7. Lowe CR. Congenital defects among children born to women under supervision or treatment for pulmonary tuberculosis. Br J Prev Soc Med 1964;18:14–6.
8. Heinonen OP, Slone D, Shapiro S. *Birth Defects and Drugs in Pregnancy*. Littleton:Publishing Sciences Group, 1977.
9. Marynowski A, Sianozecka E. Comparison of the incidence of congenital malformations in neonates from healthy mothers and from patients treated because of tuberculosis. Ginekol Pol 1972;43:713.
10. Jentgens H. Antituberkulose chimotherapie und schwangerschaft sabbruch. Prax Klin Pneumol 1973;27:479.
11. Ludford J, Doster B, Woolpert SF. Effect of isoniazid on reproduction. Am Rev Respir Dis 1973;108:1170–4.
12. Scheinhorn DJ, Angelillo VA. Antituberculosis therapy in pregnancy; risks to the fetus. West J Med 1977;127:195–8.
13. Good JT, Iseman MD, Davidson PT, Lakshminarayan S, Sahn SA. Tuberculosis in association with pregnancy. Am J Obstet Gynecol 1981;140:492–8.
14. Kingdom JCP, Kennedy DH. Tuberculous meningitis in pregnancy. Br J Obstet Gynaecol 1989;96:233–5.
15. Snider DE Jr, Layde PM, Johnson MW, Lyle MA. Treatment of tuberculosis during pregnancy. Am Rev Respir Dis 1980;122:65–79.
16. Tuman KJ, Chilcote RR, Gerkow RI, Moohr JW. Mesothelioma in child with prenatal exposure to isoniazid. Lancet 1980;2:362.
17. Hammond DC, Silidoff IJ, Robitzek EH. Isoniazid therapy in relation to later occurrence of cancer in adults and in infants. Br Med J 1967;2:792–5.
18. Eggermont E, Logghe N, Van De Casseye W, Casteels-Van Daele M, Jaeken J, Cosemans J, Verstraete M, Renaer M. Haemorrhagic disease of the newborn in the offspring of rifampicin and isoniazid treated mothers. Acta Paediatr Belg 1976;29:87–90.
19. Snider DE Jr, Powell KE. Should women taking antituberculosis drugs breast-feed? Arch Intern Med 1984;144:589–90.
20. Berlin CM Jr, Lee C. Isoniazid and acetylisoniazid disposition in human milk, saliva and plasma. Fed Proc 1979;38:426.
21. Vorherr H. Drugs excretion in breast milk. Postgrad Med 1974;56:97–104.
22. Ricci G, Copaitich T. Modalta di eliminazione dili'isoniazide somministrata per via orale attraverso il latte di donna. Rass Clin Ter 1954–5;209:53–4.
23. Committee on Drugs, American Academy of Pediatrics. Transfer of drugs and other chemicals into human milk. Pediatrics 1989;84;924–36.

Name: **ISOPROPAMIDE**

Class: **Parasympatholytic**   Risk Factor: **C**

Fetal Risk Summary

Isopropamide is an anticholinergic quaternary ammonium iodide. The Collaborative Perinatal Project monitored 50,282 mother-child pairs, 180 of which used isopropamide in the 1st trimester (1, pp. 346–353). For use anytime during pregnancy, 1,071 exposures were recorded (1, p. 439). In neither case was evidence found for an association with malformations. However, when the group of parasympatholytics were taken as a whole (2,323 exposures), a possible association with minor malformations was found (1, pp. 346–353).

Breast Feeding Summary

No data are available (see also Atropine).

Reference

1. Heinonen OP, Slone D, Shapiro S. *Birth Defects and Drugs in Pregnancy*. Littleton:Publishing Sciences Group, 1977.

Name: **ISOPROTERENOL**

Class: **Sympathomimetic**   Risk Factor: **C**

Fetal Risk Summary

No reports linking the use of isoproterenol with congenital defects have been located. Isoproterenol is teratogenic in some animal species, but human teratogenicity has not been suspected (1, 2). The Collaborative Perinatal Project monitored 50,282 mother-child pairs, 31 of which had 1st trimester exposure to isoproterenol (3, pp. 346–347). No evidence was found to suggest a relationship between large categories of major or minor malformations or to individual defects. However, an association in the 1st trimester was found between the sympathomimetic class of drugs as a whole and minor malformations (not life-threatening or major cosmetic defects), inguinal hernia, and clubfoot (3, pp. 345–356). Sympathomimetics are often administered in combination with other drugs to alleviate the symptoms of upper respiratory infections. Thus, the fetal effects of sympathomimetics, other drugs, and viruses cannot be totally separated.

Isoproterenol has been used during pregnancy to accelerate heart rhythm when high-grade atrioventricular block is present and to treat ventricular arrhythmias associated with prolonged QT intervals (4). Because of its β-adrenergic effect, the agent will inhibit contractions of the pregnant uterus (4). Of incidental interest, five term, nonlaboring pregnant women were discovered to have an increased resistance to the chronotropic effect of isoproterenol in comparison to nonpregnant women (5). One fetus had an isolated 5 beat/minute late deceleration 2 minutes after the mother received 0.25 μg of the drug (5).

Breast Feeding Summary

No data are available.

References

1. Nishimura H, Tanimura T. *Clinical Aspects of the Teratogenicity of Drugs*. Amsterdam:Excerpta Medica, 1976;231–2.
2. Shepard TH. *Catalog of Teratogenic Agents*, ed. 3. Baltimore:Johns Hopkins University Press, 1980;191.
3. Heinonen OP, Slone D, Shapiro S. *Birth Defects and Drugs in Pregnancy*. Littleton:Publishing Sciences Group, 1977.
4. Tamari I, Eldar M, Rabinowitz B, Neufeld HN. Medical treatment of cardiovascular disorders during pregnancy. Am Heart J 1982;104:1357–63.
5. DeSimone CA, Leighton BL, Norris MC, Chayen B, Menduke H. The chronotropic effect of isoproterenol is reduced in term pregnant women. Anesthesiology 1988;69:626–8.

Name: **ISOSORBIDE**

Class: **Diuretic**   Risk Factor: **C**

Fetal Risk Summary

No data are available.

Breast Feeding Summary

No data are available.

Name: **ISOSORBIDE DINITRATE**

Class: **Vasodilator**   Risk Factor: **C**

Fetal Risk Summary

See Nitroglycerin or Amyl Nitrite.

Breast Feeding Summary

No data are available.

Name: **ISOTRETINOIN**

Class: **VITAMIN**   Risk Factor: **X$_M$**

Fetal Risk Summary

Isotretinoin (Accutane) is a vitamin A isomer used for the treatment of severe, recalcitrant cystic acne. The animal teratogenicity of this drug was well documented prior to its approval for human use in 1982 (1, 2). Shortly after this approval, several publications appeared warning of the human teratogenic potential if isotretinoin was administered to women who were pregnant or who may become pregnant (3–8). In the 22 months following its introduction (September 1982–July 5, 1984), the manufacturer, the United States Food and Drug Administration (FDA), and the Centers for Disease Control (CDC), US Department of Health and Human Services received reports on 154 isotretinoin-exposed pregnancies (9). Some of these cases had been described in earlier reports (10–19). Of the 154 pregnancies, 95 were electively aborted, 12 aborted spontaneously, 26 infants were born without major defects (some may not have been exposed during the critical gestational period), and 21 had major malformations (9). Three of the 21 infants were stillborn and nine died after birth. A characteristic pattern of defects was observed in the 21 infants which closely resembled that seen in animal experiments (9). The syndrome of defects observed in these infants and in other reported cases (20–33) consists of all or part of the following:

Central nervous system:	Hydrocephalus
	Facial (VII nerve) palsy
	Posterior fossa structure defects
	Cortical and cerebellar defects
	Cortical blindness
	Optic nerve hypoplasia
	Retinal defects
	Microphthalmia
Craniofacial:	Microtia or anotia
	Low-set ears
	Agenesis or marked stenosis of external ear canals
	Micrognathia
	Small mouth
	Microcephaly
	Triangular skull
	Facial dysmorphism
	Depressed nasal bridge
	Cleft palate
	Hypertelorism
Cardiovascular:	Conotruncal malformations:
	Transposition of great vessels
	Tetralogy of Fallot
	Double-outlet right ventricle
	Truncus arteriosus communis
	Ventricular septal defect
	Atrial septal defect
	Branchial-arch mesenchymal-tissue defects:
	Interrupted or hypoplastic aortic arch
	Retroesophageal right subclavian artery
	Aortic arch hypoplasia
Thymic defects:	Ectopia, hypoplasia, or aplasia
Miscellaneous defects: (sporadic occurrence)	Spina bifida
	Nystagmus
	Hepatic abnormality
	Hydroureter
	Decreased muscle tone
	Large scrotal sac
	Simian crease
	Limb reduction (see comment below)

Other defects have been reported with isotretinoin, but in these cases exposure had either been terminated prior to conception or was outside the critical period for the defect (32). These defects are thought to be nonteratogenic or have occurred by chance (32). Similarly, three reports of anomalies in children where only the father was exposed (biliary atresia and ventricular septal defect; four-limb ectomelia and hydrocephalus; anencephaly) also probably occurred by chance (32).

A 1985 case report proposed that reduction deformities observed in all four limbs of a male infant were induced by isotretinoin (34, 35). Other evidence, however, suggested that these defects may have been secondary to amniotic bands (36).

Because isotretinoin causes central nervous system abnormalities, concern has been raised over the potential for adverse behavioral effects in infants who seemingly are normal at birth (37). Long-term studies are in progress to evaluate behavioral toxicities, such as mental retardation and learning disabilities, but have not been concluded because the exposed children are still too young for tests to produce meaningful results (38).

The teratogenic mechanism of isotretinoin and its main metabolite, 4-oxo-isotretinoin, is thought to result from an adverse effect on the initial differentiation and migration of cephalic neural crest cells (9, 39). Daily doses in the range of 0.5–1.5 mg/kg were usually ingested in cases with adverse outcome (9), but doses as low as 0.2 mg/kg or lower may also have caused teratogenicity (33, 40). The critical period of exposure is believed to be 2–5 weeks postconception, but clinically it is difficult to establish the exact dating in many cases (32). Because of the high proportion of spontaneous abortions in prospectively identified exposed women, the CDC commented that fetotoxicity may be a more common adverse outcome than liveborn infants with abnormalities (10).

The lack of reports of isotretinoin-induced abnormalities from areas other than the United States and Canada caused speculation that this was due to the use of lower doses, more restricted use in women, or later marketing of the drug (41). Several groups of investigators have responded to this, and although underdiagnosis and underreporting may contribute, the reasons are still unclear (40, 42–45).

An autosomal or X-linked recessive syndrome with features of isotretinoin-induced defects has been described in three male siblings (46). Although the mother had no history of isotretinoin or vitamin A use, the authors did not rule out a defect in vitamin A metabolism.

In a follow-up to a previous report involving 36 pregnancies, investigators noted the outcome of an additional 21 pregnancies exposed in the 1st trimester to isotretinoin (47). The outcomes of the 57 pregnancies were nine spontaneous abortions, one malformed stillborn, 10 malformed live births, and 37 normal liveborns (47). In this population, the absolute risk for a major defect in pregnancies extending to 20 weeks' gestation or longer was 23% (11 of 48) (47).

The outcome of pregnancies occurring after the discontinuation of isotretinoin was described in a 1989 article (48). Of 88 prospectively ascertained pregnancies, conception occurred in 77 within 60 days of the last dose of the drug. In 10 cases, the date of conception (defined as 14 days after the last menstrual period) occurred within 2–5 days after the last dose of isotretinoin. These 10 pregnancies ended in two spontaneous abortions and eight normal infants. Three women who had taken their last dose within 2 days of the estimated date of conception delivered normal infants. The outcomes of all 88 pregnancies were as follows: eight (9.1%) spontaneous abortions, one abnormal birth (details not provided), 75 (85.3%) normal infants, and four (4.5%) infants with congenital malformations. The defects observed were small anterior fontanelle (one case), congenital cataract with premature hypertrophic vitreous membrane (one case), congenital cataract (one case), and hypospadias (one case). The mothers had taken their last dose of isotretinoin 33, 22, 17, and 55 days prior to conception, respectively. These anomalies are not characteristic of those reported with *in utero* exposure to isotretinoin. In an additional 13 cases obtained retrospectively, five ended in spontaneous abortions, four normal infants were delivered, and four infants had congenital defects: syndactyly (one case), Down's syndrome (one case), hypoplasia of left side of heart (one case), and unknown defects (one case). In the cases of known defects, the mothers had stopped isotretinoin at least 9 months prior to conception. As with the prospective cases, the defects described in the three infants were not those typical of isotretinoin-induced anomalies. Moreover, retrospective reports are probably more likely to report abnormal outcomes and to underreport normal infants (48).

In summary, isotretinoin is a potent human teratogen. Critically important is the fact that a high percentage of the recipients of this drug are women in their childbearing years. Estimates have appeared indicating that 38% of isotretinoin users are women aged 13–19 years (13). Pregnancy must be excluded and prevented in these and other female patients before isotretinoin is prescribed. Therapy should be stopped at least 1 month prior to conception (13), but a recent report indicates that shorter intervals between the last dose of isotretinoin and conception are apparently safe (48). Fortunately, in one study the drug did not interfere with the action of oral contraceptive steroids (49).

Breast Feeding Summary

It is not known if isotretinoin or its metabolite, 4-oxo-isotretinoin, is excreted into human milk. The closely related retinoid, vitamin A, is excreted (see Vitamin A), and the presence of isotretinoin in breast milk should be expected.

References

1. Voorhees JJ, Orfanos CE. Oral retinoids. Arch Dermatol 1981;117:418–21.
2. Kamm JJ. Toxicology, carcinogenicity, and teratogenicity of some orally administered retinoids. J Am Acad Dermatol 1982;6:652–9.
3. Perry MD, McEvoy GK. Isotretinoin: new therapy for severe acne. Clin Pharm 1983;2:12–9.
4. Henderson IWD, Rice WB. Accutane. Can Med Assoc J 1983;129:682.
5. Shalita AR, Cunningham WJ, Leyden JJ, Pochi PE, Strauss JS. Isotretinoin treatment of acne and related disorders: an update. J Am Acad Dermatol 1983;9:629–38.
6. Anonymous. Update on isotretinoin (Accutane) for acne. Med Lett Drugs Ther 1983;25:105–6.
7. Conner CS. Isotretinoin: a reappraisal. Drug Intell Clin Pharm 1984;18:308–9.
8. Ward A, Brogden RN, Heel RC, Speight TM, Avery GS. Isotretinoin. A review of its pharmacological properties and therapeutic efficacy in acne and other skin disorders. Drugs 1984;28:6–37.
9. Lammer EJ, Chen DT, Hoar RM, Agnish ND, Benke PJ, Braun JT, Curry CJ, Fernhoff PM, Grix AW Jr, Lott IT, Richard JM, Sun SC. Retinoic acid embryopathy. N Engl J Med 1985;313:837–41.
10. Anonymous. Isotretinoin — a newly recognized human teratogen. MMWR 1984;33:171–3.
11. Anonymous. Update on birth defects with isotretinoin. FDA Drug Bull 1984;14:15–6.
12. Rosa FW. Teratogenicity of isotretinoin. Lancet 1983;2:513.
13. Anonymous. Adverse effects with isotretinoin. FDA Drug Bull 1983;13:21–3.

14. Braun JT, Franciosi RA, Mastri AR, Drake RM, O'Neil BL. Isotretinoin dysmorphic syndrome. Lancet 1984;1:506–7.

15. Hill RM. Isotretinoin teratogenicity. Lancet 1984;1:1465.

16. Benke PJ. The isotretinoin teratogen syndrome. JAMA 1984;251:3267–9.

17. Fernhoff PM, Lammer EJ. Craniofacial features of isotretinoin embryopathy. J Pediatr 1984;105:595–7.

18. Lott IT, Bocian M, Pribram HW, Leitner M. Fetal hydrocephalus and ear anomalies associated with maternal use of isotretinoin. J Pediatr 1984;105:597–600.

19. De La Cruz E, Sun S, Vangvanichyakorn K, Desposito F. Multiple congenital malformations associated with maternal isotretinoin therapy. Pediatrics 1984;74:428–30.

20. Stern RS, Rosa F, Baum C. Isotretinoin and pregnancy. J Am Acad Dermatol 1984;10:851–4.

21. Marwick C. More cautionary labeling appears on isotretinoin. JAMA 1984;251:3208–9

22. Zarowny DP. Accutane Roche: risk of teratogenic effects. Can Med Assoc J 1984;131:273.

23. Hall JG. Vitamin A: a newly recognized human teratogen. Harbinger of things to come? J Pediatr 1984;105:583–4.

24. Robertson R, MacLeod PM. Accutane-induced teratogenesis. Can Med Assoc J 1985;133:1147–8.

25. Willhite CC, Hill RM, Irving DW. Isotretinoin-induced craniofacial malformations in humans and hamsters. J Craniofac Genet Dev Biol 1986;2(Suppl):193–209.

26. Cohen M, Rubinstein A, Li JK, Nathenson G. Thymic hypoplasia associated with isotretinoin embryopathy. Am J Dis Child 1987;141:263–6.

27. Millan SB, Flowers FP, Sherertz EF. Isotretinoin. South Med J 1987;80:494–9.

28. Jahn AF, Ganti K. Major auricular malformations due to Accutane (isotretinoin). Laryngoscope 1987;97:832–5.

29. Bigby M, Stern RS. Adverse reactions to isotretinoin: a report from the adverse drug reaction reporting system. J Am Acad Dermatol 1988;18:543–52.

30. Anonymous. Birth defects caused by isotretinoin — New Jersey. MMWR 1988;37:171–2,177.

31. Orfanos CE, Ehlert R, Gollnick H. The retinoids: a review of their clinical pharmacology and therapeutic use. Drugs 1987;34:459–503.

32. Rosa FW, Wilk AL, Kelsey FO. Teratogen update: vitamin A congeners. Teratology 1986;33:355–64.

33. Rosa FW. Retinoic acid embryopathy. N Engl J Med 1986;315:262.

34. McBride WG. Limb reduction deformities in child exposed to isotretinoin in utero on gestation days 26–40 only. Lancet 1985;1:1276.

35. McBride WG. Isotretinoin and reduction deformities. Lancet 1985;2:503.

36. Lammer EJ, Flannery DB, Barr M. Does isotretinoin cause limb reduction defects? Lancet 1985;2:328.

37. Vorhees CV. Retinoic acid embryopathy. N Engl J Med 1986;315:262–3.

38. Lammer EJ. Retinoic acid embryopathy. In reply. N Engl J Med 1986;315:263.

39. Webster WS, Johnston MC, Lammer EJ, Sulik KK. Isotretinoin embryopathy and the cranial neural crest: an in vivo and in vitro study. J Craniofac Genet Dev Biol 1986;6:211–22.

40. Ayme S, Julian C, Gambarelli D, Mariotti B, Maurin N. Isotretinoin dose and teratogenicity. Lancet 1988;1:655.

41. Rosa F. Isotretinoin dose and teratogenicity. Lancet 1987;2:1154.

42. Robert E. Isotretinoin dose and teratogenicity. Lancet 1988;1:236.

43. Lammer EJ, Schunior A, Hayes AM, Holmes LB. Isotretinoin dose and teratogenicity. Lancet 1988;2:503–4.

44. Hope G, Mathias B. Teratogenicity of isotretinoin and etretinate. Lancet 1988;2:1143.

45. Lancaster PAL. Teratogenicity of isotretinoin. Lancet 1988;2:1254.

46. Kawashima H, Ohno I, Ueno Y, Nakaya S, Kato E, Taniguchi N. Syndrome of microtia and aortic arch anomalies resembling isotretinoin embryopathy. J Pediatr 1987;111:738–40.

47. Lammer EJ, Hayes AM, Schunior A, Holmes LB. Risk for major malformation among human fetuses exposed to isotretinoin (13-cis-retinoic acid). Teratology 1987;35:68A.

48. Dai WS, Hsu M-A, Itri LM. Safety of pregnancy after discontinuation of isotretinoin. Arch Dermatol 1989;125:363–5.

49. Orme M, Back DJ, Shaw MA, Allen WL, Tjia J, Cunliffe WJ, Jones DH. Isotretinoin and contraception. Lancet 1984;2:752–3.

Name: **ISOXSUPRINE**

Class: **Sympathomimetic (Adrenergic)**   Risk Factor: **C**

Fetal Risk Summary

No reports linking the use of isoxsuprine with congenital defects have been located. Isoxsuprine, a β-sympathomimetic, is indicated for vasodilation, but it has been used to prevent premature labor (1–6). Uterine inhibitory effects usually require high intravenous doses, which increase the risk for serious adverse effects (7, 8). Maternal heart rate increases and blood pressure decreases are usually mild at lower doses (2, 4, 6). A decrease in the incidence of neonatal respiratory distress syndrome has been observed (9). However, in one study, neonatal respiratory depression was increased if cord serum levels exceeded 10 ng/ml (10). The depression was always associated with hypotension, so the mechanism of the defect may have been related to pulmonary hypoperfusion. Neonatal toxicity is generally rare if cord levels of isoxsuprine are less than 2 ng/ml (corresponding to a drug-free interval of more than 5 hours), but levels greater than 10 ng/ml (drug-free interval of 2 hours of less) were associated with severe neonatal problems (10). These problems include hypocalcemia, hypoglycemia, ileus, hypotension and death (10–12). Hypotension and neonatal death occurred primarily in infants of 26–31 weeks' gestation, especially if cord levels exceeded 10 ng/ml, and in infants whose mothers developed hypotension or tachycardia during isoxsuprine infusion (10, 11). Neonatal ileus, up to 33% in some series, was not related to cord isoxsuprine concentrations, but hypotension and hypocalcemia were directly related, reaching 89% and 100%, respectively, when cord levels exceeded 10 ng/ml (10, 12). Fetal tachycardia is a common side effect. As compared to controls, no increase in late or variable decelerations was seen (10). In contrast to the above, infusion of isoxsuprine 30 minutes prior to cesarean section under general anesthesia was not observed to produce adverse effects in the mother, fetus, or newborn (13). Cord concentrations were not measured. Long-term evaluation of infants exposed to β-mimetics *in utero* has been reported, but not specifically for isoxsuprine (14). No harmful effects in the infants resulting from this exposure were observed.

The Collaborative Perinatal Project monitored 50,282 mother-child pairs, 54 of which were exposed to isoxsuprine during the 1st trimester (15, pp. 346–347). For use anytime during pregnancy, 858 exposures were recorded (15, p. 439). In neither case was evidence found for an association with malformations.

Breast Feeding Summary

No data are available.

References

1. Bishop EH, Woutersz TB. Isoxsuprine, a myometrial relaxant. A preliminary report. Obstet Gynecol 1961;17:442–6.
2. Hendricks CH, Cibils LA, Pose SV, Eskes TKAB. The pharmacological control of excessive uterine activity with isoxsuprine. Am J Obstet Gynecol 1961;82:1064–78.
3. Bishop EH, Woutersz TB. Arrest of premature labor. JAMA 1961;178:812–4.
4. Stander RW, Barden TP, Thompson JF, Pugh WR, Werts CE. Fetal cardiac effects of maternal isoxsuprine infusion. Am J Obstet Gynecol 1964;89:792–800.

5. Hendricks CH. The use of isoxsuprine for the arrest of premature labor. Clin Obstet Gynecol 1964;7:687–94.
6. Allen HH, Short H, Fraleigh DM. The use of isoxsuprine in the management of premature labor. Appl Ther 1965;7:544–7.
7. Anonymous. Drugs acting on the uterus. Br Med J 1964;1:1234–6.
8. Briscoe CC. Failure of oral isoxsuprine to prevent prematurity. Am J Obstet Gynecol 1966;95:885–6.
9. Kero P, Hirvonen T, Valimaki I. Perinatal isoxsuprine and respiratory distress syndrome. Lancet 1973;2:198.
10. Brazy JE, Little V, Grimm J, Pupkin M. Risk:benefit considerations for the use of isoxsuprine in the treatment of premature labor. Obstet Gynecol 1981;58:297–303.
11. Brazy JE, Pupkin MJ. Effects of maternal isoxsuprine administration on preterm infants. J Pediatr 1979;94:444–8.
12. Brazy JE, Little V, Grimm J. Isoxsuprine in the perinatal period. II. Relationships between neonatal symptoms, drug exposure, and drug concentration at the time of birth. J Pediatr 1981;98:146–51.
13. Jouppila R, Kauppila A, Tuimala R, Pakarinen A, Moilanen K. Maternal, fetal and neonatal effects of beta-adrenergic stimulation in connection with cesarean section. Acta Obstet Gynecol Scand 1980;59:489–93.
14. Freysz H, Willard D, Lehr A, Messer J. Boog G. A long term evaluation of infants who received a beta-mimetic drug while in utero. J Perinat Med 1977;5:94–9.
15. Heinonen OP, Slone D, Shapiro S. *Birth Defects and Drugs in Pregnancy*. Littleton:Publishing Sciences Group, 1977.

Name: **KANAMYCIN**

Class: **Antibiotic**   Risk Factor: **D**

Fetal Risk Summary

Kanamycin is an aminoglycoside antibiotic. At term, the drug was detectable in cord serum 15 minutes after a 500-mg intramuscular (IM) maternal dose (1). Mean cord serum levels at 3–6 hours were 6 μg/ml. Amniotic fluid levels were undetectable during the first hours, then rose during the next 6 hours to a mean value of 5.5 μg/ml. No effects on the infants were mentioned.

Eighth cranial nerve damage has been reported following *in utero* exposure to kanamycin (2, 3). In a retrospective survey of 391 mothers who had received kanamycin, 50 mg/kg, for prolonged periods during pregnancy, nine (2.3%) children were found to have hearing loss (2). Complete hearing loss in a mother and her infant was reported after the mother had been treated during pregnancy with kanamycin, 1 g IM/day for 4.5 days (3). Ethacrynic acid, an ototoxic diuretic, was also given to the mother during pregnancy.

Except for ototoxicity, no reports of congenital defects due to kanamycin have been located. Embryos were examined from five patients who aborted during the 11th–12th week of pregnancy and who had been treated with kanamycin during the 6th and 8th weeks (2). No abnormalities in the embryos were found.

Breast Feeding Summary

Kanamycin is excreted in breast milk. Milk:plasma ratios of 0.05–0.40 have been reported (4). A 1-g IM dose produced peak milk levels of 18.4 μg/ml (5). No effects were reported in the nursing infants. Since oral absorption of kanamycin is poor, ototoxicity would not be expected. However, three potential problems exist for the nursing infant: modification of bowel flora, direct effects on the infant, and interference with the interpretation of culture results if a fever workup is required. The American Academy of Pediatrics considers kanamycin to be compatible with breast feeding (6).

References

1. Good R, Johnson G. The placental transfer of kanamycin during late pregnancy. Obstet Gynecol 1971;38:60–2.
2. Nishimura H, Tanimura T. *Clinical Aspects of the Teratogenicity of Drugs*. Amsterdam:Excerpta Medica, 1976:131.
3. Jones HC. Intrauterine ototoxicity. A case report and review of literature. J Natl Med Assoc 1973;65:201–3.
4. Wilson JT. Milk/plasma ratios and contraindicated drugs. In Wilson JT, ed. *Drugs in Breast Milk*. Balgowlah, Australia:ADIS Press, 1981:79.
5. O'Brien T. Excretion of drugs in human milk. Am J Hosp Pharm 1974;31:844–54.
6. Committee on Drugs, American Academy of Pediatrics. Transfer of drugs and other chemicals into human milk. Pediatrics 1989;84:924–36.

Name: **LABETALOL**

Class: **Sympatholytic**

Risk Factor: **C$_M$**

Fetal Risk Summary

Labetalol, a combined α/β-adrenergic blocking agent, has been used for the treatment of hypertension occurring during pregnancy (1–29). The drug crosses the placenta to produce cord serum concentrations averaging 40–80% of peak maternal levels (1–5). Maternal serum and amniotic fluid concentrations are approximately equivalent 1–3 hours after a single intravenous dose (4). After oral dosing (1–42 days) in eight women, amniotic fluid concentrations of labetalol were in the same range as the plasma but lower in six of the women (6). The pharmacokinetics of labetalol in pregnant patients have been reported (7, 8). A 1988 article briefly reviewed some of the experience with labetalol in pregnancy (30).

No fetal malformations attributable to labetalol have been reported, but experience during the 1st trimester is lacking. Most reports have found no adverse effects on birth weight, head circumference, Apgar scores, or blood glucose control after *in utero* exposure to labetalol (9–13). One case of neonatal hypoglycemia has been mentioned, but the mother was also taking a thiazide diuretic (2). Offspring of mothers treated with labetalol had a significantly higher birth weight than infants of atenolol-treated mothers, 3280 g vs. 2750 g ($p < 0.001$), respectively (14). However, in a study comparing labetalol plus hospitalization to hospitalization alone for the treatment of mild preeclampsia presenting at 26–35 weeks' gestation, labetalol treatment did not improve perinatal outcome, and a significantly higher number of labetalol-exposed infants were growth retarded, 19.1% (18 of 94) vs. 9.3% (9 of 97) ($p < 0.05$), respectively (15).

Fetal heart rate is apparently unaffected by labetalol treatment of hypertensive pregnant women. However, two studies have observed newborn bradycardia in a total of five infants (16, 17). In one of these infants, bradycardia was marked (<100) and persistent (17). All five infants survived. Hypotension was noted in another infant delivered by cesarean section at 28 weeks' gestation (1). In a study examining the effects of labetalol exposure on term (37 weeks or greater) newborns, mild transient hypotension, which resolved within 24 hours, was observed in 11 infants compared to 11 matched controls (18). Maternal dosage varied from 100–300 mg three times daily with the last dose given within 12 hours of birth. The mean systolic blood pressures at 2 hours of age in exposed and nonexposed infants were 58.8 and 63.3 mm Hg ($p < 0.05$), respectively. Other measures of β-blockade—such as heart and respiratory rates, palmar sweating, blood glucose control, and metabolic and vasomotor responses to cold stress—did not differ between the groups. The investigators concluded that labetalol did not cause clinically significant β-blockade in mature newborn infants (18).

Several investigations have shown a lack of effect of labetalol treatment on uterine contractions (1–3, 16, 19–21). One study did report a higher incidence of spontaneous labor in labetalol-treated mothers (6 of 10) than in a similar group treated with methyldopa (2 of 9) (22). In another report, 3 of 31 patients treated with labetalol experienced spontaneous labor, one of whom delivered prematurely (23). The authors attributed the uterine activity to the drug because no other causes were found. However, since most trials with labetalol in hypertensive women have not shown this effect, it is questionable whether the drug has any direct effect on uterine contractility.

Labetalol does not change uteroplacental blood flow despite a drop in blood pressure (2, 4, 5, 24, 25). The lack of effect on blood flow was probably due to reduced peripheral resistance.

Labetalol apparently reduces the incidence of hyaline membrane disease in premature infants by increasing the production of pulmonary surfactant (1, 2, 4, 16, 26). The mechanism for this effect may be mediated through β_2-adrenoceptor agonist activity that the drug partially possesses (1, 2, 4, 16, 26).

Follow-up studies have been completed at 6 months of age on 10 infants exposed *in utero* to labetalol (27). All infants demonstrated normal growth and development. In addition, no ocular toxicity has been observed in newborns, even though labetalol has an affinity for ocular melanin (1, 2, 26).

In summary, the use of labetalol for the treatment of maternal hypertension does not seem to pose a risk to the fetus and may offer advantages over the use of agents with only β-blocker activity. However, one study has demonstrated intrauterine growth retardation when the drug was used for the treatment of mild preeclampsia. Although the majority of newborns have shown no adverse clinical signs after exposure except for mild transient hypotension, they should be closely observed during the first 24–48 hours for bradycardia, hypotension, and other symptoms of α/β-blockade. Long-term (>6 months) studies of infants exposed *in utero* to labetalol have not yet been conducted.

Breast Feeding Summary

Labetalol is excreted into breast milk (1, 6). In 24 lactating women, 3 days postpartum, administration of 330–800 mg/day produced a mean milk level of 33 ng/ml. No adverse effects were observed in the nursing infants. One patient, consuming 1200 mg/day, had a mean milk concentration of 600 ng/ml, but this woman did not breast feed. Three women, 6–9 days postpartum, consumed daily doses of labetalol of 600 mg, 600 mg, and 1200 mg and produced peak milk concentrations of the drug of 129 ng/ml, 223 ng/ml, and 662 ng/ml, respectively (6). Peak concentrations of labetalol in the milk occurred between 2–3 hours after a dose. Measurable plasma concentrations of labetalol were found in only one infant; 18 ng/ml at 4 hours, and 21 ng/ml at 8 hours. Although no adverse effects have been reported, nursing infants should be closely observed for bradycardia, hypotension, and other symptoms of α/β-blockade. Long-term effects of exposure to labetalol from milk have not been studied but warrant evaluation. The American Academy of Pediatrics considers labetalol to be compatible with breast feeding (31).

References

1. Michael CA. Use of labetalol in the treatment of severe hypertension during pregnancy. Br J Clin Pharmacol 1979;8(Suppl 2):211S–5S.

2. Riley AJ. Clinical pharmacology of labetalol in pregnancy. J Cardiovasc Pharmacol 1981;3(Suppl 1):S53–S9.

3. Andrejak M, Coevoet B, Fievet P, Gheerbrant JD, Comoy E, Leuillet P, Verhoest P, Boulanger JC, Vitse M, Fournier A. Effect of labetalol on hypertension and the renin-angiotensin-aldosterone and adrenergic systems in pregnancy. In Riley A, Symonds EM, eds. The Investigation of Labetalol in the Management of Hypertension in Pregnancy. Amsterdam:Excerpta Medica, 1982:77–87.

4. Lunell NO, Hjemdahl P, Fredholm BB, Lewander R, Nisell H, Nylund L, Persson B, Sarby J, Wager J, Thornstrom S. Acute effects of labetalol on maternal metabolism and uteroplacental circulation in hypertension of pregnancy. In Riley A, Symonds EM, eds. The Investigation of Labetalol in the Management of Hypertension in Pregnancy. Amsterdam:Excerpta Medica, 1982:34–45.

5. Nylund L, Lunell NO, Lewander R, Sarby B, Thornstrom S. Labetalol for the treatment of hypertension in pregnancy. Acta Obstet Gynecol Scand 1984;118(Suppl):71–3.

6. Lunell NO, Kulas J, Rane A. Transfer of labetalol into amniotic fluid and breast milk in lactating women. Eur J Clin Pharmacol 1985;28:597–9.

7. Rubin PC. Drugs in pregnancy. In Riley A, Symonds EM. eds. The Investigation of Labetalol in the Management of Hypertension in Pregnancy. Amsterdam:Excerpta Medica, 1982:28–33.

8. Rubin PC, Butters L, Kelman AW, Fitzsimons C, Reid JL. Labetalol disposition and concentration-effect relationships during pregnancy. Br J Clin Pharmacol 1983;15:465–70.

9. Lamming GD, Broughton Pipkin F, Symonds EM. Comparison of the alpha and beta blocking drug, labetalol, and methyl dopa in the treatment of moderate and severe pregnancy-induced hypertension. Clin Exp Hypertens 1980;2:865–95.

10. Lotgering FK, Derkx FMH, Wallenburg HCS. Primary hyperaldsternism in pregnancy. Am J Obstet Gynecol 1986;155:986–8.

11. Mabie WC, Gonzalez AR, Sibai BM, Amon E. A comparative trial of labetalol and hydralazine in the acute management of severe hypertension complicating pregnancy. Obstet Gynecol 1987;70:328–33.

12. Plouin P-F, Breart G, Maillard F, Papiernik E, Relier J-P. Comparison of antihypertensive efficacy and perinatal safety of labetalol and methyldopa in the treatment of hypertension in pregnancy: a randomized controlled trial. Br J Obstet Gynaecol 1988;95:868–76.

13. Pickles CJ, Symonds EM, Broughton Pipkin F. The fetal outcome in a randomized trial of labetalol versus placebo in pregnancy-induced hypertension. Br J Obstet Gynaecol 1989;96:38–43.

14. Lardoux H, Gerard J, Blazquez G, Chouty F, Flouvat B. Hypertension in pregnancy: evaluation of two beta blockers atenolol and labetalol. Eur Heart J 1983;4(Suppl G):35–40.

15. Sibai BM, Gonzalez AR, Mabie WC, Moretti M. A comparison of labetalol plus hospitalization versus hospitalization alone in the management of preeclampsia remote from term. Obstet Gynecol 1987;70:323–7.

16. Michael CA, Potter JM. A comparison of labetalol with other antihypertensive drugs in the treatment of hypertensive disease of pregnancy. In Riley A, Symonds EM. eds. The Investigation of Labetalol in the Management of Hypertension in Pregnancy. Amsterdam:Excerpta Medica, 1982:111–22.

17. Davey DA, Dommisse J, Garden A. Intravenous labetalol and intravenous dihydralazine in severe hypertension in pregnancy. In Riley A, Symonds EM, eds. The Investigation of Labetalol in the Management of Hypertension in Pregnancy. Amsterdam:Excerpta Medica, 1982:52–61.

18. MacPherson M, Broughton Pipkin F, Rutter N. The effect of maternal labetalol on the newborn infant. Br J Obstet Gynaecol 1986;93:539–42.

19. Redman CWG. A controlled trial of the treatment of hypertension in pregnancy: labetalol compared with methyldopa. In Riley A, Symonds EM, eds. The Investigation of Labetalol in the Management of Hypertension in Pregnancy. Amsterdam:Excerpta Medica, 1982:101–10.

20. Walker JJ, Crooks A, Erwin L, Calder AA. Labetalol in pregnancy-induced hypertension: fetal and maternal effects. In Riley A, Symonds EM, eds. The Investigation of Labetalol in the Management of Hypertension in Pregnancy. Amsterdam:Excerpta Medica, 1982:148–60.

21. Thulesius O, Lunell NO, Ibrahim M, Moberger B, Angilivilayil C. The effect of labetalol on contractility of human myometrial preparations. Acta Obstet Gynecol 1987;66:237–40.

22. Lamming GD, Symonds EM. Use of labetalol and methyldopa in pregnancy-induced hypertension. Br J Clin Pharmacol 1979;8(Suppl 2):217S–22S.

23. Jorge CS, Fernandes L, Cunha S. Labetalol in the hypertensive states of pregnancy. In Riley A, Symonds EM, eds. The Investigation of Labetalol in the Management of Hypertension in Pregnancy. Amsterdam:Excerpta Medica, 1982:124–30.

24. Lunell NO, Nylund L, Lewander R, Sarby B. Acute effect of an antihypertensive drug, labetalol, on uteroplacental blood flow. Br J Obstet Gynaecol 1982;89:640–4.

25. Jouppila P, Kirkinen P, Koivula A, Ylikorkala O. Labetalol does not alter the placental and fetal blood flow or maternal prostanoids in pre-eclampsia. Br J Obstet Gynaecol 1986;93:543–7.

26. Michael CA. The evaluation of labetalol in the treatment of hypertension complicating pregnancy. Br J Clin Pharmacol 1982;13(Suppl):127S–31S.

27. Symonds EM, Lamming GD, Jadoul F, Broughton Pipkin F. Clinical and biochemical aspects of the use of labetalol in the treatment of hypertension in pregnancy: comparison with methyldopa. In Riley A, Symonds EM, eds. The Investigation of Labetalol in the Management of Hypertension in Pregnancy. Amsterdam:Excerpta Medica, 1982:62–76.

28. Smith AM. Beta-blockers for pregnancy hypertension. Lancet 1983;1:708–9.

29. Walker JJ, Bonduelle M, Greer I, Calder AA. Antihypertensive therapy in pregnancy. Lancet 1983;1:932–3.

30. Frishman WH, Chesner M. Beta-adrenergic blockers in pregnancy. Am Heart J 1988;115:147–52.

31. Committee on Drugs, American Academy of Pediatrics. Transfer of drugs and other chemicals into human milk. Pediatrics 1989;84:924–36.

Name: **LACTULOSE**

Class: **Laxative/Ammonia Detoxicant**　　　　　　　　　Risk Factor: **C**

Fetal Risk Summary

No data are available.

Breast Feeding Summary

No data are available.

Name: **LAETRILE**

Class: **Unclassified/Antineoplastic**　　　　　　　　　Risk Factor: **C**

Fetal Risk Summary

Laetrile is a nonapproved agent used for the treatment of cancer. There are no studies of laetrile in pregnancy. A concern for possible gestational cyanide poisoning has been reported (1). Due to an increased amount of β-glycosidase present in the intestinal flora, the oral route would theoretically be more toxic than the parenteral route in liberation of hydrogen cyanide, which is present in various sources of laetrile (1). Long-term follow-up has been recommended because neurologic evidence of chronic cyanide exposure may not be recognizable in the infant.

Breast Feeding Summary

No data are available.

Reference

1. Peterson RG, Ruman BH. Laetrile and pregnancy. Clin Toxicol 1979;15:181–4.

Name: **LANATOSIDE C**

Class: **Cardiac Glycoside**   Risk Factor: **C**

Fetal Risk Summary

See Digitalis.

Breast Feeding Summary

See Digitalis.

Name: **LEUCOVORIN**

Class: **Vitamin**   Risk Factor: **C$_M$**

Fetal Risk Summary

Leucovorin (folinic acid) is an active metabolite of folic acid (1). It has been used for the treatment of megaloblastic anemia during pregnancy (2). See Folic Acid.

Breast Feeding Summary

Leucovorin (folinic acid) is an active metabolite of folic acid (1). See Folic Acid.

References

1. American Hospital Formulary Service. *Drug Information 1990.* Bethesda:American Society of Hospital Pharmacists, 1990:2179–81.
2. Scott JM. Folinic acid in megaloblastic anaemia of pregnancy. Br Med J 1957:2:270–2.

Name: **LEVALLORPHAN**

Class: **Narcotic Antagonist**   Risk Factor: **D**

Fetal Risk Summary

Levallorphan is a narcotic antagonist that is used to reverse respiratory depression from narcotic overdose. It has been used in combination with alphaprodine or meperidine during labor to reduce neonatal depression (1–6). Although some benefits were initially claimed, caution in the use of levallorphan during labor has been advised for the following reasons (7):

A statistically significant reduction in neonatal depression has not been demonstrated.
The antagonist also reduces analgesia.
The antagonist may increase neonatal depression if an improper narcotic-narcotic antagonist ratio is used.

As indicated above, levallorphan may cause respiratory depression in the absence of narcotics or if a critical ratio is exceeded (7). Because of these considerations, the use in pregnancy of levallorphan either alone or in combination therapy should be discouraged. If a narcotic antagonist is indicated, other agents that do not cause respiratory depression, such as naloxone, are preferred.

Breast Feeding Summary

No data are available.

References

1. Backner DD, Foldes FF, Gordon EH. The combined use of alphaprodine (Nisentil) hydrochloride and levallorphan tartrate for analgesia in obstetrics. Am J Obstet Gynecol 1957;74:271–82.
2. Roberts H, Kuck MAC. Use of alphaprodine and levallorphan during labour. Can Med Assoc J 1960;83:1088–93.
3. Roberts H, Kane KM, Percival N, Snow P, Please NW. Effects of some analgesic drugs used in childbirth. Lancet 1957;1:128–32.
4. Bullough J. Use of premixed pethidine and antagonists in obstetrical analgesia with special reference to cases in which levallorphan was used. Br Med J 1959;2:859–62.
5. Posner AC. Combined pethidine and antagonists in obstetrics. Br Med J 1960;1:124–5.
6. Bullough J. Combined pethidine and antagonists in obstetrics. Br Med J 1960;1:125.
7. Bonica JJ. Principles and Practice of Obstetric Analgesia and Anesthesia. Philadelphia:FA Davis, 1967;254–9.

Name: **LEVARTERENOL**

Class: **Sympathomimetic (Adrenergic)**   Risk Factor: **D**

Fetal Risk Summary

Levarterenol is a sympathomimetic used in emergency situations to treat hypotension. Because of the nature of its indication, experience in pregnancy is limited. Levarterenol readily crosses the placenta (1). Uterine vessels are normally maximally dilated, and they have only α-adrenergic receptors (2). Use of the α- and β-adrenergic stimulant, levarterenol, could cause constriction of these vessels and reduce uterine blood flow, thereby producing fetal hypoxia (bradycardia). Levarterenol may also interact with oxytocics or ergot derivatives to produce severe persistent maternal hypertension (2). Rupture of a cerebral vessel is possible. If a pressor agent is indicated, other drugs, such as ephedrine, should be considered.

Breast Feeding Summary

No data are available.

References

1. Morgan CD, Sandler M, Panigel M. Placental transfer of catecholamines in vitro and in vivo. Am J Obstet Gynecol 1972;112:1068–75.
2. Smith NT, Corbascio AN. The use and misuse of pressor agents. Anesthesiology 1970;33:58–101.

Name: **LEVORPHANOL**

Class: **Narcotic Analgesic**   Risk Factor: **B***

Fetal Risk Summary

No reports linking the use of levorphanol with congenital defects have been located. Use of the drug during labor should be expected to produce neonatal depression to the same degree as other narcotic analgesics (1).

[*Risk Factor D if used for prolonged periods or in high doses at term.]

Breast Feeding Summary

No data are available.

References

1. Bonica JJ. *Principles and Practice of Obstetric Analgesia and Anesthesia.* Philadelphia:FA Davis, 1967:251.

Name: **LEVOTHYROXINE**

Class: **Thyroid**   Risk Factor: **A_M**

Fetal Risk Summary

Levothyroxine (T4) is a naturally occurring thyroid hormone produced by the mother and the fetus. It is used during pregnancy for the treatment of hypothyroidism (see also Liothyronine and Thyroid). Most investigators have concluded that there is negligible transplacental passage of the drug at physiologic serum concentrations (1–6). However, maternal-fetal transfer of sufficient amounts of T4 to protect the congenital hypothryoid fetus and newborn has been demonstrated (7).

In a study of 25 neonates born with an autosomal recessive disorder that completely prevents iodination of thyroid proteins and, thus, the synthesis of T4, the thyroid hormone was measured in their cord serum in concentrations ranging from 35–70 nmol/L. Since the newborns were unable to synthesize the hormone, the T4 must have come from the mothers (7). The investigators then studied 15 newborns with thyroid agenesis and measured similar cord levels of T4. The mean serum half-life of T4 in the neonates was only 3.6 days, indicating that T4 would be below the level of detection between 8 and 19 days after birth (7). Although the amounts measured were below normal values of T4 (80–170 nmol/L), the amounts were sufficient to protect the infants initially from impaired mental development. A possible mechanism for this protection may involve increased conversion of T4 to T3 in the cerebral cortex in hypothyroid fetuses, and, when combined with a decreased rate of T3 degradation, the net effect is to normalize intracellular levels of the active thyroid hormone in the brain (7).

Several reports have described the direct administration of T4 to the fetus and amniotic fluid (5, 7–13). In almost identical cases, two fetuses were treated in the 3rd trimester with intramuscular injections of T4, 120 μg, every 2 weeks for four doses in an attempt to prevent congenital hypothyroidism (5, 9). Their mothers had been treated with radioactive iodine (I^{131}) at 13 and 13 1/2 weeks' gestation, respectively. Both newborns were hypothyroid at birth and developed respiratory stridor, but neither had physical signs of cretinism. At the time of the reports, one child had mild developmental retardation at 3 years of age (5). The second infant was stable with a tracheostomy tube in place at 6 months of age (9). In a third mother who inadvertently received I^{131} at 10–11 weeks' gestation, intra-amniotic T4, 500 μg, was given weekly during the last 7 weeks of pregnancy (10). Evidence was found that the T4 was absorbed by the fetus. A male infant was delivered who developed normally. In a study to determine the metabolic fate of T4 *in utero*, 700 μg of T4 were injected intra-amniotically 24 hours prior to delivery in five full-term healthy patients (11). Serum T4 levels were increased in all infants. Intra-amniotic T4, 200 μg, was given to eight women in whom premature delivery was inevitable or indicated to enhance fetal lung maturity (12). The patients ranged in gestational age between 29–32 weeks. No respiratory distress syndrome was found in the eight newborn infants. Delivery occurred 1–49 days after the injection. The dimensions of a large fetal goiter, secondary to propylthiouracil, were decreased but not eliminated within 5 days of an intra-amniotic 200-μg dose of T4 administered at 34.5 weeks' gestation (13). Serial lecithin:sphingomyelin (L:S) ratios before and after the injection demonstrated no effect of T4 on fetal lung maturity.

In a large prospective study, 537 mother-child pairs were exposed to levothyroxine and thyroid during the 1st trimester (14, pp. 388–400). For use anytime during pregnancy, 780 exposures were reported (14, p. 443). After 1st trimester exposure, possible associations were found with cardiovascular anomalies (nine cases), Down's syndrome (three cases), and polydactyly in blacks (three cases). Due to the small numbers involved, the statistical significance of these findings is unknown and independent confirmation is required. Maternal hypothyroidism itself has been reported to be responsible for poor pregnancy outcome (15–17). Others have not found this association, claiming that fetal development is not directly affected by maternal thyroid function (18).

Combination therapy with thyroid-antithyroid drugs was advocated at one time for the treatment of hyperthyroidism but is now considered inappropriate (see Propylthiouracil).

Breast Feeding Summary

Levothyroxine (T4) is excreted into breast milk in low concentrations. The effect of this hormone on the nursing infant is controversial (see also Liothyronine and Thyrotropin). Two reports have claimed that sufficient quantities are present to partially treat neonatal hypothyroidism (19, 20). A third study measured high T4 levels in breast-fed infants but was unsure of its significance (21). In contrast, four competing studies have found that breast feeding does not alter either T4 levels or thyroid function in the infant (22–25). Although all of the investigators, on both sides of the issue, used sophisticated available methods to arrive at their conclusions, the balance of evidence weighs in on the side of those claiming lack of effect since they have relied on increasingly refined means to measure the hormone (26–28). The reports are briefly summarized below.

In 19 healthy euthyroid mothers not taking thyroid replacement therapy, mean milk T4 concentrations in the 1st postpartum week were 3.8 ng/ml (19). Between 8–48 days, the levels rose to 42.7 ng/ml and then decreased to 11.1 ng/ml after

50 days postpartum. The daily excretion of T4 at the higher levels is about the recommended daily dose for hypothyroid infants. An infant was diagnosed as athyrotic shortly after breast feeding was stopped at age 10 months (19). Growth was at the 97th percentile during breast feeding, but the bone age remained that of a newborn. In this study, mean levels of T4 in breast milk during the last trimester (12 patients) and within 48 hours of delivery (22 patients) were 14 and 7 ng/ml, respectively. A 1983 report measured significantly greater serum levels of T4 in 22 breast-fed infants than in 25 formula-fed babies, 131.1 ng/ml vs. 118.4 ng/ml, respectively (22). The overlap between the two groups, however, cast doubt on the physiologic significance of the differences.

In 77 euthyroid mothers, measurable amounts of T4 were found in only 5 of 88 milk specimens collected over 43 months of lactation with four of the positive samples occurring within 4 days of delivery (22). Concentrations ranged from 8–13 ng/ml. A 1980 report described four exclusively breast-fed infants with congenital hypothyroidism who were diagnosed between the ages of 2–79 days (23). Breast feeding did not hinder making the diagnosis. Another 1980 research report evaluated clinical and biochemical thyroid parameters in 45 hypothyroid infants, 12 of whom were breast fed (24). No difference was detected between the breast-fed and bottle-fed babies, leading to the conclusion that breast milk did not offer protection against the effects of congenital hypothyroidism. In a 1985 study, serum concentrations of T4 were similar in breast-fed and bottle-fed infants at 5, 10, and 15 days postpartum (25).

The discrepancies described above can be partially explained by the various techniques used to measure milk T4 concentrations. Japanese researchers failed to detect milk T4 using four different methods of radioimmunoassay (RIA) (26). Using three competitive protein-binding assays, highly variable T4 levels were recovered from milk and a standard solution. Although the RIA methods were not completely reliable since recovery from a standardized solution exceeded 100% with one method, the researchers concluded that milk T4 concentrations must be very low and had no influence on the pituitary-thyroid axis of normal babies. No difficulty was encountered with measuring serum T4 levels, which were not significantly different between breast-fed and bottle-fed infants (26). Swedish investigators using RIA methods also failed to find T4 in milk (27). A second group of Swedish researchers utilized a gas chromatography-mass spectrometry technique to determine that the concentration of T4 in milk was less than 4 ng/ml (28).

In summary, levothyroxine breast milk levels, as determined by modern laboratory techniques, are apparently too low to protect a hypothyroid infant completely from the effects of the disease. The levels are also too low to interfere with neonatal thyroid screening programs (25). Breast feeding, however, probably offers better protection to infants with congenital hypothyroidism than does formula feeding.

References

1. Grumbach MM, Werner SC. Transfer of thyroid hormone across the human placenta at term. J Clin Endocrinol Metab 1956;16:1392–5.
2. Kearns JE, Hutson W. Tagged isomers and analogues of thyroxine (their transmission across the human placenta and other studies). J Nucl Med 1963;4:453–61.
3. Fisher DA, Lehman H, Lackey C. Placental transport of thyroxine. J Clin Endocrinol Metab 1964;24:393–400.

4. Fisher DA, Klein AH. Thyroid development and disorders of thyroid function in the newborn. N Engl J Med 1981;304:702–12.
5. Van Herle AJ, Young RT, Fisher DA, Uller RP, Brinkman CR III. Intrauterine treatment of a hypothyroid fetus. J Clin Endocrinol Metab 1975;40:474–7.
6. Bachrach LK, Burrow GN. Maternal-fetal transfer of thyroxine. N Engl J Med 1989;321:1549.
7. Vulsma T, Gons MH, de Vijlder JJM. Maternal-fetal transfer of thyroxine in congenital hypothyroidism due to a total organification defect or thyroid agenesis. N Engl J Med 1989;321:13–6.
8. Larsen PR. Maternal thyroxine and congenital hypothroidism. N Engl J Med 1989;321:44–6.
9. Jafek BW, Small R, Lillian DL. Congenital radioactive-iodine induced stridor and hypothyroidism. Arch Otolaryngol 1974;99:369–71.
10. Lightner ES, Fisher DA, Giles H, Woolfenden J. Intra-amniotic injection of thyroxine (T4) to a human fetus. Am J Obstet Gynecol 1977;127:487–90.
11. Klein AH, Hobel CJ, Sack J, Fisher DA. Effect of intraamniotic fluid thyroxine injection on fetal serum and amniotic fluid iodothyronine concentrations. J Clin Endocrinol Metab 1978;47:1034–7.
12. Mashiach S, Barkai G, Sach J, Stern E, Goldman B, Brish M, Serr DM. Enhancement of fetal lung maturity by intra-amniotic administration of thyroid hormone. Am J Obstet Gynecol 1978;130:289–93.
13. Weiner S, Scharf JI, Bolognese RJ, Librizzi RJ. Antenatal diagnosis and treatment of fetal goiter. J Reprod Med 1980;24:39–42.
14. Heinonen OP, Slone D, Shapiro S. *Birth Defects and Drugs in Pregnancy*. Littleton:Publishing Sciences Group, 1977.
15. Potter JD. Hypothyroidism and reproductive failure. Surg Gynecol Obstet 1980;150:251–5.
16. Pekonen F, Teramo K, Ikonen E, Osterlund K, Makinen T, Lamberg BA. Women on thyroid hormone therapy: pregnancy course, fetal outcome, and amniotic fluid thyroid hormone level. Obstet Gynecol 1984;63:635–8.
17. Man EB, Shaver BA Jr, Cooke RE. Studies of children born to women with thyroid disease. Am J Obstet Gynecol 1958;75:728–41.
18. Montoro M, Collea JV, Frasier SD, Mestman JH. Successful outcome of pregnancy in women with hypothyroidism. Ann Intern Med 1981;94:31–4.
19. Sack J, Amado O, Lunenfeld. Thyroxine concentration in human milk. J Clin Endocrinol Metab 1977;45:171–3.
20. Bode HH, Vanjonack WJ, Crawford JD. Mitigation of cretinism by breast-feeding. Pediatrics 1978;62:13–6.
21. Hahn HB Jr, Spiekerman AM, Otto WR, Hossalla DE. Thyroid function tests in neonates fed human milk. Am J Dis Child 1983;137:220–2.
22. Varma SK, Collins M, Row A, Haller WS, Varma K. Thyroxine, triiodothyronine, and reverse triiodothyronine concentrations in human milk. J Pediatr 1978;93:803–6.
23. Abbassi V, Steinour TA. Successful diagnosis of congenital hypothyroidism in four breast-fed neonates. J Pediatr 1980;97:259–61.
24. Letarte J, Guyda H, Dussault JH, Glorieux J. Lack of protective effect of breast-feeding in congenital hypothyroidism: report of 12 cases. Pediatrics 1980;65:703–5.
25. Franklin R, O'Grady C, Carpenter L. Neonatal thyroid function: comparison between breast-fed and bottle-fed infants. J Pediatr 1985;106:124–6.
26. Mizuta H, Amino N, Ichihara K, Harada T, Nose O, Tanizawa O, Miyai K. Thyroid hormones in human milk and their influence on thyroid function of breast-fed babies. Pediatr Res 1983;17:468–71.
27. Jansson L, Ivarsson S, Larsson I, Ekman R. Tri-iodothyronine and thyroxine in human milk. Acta Paediatr Scand 1983;72:703–5.
28. Moller B, Bjorkhem I, Falk O, Lantto O, Larsson A. Identification of thyroxine in human breast milk by gas chromatography-mass spectrometry. J Clin Endocrinol Metab 1983;56:30–4.

Name: **LIDOCAINE**

Class: **Local Anesthetic/Cardiac Drug**   Risk Factor: **C**

Fetal Risk Summary

Lidocaine is a local anesthetic that is also used for the treatment of cardiac ventricular arrhythmias. The majority of the information on the drug in pregnancy derives from its use as a local anesthetic during labor and delivery.

The drug rapidly crosses the placenta to the fetus, appearing in the fetal circulation within a few minutes after administration to the mother. Cord:maternal serum ratios range between 0.50–0.70 after intravenous (IV) and epidural anesthesia (1–11). In 25 women just prior to delivery, a dose of 2–3 mg/kg was given by IV infusion at a rate of 100 mg/minute (1). The mean cord:maternal serum ratio in nine patients who received 3 mg/kg was 0.55. A mean ratio of 1.32 was observed in nonacidotic newborns following local infiltration of the perineum for episiotomy (12). A similarly elevated ratio was measured in an acidotic newborn (13). The infant had umbilical venous/arterial pH values of 7.23/7.08 and a lidocaine cord:maternal serum ratio of 1.32 following epidural anesthesia. Because lidocaine is a weak base, the high ratio may have been due to ion trapping (13).

Both the fetus and the newborn are capable of metabolizing lidocaine (7, 8). The elimination half-life of lidocaine in the newborn following maternal epidural anesthesia averaged 3 hours (7). After local perineal infiltration for episiotomy, lidocaine was found in neonatal urine for at least 48 hours after delivery (12).

A number of studies have examined the effect of lidocaine on the newborn. In one report, offspring of mothers receiving continuous lumbar epidural blocks had significantly lower scores on tests of muscle strength and tone than did controls (14). Results of other tests of neurobehavior did not differ from those of controls. In contrast, four other studies failed to find adverse effects on neonatal neurobehavior following lidocaine epidural administration (9–11, 15). Continuous infusion epidural analgesia with lidocaine has been used without effect on the fetus or newborn (16).

Lidocaine may produce central nervous system depression in the newborn with high serum levels. Of eight infants with lidocaine levels greater than 2.5 μg/ml, four had Apgar scores of 6 or less (2). Three infants with levels above 3.0 μg/ml were mildly depressed at birth (2). A 1973 study observed fetal tachycardia (three cases) and bradycardia (three cases) after paracervical block with lidocaine in 12 laboring women (17). The authors were unable to determine if these effects were a direct effect of the drug. Accidental direct injection into the fetal scalp during local infiltration for episiotomy led to apnea, hypotonia, and fixed, dilated pupils 15 minutes after birth in one infant (18). Lidocaine-induced seizures occurred at 1 hour. The lidocaine concentration in the infant's serum at 2 hours was 14 μg/ml. The heart rate was 180 beats/minute. Following successful treatment, physical and neurologic examinations at 3 days and again at 7 months were normal.

Lidocaine is the treatment of choice for ventricular arrhythmias (19, 20). A 1984 report described the use of therapeutic lidocaine doses (100 mg IV injection followed by 4 mg/minute infusion) in a woman who was successfully resuscitated after a cardiac arrest at 18 weeks' gestation (21). A normal infant was delivered at 38 weeks' gestation. Neurologic development was normal at 17 months of age, but growth was below the 10th percentile.

The Collaborative Perinatal Project monitored 50,282 mother-child pairs, 293 of which had exposure to lidocaine during the 1st trimester (22, pp. 358–363). No evidence of an association with large classes of malformations was found. Greater than expected risks were found for anomalies of the respiratory tract (three cases), tumors (two cases), and inguinal hernias (eight cases), but the statistical significance is unknown and independent confirmation is required (22, pp. 358–363, 477). For use anytime during pregnancy, 947 exposures were recorded (22, pp. 440, 493). From these data, no evidence of an association with large categories of major or minor malformations or to individual defects was found.

Breast Feeding Summary

No data are available.

References

1. Shnider SM, Way EL. The kinetics of transfer of lidocaine (Xylocaine) across the human placenta. Anesthesiology 1968;29:944–50.
2. Shnider SM, Way EL. Plasma levels of lidocaine (Xylocaine) in mother and newborn following obstetrical conduction anesthesia: clinical applications. Anesthesiology 1968;29:951–8.
3. Lurie AO, Weiss JB. Blood concentrations of mepivacaine and lidocaine in mother and baby after epidural anesthesia. Am J Obstet Gynecol 1970;106:850–6.
4. Petrie RH, Paul WL, Miller FC, Arce JJ, Paul RH, Nakamura RM, Hon EH. Placental transfer of lidocaine following paracervical block. Am J Obstet Gynecol 1974;120:791–801.
5. Zador G, Lindmark G, Nilsson BA. Pudendal block in normal vaginal deliveries. Acta Obstet Gynecol Scand 1974;Suppl 34:51–64.
6. Blankenbaker WL, DiFazio CA, Berry FA Jr. Lidocaine and its metabolites in the newborn. Anesthesiology 1975;42:325–30.
7. Brown WU Jr, Bell GC, Lurie AO, Weiss JB, Scanlon JW, Alper MH. Newborn blood levels of lidocaine and mepivacaine in the first postnatal day following maternal epidural anesthesia. Anesthesiology 1975;42:698–707.
8. Kuhnert BR, Knapp DR, Kuhnert PM, Prochaska AL. Maternal, fetal, and neonatal metabolism of lidocaine. Clin Pharmacol Ther 1979;26:213–20.
9. Abboud TK, Sarkis F, Blikian A, Varakian L. Lack of adverse neurobehavioral effects of lidocaine. Anesthesiology 1982;57(Suppl):A404.
10. Kileff M, James FM III, Dewan D, Floyd H, DiFazio C. Neonatal neurobehavioral responses after epidural anesthesia for cesarean section with lidocaine and bupivacaine. Anesthesiology 1982;57(Suppl):A403.
11. Abboud TK, David S, Costandi J, Nagappala S, Haroutunian S, Yeh SY. Comparative maternal, fetal and neonatal effects of lidocaine versus lidocaine with epinephrine in the parturient. Anesthesiology 1984;61(Suppl):A405.
12. Philipson EH, Kuhnert BR, Syracuse CD. Maternal, fetal, and neonatal lidocaine levels following local perineal infiltration. Am J Obstet Gynecol 1984;149:403–7.
13. Brown WU Jr, Bell GC, Alper MH. Acidosis, local anesthetics, and the newborn. Obstet Gynecol 1976;48:27–30.
14. Scanlon JW, Brown WU Jr, Weiss JB, Alper MH. Neurobehavioral responses of newborn infants after maternal epidural anesthesia. Anesthesiology 1974;40:121–8.
15. Abboud TK, Williams V, Miller F, Henriksen EH, Doan T, Van Dorsen JP, Earl S. Comparative fetal, maternal, and neonatal responses following epidural analgesia with bupivacaine, chloroprocaine, and lidocaine. Anesthesiology 1981;55(Suppl):A315.
16. Chestnut DH, Bates JN, Choi WW. Continuous infusion epidural analgesia with lidocaine: efficacy and influence during the second stage of labor. Obstet Gynecol 1987;69:323–7.
17. Liston WA, Adjepon-Yamoah KK, Scott DB. Foetal and maternal lignocaine levels after paracervical block. Br J Anaesth 1973;45:750–4.
18. Kim WY, Pomerance JJ, Miller AA. Lidocaine intoxication in a newborn following local anesthesia for episiotomy. Pediatrics 1979;64:643–5.
19. Tamari I, Eldar M, Rabinowitz B, Neufeld HN. Medical treatment of cardiovascular disorders during pregnancy. Am Heart J 1982;104:1357–63.

20. Rotmensch HH, Elkayam U, Frishman W. Antiarrhythmic drug therapy during pregnancy. Ann Intern Med 1983;98:487–97.
21. Stokes IM, Evans J, Stone M. Myocardial infarction and cardiac arrest in the second trimester followed by assisted vaginal delivery under epidural analgesia at 38 weeks' gestation. Case report. Br J Obstet Gynaecol 1984;91:197–8.
22. Heinonen OP, Slone D, Shapiro S. *Birth Defects and Drugs in Pregnancy.* Littleton:Publishing Sciences Group, 1977.

Name: **LINCOMYCIN**

Class: **Antibiotic**   Risk Factor: **B**

Fetal Risk Summary

No reports linking the use of lincomycin with congenital defects have been located. The antibiotic crosses the placenta, achieving cord serum levels about 25% of the maternal serum level (1, 2). Multiple intramuscular injections of 600 mg did not result in accumulation in the amniotic fluid (2). No effects on the newborn were observed.

The progeny of 302 patients treated at various stages of pregnancy with oral lincomycin, 2 g/day for 7 days, were evaluated at various intervals up to 7 years after birth (3). As compared to a control group, no increases in malformations or in delayed developmental defects were observed.

Breast Feeding Summary

Lincomycin is excreted into breast milk. Six hours following oral dosing of 500 mg every 6 hours for 3 days, serum and milk levels in nine patients averaged 1.37 and 1.28 μg/ml, respectively, a milk:plasma ratio of 0.9 (1). Much lower milk:plasma ratios of 0.13–0.17 have also been reported (4). Although no adverse effects have been reported, three potential problems exist for the nursing infant: modification of bowel flora, direct effects on the infant, and interference with the interpretation of culture results if a fever workup is required.

References

1. Medina A, Fiske N, Hjelt-Harvey I, Brown CD, Prigot A. Absorption, diffusion, and excretion of a new antibiotic, lincomycin. Antimicrob Agents Chemother 1963;189–96.
2. Duignan NM, Andrews J, Williams JD. Pharmacological studies with lincomycin in late pregnancy. Br Med J 1973;3:75–8.
3. Mickal A, Panzer JD. The safety of lincomycin in pregnancy. Am J Obstet Gynecol 1975;121:1071–4.
4. Wilson JT. Milk/plasma ratios and contraindicated drugs. In Wilson JT, ed. *Drugs in Breast Milk.* Balgowlah, Australia:ADIS Press, 1981:78–9.

Name: **LINDANE**

Class: **Scabicide/Pediculicide**   Risk Factor: **B_M**

Fetal Risk Summary

Lindane (γ-benzene hexachloride) is used topically for the treatment of lice and scabies. Small amounts are absorbed through the intact skin and mucous membranes (1). No reports linking the use of this drug with toxic or congenital defects have been located, but one reference suggested that it should be used with caution due to its potential to produce neurotoxicity, convulsions, and aplastic anemia (2). Limited animal studies have not shown a teratogenic effect (3, 4). In one animal study, lindane seemed to have a protective effect when given with known teratogens (5). If treatment is required, the manufacturer recommends using lindane no more than twice during a pregnancy (6). Because of lindane's potentially serious toxicity, pyrethrins with piperonyl butoxide are recommended for the treatment of lice infestations occurring during pregnancy (see Pyrethrins with Piperonyl Butoxide).

Breast Feeding Summary

No reports describing the use of lindane in lactating women have been located. Based on theoretical considerations, the manufacturer estimates the upper limit of lindane levels in breast milk to be approximately 30 ng/ml after maternal application (E.D. Rickard, personal communication, Reed & Carnrick Pharmaceuticals, 1983). A nursing infant taking 1 liter of milk/day would thus ingest about 30 µg/day of lindane. This is in the same general range that the infant would absorb after direct topical application (E.D. Rickard, personal communication, 1983). These amounts are probably clinically insignificant.

References

1. American Hospital Formulary Service. Drug Information 1990. Bethesda:American Society of Hospital Pharmacists, 1990:2019–20.
2. Sanmiguel GS, Ferrer AP, Alberich MT, Genaoui BM. Considerociones sobre el tratamiento de la infancia y en el embarazo. Actas Dermosifilogr 1980;71:105–8.
3. Palmer AK, Cozens DD, Spicer EJF, Worden AN. Effects of lindane upon reproduction function in a 3-generation study of rats. Toxicology 1978;10:45–54.
4. Palmer AK, Bottomley AM, Worden AN, Frohberg H, Bauer A. Effect of lindane on pregnancy in the rabbit and rat. Toxicology 1978;10:239–47.
5. Shtenberg AI, Torchinski I. Adaptation to the action of several teratogens as a consequence of preliminary administration of pesticides to females. Biull Eksp Biol Med 1977;83:227–8.
6. Product information. Kwell. Reed & Carnrick Pharmaceuticals, 1990.

Name: **LIOTHYRONINE**

Class: **Thyroid**   Risk Factor: **A_M**

Fetal Risk Summary

Liothyronine (T3) is a naturally occurring thyroid hormone produced by the mother and the fetus. It is used during pregnancy for the treatment of hypothyroidism (see also Levothyroxine and Thyroid). There is little or no transplacental passage of the hormone at physiologic serum concentrations (1–3). Limited placental passage of T3 to the fetus has been demonstrated following very large doses (4, 5).

In a large prospective study, 34 mother-child pairs were exposed to liothyronine during the 1st trimester (6). No association between the drug and fetal defects was found. Maternal hypothyroidism itself has been reported to be responsible for poor pregnancy outcome (7). Others have not found this association, claiming that fetal development is not directly affected by maternal thyroid function (8).

Combination therapy with thyroid-antithyroid drugs was advocated at one time for the treatment of hyperthyroidism but is now considered inappropriate (see Propylthiouracil).

Breast Feeding Summary

Liothyronine (T3) is excreted into breast milk in low concentrations. The effect on the nursing infant is not thought to be physiologically significant, although at least one report concluded otherwise (9). An infant was diagnosed as athyrotic shortly after breast feeding was stopped at age 10 months (9). Growth was at the 97th percentile during breast feeding, but the bone age remained that of a newborn. Mean levels of T3 in breast milk during the last trimester (12 patients) and within 48 hours of delivery (22 patients) were 1.36 and 2.86 ng/ml, respectively. A 1978 study reported milk concentrations varying between 0.4–2.38 ng/ml (range 0.1–5 ng/ml) from the day of delivery to 148 days postpartum (10). No liothyronine was detected in a number of the samples. Levels in three instances, collected 16, 20, and 43 months postpartum, ranged from 0.68–4.5 ng/ml with the highest concentration measured at 20 months. From the 1st week through 148 days postdelivery, the calculated maximum amount of T3 that a nursing infant would have ingested was 2.1–2.6 µg/day, far less than the dose required to treat congenital hypothyroidism (10). However, the authors concluded this was enough to mask the symptoms of the disease without halting its progression. In a study comparing serum T3 levels between 22 breast-fed and 29 formula-fed infants, significantly higher levels were found in the breast-feeding group (11). The levels, 2.24 ng/ml and 1.79 ng/ml, were comparable to previous reports and probably were of doubtful clinical significance. A 1980 report described four exclusively breast-fed infants with congenital hypothyroidism who were diagnosed between the ages of 2–79 days (12). Breast feeding did not hinder making the diagnosis. Another 1980 research report evaluated clinical and biochemical thyroid parameters in 45 hypothyroid infants, 12 of whom were breast fed (13). No difference was detected between the breast-fed and bottle-fed babies, leading to the conclusion that breast milk does not offer protection against the effects of congenital hypothyroidism. As reported in a 1985 paper, serum concentrations of T3 were similar in breast- and bottle-fed infants at 5, 10, and 15 days postpartum (14).

Japanese researchers found a T3 milk:plasma ratio of 0.36 (15). No correlation was discovered between serum T3 and milk T3 or total daily T3 excretion. Neither was there a correlation between milk T3 levels and milk protein concentration or daily volume of milk. They concluded that breast feeding has no influence on the pituitary-thyroid axis of normal babies. A Swedish investigation measured higher levels of T3 in milk 1–3 months after delivery as compared to T3 levels in early colostrum (16). The concentrations were comparable to the studies cited above.

In summary, liothyronine breast milk concentrations are too low to protect a hypothyroid infant completely from the effects of the disease. The levels are also too low to interfere with neonatal thyroid screening programs (14).

References

1. Grumbach MM, Werner SC. Transfer of thyroid hormone across the human placenta at term. J Clin Endocrinol Metab 1956;16:1392–5.
2. Kearns JE, Hutson W. Tagged isomers and analogues of thyroxine (their transmission across the human placenta and other studies). J Nucl Med 1963;4:453–61.
3. Fisher DA, Lehman H, Lackey C. Placental transport of thyroxine. J Clin Endocrinol Metab 1964;24:393–400.
4. Raiti S, Holzman GB, Scott RI, Blizzard RM. Evidence for the placental transfer of tri-iodothyronine in human beings. N Engl J Med 1967;277:456–9.
5. Dussault J, Row VV, Lickrish G, Volpe R. Studies of serum triiodothyronine concentration in maternal and cord blood: transfer of triiodothyronine across the human placenta. J Clin Endocrinol Metab 1969; 29:595–606.
6. Heinonen OP, Slone D, Shapiro S. *Birth Defects and Drugs in Pregnancy.* Littleton:Publishing Sciences Group, 1977:388–400.
7. Potter JD. Hypothyroidism and reproductive failure. Surg Gynecol Obstet 1980;150:251–5.
8. Montoro M, Collea JV, Frasier SD, Mestman JH. Successful outcome of pregnancy in women with hypothyroidism. Ann Intern Med 1981;94:31–4.
9. Bode HH, Vanjonack WJ, Crawford JD. Mitigation of cretinism by breast-feeding. Pediatrics 1978;62:13–6.
10. Varma SK, Collins M, Row A, Haller WS, Varma K. Thyroxine, triiodothyronine, and reverse triiodothyronine concentrations in human milk. J Pediatr 1978;93:803–6.
11. Hahn HB Jr, Spiekerman AM, Otto WR, Hossalla DE. Thyroid function tests in neonates fed human milk. Am J Dis Child 1983;137:220–2.
12. Abbassi V, Steinour TA. Successful diagnosis of congenital hypothyroidism in four breast-fed neonates. J Pediatr 1980;97:259–61.
13. Letarte J, Guyda H, Dussault JH, Glorieux J. Lack of protective effect of breast-feeding in congenital hypothyroidism: report of 12 cases. Pediatrics 1980;65:703–5.
14. Franklin R, O'Grady C, Carpenter L. Nenonatal thyroid function: comparison between breast-fed and bottle-fed infants. J Pediatr 1985;106:124–6.
15. Mizuta H, Amino N, Ichihara K, Harade T, Nose O, Tanizawa O, Miyai K. Thyroid hormones in human milk and influence on thyroid function of breast-fed babies. Pediatr Res 1983;17:468–71.
16. Jansson L, Ivarsson S, Larsson I, Ekman R. Tri-iodothyronine and thyroxine in human milk. Acta Paediatr Scand 1983;72:703–5.

Name: **LIOTRIX**

Class: **Thyroid** Risk Factor: **A**

Fetal Risk Summary

Liotrix is a synthetic combination of levothyroxine and liothyronine (see Levothyroxine and Liothyronine).

Breast Feeding Summary

See Levothyroxine and Liothyronine.

Name: **LIPIDS**

Class: **Nutrient**   Risk Factor: **C**

Fetal Risk Summary

Lipids (intravenous fat emulsions) are a mixture of neutral triglycerides, primarily unsaturated fatty acids, prepared from either soybean or safflower oil. Egg yolk phospholipids are used as an emulsifier. Most fatty acids readily cross the placenta to the fetus (1, 2).

A number of reports have described the use of lipids during pregnancy in conjunction with dextrose/amino acid solutions (see Hyperalimentation, Parenteral) (3–14). However, one investigator concluded in 1977 that lipid infusions were contraindicated during pregnancy for several reasons: (a) an excessive increase in serum triglycerides, often with ketonemia, would result because of the physiologic hyperlipemia present during pregnancy, (b) premature labor would occur, and (c) placental infarctions would occur from fat deposits and cause placental insufficiency (15). A brief 1986 correspondence also stated that lipids were contraindicated due to the danger of inducing premature uterine contractions with the potential for abortion or premature delivery (16). This conclusion was based on the observation that lipids contain arachidonic acid, a precursor to prostaglandins E_2 and $F_{2\alpha}$ (16). However, another investigator concluded that concentrations of arachidonic acid must arise from decidual membranes or amniotic fluid (i.e., must be very close to the myometrium) to produce this effect (17). Fortunately, none of the complications cited above has been observed in the mothers and fetuses treated with lipids. A 1986 report described four women in whom parenteral hyperalimentation was used during pregnancy, two of whom also received lipids, and, in addition, reviewed the literature for both total parenteral nutrition and lipid use during gestation (18). These authors concluded that there was no evidence that lipid emulsions had an adverse effect on pregnancy (18).

The effect of oral administration of a triglyceride emulsion on the fetal breathing index was described in a 1982 publication (19). Six women, at 32 weeks' gestation, ingested 100 ml of the emulsion containing 67 g of triglycerides and were compared to six women, also at 32 weeks' gestation, who drank mineral water. No correlation was noted between the fetal breathing index and plasma free fatty acids, glucose, insulin, glucagon, total cortisol, free cortisol, or triglyceride levels (19).

Cardiac tamponade, resulting in maternal and fetal death, has been reported in a woman receiving central hyperalimentation with lipids for severe hyperemesis gravidarum (see Hyperalimentation, Parenteral, for details of this case) (20).

Based on limited clinical experience, intravenous lipids apparently do not pose a risk to the mother or fetus. Standard precautions, as taken with nonpregnant patients, should be followed when administering these solutions during pregnancy.

Breast Feeding Summary

No data are available.

References

1. Elphick MC, Filshie GM, Hull D. The passage of fat emulsion across the human placenta. Br J Obstet Gynaecol 1978;85:610–8.
2. Hendrickse W, Stammers JP, Hull D. The transfer of free fatty acids across the human placenta. Br J Obstet Gynaecol 1985;92:945–52.
3. Hew LR, Deitel M. Total parenteral nutrition in gynecology and obstetrics. Obstet Gynecol 1980;55:464–8.
4. Tresadern JC, Falconer GF, Turnberg LA, Irving MH. Successful completed pregnancy in a patient maintained on home parenteral nutrition. Br Med J 1983;286:602–3.
5. Tresadern JC, Falconer GF, Turnberg LA, Irving MH. Maintenance of pregnancy in a home parenteral nutrition patient. JPEN 1984;8:199–202.
6. Seifer DB, Silberman H, Catanzarite VA, Conteas CN, Wood R, Ueland K. Total parenteral nutrition in obstetrics. JAMA 1985;253;2073–5.
7. Lavin JP Jr, Gimmon Z, Miodovnik M, von Meyenfeldt M, Fischer JE. Total parenteral nutrition in a pregnant insulin-requiring diabetic. Obstet Gynecol 1982;59:660–4.
8. Rivera-Alsina ME, Saldana LR, Stringer CA. Fetal growth sustained by parenteral nutrition in pregnancy. Obstet Gynecol 1984;64:138–41.
9. Di Costanzo J, Martin J, Cano N, Mas JC, Noirclerc M. Total parenteral nutrition with fat emulsions during pregnancy—nutritional requirements: a case report. JPEN 1982;6:534–8.
10. Young KR. Acute pancreatitis in pregnancy: two case reports. Obstet Gynecol 1982;60:653–7.
11. Breen KJ, McDonald IA, Panelli D, Ihle B. Planned pregnancy in a patient who was receiving home parenteral nutrition. Med J Aust 1987;146:215–7.
12. Levine MG, Esser D. Total parenteral nutrition for the treatment of severe hyperemesis gravidarum: maternal nutritional effects and fetal outcome. Obstet Gynecol 1988;72:102–7.
13. Herbert WNP, Seeds JW, Bowes WA, Sweeney CA. Fetal growth response to total parenteral nutrition in pregnancy: a case report. J Reprod Med 1986;31:263–6.
14. Hatjis CG, Meis PJ. Total parenteral nutrition in pregnancy. Obstet Gynecol 1985;66:585–9.
15. Heller L. Parenteral nutrition in obstetrics and gynecology. In Greep JM, Soeters PB, Wesdorp RIC, et al, eds. Current Concepts in Parenteral Nutrition. The Hague:Martinus Nijhoff Medical Division, 1977:179–86.
16. Neri A. Fetal growth sustained by parenteral nutrition in pregnancy. Obstet Gynecol 1986;67:753.
17. Saldana LR. Fetal growth sustained by parenteral nutrition in pregnancy: in reply. Obstet Gynecol 1986;67:753.
18. Lee RV, Rodgers BD, Young C, Eddy E, Cardinal J. Total parenteral nutrition during pregnancy. Obstet Gynecol 1986;68:563–71.
19. Neldam S, Hornnes PJ, Kuhl C. Effect of maternal triglyceride ingestion on fetal respiratory movements. Obstet Gynecol 1982;59:640–2.
20. Greenspoon JS, Masaki DI, Kurz CR. Cardiac tamponade in pregnancy during central hyperalimentation. Obstet Gynecol 1989;73:465–6.

Name: **LITHIUM**

Class: **Tranquilizer** Risk Factor: **D**

Fetal Risk Summary

The use of lithium during the 1st trimester may be related to an increased incidence of congenital defects, particularly of the cardiovascular system. The drug freely crosses the placenta, equilibrating between maternal and cord serum (1–5). Amniotic fluid concentrations exceed cord serum levels (2). Frequent reports have described the fetal effects of lithium, the majority from data accumulated by the Lithium Baby Register (1, 6–14). The Register, founded in Denmark in 1968 and later expanded internationally, collects data on known cases of 1st trimester exposure to lithium. By 1977, the Register included 183 infants, 20 (11%) with major congenital anomalies (12). Of the 20 malformed infants, 15 involved cardiovascular defects, including 5 with the rare Ebstein's anomaly. Others have also noted the increased incidence of Ebstein's anomaly in lithium-exposed babies (15). Two new case reports bring the total number of infants with cardiovascular defects to 17, or 77% (17 of 22) of the known malformed children (16, 17). Ebstein's anomaly has been diagnosed in the fetus during the 2nd trimester by echocardiography (18). Details on 16 of the malformed infants are given below.

In 60 of the children born without malformations, follow-up comparisons with nonexposed siblings did not show an increased frequency of physical or mental anomalies (19).

Author	Case No.	Defect
Weinstein and	1	Coarctation of aorta
Goldfield (11)	2	High intraventricular septal defect
	3	Stenosis of aqueduct with hydrocephalus, spina bifida with sacral meningomyelocele, bilateral talipes equivovarus with paralysis; atonic bladder, patulous rectal sphincter and rectal prolapse (see also reference 7)
	4	Unilateral microtia
	5	Mitral atresia, rudimentary left ventricle without inlet or outlet, aorta and pulmonary artery arising from right ventricle, patent ductus arteriosus, left superior vena cava
	6	Mitral atresia
	7	Ebstein's anomaly
	8	Single umbilical artery, bilateral hypoplasia of maxilla
	9	Ebstein's anomaly
	10	Atresia of tricuspid valve
	11	Ebstein's anomaly
	12	Patent ductus arteriosus, ventricular septal defect
	13	Ebstein's anomaly
Rane et al. (16)	14	Detrocardia and situs colitus, patent ductus arteriosus, juxtaductal aortic coarctation
Weinstein (12)	15	Ebstein's anomaly
Arnon et al (17)	16	Massive tricuspid regurgitation, atrial flutter, congestive heart failure

Lithium toxicity in the newborn has been reported frequently:

Cyanosis (2, 16, 20–24)
Hypotonia (2, 10, 20–27)
Bradycardia (16, 21, 24, 26, 28)
Thyroid depression with goiter (2, 10, 27)
Atrial flutter (29)
Hepatomegaly (24)
Electrocardiogram abnormalities (T wave inversion) (21, 28)
Cardiomegaly (22, 24, 29)
Gastrointestinal bleeding (28)
Diabetes insipidus (2, 24)
Shock (24)

Most of these toxic effects are self-limiting, returning to normal in 1–2 weeks. This corresponds with the renal elimination of lithium from the infant. The serum half-life of lithium in newborns is prolonged, averaging 68–96 hours, as compared to the adult value of 10–20 hours (3, 16). The two reported cases of nephrogenic diabetes insipidus persisted for 2 months or longer (2, 24).

Fetal red blood cell choline levels are elevated during maternal therapy with lithium (30). The clinical significance of this effect on choline, the metabolic precursor to acetycholine, is unknown but may be related to the teratogenicity of lithium due to its effect on cellular lithium transport (30). In an *in vitro* study, lithium had no effect on human sperm motility (31).

In the mother, renal lithium clearance rises during pregnancy, returning to prepregnancy levels shortly after delivery (32). In four patients, the mean clearance before delivery was 29 ml/minute, declining to 15 ml/minute 6–7 weeks after delivery, a statistically significant difference ($p < 0.01$). These data emphasize the need to monitor lithium levels closely before and after pregnancy.

In summary, lithium should be avoided during pregnancy if possible, especially during the 1st trimester. Use of the drug near term may produce severe toxicity in the newborn, which is usually reversible.

Breast Feeding Summary

Lithium is excreted into breast milk (5, 21, 33, 34). Milk levels average 40% of the maternal serum concentration (21, 34). Infant serum and milk levels are approximately equal. Although no toxic effects in the nursing infant have been reported, long-term effects from this exposure have not been studied. The American Academy of Pediatrics considers lithium to be contraindicated during breast feeding (35).

References

1. Weinstein MR, Goldfield M. Lithium carbonate treatment during pregnancy: report of a case. Dis Nerv Syst 1969;30:828–32.
2. Mizrahi EM, Hobbs JF, Goldsmith DI. Nephrogenic diabetes insipidus in transplacental lithium intoxication. J Pediatr 1979;94:493–5.
3. Mackay AVP, Loose R, Glen AIM. Labour on lithium. Br Med J 1976;1:878.
4. Schou M, Amdisen A. Lithium and placenta. Am J Obstet Gynecol 1975;122:541.
5. Sykes PA, Quarrie J, Alexander FW. Lithium carbonate and breast-feeding. Br Med J 1976;2:1299.
6. Schou M, Amdisen A. Lithium in pregnancy. Lancet 1970;1:1391.
7. Aoki FY, Ruedy J. Severe lithium intoxication: management without dialysis and report of a possible teratogenic effect of lithium. Can Med Assoc J 1971;105:847–8.
8. Goldfield M, Weinstein MR. Lithium in pregnancy: a review with recommendations. Am J Psychiatry 1971;127:888–93.
9. Goldfield MD, Weinstein MR. Lithium carbonate in obstetrics: guidelines for clinical use. Am J Obstet Gynecol 1973;116:15–22.
10. Schou M, Goldfield MD, Weinstein MR, Villeneuve A. Lithium and pregnancy. I. Report from the register of lithium babies. Br Med J 1973;2:135–6.
11. Weinstein MR, Goldfield MD. Cardiovascular malformations with lithium use during pregnancy. Am J Psychiatry 1975;132:529–31.
12. Weinstein MR. Recent advances in clinical psychopharmacology. I. Lithium carbonate. Hosp Form 1977;12:759–62.
13. Linden S, Rich CL. The use of lithium during pregnancy and lactation. J Clin Psychiatry 1983;44:358–61.
14. Pitts FN. Editorial. Lithium and pregnancy. J Clin Psychiatry 1983;44:357.
15. Nora JJ, Nora AH, Toews WH. Lithium, Ebstein's anomaly, and other congenital heart defects. Lancet 1974;2:594–5.
16. Rane A, Tomson G, Bjarke B. Effects of maternal lithium therapy in a newborn infant. J Pediatr 1978;93:296–7.

17. Arnon RG, Marin-Garcia J, Peeden JN. Tricuspid valve regurgitation and lithium carbonate toxicity in a newborn infant. Am J Dis Child 1981;135:941–3.
18. Allan LD, Desai G, Tynan MJ. Prenatal echocardiographic screening for Ebstein's anomaly for mothers on lithium therapy. Lancet 1982;2:875–6.
19. Schou M. What happened later to the lithium babies? A follow-up study of children born without malformations. Acta Psychiatr Scand 1976;54:193–7.
20. Woody JN, London WL, Wilbanks GD Jr. Lithium toxicity in a newborn. Pediatrics 1971;47:94–6.
21. Tunnessen WW Jr, Hertz CG. Toxic effects of lithium in newborn infants: a commentary. J Pediatr 1972;81:804–7.
22. Piton M, Barthe ML, Laloum D, Davy J, Poilpre E, Venezia R. Acute lithium intoxication. Report of two cases: mother and her newborn. Therapie 1973;28:1123–44.
23. Wilbanks GD, Bressler B, Peete CH Jr, Cherny WB, London WL. Toxic effects of lithium carbonate in a mother and newborn infant. JAMA 1970;213:865–7.
24. Morrell P, Sutherland GR, Buamah PK, Oo M, Bain HH. Lithium toxicity in a neonate. Arch Dis Child 1983;58:539–41.
25. Silverman JA, Winters RW, Strande C. Lithium carbonate therapy during pregnancy: apparent lack of effect upon the fetus. Am J Obstet Gynecol 1971;109:934–6.
26. Strothers JK, Wilson DW, Royston N. Lithium toxicity in the newborn. Br Med J 1973;3:233–4.
27. Karlsson K, Lindstedt G, Lundberg PA, Selstam U. Transplacental lithium poisoning: reversible inhibition of fetal thyroid. Lancet 1975;1:1295.
28. Stevens D, Burman D, Midwinter A. Transplacental lithium poisoning. Lancet 1974;2:595.
29. Wilson N, Forfar JC, Godman MJ. Atrial flutter in the newborn resulting from maternal lithium ingestion. Arch Dis Child 1983;58:538–9.
30. Mallinger AG, Hanin I, Stumpf RL, Mallinger J, Kopp U, Erstling C. Lithium treatment during pregnancy: a case study of erythrocyte choline content and lithium transport. J Clin Psychiatry 1983;44:381–4.
31. Levin RM, Amsterdam JD, Winokur A, Wein AJ. Effects of psychotropic drugs on human sperm motility. Fertil Steril 1981;36:503–6.
32. Schou M, Amdisen A, Steenstrup OR. Lithium and pregnancy. II. Hazards to women given lithium during pregnancy and delivery. Br Med J 1973;2:137–8.
33. Fries H. Lithium in pregnancy. Lancet 1970;1:1233.
34. Schou M, Amdisen A. Lithium and pregnancy. III. Lithium ingestion by children breast-fed by women on lithium treatment. Br Med J 1973;2:138.
35. Committee on Drugs, American Academy of Pediatrics. Transfer of drugs and other chemicals into human milk. Pediatrics 1989;84:924–36.

Name: **LOPERAMIDE**

Class: **Antidiarrheal**   Risk Factor: **B_M**

Fetal Risk Summary

No reports linking the use of loperamide with congenital defects have been located. Animal studies have not indicated a teratogenic effect (1).

Breast Feeding Summary

Data relating to the excretion of loperamide into breast milk are lacking. One source recommends that the drug should not be used in the lactating mother (2).

References

1. Product information. Imodium. Janssen Pharmaceutica, 1990.
2. Stewart JJ. Gastrointestinal drugs. In Wilson JT, ed. *Drugs in Breast Milk*. Balgowlah, Australia:ADIS Press, 1981:71.

Name: **LORAZEPAM**

Class: **Sedative** Risk Factor: **D$_M$**

Fetal Risk Summary

Lorazepam is a benzodiazepine. No reports linking the use of lorazepam with congenital defects have been located. Other drugs in this group have been suspected of causing fetal malformations (see also Diazepam or Chlordiazepoxide). Lorazepam crosses the placenta, achieving cord levels similar to maternal serum concentrations (1–4). Placental transfer is slower than that of diazepam, but high intravenous doses may produce the "floppy infant" syndrome (2).

Lorazepam has been used in labor to potentiate the effects of narcotic analgesics (5). Although not statistically significant, a higher incidence of respiratory depression occurred in the exposed newborn infants.

Breast Feeding Summary

Lorazepam is excreted into breast milk in low concentrations (6). No effects on the nursing infant were reported, but the slight delay in establishing feeding was a cause for concern (7). In a subsequent study, 5 mg of oral lorazepam were given 1 hour before labor induction and the effects on feeding behavior were measured in the newborn infants (8). During the first 48 hours, no significant effect was observed on volume of milk consumed or duration of feeding.

References

1. de Groot G, Maes RAA, Defoort P, Thiery M. Placental transfer of lorazepam. IRCS Med Sci 1975;3:290.
2. McBride RJ, Dundee JW, Moore J, Toner W, Howard PJ. A study of the plasma concentrations of lorazepam in mother and neonate. Br J Anaesth 1979;51:971–8.
3. Kanto J, Aaltonen L, Liukko P, Maenpaa K. Transfer of lorazepam and its conjugate across the human placenta. Acta Pharmacol Toxicol (Copenh) 1980;47:130–4.
4. Kanto JH. Use of benzodiazepines during pregnancy, labour and lactation, with particular reference to pharmacokinetic considerations. Drugs 1982;23:354–80.
5. McAuley DM, O'Neill MP, Moore J, Dundee JW. Lorazepam premedication for labour. Br J Obstet Gynaecol 1982;89:149–54.
6. Whitelaw AGL, Cummings AJ, McFadyen IR. Effect of maternal lorazepam on the neonate. Br Med J 1981;282:1106–8.
7. Johnstone M. Effect of maternal lorazepam on the neonate. Br Med J 1981;282:1973.
8. Johnstone MJ. The effect of lorazepam on neonatal feeding behaviour at term. Pharmatherapeutica 1982;3:259–62.

Name: **LOXAPINE**

Class: **Tranquilizer** Risk Factor: **C**

Fetal Risk Summary

No data are available.

Breast Feeding Summary

No data are available.

Name: **LYNESTRENOL**

Class: **Progestogenic Hormone**   Risk Factor: **D**

Fetal Risk Summary

The Food and Drug Administration mandated deletion of pregnancy-related indications from all progestins because of a possible association with congenital anomalies. No reports linking the use of lynestrenol with congenital defects have been located (see Hydroxyprogesterone, Norethynodrel, Norethindrone, Medroxyprogesterone, Ethisterone). Ravn observed 16 women who had used lynestrenol for contraception and gave birth to normal infants following cessation of treatment (1). No conclusions can be made from this report. Use of progestogens during pregnancy is not recommended.

Breast Feeding Summary

See Oral Contraceptives.

Reference

1. Ravn J. Pregnancy and progeny after long-term contraceptive treatment with low-dose progestogens. Curr Med Res Opin 1975;2:616–9.

Name: **LYPRESSIN**

Class: **Pituitary Hormone, Synthetic**   Risk Factor: **C$_M$**

Fetal Risk Summary

Lypressin is a synthetic polypeptide structurally identical to the major active component of vasopressin. See Vasopressin.

Breast Feeding Summary

See Vasopressin.

Name: **LYSERGIC ACID DIETHYLAMIDE**

Class: **Hallucinogen**   Risk Factor: **C**

Fetal Risk Summary

Lysergic acid diethylamide (LSD, lysergide) is a chemical used for its hallucinogenic properties. The drug does not have a legal indication in the United States. Illicitly obtained LSD is commonly adulterated with a variety of other chemicals (e.g., amphetamines) (1, 2). In some cases, doses sold illicitly as LSD may contain little or none of the chemical; as a result, the actual amount of LSD ingested cannot be determined (1). In addition, persons consuming the hallucinogen often consume multiple abuse drugs simultaneously, such as marijuana, opiates, alcohol, amphetamines, STP (dimethyloxyamphetamine; DOM; a synthetic halluci-nogen), barbiturates, cocaine, and other prescription and nonprescription sub-stances. Further complicating the situation are the life-styles that some of these persons live, which are often not conducive to good fetal health. As a conse-quence, the effects of pure LSD on the human fetus can only be evaluated by examining those cases where the chemical was administered under strict medical supervision. These cases, however, are few in number. Most data are composed of sample populations who ingested the chemical in an unsupervised environ-ment. Correct interpretation of this latter material is extremely difficult and, al-though cited in this monograph, must be viewed cautiously.

The passage of LSD across the human placenta has not been studied. The molecular weight of the chemical, approximately 323, is low enough, however, that rapid passage to the fetus should be expected. LSD has been shown to cross the placenta in mice with early 1st trimester fetal levels averaging five times the levels measured in late gestation (3).

Concerns with fetal exposure to LSD have primarily focused on chromosomal damage (both chromatid-type and chromosome-type abnormalities), an increased risk of spontaneous abortions, and congenital malformations. These topics are discussed in the sections below.

A 1967 report was the first to claim that the use of LSD could cause chromo-somal abnormalities in human leukocytes (4). Because these abnormalities could potentially result in carcinogenic, mutagenic, and teratogenic effects in current or future generations, at least 25 studies were published in the next 7 years. These studies were the subject of three reviews published in the 1970s with all three arriving at similar conclusions (2, 5, 6). First, in the majority of studies, the addition of LSD to cells *in vitro* caused chromosomal breakage, but a dose-response rela-tionship was not always apparent. The clinical relevance of the *in vitro* studies was questionable because pure LSD was used, usually with much higher levels than could be achieved in humans, and the *in vitro* systems lacked the normal protective mechanisms of metabolism and excretion that are present in the body. Second, only a slight transitory increase in chromosome breaks was seen in a small percentage (14%) of the subjects administered pure LSD. A much higher percentage of persons (49%) consuming illicit LSD was observed to have chro-mosomal damage. The abnormalities in this latter group were probably related to the effects of multiple drug abuse and not to LSD alone. Four prospective studies found no definitive evidence that LSD damages lymphocyte chromosomes *in vivo* (2). Third, there was no evidence that the chromosome defects observed in illicit LSD users were expressed as an increased incidence of leukemias or other neo-plasia. Fourth, mutagenic changes were only observed in experimental organisms (e.g., Drosophila) when massive doses (2,000–10,000 μg/ml) were used. Be-cause of this, LSD was believed to be a weak mutagen, but mutagenicity was thought to be unlikely after exposure to any concentration used by humans (5). Finally, the reviewers found no compelling evidence for a teratogenic effect of LSD, either in animals or humans.

A 1974 investigation involving 50 psychiatric patients, who had been treated for varying intervals under controlled conditions with pure LSD, provided further con-firmation that the chemical does not cause chromosomal damage (7). Chromo-some analyses of these patients were compared with those of 50 nonexposed controls matched for age, sex, and marital status. The analysis was blinded so the investigators did not know the origin of the samples. No significant difference between the groups in chromosomal abnormalities was observed. In another 1974 reference (not included in the previously cited reviews), involving only two subjects, no evidence of chromosomal damage was found in their normal offspring (8). The two women had been treated medically with pure LSD prior to pregnancy. Thus, the predominance of evidence indicates that LSD does not induce chromosomal aberrations and, even if it did, it has no clinical significance to the fetus.

The question of whether fetal wastage could be induced by LSD exposure was investigated in a study published in 1970 (9). This investigation involved 148 pregnancies (81 patients) where either the father ($N = 60$) or the mother ($N = 21$) had ingested LSD. In 12 pregnancies, exposure occurred both before and during pregnancy. In the 136 pregnancies where the exposure occurred only prior to conception, 118 involved the administration of pure LSD (the medical group) and 18 involved both medical and illicit LSD exposure (the combined group). The spontaneous abortion rates for these two populations were 14% (17 of 118) and 28% (5 of 18), respectively. In 83 of the pregnancies, only the father had been exposed to LSD. Excluding these, the incidences of fetal loss for the medical and combined groups are 26% (11 of 43) and 40% (4 of 10), respectively. In the 12 pregnancies that occurred where LSD was consumed both before and during gestation, three were in the medical group and nine were in the combined group. The frequency of spontaneous abortions in these cases was 33% (one of three) and 56% (five of nine). In the combined sample, however, one woman accounted for five abortions and one liveborn infant. If she is excluded, the incidence of fetal wastage in the combined group is zero.

In the medical group, the number of women (12 of 46; 26%) with fetal wastage is high. However, 25 of these pregnancies occurred in women undergoing psychotherapy, and 21 occurred in an experimental setting (9). The number of spontaneous abortions in the psychotherapy group ($N = 9$) (36%) was more than twice the incidence in the experimental sample ($N = 3$) (14%). The authors speculated that the greater frequency of fetal wastage in the women undergoing psychotherapy may have been due to the greater emotional stress that often accompanies such therapy. The increased rate in the combined sample (9 of 19; 47%) was probably due to the use of multiple abuse drugs, other nondrug factors, and the inclusion of one woman with five abortions and one live birth. Exclusion of this latter patient decreases the combined sample incidence to 31% (4 of 13). Thus, although other studies examining the incidence of spontaneous abortions in LSD-exposed women have not been located, it appears unlikely that pure LSD administered in a controlled condition is an abortifacient. The increased rate of fetal wastage that was observed in the 1970 study was probably due to a combination of factors, rather than only to the ingestion of LSD.

A number of case reports have described LSD use in pregnancies ending with poor outcomes since the first report in 1967 of an exposed infant with major malformations (10–25). All of these reports, however, are biased in the respect that malformed infants exposed *in utero* to LSD are much more likely to be reported than exposed normal infants and are also more frequently reported than nonexposed malformed infants (2). Most of the reports either involved multiple drug exposures, including abuse drugs, or other drug exposures could probably be deduced because of the illicit nature of LSD. With these cautions, the reports are briefly described below.

The first mention of an anomaly observed in an infant exposed *in utero* to LSD appeared in a 1967 editorial of *The Lancet* (10). The journal, citing a report in a lay publication, briefly described a case of LSD exposure in a pregnancy that ended in a malformed infant with megacolon. Apparently, details of this case have never been published in the medical literature.

The first case report in the medical literature also appeared in 1967 and involved a female infant with unilateral fibular aplastic syndrome (11, 12). The mother had taken LSD four times between the 25th–98th days of gestation with one dose occurring during the time of most active lower limb differentiation (11). Defects in the infant, which were characteristic of the syndrome, included absence of the fibula and lateral rays of the foot, anterior bowing of the shortened tibia, shortening of the femur, and dislocated hip. A second case involving limb defects and LSD exposure was published in 1968 (13). The infant, with a right terminal transverse acheiria defect (absence of the hand), was the offspring of a woman who had taken LSD both before and during early gestation. She had also smoked marijuana throughout the pregnancy and had taken a combination product containing dicyclomine, doxylamine, and pyridoxine for 1st trimester nausea. Another infant with a terminal transverse deficit, also exposed to LSD and marijuana, was described in 1969 (14). The defect involved portions of the fingers on the left hand, syndactyly of the right hand with shortened fingers, and talipes equinovarus of the left foot. Two of these same authors described another exposed infant with amputation deformities of the third finger of the right hand and the third toe of the left foot (15). A critique of these latter three case histories concluded that the defects in the infants could have been due to amniotic band syndrome (26). Limb defects and intrauterine growth retardation were observed in an offspring of a malnourished mother who had used LSD, marijuana, methadone, and cigarettes during gestation (16). The anomalies consisted of partial adactyly of the hands and feet, syndactyly of the remaining fingers, and defective formation of the legs and forearms. In a study of 140 women using LSD and marijuana followed through 148 pregnancies, 8 of 83 liveborn infants had major defects as did 4 of 14 embryos examined after induced abortion (17). The incidence of defects in this sample was 8.1% (12 of 148) and may have been higher if the other abortuses had been examined. Only one of the liveborn infants had a limb defect (absence of both feet) combined with spina bifida occulta and hemangiomas. Defects in the other seven infants were: myelomeningocele with hydrocephalus in three babies (one with clubfoot); tetralogy of Fallot; hydrocephalus; right kidney neuroblastoma; and hydrocephalus and congestive heart failure. A limb defect was one of several anomalies found in a male infant whose mother ingested LSD both before and during gestation (18). The abnormalities included absent left arm, syndactyly, anencephaly with ectopic placenta, cleft lip and palate, coloboma of the iris, cataract, and corneal opacity with vascularization. At least one author thought the limb and cranial defects in this latter case may have been due to amniotic band syndrome (27). This opinion was contested by the original authors, who stated that the limb defects were true aplasia and not an amputation deformity (28). Similarly, they claimed that the cranial anomaly was not a form of encephalocele, which an amniotic band could have caused, but a true anencephaly (28). Congenital anomalies were observed in 11 of 120 liveborn infants in a previously cited study that examined the effects of LSD on spontaneous abortions and other pregnancy outcome (9). Nine of the 11 infants had limb defects that were, in most cases, easily correctable with either special shoes or casts. None of the 11 cases appears to be related to LSD exposure. The defects were (the number of cases and possible causes are shown in parentheses): turned-in feet (six cases; four familial, two unknown); "crimped" ureter (one case; familial); tibial rotation (two cases; two familial); pyloric stenosis (one case; possibly genetic); bone deformity of legs and deafness (one case; postrubella syndrome) (9).

Other infants with ocular defects, in addition to the case mentioned immediately above, have been described. A mother who ingested LSD, marijuana, meprobamate, amphetamines, and hydrochlorothiazide throughout pregnancy delivered an infant with generalized hypotonia, a high-pitched cry, brachycephaly with widely separated sutures, bilateral cephalohematomas, a right eye smaller than the left and with a cataract, and overlapping second and third toes (19). Two other cases of ocular defects were published in 1978 and 1980 (20, 21). In one case, a premature female infant was delivered from a 16-year-old mother who had consumed LSD, cocaine, and heroin during the 1st trimester (20). The infant, who died 1 hour after birth, had microphthalmos, intraocular cartilage, cataract, persistent hyperplastic primary vitreous, and retinal dysplasia. A hypoplastic left lung and a defect in the diaphragm were also noted. The second case involved another premature female infant born from a mother enrolled in a methadone program who also used LSD (21). The infant had left anophthalmia but no other defects.

Various other malformations have been reported after *in utero* LSD exposure (22–25). Complete exstrophy of the bladder, epispadias, widely separated pubic rami, and bilateral inguinal hernias were observed in a newborn exposed to LSD, marijuana, and mephentermine (22). The mother had consumed LSD 12–15 times during an interval extending from 2 months before conception to 2.5 months into pregnancy. A mother, who ingested LSD at the time of conception, produced a female infant with multiple defects including a short neck, left hemithorax smaller than the right, protuberant abdomen due to a severe thoracolumbar lordosis, a thoracolumbar rachischisis, craniolacunia, long fingers, clubfeet, and defects of the urinary tract and brain (23). The infant expired at age 41 days. Other drug exposures consisted of cigarettes, an estrogen preparation (type not specified) that was used unsuccessfuly to induce menstruation, and medroxyprogesterone for 1st trimester bleeding. Since the case resembled a previously described cluster of unusual defects (i.e., spondylothoracic dysplasia; Jarcho-Levin syndrome), which is due to an autosomal recessive mode of inheritance, the authors could not exclude this mechanism. In a case of a female infant with multiple anomalies compatible with trisomy 13 with D/D translocation, the mother had last used LSD 9 months prior to conception (24). She had also used marijuana, barbiturates, and amphetamines throughout gestation and, presumably, before conception. The authors theorized that the defect may have been due to LSD-induced damage to maternal germ cells prior to fertilization. A 1971 study evaluated 47 infants born of parents who had used LSD (25). Maternal use of the drug could be documented in only 30 of the cases and multiple other abuse drugs were consumed. Abnormalities observed in eight (17%) of the infants were transient hearing loss and ventricular septal defect; cortical blindness; tracheoesophageal fistula; congenital heart disease (type not specified); congenital neuroblastoma; spastic diplegia; and two infants with seizure disorders.

Two other case reports involving the combined use of LSD and marijuana with resulting adverse fetal outcomes do not appear to have any relationship to either drug (29, 30). One of these involved a report of six infants with persistent ductus arteriosus, one of whom was exposed to LSD and marijuana during early gestation (29). The history of maternal drug use was coincidenta!. The second case described an infant who died at 2.5 months of age from a bilateral *in utero* cerebral vascular accident and resulting porencephaly (30). The mother had used LSD, marijuana, alcohol, and other abuse drugs, including cocaine. This latter drug was thought to be the causative agent.

In contrast to the above reports, a large body of research has been published describing the maternal (and paternal) ingestion of LSD without apparent fetal consequences (1, 7–9, 31–36). A number of reviews have also examined the teratogenic potential of the chemical and have concluded that a causal relationship between congenital malformations and LSD does not exist (2, 5, 6, 37–45). (See reference 6 for an excellent critique of the early investigations in laboratory animals.)

In summary, the available data indicate that pure LSD does not cause chromosomal abnormalities, spontaneous abortions, or congenital malformations. There have been no cases published of fetal anomalies when only pure LSD was administered under medical supervision. Early descriptions of congenital abnormalities involved patients who had used or were using illicit LSD and are believed to be examples of reporting bias, the effects of multiple drugs, or other nondrug factors. However, long-term follow-up of exposed infants has never been reported. This is an area that warrants additional research.

Breast Feeding Summary

No reports have been located concerning the passage of lysergic acid diethylamide into breast milk. However, since the drug has a relatively low molecular weight (approximately 323), which should allow its passage into milk, and because its psychotomimetic effects are produced at extremely low concentrations, the use of LSD during lactation is contraindicated.

References

1. Warren RJ, Rimoin DL, Sly WS. LSD exposure *in utero*. Pediatrics 1970;45:466–9.
2. Matsuyama SS, Jarvik LF. Cytogenetic effects of psychoactive drugs. Mod Probl Pharmacopsychiatry 1975;10:99–132.
3. Idanpaan-Heikkila JE, Schoolar JC. LSD: autoradiographic study on the placental transfer and tissue distribution in mice. Science 1969;164:1295–7.
4. Cohen MM, Marinello MJ, Back N. Chromosomal damage in human leukocytes induced by lysergic acid diethylamide. Science 1967;155:1417–9.
5. Dishotsky NI, Loughman WD, Mogar RE, Lipscomb WR. LSD and genetic damage: is LSD chromosome damaging, carcinogenic, mutagenic, or teratogenic? Science 1971;172:431–40.
6. Long SY. Does LSD induce chromosomal damage and malformations? A review of the literature. Teratology 1972;6:75–90.
7. Robinson JT, Chitham RG, Greenwood RM, Taylor JW. Chromosome aberrations and LSD: a controlled study in 50 psychiatric patients. Br J Psychiatry 1974;125:238–44.
8. Fernandez J, Brennan T, Masterson J, Power M. Cytogenetic studies in the offspring of LSD users. Br J Psychiatry 1974;124:296–8.
9. McGlothlin WH, Sparkes RS, Arnold DO. Effect of LSD on human pregnancy. JAMA 1970;212:1483–7.
10. Anonymous. Hallucinogen and teratogen? Lancet 1967;2:504–5.
11. Zellweger H, McDonald JS, Abbo G. Is lysergic-acid diethylamide a teratogen? Lancet 1967;2:1066–8.
12. Zellweger H, McDonald JS, Abbo G. Is lysergide a teratogen? Lancet 1967;2:1306.

13. Hecht F, Beals RK, Lees MH, Jolly H, Roberts P. Lysergic-acid-diethylamide and cannabis as possible teratogens in man. Lancet 1968;2:1087.

14. Carakushansky G, Neu RL, Gardner LI. Lysergide and cannabis as possible teratogens in man. Lancet 1969;1:150–1.

15. Assemany SR, Neu RL, Gardner LI. Deformities in a child whose mother took L.S.D. Lancet 1970;1:1290.

16. Jeanbart P, Berard MJ. A propos d'un cas personnel de malformations congenitales possiblement dues au LSD-25: revue de la litterature. Union Med Can 1971;100:919–29.

17. Jacobson CB, Berlin CM. Possible reproductive detriment in LSD users. JAMA 1972;222:1367–73.

18. Apple DJ, Bennett TO. Multiple systemic and ocular malformations associated with maternal LSD usage. Arch Ophthalmol 1974;92:301–3.

19. Bogdanoff B, Rorke LB, Yanoff M, Warren WS. Brain and eye abnormalities: possible sequelae to prenatal use of multiple drugs including LSD. Am J Dis Child 1972;123:145–8.

20. Chan CC, Fishman M, Egbert PR. Multiple ocular anomalies associated with maternal LSD ingestion. Arch Ophthalmol 1978;96:282–4.

21. Margolis S, Martin L. Anophthalmia in an infant of parents using LSD. Ann Ophthalmol 1980;12:1378–81.

22. Gelehrter TD. Lysergic acid diethylamide (LSD) and exstrophy of the bladder. J Pediatr 1970;77:1065–6.

23. Eller JL, Morton JM. Bizarre deformities in offspring of user of lysergic acid diethylamide. N Engl J Med 1970;283:395–7.

24. Hsu LY, Strauss L, Hirschhorn K. Chromosome abnormality in offspring of LSD user: D trisomy with D/D translocation. JAMA 1970;211:987–90.

25. Dumars KW Jr. Parental drug usage: effect upon chromosomes of progeny. Pediatrics 1971;47:1037–41.

26. Blanc WA, Mattison DR, Kane R, Chauhan P. L.S.D., intrauterine amputations, and amniotic-band syndrome. Lancet 1971;2:158–9.

27. Holmes LB. Ocular malformations associated with maternal LSD usage. Arch Ophthalmol 1975;93:1061.

28. Apple DJ. Ocular malformations associated with maternal LSD usage: in reply. Arch Ophthalmol 1975;93:1061.

29. Brown R, Pickering D. Persistent transitional circulation. Arch Dis Child 1974;49:883–5.

30. Tenorio GM, Nazvi M, Bickers GH, Hubbird RH. Intrauterine stroke and maternal polydrug abuse. Clin Pediatr 1988;27:565–7.

31. Cohen MM, Hirschhorn K, Frosch WA. In vivo and in vitro chromosomal damage induced by LSD-25. N Engl J Med 1967;277:1043–9.

32. Sato H, Pergament E. Is lysergide a teratogen? Lancet 1968;1:639–40.

33. Egozcue J, Irwin S, Maruffo CA. Chromosomal damage in LSD users. JAMA 1968;204:214–8.

34. Cohen MM, Hirschhorn K, Verbo S, Frosch WA, Groeschel MM. The effect of LSD-25 on the chromosomes of children exposed in utero. Pediatr Res 1968;2:486–92.

35. Hulten M, Lindsten J, Lidberg L, Ekelund H. Studies on mitotic and meiotic chromosomes in subjects exposed to LSD. Ann Genet (Paris) 1968;11:201–10.

36. Aase JM, Laestadius N, Smith DW. Children of mothers who took L.S.D. in pregnancy. Lancet 1970;2:100–1.

37. Hoffer A. Effect of LSD on chromosomes. Can Med Assoc J 1968;98:466.

38. Smart RG, Bateman K. The chromosomal and teratogenic effects of lysergic acid diethylamide: a review of the current literature. Can Med Assoc J 1968;99:805–10.

39. Rennert OM. Drug-induced somatic alterations. Clin Obstet Gynecol 1975;18:185–98.

40. Glass L, Evans HE. Perinatal drug abuse. Pediatr Ann 1979;8:84–92.

41. VanBlerk GA, Majerus TC, Myers RAM. Teratogenic potential of some psychopharmacologic drugs: a brief review. Int J Gynaecol Obstet 1980;17:399–402.

42. Chernoff GF, Jones KL. Fetal preventive medicine: teratogens and the unborn baby. Pediatr Ann 1981;10:210–7.

43. Stern L. In vivo assessment of the teratogenic potential of drugs in humans. Obstet Gynecol 1981;58:3S–8S.

44. Lee CC, Chiang CN. Maternal-fetal transfer of abused substances: pharmacokinetic and pharmacodynamic data. Natl Inst Drug Abuse Res Monogr Ser 1985;60:110–47.

45. McLane NJ, Carroll DM. Ocular manifestations of drug abuse. Surv Ophthalmol 1986;30:298–313.

Name: ***l*-LYSINE**

Class: **AMINO ACID**   Risk Factor: **C**

Fetal Risk Summary

l-Lysine is an essential amino acid that has been occasionally used for the treatment and prophylaxis of herpes simplex infections (the effectiveness of this indication is questionable). No reports on the use of the commercial formulation in human pregnancy have been located.

l-Lysine is actively transported across the human placenta to the fetus with a steady-state fetal:maternal ratio of approximately 1.6:1 (1, 2). Fetal tissues retain most of the essential amino acids, including *l*-lysine, in preference to the nonessential amino acids (3).

One published case has been located that described a woman with familial hyperlysinemia due to deficiency of the enzymes lysine ketoglutarate reductase and saccharopine dehydrogenase (4). The woman gave birth to a normal child. No details of the pregnancy or the child were provided other than that the child was normal. Serum lysine levels, which were regularly above 10 mg/100 ml and may have been as high as 20 mg/100 ml or more when the disorder was detected, were not measured during the pregnancy or in the baby.

Breast Feeding Summary

No data are available.

References

1. Schneider H, Mohlen KH, Dancis J. Transfer of amino acids across the in vitro perfused human placenta. Pediatr Res 1979;13:236–40.
2. Schneider H, Mohlen KH, Challier JC, Dancis J. Transfer of glutamic acid across the human placenta perfused in vitro. Br J Obstet Gynaecol 1979;86:299–306.
3. Velazquez A, Rosado A, Bernal A, Noriega L, Arevalo N. Amino acid pools in the feto-maternal system. Biol Neonate 1976;29:28–40.
4. Dancis J, Hutzler J, Ampola MG, Shih VE, van Gelderen HH, Kirby LT, Woody NC. The prognosis of hyperlysinemia: an interim report. Am J Hum Genet 1983;35:438–42.

Name: **MAGNESIUM SULFATE**

Class: **Anticonvulsant/Cathartic**   Risk Factor: **B**

Fetal Risk Summary

Magnesium sulfate ($MgSO_4$) is commonly used as an anticonvulsant for toxemia and as a tocolytic agent for premature labor during the last half of pregnancy. Concentrations of magnesium, a natural constituent of human serum, are readily increased in both the mother and fetus following maternal therapy with cord serum levels ranging from 70–100% of maternal concentrations (1–6). Elevated levels in the newborn may persist for up to 7 days with an elimination half-life of 43.2 hours (2). The elimination rate is the same in premature and full-term infants (2). Intravenous magnesium sulfate did not cause lower Apgar scores in a study of women treated for pregnancy-induced hypertension, although the magnesium levels in the newborns reflected hypermagnesemia (6). The mean cord magnesium level, 5.3 mEq/100 ml, was equal to the mean maternal serum level.

No reports linking the use of magnesium sulfate with congenital defects have been located. The Collaborative Perinatal Project monitored 50,282 mother-child pairs, 141 of which had exposure to magnesium sulfate during pregnancy (7). No evidence was found to suggest a relationship to congenital malformations.

In a 1987 report, 17 women, who had been successfully treated with intravenous magnesium sulfate for preterm labor, were given 1 g of magnesium gluconate every 4 hours after the intravenous (IV) magnesium had been discontinued (8). A mean serum magnesium level before any therapy was 1.44 mg/100 ml. Two hours after an oral dose (12–24 hours after discontinuation of IV magnesium), the mean magnesium serum level was 2.16 mg/100 ml, a significant increase ($p < 0.05$). A group of 568 women was randomly assigned to receive either 15 mmol of magnesium-aspartate hydrochloride ($N = 278$) or 13.5 mmol of aspartic acid ($N = 290$) per day (9). Therapy was started as early as possible in the pregnancies, but not later than 16 weeks' gestation. Women receiving the magnesium tablets had fewer hospitalizations ($p < 0.05$), fewer preterm deliveries, and less frequent referral of the newborn to the neonatal intensive care unit ($p < 0.01$) (9). In a double blind randomized, controlled clinical study, 374 young women (mean age approximately 18 years) were treated with either 365 mg of elemental magnesium/day (provided by six tablets of magnesium-aspartate hydrochloride each containing 60.8 mg of elemental magnesium) ($N = 185$) or placebo tablets containing aspartic acid only ($N = 189$) (10). Treatment began at approximately a mean gestational age of 18 weeks (range 13–24 weeks). In addition, both groups received prenatal vitamins containing 100 mg of elemental magnesium. In contrast to the reference cited above, the magnesium therapy did not improve the outcome of the pregnancies as judged by the nonsignificant differences between the groups in incidences of preeclampsia, fetal growth retardation, preterm labor, birth weight, gestational age at delivery, or number of infants admitted to the special care unit (10).

Most studies have been unable to find a correlation between cord serum magnesium levels and newborn condition (2, 5, 11–15). In a study of 7000 offspring of mothers treated with MgSO$_4$ for toxemia, no adverse effects from the therapy were noted in fetuses or newborns (5). Other studies have also observed a lack of toxicity (16, 17). A 1983 investigation of women at term with pregnancy-induced hypertension compared newborns of magnesium-treated mothers with newborns of untreated mothers (15). No differences in neurologic behavior were observed between the two groups except that exposed infants had decreased active tone of the neck extensors on the 1st day after birth.

Newborn depression and hypotonia have been reported as effects of maternal magnesium therapy in some series but intrauterine hypoxia could not always be eliminated as a potential cause or contributing factor (2, 11, 12, 18–20). In a study reporting on the effects of IV magnesium on Apgar scores, the most common negative score was assigned for color, rather than for muscle tone (6).

A 1971 report described two infants with magnesium levels above 8 mg/100 ml who were severely depressed at birth (13). Spontaneous remission of toxic symptoms occurred after 12 hours in one infant, but the second had residual effects of anoxic encephalopathy. In a 1982 study, activities requiring sustained muscle contraction, such as head lag, ventral suspension, suck reflex, and cry response, were impaired up to 48 hours after birth in infants exposed *in utero* to magnesium (14). A hypertensive woman, treated with 11 g of magnesium sulfate within 3.5 hours of delivery, gave birth to a depressed infant without spontaneous respirations, movement, or reflexes (21). An exchange transfusion at 24 hours reversed the condition. In another study, decreased gastrointestinal motility, ileus, hypotonia, and patent ductus arteriosus occurring in the offspring of mothers with severe hypertension were thought to be due to maternal drug therapy, including magnesium sulfate (22). However, the authors could not relate their findings to any particular drug or drugs and could not completely eliminate the possibility that the effects were due to the severe maternal disease.

A mild decrease in cord calcium concentrations has been reported in mothers treated with magnesium (3, 13, 15). In contrast, a 1980 study reported elevated calcium levels in cord blood following magnesium therapy (4). No newborn symptoms were associated with either change in serum calcium concentrations. However, long-term maternal tocolysis with IV magnesium sulfate may cause injury to the newborn as described below.

In an investigation of five newborn infants whose mothers had been treated with IV magnesium sulfate for periods ranging from 5–14 weeks, radiographic bony abnormalities were noted in two of the infants (18). One of the mothers, a class C diabetic who had been insulin dependent for 12 years, was treated with IV magnesium, beginning at 21 weeks' gestation, for 14 weeks. A 2030-g female infant was delivered vaginally at 35 weeks' gestation following spontaneous rupture of the mother's membranes. The maternal histories of this and another case treated for 6 weeks were described in 1986 (19). The infant had frank rachitic changes of the long bones and the calvaria. Serum calcium at 6 hours of age was normal. She was treated with IV calcium gluconate for 3 days, then given bottle feedings without additional calcium or vitamin D. Scout films for an intravenous pyelogram taken at 4 months of age because of a urinary tract infection showed no bony abnormalities. Growth over the first 3 years has been consistently at the 3rd percentile for height, weight, and head circumference. Dental enamel hypoplasia, especially of the central upper incisors, was the only physical abnormality noted at 3 years of age. The second infant's mother had been treated with IV magnesium for 9 weeks beginning at 25 weeks' gestation. The 2190-g female infant was delivered vaginally at 34 weeks because of spontaneous rupture of membranes. Hypocalcemia (5.8 mg/100 ml, normal 6.0–10.0 mg/100 ml) was measured at 6 hours of age. A chest radiograph taken on the 1st day revealed lucent bands at the distal ends of the metaphyses (18). She was treated with IV calcium for 5 days and then given bottle feedings without additional calcium or vitamin D. A scout film for an intravenous pyelogram at 5 months of age showed no bony abnormalities. In the remaining three cases, the mothers had been treated with IV magnesium for 4–6 weeks and their infants were normal on examination. The authors hypothesized that the fetal hypermagnesemia produced by the long-term maternal administration of magnesium caused a depression of parathyroid hormone release that resulted in fetal hypocalcemia (18).

In another study of long-term IV magnesium tocolysis, 22 women were treated for an average of 26.3 ± 19.2 days (maximum duration in any patient was 75 days) (20). Two infants delivered from this group were noted to have wide-spaced fontanelles and parietal bone thinning. These effects returned to normal with time. A third newborn, delivered from a mother belonging to an intermediate group treated with IV magnesium for an average of 6.3 ± 1.9 days, suffered a parietal bone fracture during an instrumental delivery and developed spastic quadriplegia (20). The authors could not determine if bone thinning secondary to magnesium contributed to the complication.

Clinically significant drug interactions have been reported, one in a newborn and three in mothers, after maternal administration of $MgSO_4$. In one case, an interaction between in utero acquired magnesium and gentamicin was reported in a newborn 24 hours after birth (23, 24). The mother had received 24 g of $MgSO_4$ during the 32 hours preceding birth of a neurologically depressed female infant. Gentamicin, 2.5 mg/kg intramuscularly every 12 hours, was begun at 12 hours of age for presumed sepsis. The infant developed respiratory arrest following the second dose of gentamicin, which resolved after the antibiotic was stopped. Animal experiments confirmed the interaction. The maternal cases involved an interaction between magnesium and nifedipine (25, 26). One report described two women who were hospitalized at 30 and 32 weeks' gestation, respectively, for hypertension (25). In both cases, oral methyldopa 2 g and intravenous $MgSO_4$ 20 g daily were ineffective in lowering the mother's blood pressure. Oral nifedipine 10 mg was given and a marked hypotensive response occurred 45 minutes later. The blood pressures before nifedipine in the women were 150/110 and 140/105 mm Hg, respectively, then decreased to 80/50 and 90/60 mm Hg, respectively, after administration of the calcium channel blocker. Blood pressure returned to previous levels 25–30 minutes later. Both infants were delivered following the hypotensive episodes, but only one survived. In the third maternal case, a woman, in premature labor at 32 weeks' gestation, was treated with oral nifedipine 60 mg over 3 hours, then 20 mg every 8 hours (26). Because uterine contractions returned, intravenous $MgSO_4$ was begun 12 hours later followed by the onset of pronounced muscle weakness after 500 mg had been administered. Her symptoms included jerky movements of the extremities, difficulty in swallowing, paradoxical respirations, and an inability to lift her head from the pillow. The magnesium was stopped and the symptoms resolved over the next 25 minutes. The reaction was attributed to nifedipine potentiation of the neuromuscular blocking action of magnesium.

Maternal hypothermia with maternal and fetal bradycardia apparently due to IV magnesium sulfate has been reported (27). The 30-year-old woman, at about 31 weeks' gestation, was being treated for premature labor. She had received a single, 12-mg intramuscular dose of betamethasone at the same time that magnesium therapy was started. Her oral temperature fell from 99.8°F to 97°F 2 hours after the infusion had been increased from 2 g/hour to 3 g/hour. Twelve hours after admission to the hospital, her heart rate fell to 64 beats/minute (baseline 80 beats/minute) while the fetal heart rate decreased to 110 beats/minute (baseline 140–150 beats/minute). A rectal temperature at this time was 95.8°F and the patient complained of lethargy and diplopia. Her serum magnesium level was 6.6 mg/100 ml. Magnesium therapy was discontinued and all signs and symptoms returned to baseline values within 6 hours. Neither the mother nor the fetus suffered adversely from the effects attributed to magnesium.

In summary, the administration of magnesium sulfate to the mother for anticonvulsant or tocolytic effects does not usually pose a risk to the fetus or newborn. Long-term infusions of magnesium may be associated with sustained hypocalcemia in the fetus resulting in congenital rickets. Neonatal neurologic depression may occur with respiratory depression, muscle weakness, and loss of reflexes. The toxicity is not usually correlated with cord serum magnesium levels. Offspring of mothers treated with this drug close to delivery should be closely observed for signs of toxicity during the first 24–48 hours after birth. Caution is also advocated with the use of aminoglycoside antibiotics during this period.

Breast Feeding Summary

Magnesium salts may be encountered by nursing mothers using over-the-counter laxatives. A study in which 50 mothers received an emulsion of magnesium and liquid petrolatum or mineral oil found no evidence of changes or frequency of stools in nursing infants (28). In 10 preeclamptic patients receiving magnesium sulfate, 1 g/hour intravenously during the first 24 hours after delivery, magnesium levels in breast milk were 64 µg/ml as compared to 48 µg/ml in nontreated controls (29). Twenty-four hours after stopping the drug, milk levels in treated and nontreated patients were 38 and 32 µg/ml, respectively. By 48 hours, the levels were identical in the two groups. Milk:plasma ratios were 1.9 and 2.1 in treated and nontreated patients, respectively. The American Academy of Pediatrics considers magnesium sulfate to be compatible with breast feeding (30).

References

1. Chesley LC, Tepper I. Plasma levels of magnesium attained in magnesium sulfate therapy for preeclampsia and eclampsia. Surg Clin North Am 1957;37:353–67.
2. Dangman BC, Rosen TS. Magnesium levels in infants of mothers treated with MgSO₄. Pediatr Res 1977;11:415 (Abstract #262).
3. Cruikshank DP, Pitkin RM, Reynolds WA, Williams GA, Hargis GK. Effects of magnesium sulfate treatment on perinatal calcium metabolism. I. Maternal and fetal responses. Am J Obstet Gynecol 1979;134:243–9.
4. Donovan EF, Tsang RC, Steichen JJ, Strub RJ, Chen IW, Chen M. Neonatal hypermagnesemia: effect on parathyroid hormone and calcium homeostasis. J Pediatr 1980;96:305–10.

5. Stone SR, Pritchard JA. Effect of maternally administered magnesium sulfate on the neonate. Obstet Gynecol 1970;35:574–7.
6. Pruett KM, Kirshon B, Cotton DB, Adam K, Doody KJ. The effects of magnesium sulfate therapy on Apgar scores. Am J Obstet Gynecol 1988;159:1047–8.
7. Heinonen OP, Slone D, Shapiro S. *Birth Defects and Drugs in Pregnancy*. Littleton:Publishing Sciences Group, 1977:440.
8. Martin RW, Gaddy DK, Martin JN Jr, Lucas JA, Wiser WL, Morrison JC. Tocolysis with oral magnesium. Am J Obstet Gynecol 1987;156:433–4.
9. Spatling L, Spatling G. Magnesium supplementation in pregnancy: a double-blind study. Br J Obstet Gynaecol 1988;95:120–5.
10. Sibai BM, Villar L. MA, Bray E. Magnesium supplementation during pregnancy: a double-blind randomized controlled clinical trial. Am J Obstet Gynecol 1989;161:115–9.
11. Lipsitz PJ, English IC. Hypermagnesemia in the newborn infant. Pediatrics 1967;40:856–62.
12. Lipsitz PJ. The clinical and biochemical effects of excess magnesium in the newborn. Pediatrics 1971;47:501–9.
13. Savory J, Monif GRG. Serum calcium levels in cord sera of the progeny of mothers treated with magnesium sulfate for toxemia of pregnancy. Am J Obstet Gynecol 1971;110:556–9.
14. Rasch DK, Huber PA, Richardson CJ, L'Hommedieu CS, Nelson TE, Reddi R. Neurobehavioral effects of neonatal hypermagnesemia. J Pediatr 1982;100:272–6.
15. Green KW, Key TC, Coen R, Resnik R. The effects of maternally administered magnesium sulfate on the neonate. Am J Obstet Gynecol 1983;146:29–33.
16. Sibai BM, Lipshitz J, Anderson GD, Dilts PV Jr. Reassessment of intravenous $MgSO_4$ therapy in preeclampsia-eclampsia. Obstet Gynecol 1981;57:199–202.
17. Hutchinson HT, Nichols MM, Kuhn CR, Vasicka A. Effects of magnesium sulfate on uterine contractility, intrauterine fetus, and infant. Am J Obstet Gynecol 1964;88:747–58.
18. Lamm CI, Norton KI, Murphy RJC, Wilkins IA, Rabinowitz JG. Congenital rickets associated with magnesium sulfate infusion for tocolysis. J Pediatr 1988;113:1078–82.
19. Wilkins IA, Goldberg JD, Phillips RN, Bacall CJ, Chervenak FA, Berkowitz RL. Long-term use of magnesium sulfate as a tocolytic agent. Obstet Gynecol 1986;67:38S–40S.
20. Dudley D, Gagnon D, Varner M. Long-term tocolysis with intravenous magnesium sulfate. Obstet Gynecol 1989;73:373–8.
21. Brady JP, Williams HC. Magnesium intoxication in a premature infant. Pediatrics 1967;40:100–3.
22. Brazy JE, Grimm JK, Little VA. Neonatal manifestations of severe maternal hypertension occurring before the thirty-sixth week of pregnancy. J Pediatr 1982;100:265–71.
23. L'Hommedieu CS, Nicholas D, Armes DA, Jones P, Nelson T, Pickering LK. Potentiation of magnesium sulfate-induced neuromuscular weakness by gentamicin, tobramycin, and amikacin. J Pediatr 1983;102:629–31.
24. L'Hommedieu CS, Huber PA, Rasch DK. Potentiation of magnesium-induced neuromuscular weakness by gentamicin. Crit Care Med 1983;11:55–6.
25. Waisman GD, Mayorga LM, Camera MI, Vignolo CA, Martinotti A. Magnesium plus nifedipine: potentiation of hypotensive effect in preeclampsia? Am J Obstet Gynecol 1988;159:308–9.
26. Snyder SW, Cardwell MS. Neuromuscular blockade with magnesium sulfate and nifedipine. Am J Obstet Gynecol 1989;161:35–6.
27. Rodis JF, Vintzileos AM, Campbell WA, Deaton JL, Nochimson DJ. Maternal hypothermia: an unusual complication of magnesium sulfate therapy. Am J Obstet Gynecol 1987;156:435–6.
28. Baldwin WF. Clinical study of senna administration to nursing mothers: assessment of effects on infant bowel habits. Can Med Assoc J 1963;89:566–8.
29. Cruikshank DP, Varner MW, Pitkin RM. Breast milk magnesium and calcium concentrations following magnesium sulfate treatment. Am J Obstet Gynecol 1982;143:685–8.
30. Committee on Drugs, American Academy of Pediatrics. Transfer of drugs and other chemicals into human milk. Pediatrics 1989;84:924–36.

Name: **MANDELIC ACID**

Class: **Urinary Germicide**

Risk Factor: **C**

Fetal Risk Summary

Mandelic acid is available as a single agent and in combination with methenamine (see also Methenamine). The Collaborative Perinatal Project reported 30 1st trimester exposures for this drug (1, pp. 299, 302). For use anytime in pregnancy, 224 exposures were recorded (1, p. 435). Only in the latter group was a possible association with malformations found. The statistical significance of this association is not known. Independent confirmation is required.

Breast Feeding Summary

Mandelic acid is excreted into breast milk. In six mothers given 12 g/day, milk levels averaged 550 μg/ml (2). The drug was found in the urine of all infants. It was estimated that an infant would receive an average dose of 86 mg/kg/day by this route. The significance of this amount is not known.

References

1. Heinonen OP, Slone D, Shapiro S. *Birth Defects and Drugs in Pregnancy.* Littleton:Publishing Sciences Group, 1977.
2. Berger H. Excretion of mandelic acid in breast milk. Am J Dis Child 1941;61:256–61.

Name: **MANNITOL**

Class: **Diuretic**

Risk Factor: **C**

Fetal Risk Summary

Mannitol is an osmotic diuretic. No reports of its use in pregnancy following intravenous administration have been located. Mannitol, given by intra-amniotic injection, has been used for the induction of abortion (1).

Breast Feeding Summary

No data are available.

Reference

1. Craft IL, Mus BD. Hypertonic solutions to induce abortions. Br Med J 1971;2:49.

Name: **MAPROTILINE**
Class: **Antidepressant**   Risk Factor: **B_M**

Fetal Risk Summary

No reports linking the use of maprotiline with congenital defects have been located. Animal studies have failed to demonstrate teratogenicity, carcinogenicity, mutagenicity, or impairment of fertility (1).

Breast Feeding Summary

Maprotiline is excreted into breast milk (2). Milk:plasma ratios of 1.5 and 1.3 have been reported following a 100-mg single dose and 150 mg in divided doses for 120 hours. Multiple dosing resulted in milk concentrations of unchanged maprotiline of 0.2 µg/ml. Although this amount is low, the significance to the nursing infant is not known.

References

1. Product information. Ludiomil. CIBA, 1990.
2. Reiss W. The relevance of blood level determinations during the evaluation of maprotiline in man. In Murphy JE, ed. *Research and Clinical Investigation in Depression.* Northampton, England:Cambridge Medical Publications, 1980;19–38.

Name: **MARIJUANA**
Class: **Hallucinogen**   Risk Factor: **C**

Fetal Risk Summary

Marijuana (cannabis; hashish) is a natural substance that is smoked for its hallucinogenic properties. (One marijuana cigarette is commonly referred to as a "joint.") Hashish is a potent concentrated form of marijuana. The main psychoactive ingredient, Δ-9-tetrahydrocannabinol (Δ-9-THC, THC), is also available in a commercial oral formulation (dronabinol) for use as an antiemetic agent. Natural preparations of marijuana may vary widely in their potency and, and except for the commercial preparation, no standardization exists either for the THC content or for the presence of contaminants. Only the commercially available oral formulation can be legally used in the United States.

The use of marijuana by pregnant women is common. Most investigators have reported incidences of 3–16% (1–17). Other researchers have proposed that even these figures represent under reporting, especially in the 1st month when pregnancy may not be suspected (18–20). Because of the illicit nature of marijuana, many women will simply not admit to its use (4, 8). Data from the Ottawa Prenatal Prospective Study in Canada indicated that 20% of their patients used marijuana during the year prior to pregnancy with the incidence declining to about one-half this figure after the women knew they were pregnant (13). In addition, heavy marijuana usage (more than five joints/week or the use of hashish), when compared with alcohol or nicotine usage, was the least reduced of the three agents during pregnancy (21).

Even though the usage of marijuana by pregnant women is common, the effects of this usage on the pregnancies and the fetuses are still unclear. Part of this problem is attributable to the close association between marijuana, alcohol, nicotine, other abuse drugs, and life-styles that may increase perinatal risk (1–3, 6, 7). Separating the effects of these agents by statistical methods becomes a major task of almost all studies. The results of this separation have produced sufficient data, however, to allow classification of the major concerns surrounding exposure to marijuana during pregnancy. These concerns are:

Placental passage of Δ-9-THC
Pregnancy complications
   Length of gestation
   Quality and duration of labor
   Effect on maternal hormone levels
Fetal/newborn complications
   In utero growth retardation
   Congenital anomalies
   Neurobehavioral complications in newborn
   Induction of leukemia in childhood

Δ-9-THC and a metabolite, 9-carboxy-THC, cross the placenta to the fetus at term (4, 22). Data for other periods of gestation and for other metabolites are not available. A 1982 study found measurable amounts of 9-carboxy-THC, but not THC, in two cord blood samples but did not quantify the concentrations (4). In a study of 10 women who daily smoked up to five marijuana cigarettes, maternal serum samples were drawn 10–20 minutes before corresponding cord blood samples (22). The time interval between last exposure and sampling ranged from 5–26 hours. This is well beyond the time of peak THC levels that occur 3–8 minutes after beginning to smoke (23). Maternal levels of THC were below the limit of sensitivity (0.2 ng/ml) in five samples and ranged from 0.4–6 ng/ml in the others. Measurable cord blood concentrations of THC were found in three samples and varied between 0.3–1.0 ng/ml. The maternal plasma:cord blood ratios for these three samples were 2.7, 4, and 6, respectively. The metabolite, 9-carboxy-THC, was measured in all maternal and cord blood samples, ranging between 2.3–125 ng/ml and 0.4–18 ng/ml, respectively. Plasma:cord blood ratios for the metabolite varied from 1.7–7.8.

Marijuana-induced complications of pregnancy are controversial, with different studies producing conflicting results. One of these areas of controversy involves the effect of marijuana on length of gestation. A 1980 prospective study of 291 women found no relationship between maternal use of marijuana and gestational length (3). Similar results were reported from two studies, one in 1982 involving 1,690 women (24) and one in 1989 with 1,226 women (25). Of interest, marijuana use by the women in the later study was confirmed with urine assays (25). A significantly ($p < 0.001$) shorter gestational period was found in 1,246 users in a retrospective study of 12,424 pregnancies, but this difference disappeared when the data were controlled for nicotine exposure, demographic characteristics, and medical and obstetric histories (9).

In contrast to the above reports, three groups of investigators have associated regular marijuana use with shorter gestations (1, 10, 14) and one group with longer gestations (26). In 36 women using marijuana two or more times/week, 9 (25%) delivered prematurely, a rate much higher than the 5.1% for users of marijuana one time or less/week and the 5.6% for nonusers (1). Investigation of 583 women who delivered single live births, a continuation of the 1980 study mentioned above, now revealed that heavy use of marijuana (more than five marijuana cigarettes/week) was significantly ($p = 0.008$) associated with a reduction of 0.8 week in gestational length after adjustment for the mother's prepregnancy weight (10). A total of 84 (14.4%) used marijuana in this population, 18 of whom were classified as heavy users. A large prospective study of 3857 pregnancies ending in singleton live births found that regular marijuana use (two to three times/month or more) was associated with an increased risk of preterm (<37 weeks) delivery for white women but not for nonwhite women (14). For the white 122 regular users, 8.2% delivered prematurely compared with 3.8% of 105 occasional users (one marijuana cigarette or less/month) and 4.0% of 2778 nonusers. In the nonwhite groups, the incidences of shortened gestation for the 86 regular, 53 occasional, and 706 nonusers were 10.5%, 11.3%, and 8.8%, respectively. In a population of lower socioeconomic status women, the total amount of marijuana used during pregnancy was positively correlated with an average 2 days prolongation of gestation (26). However, the authors of this study noted that their evidence for a longer gestational period was weak in terms of magnitude.

A second pregnancy complication examined frequently is the effect of marijuana on the quality and duration of labor. No association between marijuana and duration of labor, including precipitate labor and the type of presentation at birth, was found in the Ottawa Prenatal Prospective Study (3, 5, 8) or in another study (26). In contrast, other investigators found a significant difference ($p < 0.01$) in precipitate labor (<3 hours total) between users (29%) and nonusers (3%)(4, 27). Although not significant, 31% of users (11 of 35) had prolonged, protracted, or arrested labor as compared to 19% (7 of 36) nonusers (4, 27). Because of the dysfunctional labor, 57% of the newborn infants in the user group had meconium staining vs. 25% among nonusers ($p = 0.05$), a situation that probably resulted in the observation that 41% of newborn infants of users required resuscitation compared to 21% of infants of nonusers. Adjustment of the data for race, income, smoking, alcohol use, and first physician visit did not change the findings. A second study by these latter investigators using a different group of patients produced similar results in the incidence of dysfunctional labor, precipitate labor, and meconium staining, but the differences between users and nonusers were not significant (7).

In nonhuman primates, marijuana disrupts the menstrual cycle by inhibiting ovulation through its effects on the pituitary trophic hormones (luteinizing hormone and follicle-stimulating hormone), prolactin, and resulting decreases in estrogen and progesterone levels (16). Tolerance to these effects has been reported (16). Similar effects have been observed in human clinical studies (16).

Thirteen pregnant women, who were regular users of marijuana (once/month to four times/day), were matched with controls (28). No effect of this exposure was measured on the levels of human chorionic gonadotropin (hCG), pregnancy-specific β-1-glycoprotein, placental lactogen, progesterone, 17-hydroxyprogesterone, estradiol, and estiol.

Concerns with the fetal complications arising from maternal marijuana use center around the effects on *in utero* growth retardation, structural anomalies, and neurobehavioral complications in the newborn infant. A recent report has now indicated that induction of leukemia in childhood must also be considered. As with pregnancy complications, conflicting reports are common.

Data of the Ottawa Prenatal Prospective Study indicated no significant reduction in birth weight or head circumference (after adjustment for other factors) in babies of marijuana users (3, 5, 8, 10, 13). Compared to infants of nonusers, birth weight actually increased by an average of 67 g in irregular users (one marijuana cigarette/week or less) and 117 g in moderate users (two to five/week), whereas heavy use (more than five/week) was associated with a nonsignificant reduction of 52 g (10). Other studies have observed no effect on growth after adjustment of their data (1, 7, 9, 26, 29). However, in one study, a reduction of 0.55 cm in infant length, but not head circumference, was correlated with maternal use of three marijuana cigarettes/day in the 1st trimester (26). Use during the remainder of pregnancy or the total amount smoked during pregnancy did not significantly affect the infants' length or head circumference.

Positive correlations with reduced *in utero* growth (after adjustment) have been reported by a number of researchers. In one study, use of less than three joints/week was associated with a decrease in birth weight of 95 g compared to that of controls, and use of three or more cigarettes/week was associated with a reduction of 139 g (24, 30). Both weight reductions were significant ($p < 0.01$). Some of these same researchers published a related study in 1989 involving Boston-area women enrolled in an investigation between 1984–1987 (25). Their findings indicated that marijuana use during pregnancy, when confirmed by positive urine assays, was independently associated with impaired fetal growth, and that the effects of cocaine abuse were additive but not synergistic (25). However, they could not demonstrate a cause-and-effect relationship with marijuana because of other factors, such as the markedly elevated blood levels of carbon monoxide that occur with marijuana use (blood carboxyhemoglobin levels after smoking marijuana are about five times those observed after smoking tobacco) (25). Of 1226 mothers who were studied, 331 (27%) used marijuana during gestation as determined by history and positive urine assay. Only 278 (84%) of these would have been detected by history alone. After controlling for potentially confounding variables (e.g., tobacco, alcohol, opiates, certain diseases, and obstetric factors), infants of marijuana users with positive urine assays ($N = 202$) were compared with infants of nonusers ($N = 895$) and found to have statistically significant differences in birth weight (reduction of 79 g; $p = 0.04$) and length (reduction of 0.52 cm; $p = 0.02$). Head circumference was reduced by 0.19 cm but the difference was not significant ($p = 0.15$). The birth weight and length measurements did not differ statistically if only self-reported marijuana use was considered, demonstrating the importance of a biologic marker in studies involving this drug.

Another study, conducted from 1975–1983 in two phases, found decreased birth weight only in the second phase (17). The two phases, involving 1434 and 1381 patients, respectively, differed primarily in their assessment of marijuana use early in pregnancy. In the first phase, 9.3% used marijuana, with consumption of two to four joints/month associated with a significant increase in birth weight. No trend was observed with more or less frequent use. The second phase, with 10.3% users, found weight reductions in all classifications of marijuana exposure: 127 g for two to three joints/week, 143 g for four to six joints/week, and 230 g for daily use (17). The authors speculated that the difference between the groups may have been due to the use of other abuse drugs (e.g., cocaine) or changes in the composition or contaminants of marijuana. Regular use (two to three times/month or more) of marijuana was correlated with an increased risk of low-birth-weight (<2500 g) and small-for-gestational-age (SGA) infants in whites only in a 1986 study (14). Compared to 3490 nonusers, where the risks of low-birth-weight and SGA infants were 2.7% and 4.9%, respectively, regular use ($N = 122$) was associated with rates of 8.2% and 12.5%, respectively. In 845 nonwhites, no differences between users and nonusers were observed. Examination of 462 infants, 16% of whom were exposed to marijuana and alcohol during early gestation, found a significant correlation between maternal marijuana use and decreased body length at 8 months of age (11). Body weight and head circumference were not significantly affected.

In three case reports on the same five infants, low birth weight (all <2500 g) with reduced head circumference and length were observed (31–33). Two of the infants were premature (<37 weeks). The mothers of these infants smoked 2–14 marijuana cigarettes/day during pregnancy with one also using alcohol, cocaine and nicotine, and two others using nicotine.

Animal research in the 1960s and 1970s yielded inconclusive evidence on the teratogenicity of marijuana and its active ingredients unless high doses were used in certain species (34–37). In humans, most investigators and reviewers have concluded either that marijuana does not produce structural defects or that insufficient data exist to reach any conclusion (1, 13, 25, 26, 29, 38–49). However, one reviewer cautioned that marijuana-induced birth defects could be rare and easily missed (48), and another observed that marijuana could potentiate known teratogens by lowering the threshold for their effects (42). A previously mentioned study that used urine assays to document marijuana exposure found that the drug was not associated with minor (either singly or as a constellation of three) or major congenital anomalies (25).

Because marijuana use is so common in women during pregnancy, and because of its frequent association with alcohol and other abuse drugs, it is not surprising that a number of studies and case reports have described congenital malformations in infants whose mothers were smoking marijuana. With some exceptions, the majority of these investigators did not attribute the observed defects to marijuana, but they are chronicled here mainly for a complete record.

Frequent references have described the combined maternal use of marijuana and lysergic acid diethylamide (LSD) in cases ending with poor fetal outcome. A 1968 report described an infant with right terminal transverse acheiria (absence of hand) (50). The mother had taken LSD early in gestation before she knew she was pregnant. She had also smoked marijuana throughout the pregnancy and had taken a combination product containing dicyclomine, doxylamine, and pyridoxine for 1st trimester nausea. A second infant with a terminal transverse deficit, and who was also exposed to the two hallucinogens, was described in 1969 (51). The defect involved portions of fingers of the left hand. Syndactyly of the right hand with shortened fingers and talipes equinovarus of the left foot were also present. A critique of these case reports and others concluded that the defects in the two infants may have been due to amniotic band syndrome (52). Complete exstrophy of the bladder, epispadias, widely separated pubic rami, and bilateral inguinal hernias were observed in a newborn exposed to LSD, marijuana, and mephentermine (53). Marijuana was allegedly used only twice by the mother. In another case, a female infant with multiple anomalies compatible with trisomy 13 with D/D translocation was delivered from a 22-year-old mother who had last used LSD 9 months prior to conception (54). The mother used marijuana, barbiturates and amphetamines throughout gestation and, presumably, before conception. The authors speculated that the defect may have been due to LSD-induced damage of maternal germ cells prior to fertilization. A 1972 case report described an infant with multiple eye and central nervous system defects consisting of brachycephaly with widely separated sutures, bilateral cephalohematomas, a right eye smaller than the left, a possible cataract, and multiple brain anomalies (55). The mother had taken marijuana, LSD, and other drugs throughout pregnancy. In a study of 140 women using LSD and marijuana followed through 148 pregnancies, 8 of 83 liveborn infants had major defects as did 4 of 14 embryos examined after induced abortion (56). The incidence of defects in this sample is high (8.1%), but many of the women were using multiple other abuse drugs and had life-styles that probably were not conducive to good fetal health. Two other reports involving the combined use of marijuana and LSD with resulting adverse fetal outcomes do not appear to have any relationship to either drug (57, 58). One of these involved a report of six cases of persistent ductus arteriosus, one of which was exposed to marijuana *in utero* (57). The history of maternal marijuana use was coincidental. The second case described an infant who died at 2.5 months of age from a bilateral *in utero* cerebral vascular accident and resulting porencephaly (58). The mother had used marijuana, LSD, alcohol, and other abuse drugs, including cocaine. This latter drug was thought to be the causative agent.

In one of two fatal cases of congenital hypothalamic hamartoblastoma tumor, an infant exposed to marijuana also had congenital heart disease and skeletal anomalies suggestive of the Ellis-von Creveld syndrome (i.e., chondroectodermal dysplasia syndrome) (59). In addition to marijuana, the mother had used cocaine and methaqualone during early pregnancy, but the authors did not attribute the defects to a particular agent. In a report of an infant with a random pattern of amputations and constrictions consistent with the amniotic band sequence, the mother's occasional use of marijuana was coincidental (60).

In contrast to the above case reports, where marijuana use during the pregnancies was apparently not related to fetal outcome, two studies have reported possible associations with the drug (9, 24) and one case report found defects similar to those reported in one of the studies (31–33). However, in both studies, marijuana usage in pregnancy was poorly quantified (9). Additionally, a third study observed severe minor facial defects only in the offspring of heavy users (61). In a study of 1,690 mother-child pairs, women who smoked marijuana, but who only drank small amounts of alcohol, were five times more likely than nonusers to deliver an infant with features compatible with the fetal alcohol syndrome (see Ethanol) (24). The relative risk for this defect in marijuana users was 12.7 compared to 2.0 in nonusers. In a series of case reports, five infants were described with congenital defects suggestive of the fetal alcohol syndrome (31–33). In addition to daily marijuana use by the mothers, one used alcohol, cocaine, and nicotine; two used nicotine only; and two denied the use of other drugs (31). In a large study involving 12,424 women of whom 1,246 (10%) used marijuana during pregnancy, a crude association between one or more major malformations and marijuana usage was discovered; no association was found with minor malformations (9). Logistic regression was used to control confounding variables, and although the odds ratio

(1.36) was suggestive, the association between marijuana and the defects was not significant. The third study compared 25 marijuana users with 25 closely matched nonusing controls in a search for minor anomalies (61). Infants were examined at a mean age of 28.8 months. No relationship between the drug use and minor malformations was found, but the authors could not exclude the existence of a possible relationship at birth since some minor anomalies disappear with age. Of interest, three infants had severe epicanthal folds, three had true ocular hypertelorism, and all were the offspring of heavy (more than five joints/week) users (61).

Strabismus was diagnosed in 24% (7 of 29) of the infants delivered from mothers maintained on methadone throughout pregnancy in a 1987 report (62). This percentage was approximately four to eight times the expected incidence of the eye defect in the general population. Two (29%) of the seven infants were also exposed *in utero* to marijuana vs. three (14%) of the nonaffected infants. While use of other abuse drugs was common, the authors attributed the eye condition to low birth weight and, possibly, an unknown contribution from methadone. However, in the Ottawa Prenatal Prospective Study, 35% of the marijuana-exposed infants compared to 6% of the controls had more than one of the following eye problems: myopia, strabismus, abnormal oculomotor functioning, or unusual discs ($p < 0.008$) (13). The examiner was blinded to the prenatal histories of the infants.

Significant alterations in neurobehavior in offspring of regular marijuana users were noted in the Ottawa Prenatal Prospective Study (3, 5, 13, 15). After adjustment for nicotine and alcohol use, *in utero* exposure to marijuana was associated with increased tremors and exaggerated startles, both spontaneous and in response to minimal stimuli (13, 15). Decreased visual responses, including poorer visual habituation to light, were also observed in these infants. In addition, a slight increase in irritability was noted. In early data from the Ottawa group, a distinctive shrill, high-pitched, cat-like cry, reminiscent of the cry considered to be symptomatic of drug withdrawal, was heard from a large number of the offspring of regular users (3). No differences were noted between exposed and nonexposed infants in terms of lateralization, muscle tone, hand-to-mouth behavior, general activity, alertness, or lability of states (3). On follow-up examinations, the abnormalities in neonatal neurobehavior apparently did not result in poorer performance on cognitive and motor tests at 18 and 24 months (13). The investigators cautioned that they were unable to determine if the follow-up results were truly indicative of a return to normal or due to insensitivity of the available tests (13). A 1984 report examining maternal drinking and neonatal withdrawal found that marijuana use had no effect on the signs of withdrawal in their patients (63). In another study, no increase in startles, tremors, or other neurobehavioral measures at birth was noted in exposed infants (26). Marijuana exposure also had no effect on muscle tone. Evaluation at 1 year of age found no significant differences in growth or in mental and motor development between infants exposed *in utero* to either none or varying amounts of the drug (26).

The development of leukemia in children exposed to marijuana during gestation has been suggested in a 1989 report (64). In a multicenter study conducted between 1980–1984 by the Childrens Cancer Study Group, *in utero* marijuana exposure was significantly related to the development of acute nonlymphoblastic leukemia (ANLL). Of the 204 cases that were analyzed, marijuana use was found in

10 mothers, only one of whom used other (LSD) mind-altering drugs. An eleventh case mother used methadone. Only one of the 203 closely matched healthy controls were exposed to abuse drugs. The 10-fold risk induced by marijuana exposure was statistically significant ($p = 0.005$). The mean age of ANLL diagnosis was significantly younger in the exposed children than in nonexposed children, 37.7 months vs. 96.1 months, respectively ($p = 0.007$). Based on the French-American-British system of classification, the morphology of the leukemias also differed significantly with 70% of the exposed cases presenting with monocytic (M5) or myelomonocytic (M4) morphology compared to 31% of the nonexposed cases ($p = 0.02$). Additionally, only 10% of the exposed children had M1 or M2 (myelocytic) morphology vs. 58% of the nonexposed children ($p = 0.02$). The authors were able to exclude reporting bias but could not exclude the possibility that the association was due to other factors, such as the presence of herbicides or pesticides on the marijuana.

Early concerns (65, 66) that marijuana-induced chromosome damage could eventually lead to congenital defects have been largely laid to rest (39, 48, 49). The clinical significance of any drug-induced chromosomal abnormality is doubtful (48). Finally, heavy marijuana use in males has been associated with decreased sperm production (16, 66). However, the clinical significance of this finding has been questioned since there is no evidence that the reduction in sperm counts is related to infertility (16, 66).

In summary, the use of marijuana in pregnancy has produced conflicting reports on the length of gestation, the quality and duration of labor, fetal growth, congenital defects, and neurobehavior in the newborn. These effects have been the subject of a number of reviews (16, 35, 36, 38–42, 45–49, 67, 68). Research using urine assays to document maternal marijuana use indicates that the drug is associated with reduced fetal growth (weight and length) but not with gestational length (25). Moreover, this growth retardation is independent of the effects of cocaine, with the effects being additive rather than synergistic. The possible association of *in utero* marijuana exposure with acute nonlymphoblastic leukemia in children should be a major concern of any woman who chooses to use this drug during pregnancy. No pattern of malformations has been observed that could be considered characteristic of *in utero* marijuana exposure. In most studies, the use of marijuana is closely associated with the use of nicotine and alcohol, and the abuse of other drugs, both prescription and illicit, occurs frequently. In addition, failure to account for the varying concentrations of Δ-9-THC contained in the natural product, the presence of contaminants, and the underreporting of maternal marijuana use could very well have changed the findings of many studies. Based on this information, it is probable that some of the effects observed in offspring of marijuana users are the result of a combination of such factors as drug use, lifestyles, socioeconomic status, maternal diseases and nutrition, and other unidentified elements. The effects on fetal growth and the reported association with childhood leukemia may be due to marijuana or to factors closely related to the use of the drug. Additional research, especially long-term studies on exposed infants, are required before final conclusions can be reached.

Breast Feeding Summary

Δ-9-Tetrahydrocannabinol (Δ-9-THC; THC), the main active ingredient of marijuana (cannabis, hashish), is excreted into breast milk (26, 42, 69, 70). Analysis of

THC and two metabolites, 11-hydroxy-THC and 9-carboxy-THC, were conducted on the milk of two women who had been nursing for 7 and 8 months, respectively, and who smoked marijuana frequently (69). A THC concentration of 105 ng/ml, but no metabolites, was found in the milk of the woman smoking one pipe of marijuana daily. In the second woman, who smoked seven pipes/day, concentrations of THC, 11-hydroxy-THC, and 9-carboxy-THC were 340 ng/ml, 4 ng/ml, and none, respectively. The analysis was repeated in the second mother, approximately 1 hour after the last use of marijuana, using simultaneously obtained samples of milk and plasma. Concentrations (in ng/ml) of the active ingredient and metabolites in milk and plasma (ratios shown in parenthesis) were 60.3 and 7.2 (8.4), 1.1 and 2.5 (0.4), and 1.6 and 19 (0.08), respectively. The marked differences in THC found between the milk samples was thought to be due to the amount of marijuana smoked and the interval between smoking and sample collection. A total fecal sample from the infant yielded levels of 347 ng of THC, 67 ng of 11-hydroxy-THC, and 611 ng of 9-carboxy-THC. Due to the large concentration of metabolites, the authors interpreted this as evidence that the nursing infant was absorbing and metabolizing the THC from the milk. In spite of the evidence that the fat-soluble THC was concentrated in breast milk, both nursing infants were developing normally.

In animals, THC decreases the amount of milk produced by suppressing the production of prolactin and, possibly, by a direct action on the mammary glands (42). While data on this effect are not available in humans, maternal marijuana use does not seem grossly to affect the nursing infant (26). In 27 infants evaluated at 1 year of age, who were exposed to marijuana via the milk, compared to 35 nonexposed infants, no significant differences were found in terms of age at weaning, growth, and mental or motor development (26).

Although no adverse effects of marijuana exposure from breast milk have been reported, follow-up of these infants is inadequate. At the present time, the long-term effects of this exposure are unknown and additional research to determine these effects, if any, is warranted (70). The American Academy of Pediatrics considers the use of marijuana during breast feeding to be contraindicated (71).

References

1. Gibson GT, Baghurst PA, Colley DP. Maternal alcohol, tobacco and cannabis consumption and the outcome of pregnancy. Aust NZ J Obstet Gynaecol 1983;23:15–9.
2. Fried PA, Watkinson B, Grant A, Knights RM. Changing patterns of soft drug use prior to and during pregnancy: a prospective study. Drug Alcohol Depend 1980;6:323–43.
3. Fried PA. Marihuana use by pregnant women: neurobehavioral effects in neonates. Drug Alcohol Depend 1980;6:415–24.
4. Greenland S, Staisch KJ, Brown N, Gross SJ. The effects of marijuana use during pregnancy. I. A preliminary epidemiologic study. Am J Obstet Gynecol 1982;143:408–13.
5. Fried PA. Marihuana use by pregnant women and effects on offspring: an update. Neurobehav Toxicol Teratol 1982;4:451–4.
6. Rayburn W, Wible-Kant J, Bledsoe P. Changing trends in drug use during pregnancy. J Reprod Med 1982;27:569–75.
7. Greenland S, Richwald GA, Honda GD. The effects of marijuana use during pregnancy. II. A study in a low-risk home-delivery population. Drug Alcohol Depend 1983;11:359–66.
8. Fried PA, Buckingham M, Von Kulmiz P. Marijuana use during pregnancy and perinatal risk factors. Am J Obstet Gynecol 1983;146:992–4.
9. Linn S, Schoenbaum SC, Monson RR, Rosner R, Stubblefield PC, Ryan KJ. The association of marijuana use with outcome of pregnancy. Am J Public Health 1983;73:1161–4.

10. Fried PA, Watkinson B, Willan A. Marijuana use during pregnancy and decreased length of gestation. Am J Obstet Gynecol 1984;150:23–7.
11. Barr HM, Streissguth AP, Martin DC, Herman CS. Infant size at 8 months of age: relationship to maternal use of alcohol, nicotine, and caffeine during pregnancy. Pediatrics 1984;74:336–41.
12. Zuckerman BS, Hingson RW, Morelock S, Amaro H, Frank D, Sorenson JR, Kayne HL, Timperi R. A pilot study assessing maternal marijuana use by urine assay during pregnancy. Natl Inst Drug Abuse Res Monogr Ser 1985;57:84–93.
13. Fried PA. Postnatal consequences of maternal marijuana use. Natl Inst Drug Abuse Res Monogr Ser 1985;59:61–72.
14. Hatch EE, Bracken MB. Effect of marijuana use in pregnancy on fetal growth. Am J Epidemiol 1986;124:986–93.
15. Fried PA, Makin JE. Neonatal behavioural correlates of prenatal exposure to marihuana, cigarettes and alcohol in a low risk population. Neurotoxicol Teratol 1987;9:1–7.
16. Smith CG, Asch RH. Drug abuse and reproduction. Fertil Steril 1987;48:355–73.
17. Kline J, Stein Z, Hutzler M. Cigarettes, alcohol and marijuana: varying associations with birthweight. Int J Epidemiol 1987;16:44–51.
18. Day NL, Wagener DK, Taylor PM. Measurement of substance use during pregnancy: methodologic issues. Natl Inst Drug Abuse Res Monogr Ser 1985;59:36–47.
19. Hingson R, Zuckerman B, Amaro H, Frank DA, Kayne H, Sorenson JR, Mitchell J, Parker S, Morelock S, Timperi R. Maternal marijuana use and neonatal outcome: uncertainty posed by self-reports. Am J Public Health 1986;76:667–9.
20. Little RE, Uhl CN, Labbe RF, Abkowitz JL, Phillips ELR. Agreement between laboratory tests and self-reports of alcohol, tobacco, caffeine, marijuana and other drug use in post-partum women. Soc Sci Med 1986;22:91–8.
21. Fried PA, Barnes MV, Drake ER. Soft drug use after pregnancy compared to use before and during pregnancy. Am J Obstet Gynecol 1985;151:787–92.
22. Blackard C, Tennes K. Human placental transfer of cannabinoids. N Engl J Med 1984;311:797.
23. Busto U, Bendayan R, Sellers EM. Clinical pharmacokinetics of non-opiate abused drugs. Clin Pharmacokinet 1989;16:1–26.
24. Hingson R, Alpert JJ, Day N, Dooling E, Kayne H, Morelock S, Oppenheimer E, Zuckerman B. Effects of maternal drinking and marijuana use on fetal growth and development. Pediatrics 1982;70:539–46.
25. Zuckerman B, Frank DA, Hingson R, Amaro H, Levenson SM, Kayne H, Parker S, Vinci R, Aboagye K, Fried LE, Cabral H, Timperi R, Bauchner H. Effects of maternal marijuana and cocaine use on fetal growth. N Engl J Med 1989;320:762–8.
26. Tennes K, Avitable N, Blackard C, Boyles C, Hassoun B, Holmes L, Kreye M. Marijuana: prenatal and postnatal exposure in the human. Natl Inst Drug Abuse Res Monogr Ser 1985;59:48–60.
27. Greenland S, Staisch KJ, Brown N, Gross SJ. Effects of marijuana on human pregnancy, labor, and delivery. Neurobehav Toxicol Teratol 1982;4:447–50.
28. Braunstein GD, Buster JE, Soares JR, Gross SJ. Pregnancy hormone concentrations in marijuana users. Life Sci 1983;33:195–9.
29. Rosett HL, Weiner L, Lee A, Zuckerman B, Dooling E, Oppenheimer E. Patterns of alcohol consumption and fetal development. Obstet Gynecol 1983;61:539–46.
30. Zuckerman B, Alpert JJ, Dooling E, Oppenheimer E, Hingson R, Day N, Rosett H. Substance abuse during pregnancy and newborn size. Pediatr Res 1980;15:524.
31. Qazi QH, Mariano E, Milman DH, Beller E, Crombleholme W. Abnormalities in offspring associated with prenatal marihuana exposure. Dev Pharmacol Ther 1985;8:141–8.
32. Qazi QH, Mariano E, Beller E, Milman DH, Crombleholme W. Abnormalities in offspring associated with prenatal marihuana exposure. Pediatr Res 1983;17:153A.
33. Qazi QH, Milman DH. Nontherapeutic use of psychoactive drugs. N Engl J Med 1983;309:797–8.
34. Abel EL. Prenatal exposure to cannabis: a critical review of effects on growth, development, and behavior. Behav Neural Biol 1980;29:137–56.
35. VanBlerk GA, Majerus TC, Myers RAM. Teratogenic potential of some psychopharmacologic drugs: a brief review. Int J Gynaecol Obstet 1980;17:399–402.
36. Lee CC, Chiang CN. Maternal-fetal transfer of abused substances: pharmacokinetic and pharmacodynamic data. Natl Inst Drug Abuse Res Monogr Ser 1985;60:110–47.
37. Shepard TH. *Catalog of Teratogenic Agents*, 5th ed. Baltimore:Johns Hopkins University Press, 1986:353–6.
38. Rennert OM. Drug-induced somatic alterations. Clin Obstet Gynecol 1975;18:185–98.

39. Matsuyama S, Jarvik L. Effects of marihuana on the genetic and immune systems. Natl Inst Drug Abuse Res Monogr Ser 1977;14:179–93.
40. Nahas GG. Current status of marijuana research: symposium on marijuana held July 1978 in Reims, France. JAMA 1979;242:2775–8.
41. Glass L, Evans HE. Perinatal drug abuse. Pediatr Ann 1979;8:84–92.
42. Harclerode J. The effect of marijuana on reproduction and development. Natl Inst Drug Abuse Res Monogr Ser 1980;31:137–66.
43. Chernoff GF, Jones KL. Fetal preventive medicine: teratogens and the unborn baby. Pediatr Ann 1981;10:210–7.
44. Stern L. In vivo assessment of the teratogenic potential of drugs in humans. Obstet Gynecol 1981;58:3S–8S.
45. Shy KK, Brown ZA. Maternal and fetal well-being. West J Med 1984;141:807–15.
46. Tennes K. Effects of marijuana on pregnancy and fetal development in the human. Natl Inst Drug Abuse Res Monogr Ser 1984;44:115–23.
47. Mullins CL, Gazaway PM III. Alcohol and drug use in pregnancy: a case for management. Md Med J 1985;34:991–6.
48. Hollister LE. Health aspects of cannabis. Pharmacol Rev 1986;38:1–20.
49. O'Connor MC. Drugs of abuse in pregnancy—an overview. Med J Aust 1987;147:180–3.
50. Hecht F, Beals RK, Lees MH, Jolly H, Roberts P. Lysergic-acid-diethylamide and cannabis as possible teratogens in man. Lancet 1968;2:1087.
51. Carakushansky G, Neu RL, Gardner LI. Lysergide and cannabis as possible teratogens in man. Lancet 1969;1:150–1.
52. Blanc WA, Mattison DR, Kane R, Chauhan P. L.S.D., intrauterine amputations, and amniotic-band syndrome. Lancet 1971;2:158–9.
53. Gelehrter TD. Lysergic acid diethylamide (LSD) and exstrophy of the bladder. J Pediatr 1970;77:1065–6.
54. Hsu LY, Strauss L, Hirschorn K. Chromosome abnormality in offspring of LSD user. JAMA 1970;211:987–90.
55. Bogdanoff B, Rorke LB, Yanoff M, Warren WS. Brain and eye abnormalities. Am J Dis Child 1972;123:145–8.
56. Jacobson CB, Berlin CM. Possible reproductive detriment in LSD users. JAMA 1972;222:1367–73.
57. Brown R, Pickering D. Persistent transitional circulation. Arch Dis Child 1974;49:883–5.
58. Tenorio GM, Nazvi M, Bickers GH, Hubbird RH. Intrauterine stroke and maternal polydrug abuse. Clin Pediatr 1988;27:565–7.
59. Huff DS, Fernandes M. Two cases of congenital hypothalamic hamartoblastoma, polydactyly, and other congenital anomalies (Pallister-Hall syndrome). N Engl J Med 1982;306:430–1.
60. Lage JM, VanMarter LJ, Bieber FR. Questionable role of amniocentesis in the etiology of amniotic band formation. A case report. J Reprod Med 1988;33:71–3.
61. O'Connell CM, Fried PA. An investigation of prenatal cannabis exposure and minor physical anomalies in a low risk population. Neurobehav Toxicol Teratol 1984;6:345–50.
62. Nelson LB, Ehrlich S, Calhoun JH, Matteucci T, Finnegan LP. Occurrence of strabismus in infants born to drug-dependent women. Am J Dis Child 1987;141:175–8.
63. Coles CD, Smith IE, Fernhoff PM, Falek A. Neonatal ethanol withdrawal: characteristics in clinically normal, nondysmorphic neonates. J Pediatr 1984;105:445–51.
64. Robison LL, Buckley JD, Daigle AE, Wells R, Benjamin D, Arthur DC, Hammond GD. Maternal drug use and risk of childhood nonlymphoblastic leukemia among offspring: an epidemiologic investigation implicating marijuana (a report from the Childrens Cancer Study Group). Cancer 1989;63:1904–11.
65. Stenchever MA, Kunysz TJ, Allen MA. Chromosome breakage in users of marihuana. Am J Obstet Gynecol 1974;118:106–13.
66. Matsuyama SS, Jarvik LF. Cytogenetic effects of psychoactive drugs. Mod Probl Pharmacopsychiatry 1975;10:99–132.
67. Abel EL. Marihuana and sex: a critical survey. Drug Alcohol Depend 1981;8:1–22.
68. Nahas GG. Cannabis: toxicological properties and epidemiological aspects. Med J Aust 1986;145:82–7.
69. Perez-Reyes M, Wall ME. Presence of delta-9-tetrahydrocannabinol in human milk. N Engl J Med 1982;307:819–20.
70. Arena JM. Drugs and chemicals excreted in breast milk. Pediatr Ann 1980;9:452–7.

71. Committee on Drugs, American Academy of Pediatrics. Transfer of drugs and other chemicals into human milk. Pediatrics 1989;84:924–36.

Name: **MAZINDOL**

Class: **Central Stimulant/Anorectant**   Risk Factor: **C**

Fetal Risk Summary

No data are available.

Breast Feeding Summary

No data are available.

Name: **MEBANAZINE**

Class: **Antidepressant**   Risk Factor: **C**

Fetal Risk Summary

No data are available (see Phenelzine).

Breast Feeding Summary

No data are available (see Phenelzine).

Name: **MEBENDAZOLE**

Class: **Anthelmintic**   Risk Factor: **C$_M$**

Fetal Risk Summary

Mebendazole is a synthetic anthelmintic agent. Although an animal teratogen, no reports of human teratogenicity due to mebendazole have been located. One manufacturer has reports of mebendazole exposure in 170 pregnancies going to term without an identifiable teratogenic risk (1). An earlier manufacturer knew of only one malformation, a digital reduction of one hand, in 112 infants exposed *in utero* to the drug (2).

During a 1984 outbreak of trichinosis (*Trichinella spiralis*) in Lebanon, four pregnant patients were treated with mebendazole and corticosteroids (3). Two women, both in the 1st trimester, had miscarriages. The authors did not comment if this was due to the disease or the drug. Neither fetus was examined. The remaining two patients, both in the 3rd trimester, delivered healthy infants. In a separate case, a pregnant patient, also with trichinosis, was treated with mebendazole and delivered a normal infant (4). The period of pregnancy when the infection and treatment occurred was not specified.

A 1985 review of intestinal parasites and pregnancy concluded that treatment of the pregnant patient should only be considered if the "parasite is causing clinical disease or may cause public health problems" (5). When indicated, mebendazole was recommended for the treatment of *Trichuris trichiura* (whipworm) occurring during pregnancy (5). A 1986 review recommended mebendazole therapy, when indicated, for the treatment of *Ascaris lumbricoides* (roundworm) and *Enterobius vermicularis* (threadworm) (6).

Breast Feeding Summary

No data have been located on the passage of mebendazole into human milk. One nursing woman, in her 10th week of lactation, was treated with mebendazole (100 mg twice daily for 3 days) for a roundworm infection (7). Immediately prior to this she had been treated for 7 days with metronidazole for genital *Trichomonas vaginalis*. Milk production decreased markedly on the 2nd day of mebendazole therapy and stopped completely within 1 week. Although no mechanism was suggested, the author concluded that the halt in lactation was mebendazole-induced.

References

1. Product information. Vermox. Janssen Pharmaceutica, Inc., 1990.
2. Shepard TH. *Catalog of Teratogenic Agents*, 5th ed. Baltimore:Johns Hopkins University Press, 1986:911.
3. Blondheim DS, Klein R, Ben-Dror G, Schick G. Trichinosis in southern Lebanon. Isr J Med Sci 1984;20:141–4.
4. Draghici O, Vasadi T, Draghici G, Codrea A, Mihuta A, Dragan S, Biro S, Mocuja D, Mihuja S. Comments with reference to a trichinellosis focus. Rev Ig (Bacteriol) 1976;21:99–104.
5. D'Alauro F, Lee RV, Pao-In K, Khairallah M. Intestinal parasites and pregnancy. Obstet Gynecol 1985;66:639–43.
6. Ellis CJ. Antiparasitic agents in pregnancy. Clin Obstet Gynecol 1986;13:269–75.
7. Rao TS. Does mebendazole inhibit lactation? NZ Med J 1983;96:589–90.

Name: **MECHLORETHAMINE**

Class: **Antineoplastic**   Risk Factor: **D**

Fetal Risk Summary

Mechlorethamine is an alkylating antineoplastic agent. The drug has been used in pregnancy, usually in combination with other antineoplastic drugs. Most reports have not shown an adverse effect in the fetus even when mechlorethamine was given during the 1st trimester (1–5). Two malformed infants have resulted following 1st trimester use of mechlorethamine (6, 7):

Oligodactyly of both feet with webbing of third and fourth toes, four metatarsals on left, three on right, bowing of right tibia, cerebral hemorrhage (6)
Malformed kidneys—markedly reduced size and malpositioned (7)

Data from one review indicated that 40% of the infants exposed to anticancer drugs were of low birth weight (3). Long-term studies of growth and mental development in offspring exposed to mechlorethamine during the 2nd trimester, the period of neuroblast multiplication, have not been conducted (8).

Ovarian function has been evaluated in 27 women previously treated with mechlorethamine and other antineoplastic drugs (9). Excluding three patients who received pelvic radiation, 13 (54%) maintained regular cyclic menses and, overall, 13 normal children were born after therapy. Other successful pregnancies have been reported following combination chemotherapy with mechlorethamine (10–16). Ovarian failure is apparently often gradual in onset and is age related (9). Mechlorethamine therapy in males has been observed to produce testicular germinal cell depletion and azoospermia (14, 15, 17, 18).

Occupational exposure of the mother to antineoplastic agents during pregnancy may present a risk to the fetus. A position statement from the National Study Commission on Cytotoxic Exposure and a research article involving some antineoplastic agents are presented in the monograph for cyclophosphamide (see Cyclophosphamide).

Breast Feeding Summary

No data are available.

References

1. Hennessy JP, Rottino A. Hodgkin's disease in pregnancy with a report of twelve cases. Am J Obstet Gynecol 1952;63:756–64.
2. Riva HL, Andreson PS, O'Grady JW. Pregnancy and Hodgkin's disease: a report of eight cases. Am J Obstet Gynecol 1953;66:866–70.
3. Nicholson HO. Cytotoxic drugs in pregnancy: review of reported cases. J Obstet Gynaecol Br Commonw 1968;75:307–12.
4. Jones RT, Weinerman ER. MOPP (nitrogen mustard, vincristine, procarbazine, and prednisone) given during pregnancy. Obstet Gynecol 1979;54:477–8.
5. Johnson IR, Filshie GM. Hodgkin's disease diagnosed in pregnancy: case report. Br J Obstet Gynaecol 1977;84:791–2.
6. Garrett MJ. Teratogenic effects of combination chemotherapy. Ann Intern Med 1974;80:667.
7. Mennuti MT, Shepard TH, Mellman WJ. Fetal renal malformation following treatment of Hodgkin's disease during pregnancy. Obstet Gynecol 1975;46:194–6.
8. Dobbing J. Pregnancy and leukaemia. Lancet 1977;1:1155.
9. Schilsky RL, Sherins RJ, Hubbard SM, Wesley MN, Young RC, DeVita VT Jr. Long-term follow-up of ovarian function in women treated with MOPP chemotherapy for Hodgkin's disease. Am J Med 1981;71:552–6.
10. Ross GT. Congenital anomalies among children born of mothers receiving chemotherapy for gestational trophoblastic neoplasms. Cancer 1976;37:1043–7.
11. Johnson SA, Goldman JM, Hawkins DF. Pregnancy after chemotherapy for Hodgkin's disease. Lancet 1979;2:93.
12. Whitehead E, Shalet SM, Blackledge G, Todd I, Crowther D, Beardwell CG. The effect of combination chemotherapy on ovarian function in women treated for Hodgkin's disease. Cancer 1983;52:988–993.
13. Andrieu JM, Ochoa-Molina ME. Menstrual cycle, pregnancies and offspring before and after MOPP therapy for Hodgkin's disease. Cancer 1983;52:435–8.
14. Dein RA, Mennuti MT, Kovach P, Gabbe SG. The reproductive potential of young men and women with Hodgkin's disease. Obstet Gynecol Surv 1984;39:474–82.
15. Schilsky RL, Lewis BJ, Sherins RJ, Young RC. Gonadal dysfunction in patients receiving chemotherapy for cancer. Ann Intern Med 1980;93:109–14.
16. Shalet SM, Vaughan Williams CA, Whitehead E. Pregnancy after chemotherapy induced ovarian failure. Br Med J 1985;290:898.
17. Sherins RJ, Olweny CLM, Ziegler JL. Gynecomastia and gonadal dysfunction in adolescent boys treated with combination chemotherapy for Hodgkin's disease. N Engl J Med 1978;299:12–6.
18. Sherins RJ, DeVita VT Jr. Effect of drug treatment for lymphoma on male reproductive capacity: studies of men in remission after therapy. Ann Intern Med 1973;79:216–20.

Name: **MECLIZINE**

Class: **Antihistamine/Antiemetic**   Risk Factor: **B**$_M$

Fetal Risk Summary

Meclizine is a piperazine antihistamine that is frequently used as an antiemetic (see also Buclizine and Cyclizine). The drug is teratogenic in animals but apparently not in humans. Since late 1962, the question of meclizine's effect on the fetus has been argued in numerous citations, the bulk of which are case reports and letters (1–27). Three studies involving large numbers of patients have concluded that meclizine is not a human teratogen (28–30).

The Collaborative Perinatal Project (CPP) monitored 50,282 mother-child pairs, 1,014 of which had exposure to meclizine in the 1st trimester (28, p. 328). For use anytime during pregnancy, 1,463 exposures were recorded (28, p. 437). In neither case was evidence found to suggest a relationship to large categories of major or minor malformations. Several possible associations with individual malformations were found, but their statistical significance is unknown (28, pp. 328, 437, 475). Independent confirmation is required to determine the actual risk.

Respiratory defects (7 cases)
Eye and ear defects (7 cases)
Inguinal hernia (18 cases)
Hypoplasia cordis (3 cases)
Hypoplastic left heart syndrome (3 cases)

The CPP study indicated a possible relationship to ocular malformations, but the authors warned that the results must be interpreted with extreme caution (31). The Food and Drug Administration's Over-the-counter Laxative Panel, acting on the data from the CPP study, concluded that meclizine was not teratogenic (32). A second large prospective study covering 613 1st trimester exposures supported these negative findings (29). No harmful effects were found in the exposed offspring as compared to the total sample. Finally, in a 1971 report, significantly fewer infants with malformations were exposed to antiemetics in the 1st trimester as compared to controls (30). Meclizine was the third most commonly used antiemetic.

An association between exposure during the last 2 weeks of pregnancy to antihistamines in general and retrolental fibroplasia in premature infants has been reported. See Brompheniramine for details.

Breast Feeding Summary

No data are available.

References

1. Watson GI. Meclozine ("Ancoloxin") and foetal abnormalities. Br Med J 1962;2:1446.
2. Smithells RW. "Ancoloxin" and foetal abnormalities. Br Med J 1962;2:1539.
3. Diggorg PLC, Tomkinson JS. Meclozine and foetal abnormalities. Lancet 1962;2:1222.
4. Carter MP, Wilson FW. "Ancoloxin" and foetal abnormalities. Br Med J 1962;2:1609.
5. Macleod M. "Ancoloxin" and foetal abnormalities. Br Med J 1962;2:1609.
6. Lask S. "Ancoloxin" and foetal abnormalities. Br Med J 1962;2:1609.
7. Leck IM. "Ancoloxin" and foetal abnormalities. Br Med J 1962;2:1610.
8. McBride WG. Drugs and foetal abnormalities. Br Med J 1962;2:1681.

9. Fagg CG. "Ancoloxin" and foetal abnormalities. Br Med J 1962;2:1681.
10. Barwell TE. "Ancoloxin" and foetal abnormalities. Br Med J 1962;2:1681–2.
11. Woodall J. "Ancoloxin" and foetal abnormalities. Br Med J 1962;2:1682.
12. McBride WG. Drugs and congenital abnormalities. Lancet 1962;2:1332.
13. Lenz W. Drugs and congenital abnormalities. Lancet 1962;2:1332–3.
14. David A, Goodspeed AH. "Ancoloxin" and foetal abnormalities. Br Med J 1963;1:121.
15. Gallagher C. "Ancoloxin" and foetal abnormalities. Br Med J 1963;1:121–2.
16. Watson GI. "Ancoloxin" and foetal abnormalities. Br Med J 1963;1:122.
17. Mellin GW, Katzenstein M. Meclozine and foetal abnormalities. Lancet 1963;1:222–3.
18. Salzmann KD. "Ancoloxin" and foetal abnormalities. Br Med J 1963;1:471.
19. Burry AF. Meclozine and foetal abnormalities. Br Med J 1963;1:1476.
20. Smithells RW, Chinn ER. Meclozine and feotal abnormalities. Br Med J 1963;1:1678.
21. O'Leary JL, O'Leary JA. Nonthalidomide ectromelia. Report of a case study. Obstet Gynecol 1964;23:17–20.
22. Smithells RW, Chinn ER. Meclozine and foetal malformations: a prospective study. Br Med J 1964;1:217–8.
23. Pettersson F. Meclozine and congenital malformations. Lancet 1964;1:675.
24. Yerushalmy J, Milkovich L. Evaluation of the teratogenic effect of meclizine in man. Am J Obstet Gynecol 1965;93:553–62.
25. Sadusk JF Jr, Palmisano PA. Teratogenic effect of meclizine, cyclizine, and chlorcyclizine. JAMA 1965;194:987–9.
26. Lenz W. Malformations caused by drugs in pregnancy. Am J Dis Child 1966;112:99–106.
27. Lenz W. How can the teratogenic action of a factor be established in man? South Med J 1971;64(Suppl 1):41–7.
28. Heinonen OP, Slone D, Shapiro S. Birth Defects and Drugs in Pregnancy. Littleton:Publishing Sciences Group, 1977.
29. Milkovich L, Van den Berg BJ. An evaluation of the teratogenicity of certain antinauseant drugs. Am J Obstet Gynecol 1976;125:244–8.
30. Nelson MM, Forfar JO. Associations between drugs administered during pregnancy and congenital abnormalities of the fetus. Br Med J 1971;1:523–7.
31. Shapiro S, Kaufman DW, Rosenberg L, Slone D, Monson RR, Siskind V, Heinonen OP. Meclizine in pregnancy in relation to congenital malformations. Br Med J 1978;1:483.
32. Anonymous. Pink Sheets. Meclizine, cyclizine not teratogenic. FDC Rep 1974;2.

Name: **MECLOFENAMATE**

Class: **Nonsteroidal Anti-inflammatory** Risk Factor: **B***

Fetal Risk Summary

No reports linking the use of meclofenamate with congenital defects have been located. Theoretically, meclofenamate, a prostaglandin synthetase inhibitor, could cause constriction of the ductus arteriosus *in utero* (1). Persistent pulmonary hypertension of the newborn should also be considered (2). Drugs in this class have been shown to inhibit labor and prolong pregnancy (2).

[*Risk Factor D if used in the 3rd trimester.]

Breast Feeding Summary

No data are available.

References

1. Levin DL. Effects of inhibition of prostaglandin synthesis on fetal development, oxygenation, and the fetal circulation. Semin Perinatol 1980;4:35–44.

2. Fuchs F. Prevention of prematurity. Am J Obstet Gynecol 1976;126:809–20.

Name: **MEDROXYPROGESTERONE**

Class: **Progestogenic Hormone**   Risk Factor: **D**

Fetal Risk Summary

The Food and Drug Administration mandated deletion of pregnancy-related indications from all progestins because of a possible association with congenital anomalies. Fourteen cases of ambiguous genitalia of the fetus have been reported to the FDA, although the literature is more supportive of the 19-nortestosterone derivatives (see Norethindrone, Norethynodrel) (1). The Collaborative Perinatal Project monitored 866 mother-child pairs with 1st trimester exposure to progestational agents, including 130 with exposure to medroxyprogesterone (2, p. 389). An increase in the expected frequency of cardiovascular defects and hypospadias was observed for the progestational agents as a group (2, p. 394). The cardiovascular defects included a ventricular septal defect and tricuspid atresia (3). Re-evaluation of these data in terms of timing of exposure, vaginal bleeding in early pregnancy, and previous maternal obstetric history, however, failed to support an association between female sex hormones and cardiac malformations (4). Other studies have also failed to find any relationship with nongenital malformations (5, 6).

A 1985 study described 2754 infants born to mothers who had vaginal bleeding during the 1st trimester (7). Of the total group, 1608 of the newborns were delivered from mothers treated during the 1st trimester with either oral medroxyprogesterone (20–30 mg/day), 17-hydroxyprogesterone (500 mg/week by injection), or a combination of the two. Medroxyprogesterone was used exclusively in 1274 (79.2%) of the study group. The control group consisted of 1146 infants delivered from mothers who bled during the 1st trimester but who were not treated. There were no differences between the study and control groups in the overall rate of malformations (120 vs. 123.9/1000, respectively) or in the rate of major malformations (63.4 vs. 71.5/1000, respectively). Another 1985 study compared 988 infants exposed *in utero* to various progesterones to a matched cohort of 1976 unexposed controls (8). Only 60 infants were exposed to medroxyprogesterone. No association between progestins, primarily progesterone and 17-hydroxyprogesterone, and fetal malformations was discovered.

Breast Feeding Summary

Medroxyprogesterone has not been shown to affect lactation adversely (9, 10). A 1981 review concluded that use of the drug by the mother would not have a significant effect on the nursing infant (11). Milk production and duration of lactation may be increased if the drug is given in the puerperium. If breast feeding is desired, medroxyprogesterone may be used safely. The American Academy of Pediatrics considers medroxyprogesterone to be compatible with breast feeding (12).

References

1. Dayan E, Rosa FW. Fetal ambiguous genitalia associated with sex hormones use early in pregnancy. Food and Drug Administration, Division of Drug Experience. ADR Highlights 1981:1–14.
2. Heinonen OP, Slone D, Shapiro S. *Birth Defects and Drugs in Pregnancy.* Littleton:Publishing Sciences Group, 1977.
3. Heinonen OP, Slone D, Monson RR, Hook EB, Shapiro S. Cardiovascular birth defects and antenatal exposure to female sex hormones. N Engl J Med 1977;296:67–70.
4. Wiseman RA, Dodds-Smith IC. Cardiovascular birth defects and antenatal exposure to female sex hormones: a reevaluation of some base data. Teratology 1984;30:359–70.
5. Wilson JG, Brent RL. Are female sex hormones teratogenic? Am J Obstet Gynecol 1981;141:567–80.
6. Dahlberg K. Some effects of depo-medroxyprogesterone acetate (DMPA): observations in the nursing infant and in the long-term user. Int J Gynaecol Obstet 1982;20:43–8.
7. Katz Z, Lancet M, Skornik J, Chemke J, Mogilner BM, Klinberg M. Teratogenicity of progestogens given during the first trimester of pregnancy. Obstet Gynecol 1985;65:775–80.
8. Resseguie LJ, Hick JF, Bruen JA, Noller KL, O'Fallon WM, Kurland LT. Congenital malformations among offspring exposed *in utero* to progestins, Olmsted County, Minnesota, 1936–74. Fertil Steril 1985;43:514–9.
9. Guiloff E, Ibarra-Polo A, Zanartu J, Toscanini C, Mischler TW, Gomez-Rogers C. Effect of contraception on lactation. Am J Obstet Gynecol 1974;118:42–5.
10. Karim M, Ammar R, El Mahgoub S, El Ganzoury B, Fikri F, Abdou Z. Injected progesterone and lactation. Br Med J 1971;1:200–3.
11. Schwallie PC. The effect of depot-medroxyprogesterone acetate on the fetus and nursing infant: a review. Contraception 1981;23:375–86.
12. Committee on Drugs, American Academy of Pediatrics. Transfer of drugs and other chemicals into human milk. Pediatrics 1989;84:924–36.

Name: **MELPHALAN**

Class: **Antineoplastic**   Risk Factor: **D$_M$**

Fetal Risk Summary

No reports linking the use of melphalan with congenital defects have been located. Melphalan is mutagenic as well as carcinogenic (1–8). These effects have not been described in infants following *in utero* exposure. Although there are no supportive data to suggest a teratogenic effect, melphalan is structurally similar to other alkylating agents that have produced defects (see Chlorambucil, Mechlorethamine, Cyclophosphamide).

Data from one review indicated that 40% of the infants exposed to anticancer drugs were of low birth weight (9). Long-term studies of growth and mental development in offspring exposed to melphalan and other antineoplastic drugs during the 2nd trimester, the period of neuroblast multiplication, have not been conducted (10).

Melphalan has caused suppression of ovarian function resulting in amenorrhea (10–13). These effects should be considered prior to administering the drug to patients in their reproductive years. However, in 436 long-term survivors treated with chemotherapy between 1958–1978 for gestational trophoblastic tumors, 15 received melphalan as part of their treatment regimens (14). Three of these women had at least one live birth (mean melphalan dose 18 mg; maximum dose

24 mg), and the remaining 12 did not attempt to conceive. Complete details of this study are discussed in the monograph for methotrexate (see Methotrexate).

Occupational exposure of the mother to antineoplastic agents during pregnancy may present a risk to the fetus. A position statement from the National Study Commission on Cytotoxic Exposure and a research article on some antineoplastic agents are presented in the monograph for cyclophosphamide (see Cyclophosphamide).

Breast Feeding Summary

No data are available.

References

1. Sharpe HB. Observations on the effect of therapy with nitrogen mustard or a derivative on chromosomes of human peripheral blood lymphocytes. Cell Tissue Kinet 1971;4:501–4.
2. Kyle RA, Pierre RV, Bayrd ED. Multiple myeloma and acute myelomonocytic leukemia. N Engl J Med 1970;283:1121–5.
3. Kyle RA. Primary amyloidosis in acute leukemia associated with melphalan. Blood 1974;44:333–7.
4. Burton IE, Abbott CR, Roberts BE, Antonis AH. Acute leukemia after four years of melphalan treatment for melanoma. Br Med J 1976;1:20.
5. Peterson HS. Erythroleukemia in a melphalan treated patient with primary macroglobulinaemia. Scand J Haematol 1973;10:5–11.
6. Stavem P, Harboe M. Acute erythroleukaemia in a patient treated with melphalan for the cold agglutinin syndrome. Scand J Haematol 1971;8:375–9.
7. Einhorn N. Acute leukemia after chemotherapy (melphalan). Cancer 1978;41:444–7.
8. Reimer RR, Hover R, Fraumen JF, Young RC. Acute leukemia after alkylating agent therapy of ovarian cancer. N Engl J Med 1977;297:177–81.
9. Nicholson HO. Cytotoxic drugs in pregnancy: review of reported cases. J Obstet Gynaecol Br Commonw 1968;75:307–12.
10. Dobbing J. Pregnancy and leukaemia. Lancet 1977;1:11–15.
11. Rose DP, David PE. Ovarian function in patients receiving adjuvant chemotherapy for breast cancer. Lancet 1977;1:1174–6.
12. Ahmann DL. Repeated adjuvant chemotherapy with phenylalanine mustard or 5-fluorouracil, cyclophosphamide and prednisone with or without radiation. Lancet 1978;1:893–6.
13. Schilsky RL, Lewis BJ, Sherins RJ, Young RC. Gonadal dysfunction in patients receiving chemotherapy for cancer. Ann Intern Med 1980;93:109–14.
14. Rustin GJS, Booth M, Dent J, Salt S, Rustin F, Bagshawe KD. Pregnancy after cytotoxic chemotherapy for gestational trophoblastic tumours. Br Med J 1984;288:103–6.

Name: **MENADIONE**

Class: **Vitamin**   Risk Factor: **C*$_M$**

Fetal Risk Summary

Menadione (vitamin K_3) is a synthetic, fat-soluble form of vitamin K used to prevent hypoprothombinemia due to vitamin K deficiency (1). The water-soluble derivative of menadione, menadiol sodium phosphate, also known as vitamin K_3, is available for parenteral use.

Vitamin K_1 occurs naturally in a variety of foods and is synthesized by the normal intestinal flora (see Phytonadione) (1). Administration of vitamin K during pregnancy is usually not required unless the mother develops hypoprothrombinemia or is taking certain drugs that may produce severe vitamin K deficiency in the fetus resulting in hemorrhagic disease of the newborn (e.g., anticonvulsants, warfarin, rifampin, isoniazid). Early attempts to prevent maternal-induced hemorrhagic disease of the newborn by administering vitamin K_3 to the mother shortly before delivery often resulted in marked hyperbilirubinemia and kernicterus in the newborn, especially in premature infants (2–5). Several large reviews have described the relationship between vitamin K and bilirubin and have discussed the toxicity of the vitamin K analogues (2–5). Because menadione and menadiol may produce newborn toxicity, phytonadione is considered the drug of choice for administration during pregnancy or to the newborn (6, 7).

[*Risk Factor X if used in 3rd trimester or close to delivery.]

Breast Feeding Summary

See Phytonadione.

References

1. American Hospital Formulary Service. *Drug Information 1990*. Bethesda:American Society of Hospital Pharmacists, 1990:2135–6.
2. Lane PA, Hathaway WE. Vitamin K in infancy. J Pediatr 1985;106:351–9.
3. Payne NR, Hasegawa DK. Vitamin K deficiency in newborns: a case report in α-1-antitrypsin deficiency and a review of factors predisposing to hemorrhage. Pediatrics 1984;73:712–6.
4. Wynn RM. The obstetric significance of factors affecting the metabolism of bilirubin, with particular reference to the role of vitamin K. Obstet Gynecol Surv 1963;18:333–54.
5. Finkel MJ. Vitamin K_1 and the vitamin K analogues. J Clin Pharmacol Therap 1961;2:795–814.
6. Committee on Nutrition, American Academy of Pediatrics. Vitamin K compounds and the water-soluble analogues. Pediatrics 1961;28:501–7.
7. Committee on Nutrition, American Academy of Pediatrics. Vitamin and mineral supplement needs in normal children in the United States. Pediatrics 1980;66:1015–21.

Name: **MEPENZOLATE**

Class: **Parasympatholytic (Anticholinergic)**   Risk Factor: **C**

Fetal Risk Summary

Mepenzolate is an anticholinergic quaternary ammonium bromide. In a large prospective study, 2323 patients were exposed to this class of drugs during the 1st trimester, 1 of whom took mepenzolate (1). A possible association was found between the total group and minor malformations.

Breast Feeding Summary

No data are available (see also Atropine).

Reference

1. Heinonen OP, Slone D, Shapiro S. *Birth Defects and Drugs in Pregnancy*. Littleton:Publishing Sciences Group, 1977:346–53.

Name: **MEPERIDINE**
Class: **Narcotic Analgesic**   Risk Factor: **B***

Fetal Risk Summary

Fetal problems have not been reported from the therapeutic use of meperidine in pregnancy except when it has been given during labor. Like all narcotics, maternal and neonatal addiction are possible from inappropriate use. Neonatal depression, at times fatal, has historically been the primary concern following obstetric meperidine analgesia. Controversy has now arisen over the potential long-term adverse effects resulting from this use.

Meperidine's placental transfer is very rapid, appearing in cord blood within 2 minutes following intravenous administration (1). It is detectable in amniotic fluid 30 minutes after intramuscular (IM) injection (2). Cord blood concentrations average 70–77% (range 45–106%) of maternal plasma levels (3, 4). The drug has been detected in the saliva of newborns for 48 hours following maternal administration during labor (5). Concentrations in pharyngeal aspirates were higher than in either arterial or venous cord blood.

Respiratory depression in the newborn following use of the drug in labor is time and dose dependent. The incidence of depression increases markedly if delivery occurs 60 minutes or longer after injection, reaching a peak around 2–3 hours (6, 7). Whether this depression is due to metabolites of meperidine (e.g., normeperidine) or the drug itself is currently not known (2, 8–10). However, recent work suggests that these effects are related to unmetabolized meperidine and not to normeperidine (7).

Impaired behavioral response and EEG changes persisting for several days have been observed (11, 12). These persistent effects may be partially explained by the slow elimination of meperidine and normeperidine from the neonate over several days (13, 14). One group of investigators related depressed attention and social responsiveness during the first 6 weeks of life to high cord blood levels of meperidine (15). An earlier study reported long-term follow-up of 70 healthy neonates born to mothers who had received meperidine within 2 hours of birth (16, 17). Psychologic and physical parameters at age 5 years were similar in both exposed and control groups. Academic progress and behavior during the 3rd and 4th years in school were also similar.

The Collaborative Perinatal Project monitored 50,282 mother-child pairs, 268 of which had 1st trimester exposure to meperidine (18, pp. 287–295). For use anytime during pregnancy, 1,100 exposures were recorded (18, p. 434). No evidence was found to suggest a relationship to large categories of major or minor malformations. A possible association between the use of meperidine in the 1st trimester and inguinal hernia was found based on six cases (18, p. 471). The statistical significance of this association is unknown and independent confirmation is required.

[*Risk Factor D if used for prolonged periods or in high doses at term.]

Breast Feeding Summary

Meperidine is excreted into breast milk (19, 20). In a group of mothers who had received meperidine during labor, the breast-fed infants had higher saliva levels of the drug for up to 48 hours after birth than a similar group that was bottle-fed (5). In nine nursing mothers, a single 50-mg IM dose produced peak levels of 0.13 µg/ml at 2 hours (20). After 24 hours, the concentrations decreased to 0.02 µg/ml. Average milk:plasma ratios for the nine patients were greater than 1.0. No adverse effects in nursing infants were reported in any of the above studies. In their 1983 statement on drugs in breast milk, the American Academy of Pediatrics classified meperidine as compatible with breast feeding (21). However, the drug was not mentioned in the 1989 revision of their statment.

References

1. Crawford JS, Rudofsky S. The placental transmission of pethidine. Br J Anaesth 1965;37:929–33.
2. Szeto HH, Zervoudakis IA, Cederquist LL, Inturrise CE. Amniotic fluid transfer of meperidine from maternal plasma in early pregnancy. Obstet Gynecol 1978;52:59–62.
3. Apgar V, Burns JJ, Brodie BB, Papper EM. The transmission of meperidine across the human placenta. Am J Obstet Gynecol 1952;64:1368–70.
4. Shnider SM, Way EL, Lord MJ. Rate of appearance and disappearance of meperidine in fetal blood after administration of narcotic to the mother. Anesthesiology 1966;27:227–8.
5. Freeborn SF, Calvert RT, Black P, MacFarlane T, D'Souza SW. Saliva and blood pethidine concentrations in the mother and the newborn baby. Br J Obstet Gynaecol 1980;87:966–9.
6. Morrison JC, Wiser WL, Rosser SI, et al. Metabolites of meperidine related to fetal depression. Am J Obstet Gynecol 1973;115:1132–7.
7. Belfrage P, Boreus LO, Hartvig P, Irestedt L, Raabe N. Neonatal depression after obstetrical analgesia with pethidine. The role of the injection-delivery time interval and the plasma concentrations of pethidine and norpethidine. Acta Obstet Gynecol Scand 1981;60:43–9.
8. Morrison JC, Whybrew WD, Rosser SI, Bucovaz ET, Wiser WL, Fish SA. Metabolites of meperidine in the fetal and maternal serum. Am J Obstet Gynecol 1976;126:97–1002.
9. Clark RB, Lattin DL. Metabolites of meperidine in serum. Am J Obstet Gynecol 1978;130:113–5.
10. Morrison JC. Reply to Drs. Clark and Lattin. Am J Obstet Gynecol 1978;130:115–7.
11. Borgstedt AD, Rosen MG. Medication during labor correlated with behavior and EEG of the newborn. Am J Dis Child 1968;115:21–4.
12. Hodgkinson R, Bhatt M, Wang CN. Double-blind comparison of the neurobehaviour of neonates following the administration of different doses of meperidine to the mother. Can Anaesth Soc J 1978;25:405–11.
13. Cooper LV, Stephen GW, Aggett PJA. Elimination of pethidine and bupivacaine in the newborn. Arch Dis Child 1977;52:638–41.
14. Kuhnert BR, Kuhnert PM, Prochaska AL, Sokol RJ. Meperidine disposition in mother, neonate and nonpregnant females. Clin Pharmacol Ther 1980;27:486–91.
15. Belsey EM, Rosenblatt DB, Lieberman BA, et al. The influence of maternal analgesia on neonatal behaviour. I. Pethidine. Br J Obstet Gynaecol 1981;88:398–406.
16. Buck C, Gregg R, Stavraky K, Subrahmaniam K, Brown J. The effect of single prenatal and natal complications upon the development of children of mature birthweight. Pediatrics 1969;43:942–55.
17. Buck C. Drugs in pregnancy. Can Med Assoc J 1975;112:1285.
18. Heinonen O, Slone D, Shapiro S. *Birth Defects and Drugs in Pregnancy*. Littleton:Publishing Sciences Group, 1977.
19. Vorherr H. Drug excretion in breast milk. Postgrad Med 1974;56:97–104.
20. Peiker G, Muller B, Ihn W, Noschel H. Excretion of pethidine in mother's milk. Zentralbl Gynaekol 1980;102:537–41.
21. Committee on Drugs, American Academy of Pediatrics. The transfer of drugs and other chemicals into human breast milk. Pediatrics 1983;72:375–83.

Name: **MEPHENTERMINE**

Class: **Sympathomimetic (Adrenergic)**   Risk Factor: **C**

Fetal Risk Summary

Mephentermine is a sympathomimetic used in emergency situations to treat hypotension. Because of the nature of its indication, experience in pregnancy with mephentermine is limited. Mephentermine's primary action is to increase cardiac output due to enhanced cardiac contraction and, to a lesser extent, from peripheral vasoconstriction (1). Its effect on uterine blood flow should be minimal (1).

A newborn infant with complete exstrophy of the bladder, epispadias, widely separated pubic rami, and bilateral inguinal hernias was described in a 1970 publication (2). The infant's mother, a 19-year-old woman, had used lysergic acid diethylamide (LSD) on at least 12–15 occasions during the 2 months prior to conception and during the first 2.5 months of pregnancy. In addition, she had smoked marijuana twice and had ingested mephentermine sulfate once during the above interval. The etiology of the defects observed in the infant is unknown.

Breast Feeding Summary

No data are available.

References

1. Smith NT, Corbascio AN. The use and misuse of pressor agents. Anesthesiology 1970;33:58–101.
2. Gelehrter TD. Lysergic acid diethylamide (LSD) and exstrophy of the bladder. J Pediatr 1970;77:1065–6.

Name: **MEPHENYTOIN**

Class: **Anticonvulsant**   Risk Factor: **C**

Fetal Risk Summary

Mephenytoin is a hydantoin anticonvulsant similar to phenytoin (see Phenytoin). The drug is infrequently prescribed because of the greater incidence of serious side effects as compared with phenytoin (1). There have been reports of 12 infants with 1st trimester exposure to mephenytoin (2–5). No evidence of adverse fetal effects was found.

Breast Feeding Summary

No data are available.

References

1. Rall TW, Shleifer LS. Drugs effective in the treatment of the epilepsies. In Goodman AG, Goodman LS, Gilman A, eds. *The Pharmacological Basis of Therapeutics*, ed. 6. New York:Macmillan Publishing, 1980:456.
2. Fedrick J. Epilepsy and pregnancy: a report from the Oxford Linkage Study. Br Med J 1973;2:442–8.

3. Heinonen O, Slone D, Shapiro S. *Birth Defects and Drugs in Pregnancy*. Littleton:Publishing Sciences Group, 1977:358–9.
4. Annegers JF, Elveback LR, Hauser WA, Kurland LT. Do anticonvulsants have a teratogenic effect? Arch Neurol 1974;31:364–73.
5. Speidel BD, Meadow SR. Maternal epilepsy and abnormalities of the fetus and newborn. Lancet 1972;2:839–43.

Name: **MEPHOBARBITAL**

Class: **Anticonvulsant/Sedative** Risk Factor: **D**

Fetal Risk Summary

No reports linking the use of mephobarbital with congenital defects have been located. The drug is demethylated by the liver to phenobarbital (see Phenobarbital). The Collaborative Perinatal Project monitored 50,282 mother-child pairs, eight of which had 1st trimester exposure to mephobarbital (1). No evidence was found to suggest a relationship to large categories of major or minor malformations or to individual defects. Hemorrhagic disease and barbiturate withdrawal in the newborn are theoretically possible, although they have not been reported with mephobarbital.

Breast Feeding Summary

See Phenobarbital.

Reference

1. Heinonen O, Slone D, Shapiro S. *Birth Defects and Drugs in Pregnancy*. Littleton:Publishing Sciences Group, 1977:336.

Name: **MEPINDOLOL**

Class: **Sympatholytic (β-Adrenergic Blocker)** Risk Factor: **C**

Fetal Risk Summary

Mepindolol is a nonselective β-adrenergic blocking agent. No reports of its use in pregnancy have been located. The use near delivery of some agents in this class has resulted in persistent β-blockade in the newborn (see Acebutolol, Atenolol, and Nadolol). Thus, newborns exposed *in utero* to mepindolol should be closely observed during the first 24–48 hours after birth for bradycardia and other symptoms. The long-term effects of *in utero* exposure to β-blockers have not been studied but warrant evaluation.

Breast Feeding Summary

Mepindolol is excreted into breast milk (1). Following a 20-mg dose, mean milk concentrations in five mothers at 2 and 6 hours were 18 and 16 ng/ml, respectively, with a milk:plasma ratio at 2 hours of 0.35. Continuous dosing of 20 mg daily for 5 days produced milk levels at 2 and 6 hours of 22 and 33 ng/ml. The milk:plasma ratio at 6 hours was 0.61. At a detection limit of 1 ng/ml, mepindolol could be found in the serum of only one of the five breast-fed infants. Although no adverse effects were observed, nursing infants should be closely watched for bradycardia and other signs and symptoms of β-blockade. Long-term effects of exposure to β-blockers from milk have not been studied but warrant evaluation.

Reference

1. Krause W, Stoppelli I, Milia S, Rainer E. Transfer of mepindolol to newborns by breast-feeding mothers after single and repeated daily doses. Eur J Clin Pharmacol 1982;22:53–5.

Name: **MEPROBAMATE**

Class: **Sedative**   Risk Factor: **D**

Fetal Risk Summary

Meprobamate use in pregnancy has been associated with an increased risk of congenital anomalies (1.9–12.1%) (1, 2). In one study of 395 patients, eight defects were observed (1):

Congenital heart disease (two with multiple other defects) (five cases)
Down's syndrome (one case)
Deafness (partial) (one case)
Deformed elbows and joints (one case)

One other report described congenital heart defects in a newborn exposed to meprobamate (3). The mother of this patient was treated very early in the 1st trimester with meprobamate and propoxyphene:

Omphalocele, defective anterior abdominal wall, defect in diaphragm, congenital heart disease with partial ectopic cordis secondary to sternal cleft, dysplastic hips

Multiple defects of the eye and central nervous system were observed in a newborn exposed to multiple drugs, including meprobamate and LSD (4).

The Collaborative Perinatal Project monitored 50,282 mother-child pairs, 356 of which were exposed in the 1st trimester to meprobamate (5, 6). No association of meprobamate with large classes of malformations or to individual defects was found. Others have also failed to find a relationship between the use of meprobamate and congenital malformations (7).

Since few indications exist for this drug in the pregnant woman, it should be used with extreme caution, if at all, during pregnancy. Use during the first 6 weeks of pregnancy may be correlated with an increased risk for fetal malformations.

Breast Feeding Summary

Meprobamate is excreted into breast milk (8). Milk concentrations are 2–4 times that of maternal plasma (8, 9). The effect on the nursing infant is not known.

References

1. Milkovich L, van den Berg BJ. Effects of prenatal meprobamate and chlordiazepoxide hydrochloride on human embryonic and fetal development. N Engl J Med 1974;291:1268–71.
2. Crombie DL, Pinsent RJ, Fleming DM, Rumeau-Rouguette C, Goujard J, Huel G. Fetal effects of tranquilizers in pregnancy. N Engl J Med 1975;293:198–9.
3. Ringrose CAD. The hazard of neurotropic drugs in the fertile years. Can Med Assoc J 1972;106:1058.
4. Bogdanoff B, Rorke LB, Yanoff M, Warren WS. Brain and eye abnormalities: possible sequelae to prenatal use of multiple drugs including LSD. Am J Dis Child 1972;123:145–8.
5. Heinonen OP, Slone D, Shapiro S. *Birth Defects and Drugs in Pregnancy*. Littleton:Publishing Sciences Group, 1977:336–7.
6. Hartz SC, Heinonen OP, Shapiro S, Siskind V, Slone D. Antenatal exposure to meprobamate and chlordiazepoxide in relation to malformations, mental development, and childhood mortality. N Engl J Med 1975;292:726–8.
7. Belafsky HA, Breslow S, Hirsch LM, Shangold JE, Stahl MB. Meprobamate during pregnancy. Obstet Gynecol 1969;34:378–86.
8. Product information. Miltown. Wallace, 1985.
9. Wilson JT, Brown RD, Cherek DR, Dailey JW, Hilman B, Jobe PC, Manno BR, Manno JE, Redetzki HM, Stewart JJ. Drug excretion in human breast milk: principles, pharmacokinetics and projected consequences. Clin Pharmacokinet 1980;5:1–66.

Name: **MERCAPTOPURINE**

Class: **Antineoplastic** Risk Factor: **D**

Fetal Risk Summary

Mercaptopurine (6-MP) is an antimetabolite antineoplastic agent. References citing the use of mercaptopurine in 79 human pregnancies have been located, including 34 cases in which the drug was used in the 1st trimester (1–21). Excluding those pregnancies that ended in abortion or stillbirths, congenital abnormalities were observed in only one infant (10). Defects noted in the infant were cleft palate, microphthalmia, hypoplasia of the ovaries and thyroid gland, corneal opacity, cytomegaly, and intrauterine growth retardation. The anomalies were attributed to busulfan. Neonatal toxicity due to combination chemotherapy was observed in three other infants: pancytopenia (6), microangiopathic hemolytic anemia (9), and transient severe bone marrow hypoplasia (12). In the latter case, administration of mercaptopurine was stopped 3.5 weeks prior to delivery because of severe maternal myelosuppression. No chemotherapy was given during this period and her peripheral blood counts were normal during the final 2 weeks of her pregnancy (12).

In another case, a 34-year-old woman with acute lymphoblastic leukemia was treated with multiple antineoplastic agents from 22 weeks' gestation until delivery of a healthy female infant 18 weeks later (14). Mercaptopurine was administered throughout the 3rd trimester. Chromosome analysis of the newborn revealed a normal karyotype (46X,X) but with gaps and a ring chromosome. The clinical significance of these findings is unknown, but since these abnormalities may persist for several years, the potential existed for an increased risk of cancer, as well as for a risk of genetic damage in the next generation (14).

Data from one review indicated that 40% of the infants exposed to anticancer drugs were of low birth weight (2). This finding was not related to the timing of exposure. In addition, except in a few cases, long-term studies of growth and mental development in infants exposed to mercaptopurine during the 2nd trimester, the period of neuroblast multiplication, have not been conducted (22). However, growth and development were normal in 13 infants (one set of twins) followed for 6 months to 10 years (12, 15, 16, 18–21).

Severe oligospermia has been described in a 22-year-old male receiving sequential chemotherapy of cyclophosphamide, methotrexate, and mercaptopurine for leukemia (23). After treatment was stopped, the sperm count returned to normal and the patient fathered a healthy female child. Others have also observed reversible testicular dysfunction (24).

Ovarian function in females exposed to mercaptopurine does not seem to be affected adversely (25–29). An investigator noted in 1980 that long-term analysis of human reproduction following mercaptopurine therapy had not been reported (30). However, a brief 1979 correspondence described the reproductive performance of 314 women after treatment of gestational trophoblastic tumors, 159 of whom had conceived with a total of 218 pregnancies (28). Excluding the 17 women still pregnant at the time of the report, 38 (79%) of 48 women, exposed to mercaptopurine as part of their therapy, delivered live, term infants. A more detailed report of these and additional patients was published in 1984 (31). This latter study, and another published in 1988 (32), both involving women treated for gestational trophoblastic neoplasms, are discussed in the sections below.

In 436 long-term survivors treated with chemotherapy between 1958–1978, 95 (22%) received mercaptopurine as part of their treatment regimens (31). Of the 95 women, 33 (35%) had at least one live birth (numbers given in parentheses refer to mean/maximum mercaptopurine dose in grams) (5.9/30.0), 3 (3%) conceived but had no live births (5.3/14.0), 3 (3%) failed to conceive (1.3/2.0), and 56 (59%) did not try to conceive (5.4/30.0). Additional details, including congenital anomalies observed, are described in the monograph for methotrexate (see Methotrexate).

A 1988 report described the reproductive results of 265 women who had been treated from 1959–1980 for gestational trophoblastic disease (32). Single agent chemotherapy was administered to 91 women, including 26 cases in which mercaptopurine was the only agent used, while sequential (single agent) and combination therapy was administered to 67 and 107 women, respectively. Of the total group, 241 were exposed to pregnancy and 205 (85%) of these women conceived, with a total of 355 pregnancies. The time interval between recovery and pregnancy was 1 year or less (8.5%), 1–2 years (32.1%), 2–4 years (32.4%), 4–6 years (15.5%), 6–8 years (7.3%), 8–10 years (1.4%), and more than 10 years (2.8%). A total of 303 (four sets of twins) liveborn infants resulted from the 355 pregnancies, three of whom had congenital malformations: anencephaly, hydrocephalus, and congenital heart disease (one in each case). No gross developmental abnormalities were observed in the dead fetuses. Cytogenetic studies were conducted on the peripheral lymphocytes of 94 children and no significant chromosomal abnormalities were noted. Moreover, follow-up of the children, more than 80% of the group older than 5 years of age (the oldest was 25 years), revealed normal development. The reproductive histories and pregnancy outcomes of the treated women were comparable to those of the normal population (32).

Occupational exposure of the mother to antineoplastic agents during pregnancy may present a risk to the fetus. A position statement from the National Study Commission on Cytotoxic Exposure and a research article involving some antineoplastic agents are presented in the monograph for cyclophosphamide (see Cyclophosphamide).

Breast Feeding Summary

No data are available.

References

1. Moloney WC. Management of leukemia in pregnancy. Ann NY Acad Sci 1964;114:857–67.
2. Nicholson HO. Cytotoxic drugs in pregnancy: review of reported cases. J Obstet Gynaecol Br Commonw 1968;75:307–12.
3. Gililland J, Weinstein L. The effects of cancer chemotherapeutic agents on the developing fetus. Obstet Gynecol Surv 1983;38:6–13.
4. Wegelius R. Successful pregnancy in acute leukaemia, Lancet 1975;2:1301.
5. Nicholson HO. Leukaemia and pregnancy: a report of five cases and discussion of management. J Obstet Gynaecol Br Commonw 1968;75:517–20.
6. Pizzuto J, Aviles A, Noriega L, Niz J, Morales M, Romero F. Treatment of acute leukemia during pregnancy: presentation of nine cases. Cancer Treat Rep 1980;64:679–83.
7. Burnier AM. Discussion. In Plows CW. Acute myelomonocytic leukemia in pregnancy: report of a case. Am J Obstet Gynecol 1982;143:41–3.
8. Dara P, Slater LM, Armentrout SA. Successful pregnancy during chemotherapy for acute leukemia. Cancer 1981;47:845–6.
9. McConnell JF, Bhoola R. A neonatal complication of maternal leukemia treated with 6-mercaptopurine. Postgrad Med J 1973;49:211–3.
10. Diamond J, Anderson MM, McCreadie SR. Transplacental transmission of busulfan (Myleran) in a mother with leukemia: production of fetal malformation and cytomegaly. Pediatrics 1960;25:85–90.
11. Khurshid M, Saleem M. Acute leukaemia in pregnancy. Lancet 1978;2:534–5.
12. Okun DB, Groncy PK, Sieger L, Tanaka KR. Acute leukemia in pregnancy: transient neonatal myelosuppression after combination chemotherapy in the mother. Med Pediatr Oncol 1979;7:315–9.
13. Doney KC, Kraemer KG, Shepard TH. Combination chemotherapy for acute myelocytic leukemia during pregnancy: three case reports. Cancer Treat Rep 1979;63:369–71.
14. Schleuning M, Clemm C. Chromosomal aberrations in a newborn whose mother received cytotoxic treatment during pregnancy. N Engl J Med 1987;317:1666–7.
15. Turchi JJ, Villasis C. Anthracyclines in the treatment of malignancy in pregnancy. Cancer 1988;61:435–40.
16. Feliu J, Juarez S, Ordonez A, Garcia-Paredes ML, Gonzalez-Baron M, Montero JM. Acute leukemia and pregnancy. Cancer 1988;61:580–4.
17. Haerr RW, Pratt AT. Multiagent chemotherapy for sarcoma diagnosed during pregnancy. Cancer 1985;56:1028–33.
18. Frenkel EP, Meyers MC. Acute leukemia and pregnancy. Ann Intern Med 1960;53:656–71.
19. Loyd HO. Acute leukemia complicated by pregnancy. JAMA 1961;178:1140–3.
20. Lee RA, Johnson CE, Hanlon DG. Leukemia during pregnancy. Am J Obstet Gynecol 1962;84:455–8.
21. Coopland AT, Friesen WJ, Galbraith PA. Acute leukemia in pregnancy. Am J Obstet Gynecol 1969;105:1288–9.
22. Dobbing J. Pregnancy and leukaemia. Lancet 1977;1:1155.
23. Hinkes E, Plotkin D. Reversible drug-induced sterility in a patient with acute leukemia. JAMA 1973;223:1490–1.
24. Lendon M, Palmer MK, Hann IM, Shalet SM, Jones PHM. Testicular histology after combination chemotherapy in childhood for acute lymphoblastic leukaemia. Lancet 1978;2:439–41.
25. Schilsky RL, Lewis BJ, Sherins RJ, Young RC. Gonadal dysfunction in patients receiving chemotherapy for cancer. Ann Intern Med 1980;93:109–14.
26. Gasser C. Long-term survival (cures) in childhood acute leukemia. Paediatrician 1980;9:344–57.

27. Bacon C, Kernahan J. Successful pregnancy in acute leukaemia. Lancet 1975;2:515.
28. Walden PAM, Bagshawe KD. Pregnancies after chemotherapy for gestational trophoblastic tumours. Lancet 1979;2:1241.
29. Sanz MH, Rafecas FJ. Successful pregnancy during chemotherapy for acute promyelocytic leukemia. N Engl J Med 1982;306:939.
30. Steckman ML. Treatment of Chohn's disease with 6-mercaptopurine: what effects on fertility? N Engl J Med 1980;303:817.
31. Rustin GJS, Booth M, Dent J, Salt S, Rustin F, Bagshawe KD. Pregnancy after cytotoxic chemotherapy for gestational trophoblastic tumours. Br Med J 1984;288:103–6.
32. Song H, Wu P, Wang Y, Yang X, Dong S. Pregnancy outcomes after successful chemotherapy for choriocarcinoma and invasive mole: long-term follow-up. Am J Obstet Gynecol 1988;158:538–45.

Name: **MESORIDAZINE**

Class: **Tranquilizer**   Risk Factor: **C**

Fetal Risk Summary

Mesoridazine is a piperidyl phenothiazine. Phenothiazines readily cross the placenta (1). No specific information on its use in pregnancy has been located. Although occasional reports have attempted to link various phenothiazine compounds with congenital malformations, the bulk of the evidence indicates that these drugs are safe for the mother and fetus (see Chlorpromazine).

Breast Feeding Summary

No reports describing the excretion of mesoridazine into breast milk have been located. The American Academy of Pediatrics classifies mesoridazine as an agent whose effect on the nursing infant is unknown but may be of concern (2).

References

1. Moya F, Thorndike V. Passage of drugs across the placenta. Am J Obstet Gynecol 1962;84:1778–98.
2. Committee on Drugs, American Academy of Pediatrics. Transfer of drugs and other chemicals into human milk. Pediatrics 1989;84:924–36.

Name: **MESTRANOL**

Class: **Estrogenic Hormone**   Risk Factor: **X**

Fetal Risk Summary

Mestranol is the 3-methyl ester of ethinyl estradiol. Mestranol is used frequently in combination with progestins for oral contraception (see Oral Contraceptives). Congenital malformations attributed to the use of mestranol alone have not been reported. The Collaborative Perinatal Project monitored 614 mother-child pairs with 1st trimester exposure to estrogenic agents (including 179 with exposure to mestranol) (1, pp. 389, 391). An increase in the expected frequency of cardiovascular defects, eye and ear anomalies, and Down's syndrome was found for estrogens as a group but not for mestranol (1, pp. 389, 391, 395). Re-evaluation of these data in terms of timing of exposure, vaginal bleeding in early pregnancy, and previous maternal obstetric history, however, failed to support an association between estrogens and cardiac malformations (2). An earlier study also failed to find any relationship with nongenital malformations (3). The use of estrogenic hormones during pregnancy is contraindicated.

Breast Feeding Summary

Estrogens are frequently used for suppression of postpartum lactation (4). Doses of 100–150 µg of ethinyl estradiol (equivalent to 160–240 µg of mestranol) for 5–7 days are used (4). Mestranol, when used in oral contraceptives with doses of 30–80 µg, has been associated with decreased milk production, lower infant weight gain, and decreased composition of nitrogen and protein content of human milk (5–7). The magnitude of these changes is low. However, the changes in milk production and composition may be of nutritional importance in malnourished mothers. If breast feeding is desired, the lowest dose of oral contraceptives should be chosen. Monitoring of infant weight gain and the possible need for nutritional supplementation should be considered (see Oral Contraceptives).

References

1. Heinonen OP, Slone D, Shapiro S. *Birth Defects and Drugs in Pregnancy*. Littleton:Publishing Sciences Group, 1977.
2. Wiseman RA, Dodds-Smith IC. Cardiovascular birth defects and antenatal exposure to female sex hormones: a reevaluation of some base data. Teratology 1984;30:359–70.
3. Wilson JG, Brent RL. Are female sex hormones teratogenic? Am J Obstet Gynecol 1981;141:567–80.
4. Gilman AG, Goodman LS, Gilman A. *The Pharmacological Basis of Therapeutics*. New York:MacMillan, 1980:1431.
5. Kora SJ. Effect of oral contraceptives on lactation. Fertil Steril 1969;20:419–23.
6. Miller GH, Hughs LR. Lactation and genital involution effects of a new low-dose oral contraceptive on breast-feeding mothers and their infants. Obstet Gynecol 1970;35:44–50.
7. Lonnerdal B, Forsum E, Hambraeus L. Effect of oral contraceptives on composition and volume of breast milk. Am J Clin Nutr 1980;33:816–24.

Name: **METAPROTERENOL**

Class: **Sympathomimetic (Adrenergic)**　　　　　　　　　Risk Factor: **C$_M$**

Fetal Risk Summary

No reports linking the use of metaproterenol with congenital defects have been located. Metaproterenol, a β-sympathomimetic, has been used to prevent premature labor (1–3). Its use for this purpose has been largely assumed by ritodrine, albuterol, or terbutaline. Like all β-mimetics, metaproterenol causes maternal and, to a lesser degree, fetal tachycardia. Maternal hypotension, hyperglycemia, and neonatal hypoglycemia should be expected (see also Ritodrine, Albuterol, and Terbutaline). Long-term evaluation of infants exposed *in utero* to β-mimetics has been reported, but not specifically for metaproterenol (4). No harmful effects in the infants were observed.

Breast Feeding Summary

No data are available.

References

1. Baillie P, Meehan FP, Tyack AJ. Treatment of premature labour with orciprenaline. Br Med J 1970;4:154–5.
2. Tyack AJ, Baillier P, Meehan FP. In-vivo response of the human uterus to orciprenaline in early labour. Br Med J 1971;2:741–3.
3. Zilianti M, Aller J. Action of orciprenaline on uterine contractility during labor, maternal cardiovascular system, fetal heart rate, and acid-base balance. Am J Obstet Gynecol 1971;109:1073–9.
4. Freysz H, Willard D, Lehr A, Messer J, Boog G. A long term evaluation of infants who received a beta-mimetic drug while in utero. J Perinat Med 1977;5:94–9.

Name: **METARAMINOL**

Class: **Sympathomimetic (Adrenergic)**   Risk Factor: **D**

Fetal Risk Summary

Metaraminol is a sympathomimetic used in emergency situations to treat hypotension. Because of the nature of its indications, experience in pregnancy with metaraminol is limited. Uterine vessels are normally maximally dilated and they have only α-adrenergic receptors (1). Use of the predominantly α-adrenergic stimulant, metaraminol, could cause constriction of these vessels and reduce uterine blood flow, thereby producing fetal hypoxia (bradycardia). Metaraminol may also interact with oxytocics or ergot derivatives to produce severe persistent maternal hypertension (1). Rupture of a cerebral vessel is possible. If a pressor agent is indicated, other drugs such as ephedrine should be considered.

Breast Feeding Summary

No data are available.

Reference

1. Smith NT, Corbascio AN. The use and misuse of pressor agents. Anesthesiology 1970;33:58–101.

Name: **METHACYCLINE**

Class: **Antibiotic**   Risk Factor: **D**

Fetal Risk Summary

See Tetracycline.

Breast Feeding Summary

See Tetracycline.

Name: **METHADONE**

Class: **Narcotic Analgesic**   Risk Factor: **B***

Fetal Risk Summary

Methadone use in pregnancy is almost exclusively related to the treatment of heroin addiction. No increase in congenital defects has been observed. However, since these patients normally consume a wide variety of drugs, it is not possible to separate completely the effects of methadone from the effects of other agents. Neonatal narcotic withdrawal and low birth weight seem to be the primary problems.

Withdrawal symptoms occur in approximately 60–90% of the infants (1–6). One study concluded that the intensity of withdrawal was increased if the daily maternal dosage exceeded 20 mg (5). When withdrawal symptoms do occur, they normally start within 48 hours after delivery, but a small percentage may be delayed up to 7–14 days (1). One report observed initial withdrawal symptoms appearing up to 28 days after birth, but the authors do not mention if mothers of these infants were breast feeding (6). Methadone concentrations in breast milk are reported to be sufficient to prevent withdrawal in addicted infants (See Breast Feeding Summary below). Some authors believe methadone withdrawal is more intense than that occurring with heroin (1). Less than one-third of symptomatic infants require therapy (1–5). A lower incidence of hyaline membrane disease is seen in infants exposed *in utero* to chronic methadone and may be due to elevated blood levels of prolactin (7).

Infants of drug-addicted mothers are often small for gestational age. In some series, one-third or more of the infants weigh less than 2500 g (1, 2, 4). The newborn of methadone addicts may have a higher birth weight than comparable offspring of heroin addicts for reasons that remain unclear (4).

Other problems occurring in the offspring of methadone addicts are increased mortality, sudden infant death syndrome (SIDS), jaundice, and thrombocytosis. A correlation between drug addiction and SIDS has been suggested with 20 cases (2.8%) in a group of 702 infants, but the data could not attribute the increase to a single drug (8, 9). Another study of 313 infants of methadone-addicted mothers reported 2 cases (0.6%) of SIDS, an incidence similar to the overall experience of that location (4). In one study, a positive correlation was found between severity of neonatal withdrawal and the incidence of SIDS (9). Maternal withdrawal during pregnancy has been observed to produce a marked response of the fetal adrenal glands and sympathetic nervous system (10). An increased stillborn and neonatal mortality rate has also been reported (11). Both reports recommend against detoxification of the mother during gestation. Jaundice is comparatively infrequent in both heroin- and methadone-exposed newborns. However, a higher rate of severe hyperbilirubinemia in methadone infants than in a comparable group of heroin infants has been observed (1). Thrombocytosis developing in the 2nd week of life, with some platelet counts exceeding 1,000,000/mm^3 and persisting for over 16 weeks, has been reported (12). The condition was not related to withdrawal symptoms or neonatal treatment. Some of these infants also had increased circulating platelet aggregates.

Respiratory depression is not a significant problem, and Apgar scores are comparable to those of a nonaddicted population (1–5). Long-term effects on the behavior and gross motor development skills are not known.

[*Risk Factor D if used for prolonged periods or in high doses at term.]

Breast Feeding Summary

Methadone enters breast milk in concentrations approaching plasma levels and may prevent withdrawal symptoms in addicted infants. One study reported an average milk concentration in 10 patients of 0.27 µg/ml, representing an average milk:plasma ratio of 0.83 (13). The same investigators earlier reported levels ranging from 0.17–5.6 µg/ml in the milk of mothers on methadone maintenance (2). At least one infant death has been attributed to methadone obtained through breast milk (14). However, a recent report claimed that methadone enters breast milk in very low quantities that are clinically insignificant (15). The American Academy of Pediatrics considers methadone to be compatible with breast feeding with no adverse effects reported in the nursing infant when the mother was consuming 20 mg/24 hours or less (16).

References

1. Zelson C, Lee SJ, Casalino M. Neonatal narcotic addiction. N Engl J Med 1973;289:1216–20.
2. Blinick G, Jerez E, Wallach RC. Methadone maintenance, pregnancy and progeny. JAMA 1973;225:477–9.
3. Strauss ME, Andresko M, Stryker JC, Wardell JN, Dunkel LD. Methadone maintenance during pregnancy: pregnancy, birth and neonate characteristics. Am J Obstet Gynecol 1974;120:895–900.
4. Newman RG, Bashkow S, Calko D. Results of 313 consecutive live births of infants delivered to patients in the New York City methadone maintenance program. Am J Obstet Gynecol 1975;121:233–7.
5. Ostrea EM, Chavez CJ, Strauss ME. A study of factors that influence the severity of neonatal narcotic withdrawal. J Pediatr 1976;88:642–5.
6. Kandall SR, Gartner LM. Delayed presentation of neonatal methadone withdrawal. Pediatr Res 1973;7:320.
7. Parekh A, Mukherjee TK, Jhaveri R, Rosenfeld W, Glass L. Intrauterine exposure to narcotics and cord blood prolactin concentrations. Obstet Gynecol 1981;57:447–9.
8. Pierson PS, Howard P, Kleber HD. Sudden deaths in infants born to methadone-maintained addicts. JAMA 1972;220:1733–4.
9. Chavez CJ, Ostrea EM, Stryker JC, Smialek Z. Sudden infant death syndrome among infants of drug-dependent mothers. J Pediatr 1979;95:407–9.
10. Zuspan FP, Gumpel JA, Mejia-Zelaya A, Madden J, David R. Fetal stress from methadone withdrawal. Am J Obstet Gynecol 1975;122:43–6.
11. Rementeria JL, Nunag NN. Narcotic withdrawal in pregnancy: stillbirth incidence with a case report. Am J Obstet Gynecol 1973;116:1152–6.
12. Burstein Y, Giardina PJV, Rausen AR, Kandall SR, Siljestrom K, Peterson CM. Thrombocytosis and increased circulating platelet aggregates in newborn infants of polydrug users. J Pediatr 1979;94:895–9.
13. Blinick G, Inturrisi CE, Jerez E, Wallach RC. Methadone assays in pregnant women and progeny. Am J Obstet Gynecol 1975;121:617–21.
14. Smialek JE, Monforte JR, Aronow R, Spitz WU. Methadone deaths in children—a continuing problem. JAMA 1977;238:2516–7.
15. Anonymous. Methadone in breast milk. Med Lett Drugs Ther 1979;21:52.
16. Committee on Drugs, American Academy of Pediatrics. Transfer of drugs and other chemicals into human milk. Pediatrics 1989;84:924–36.

Name: **METHAMPHETAMINE**

Class: **Central Stimulant**   Risk Factor: C_M

Fetal Risk Summary

See Amphetamine.

Breast Feeding Summary

See Amphetamine.

Name: **METHANTHELINE**

Class: **Parasympatholytic (Anticholinergic)**   Risk Factor: **C**

Fetal Risk Summary

Methantheline is an anticholinergic quaternary ammonium bromide. In a large prospective study, 2323 patients were exposed to this class of drugs during the 1st trimester, 2 of whom took methantheline (1). A possible association was found between the total group and minor malformations.

Breast Feeding Summary

No data are available (see also Atropine).

Reference

1. Heinonen OP, Slone D, Shapiro S. *Birth Defects and Drugs in Pregnancy*. Littleton:Publishing Sciences Group, 1977:346–53.

Name: **METHAQUALONE**

Class: **Hypnotic**   Risk Factor: **D**

Fetal Risk Summary

No reports linking the use of methaqualone with congenital defects have been located. One manufacturer was not aware of any adverse effects following 1st trimester use (R.R. Smith, personal communication, William H. Rorer, Inc., 1972). The autopsy of a 6-day-old infant found a congenital hypothalamic hamartoblastoma and multiple malformations (1). The baby had been exposed to methaqualone, marijuana, and cocaine early in gestation but the correlation to any of these agents is unknown. Methaqualone is often used as an illicit abuse drug. Separating fetal effects from adulterants or other drugs is not possible. Due to the abuse potential, methaqualone is not recommended during pregnancy.

Breast Feeding Summary

No data are available.

Reference

1. Huff DS, Fernandes M. Two cases of congenital hypothalamic hamartoblastoma, polydactyly, and other congenital anomalies (Pallister-Hall syndrome). N Engl J Med 1982;306:430–1.

Name: **METHARBITAL**

Class: **Anticonvulsant/Sedative**   Risk Factor: **D**

Fetal Risk Summary

No reports linking the use of metharbital with congenital defects have been located. Metharbital is demethylated to barbital by the liver (see also Phenobarbital).

Breast Feeding Summary

Metharbital's metabolite, barbital, has been demonstrated in breast milk in trace amounts (1). No reports linking the use of metharbital with adverse effects in the nursing infant have been located.

Reference

1. Kwit NT, Hatcher RA. Excretion of drugs in milk. Am J Dis Child 1935;40:900–4.

Name: **METHAZOLAMIDE**

Class: **Carbonic Anhydrase Inhibitor**   Risk Factor: **C**

Fetal Risk Summary

Methazolamide is a carbonic anhydrase inhibitor used in glaucoma to lower intraocular pressure. No reports describing the use of methazolamide in human pregnancy have been located. The drug is teratogenic in some animal species (1). (See also Acetazolamide.)

Breast Feeding Summary

No data are available.

Reference

1. Product information. Neptazane. Lederle Laboratories, 1988.

Name: **METHDILAZINE**

Class: **Antihistamine**   Risk Factor: **C**

Fetal Risk Summary

No data are available. See Promethazine for representative agent in this class.

Breast Feeding Summary

No data are available.

Name: **METHENAMINE**

Class: **Urinary Germicide**   Risk Factor: **C$_M$**

Fetal Risk Summary

Methenamine, in either the mandelate or hippurate salt form, is used for chronic suppressive treatment of bacteriuria. In two studies, the mandelate form was given to 120 patients and the hippurate to 70 patients (1, 2). No increases in congenital defects or other problems as compared to controls were observed. The Collaborative Perinatal Project reported 49 1st trimester exposures to methenamine (3, pp. 299, 302). For use anytime in pregnancy, 299 exposures were recorded (3, p. 435). Only in the latter group was a possible association with malformations found. The statistical significance of this is not known. Independent confirmation is required.

Methenamine interferes with the determination of urinary estrogen (4). Urinary estrogen was formerly used to assess the condition of the fetoplacental unit, depressed levels being associated with fetal distress. This assessment is now made by measuring unconjugated estriol, which is not affected by methenamine.

Breast Feeding Summary

Methenamine is excreted into breast milk. Peak levels occur at 1 hour (5). No adverse effects on the nursing infant have been reported.

References

1. Gordon SF. Asymptomatic bacteriuria of pregnancy. Clin Med 1972;79:22–4.
2. Furness ET, McDonald PJ, Beasley NV. Urinary antiseptics in asymptomatic bacteriuria of pregnancy. NZ Med J 1975;81:417–9.
3. Heinonen OP, Slone D, Shapiro S. *Birth Defects and Drugs in Pregnancy*. Littleton:Publishing Sciences Group, 1977.
4. Kivinen S, Tuimala R. Decreased urinary oestriol concentrations in pregnant women during hexamine hippurate treatment. Br Med J 1977;2:682.
5. Sapeika N. The excretion of drugs in human milk—a review. J Obstet Gynaecol Br Emp 1947;54:426–31.

Name: **METHICILLIN**

Class: **Antibiotic**   Risk Factor: **B$_M$**

Fetal Risk Summary

Methicillin is a penicillin antibiotic (see also Penicillin G). The drug rapidly crosses the placenta into the fetal circulation and amniotic fluid (1, 2). Following a 500-mg intravenous dose over 10–15 minutes, peak levels of 13.0 and 10.5 µg/ml were measured in maternal and fetal serums, respectively, at 30 minutes (1). Equilibration occurred between the two serums within 1 hour. No effects were reported in the infants.

No reports linking the use of methicillin with congenital defects have been located. The Collaborative Perinatal Project monitored 50,282 mother-child pairs, 3,546 of which had 1st trimester exposure to penicillin derivatives (3, pp. 297–313). For use anytime during pregnancy, 7,171 exposures were recorded (3, p. 435). In neither case was evidence found to suggest a relationship to large categories of major or minor malformations or to individual defects.

Breast Feeding Summary

No data are available (see Penicillin G).

References

1. Depp R, Kind A, Kirby W, Johnson W. Transplacental passage of methicillin and dicloxacillin into the fetus and amniotic fluid. Am J Obstet Gynecol 1970;107:1054–7.
2. MacAulay M, Molloy W, Charles D. Placental transfer of methicillin. Am J Obstet Gynecol 1973;115:58–65.
3. Heinonen OP, Slone D, Shapiro S. *Birth Defects and Drugs in Pregnancy*. Littleton:Publishing Sciences Group, 1977.

Name: **METHIMAZOLE**

Class: **Antithyroid**   Risk Factor: **D**

Fetal Risk Summary

Nine cases of scalp defects (aplasia cutis) in newborns exposed *in utero* to methimazole or carbimazole (converted *in vivo* to methimazole) have been reported (1–3). In two of the nine infants, umbilical defects (patent urachus in one; patent vitelline duct in another) were also observed, suggesting to one investigator, because of the rarity of these defects, that the combination of anomalies represented a possible malformation syndrome (3). In contrast, a 1987 report examined the records of 49,091 live births for cases of congenital skin defects (4). Twenty-five (0.05%) such cases were discovered, 13 (0.03%) of which were confined to the scalp. In the sample of 48,057 women, 24 were treated with methimazole or carbimazole during the 1st trimester, but none of these mothers produced children with the skin defects. The authors concluded that they could not exclude an association between the therapy and scalp defects, but if it existed, it was a weak association (4).

Defects observed in two infants exposed to the antithyroid agents in two other reports were imperforate anus (2) and transposition of the great arteries (died at 3 days of age) (5). In a large prospective study, 25 patients were exposed to one or more noniodide thyroid suppressants during the 1st trimester, nine of whom took methimazole (6). From the total group, four children with nonspecified malformations were found, suggesting that the drugs may be teratogenic. However, since 16 of the group took other antithyroid drugs, the relationship between methimazole and the anomalies cannot be determined. In a study of 25 infants exposed to carbimazole, two were found to have defects: bilateral congenital cataracts, and partial adactyly of the right foot (7). Because no pattern of malformations has emerged from these reports, it appears that these malformations were not associated with the drug therapy. In addition, other reports have described the use of methimazole and carbimazole during pregnancy without fetal anomalies (8–22).

A 1984 report described the relationship between maternal Graves' disease and major structural malformations of external organs, including the oral cavity, in 643 newborns (23). Of 167 newborns delivered from mothers who were hyperthyroid during gestation, 117 were exposed *in utero* to methimazole. In 50 newborns, the mothers received no treatment, other than subtotal thyroidectomy before and/ or during pregnancy. The incidences of anomalies in these two groups were 1.7% (2 of 117) and 6.0% (3 of 50), respectively. For 476 neonates the mothers were euthyroid during gestation, with 126 receiving treatment with methimazole and 350 receiving no treatment (other than surgery). No malformations were observed in the methimazole-exposed infants and only one (0.3%; 1 of 350) occurred in the patients not receiving drug therapy. The difference in malformation rates between the nonexposed neonates in the hyperthyroid and euthyroid groups was significant (6% vs. 0.3%, $p < 0.01$). Similarly, the difference between the two groups in total malformations, 3% (5 of 167) vs. 0.2% (1 of 476) was also significant ($p < 0.01$). The defects observed were malformation of the earlobe (methimazole-exposed, hyperthyroid), omphalocele (methimazole-exposed, hyperthyroid), imperforate anus (hyperthyroid), anencephaly (hyperthyroid), harelip (hyperthyroid), and polydactyly (euthyroid). The authors concluded that the disease itself causes congenital malformations and that the use of methimazole lessened the risk for adverse outcome.

Methimazole readily crosses the placenta to the fetus. Two patients undergoing 2nd trimester therapeutic abortions were given a single 10-mg ^{35}S-labeled oral dose 2 hours before pregnancy termination (24). Fetal:maternal serum ratios were 0.72 and 0.81, representing 0.22% and 0.24% of the administered dose. In the same study, three patients at 14, 14, and 20 weeks' gestation were given an equimolar dose of carbimazole (16.6 mg). Fetal:maternal serum ratios were 0.80–1.09 with 0.17%–0.87% of the total radioactivity in the fetus. The highest serum and tissue levels were found in the 20-week-old fetus.

Several reports have studied pregnancies complicated by Graves' disease and the effects of methimazole and carbimazole on maternal and fetal thyroid indexes (19, 25–28). In separate pregnancies in a mother with Graves' disease, fetal thyrotoxicosis was treated with 20–40 mg/day of carbimazole with successful resolution of fetal tachycardia in both cases and disappearance of fetal goiter in the first infant (19). A woman with hyperthyroidism was treated with a partial thyroidectomy prior to pregnancy (26). She subsequently had four pregnancies, all of which were complicated by fetal hyperthyroidism. No antithyroid therapy was administered during her first two pregnancies. The first ended in a late stillborn, and the second resulted in a child with skull deformities. Both adverse outcomes were compatible with fetal hyperthyroidism. Carbimazole was administered in the next two pregnancies and both resulted in normal infants.

Treatment of maternal hyperthyroidism may result in mild fetal hypothyroidism due to increased levels of fetal pituitary thyrotropin (13, 16, 27, 29). This usually resolves within a few days without treatment (16). An exception to this occurred in one newborn exposed to 30 mg of carbimazole daily to term who appeared normal at birth but who developed hypothyroidism evident at 2 months of age with subsequent mental retardation (8).

Small, usually nonobstructing, goiters in the newborn have been reported frequently with propylthiouracil (see Propylthiouracil). Only two goiters have been reported in carbimazole-exposed newborns and none with methimazole (5). Long-term follow-up of 25 children exposed *in utero* to carbimazole has shown normal growth and development (7).

Combination therapy with thyroid-antithyroid drugs was advocated at one time but is now considered inappropriate (see also Propylthiouracil) (14, 18, 29, 30). Two reasons contributed to this change: (a) use of thyroid hormones may require higher doses of the antithyroid drug to be used, and (b) placental transfer of levothroxine and liothyronine is minimal and not sufficient to reverse fetal hypothyroidism (see also Levothyroxine and Liothyronine) (16).

Due to the possible association with aplasia cutis and passage of methimazole into breast milk, many experts consider propylthiouracil to be the drug of choice for the medical treatment of hyperthyroidism during pregnancy. If methimazole or carbimazole is used, the smallest possible dose to control the maternal disease should be given (5, 29). One review recommended that the dosage should be adjusted to maintain the maternal free thyroxine levels in a mildly thyrotoxic range (28).

Breast Feeding Summary

Methimazole is excreted into breast milk (31–35). In a patient given 10 mg of radiolabeled carbimazole (converted *in vivo* to methimazole), the milk:plasma ratio was a fairly constant 1.05 over 24 hours (25). This represented about 0.47% of the given radioactive dose. In a second study, a patient was administered 2.5 mg of methimazole every 12 hours (32). The mean milk:plasma ratio was 1.16, representing 16–39 μg of methimazole in the daily milk supply. Extrapolation of these results to a daily dose of 20 mg indicated that approximately 3 mg/day would be excreted into the milk (32). Five lactating women were given 40 mg of carbimazole, producing a mean milk:plasma ratio at 1 hour of 0.72 (33). For the 8-hour period after dosing, the milk:plasma ratio was 0.98. A new radioimmunoassay was used to measure methimazole milk levels after a single 40-mg oral dose in four lactating women (34). The mean milk:plasma ratio during the first 8 hours was 0.97, with 70 μg excreted in the milk.

A 1987 publication described the results of carbimazole therapy in a woman breast feeding twins (35). Two months after delivery, the mother was started on carbimazole, 30 mg/day. The dose was decreased as she became euthyroid. Three paired milk:plasma levels revealed ratios of 0.30–0.70. The mean free methimazole concentration in milk, determined between 2–16 weeks of therapy, was 43 ng/ml (range 0–92 ng/ml). Peak milk levels occurred 2–4 hours after a dose. Mean plasma levels in the twins were 45 ng/ml (range 0–105 ng/ml) and 52 ng/ml (range 0–156 ng/ml), respectively, with the highest concentrations occurring while the mother was taking 30 mg/day. No evidence of thyroid suppression was found clinically or after thyroid function tests in the nursing twins. A similar lack of effect was observed during a 3-week study of 11 infants whose mothers were taking 5–15 mg/day of carbimazole (36).

Because the amounts found in the above studies may cause thyroid dysfunction in the nursing infant, methimazole and carbimazole have, in the past, been considered contraindicated during lactation. If antithyroid drug therapy was required, propylthiouracil (PTU) was considered the treatment of choice, partially because PTU is ionized at physiologic pH and because 80% of the drug is protein bound (37). Methimazole is neither ionized nor protein bound (37). However, recent recommendations now state that small doses (e.g., 10–15 mg or less/day) do not pose a major risk to the nursing infant if thyroid function is monitored at frequent (e.g., weekly or biweekly) intervals (36, 37). PTU is, however, still considered the treatment of choice by some (37). The American Academy of Pediatrics considers methimazole and carbimazole to be compatible with breast feeding (38).

References

1. Milham S Jr, Elledge W. Maternal methimazole and congenital defects in children. Teratology 1972;5:125.
2. Mujtaba Q, Burrow GN. Treatment of hyperthyroidism in pregnancy with propylthiouracil and methimazole. Obstet Gynecol 1975;46:282–6.
3. Milham S Jr. Scalp defects in infants of mothers treated for hyperthyroidism with methimazole or carbimazole during pregnancy. Teratology 1985;32:321.
4. Van Dijke CP, Heydendael RJ, De Kleine MJ. Methimazole, carbimazole, and congenital skin defects. Ann Intern Med 1987;106:60–1.
5. Sugrue D, Drury MI. Hyperthyroidism complicating pregnancy: results of treatment by antithyroid drugs in 77 pregnancies. Br J Obstet Gynaecol 1980;87:970–5.
6. Heinonen OP, Slone D, Shapiro S. *Birth Defects and Drugs in Pregnancy*. Littleton:Publishing Sciences Group, 1977:388–400.
7. McCarroll AM, Hutchinson M, McAuley R, Montgomery DAD. Long-term assessment of children exposed in utero to carbimazole. Arch Dis Child 1976;51:532–6.
8. Hawe P, Francis HH. Pregnancy and thyrotoxicosis. Br Med J 1962;2:817–22.
9. Herbst AL. Selenkow HA. Combined antithyroid-thyroid therapy of hyperthyroidism in pregnancy. Obstet Gynecol 1963;21:543–50.
10. Reveno WS, Rosenbaum H. Observation on the use of antithyroid drugs. Ann Intern Med 1964;60:982–9.
11. Herbst AL, Selenkow HA. Hyperthyroidism during pregnancy. N Engl J Med 1965;273:627–33.
12. Talbert LM, Thomas CG Jr, Holt WA, Rankin P. Hyperthyroidism during pregnancy. Obstet Gynecol 1970;36:779–85.
13. Refetoff S, Ochi Y, Selenkow HA, Rosenfield RL. Neonatal hypothyroidism and goiter in one infant of each of two sets of twins due to maternal therapy with antithyroid drugs. J Pediatr 1974;85:240–4.
14. Mestman JH, Manning PR, Hodgman J. Hyperthyroidism and pregnancy. Ann Intern Med 1974;134:434–9.
15. Ramsay I. Attempted prevention of neonatal thyrotoxicosis. Br Med J 1976;2:1110.
16. Low L, Ratcliffe W, Alexander W. Intrauterine hypothyroidism due to antithyroid-drug therapy for thyrotoxicosis during pregnancy. Lancet 1978;2:370–1.
17. Robinson PL, O'Mullane NH, Alderman B. Prenatal treatment of fetal thyrotoxicosis. Br Med J 1979;1:383–4.
18. Kock HCLV, Merkus JMWM. Graves' disease during pregnancy. Eur J Obstet Gynecol Reprod Biol 1983;14:323–30.
19. Pekonen F, Teramo K, Makinen T, Ikonen E, Osterlund K, Lamberg BA. Prenatal diagnosis and treatment of fetal thyrotoxicosis. Am J Obstet Gynecol 1984;150:893–4.
20. Jeffcoate WJ, Bain C. Recurrent pregnancy-induced thyrotoxicosis presenting as hyperemesis gravidarum. Case report. Br J Obstet Gynaecol 1985;92:413–5.
21. Johnson IR, Filshie GM. Hodgkin's disease diagnosed in pregnancy: case report. Br J Obstet Gynaecol 1977;84:791–2.
22. Ramsay I, Kaur S, Krassas G. Thyrotoxicosis in pregnancy: results of treatment by antithyroid drugs combined with T4. Clin Endocrinol (Oxf) 1983;18:73–85.
23. Momotani N, Ito K, Hamada N, Ban Y, Nishikawa Y, Mimura T. Maternal hyperthyroidism and congenital malformation in the offspring. Clin Endocrinol (Oxf) 1984;20:695–700.
24. Marchant B, Brownlie EW, Hart DM, Horton PW, Alexander WD. The placental transfer of propylthiouracil, methimazole and carbimazole. J Clin Endocrinol Metab 1977;45:1187–93.

25. Hardisty CA, Munro DS. Serum long acting thyroid stimulator protector in pregnancy complicated by Graves' disease. Br Med J 1983;286:934–5.
26. Cove DH, Johnston P. Fetal hyperthyroidism: experience of treatment in four siblings. Lancet 1985;1:430–2.
27. Burrow GN. The management of thyrotoxicosis in pregnancy. N Engl J Med 1985;313:562–5.
28. Momotani N, Noh J, Oyanagi H, Ishikawa N, Ito K. Antithyroid drug therapy for Graves' disease during pregnancy: optimal regimen for fetal thyroid status. N Engl J Med 1986;315:24–8.
29. Burr WA. Thyroid disease. Clin Obstet Gynecol 1981;8:341–51.
30. Anonymous. Transplacental passage of thyroid hormones. N Engl J Med 1967;277:486–7.
31. Low LCK, Lang J, Alexander WD. Excretion of carbimazole and propylthiouracil in breast milk. Lancet 1979;2:1011.
32. Tegler L, Lindstrom B. Antithyroid drugs in milk. Lancet 1980;2:591.
33. Johansen K, Andersen AN, Kampmann JP, Hansen JM, Mortensen HB. Excretion of methimazole in human milk. Eur J Clin Pharmacol 1982;23:339–41.
34. Cooper DS, Bode HH, Nath B, Saxe V, Malcof F, Ridgway EC. Methimazole in man: studies using a newly developed radioimmunoassay for methimazole. J Clin Endocrinol Metab 1984;58:473–9.
35. Rylance GW, Woods CG, Donnelly MC, Oliver JS, Alexander WD. Carbimazole and breastfeeding. Lancet 1987;1:928.
36. Lamberg BA, Ikonen E, Osterlund K, Teramo K, Pekonen F, Peltola J, Valimaki M. Antithyroid treatment of maternal hyperthyroidism during lactation. Clin Endocrinol 1984;21:81–7.
37. Cooper DS. Antithyroid drugs: to breast-feed or not to breast-feed. Am J Obstet Gynecol 1987;157:234–5.
38. Committee on Drugs, American Academy of Pediatrics. Transfer of drugs and other chemicals into human milk. Pediatrics 1989;84:924–36.

Name: **METHIXENE**

Class: **Parasympatholytic**   Risk Factor: **C**

Fetal Risk Summary

Methixene is an anticholinergic agent. No reports of its use in pregnancy have been located (see also Atropine).

Breast Feeding Summary

No data are available (see also Atropine).

Name: **METHOTREXATE**

Class: **Antineoplastic**   Risk Factor: **D**

Fetal Risk Summary

Methotrexate is a folic acid antagonist. References describing the use of this antineoplastic agent in 26 pregnancies, 10 in the 1st trimester, have been located (1–16). Three of the 10 1st trimester exposures resulted in malformed infants (2, 3, 6). Methotrexate-induced congenital defects are similar to those produced by another folic acid antagonist, aminopterin (see also Aminopterin) (6). Two infants had the following anomalies:

Absence of lambdoid and coronal sutures, oxycephaly, absence of frontal bone, low-set ears, hypertelorism, dextroposition of heart, absence of digits on feet, growth retardation, very wide posterior fontanel, hypoplastic mandible, multiple anomalous ribs (2)

Oxycephaly due to absent coronal sutures, large anterior fontanel, depressed/wide nasal bridge, low-set ears, long webbed fingers, wide-set eyes (3)

Possible retention of methotrexate in maternal tissues prior to conception was suggested as the cause of a rare pulmonary disorder in a newborn, desquamating fibrosing alveolitis (17). The infant's mother had conceived within 6 months of completing treatment with the antineoplastic. (Note: A later publication from these investigators, that included this case, noted that the newborn was conceived within 2 months of treatment termination (see reference 29). In addition, a sister of the infant born 3 years later developed the same disorder, while a third child born from the mother 1 year later developed normally.) Previous studies have shown that methotrexate may persist for prolonged periods in human tissues (18). However, conception occurred 3 months after discontinuance of therapy in one case (19), after 6 months in a second (13), and after 7 months in a third (20). Four (one set of twins) normal infants resulted from these latter pregnancies. Thus, the association between methotrexate and the pulmonary disorder is unknown.

Two cases of severe newborn myelosuppression have been reported after methotrexate use in pregnancy. In one case, pancytopenia was discovered in a 1000-g male newborn after exposure to six different antineoplastic agents, including methotrexate, in the 3rd trimester (4). The second infant, delivered at 31 weeks' gestation, was exposed to methotrexate only during the 12th week of pregnancy (9). The severe bone marrow hypoplasia was most likely due to the use of mercaptopurine near delivery.

Data from one review indicated that 40% of the infants exposed to cytotoxic drugs were of low birth weight (1). This finding was not related to the timing of the exposure. Long-term studies of growth and mental development in offspring exposed to antineoplastic agents during the 2nd trimester, the period of neuroblast multiplication, have not been conducted (21, 22). Several studies, however, have followed individual infants for periods ranging from 2–84 months and have not discovered any problems (9–13, 15, 16).

Methotrexate crosses the placenta to the fetus (14). A 34-year-old mother was treated with multiple antineoplastic agents for acute lymphoblastic leukemia beginning in her 22nd week of pregnancy. Weekly intrathecal methotrexate (10 mg^2) was administered from approximately 26–29 weeks' gestation, then the dose was increased to 20 mg/m^2 weekly until delivery at 40 weeks' gestation. Methotrexate levels in cord serum and red cells were 1.86×10^{-9} M, and 2.6×10^{-9} M/g of hemoglobin, respectively, with 29% as the polyglutamate metabolite.

In the case described above, chromosome analysis of the newborn revealed a normal karyotype (46,XX), but with gaps and a ring chromosome (14). The clinical significance of these findings is unknown, but because these abnormalities may persist for several years, the potential existed for an increased risk of cancer as well as for a risk of genetic damage in the next generation (14).

Successful pregnancies have followed the use of methotrexate prior to conception (13, 17, 19, 20, 23–29). Apparently, ovarian and testicular dysfunction are reversible (22, 30–33). Two studies, one in 1984 and one in 1988, both involving women treated for gestational trophoblastic neoplasms, have analyzed reproductive function after methotrexate therapy and are described below (29, 34).

In 438 long-term survivors treated with chemotherapy between 1958–1978, 436 received methotrexate either alone or in combination with other antineoplastic agents (29). This report was a continuation of a brief 1979 correspondence that discussed some of the same patients (17). The mean duration of chemotherapy was 4 months with a mean interval from completion of therapy to the first pregnancy of 2.7 years. Conception occurred within 1 year of therapy completion in 45 women, resulting in 31 live births, one anencephalic stillbirth, seven spontaneous abortions, and six elective abortions. Of the 436 women, 187 (43%) had at least one live birth (numbers given in parentheses refer to mean/maximum methotrexate dose in grams when used alone; mean/maximum dose in grams when used in combination) (1.26/6.0; 1.22/6.8), 23 (5%) had no live births (1.56/2.6; 1.33/6.5), 7 (2%) failed to conceive (1.30/1.6; 1.95/4.5), and 219 (50%) did not try to conceive (1.10/2.0; 2.20/34.5). The average ages at the end of treatment in the four groups were 24.9, 24.4, 24.4, and 31.5 years, respectively. Congenital abnormalities noted were anencephaly (two), spina bifida (one), tetralogy of Fallot (one), talipes equinovarus (one), collapsed lung (one), umbilical hernia (one), desquamative fibrosing alveolitis (one; same case as described above), asymptomatic heart murmur (one), and mental retardation (one). An eleventh child had tachycardia but developed normally after treatment. One case of sudden infant death syndrome occurred in a female infant at 4 weeks of age. None of these outcomes differed statistically from that expected in a normal population (29).

The 1988 report described the reproductive results of 265 women who had been treated from 1959–1980 for gestational trophoblastic disease (34). Single agent chemotherapy was administered to 91 women, only two of whom received methotrexate. Sequential (single agent) and combination therapy were administered to 67 and 107 women, respectively, but the individual agents used were not specified. Further details of this study are provided in the monograph for mercaptopurine (see Mercaptopurine).

The long-term effects of combination chemotherapy on menstrual and reproductive function have also been described in women treated for malignant ovarian germ cell tumors (35). Only two of the 40 women treated received methotrexate. The results of this study are discussed in the monograph for cyclophosphamide (see Cyclophosphamide).

A 34-year-old man, being treated with oral methotrexate for Reiter's syndrome, fathered a normal full-term female infant (36). The man had been receiving intermittent treatment with the drug for approximately 5 years and continuously for 5 months prior to conception.

Occupational exposure of the mother to antineoplastic agents during pregnancy may present a risk to the fetus. A position statement from the National Study Commission on Cytotoxic Exposure and a research article involving some antineoplastic agents are presented in the monograph for cyclophosphamide (see Cyclophosphamide).

Breast Feeding Summary

Methotrexate is excreted into breast milk in low concentrations (37). After a dose of 22.5 mg/day, milk concentrations of 6×10^{-9} M (0.26 μg/dl) have been measured with a milk:plasma ratio of 0.08. The significance of this small amount is not known. However, because the drug may accumulate in neonatal tissues, breast feeding is not recommended. The American Academy of Pediatrics considers methotrexate to be contraindicated during breast feeding because of several potential problems, including immune suppression, neutropenia, adverse effects on growth, and carcinogenesis (38).

References

1. Nicholson HO. Cytotoxic drugs in pregnancy: review of reported cases. J Obstet Gynaecol Br Commonw 1968;75:307–12.
2. Milunsky A, Graef JW, Gaynor MF. Methotrexate-induced congenital malformations. J Pediatr 1968;72:790–5.
3. Powell HR, Ekert H. Methotrexate-induced congenital malformations. Med J Aust 1971;2:1076–7.
4. Pizzuto J, Aviles A, Noriega L, Niz J, Morales M, Romero F. Treatment of acute leukemia during pregnancy: presentation of nine cases. Cancer Treat Rep 1980;64:679–83.
5. Dara P, Slater LM, Armentrout SA. Successful pregnancy during chemotherapy for acute leukemia. Cancer 1981;47:845–6.
6. Warkany J. Teratogenicity of folic acid antagonists. Cancer Bull 1981;33:76–7.
7. Burnier AM. Discussion. In Plows CW. Acute myelomonocytic leukemia in pregnancy: report of a case. Am J Obstet Gynecol 1982;143:41–3.
8. Khurshid M, Saleem M. Acute leukaemia in pregnancy. Lancet 1978;2:534–5.
9. Okun DB, Groncy PK, Sieger L, Tanaka KR. Acute leukemia in pregnancy: transient neonatal myelosuppression after combination chemotherapy in the mother. Med Pediatr Oncol 1979;7:315–9.
10. Doney KC, Kraemer KG, Shepard TH. Combination chemotherapy for acute myelocytic leukemia during pregnancy: three case reports. Cancer Treat Rep 1979;63:369–71.
11. Karp GI, von Oeyen P, Valone F, Khetarpal VK, Israel M, Mayer RJ, Frigoletto FD, Garnick MB. Doxorubicin in pregnancy; possible transplacental passage. Cancer Treat Rep 1983;67:773–7.
12. Feliu J, Juarez S, Ordonez A, Garcia-Paredes ML, Gonzalez-Baron M, Montero JM. Acute leukemia and pregnancy. Cancer 1988;61:580–4.
13. Turchi JJ, Villasis C. Anthracyclines in the treatment of malignancy in pregnancy. Cancer 1988;61:435–40.
14. Schleuning M, Clemm C. Chromosomal aberrations in a newborn whose mother received cytotoxic treatment during pregnancy. N Engl J Med 1987;317:1666–7.
15. Frenkel EP, Meyers MC. Acute leukemia and pregnancy. Ann Intern Med 1960;53:656–71.
16. Coopland AT, Friesen WJ, Galbraith PA. Acute leukemia in pregnancy. Am J Obstet Gynecol 1969;105:1288–9.
17. Walden PAM, Bagshawe KD. Pregnancies after chemotherapy for gestational trophoblastic tumours. Lancet 1979;2:1241.
18. Charache S, Condit PT, Humphreys SR. Studies on the folic acid vitamins. IV. The persistence of amethopterin in mammalian tissues. Cancer 1960;13:236–40.
19. Barnes AB, Link DA. Childhood dermatomyositis and pregnancy. Am J Obstet Gynecol 1983;146:335–6.
20. Sivanesaratnam V, Sen DK. Normal pregnancy after successful treatment of choriocarcinoma with cerebral metastases: a case report. J Reprod Med 1988;33:402–3.
21. Dobbing J. Pregnancy and leukaemia. Lancet 1977;1:1155.
22. Schilsky RL, Lewis BJ, Sherins RJ, Young RC. Gonadal dysfunction in patients receiving chemotherapy for cancer. Ann Intern Med 1980;93:109–14.
23. Bacon C, Kernahan J. Successful pregnancy in acute leukaemia. Lancet 1975;2:515.
24. Wegelius R. Successful pregnancy in acute leukaemia. Lancet 1975;2:1301.
25. Ross GT. Congenital anomalies among children born of mothers receiving chemotherapy for gestational trophoblastic neoplasms. Cancer 1976;37:1043–7.
26. Gasser C. Long-term survival (cures) in childhood acute leukemia. Paediatrician 1980;9:344–57.
27. Sanz MA, Rafecas FJ. Successful pregnancy during chemotherapy for acute promyelocytic leukemia. N Engl J Med 1982;306:939.
28. Deeg HJ, Kennedy MS, Sanders JE, Thomas ED, Storb R. Successful pregnancy after marrow transplantation for severe aplastic anemia and immunosuppression with cyclosporine. JAMA 1983;250:647.

29. Rustin GJS, Booth M, Dent J, Salt S, Rustin F, Bagshawe KD. Pregnancy after cytotoxic chemotherapy for gestational trophoblastic tumours. Br Med J 1984;288:103–6.
30. Hinkes E, Plotkin D. Reversible drug-induced sterility in a patient with acute leukemia. JAMA 1973;223:1490–1.
31. Sherins RJ, DeVita VT Jr. Effect of drug treatment for lymphoma on male reproductive capacity. Ann Intern Med 1973;79:216–20.
32. Lendon M, Palmer MK, Hann IM, Shalet SM, Jones PHM. Testicular histology after combination chemotherapy in childhood for acute lymphoblastic leukaemia. Lancet 1978;2:439–41.
33. Evenson DP, Arlin Z, Welt S, Claps ML, Melamed MR. Male reproductive capacity may recover following drug treatment with the L-10 protocol for acute lymphocytic leukemia. Cancer 1984;53:30–6.
34. Song H, Wu P, Wang Y, Yang X, Dong S. Pregnancy outcomes after successful chemotherapy for choriocarcinoma and invasive mole: long-term follow-up. Am J Obstet Gynecol 1988;158:538–45.
35. Gershenson DM. Menstrual and reproductive function after treatment with combination chemotherapy for malignant ovarian germ cell tumors. J Clin Oncol 1988;6:270–5.
36. Perry WH. Methotrexate and teratogenesis. Arch Dermatol 1983;119:874.
37. Johns DG, Rutherford LD, Keighton PC, Vogel CL. Secretion of methotrexate into human milk. Am J Obstet Gynecol 1972;112:978–80.
38. Committee on Drugs, American Academy of Pediatrics. Transfer of drugs and other chemicals into human milk. Pediatrics 1989;84:924–36.

Name: **METHOTRIMEPRAZINE**

Class: **Sedative/Analgesic**   Risk Factor: **C**

Fetal Risk Summary

Methotrimeprazine, a propylamino phenothiazine in the same class as chlorpromazine, is used primarily as a sedative and analgesic. Although specific data are not available, other phenothiazines readily cross the placenta and methotrimeprazine should be expected to enter the fetus.

Methotrimeprazine has been used for obstetric analgesia (1, 2). The drug does not affect the force, duration, and frequency of uterine contractions nor does it affect fetal heart tones (1, 2). The manufacturer, however, has unsubstantiated data on file that methotrimeprazine may increase the rate of cervical dilation (2). No adverse effects were observed in over 800 newborns exposed to the drug during labor (2).

In a prospective study that compared 315 women consuming phenothiazines during the 1st trimester with 11,099 nonexposed controls, malformations were observed in 11 exposed infants (3.5%) vs. 178 controls (1.6%) ($p < 0.01$) (3). In the phenothiazine group, methotrimeprazine was taken by 18 women, 2 of whom delivered children with defects, one with hydrocephalus and one with a cardiac malformation (type not specified).

A cause-and-effect relationship between methotrimeprazine and the defects cannot be determined from this study. However, other phenothiazines are generally considered safe for both mother and fetus if used occasionally in low doses (e.g., see Chlorpromazine) and methotrimeprazine can probably be classified similarly. Other reviewers have also concluded that the phenothiazines are not teratogenic (4, 5).

Breast Feeding Summary

No data are available.

References

1. DeKornfeld TJ, Pearson JW, Lasagna L. Methotrimeprazine in the treatment of labor pain. N Engl J Med 1964;270:391–4.
2. Levoprome: methotrimeprazine parenteral. Lederle Laboratories, December 1966:15.
3. Rumeau-Rouquette C, Goujard J, Huel G. Possible teratogenic effect of phenothiazines in human beings. Teratology 1976;15:57–64.
4. Ayd FJ Jr. Children born of mothers treated with chlorpromazine during pregnancy. Clin Med 1964;71:1758–63.
5. Ananth J. Congenital malformations with psychopharmacologic agents. Compr Psychiatry 1975;16:437–45.

Name: **METHOXAMINE**

Class: **Sympathomimetic**   Risk Factor: **C$_M$**

Fetal Risk Summary

Methoxamine is a sympathomimetic used in emergency situations to treat hypotension. Because of the nature of its indications, experience in pregnancy with methoxamine is limited. Uterine vessels are normally maximally dilated and they have only α-adrenergic receptors (1). Use of the predominantly α-adrenergic stimulant, methoxamine, could cause constriction of these vessels and reduce uterine blood flow, thereby producing fetal hypoxia and bradycardia. Methoxamine may also interact with oxytocics or ergot derivatives to produce severe persistent maternal hypertension (1). Rupture of a cerebral vessel is possible. If a pressor agent is indicated, other drugs, such as ephedrine, should be considered.

Breast Feeding Summary

No data are available.

Reference

1. Smith NT, Corbascio AN. The use and misuse of pressor agents. Anesthesiology 1970;33:58–101.

Name: **METHSCOPOLAMINE**

Class: **Parasympatholytic (Anticholinergic)**   Risk Factor: **C**

Fetal Risk Summary

Methscopolamine is an anticholinergic quaternary ammonium bromide derivative of scopolamine (see also Scopolamine). In a large prospective study, 2323 patients were exposed to this class of drugs during the 1st trimester, two of whom took methscopolamine (1). A possible association was found between the total group and minor malformations.

Breast Feeding Summary

No data are available (see also Atropine).

Reference

1. Heinonen OP, Slone D, Shapiro S. *Birth Defects and Drugs in Pregnancy*. Littleton:Publishing Sciences Group, 1977:346–53.

Name: **METHSUXIMIDE**

Class: **Anticonvulsant**   Risk Factor: **C**

Fetal Risk Summary

Methsuximide is a succinimide anticonvulsant used in the treatment of petit mal epilepsy. The use of methsuximide during the 1st trimester has been reported in only five pregnancies (1, 2). No evidence of adverse fetal effects was found. Methsuximide has a much lower teratogenic potential than the oxazolidinedione class of anticonvulsants (see Trimethadione) (3, 4). The succinimide anticonvulsants should be considered the anticonvulsants of choice for the treatment of petit mal epilepsy during the 1st trimester (see Ethosuximide).

Breast Feeding Summary

No data are available.

References

1. Annegers JF, Elveback LR, Hauser WA, Kurland LT. Do anticonvulsants have a teratogenic effect? Arch Neurol 1974;31:364–73.
2. Heinonen OP, Slone D, Shapiro S. *Birth Defects and Drugs in Pregnancy*. Littleton:Publishing Sciences Group, 1977:358–9.
3. Fabro S, Brown NA. Teratogenic potential of anticonvulsants. N Engl J Med 1979;300:1280–1.
4. The National Institutes of Health. Anticonvulsants found to have teratogenic potential. JAMA 1981;241:36.

Name: **METHYCLOTHIAZIDE**

Class: **Diuretic**   Risk Factor: **D**

Fetal Risk Summary

See Chlorothiazide.

Breast Feeding Summary

See Chlorothiazide.

Name: **METHYLDOPA**

Class: **Antihypertensive**   Risk Factor: **C**

Fetal Risk Summary

Methyldopa crosses the placenta and achieves fetal concentrations similar to the maternal serum concentration (1–3). The Collaborative Perinatal Project monitored only one mother-child pair in which 1st trimester exposure to methyldopa was recorded (4). No abnormalities were found. A decrease in intracranial volume has been reported after 1st trimester exposure to methyldopa (5, 6). Children evaluated at 4 years of age showed no association between small head size and retarded mental development (7). Review of 1157 hypertensive pregnancies demonstrated no adverse effects from methyldopa administration (8–20). A reduced systolic blood pressure of 4–5 mm Hg in 24 infants for the first 2 days after delivery has been reported (21). This mild reduction in blood pressure was not considered significant. An infant born with esophageal atresia with fistula, congenital heart disease, absent left kidney, and hypospadias was exposed to methyldopa throughout gestation (22). The mother also took clomiphene early in the 1st trimester.

Breast Feeding Summary

Methyldopa is excreted into breast milk in small amounts. In four lactating women taking 750–2000 mg/day, milk levels of free and conjugated methyldopa ranged from 0.1–0.9 μg/ml (1). A milk:plasma ratio could not be determined since simultaneous plasma levels were not obtained. The American Academy of Pediatrics considers methyldopa to be compatible with breast feeding (23).

References

1. Jones HMR, Cummings AJ. A study of the transfer of α-methyldopa to the human foetus and newborn infant. Br J Clin Pharmacol 1978;6:432–4.
2. Jones HMR, Cummings AJ, Setchell KDR, Lawson AM. Pharmacokinetics of methyldopa in neonates. Br J Clin Pharmacol 1979;8:433–40.
3. Cummings AJ, Whitelaw AGL. A study of conjugation and drug elimination in the human neonate. Br J Clin Pharmacol 1981;12:511–5.
4. Heinonen OP, Slone D, Shapiro S. *Birth Defects and Drugs in Pregnancy*. Littleton:Publishing Sciences Group, 1977:372.
5. Myerscough PR. Infant growth and development after treatment of maternal hypertension. Lancet 1980;1:883.
6. Moar VA, Jefferies MA, Mutch LMM, Dunsted MK, Redman CWG. Neonatal head circumference and the treatment of maternal hypertension. Br J Obstet Gynaecol 1978;85:933–7.
7. Dunsted M, Moar VA, Redman CWG. Infant growth and development following treatment of maternal hypertension. Lancet 1980;1:705.
8. Redman CWG, Beilin LJ, Bonnar J, Ounsted MK. Fetal outcome in trial of antihypertensive treatment in pregnancy. Lancet 1976;2:753–6.
9. Hamilton M, Kopelman H. Treatment of severe hypertension with methyldopa. Br Med J 1963;1:151–5.
10. Abramowsky CR, Vegas ME, Swinehart G, Gyves MT. Decidual vasculopathy of the placenta in lupus erythematosus. N Engl J Med 1980;303:668–72.
11. Gallery EDM, Sounders DM, Hunyor SN, Gyory AZ. Randomised comparison of methyldopa and oxprenolol for treatment of hypertension in pregnancy. Br Med J 1979;1:1591–4.
12. Gyory AZ, Gallery ED, Hunyor SN. Effect of treatment of maternal hypertension with oxprenolol and α-methyldopa on plasma volume, placental and birth weights. Eighth World Congress of Cardiology, Tokyo, 1978; abstract No. 1098.

13. Arias F, Zamora J. Antihypertensive treatment and pregnancy outcome in patients with mild chronic hypertension. Obstet Gynecol 1979;53:489–94.

14. Redman CWG, Beilin LJ, Bonnar J. A trial of hypotensive treatment in pregnancy. Clin Sci Mol Med 1975;49:3–4.

15. Tcherdakoff P, Milliez P. Traitement de l'hypertension arterielle par alphamethyldopa au cours de lo grossesse. Proc Premier Symposium National, Hypertension Arterielle, Cannes, 1970:207–9.

16. Lselve A, Berger R, Vial JY, Gaillard MF. Alpha-methyldopa/Aldomet and reserpine/Serpasil: treatment of pregnancy hypertensions. J Med Lyon 1968;1369–75.

17. Leather HM, Humphreys DM, Baker P, Chadd MA. A controlled trial of hypotensive agents in hypertension in pregnancy. Lancet 1968;2:488–90.

18. Hamilton H. Some aspects of the long-term treatment of severe hypertension with methyldopa. Postgrad Med J 1968;44:66–9.

19. Skacel K, Sklendvsky A, Gazarek F, Matlocha Z, Mohapl M. Therapeutic use of alpha-methyldopa in cases of late toxemia of pregnancy. Cesk Gynecol 1967;32:78–80.

20. Kincaid-Smith P, Bullen M. Prolonged use of methyldopa in severe hypertension in pregnancy. Br Med J 1966;1:274–6.

21. Whitelaw A. Maternal methyldopa treatment and neonatal blood pressure. Br Med J 1981;283:471.

22. Ylikorkala O. Congenital anomalies and clomiphene. Lancet 1975;2:1262–3.

23. Committee on Drugs, American Academy of Pediatrics. Transfer of drugs and other chemicals into human milk. Pediatrics 1989;84:924–36.

Name: METHYLENE BLUE

Class: **Urinary Germicide/Diagnostic Dye**   Risk Factor: **C*M**

Fetal Risk Summary

Methylene blue may be administered orally for its weak urinary germicide properties or injected into the amniotic fluid to diagnose premature rupture of the membranes. For oral dosing, nine exposures in the 1st trimester have been reported (1, p. 299). No congenital abnormalities were observed. For use anytime during pregnancy, 46 exposures were reported (1, pp. 434–435). A possible association with malformations was found, but the statistical significance is not known.

Diagnostic intra-amniotic injection of methylene blue has resulted in hemolytic anemia, hyperbilirubinemia, and methemoglobinemia in the newborn (2–10). Doses of the dye in most reports ranged from 10–70 mg, but in one case, 200 mg were injected into the amniotic cavity (7). Deep blue staining of the newborn may occur after injection of the agent into the amniotic fluid (7–9). One author suggested that smaller doses, such as 1.6 mg, would be adequate to confirm the presence of ruptured membranes without causing hemolysis (2).

In a 1989 report, 1 ml of a 1% solution (10 mg) was used to diagnose suspected membrane rupture in a woman with premature labor at 26 weeks of gestation (11). A 920-g girl was born 18 hours later who was stained a deep blue. The clinical assessment of hypoxia was impaired by the skin color as was pulse oximetry. A transcutaneous oxygen monitor was eventually used to measure arterial blood gas so that ventilator therapy could be regulated. No evidence of hemolysis was observed. The bluish tinge persisted for more than 2 weeks in spite of frequent baths.

Inadvertent intrauterine injection in the 1st trimester has been reported (12). No adverse effects were reported in the full term neonate.

[*Risk Factor D if injected intra-amniotically.]

Breast Feeding Summary

No data are available.

References

1. Heinonen OP, Slone D, Shapiro S. *Birth Defects and Drugs in Pregnancy*. Littleton:Publishing Sciences Group, 1977.
2. Plunkett GD. Neonatal complications. Obstet Gynecol 1973;41:476–7.
3. Cowett RM, Hakanson DO, Kocon RW, Oh W. Untoward neonatal effect of intraamniotic administration of methylene blue. Obstet Gynecol 1976;48:74s–5s.
4. Kirsch IR, Cohen HJ. Heinz body hemolytic anemia from the use of methylene blue in neonates. J Pediatr 1980;96:276–8.
5. Crooks J. Haemolytic jaundice in a neonate after intra-amniotic injection of methylene blue. Arch Dis Child 1982;57:872–3.
6. McEnerney JK. McEnerney LN. Unfavorable neonatal outcome after intraamniotic injection of methylene blue. Obstet Gynecol 1983;61:35S–6S.
7. Serota FT, Bernbaum JC, Schwartz E. The methylene-blue baby. Lancet 1979;2:1142–3.
8. Vincer MJ, Allen AC, Evans JR, Nwaesei C, Stinson DA. Methylene-blue-induced hemolytic anemia in a neonate. Can Med Assoc J 1987;136:503–4.
9. Spahr RC, Salsburey DJ, Krissberg A, Prin W. Intraamniotic injection of methylene blue leading to methemoglobinemia in one of twins. Int J Gynaecol Obstet 1980;17:477–8.
10. Poinsot J, Guillois B, Margis D, Carlhant D, Boog G, Alix D. Neonatal hemolytic anemia after intra-amniotic injection of methylene blue. Arch Fr Pediatr 1988;45:657–60.
11. Troche BI. The methylene-blue baby. N Engl J Med 1989;320:1756–7.
12. Katz Z, Lancet M. Inadvertent intrauterine injection of methylene blue in early pregnancy. N Engl J Med 1981;304:1427.

Name: **METHYLPHENIDATE**

Class: **Central Stimulant**   Risk Factor: **C**

Fetal Risk Summary

No reports linking the use of methylphenidate with congenital defects have been located. The Collaborative Perinatal Project monitored 3082 mother-child pairs with exposure to sympathomimetic drugs, 11 of which were exposed to methylphenidate (1). No evidence for an increased malformation rate was found.

Breast Feeding Summary

No data are available.

Reference

1. Heinonen OP, Slone D, Shapiro S. *Birth Defects and Drugs in Pregnancy*. Littleton:Publishing Sciences Group, 1977:346–7.

Name: **METOCLOPRAMIDE**

Class: **Antiemetic**   Risk Factor: **B$_M$**

Fetal Risk Summary

Metoclopramide has been used during pregnancy as an antiemetic and to decrease gastric emptying time (1–19). No congenital malformations or other fetal/newborn adverse effects have been observed. Except for the one study noted below, long-term evaluation of infants exposed *in utero* to metoclopramide has not been reported.

Metoclopramide crosses the placenta at term (1–3). Cord:maternal plasma ratios were 0.57–0.84 after intravenous doses just prior to cesarean section. Placental transfer during other stages of pregnancy has not been studied.

Four reports have described the use of metoclopramide for the treatment of nausea and vomiting occurring in early pregnancy (4–6, 19). Administration of the drug in two of these studies began at 7–8 weeks' gestation (4, 5). The exact timing of pregnancy was not specified in the third report. Daily doses ranged between 10–60 mg. Metoclopramide was as effective as other antiemetics for this indication and superior to placebo (7, 8). Normal infant development for up to 4 years was mentioned in one study, but no details were provided (6).

In a fourth case of metoclopramide use for nausea and vomiting, the drug was started at 10 weeks' gestation (19). Dosage was not specified. At 18 weeks, after 8 weeks of therapy, the patient developed a neuropsychiatric syndrome with acute asymmetrical axonal motor-sensory polyneuropathy and marked anxiety, depression, irritability, and memory and concentration difficulties (19). Acute porphyria was diagnosed based on the presence of increased porphyrin precursors in the patient's urine. Metoclopramide was discontinued and the patient was treated with a high-carbohydrate diet. Eventually, a normal, 3500-g infant was delivered at term. The woman recovered except for slight residual weakness in the lower extremities. The investigators speculated that the pregnancy itself, the starvation, the drug, or a combination of these may have precipitated the acute attack (19).

Several studies have examined the effect of metoclopramide on gastric emptying time during labor for the prevention of Mendelson's syndrome (i.e., pulmonary aspiration of acid gastric contents and resulting chemical pneumonitis and pulmonary edema) (1, 3, 9–15). Gastroesophageal reflux was decreased as was the gastric emptying time. The drug was effective in preventing vomiting during anesthesia. No effects were noted on the course of labor or the fetus. Apgar scores and results of neurobehavioral tests did not differ from those of controls (1, 3, 9, 15) nor did newborn heart rates or blood pressures (1).

The effect of metoclopramide on maternal and fetal prolactin secretion during pregnancy and labor has been studied (2, 16, 17). The drug is a potent stimulator of prolactin release from the anterior pituitary by antagonism of hypothalamic dopaminergic receptors. However, transplacentally acquired metoclopramide did not cause an increased prolactin release from the fetal pituitary nor did maternal prolactin cross the placenta to the fetus (2, 16). In another study, 10 mg of intravenous metoclopramide administered during labor did not affect the levels of maternal or fetal thyroid-stimulating hormone or thyroid hormones (18).

Breast Feeding Summary

Metoclopramide is excreted into human breast milk. Accumulation, due to ion trapping of the drug in the more acidic (as compared to plasma) milk, occurs with milk:plasma ratios of 1.8–1.9 after steady-state conditions are reached (20–22).

Several studies have examined the effect of metoclopramide as a lactation stimulant in women with inadequate or decreased milk production (20–30). One study involved 23 women who had delivered prematurely (mean gestational length, 30.4 weeks) (30). The drug, by stimulating the release of prolactin from the anterior pituitary, was effective in increasing milk production with doses of 20–45 mg/day (8, 21–30). Doses of 15 mg/day were not effective (26). In one study, metoclopramide caused a shift in the amino acid composition of milk, suggesting an enhanced rate of transition from colostrum to mature milk (27). No effect on the serum levels of prolactin, thyroid-stimulating hormone, or free thyroxin was observed in nursing infants in a 1985 study of 11 women with lactational insufficiency (28).

The total daily dose that would be consumed by a nursing infant during the maternal use of 30 mg/day has been estimated to be 1–45 μg/kg/day (20–22). This is much less the maximum daily dose of 500 μg/kg recommended in infants (8) or the 100 μg/kg/day dosage that has been given to premature infants (31). Metoclopramide was detected in the plasma of one of five infants whose mothers were taking 10 mg three times daily (21, 22). Adverse effects have been observed in only two infants—both with mild intestinal discomfort (25, 26). In one case the mother was consuming 30 mg/day (25) and in the other, 45 mg/day (26).

In summary, metoclopramide apparently does not present a risk to the nursing infant with maternal doses of 45 mg/day or less. One review has stated that the drug should not be used during breast feeding because of the potential risks to the neonate (32), but there are no published studies to substantiate this caution. Although no adverse effects in the nursing infant have been reported, the American Academy of Pediatrics considers the use of metoclopramide during lactation to be of concern because of the potent central nervous system effects that the drug is capable of producing (33).

References

1. Bylsma-Howell M, Riggs KW, McMorland GH, Rurak DW, Ongley R, McErlane B, Price JDE, Axelson JE. Placental transport of metoclopramide: assessment of maternal and neonatal effects. Can Anaesth Soc J 1983;30:487–92.
2. Arvela P, Jouppila R, Kauppila A, Pakarinen A, Pelkonen O, Tuimala R. Placental transfer and hormonal effects of metoclopramide. Eur J Clin Pharmacol 1983;24:345–8.
3. Cohen SE, Jasson J, Talafre M-L, Chauvelot-Moachon L, Barrier G. Does metoclopramide decrease the volume of gastric contents in patients undergoing cesarean section? Anesthesiology 1984;61:604–7.
4. Lyonnet R, Lucchini G. Metoclopramide in obstetrics. J Med Chir Prat 1967;138:352–5.
5. Sidhu MS, Lean TH. The use of metoclopramide (Maxolon) in hyperemesis gravidarum. Proc Obset Gynaecol Soc Singapore 1970;1:1–4.
6. Martynshin MYA, Arkhengel'skii AE. Experience in treating early toxicoses of pregnancy with metoclopramide. Akush Ginekol 1981;57:44–5.
7. Pinder RM, Brogden RN, Sawyer PR, Speight TM, Avery GS. Metoclopramide: a review of its pharmacological properties and clinical use. Drugs 1976;12:81–131.
8. Harrington RA, Hamilton CW, Brogden RN, Linkewich JA, Romankiewicz JA, Heel RC. Metoclopramide: an update review of its pharmacological properties and clinical use. Drugs 1983;25:451–94.

9. McGarry JM. A double-blind comparison of the anti-emetic effect during labour of metoclopramide and perphenazine. Br J Anaesth 1971;43:613–5.
10. Howard FA, Sharp DS. Effect of metoclopramide on gastric emptying during labour. Br Med J 1973;1:446–8.
11. Brock-Utne JG, Dow TGB, Welman S, Dimopoulos GE, Moshal MG. The effect of metoclopramide on the lower oesophageal sphincter in late pregnancy. Anaesth Intensive Care 1978;6:26–9.
12. Hey VMF, Ostick DG. Metoclopramide and the gastro-oesophageal sphincter. Anaesthesia 1978;33:462–5.
13. Feeney JG. Heartburn in pregnancy. Br Med J 1982;284:1138–9.
14. Murphy DF, Nally B, Gardiner J, Unwin A. Effect of metoclopramide on gastric emptying before elective and emergency caesarean section. Br J Anaesth 1984;56:1113–6.
15. Vella L, Francis D, Houlton P, Reynolds F. Comparison of the antiemetics metoclopramide and promethazine in labour. Br Med J 1985;290:1173–5.
16. Messinis IE, Lolis DE, Dalkalitsis N, Kanaris C, Souvatzoglou A. Effect of metoclopramide on maternal and fetal prolactin secretion during labor. Obstet Gynecol 1982;60:686–8.
17. Bohnet HG, Kato K. Prolactin secretion during pregnancy and puerperium: response to metoclopramide and interactions with placental hormones. Obstet Gynecol 1985;65:789–92.
18. Roti E, Robuschi G, Emanuele R, d'Amato L, Gnudi A, Fatone M, Benassi L, Foscolo MS, Gualerzi C, Braverman LE. Failure of metoclopramide to affect thyrotropin concentration in the term human fetus. J Clin Endocrinol Metab 1983;56:1071–5.
19. Milo R, Neuman M, Klein C, Caspi E, Arlazoroff A. Acute intermittent porphyria in pregnancy. Obstet Gynecol 1989;73:450–2.
20. Lewis PJ, Devenish C, Kahn C. Controlled trial of metoclopramide in the initiation of breast feeding. Br J Clin Pharmacol 1980;9:217,219.
21. Pelkonen O, Arvela P, Kauppila A, Koivisto M, Kivinen S, Ylikorkala O. Metoclopramide in breast milk and newborn. Acta Physiol Scand 1982;(Suppl 502):62 (Abstract).
22. Kauppila A, Arvela P, Koivisto M, Kivinen S, Ylikorkala O, Pelkonen O. Metoclopramide and breast feeding: transfer into milk and the newborn. Eur J Clin Pharmacol 1983;25:819–23.
23. Sousa PLR. Metoclopramide and breast-feeding. Br Med J 1975;1:512.
24. Guzman V, Toscano G, Canales ES, Zarate A. Improvement of defective lactation by using oral metoclopramide. Acta Obstet Gynecol Scand 1979;58:53–5.
25. Kauppila A, Kivinen S, Ylikorkala O. Metoclopramide increases prolactin release and milk secretion in puerperium without stimulating the secretion of thyrotropin and thyroid hormones. J Clin Endocrinol Metab 1981;52:436–9.
26. Kauppila A, Kivinen S, Ylikorkala O. A dose response relation between improved lactation and metoclopramide. Lancet 1981;1:1175–7.
27. de Gezelle H, Ooghe W, Thiery M, Dhont M. Metoclopramide and breast milk. Eur J Obstet Gynecol Reprod Biol 1983;15:31–6.
28. Kauppila A, Anunti P, Kivinen S, Koivisto M, Ruokonen A. Metoclopramide and breast feeding: efficacy and anterior pituitary responses of the mother and the child. Eur J Obstet Gynecol Reprod Biol 1985;19:19–22.
29. Gupta AP, Gupta PK. Metoclopramide as a lactogogue. Clin Pediatr 1985;24:269–72.
30. Ehrenkranz RA, Ackerman BA. Metoclopramide effect on faltering milk production by mothers of premature infants. Pediatrics 1986;78:614–20.
31. Sankaran K, Yeboah E, Bingham WT, Ninan A. Use of metoclopramide in preterm infants. Dev Pharmacol Ther 1982;5:114–9.
32. Lewis JH, Weingold AB, The Committee on FDA-Related Matters, American College of Gastroenterology. The use of gastrointestinal drugs during pregnancy and lactation. Am J Gastroenterol 1985;80:912–23.
33. Committee on Drugs, American Academy of Pediatrics. Transfer of drugs and other chemicals into human milk. Pediatrics 1989;84:924–36.

Name: **METOLAZONE**

Class: **Diuretic** Risk Factor: **D**

Fetal Risk Summary

Metolazone is structurally related to the thiazide diuretics. See Chlorothiazide.

Breast Feeding Summary

See Chlorothiazide.

Name: **METOPROLOL**

Class: **Sympatholytic (β-Adrenergic Blocker)** Risk Factor: **B$_M$**

Fetal Risk Summary

Metoprolol, a cardioselective β-adrenergic blocking agent, has been used during pregnancy for the treatment of maternal hypertension and tachycardia (1–10). The drug readily crosses the placenta, producing approximately equal concentrations of metoprolol in maternal and fetal serum at delivery (1–3). The serum half-lives of metoprolol determined in five women during the 3rd trimester and repeated 3–5 months after delivery were similar, 1.3 vs. 1.7 hours, respectively, but peak levels during pregnancy were only 20–40% of those measured later (4). Neonatal serum levels of metoprolol increase up to 4-fold in the first 2–5 hours after birth then decline rapidly over the next 15 hours (2, 3).

No fetal malformations attributable to metoprolol have been reported, but experience during the 1st trimester is limited. Twins, exposed throughout gestation to metoprolol 200 mg/day plus other antihypertensive agents for severe maternal hypertension, were reported to be doing well at 10 months of age (7). In a 1978 study, 101 hypertensive pregnant patients treated with metoprolol alone (57 patients) or combined with hydralazine (44 patients) were compared to 97 patients treated with hydralazine alone (1). The duration of pregnancy at the start of antihypertensive treatment was 34.1 weeks (range 13–41) for the metoprolol group and 32.5 weeks (range 12–40) for the hydralazine group. The metoprolol group experienced a lower rate of perinatal mortality (2% vs. 8%) and a lower incidence of intrauterine growth retardation (11.7% vs. 16.3%). No signs or symptoms of β-blockade were noted in the fetuses or newborns in this or other studies (1, 2, 5).

The use of metoprolol in a pregnant patient with pheochromocytoma has been reported (5). High blood pressure had been controlled with prazosin, an α-adrenergic blocking agent, but the onset of maternal tachycardia required the addition of metoprolol during the last few weeks of pregnancy. No adverse effects were observed in the newborn.

The acute effects of metoprolol on maternal hemodynamics have been studied (11). Nine women at a mean gestational age of 36.7 ± 3.0 weeks with a diagnosis of pregnancy-induced hypertension were given a single oral dose of 100 mg of metoprolol. Statistically significant ($p < 0.01$) decreases were observed in maternal heart rate, systolic and diastolic blood pressure, and cardiac output. No significant change was noted in mean blood volume or intervillous blood flow. An improvement was observed in four women for the latter parameter, but a reduction occurred in another four. The intervillous blood flow did not change in the ninth patient.

Although the use of metoprolol for maternal disease does not seem to pose a risk to the fetus, the long-term effects of *in utero* exposure to β-blockers have not been studied. Persistent β-blockade has been observed in newborns exposed near delivery to other members of this class (see Acebutolol, Atenolol, and Nadolol). Thus, newborns exposed *in utero* to metoprolol should be closely observed during the first 24–48 hours after birth for bradycardia and other symptoms.

Breast Feeding Summary

Metoprolol is concentrated in breast milk (1, 3, 12–14). Milk concentrations are approximately three times those found simultaneously in the maternal serum (reported range 2.0–3.7). No adverse effects have been observed in nursing infants exposed to metoprolol in milk. Based on calculations from a 1984 study, a mother ingesting 200 mg/day of metoprolol would only provide about 225 µg in a liter of her milk (3). To minimize this exposure even further, one reference suggested waiting 3–4 hours after a dose to breast feed (14). Although these levels are probably clinically insignificant, nursing infants should be closely observed for signs or symptoms of β-blockade. The long-term effects of exposure to β-blockers from milk have not been studied but warrant evaluation. The American Academy of Pediatrics considers the drug to be compatible with breast feeding (15).

References

1. Sandstrom B. Antihypertensive treatment with the adrenergic beta-receptor blocker metoprolol during pregnancy. Gynecol Invest 1978;9:195–204.
2. Lundborg P, Agren G, Ervik M, Lindeberg S, Sandstrom B. Disposition of metoprolol in the newborn. Br J Clin Pharmacol 1981;12:598–600.
3. Lindeberg S, Sandstrom B, Lundborg P, Regardh CG. Disposition of the adrenergic blocker metoprolol in the late-pregnant woman, the amniotic fluid, the cord blood and the neonate. Acta Obstet Gynecol Scand 1984;118(Suppl):61–4.
4. Hogstedt S, Lindberg B, Rane A. Increased oral clearance of metoprolol in pregnancy. Eur J Clin Pharmacol 1983;24:217–20.
5. Venuto R, Burstein P, Schneider R. Pheochromocytoma: antepartum diagnosis and management with tumor resection in the puerperium. Am J Obstet Gynecol 1984;150:431–2.
6. Robson DJ, Jeeva Ray MV, Storey GAC, Holt DW. Use of amiodarone during pregnancy. Postgrad Med J 1985;61:75–7.
7. Coen G, Cugini P, Gerlini G, Finistauri D, Cinotti GA. Successful treatment of long-lasting severe hypertension with captopril during a twin pregnancy. Nephron 1985;40:498–500.
8. Gallery EDM. Hypertension in pregnant women. Med J Aust 1985;143:23–7.
9. Hogstedt S, Lindeberg S, Axelsson O, Lindmark G, Rane A, Sandstrom B, Lindberg BS. A prospective controlled trial of metoprolol-hydralazine treatment in hypertension during pregnancy. Acta Obstet Gynecol Scand 1985;64:505–10.
10. Frishman WH, Chesner M. Beta-adrenergic blockers in pregnancy. Am Heart J 1988;115:147–52.
11. Suonio S, Saarikoski S, Tahvanainen K, Paakkonen A, Olkkonen H. Acute effects of dihydralazine mesylate, furosemide, and metoprolol on maternal hemodynamics in pregnancy-induced hypertension. Am J Obstet Gynecol 1985;155:122–5.
12. Sandstrom B, Regardh CG. Metoprolol excretion into breast milk. Br J Clin Pharmacol 1980;9:518–9.
13. Liedholm H, Melander A, Bitzen PO, Helm G, Lonnerholm G, Mattiasson I, Nilsson B. Accumulation of atenolol and metoprolol in human breast milk. Eur J Clin Pharmacol 1981;20:229–31.

14. Kulas J, Lunell NO, Rosing U, Steen B, Rane A. Atenolol and metoprolol. A comparison of their excretion into human breast milk. Acta Obstet Scand 1984;118(Suppl):65–9.
15. Committee on Drugs, American Academy of Pediatrics. Transfer of drugs and other chemicals into human milk. Pediatrics 1989;84;924–36.

Name: **METRIZAMIDE**

Class: **Diagnostic**   Risk Factor: **D**

Fetal Risk Summary

Metrizamide contains a high concentration of organically bound iodine. See Diatrizoate for possible effects on the fetus and newborn.

Breast Feeding Summary

Metrizamide is excreted into milk in small quantities (1). A woman was injected with 5.06 g of metrizamide into the subarachnoid space. Milk levels increased linearly with time, but only 1.1 mg (0.02%) of the dose was recovered in 44.3 hours. This amount of contrast media probably does not pose a risk to the nursing infant. The American Academy of Pediatrics considers metrizamide to be compatible with breast feeding (2).

References

1. Ilett KF, Hackett LP, Paterson JW, McCormick CC. Excretion of metrizamide in milk. Br J Radiol 1981;54:537–8.
2. Committee on Drugs, American Academy of Pediatrics. Transfer of drugs and other chemicals into human milk. Pediatrics 1989;84:924–36.

Name: **METRIZOATE**

Class: **Diagnostic**   Risk Factor: **D**

Fetal Risk Summary

Metrizoate has been used for phlebography during pregnancy for the diagnosis of deep vein thrombosis (1). Seventeen pregnant women were given either metrizoate or iothalamate at various stages of gestation. Two patients, one exposed in the 1st trimester and one in the 2nd trimester, were diagnosed as having thrombosis and were treated with heparin. While the baby of the mother exposed in the 2nd trimester was normal, the other newborn had hyperbilirubinemia and undescended testis. The relationship between the diagnostic agents and the defect is unknown.

   Use of organically bound iodine preparations near term has resulted in hypothyroidism in some newborns (see Diatrizoate). Appropriate measures should be taken to treat neonatal hypothyroidism if diagnostic tests with metrizoate are required close to delivery.

Breast Feeding Summary

See Potassium Iodide.

Reference

1. Kierkegaard A. Incidence and diagnosis of deep vein thrombosis associated with pregnancy. Acta Obstet Gynecol Scand 1983;62:239–43.

Name: **METRONIDAZOLE**

Class: **Antiprotozoal/Antibacterial**   Risk Factor: **B$_M$**

Fetal Risk Summary

Metronidazole possesses trichomonicidal and amebicidal activity as well as effectiveness against certain bacteria. The drug crosses the placenta to the fetus throughout gestation with a cord:maternal plasma ratio at term of approximately 1.0 (1–3). The pharmacokinetics of metronidazole in pregnant women have been reported (4, 5).

The use of metronidazole in pregnancy is controversial. The drug is mutagenic in bacteria and carcinogenic in rodents, and although these properties have never been shown in humans, concern for these toxicities have led some to advise against the use of metronidazole in pregnancy (6, 7). To date, no association with human cancer has been proven (7, 8).

Several studies, individual case reports, and reviews have described the safe use of metronidazole during pregnancy (9–22). Included among these is a 1972 review summarizing 20 years of experience with the drug and involving 1469 pregnant women, 206 of whom were treated during the 1st trimester (22). No association with congenital malformations, abortions, or stillbirths was found. Some investigations, however, have found an increased risk when the agent was used early in pregnancy (8, 23–25).

The Collaborative Perinatal Project monitored 50,282 mother-child pairs, 31 of which had 1st trimester exposure to metronidazole (23). A possible association with malformations was found (relative risk 2.02) based on defects in four children. The statistical significance of this finding is unknown. Independent confirmation is required to determine the actual risk. In a 1979 report, metronidazole was used in 57 pregnancies including 23 during the 1st trimester (8). Three of the 1st trimester exposures ended in spontaneous abortion (a normal incidence), and in the remaining 20 births, there were five congenital anomalies: hydrocele (two), congenital dislocated hip (female twin), metatarsus varus, and mental retardation (both parents mentally retarded). Analysis of the data is not possible because of the small numbers and possible involvement of genetic factors (8).

Two mothers, treated with metronidazole during the 5th–7th weeks of gestation for amebiasis, gave birth to infants with midline facial defects (24). Diiodohydroxyquinoline was also used in one of the pregnancies. One of the infants had holotelencephaly and one had unilateral cleft lip and palate. In another case report, a mother treated for trichomoniasis during between the 6th–7th weeks of gestation gave birth to a male infant with a cleft of the hard and soft palate, optic atrophy, a hypoplastic, short philtrum, and a Sydney crease on the left hand (25).

The mother was also taking an antiemetic medication (Bendectin) on an "as needed" basis. Chromosome analysis of the infant was normal. The relationship between metronidazole and the defects described above is unknown.

As of May 1987, the Food and Drug Administration had received reports of 27 adverse outcomes with metronidazole: spontaneous abortions (three), brain defects (six), limb defects (five), genital defects (four), unspecified defects (three), and one each of craniostenosis, peripheral neuropathy, ventricular septal defect, retinoblastoma, obstructive uropathy, and a chromosomal defect (26). In this same report, the authors, from data obtained from the Michigan Medicaid program between 1980–1983, cited 1,020 other cases where metronidazole use in the 1st trimester for treatment of vaginitis was not linked with birth defects. In an additional 63 cases, use of the agent for this indication was linked to a birth defect diagnoses. Based on these data, the estimated relative risk of a birth defect was 0.92 (95% confidence limits 0.7–1.2) (26). Of the 122 infants with oral clefts, none was exposed to metronidazole. An estimated relative risk for spontaneous abortion of 1.67 (95% confidence limits 1.4–2.0) was determined from 135 exposures among 4,264 spontaneous abortions compared to 1,020 exposures among 55,736 deliveries.

Metronidazole, which is not an animal teratogen, has been shown to markedly potentiate the fetotoxicity and teratogenicity of alcohol in mice (27). Human studies of this possible clinically significant interaction have not been reported.

In summary, the available reports have arrived at conflicting conclusions on the safety of metronidazole in pregnancy. It is not possible to assess the risk to the fetus until additional data have been collected. The long-term risks from exposure to this drug, including the potential for cancer, have not been completely evaluated. The manufacturer and the Centers for Disease Control (CDC) consider metronidazole to be contraindicated during the 1st trimester in patients with trichomoniasis (28, 29). Use for trichomoniasis during the 2nd and 3rd trimesters may be acceptable if alternate therapies have failed (28, 29). Single dose therapy should be avoided (29). For other indications, the risk:benefit ratio must be carefully weighed prior to the use of metronidazole, especially in the 1st trimester.

Breast Feeding Summary

Metronidazole is excreted into breast milk. Following a single 2-g oral dose in three patients, peak milk concentrations in the 50–60 µg/ml range were measured at 2–4 hours (30). With normal breast feeding, infants would have received about 25 mg of metronidazole over the next 48 hours. By interrupting feedings for 12 hours, infant exposure to the drug would have been reduced to 9.8 mg, or 3.5 mg if feeding had been stopped for 24 hours (30).

In women treated with divided oral doses of either 600 or 1200 mg/day, the mean milk levels were 5.7 and 14.4 µg/ml, respectively (31). The milk:plasma ratios in both groups were approximately 1.0. The mean plasma concentrations in the exposed infants were about 20% of the maternal plasma drug level. Eight women treated with metronidazole rectal suppositories, 1 g every 8 hours, produced a mean milk drug level of 10 µg/ml with maximum concentrations of 25 µg/ml (32).

One report described diarrhea and secondary lactose intolerance in a breast-fed infant whose mother was receiving metronidazole (33). The relationship between the drug and the events is unknown. Except for this one case, no reports of adverse effects in metronidazole-exposed nursing infants have been located. However, since the drug is mutagenic and carcinogenic in some test species (see Fetal Risk Summary), unnecessary exposure to metronidazole should be avoided. A single, 2-g oral dose has been recommended by the Centers for Disease Control if metronidazole is used for trichomoniasis during lactation (28). If this dose is given, the American Academy of Pediatrics recommends discontinuing breast feeding for 12–24 hours to allow excretion of the drug (34).

References

1. Amon K, Amon I, Huller H. Maternal-fetal passage of metronidazole. In *Advances in Antimicrobial and Antineoplastic Chemotherapy*. Proceedings of the VII International Congress of Chemotherapy, Prague, 1971:113–5.
2. Heisterberg L. Placental transfer of metronidazole in the first trimester of pregnancy. J Perinat Med 1984;12:43–5.
3. Karhunen M. Placental transfer of metronidazole and tinidazole in early human pregnancy after a single infusion. Br J Clin Pharmacol 1984;18:254–7.
4. Amon I, Amon K, Franke G, Mohr C. Pharmacokinetics of metronidazole in pregnant women. Chemotherapy 1981;27:73–9.
5. Visser AA, Hundt HKL. The pharmacokinetics of a single intravenous dose of metronidazole in pregnant patients. J Antimicrob Chemother 1984;13:279–83.
6. Anonymous. Is Flagyl dangerous? Med Lett Drugs Ther 1975;17:53–4.
7. Finegold SM. Metronidazole. Ann Intern Med 1980;93:585–7.
8. Beard CM, Noller KL, O'Fallon WM, Kurland LT, Dockerty MB. Lack of evidence for cancer due to use of metronidazole. N Engl J Med 1979;301:519–22.
9. Gray MS. Trichomonas vaginalis in pregnancy: the results of metronidazole therapy on the mother and child. J Obstet Gynaecol Br Commonw 1961;68:723–9.
10. Robinson SC, Johnston DW. Observations on vaginal trichomoniasis. II. Treatment with metronidazole. Can Med Assoc J 1961;85:1094–6.
11. Luthra R, Boyd JR. The treatment of trichomoniasis with metronidazole. Am J Obstet Gynecol 1962;83:1288–93.
12. Schram M, Kleinman H. Use of metronidazole in the treatment of trichomoniasis. Am J Obstet Gynecol 1962;83:1284–7.
13. Andrews MC, Andrews WC. Systemic treatment of trichomonas vaginitis. South Med J 1963;56:1214–8.
14. Zacharias LF, Salzer RB, Gunn JC, Dierksheide EB. Trichomoniasis and metronidazole. Am J Obstet Gynecol 1963;86:748–52.
15. Kotcher E, Frick CA, Giesel LO, Jr. The effect of metronidazole on vaginal microbiology and maternal and neonatal hematology. Am J Obstet Gynecol 1964;88:184–9.
16. Scott-Gray M. Metronidazole in obstetric practice. J Obstet Gynaecol Br Commonw 1964;71:82–5.
17. Perl G. Metronidazole treatment of trichomoniasis in pregnancy. Obstet Gynecol 1965;25:273–6.
18. Peterson WF, Stauch JE, Ryder CD. Metronidazole in pregnancy. Am J Obstet Gynecol 1966;94:343–9.
19. Robinson SC, Mirchandani G. Trichomonas vaginalis. V. Further observations on metronidazole (Flagyl) (including infant follow-up). Am J Obstet Gynecol 1965;93:502–5.
20. Mitchell RW, Teare AJ. Amoebic liver abscess in pregnancy. Case reports. Br J Obstet Gynaecol 1984;91:393–5.
21. Morgan I. Metronidazole treatment in pregnancy. Int J Gynaecol Obstet 1978;15:501–2.
22. Berget A, Weber T. Metronidazole and pregnancy. Ugeskr Laeger 1972;134:2085–9. As cited in Shepard TH. *Catalog of Teratogenic Agents*, 3rd ed. Baltimore:Johns Hopkins University Press, 1980:228.
23. Heinonen OP, Slone D, Shapiro S. *Birth Defects and Drugs in Pregnancy*. Littleton:Publishing Sciences Group, 1977:298, 299, 302.
24. Cantu JM, Garcia-Cruz D. Midline facial defect as a teratogenic effect of metronidazole. Birth Defects 1982;18:85–8.
25. Greenberg F. Possible metronidazole teratogenicity and clefting. Am J Med Genet 1985;22:825.

26. Rosa FW, Baum C, Shaw M. Pregnancy outcomes after first-trimester vaginitis drug therapy. Obstet Gynecol 1987;69:751–5.
27. Damjanov I. Metronidazole and alcohol in pregnancy. JAMA 1986;256:472.
28. American Hospital Formulary Service. *Drug Information 1990*. Bethesda:American Society of Hospital Pharmacists, 1990:453–8.
29. Product information. Flagyl. Searle and Company, 1990.
30. Erickson SH, Oppenheim GL, Smith GH. Metronidazole in breast milk. Obstet Gynecol 1981;57:48–50.
31. Heisterberg L, Branebjerg PE. Blood and milk concentrations of metronidazole in mothers and infants. J Perinat Med 1983;11:114–20.
32. Moore B, Collier J. Drugs and breast-feeding. Br Med J 1979;2:211.
33. Clements CJ. Metronidazole and breast feeding. NZ Med J 1980;92:329.
34. Committee on Drugs, American Academy of Pediatrics. Transfer of drugs and other chemicals into human milk. Pediatrics 1989;84:924–36.

Name: **MICONAZOLE**

Class: **Antifungal Antibiotic** Risk Factor: **C$_M$**

Fetal Risk Summary

Miconazole is normally used as a topical antifungal agent. Small amounts are absorbed from the vagina (1). Use in pregnant patients with vulvovaginal candidiasis (moniliasis) has not been associated with an increase in congenital malformations (1–7). Effects following intravenous use are unknown.

In data obtained from the Michigan Medicaid program between 1980–1983, a total of 2,092 women were exposed to miconazole during the 1st trimester from a total sample of 97,775 deliveries not linked to a birth defect diagnosis (8). Of 6,564 deliveries linked to such a diagnosis, miconazole was used in 144 cases. The estimated relative risk for birth defects from these data was 1.02 (95% confidence limits 0.9–1.2). An estimated relative risk for spontaneous abortions of 1.38 (95% confidence limits 1.2–1.5) was calculated based on 250 miconazole exposures among 4,264 abortions compared with 2,236 1st trimester exposures among 55,736 deliveries (8). Moreover, no association was found between miconazole use and oral clefts, spina bifida, or cardiovascular defects. Although the relative risks for total birth defects or the three specific defects were not increased, the authors could not exclude the possibility of an association with other specific defects (8).

Breast Feeding Summary

No data are available.

References

1. Product information. Monistat. Ortho Pharmaceutical, 1990.
2. Culbertson C. Monistat: a new fungicide for treatment of vulvovaginal candidiasis. Am J Obstet Gynecol 1974;120:973–6.
3. Wade A, ed. *Martindale. The Extra Pharmacopoeia*, ed. 27. London:Pharmaceutical Press, 1977:648.
4. Davis JE, Frudenfeld JH, Goddard JL. Comparative evaluation of Monistat and Mycostatin in the treatment of vulvovaginal candidiasis. Obstet Gynecol 1974;44:403–6.

5. Wallenburg HCS, Wladimiroff JW. Recurrence of vulvovaginal candidosis during pregnancy. Comparison of miconazole vs nystatin treatment. Obstet Gynecol 1976;48:491–4.
6. McNellis D, McLeod M, Lawson J, Pasquale SA. Treatment of vulvovaginal candidiasis in pregnancy: a comparative study. Obstet Gynecol 1977;50:674–8.
7. Weisberg M. Treatment of vaginal candidiasis in pregnant women. Clin Therap 1986;8:563–7.
8. Rosa FW, Baum C, Shaw M. Pregnancy outcomes after first-trimester vaginitis drug therapy. Obstet Gynecol 1987;69:751–5.

Name: **MINERAL OIL**

Class: **Laxative**   Risk Factor: **C**

Fetal Risk Summary

Mineral oil is an emollient laxative. The drug is generally considered nonabsorbable. Chronic use may lead to decreased absorption of fat-soluble vitamins.

Breast Feeding Summary

No data are available.

Name: **MINOCYCLINE**

Class: **Antibiotic**   Risk Factor: **D**

Fetal Risk Summary

See Tetracycline.

Breast Feeding Summary

See Tetracycline.

Name: **MINOXIDIL**

Class: **Antihypertensive**   Risk Factor: **C$_M$**

Fetal Risk Summary

Minoxidil is a potent antihypertensive peripheral vasodilator. Information on its use in human pregnancy is very limited, with only four occurrences of fetal exposure located in the medical literature (1–3).

In one case, minoxidil was used throughout gestation, and no effect of this exposure was seen in the healthy newborn (1). A second case involved a mother with a history of renal artery stenosis and malignant hypertension who was treated throughout gestation with minoxidil, captopril, and propranolol (2). Three of her four previous pregnancies had ended in midgestation stillbirths. The most recent stillbirth, her fourth pregnancy, involved a 500-g male infant with low-set ears but no gross anomalies. The mother had been treated with the above regimen plus furosemide. In her second pregnancy, she had been treated only with hydrochlorothiazide, and she had delivered a normal term infant. No information was available on the first and third pregnancies, both of which ended in stillbirths. In her current pregnancy, daily doses of the three drugs were 10 mg, 50 mg, and 160 mg, respectively. The infant, delivered by cesarean section at 38 weeks' gestation, had multiple abnormalities, including an omphalocele (repaired on the 2nd day), pronounced hypertrichosis of the back and extremities, depressed nasal bridge, low-set ears, micrognathia, bilateral fifth finger clinodactyly, undescended testes, a circumferential midphallic constriction, a large ventriculoseptal defect, and a brain defect consisting of slightly prominent sulci, especially the basal cisterns and interhemispheric fissure. Growth retardation was not evident, but the weight (3170 g, 60th percentile), length (46 cm, 15th percentile), and head circumference (32.5 cm, 25th percentile) were disproportionate. Neurologic, skeletal, and kidney examinations were normal. Marked hypotension (30–50 mm Hg systolic) was present, which resolved after 24 hours. Heart rate, blood glucose, and renal function were normal. The infant's hospital course was marked by failure to thrive, congestive heart failure, prolonged physiologic jaundice, and eight episodes of hyperthermia (>38.5°C without apparent cause) between 2–6 weeks of age. The hypertrichosis, which was much less prominent at 2 months of age, is a known side effect of minoxidil therapy in both children and adults, and the condition in this infant was thought to be due to that drug (2). The etiology of the other defects could not be determined, but a chromosome abnormality was excluded based on a normal male karyotype (46X,Y) determined after a midgestation amniocentesis.

Two additional cases of *in utero* exposure to minoxidil were reported to the Food and Drug Administration and published in 1987 (3). The first infant was the product of a 32 weeks' gestation in a 22-year-old woman with severe uncontrolled renal hypertension who was treated during pregnancy with minoxidil, methyldopa, hydralazine, furosemide, and phenobarbital. The 1770-g infant died of congenital heart disease the day after delivery. Defects noted at autopsy were transposition of the great vessels and pulmonic bicuspid valvular stenosis. Hypertrichosis was not observed. No conclusions can be drawn on the etiology of the cardiac defects. The second infant, delivered near term and weighing 3220 g, was exposed throughout gestation to minoxidil (5 mg/day) plus metoprolol (100 mg/day) and prazosin (20 mg/day). The mother had severe hypertension secondary to chronic nephritis. Hypertrichosis was evident in both the mother and the newborn, but no other abnormalities were noted in the infant. The excessive hair growth, which was longest in the sacral area, gradually disappeared over the following 2–3 months. Normal development was noted at 2 years of age.

Breast Feeding Summary

Minoxidil is excreted into breast milk (1). Levels in the milk ranged from 41.7 ng/ml (1 hour) to 0.3 ng/ml (12 hours), with milk:plasma ratios during this interval varying from 0.67–1.0. No adverse effects were observed in the infant. The American Academy of Pediatrics considers minoxidil to be compatible with breast feeding (4).

References

1. Valdivieso A, Valdes G, Spiro TE, Westerman RL. Minoxidil in breast milk. Ann Intern Med 1985;102:135.
2. Kaler SG, Patrinos ME, Lambert GH, Myers TF, Karlman R, Anderson CL. Hypertrichosis and congenital anomalies associated with maternal use of minoxidil. Pediatrics 1987;79:434–6.
3. Rosa FW, Idanpaan-Heikkila J, Asanti R. Fetal minoxidil exposure. Pediatrics 1987;80:120.
4. Committee on Drugs, American Academy of Pediatrics. Transfer of drugs and other chemicals into human milk. Pediatrics 1989;84:924–36.

Name: **MOLINDONE**

Class: **Tranquilizer**   Risk Factor: **C**

Fetal Risk Summary

Molindone is an antipsychotic drug. The only reported use of it in pregnancy was in a woman who gave birth at term to normal twin boys (1). The mother had ingested 9800 mg of molindone during her 9-month pregnancy. No abnormalities in physical or mental development were noted in their first 20 years of life.

Breast Feeding Summary

No data are available.

Reference

1. Ayd FJ Jr. Moban: the first of a new class of neuroleptics. In Ayd FJ Jr., ed. *Rational Psychopharmacotherapy and the Right to Treatment*. Baltimore:Ayd Medical Communications, 1975:91–106.

Name: **MORPHINE**

Class: **Narcotic Analgesic**   Risk Factor: **B***

Fetal Risk Summary

No reports linking the therapeutic use of morphine with major congenital defects have been located. Bilateral horizontal nystagmus persisting for 1 year was reported in one addicted newborn (1). Like all narcotics, placental transfer of morphine is very rapid (2, 3). Maternal addiction with subsequent neonatal withdrawal is well known following illicit use (see also Heroin) (1, 4, 5). Morphine was widely used in labor until the 1940s, when it was largely displaced by meperidine. Clinical impressions that meperidine caused less respiratory depression in the newborn were apparently confirmed (6, 7). Other clinicians reported no difference between narcotics in the degree of neonatal depression when equianalgesic intravenous doses were used (3). Epidural use of morphine has been reported in women in labor but with unsatisfactory analgesic effects (8). The intrathecal route, however, has provided safe and effective analgesia without fetal or newborn toxicity (9–11).

The Collaborative Perinatal Project monitored 50,282 mother-child pairs, 70 of which had 1st trimester exposure to morphine (12, pp. 287–295). For use anytime during pregnancy, 448 exposures were recorded (12, p. 434). No evidence was found to suggest a relationship to large categories of major or minor malformations. A possible association with inguinal hernia (10 cases) after anytime use was observed (12, p. 484). The statistical significance of this association is unknown and independent confirmation is required.

[*Risk Factor D if used for prolonged periods or in high doses at term.]

Breast Feeding Summary

Only trace amounts of morphine enter breast milk. The significance is unknown (13–15). The American Academy of Pediatrics considers morphine to be compatible with breast feeding (16).

References

1. Perlstein MA. Congenital morphinism. A rare cause of convulsions in the newborn. JAMA 1947;135:633.
2. Fisher DE, Paton JB. The effect of maternal anesthetic and analgesic drugs on the fetus and newborn. Clin Obstet Gynaecol 1974;17:275–87.
3. Bonica JJ. *Principles and Practice of Obstetric Analgesia and Anesthesia.* Philadelphia:FA Davis, 1967:247.
4. McMullin GP, Mobarak AN. Congenital narcotic addiction. Arch Dis Child 1970;45:140–1.
5. Cobrinik RW, Hodd RT Jr, Chusid E. The effect of maternal narcotic addiction on the newborn infant. Pediatrics 1959;24:288–304.
6. Gilbert G, Dixon AB. Observations on Demerol as an obstetric analgesic. Am J Obstet Gynecol 1943;45:320–6.
7. Way WL, Costley EC, Way EL. Respiratory sensitivity of the newborn infant to meperidine and morphine. Clin Pharmacol Ther 1965;6:454–61.
8. Nybell-Lindahl G, Carlsson C, Ingemarsson I, Westgren M, Paalzow L. Maternal and fetal concentrations of morphine after epidural administration during labor. Am J Obstet Gynecol 1981;139:20–1.
9. Baraka A, Noueihid R, Hajj S. Intrathecal injection of morphine for obstetric analgesia. Anesthesiology 1981;54:136–40.
10. Bonnardot JP, Maillet M, Colau JC, Millot F, Deligne P. Maternal and fetal concentration of morphine after intrathecal administration during labour. Br J Anaesth 1982;54:487–9.
11. Brizgys RV, Shnider SM. Hyperbaric intrathecal morphine analgesia during labor in a patient with Wolff-Parkinson-White syndrome. Obstet Gynecol 1984;64:44S–6S.
12. Heinonen OP, Slone D, Shapiro S. *Birth Defects and Drugs in Pregnancy.* Littleton:Publishing Sciences Group, 1977.
13. Terwilliger WG, Hatcher RA. The elimination of morphine and quinine in human milk. Surg Gynecol Obstet 1934;58:823–6.
14. Kwit NT, Hatcher RA. Excretion of drugs in milk. Am J Dis Child 1935;49:900–4.
15. Anonymous. Drugs in breast milk. Med Lett Drugs Ther 1979;21:21–4.
16. Committee on Drugs, American Academy of Pediatrics. Transfer of drugs and other chemicals into human milk. Pediatrics 1989;84:924–36.

Name: **MOXALACTAM**

Class: **Antibiotic**   Risk Factor: **C$_M$**

Fetal Risk Summary

Moxalactam is a cephalosporin antibiotic. No controlled studies on its use in pregnancy have been located. The drug crosses the placenta to the fetus, producing a mean peak level at 1 hour in the cord blood of 38.4 μg/ml following a 1-g intravenous dose (R. Kammer, personal communication, Eli Lilly and Company, 1985). Peak amniotic fluid levels of 10.3 μg/ml occurred at 7.5 hours.

Breast Feeding Summary

Moxalactam is excreted into breast milk (1). In eight women receiving 2 g every 8 hours, mean daily concentrations of the antibiotic varied from 1.56–3.66 mg/ml, representing a daily dose of 0.86–2.01 mg. Since moxalactam is acid stable, the authors cautioned that colonization of the infant's bowel with gram-positive organisms could occur, resulting in a risk for enterocolitis (1). Due to this theoretical risk, they advised against breast feeding if the mother was being treated with moxalactam. The American Academy of Pediatrics considers moxalactam to be compatible with breast feeding (2).

References

1. Miller RD, Keegan KA, Thrupp LD, Brann J. Human breast milk concentration of moxalactam. Am J Obstet Gynecol 1984;148:348–9.
2. Committee on Drugs, American Academy of Pediatrics. Transfer of drugs and other chemicals into human milk. Pediatrics 1989;84:924–36.

Name: **NADOLOL**

Class: **Sympatholytic (β-Adrenergic Blocker)**   Risk Factor: **C$_M$**

Fetal Risk Summary

Nadolol is a nonselective β-adrenergic blocking agent used for hypertension and angina pectoris. Only one reported case of its use in pregnancy has been located (1). A mother with IgA nephropathy and hypertension was treated throughout pregnancy with nadolol, 20 mg/day, plus a diuretic (triamterene/hydrochlorothiazide) and thyroid. The infant, delivered by emergency cesarean section at 35 weeks gestation, was growth retarded and exhibited tachypnea (68 breaths/minute) and mild hypoglycemia (20 mg/100 ml). Depressed respirations (23 breaths/minute), slowed heart rate (112 beats/minute), and hypothermia (96.5°) occurred at 4.5 hours of age. The lowered body temperature responded to warming, but the cardiorespiratory depression, with brief episodes of bradycardia, persisted for 72 hours. Nadolol serum concentrations in cord blood and in the infant at 12 and 38 hours after delivery were 43, 145, and 80 ng/ml, respectively.

The etiology of some or all of the effects observed in this infant may have been β-blockade (1). However, maternal disease could not be excluded as the sole or contributing factor behind the intrauterine growth retardation and hypoglycemia (1). In addition, hydrochlorothiazide may have contributed to the low blood glucose (see Chlorothiazide).

The authors identified several characteristics of nadolol in the adult that could potentially increase its toxicity in the fetus and newborn, including a long serum half-life (17–24 hours), lack of metabolism (excreted unchanged by the kidneys), and low protein binding (30%) (1). Because of these factors, other β-blockers may be safer for use during pregnancy, although persistent β-blockade has also been observed with acebutolol and atenolol. As with other agents in this class, long-term effects of *in utero* β-blockade have not been studied but warrant evaluation.

Breast Feeding Summary

Nadolol is excreted into breast milk (1, 2). A mother taking 20 mg of nadolol/day had a concentration in her milk of 146 ng/ml 38 hours after delivery (1). In 12 lactating women ingesting 80 mg once daily for 5 days, mean steady-state levels of nadolol, approximately 357 ng/ml, were attained at 3 days. This level was approximately 4.6 times higher than simultaneously measured maternal serum levels (2). By calculation, a 5-kg infant would have received 2–7% of the adult therapeutic dose, but the infants were not allowed to breast feed (2).

Because experience is lacking, nursing infants of mothers consuming nadolol should be closely observed for symptoms of β-blockade. Long-term effects of exposure to β-blockers from milk have not been studied but warrant evaluation. The

American Academy of Pediatrics considers nadolol to be compatible with breast feeding (3).

References

1. Fox RE, Marx C, Stark AR. Neonatal effects of maternal nadolol therapy. Am J Obstet Gynecol 1985;152:1045–6.
2. Devlin RG, Duchin KL, Fleiss PM. Nadolol in human serum and breast milk. Br J Clin Pharmacol 1981;12:393–6.
3. Committee on Drugs, American Academy of Pediatrics. Transfer of drugs and other chemicals into human milk. Pediatrics 1989;84:924–36.

Name: **NAFCILLIN**

Class: **Antibiotic**   Risk Factor: **B**

Fetal Risk Summary

Nafcillin is a pencillin antibiotic (see also Pencillin G). No reports linking its use with congenital defects have been located. The Collaborative Perinatal Project monitored 50,282 mother-child pairs, 3,546 of which had 1st trimester exposure to pencillin derivatives (1, pp. 297–313). For use anytime during pregnancy, 7,171 exposures were recorded (1, p. 435). In neither case was evidence found to suggest a relationship to large categories of major or minor malformations or to individual defects.

Breast Feeding Summary

No data are available (see Pencillin G).

Reference

1. Heinonen OP, Slone D, Shapiro S. *Birth Defects and Drugs in Pregnancy*. Littleton:Publishing Sciences Group, 1977.

Name: **NALBUPHINE**

Class: **Analgesic**   Risk Factor: **B***

Fetal Risk Summary

No congenital defects have been reported in humans or in experimental animals following the use of nalbuphine in pregnancy (1). Nalbuphine has both narcotic agonist and antagonist effects. Prolonged use during pregnancy could theoretically result in fetal addiction with subsequent withdrawal in the newborn (see also Pentazocine). Use of the drug in labor produces neonatal respiratory depression comparable to that produced by meperidine (1).

Nalbuphine crosses the placenta to the fetus (2). The cord:maternal serum ratio in five women in active labor given 20 mg as an intravenous bolus ranged from 0.37–6.03. A sixth patient given 15 mg had a ratio of 1.24. Umbilical cord concentrations of nalbuphine obtained 3–10 hours after a dose varied from "not detectable" to 46 ng/ml. The terminal half-life of the drug in the mothers was 2.4 ± 0.4 hours.

A sinusoidal fetal heart rate pattern was observed after a 10-mg intravenous dose administered to a woman in labor at 42 weeks' gestation (3). The sinusoidal pattern persisted for at least 2.25 hours, and periodic late decelerations became evident. A cesarean section was performed to deliver a healthy baby girl with Apgar scores of 8 and 9 at 1 and 5 minutes, respectively. The infant did well following delivery. The authors attributed the persistent sinusoidal pattern to the prolonged plasma half-life in adults (3).

[*Risk Factor D if used for prolonged periods or in high doses at term.]

Breast Feeding Summary

No data are available.

References

1. Miller RR. Evaluation of nalbuphine hydrochloride. Am J Hosp Pharm 1980;37:942–9.
2. Wilson SJ, Errick JK, Balkon J. Pharmacokinetics of nalbuphine during parturition. Am J Obstet Gynecol 1986;155:340–4.
3. Feinstein SJ, Lodeiro JG, Vintzileos AM, Campbell WA, Montgomery JT, Nochimson DJ. Sinusoidal fetal heart rate pattern after administration of nalbuphine hydrochloride: a case report. Am J Obstet Gynecol 1986;154:159–60.

Name: **NALIDIXIC ACID**

Class: **Urinary Germicide**　　　　　　　　　　　　　　　Risk Factor: **B**

Fetal Risk Summary

No reports linking the use of nalidixic acid with congenital defects have been located. Chromosome damage was not observed in human leukocytes cultured with varying concentrations of the drug (1). One author cautioned that the drug should be avoided in late pregnancy since it may produce hydrocephalus (2). However, a subsequent report examined the newborns of 63 patients treated with nalidixic acid at various stages of gestation (3). No defects attributable to the drug or intracranial hypertension were observed.

Breast Feeding Summary

Nalidixic acid is excreted into breast milk in low concentrations. Hemolytic anemia was reported in one infant with glucose-6-phosphate dehydrogenase deficiency whose mother was taking 1 g four times a day (4). Milk levels were not measured in this case, but the author noted data from the manufacturer where milk levels from four women taking a similar dose were found to be 4 μg/ml. The milk:plasma ratio has been reported as 0.08–0.13 (5). These quantities are normally considered insignificant (6). Although noting the single case of hemolytic anemia described above, the American Academy of Pediatrics considers nalidixic acid to be compatible with breast feeding (7).

References

1. Stenchever MA, Powell W, Jarvis JA. Effect of nalidixic acid on human chromosome integrity. Am J Obstet Gynecol 1970;107:329–30.
2. Asscher AW. Diseases of the urinary system. Urinary tract infections. Br Med J 1977;1:1332.
3. Murray EDS. Nalidixic acid in pregnancy. Br Med J 1981;282:224.
4. Belton EM, Jones RV. Hemolytic anemia due to nalidixic acid. Lancet 1965;2:691.
5. Wilson JT. Milk/plasma ratios and contraindicated drugs. In Wilson JT, ed. *Drugs in Breast Milk*. Balgowlah, Australia:ADIS Press, 1981:78–9.
6. Takyi BE. Excretion of drugs in human milk. J Hosp Pharm 1970;28:317–25.
7. Committee on Drugs, American Academy of Pediatrics. Transfer of drugs and other drugs into human milk. Pediatrics 1989;84:924–36.

Name: **NALORPHINE**

Class: **Narcotic Antagonist**   Risk Factor: **D**

Fetal Risk Summary

Nalorphine is a narcotic antagonist that is used to reverse respiratory depression from narcotic overdose. It has been used either alone or in combination with meperidine or morphine during labor to reduce neonatal depression (1–6). Nalorphine has also been given to the newborn to prevent neonatal asphyxia (3, 7). Although some benefits were initially claimed, caution in the use of nalorphine during labor has been advised for the following reasons: (a) a statistically significant reduction in neonatal depression has not been demonstrated; (b) the antagonist reduces analgesia; (c) the antagonist may increase neonatal depression if an improper narcotic-narcotic antagonist ratio is used (8).

An adverse effect on fetal cord blood pH, pCO_2, and base deficit was shown when nalorphine was given in combination with meperidine during labor (9). As indicated above, nalorphine may cause respiratory depression in the absence of narcotics or if the critical ratio is exceeded (8). Because of these considerations, the use of nalorphine either alone or in combination therapy in pregnancy should be discouraged. If a narcotic antagonist is indicated, other agents that do not cause respiratory depression, such as naloxone, are preferred.

Breast Feeding Summary

No data are available.

References

1. Cappe BE, Himel SZ, Grossman F. Use of a mixture of morphine and N-allynormorphine as an analgesic. Am J Obstet Gynecol 1953;66:1231–4.
2. Echenhoff JE, Hoffman GL, Funderburg LW. N-Allynormorphine: an antagonist to neonatal narcosis produced by sedation of the parturient. Am J Obstet Gynecol 1953;65:1269–75.
3. Echenhoff JE, Funderburg LW. Observations in the use of the opiate antagonists nalorphine and levallorphan. Am J Med Sci 1954;228:546–53.
4. Baker FJ. Pethidine and nalorphine in labor. Anaesthesia 1957;12:282–92.
5. Gordon DWS, Pinker GD. Increased pethidine dosage in obstetrics associated with the use of nalorphine. J Obstet Gynaecol Br Commonw 1958;65:606–11.
6. Bullough J. Use of premixed pethidine and antagonists in obstetrical analgesia with special reference to cases in which levallorphan was used. Br Med J 1959;2:859–62.

7. Paterson S, Prescott F. Nalorphine in prevention of neonatal asphyxia due to maternal sedation with pethidine. Lancet 1954;1:490–3.
8. Bonica JJ. *Principles and Practice of Obstetric Analgesia and Anesthesia.* Philadelphia:FA Davis, 1967:254–9.
9. Hounslow D, Wood C, Humphrey M, Chang A. Intrapartum drugs and fetal blood pH and gas status. J Obstet Gynaecol Br Commonw 1973;80:1007–12.

Name: **NALOXONE**

Class: **Narcotic Antagonist**

Risk Factor: **B$_M$**

Fetal Risk Summary

Naloxone is a narcotic antagonist that is used to reverse the effects of narcotic overdose. The drug has no intrinsic respiratory depressive actions or other narcotic effects of its own (1). Naloxone has been shown to cross the placenta, appearing in fetal blood 2 minutes after a maternal dose and gradually increasing over 10–30 minutes (2).

In three reports, naloxone was given to mothers in labor after the administration of meperidine (3–5). One study found that 18–40 μg/kg (maternal weight) given intravenously provided the best results in comparison with controls who did not receive meperidine or naloxone (4). In measurements of newborn neurobehavior, groups treated in labor with either meperidine or meperidine plus naloxone (0.4 mg) were compared with a nontreated control group (5). The control group scored better in the 1st 24 hours than either of the treated groups and, after 2 hours, no difference was found between meperidine or meperidine plus naloxone-treated patients. Women in active labor received 1.0 mg of morphine intrathecally followed in 1 hour by a 0.4-mg intravenous bolus of naloxone plus 0.6 mg/hour or placebo as constant infusion for 23 hours (6). A reduction in some morphine-induced maternal side effects was seen with naloxone, but no significant differences with placebo were found for fetal heart rate or variability, Apgar scores, umbilical venous and arterial gasses, neonatal respirations, or neurobehavioral examination scores. Cord:maternal serum ratio for naloxone was 0.50. Naloxone has also been safely given to newborns within a few minutes of delivery (7–12).

Naloxone has been used at term to treat fetal heart rate baselines with low beat-to-beat variability not due to maternally administered narcotics (13). This use was based on the assumption that the heart rate patterns were due to elevated fetal endorphins. In one case, however, naloxone may have enhanced fetal asphyxia, leading to fatal respiratory failure in the newborn (13). Based on the above data, naloxone should not be given to the mother just prior to delivery to reverse the effects of narcotics in the fetus or newborn unless narcotic toxicity is evident. Information on its fetal effects during pregnancy, other than labor, are not available.

In a study of the effects of naloxone on fetal behavior, 54 pregnant women with gestational ages between 37–39 weeks were evenly divided into two groups (14). One group received 0.4 mg of naloxone while the other received an equal volume of saline placebo. In the group receiving naloxone, significant increases were observed in the number, duration, and amplitude of fetal heart rate accelerations.

Significant increases were also observed in the number of fetal body movements and the percentage of time spent breathing. Moreover, significantly more fetuses exposed to naloxone were actively awake than those not exposed. The investigators attributed their findings to reversal of the effects of fetal endorphins.

Breast Feeding Summary

No data are available.

References

1. Jaffe JH, Martin WR. Opoid analgesics and antagonists. In Gilman AG, Goodman LS, Gilman A, eds. *The Pharmacological Basis of Therapeutics*, ed 6. New York:MacMillan, 1980:522–5.
2. Finster M, Gibbs C, Dawes GS, et al. Placental transfer of meperidine (Demerol) and naloxone (Narcan). Presented at the Annual Meeting of the American Society of Anesthesiologists, Boston, October 4, 1972. In Clark RB, Beard AG, Greifenstein FE, Barclay DL. South Med J 1976;69:570–5.
3. Clark RB. Transplacental reversal of meperidine depression in the fetus by naloxone. J Arkansas Med Soc 1971;68:128–30.
4. Clark RB, Beard AG, Greifenstein FE, Barclay DL. Naloxone in the parturient and her infant. South Med J 1976;69:570–5.
5. Hodgkinson R, Bhatt M, Grewal G, Marx GF. Neonatal neurobehavior in the first 48 hours of life: effect of the administration of meperidine with and without naloxone in the mother. Pediatrics 1978;62:294–8.
6. Brookshire GL, Shnider SM, Abboud TK, Kotelko DM, Nouiehed R, Thigpen JW, Khoo SS, Raya JA, Foutz SE, Brizgys RV. Effects of naloxone on the mother and neonate after intrathecal morphine for labor analgesia. Anesthesiology 1983;59:A417.
7. Evans JM, Hogg MIJ, Rosen M. Reversal of narcotic depression in the neonate by naloxone. Br Med J 1976;2:1098–1100.
8. Wiener PC, Hogg MIJ, Rosen M. Effects of naloxone on pethidine-induced neonatal depression. II. Intramuscular naloxone. Br Med J 1977;2:229–31.
9. Wiener PC, Hogg MIJ, Rosen M. Effects of naloxone on pethidine-induced neonatal depression. I. Intravenous naloxone. Br Med J 1977;2:228–9.
10. Gerhardt T, Bancalari E, Cohen H, Rocha LF. Use of naloxone to reverse narcotic respiratory depression in the newborn infant. J Pediatr 1977;90:1009–12.
11. Bonta BW, Gagliardi JV, Williams V, Warshaw JB. Naloxone reversal of mild neurobehavioral depression in normal newborn infants after routine obstetric analgesia. J Pediatr 1979;94:102–5.
12. Welles B, Belfrage P, de Chateau P. Effects of naloxone on newborn infant behavior after maternal analgesia with pethidine during labor. Acta Obstet Gynecol Scand 1984;63:617–9.
13. Goodlin RC. Naloxone and its possible relationship to fetal endorphin levels and fetal distress. Am J Obstet Gynecol 1981;139:16–9.
14. Arduini D, Rizzo G, Dell'Acqua S, Mancuso S, Romanini C. Effect of naloxone on fetal behavior near term. Am J Obstet Gynecol 1987;156:474–8.

Name: **NAPROXEN**

Class: **Nonsteroidal Anti-inflammatory**   Risk Factor: **B*ₘ**

Fetal Risk Summary

Naproxen is a potent inhibitor of prostaglandin synthetase. Drugs in this class have been shown to inhibit labor and to prolong the length of pregnancy (1). Naproxen readily crosses the placenta to the fetal circulation (2, 3). In a mother treated with 250 mg of naproxen every 8 hours for four doses, cord blood levels in twins 5 hours after the last dose were 59.5 and 68 µg/ml, respectively (3). Prostaglandin synthetase inhibitors may cause constriction of the ductus arteriosus *in utero,* which may result in primary pulmonary hypertension of the newborn (4, 5). The dose, duration, and period of gestation are important determinants of these effects. Most studies of nonsteroidal anti-inflammatory agents used as tocolytics have indicated that the fetus is relatively resistant to premature closure of the ductus before the 34th or 35th week of gestation (see Indomethacin). However, three fetuses (one set of twins) exposed to naproxen at 30 weeks for 2–6 days in an unsuccessful attempt to halt premature labor had markedly decreased plasma concentrations of prostaglandin E (3, 6). Primary pulmonary hypertension of the newborn with severe hypoxemia, increased blood clotting times, hyperbilirubinemia, and impaired renal function were observed in the newborns. One infant died 4 days after birth, probably due to subarachnoid hemorrhage. Autopsy revealed a short and constricted ductus arteriosus. Use in other patients for premature labor at 34 weeks or earlier did not result in neonatal problems (7, 8). Because of the potential newborn toxicity, naproxen should not be used late in the 3rd trimester (2, 3, 9).

[*Risk Factor D if used in 3rd trimester or near delivery.]

Breast Feeding Summary

Naproxen passes into breast milk in very small quantities. The milk:plasma ratio is approximately 0.01 (2). Following 250 or 375 mg twice daily, maximum milk levels were found 4 hours after a dose and ranged from 0.7–1.25 µg/ml and 1.76–2.37 µg/ml, respectively (10, 11). The total amount of naproxen excreted in the infant's urine was 0.26% of the mother's dose. The effect on the infant from these amounts is unknown. In their 1983 statement, the American Academy of Pediatrics considered naproxen to be compatible with breast feeding (12). However, the agent was not listed in the 1989 revision of that statement.

References

1. Fuchs F. Prevention of prematurity. Am J Obstet Gynecol 1976;126:809–20.
2. Product information. Naprosyn. Syntex Laboratories, 1990.
3. Wilkinson AR. Naproxen levels in preterm infants after maternal treatment. Lancet 1980;2:591–2.
4. Levin DL. Effects of inhibition of prostaglandin synthesis on fetal development, oxygenation, and the fetal circulation. Semin Perinatol 1980;4:35–44.
5. Rudolph AM. The effects of nonsteroidal antiinflammatory compounds on fetal circulation and pulmonary function. Obstet Gynecol 1981;58(Suppl):63s–7s.
6. Wilkinson AR, Aynsley-Green A, Mitchell MD. Persistent pulmonary hypertension and abnormal prostaglandin E levels in preterm infants after maternal treatment with naproxen. Arch Dis Child 1979;54:942–5.
7. Gerris J, Jonckheer M, Sacre-Smits L. Acute hyperthyroidism during pregnancy: a case report and critical analysis. Eur J Obstet Gynecol Reprod Biol 1981;12:271–80.
8. Wiqvist N, Kjellmer I, Thiringer K, Ivarsson E, Karlsson K. Treatment of premature labor by prostaglandin synthetase inhibitors. Acta Biol Med Germ 1978;37:923–30.
9. Anonymous. PG-synthetase inhibitors in obstetrics and after. Lancet 1980;2:185–6.
10. Jamali F, Tam YK, Stevens RD. Naproxen excretion in breast milk and its uptake by suckling infant. Drug Intell Clin Pharm 1982;16:475 (Abstr).
11. Jamali F, Stevens DRS. Naproxen excretion in milk and its uptake by the infant. Drug Intell Clin Pharm 1983;17:910–11.
12. Committee on Drugs, American Academy of Pediatrics. The transfer of drugs and other chemicals into human breast milk. Pediatrics 1983;72:375–83.

Name: **NEOMYCIN**

Class: **Antibiotic**   Risk Factor: **C**

Fetal Risk Summary

Neomycin is an aminoglycoside antibiotic. No reports describing its passage across the placenta to the fetus have been located, but this should be expected (see other aminoglycosides Amikacin, Gentamicin, Kanamycin, Streptomycin, and Tobramycin).

Ototoxicity, which is known to occur after oral, topical, and parenteral neomycin therapy, has not been reported as an effect of *in utero* exposure. However, eighth cranial nerve toxicity in the fetus is well known following exposure to kanamycin and streptomycin and may potentially occur with neomycin.

Oral neomycin therapy, 2 g daily, depresses urinary estrogen excretion, apparently by inhibiting steroid conjugate hydrolysis in the gut (1). The fall in estrogen excretion resembles the effect produced by ampicillin but occurs about 2 days later. Urinary estriol was formerly used to assess the condition of the fetoplacental unit, depressed levels being associated with fetal distress. This assessment is now made by measuring plasma conjugated estriol, which is not usually affected by neomycin.

No reports linking the use of neomycin to congenital defects have been located. The Collaborative Perinatal Project monitored 50,282 mother-child pairs, 30 of which had 1st trimester exposure to neomycin (2). No evidence was found to suggest a relationship to large categories of major or minor malformations or to individual defects.

Breast Feeding Summary

No data are available.

References

1. Pulkkinen M, Willman K. Reduction of maternal estrogen excretion by neomycin. Am J Obstet Gynecol 1973;115:1153.
2. Heinonen OP, Slone D, Shapiro S. *Birth Defects and Drugs in Pregnancy.* Littleton:Publishing Sciences Group, 1977:297–301.

Name: **NEOSTIGMINE**

Class: **Parasympathomimetic (Cholinergic)**   Risk Factor: **C$_M$**

Fetal Risk Summary

Neostigmine is a quaternary ammonium compound with anticholinesterase activity used in the diagnosis and treatment of myasthenia gravis. Because it is ionized at physiologic pH, it would not be expected to cross the placenta in significant amounts. Use of the drug during pregnancy, including the 1st trimester, has been reported for the treatment of maternal myasthenia gravis (1–10). One study reported 22 exposures to neostigmine in the 1st trimester (1). No relationship to congenital defects was found. A 1973 study described the use of 0.5 mg orally/

day for 3 days in 27 pregnant patients (5–14 weeks) (2). One patient aborted and 26 went to term without complications. McNall considers neostigmine to be one of the drugs of choice for pregnant patients with myasthenia gravis (3). She also cautioned that intravenous anticholinesterases should not be used in pregnancy for fear of inducing premature labor and suggests that intramuscular neostigmine be used in place of intravenous edrophonium for diagnostic purposes. Other investigators have reported the safe use of neostigmine for myasthenia gravis in pregnancy (4–6).

Transient muscular weakness has been observed in about 20% of newborns of mothers with myasthenia gravis (9). The neonatal myasthenia is due to transplacental passage of anti-acetylcholine receptor immunoglobulin G antibodies (9).

Breast Feeding Summary

Because it is ionized at physiologic pH, neostigmine apparently is not excreted into breast milk (10, 11). However, pyridostigmine, another quaternary ammonium compound, is found in breast milk as determined by modern analytical techniques (see Pyridostigmine). Thus, the passage of neostigmine from maternal plasma to milk cannot be totally excluded at the present time.

References

1. Heinonen OP, Slone D, Shapiro S. *Birth Defects and Drugs in Pregnancy*. Littleton:Publishing Sciences Group, 1977:345–56.
2. Brunclik V, Hauser GA. Short-term therapy in secondary amenorrhea. Ther Umsch 1973;30:496–502.
3. McNall PG, Jafarnia MR. Management of myasthenia gravis in the obstetrical patient. Am J Obstet Gynecol 1965;92:518–25.
4. Foldes FF, McNall PG. Myasthenia gravis: a guide for anesthesiologists. Anesthesiology 1962;23:837–72.
5. Chambers DC, Hall JE, Boyce J. Myasthenia gravis and pregnancy. Obstet Gynecol 1967;29:597–603.
6. Hay DM. Myasthenia gravis and pregnancy. J Obstet Gynaecol Br Commonw 1969;76:323–9.
7. Blackhall MI, Buckley GA, Roberts DV, Roberts JB, Thomas BH, Wilson A. Drug-induced neonatal myasthenia. J Obstet Gynaecol Br Commonw 1969;76:157–62.
8. Eden RD, Gall SA. Myasthenia gravis and pregnancy: a reappraisal of thymectomy. Obstet Gynecol 1983;62:328–33.
9. Plauche WC. Myasthenia gravis in pregnancy: an update. Am J Obstet Gynecol 1979;135:691–7.
10. Fraser D, Turner JWA. Myastenia gravis and pregnancy. Proc R Soc Med 1963;56:379–81.
11. Wilson JT. Pharmacokinetics of drug excretion. In Wilson JT, ed. *Drugs in Breast Milk*. Balgowlah, Australia:ADIS Press, 1981:17.

Name: **NIACIN**

Class: **Vitamin** Risk Factor: **A***

Fetal Risk Summary

Niacin, a B complex vitamin, is converted in humans to niacinamide, the active form of vitamin B_3. See Niacinamide.

[*Risk Factor C if used in doses above the RDA.]

Breast Feeding Summary

See Niacinamide.

Name: **NIACINAMIDE**

Class: **Vitamin**   Risk Factor: **A***

Fetal Risk Summary

Niacinamide, a water-soluble B complex vitamin, is an essential nutrient required for lipid metabolism, tissue respiration, and glycogenolysis (1). Both niacin, which is converted to niacinamide *in vivo*, and niacinamide are available commercially and are collectively known as vitamin B_3. The American recommended daily allowance for niacinamide in pregnancy is 15–17 mg (2).

Only two reports have been located that link niacinamide with maternal or fetal complications. A 1948 study observed an association between niacinamide deficiency and pregnancy-induced-hypertension (PIH) (3). Other B complex vitamins have also been associated with this disease, but any relationship between vitamins and PIH is controversial (see other B complex vitamins). One patient with hyperemesis gravidarum presented with neuritis, reddened tongue, and psychosis (4). She was treated with 100 mg of niacin plus other B complex vitamins, resulting in the rapid disappearance of her symptoms. The authors attributed her response to the niacin.

Niacinamide is actively transported to the fetus (5, 6). Higher concentrations are found in the fetus and newborn than in the mother (6–9). Deficiency of niacinamide in pregnancy is uncommon except in women with poor nutrition (7, 8). At term, mean niacinamide values in 174 mothers were 3.9 μg/ml (range 2.0–7.2) and in their newborns 5.8 μg/ml (range 3.0–10.5) (7). Conversion of the amino acid, tryptophan, to niacin and then to niacinamide is enhanced in pregnancy (10).

[*Risk Factor C if used in doses above the RDA.]

Breast Feeding Summary

Niacin, the precursor to niacinamide, is actively excreted in human breast milk (11). Reports on the excretion of niacinamide in milk have not been located, but it is probable that it also is actively transferred. In a study of lactating women with low nutritional status, supplementation with niacin in doses of 2.0–60.0 mg/day resulted in mean milk concentrations of 1.17–2.75 μg/ml (11). Milk concentrations were directly proportional to dietary intake. A 1983 English study measured niacin levels in pooled human milk obtained from preterm (26 mothers: 29–34 weeks) and term (35 mothers: 39 weeks or longer) patients (12). Preterm milk rose from 0.65 μg/ml (colostrum) to 2.05 μg/ml (16–196 days) while term milk increased over the same period from 0.50 μg/ml to 1.82 μg/ml.

The American recommended daily allowance (RDA) for niacinamide during lactation is 18–20 mg (2). If the diet of the lactating woman adequately supplies this amount, supplementation with niacinamide is not needed. Maternal supplementation with the RDA for niacinamide is recommended for those patients with inadequate nutritional intake.

References

1. American Hospital Formulary Service. *Drug Information 1990*. Bethesda:American Society of Hospital Pharmacists, 1990:2113–4.
2. *Recommended Dietary Allowances*, 9th ed. Washington:National Academy of Sciences, 1980.
3. Hobson W. A dietary and clinical survey of pregnant women with particular reference to toxaemia of pregnancy. J Hyg 1948;46:198–216.
4. Hart BF, McConnell WT. Vitamin B factors in toxic psychosis of pregnancy and the puerperium. Am J Obstet Gynecol 1943;46:283.
5. Hill EP, Longo LD. Dynamics of maternal-fetal nutrient transfer. Fed Proc 1980;39:239–44.
6. Kaminetzky HA, Baker H, Frank O, Langer A. The effects of intravenously administered water-soluble vitamins during labor in normovitaminemic and hypovitaminemic gravidas on maternal and neonatal blood vitamin levels at delivery. Am J Obstet Gynecol 1974;120:697–703.
7. Baker H, Frank O, Thomson AD, Langer A, Munves ED, De Angelis B, Kaminetzky HA. Vitamin profile of 174 mothers and newborns at parturition. Am J Clin Nutr 1975;28:59–65.
8. Baker H, Frank O, Deangelis B, Feingold S, Kaminetzky HA. Role of placenta in maternal-fetal vitamin transfer in humans. Am J Obstet Gynecol 1981;141:792–6.
9. Baker H, Thind IS, Frank O, DeAngelis B, Caterini H, Lquria DB. Vitamin levels in low-birth-weight newborn infants and their mothers. Am J Obstet Gynecol 1977;129:521–4.
10. Wertz AW, Lojkin ME, Bouchard BS, Derby MB. Tryptophan-niacin relationships in pregnancy. Am J Nutr 1958;64:339–53.
11. Deodhar AD, Rajalakshmi R, Ramakrishnan CV. Studies on human lactation. Part III. Effect of dietary vitamin supplementation on vitamin contents of breast milk. Acta Paediatr Scand 1964;53:42–8.
12. Ford JE, Zechalko A, Murphy J, Brooke OG. Comparison of the B vitamin composition of milk from mothers of preterm and term babies. Arch Dis Child 1983;58:367–72.

Name: **NIALAMIDE**

Class: **Antidepressant**   Risk Factor: **C**

Fetal Risk Summary

No data are available (see Phenelzine).

Breast Feeding Summary

No data are available (see Phenelzine).

Name: **NICOTINYL ALCOHOL**

Class: **Vasodilator**   Risk Factor: **C**

Fetal Risk Summary

Nicotinyl alcohol is converted in the body to niacin, the active form. Only one report of its use in pregnancy has been located. The Collaborative Perinatal Project recorded one 1st trimester exposure to nicotinyl alcohol plus 14 other patients exposed to other vasodilators (1). From this small group of 15 patients, 4 malformed children were produced, a statistically significant incidence ($p < 0.02$). It was not stated if nicotinyl alcohol was taken by a mother of one of the affected infants. Although the data serve as a warning, the number of patients is so small that conclusions as to the relative safety of this drug in pregnancy cannot be made.

Breast Feeding Summary

No data are available.

Reference

1. Heinonen OP, Slone D, Shapiro S. *Birth Defects and Drugs in Pregnancy*. Littleton:Publishing Sciences Group, 1977:371–3.

Name: **NICOUMALONE**

Class: **Anticoagulant**   Risk Factor: **D**

Fetal Risk Summary

See Coumarin Derivatives.

Breast Feeding Summary

See Coumarin Derivatives.

Name: **NIFEDIPINE**

Class: **Cardiac Drug**   Risk Factor: **C$_M$**

Fetal Risk Summary

The use of nifedipine, a calcium channel-blocking agent, during pregnancy is controversial. Studies in pregnant sheep with intravenous infusions of the drug indicate that a progressive decrease in mean maternal arterial blood pressure occurs without a significant alteration of uterine vascular resistance (1). The hypotensive effect of nifedipine resulted in a decrease in uterine blood flow and fetal arterial oxygen content. Other investigators have reported similar results in animals with other calcium channel blockers (2). Although these studies indicated the potential problems with nifedipine, the investigators cautioned that their findings were preliminary and needed to be confirmed in humans (1, 3).

A human study was reported in 1988 in which nine hypertensive pregnant women in the 3rd trimester were treated with 5 mg of nifedipine sublingually and compared to nine hypertensive women treated with placebo (4). The women were randomly assigned to the two groups but treatment was not blinded. Both maternal arterial blood pressure and uterine artery perfusion pressure were significantly lowered by nifedipine, but no apparent reduction in uteroplacental blood flow was detected. The investigators interpreted their findings as suggestive of a relative uterine vasodilation and a relative decrease in uterine vascular resistance which was proportional to the decrease in blood pressure.

Nifedipine has been used during the 2nd and 3rd trimesters for the treatment of severe hypertension (5). No fetal heart rate changes were observed after reduction of maternal blood pressure or other adverse effects in the fetus or newborn. In a 1987 study, 22 women suffering from severe hypertension with various etiologies (4 gestational, 17 essential, 1 renal, and 1 systemic lupus erythematosus) who failed to respond to first-line therapy had slow-release nifedipine, 40–120 mg/ day, added to their regimens (6). In an additional patient, nifedipine, 40 mg/day, was used as initial therapy. For 22 of the women, nifedipine was combined with other antihypertensive therapy (atenolol 11, methyldopa 4, atenolol plus methyldopa 4, and atenolol plus hydralazine 3). Good blood pressure control was obtained in 20 women. The mean duration of therapy was 8.75 weeks (range 1– 24 weeks). There were three perinatal deaths (rate 130/1000), but none could be attributed to drug therapy. The mean gestational age at delivery was 35 weeks (range 29–39 weeks), and 15 (71%) of the 21 liveborn infants were delivered by cesarean section. A high percentage of the 22 infants with accessible data were growth retarded; 9 (41%) had birth weights at or below the 3rd percentile, and 20 (91%) were at or below the 10th percentile for body weight. The investigators could not determine if this outcome was due to the severe maternal disease, drug therapy, or a combination of both (6).

Nifedipine has been used as a tocolytic agent. An *in vitro* study using pregnant human myometrium found that nifedipine caused a dose-related decrease in contraction strength and lengthened the period of contraction in a non-dose-related manner (7). In three studies totaling 31 women, nifedipine was used for this purpose (8–10). In one patient, nifedipine, 20 mg three times daily combined with terbutaline, was given for a total of 55 days (9). A study involving 60 women in presumed early labor was reported in 1986 (10). Women were included in this open trial if they had a singleton pregnancy, intact membranes, were between 20– 35 weeks' gestation, were contracting at least once every 10 minutes, and their cervix was less than 4 cm dilated. Included among the various exclusions were a history of midtrimester abortion or previous preterm delivery. The women were equally divided into three groups; nifedipine, ritodrine, and no treatment. Nifedipine dosage was 30 mg orally followed by 20 mg every 8 hours for 3 days. Ritodrine was initially administered as a standard intravenous infusion followed by 48 hours of oral therapy. The days from presentation to delivery in the nifedipine, ritodrine, and no treatment groups were 36.3, 25.1, and 19.3 ($p < 0.001$ nifedipine compared to the other two groups), respectively (10). No complications of the therapy were found in any of the infants from the three studies. Two of the studies (8, 9) conducted follow-up examinations of the infants at 5–12 months of age and all were alive and well.

Two apparently clinically significant drug interactions when nifedipine and magnesium were used concurrently have been reported (11, 12). A woman, at 32 weeks' gestation in premature labor, was treated with 60 mg of nifedipine orally over 3 hours followed by 20 mg every 8 hours. Uterine contractions returned 12 hours later and intravenous magnesium sulfate was started followed by the onset of pronounced muscle weakness after 500 mg had been administered. Her symptoms consisted of jerky movements of the extremities, difficulty in swallowing, paradoxical respirations, and an inability to raise her head from the pillow (11). The muscle weakness resolved 25 minutes after the magnesium was stopped. The effects were attributed to nifedipine potentiation of the neuromuscular blocking action of magnesium. In a second report, two women were hospitalized for hypertension at 30 and 32 weeks' gestation, respectively (12). In both cases, oral methyldopa 2 g and intravenous magnesium sulfate 20 g daily were ineffective in lowering the mother's blood pressure. Oral nifedipine 10 mg was given, and a marked hypotensive response occurred 45 minutes later. The blood pressures before nifedipine were 150/110 and 140/105 mm Hg, respectively, then decreased to 80/50 and 90/60 mm Hg, respectively, after administration of the calcium channel blocker. The blood pressures returned to the previous levels 25–30 minutes later. Both infants were delivered following the hypotensive episodes, but only one survived.

The pharmacokinetics of nifedipine in pregnant women have been studied (13).

In summary, the experience with nifedipine in human pregnancy is limited, although the agent has been used for tocolysis and as an antihypertensive agent in pregnant women. Severe adverse reactions have occurred when the drug was combined with intravenous magnesium sulfate. Moreover, intravenous nifedipine in pregnant rhesus monkeys has been associated with fetal hypoxemia and acidosis (14). As a consequence of this and other animal studies, nifedipine should probably be reserved for women with severe hypertension who are unresponsive to standard therapy or in controlled trials until this toxicity has been studied more carefully.

Breast Feeding Summary

Nifedipine is excreted into human breast milk (15). A woman with persistent hypertension after premature delivery at 26 weeks' gestation was treated with nifedipine 30 mg every 8 hours for 48 hours, then 20 mg every 8 hours for 48 hours, then 10 mg every 8 hours for 36 hours. Concentrations of the drug in milk were related to dosage and the time interval between the dose and milk collection. Peak concentrations and time of occurrence were 53.35 ng/ml 30 minutes after 30 mg, 16.35 ng/ml 1 hour after 20 mg, and 12.89 ng/ml 30 minutes after 10 mg. The estimated milk half-lives after the three doses were 2.4 hours (30 mg), 3.1 hours (20 mg), and 1.4 hours (10 mg). In comparison to controls, nifedipine had no effect on milk composition. The authors concluded that these amounts, representing less than 5% of a therapeutic dose, posed little risk to a nursing infant. If desired, delaying breast feeding by 3–4 hours after a dose would significantly decrease the amount of drug ingested by the infant (15).

References

1. Harake B, Gilbert RD, Ashwal S, Power GG. Nifedipine: effects on fetal and maternal hemodynamics in pregnant sheep. Am J Obstet Gynecol 1987;157:1003–8.
2. Holbrook RH Jr. Effects of calcium antagonists during pregnancy. Am J Obstet Gynecol 1989;160:1018.
3. Gilbert RD. Effects of calcium antagonists during pregnancy. Reply. Am J Obstet Gynecol 1989;160:1018–9.
4. Lindow SW, Davies N, Davey DA, Smith JA. The effect of sublingual nifedipine on uteroplacental blood flow in hypertensive pregnancy. Br J Obstet Gynaecol 1988;95:1276–81.
5. Walters BNJ, Redman CWG. Treatment of severe pregnancy-associated hypertension with the calcium antagonist nifedipine. Br J Obstet Gynaecol 1984;91:330–6.
6. Constantine G, Beevers DG, Reynolds AL, Luesley DM. Nifedipine as a second line antihypertensive drug in pregnancy. Br J Obstet Gynaecol 1987;94;1136–42.

7. Bird LM, Anderson NC Jr, Chandler ML, Young RC. The effects of aminophylline and nifedipine on contractility of isolated pregnant human myometrium. Am J Obstet Gynecol 1987;157:171–7.
8. Ulmsten U, Andersson K-E, Wingerup L. Treatment of premature labor with the calcium antagonist nifedipine. Arch Gynecol 1980;229:1–5.
9. Kaul AF, Osathanondh R, Safon LE, Frigoletto FD Jr, Friedman PA. The management of preterm labor with the calcium channel-blocking agent nifedipine combined with the β-mimetic terbutaline. Drug Intell Clin Pharm 1985;19:369–71.
10. Read MD, Wellby DE. The use of a calcium antagonist (nifedipine) to suppress preterm labour. Br J Obstet Gynaecol 1986;93:933–7.
11. Snyder SW, Cardwell MS. Neuromuscular blockade with magnesium sulfate and nifedipine. Am J Obstet Gynecol 1989;161:35–6.
12. Waisman GD, Mayorga LM, Camera MI, Vignolo CA, Martinotti A. Magnesium plus nifedipine: potentiation of hypotensive effect in preeclampsia? Am J Obstet Gynecol 1988;159:308–9.
13. O'Neill S, Osathanondh R, Kaul AF, Scavone JM, Bromley BS, Malin MA. The pharmacokinetics of nifedipine in pregnant women. Drug Intell Clin Pharm 1986;20:460–1 (Abstract).
14. Ducsay CA, Cook MJ, Veille JC, Novy MJ. Nifedipine tocolysis in pregnant rhesus monkeys: maternal and fetal cardiorespiratory effects. Abstract No. 79, Society of Perinatal Obstetricians Annual Meeting, Las Vegas, Nevada, February, 1985.
15. Ehrenkranz RA, Ackerman BA, Hulse JD. Nifedipine transfer into human milk. J Pediatr 1989;114:478–80.

Name: **NITROFURANTOIN**

Class: **Urinary Germicide**   Risk Factor: **B**

Fetal Risk Summary

No reports linking the use of nitrofurantoin with congenital defects have been located. One manufacturer (Norwich-Eaton Laboratories) has collected over 1700 case histories describing the use of this drug during various stages of pregnancy (95 references) (personal communication, 1981). None of the reports observed deleterious effects on the fetus. In a published study, a retrospective analysis of 91 pregnancies in which nitrofurantoin was used yielded no evidence of fetal toxicity (1). Other studies have also supported the safety of this drug in pregnancy (2).

Nitrofurantoin is capable of inducing hemolytic anemia in glucose-6-phosphate dehydrogenase-deficient patients and in patients whose red blood cells are deficient in reduced glutathione (3). Since the red blood cells of newborns are deficient in reduced glutathione, the manufacturer's package insert (Norwich-Eaton) carries a warning against use of the drug at term. However, hemolytic anemia in the newborn as a result of *in utero* exposure to nitrofurantoin has not been reported.

Nitrofurantoin has been reported to cause discoloration of the primary teeth when given to an infant; by implication, this could occur from *in utero* exposure (4). However, the fact that the baby was also given a 14-day course of tetracycline and the lack of other confirming reports makes the likelihood for a causal relationship remote (5).

When given orally in high doses of 10 mg/kg/day to young males, nitrofurantoin may produce slight to moderate transient spermatogenic arrest (6). The lower doses used clinically do not seem to have this effect.

Breast Feeding Summary

Nitrofurantoin is excreted into breast milk in very low concentrations. The drug could not be detected in 20 samples from mothers receiving 100 mg four times daily (7). In a second study, nine mothers were given 100 mg every 6 hours for 1 day, then either 100 mg or 200 mg the next morning (8). Only two of the four patients receiving the 200-mg dose excreted measurable amounts of nitrofurantoin, 0.3–0.5 μg/ml. Although these amounts are negligible, the authors cautioned that infants with glucose-6-phosphate dehydrogenase deficiency may develop hemolytic anemia from this exposure. The American Academy of Pediatrics considers nitrofurantoin to be compatible with breast feeding (9).

References

1. Hailey FJ, Fort H, Williams JC, Hammers B. Foetal safety of nitrofurantoin macrocrystals therapy during pregnancy: a retrospective analysis. J Int Med Res 1983;11:364–9.
2. Lenke RR, VanDorsten JP, Schifrin BS. Pyelonephritis in pregnancy: a prospective randomized trial to prevent recurrent disease evaluating suppressive therapy with nitrofurantoin and close surveillance. Am J Obstet Gynecol 1983;146:953–7.
3. Powell RD, DeGowin RL, Alving AS. Nitrofurantoin-induced hemolysis. J Lab Clin Med 1963;62:1002–3.
4. Ball JS, Ferguson AN. Permanent discoloration of primary dentition by nitrofurantoin. Br Med J 1962;2:1103.
5. Duckworth R, Swallow JN. Nitrofurantoin and teeth. Br Med J 1962;2:1617.
6. Nelson WO, Bunge RG. The effect of therapeutic dosages of nitrofurantoin (Furadantin) upon spermatogenesis in man. J Urol 1957;77:275–81.
7. Hosbach RE, Foster RB. Absence of nitrofurantoin from human milk. JAMA 1967;202:1057.
8. Varsano I, Fischl J, Shochet SB. The excretion of orally ingested nitrofurantoin in human milk. J Pediatr 1973;82:886–7.
9. Committee on Drugs, American Academy of Pediatrics. Transfer of drugs and other chemicals into human milk. Pediatrics 1989;84:924–36.

Name: **NITROGLYCERIN**

Class: **Vasodilator**   Risk Factor: C_M

Fetal Risk Summary

Nitroglycerin is a rapid acting, short duration vasodilator used primarily for the treatment or prevention of angina pectoris. Due to the nature of its indication, experience in pregnancy is limited. The drug has been used to control severe hypertension during cesarean section (1, 2). No hypotension or other effects of the drug were observed in the newborn infants. Use of nitroglycerin sublingually for angina during pregnancy without fetal harm has also been reported (3). The Collaborative Perinatal Project recorded 7 1st trimester exposures to nitroglycerin and amyl nitrite plus 8 other patients exposed to other vasodilators (4). From this small group of 15 patients, 4 malformed children were produced, a statistically significant incidence ($p < 0.02$). The data did not indicate if nitroglycerin was taken by any of the mothers of the affected infants. Due to the lack of specific information and the small number of patients, no conclusions as to the relative safety of nitroglycerin in pregnancy can be made.

The use of intravenous nitroglycerin in pregnancy-induced hypertension has been published (5, 6). In three patients, nitroglycerin infusion was effective in rapidly correcting the hemodynamic disturbances in pregnancy-induced hypertension complicated by hydrostatic pulmonary edema, but a rapid improvement in arterial oxygenation did not occur (5). In another study by these same investigators, the effectiveness of nitroglycerin to decrease blood pressure in six women with pregnancy-induced hypertension was dependent on the patient's volume status (6). When volume expansion was combined with nitroglycerin therapy, a marked resistance to the hypotensive effect of the drug was observed. In two of the women treated with nitroglycerin alone, significant reductions in blood pressure occurred, resulting in fetal heart rate changes including late decelerations and bradycardia. Recovery occurred after nitroglycerin therapy was terminated and then restarted at a lower dose. In three other fetuses, a loss of beat-to-beat variability (average variability <5 beats/minute) was noted. Therapy was continued and no abnormalities were observed in the umbilical blood gasses or Apgar scores.

Breast Feeding Summary

No data are available.

References

1. Snyder SW, Wheeler AS, James FM III. The use of nitroglycerin to control severe hypertension of pregnancy during cesarean section. Anesthesiology 1979;51:563–4.
2. Hood DD, Dewan DM, James FM III, Bogard TD, Floyd HM. The use of nitroglycerin in preventing the hypertensive response to tracheal intubation in severe preeclamptics. Anesthesiology 1983;59:A423.
3. Diro M, Beydown SN, Jaramillo B, O'Sullivan MJ, Kieval J. Successful pregnancy in a woman with a left ventricular cardiac aneurysm: a case report. J Reprod Med 1983;28:559–63.
4. Heinonen OP, Slone D, Shapiro S. *Birth Defects and Drugs in Pregnancy.* Littleton:Publishing Sciences Group, 1977:371–3.
5. Cotton DB, Jones MM, Longmire S, Dorman KF, Tessem J, Joyce TH III. Role of intravenous nitroglycerin in the treatment of severe pregnancy-induced hypertension complicated by pulmonary edema. Am J Obstet Gynecol 1986;154:91–3.
6. Cotton DB, Longmire S, Jones MM, Dorman KF, Tessem J, Joyce TH III. Cardiovascular alterations in severe pregnancy-induced hypertension: effects of intravenous nitroglycerin coupled with blood volume expansion. Am J Obstet Gynecol 1986;154:1053–9.

Name: **NONOXYNOL-9/OCTOXYNOL-9**

Class: **Vaginal Spermicides**   Risk Factor: **C**

Fetal Risk Summary

Nonoxynol-9 and octoxynol-9 are vaginal spermicides used to prevent conception. These agents, applied intravaginally, act by inactivating sperm after direct contact. Although human data are lacking, in animals nonoxynol-9 rapidly crosses the vaginal wall into the systemic circulation (1). Octoxynol should also be expected to act in a similar manner. The use of vaginal spermicides just prior to conception or inadvertently during the early stages of pregnancy has led to investigations of their effects on the fetus. The effects studied include congenital malformations, spontaneous abortion, low birth weight, stillbirth, sex ratio at birth, frequency of multiple births, and premature delivery.

A causal relationship between vaginal spermicides and congenital abnormalities was first tentatively proposed in a 1981 study comparing 763 spermicide users and 3902 nonuser controls (2). The total number of infants with malformations was low: 17 (2.2%) in the exposed group and 39 (1.0%) in the nonexposed group. Malformations thought to be associated with spermicide use were limb reduction deformities (three cases), neoplasms (two cases), chromosomal abnormalities (Down's syndrome) (three cases), and hypospadias (two cases). An earlier investigation, published in 1977, had concluded there was no causal relationship between spermicides and congenital defects, although there was an increased incidence of limb reduction defects in infants of users (11 of 93) as compared to nonusers (8 of 186) (3). Three reports appeared in 1982 that suggested a possible relationship between spermicide use and congenital malformations (4–6). In a case-control study conducted by one of the co-authors of the 1981 investigation, a positive association with Down's syndrome was proposed when in a group of 16 affected infants, four were from users of spermicides (4). In another case-control study, increased risk ratios after spermicide use, although not statistically significant, were reported for limb reduction defects (relative risk 2.00; six infants) and hypospadias (relative risk 4.00; eight infants) (5). Finally, an English study observed, among other defects, two cases each of hypospadias, limb reduction deformity, and Down's syndrome among infants of 1103 spermicide users (6). The authors stated that their data were not conclusive, but the occurrence rates of these particular defects were higher than those observed in a comparative nonuser group.

Several criticisms have been directed at the original 1981 study (7–10). First, an infant was presumed exposed if the mother had a prescription filled at a designated pharmacy within 600 days of delivery. No attempt was made to ascertain actual use of the product or if the mothers, either users or nonusers, had purchased a spermicide without a prescription (7–9). In a subsequent correspondence, all of the study's exposed cases of limb reduction deformity (three cases), Down's syndrome (three cases), and neoplasm (two cases) were re-examined in terms of the exact timing of spermicide use (10). The data suggested that spermicides were not used near the time of conception in these cases. However, this does not eliminate the possibility that spermicides may act directly on the ovum prior to conception (11). Second, the four types of malformations lack a common etiology and time of occurrence (9). Even a single type of defect, such as limb reduction deformity, has a varied etiology (9). Third, the total number of infants with malformations was low (2.2% vs. 1.0%). Since these values are comparable to the 2–5% reported incidence of major malformations in hospital-based studies, the apparent association may have been due to a lower than expected rate of defects in the nonexposed group rather than an increase in the exposed infants (7, 9). Fourth, no confounding variables other than maternal age were adjusted (9).

A number of investigators have been unable to reproduce the results published in 1981 (8, 12–19). In a study examining 188 infants with chromosomal abnormalities or limb reduction defects, no relationship between periconceptional use of spermicides and these defects were observed (8). No association between spermicide use at conception and any congenital malformation was observed in a study comparing 1,427 cases with 3,001 controls (12). In a prospective study of 34,660 women controlled for age, time in pregnancy, concentration of spermicide used, and other confounding variables, the malformation rate of spermicide users was no greater than in users of other contraceptive methods (13–15). A cohort study, the Collaborative Perinatal Project involving 50,282 mother-child pairs, found no greater risk for limb reduction deformities, neoplasm, Down's syndrome, or hypospadias in children exposed *in utero* to spermicides (16). One group of investigators interviewed 12,440 women during delivery and found no relationship between the last contraceptive method used and congenital malformations (17). Spermicides were the last contraceptive method used by 3,891 (31%) of the women. A 1987 case-control study of infants with Down's syndrome ($N = 265$), hypospadias ($N = 396$), limb reduction defects ($N = 146$), neoplasms ($N = 116$), or neural tube defects ($N = 215$) compared to 3,442 control infants with a wide variety of other defects was unable to establish any causal relationship to maternal spermicide use (18). The authors investigated spermicide usage at three different time intervals—preconceptional (1 month before to 1 month after the last menstrual period), first trimester (first 4 lunar months), and any use during life-time—without producing a positive association. A similar study, involving 13,729 women who had produced 154 fetuses with trisomy, 98 with trisomy 21 (i.e., Down's syndrome), also failed to find any association with spermicides (19). In addition, a letter correspondence from one researcher argued that an association between vaginal spermicides, or any environmental risk factor for that matter, and trisomies was implausible based on an understanding of the origin of these defects (20).

An association between vaginal spermicides and spontaneous abortions was found in five studies (21–25). A strong association was found among subjects who had obtained a spermicide within 12 weeks of conception (21). Another study demonstrated approximately twice the rate of spontaneous abortions in women who continued to use spermicides after conception compared to users before or close to the time of conception (22). However, a 1985 critique concluded that both sets of investigators had seriously biased their results by failing to adjust for potentially confounding variables (9). In a study involving women aborting spontaneously before the 28th week of gestation and controls delivering after the 28th week, women who used spermicides at the time of conception demonstrated a 5-fold increase in chromosomal anomalies upon karyotype examinations in 929 cases (23). Although no association between spermicide use and chromosomally normal abortion was found in a study involving 6,339 women, spermicide use of more than 1 year was more common in cases aborting trisomic conception than in controls (24). In an earlier report, the same authors observed an odds ratio of 4.8 for the association between abortuses with anomalies and unexposed controls (25). Two of these latter studies (23, 25) did not adjust for confounding variables.

Three studies have found no association with spontaneous abortions (6, 14, 26). No significant risk for spontaneous abortion was observed in a large cohort study involving 17,032 subjects (6) or in another study examining periconceptional spermicide use (14). In a well-designed, large prospective study involving 32,123 subjects, spermicide use prior to conception was associated with a significant reduction in spontaneous abortion during the second trimester (26).

Three studies found no association between spermicide use and birth weight (6, 14, 22), and one study did find such an association (5). In this latter investigation, spermicide use after the last menstrual period was significantly associated with a lower mean birth weight among female infants of both smoking and non-smoking mothers. For male births, an association with lower birth weight was found only when the mothers smoked. The authors were unable to determine if these relationships were causal. Spermicide use before the last menstrual period had no effect on birth weight.

Under miscellaneous effects, a case-control study of 73 nontraumatic stillbirths found no relationship with the use of vaginal spermicides (27). No association between sex ratio at birth or frequency of multiple births and spermicides was found in one study (6). However, in a 1976 national survey, female births were approximately 25% higher among women using spermicides near the time of conception compared to nonusers, a statistically significant difference (22). Finally, a 1985 study found no evidence of a relationship between spermicide use and preterm delivery (14).

In summary, the currently available evidence does not indicate that the use of vaginal spermicides, either before or during early pregnancy, poses a major risk of congenital malformations to the fetus. If a risk does exist, it must be small. Three authors of the original 1981 paper reporting a relationship between spermicides and congenital defects have commented that available data now argue against a causal association (28). In addition, the Food and Drug Administration has issued a statement that spermicides do not cause birth defects (29). There is also controversy on whether the 1981 study should have been published (30, 31). The data for spontaneous abortions, low birth weight, stillbirths, sex ratios at birth, frequency of multiple births, and premature delivery also indicate it is unlikely that these factors are influenced by spermicide use.

Breast Feeding Summary

Although human data are lacking, nonoxynol-9 is rapidly excreted into the milk of lactating rats (1). Similar excretion in humans should be expected for both nonoxynol-9 and octoxynol-9. If excretion does occur, the effect on the nursing infant is unknown.

References

1. Chvapil M, Eskelson CD, Stiffel V, Owen JA, Droegemueller W. Studies on nonoxynol-9. II. Intravaginal absorption, distribution, metabolism and excretion in rats and rabbits. Contraception 1980;22:325–39.
2. Jick H, Walker AM, Rothman KJ, Hunter JR, Holmes LB, Watkins RN, D'Ewart DC, Danford A, Madsen S. Vaginal spermicides and congenital disorders. JAMA 1981;245:1329–32.
3. Smith ESO, Dafoe CS, Miller JR, Banister P. An epidemiological study of congenital reduction deformities of the limbs. Br J Prev Soc Med 1977;31:39–41.
4. Rothman KJ. Spermicide use and Down's syndrome. Am J Public Health 1982;72:399–401.
5. Polednak AP, Janerich DT, Glebatis DM. Birth weight and birth defects in relation to maternal spermicide use. Teratology 1982;26:27–38.
6. Huggins G, Vessey M, Flavel R, Yeates D, McPherson K. Vaginal spermicides and outcome of pregnancy: findings in a large cohort study. Contraception 1982;25:219–30.
7. Oakley GP Jr. Spermicides and birth defects. JAMA 1982;247:2405.
8. Cordero JF, Layde PM. Vaginal spermicides, chromosomal abnormalities and limb reduction defects. Fam Plann Perspect 1983;15:16–8.
9. Bracken MB. Spermicidal contraceptives and poor reproductive outcomes: the epidemiologic evidence against an association. Am J Obstet Gynecol 1985;151:552–6.
10. Watkins RN. Vaginal spermicides and congenital disorders: the validity of a study. JAMA 1986;256:3095.

11. Jick H, Walker A, Rothman KJ. Vaginal spermicides and congenital disorders: the validity of a study—in reply. JAMA 1986;256:3095–6.
12. Bracken MB, Vita K. Frequency of non-hormonal contraception around conception and association with congenital malformations in offspring. Am J Epidemiol 1983;117:281–91.
13. Mills JL, Harley EE, Reed GF, Berendes HW. Are spermicides teratogenic? JAMA 1982;248:2148–51.
14. Mills JL, Reed GF, Nugent RP, Harley EE, Berendes HW. Are there adverse effects of periconceptional spermicide use? Fertil Steril 1985;43:442–6.
15. Harlap S, Shiono PH, Ramcharan S. Congenital abnormalities in the offspring of women who used oral and other contraceptives around the time of conception. Int J Fertil 1985;30:39–47.
16. Shapiro S, Slone D, Heinonen OP, Kaufman DW, Rosenberg L, Mitchell AA, Helmrich SP. Birth defects and vaginal spermicides. JAMA 1982;247:2381–4.
17. Linn S, Schoenbaum SC, Monson RR, Rosner B, Stubblefield PG, Ryan KJ. Lack of association between contraceptive usage and congenital malformations in offspring. Am J Obstet Gynecol 1983;147:923–8.
18. Louik C, Mitchell AA, Werler MM, Hanson JW, Shapiro S. Maternal exposure to spermicides in relation to certain birth defects. N Engl J Med 1987;317:474–8.
19. Warburton D, Neugut RH, Lustenberger A, Nicholas AG, Kline J. Lack of association between spermicide use and trisomy. N Engl J Med 1987;317:478–82.
20. Bracken MB. Vaginal spermicides and congenital disorders: study reassessed, not retracted. JAMA 1987;257:2919.
21. Jick H, Shiota K, Shepard TH, Hunter JR, Stergachis A, Madsen S, Porter JB. Vaginal spermicides and miscarriage seen primarily in the emergency room. Teratogenesis Carcinog Mutagen 1982;2:205–10.
22. Scholl TO, Sobel E, Tanfer K, Soefer EF, Saidman B. Effects of vaginal spermicides on pregnancy outcome. Fam Plann Perspect 1983;15:244,249–50.
23. Warburton D, Stein Z, Kline J, Strobino B. Environmental influences on rates of chromosome anomalies in spontaneous abortions. Am J Hum Genet 1980;32:92A (Abstract).
24. Strobino B, Kline J, Lai A, Stein Z, Susser M, Warburton D. Vaginal spermicides and spontaneous abortion of known karyotype. Am J Epidemiol 1986;123:431–43.
25. Strobino B, Kline J, Stein Z, Susser M, Warburton D. Exposure to contraceptive creams, jellies and douches and their effect on the zygote. Am J Epidemiol 1980;112:434 (Abstract).
26. Harlap S, Shiono PH, Ramcharan S. Spontaneous foetal losses in women using different contraceptives around the time of conception. Int J Epidemiol 1980;9:49–56.
27. Porter JB, Hunter-Mitchell J, Jick H, Walker AM. Drugs and stillbirth. Am J Public Health 1986;76:1428–31.
28. Jick H, Walker AM, Rothman KJ. The relation between vaginal spermicides and congenital disorders—in reply. JAMA 1987;258:2066.
29. Anonymous. Data do not support association between spermicides, birth defects. FDA Drug Bull 1986;16:21.
30. Mills JL. Reporting provocative results; can we publish "hot" papers without getting burned? JAMA 1987;258:3428–9.
31. Holmes LB. Vaginal spermicides and congenital disorders: the validity of a study—in reply. JAMA 1986;256:3096.

Name: **NORETHINDRONE**

Class: **Progestogenic Hormone**   Risk Factor: X_M

Fetal Risk Summary

Norethindrone is a progestogen derived from 19-nortestosterone. It is used in oral contraceptives and hormonal pregnancy tests (no longer available in the United States). Masculinization of the female fetus has been associated with norethindrone (1–3). One researcher observed an 18% incidence of masculinization of

female infants born to mothers given norethindrone (2). A more conservative estimate for the incidence of masculinization due to synthetic progestogens has been
reported as 0.3% (4). The Collaborative Perinatal Project monitored 866 mother-
child pairs with 1st trimester exposure to progestational agents (including 132 with
exposure to norethindrone) (5, pp. 389, 391). Evidence of an increased risk of
malformation was found for norethindrone. An increase in the expected frequency
of cardiovascular defects and hypospadias was also observed for progestational
agents as a group (5, p. 394; 6). Re-evaluation of these data in terms of timing of
exposure, vaginal bleeding in early pregnancy, and previous maternal obstetric
history, however, failed to support an association between female sex hormones
and cardiac malformations (7). An earlier study also failed to find any relationship
with nongenital malformations (3). One investigator observed two infants with
malformations exposed to norethindrone (8). The congenital defects included
spina bifida and hydrocephalus. The relationship between norethindrone and the
anomalies is unknown.

Breast Feeding Summary

Norethindrone exhibits a dose-dependent suppression of lactation (9). Lower infant weight gain, decreased milk production, and decreased composition of nitrogen and protein content of human milk have been associated with norethindrone
and estrogenic agents (10–13). The magnitude of these changes is low. However,
the changes in milk production and composition may be of nutritional importance
in malnourished mothers. If breast feeding is desired, the lowest dose of oral contraceptives should be chosen. Monitoring of infant weight gain and the possible
need for nutritional supplementation should be considered. The American Academy of Pediatrics considers norethindrone to be compatible with breast feeding
(14).

References

1. Hagler S, Schultz A, Hankin H, Kunstadter RN. Fetal effects of steroid therapy during pregnancy.
   Am J Dis Child 1963;106:586–90.
2. Jacobson BD. Hazards of norethindrone therapy during pregnancy. Am J Obstet Gynecol
   1962;84:962–8.
3. Wilson JG, Brent RL. Are female sex hormones teratogenic? Am J Obstet Gynecol
   1981;141:567–80.
4. Bongiovanni AM, McFadden AJ. Steroids during pregnancy and possible fetal consequences.
   Fertil Steril 1960;11:181–4.
5. Heinonen OP, Slone D, Shapiro S. *Birth Defects and Drugs in Pregnancy.* Littleton:Publishing
   Sciences Group, 1977.
6. Heinonen OP, Slone D, Monson RR, Hook EB, Shapiro S. Cardiovascular birth defects and antenatal exposure to female sex hormones. N Engl J Med 1977;296:67–70.
7. Wiseman RA, Dodds-Smith IC. Cardiovascular birth defects and antenatal exposure to female
   sex hormones: a reevaluation of some base data. Teratology 1984;30:359–70.
8. Dillon S. Congenital malformations and hormones in pregnancy. Br Med J 1976;2:1446.
9. Guiloff E, Ibarra-Polo A, Zanartu J, Toscanini C, Mischler TW, Gomez-Rogers C. Effect of contraception on lactation. Am J Obstet Gynecol 1974;118:42–5.
10. Karim M, Ammarr R, El-Mahgoubh S, El-Ganzoury B, Fikri F, Abdou I. Injected progestogen and
    lactation. Br Med J 1971;1:200–3.
11. Kora SJ. Effect of oral contraceptives on lactation. Fertil Steril 1969;20:419–23.
12. Miller GH, Hughes LR. Lactation and genital involution effects of a new low-dose oral contracep-
    tive on breast-feeding mothers and their infants. Obstet Gynecol 1970;35:44–50.
13. Lonnerdal B, Forsum E, Hambraeus L. Effect of oral contraceptives on composition and volume of
    breast milk. Am J Clin Nutr 1980;33:816–24.

14. Committee on Drugs, American Academy of Pediatrics. Transfer of drugs and other chemicals into human milk. Pediatrics 1989;84:924–36.

Name: **NORETHYNODREL**

Class: **Progestogenic Hormone**   Risk Factor: X_M

Fetal Risk Summary

Norethynodrel is a progestogen derived from 19-nortestosterone. It is used in oral contraceptive agents and hormonal pregnancy tests (no longer available in the United States). Masculinization of the female infant has been associated with norethynodrel (1, 2). The Collaborative Perinatal Project monitored 866 mother-child pairs with 1st trimester exposure to progestational agents (including 154 with exposure to norethynodrel) (3, pp. 389, 391). Fetuses exposed to norethynodrel were not at an increased risk for malformation. However, an increase in the expected frequency of cardiovascular defects and hypospadias was observed for progestational agents as a group (3, p. 394; 4). Re-evaluation of these data in terms of timing of exposure, vaginal bleeding in early pregnancy, and previous maternal obstetric history, however, failed to support an association between female sex hormones and cardiac malformations (5). An earlier study also failed to find any relationship with nongenital malformations (1). One investigator observed three infants, exposed to norethynodrel and mestranol during the 1st trimester, who had congenital defects, including atrial and ventricular septal defects (one infant), hypospadias (one infant), and inguinal hernias (two infants) (6). The relationship between the anomalies and the exposure to the hormones is unknown.

Breast Feeding Summary

Norethynodrel exhibits a dose-dependent suppression of lactation (7). Lower infant weight gain, decreased milk production, and decreased composition of nitrogen and protein content of human milk have been associated with similar synthetic progestogens and estrogen products (see Norethindrone, Mestranol, Ethinyl Estradiol, Oral Contraceptives) (8–10). The magnitude of these changes is low. However, the changes in milk production and composition may be of nutritional importance in malnourished mothers. If breast feeding is desired, the lowest dose of oral contraceptives should be chosen. Monitoring of infant weight gain and the possible need for nutritional supplementation should be considered. The American Academy of Pediatrics considers norethynodrel to be compatible with breast feeding (11).

References

1. Wilson JG, Brent RL. Are female sex hormones teratogenic? Am J Obstet Gynecol 1981;141:567–80.
2. Hagler S. Schultz A, Hankin H, Kunstadter RN. Fetal effects of steroid therapy during pregnancy. Am J Dis Child 1963;106:586–90.
3. Heinonen OP, Slone D, Shapiro S. *Birth Defects and Drugs in Pregnancy*. Littleton:Publishing Sciences Group, 1977.
4. Heinonen OP, Slone D, Monson RR, Hook EB, Shapiro S. Cardiovascular birth defects and antenatal exposure to female hormones. N Engl J Med 1977;296:67–70.

5. Wiseman RA, Dodds-Smith IC. Cardiovascular birth defects and antenatal exposure to female sex hormones: a reevaluation of some base data. Teratology 1984;30:359–70.
6. Dillon S. Congenital malformations and hormones in pregnancy. Br Med J 1976;2:1446.
7. Guiloff E, Ibarra-Polo A, Zanartu J, Toscanini C, Mischler TW, Gomez-Rogers C. Effect of contraception on lactation. Am J Obstet Gynecol 1974;118:42–5.
8. Kora SJ. Effect of oral contraceptives on lactation. Fertil Steril 1969;20:419–23.
9. Miller GH, Hughes LR. Lactation and genital involution effects of a new low-dose oral contraceptive on breast-feeding mothers and their infants. Obstet Gynecol 1970;35:44–50.
10. Lonnerdal B, Forsum E, Hambraeus L. Effect of oral contraceptives on composition and volume of breast milk. Am J Clin Nutr 1980;33:816–24.
11. Committee on Drugs, American Academy of Pediatrics. Transfer of drugs and other chemicals into human milk. Pediatrics 1989;84:924–36.

Name: **NORGESTREL**

Class: **Progestogenic Hormone**   Risk Factor: **X$_M$**

Fetal Risk Summary

Norgestrel is commonly used as an oral contraceptive either alone or in combination with estrogens (see Oral Contraceptives).

Breast Feeding Summary

No data are available (see Oral Contraceptives).

Name: **NORTRIPTYLINE**

Class: **Antidepressant**   Risk Factor: **D**

Fetal Risk Summary

Limb reduction anomalies have been reported with nortriptyline (1, 2). However, one of these children was not exposed until after the critical period for limb development (3). The second infant was also exposed to sulfamethizole and heavy cigarette smoking (1). Evaluation of data from 86 patients with 1st trimester exposure to amitriptyline, the active precursor of nortriptyline, does not support the drug as a major cause of congenital limb deformities (see Amitriptyline). Urinary retention in the neonate has been associated with maternal use of nortriptyline (4).

Breast Feeding Summary

Nortriptyline is excreted into breast milk in low concentrations (5–8). A milk level in one patient was 59 ng/ml, representing a milk:serum ratio of 0.7 (6). A second patient was treated with nortriptyline 100 mg daily during the 2nd and 3rd trimesters, then stopped 2 weeks prior to an elective cesarean section (8). Treatment was restarted at 125 mg every night on the 1st postpartum day, then decreased to 75 mg nightly over the next 7 weeks. The mother was also receiving flupenthixol. Milk concentrations of nortriptyline, measured 11–13.5 hours after a dose on postpartum days 6 (four samples), 20 (two samples), and 48 (two samples), ranged from 90–404 ng/ml, mean 230 ng/ml. The milk:serum ratios for these samples ranged from 0.87–3.71, mean 1.62. No effects of the drug exposure were observed in the nursing infant, who had normal motor development over the first 4 months (8). Infant serum concentrations were not determined. However, nortriptyline was not detected in the serum of other breast-fed infants when their mothers were taking the drug (6, 7). The significance of chronic exposure of the nursing infant to the antidepressant is unknown, but concern was expressed about the effects of long-term exposure on the infant's neurobehavioral mechanisms (8).

References

1. Bourke GM. Antidepressant teratogenicity? Lancet 1974;1:98.
2. McBride WG. Limb deformities associated with iminobenzyl hydrochloride. Med J Aust 1972;1:492.
3. Australian Drug Evaluation Committee. Tricyclic antidepressants and limb reduction deformities. Med J Aust 1973;1:768–9.
4. Shearer WT, Schreiner RL, Marshall RE. Urinary retention in a neonate secondary to maternal ingestion of nortriptyline. J Pediatr 1972;81:570–2.
5. Bader TF, Newman K. Amitriptyline in human breast milk and the nursing infant's serum. Am J Psychiatry 1980;137:855–6.
6. Erickson SH, Smith GH, Heidrich F. Tricyclics and breast feeding. Am J Psychiatry 1979;136:1483.
7. Brixen-Rasmussen L, Halgrener J, Jorgensen A. Amitriptyline and nortriptyline excretion in human breast milk. Psychopharmacology (Berlin) 1982;76:94–5.
8. Matheson I, Skjaeraasen J. Milk concentrations of flupenthixol, nortriptyline and zuclopenthixol and between-breast differences in two patients. Eur J Clin Pharmacol 1988;35;217–20.

Name: **NOVOBIOCIN**

Class: **Antibiotic**   Risk Factor: **C**

Fetal Risk Summary

No reports linking the use of novobiocin with congenital defects have been located. One study listed 21 patients exposed to the drug in the 1st trimester (1). No association with malformations was found. Since novobiocin may cause jaundice due to inhibition of glucuronyl transferase, its use near term is not recommended (2).

Breast Feeding Summary

Novobiocin is excreted into breast milk. Concentrations up to 7 µg/ml have been reported with milk:plasma ratios of 0.1–0.25 (3, 4). While adverse effects have not been reported, three potential problems exist for the nursing infant: modification of bowel flora, direct effects on the infant, and interference with the interpretation of culture results if a fever workup is required.

References

1. Heinonen OP, Slone D, Shapiro S. *Birth Defects and Drugs in Pregnancy*. Littleton:Publishing Sciences Group, 1977:297, 301.
2. Weistein L. Antibiotics. IV. Miscellaneous antimicrobial, antifungal, and antiviral agents. In Goodman LS, Gilman A, eds. *The Pharmacological Basis of Therapeutics*, ed. 4. New York:MacMillan, 1970:1292.

3. Knowles JA. Excretion of drugs in milk—a review. J Pediatr 1965;66:1068–82.
4. Anderson PO. Drugs and breast feeding—a review. Drug Intell Clin Pharm 1977;11:208–23.

Name: **NYLIDRIN**

Class: **Vasodilator**   Risk Factor: **C_M**

Fetal Risk Summary

Nylidrin is a β-adrenergic receptor stimulant used as a vasodilator in the United States. The drug has been studied in Europe as a tocolytic agent for premature labor and for the treatment of hypertension in pregnancy (1–7). Systolic blood pressure is usually unchanged, with a fall in total peripheral resistance greater than the decrease in diastolic pressure (8, 9). Although maternal hyperglycemia has been observed, especially in diabetic patients, this or other serious adverse effects were not reported in the above studies in mothers or in newborns.

Breast Feeding Summary

No data are available.

References

1. Neubuser D. Comparative investigation of two inhibitors of labour (TV 399 and buphenin). Geburtshilfe Fraunheilkd 1972;32:781–6.
2. Castren O, Gummerus M, Saarikoski S. Treatment of imminent premature labour. Acta Obstet Gynecol Scand 1975;54:95–100.
3. Gummerus M. Prevention of premature birth with nylidrin and verapamil. Z Geburtshilfe Perinatol 1975;179:261–6.
4. Wolff F, Bolte A, Berg R. Does an additional administration of acetylsalicylic acid reduce the requirement of betamimetics in tocolytic treatment? Geburtshilfe Fraunheilkd 1981;41:293–6.
5. Hofer U, Ammann K. The oral tocolytic longtime therapy and its effects on the child. Ther Umsch 1978;35:417–21.
6. Retzke VU, Schwarz R, Lanckner W, During R. Dilatol for hypertension therapy in pregnancy. Zentralbl Gynaekol 1979;101:1034–8.
7. During VR, Mauch I. Effects of nylidrin (Dilatol) on blood pressure of hypertensive patients in advanced pregnancy. Zentralbl Gynaekol 1980;102:193–8.
8. Retzke VU, Schwarz R, Barten G. Cardiovascular effects of nylidrin (Dilatol) in pregnancy. Zentralbl Gynaekol 1976;98:1059–65.
9. During VR, Reincke R. Action of nylidrin (Dilatol) on utero-placental blood supply. Zentralbl Gynaekol 1981;103:214–9.

Name: **NYSTATIN**

Class: **Antifungal Antibiotic**   Risk Factor: **B**

Fetal Risk Summary

Nystatin is poorly absorbed after oral administration and from intact skin and mucous membranes. The Collaborative Perinatal Project found a possible association with congenital malformations after 142 1st trimester exposures, but this was probably due to its use as an adjunct to tetracycline therapy (1, p. 313). No association was found following 230 exposures anytime in pregnancy (1, p. 435). Other investigators have reported its safe use in pregnancy (2–5).

Breast Feeding Summary

Since nystatin is poorly absorbed, if at all, serum and milk levels would not occur.

References

1. Heinonen OP, Slone D, Shapiro S. *Birth Defects and Drugs in Pregnancy*. Littleton:Publishing Sciences Group, 1977.
2. Culbertson C. Monistat: a new fungicide for treatment of vulvovaginal candidiasis. Am J Obstet Gynecol 1974;120:973–6.
3. David JE, Frudenfeld JH, Goddard JL. Comparative evaluation of Monistat and Mycostatin in the treatment of vulvovaginal candidiasis. Obstet Gynecol 1974;44:403–6.
4. Wallenburg HCS, Wladimiroff JW. Recurrence of vulvovaginal candidosis during pregnancy. Comparison of miconazole vs nystatin treatment. Obstet Gynecol 1976;48:491–4.
5. Rosa FW, Baum C, Shaw M. Pregnancy outcomes after first-trimester vaginitis drug therapy. Obstet Gynecol 1987;69:751–5.

Name: **OLEANDOMYCIN**

Class: **Antibiotic**   Risk Factor: **C**

Fetal Risk Summary

No reports linking the use of oleandomycin or its triacetyl ester, troleandomycin, with congenital defects have been located. One study listed nine patients exposed to the drugs in the 1st trimester (1). No association with malformations was found.

Breast Feeding Summary

No data are available.

Reference

1. Heinonen OP, Slone D, Shapiro S. *Birth Defects and Drugs in Pregnancy*. Littleton:Publishing Sciences Group, 1977:297, 301.

Name: **OPIPRAMOL**

Class: **Antidepressant**   Risk Factor: **D**

Fetal Risk Summary

No data are available (see Imipramine).

Breast Feeding Summary

No data are available (see Imipramine).

Name: **OPIUM**

Class: **Narcotic Antidiarrheal**   Risk Factor: **B***

Fetal Risk Summary

The effects of opium are due to morphine (see Morphine). The Collaborative Perinatal Project monitored 50,282 mother-child pairs, 36 of which had 1st trimester exposure to opium (1, pp. 287–295). For use anytime during pregnancy, 181 exposures were recorded (1, p. 424). Although these numbers are small, a possible relationship may exist between the use of this drug and major and minor malformations. Further, a possible association with inguinal hernia (seven cases) after anytime use was observed (1, p. 485). The statistical significance of these associations is unknown and independent confirmation is required.

Narcotic withdrawal was observed in a newborn whose mother was treated for regional ileitis with deodorized tincture of opium during the 2nd and 3rd trimesters (2). Symptoms of withdrawal in the infant began at 48 hours of age.

[*Risk Factor D if used for prolonged periods or in high doses at term.]

Breast Feeding Summary

See Morphine.

References

1. Heinonen OP, Slone D, Shapiro S. *Birth Defects and Drugs in Pregnancy*. Littleton:Publishing Sciences Group, 1977.
2. Fisch GR, Henley WL. Symptoms of narcotic withdrawal in a newborn infant secondary to medical therapy of the mother. Pediatrics 1961;28:852–3.

Name: **ORAL CONTRACEPTIVES**

Class: **Estrogenic/Progestogenic Hormones**   Risk Factor: **X**

Fetal Risk Summary

Oral contraceptives contain a 19-nortestosterone progestin and a synthetic estrogen (see Mestranol, Norethindrone, Norethynodrel, Ethinyl Estradiol, Progesterone, Hydroxyprogesterone, Ethisterone). Because oral contraceptives are primarily combination products, it is difficult to separate entirely the fetal effects of progestogens and estrogens. Two groups of investigators have reviewed the effects of these hormones on the fetus (133 references) (1, 2). Several potential problems were discussed: congenital heart defects, central nervous system defects, limb reduction malformations, general malformations, and modified development of sexual organs. Except for the latter category, no firm evidence has appeared that establishes a causal relationship between oral contraceptives and various congenital anomalies. The acronym VACTERL (Vertebral, Anal, Cardiac, Tracheal, Esophageal, Renal or Radial, and Limb) has been used to describe the fetal malformations produced by oral contraceptives or the related hormonal pregnancy test preparations (no longer available in the United States) (2, 3). The use of this acronym should probably be abandoned in favor of more conventional terminology as a large variety of malformations have been reported with estrogen-progestogen-containing products (1–11). The Population Council estimates that even if the study findings for VACTERL malformations are accurate, such abnormalities would occur in only 0.07% of the pregnancies exposed to oral contraceptives (12). Some reviewers have concluded that the risk to the fetus for nongenital malformations after *in utero* exposure to these agents is small, if indeed it exists at all (2).

In contrast to the above, the effect of estrogens and some synthetic progestogens on the development of the sexual organs is well established (2). Masculinization of the female infant has been associated with norethindrone, norethynodrel, hydroxyprogesterone, medroxyprogesterone, and diethylstilbestrol (2, 13,

14). The incidence of masculinization of female infants exposed to synthetic progestogens is reported to be approximately 0.3% (15). Pseudohermaphroditism in the male infant is not a problem, due to the low doses of estrogen employed in oral contraceptives (14).

Increased serum bilirubin in neonates of mothers taking oral contraceptives or progestogens before and after conception has been observed (16). Icterus occasionally reached clinically significant levels in infants whose mothers were exposed to the progestogens.

Concern that oral contraceptives may be a risk factor for preeclampsia has been suggested on the basis of the known effects of oral contraceptives on blood pressure (17). However, a retrospective controlled review of 341 patients found no association between this effect and the drugs (17).

Possible interactions between oral contraceptives and tetracycline, rifampin, ampicillin, or chloramphenicol resulting in pregnancy have been reported (18–25). The mechanism for this interaction may involve the interruption of the enterohepatic circulation of contraceptive steroids by inhibiting gut hydrolysis of steroid conjugates, resulting in lower concentrations of circulating steroids.

Breast Feeding Summary

Use of oral contraceptives during lactation has been associated with shortened duration of lactation, decreased infant weight gain, decreased milk production, and decreased composition of nitrogen and protein content of milk (26–29). The American Academy of Pediatrics has reviewed this subject (30) (37 references). Although the magnitude of these changes is low, the changes in milk production and composition may be of nutritional importance in malnourished mothers.

In general, progestin-only contraceptives demonstrate no consistent alteration of breast milk composition, volume, or duration of lactation (30). The composition and volume of breast milk will vary considerably even in the absence of steroidal contraceptives (29). Both estrogens and progestins cross into milk. An infant consuming 600 ml of breast milk daily from a mother using contraceptives containing 50 μg of ethinyl estradiol will probably receive a daily dose in the range of 10 ng (30). This is in the same range as the amount of natural estradiol received by infants of mothers not using oral contraceptives. Progestins also pass into breast milk, although naturally occurring progestins have not been identified. One study estimated 0.03 μg, 0.15 μg, and 0.3 μg of d-norgestrel/600 ml of milk from mothers receiving 30 μg, 150 μg, and 250 μg of the drug, respectively (31). A milk:plasma ratio of 0.15 for norgestrel was calculated by the authors (31). A ratio of 0.16 has been calculated for lynestrol (31, 32).

Reports of adverse effects are lacking except for one child with mild breast tenderness and hypertrophy who was exposed to large doses of estrogen (30). If breast feeding is desired, the lowest effective dose of oral contraceptives should be chosen. Infant weight gain should be monitored, and the possible need for nutritional supplements should be considered. The American Academy of Pediatrics considers combination oral contraceptives to be compatible with breast feeding (33).

References

1. Ambani LM, Joshi NJ, Vaidya RA, Devi PK. Are hormonal contraceptives teratogenic? Fertil Steril 1977;28:791–7.

2. Wilson JG, Brent RL. Are female sex hormones teratogenic? Am J Obstet Gynecol 1981;141:567–80.
3. Corcoran R, Entwistle GC. VACTERL congenital malformations and the male fetus. Lancet 1975;2:981–2.
4. Nora JJ, Nora AH. Can the pill cause birth defects. N Engl J Med 1974;294:731–2.
5. Kasan PN, Andrews J. Oral contraceptives and congenital abnormalities. Br J Obstet Gynaecol 1980;87:545–51.
6. Kullander S, Kallen B. A prospective study of drugs and pregnancy. Acta Obstet Gynecol Scand 1976;55:221–4.
7. Oakley GP, Flynt JW. Hormonal pregnancy test and congenital malformations. Lancet 1973;2:256–7.
8. Savolainen E, Saksela E, Saxen L. Teratogenic hazards of oral contraceptives analyzed in a national malformation register. Am J Obstet Gynecol 1981;140:521–4.
9. Frost O. Tracheo-oesophageal fistula associated with hormonal contraception during pregnancy. Br Med J 1976;3:978.
10. Redline RW, Abramowsky CR. Transposition of the great vessels in an infant exposed to massive doses of oral contraceptives. Am J Obstet Gynecol 1981;141:468–9.
11. Farb HF, Thomason J, Carandang FS, Sampson MB, Spellacy WH. Anencephaly twins and HLA-B27. J Reprod Med 1980;25:166–9.
12. Department of Medical and Public Affairs. *Population Reports*. Washington:The George Washington University Medical Center, 1975;2:A29–51.
13. Bongiovanni AM, DiGeorge AM, Grumbach MM. Masculinization of the female infant associated with estrogenic therapy alone during gestation: four cases. J Clin Endocrinol Metab 1959;19:1004–11.
14. Hagler S, Schultz A, Hankin H, Kunstadter RH. Fetal effects of steroid therapy during pregnancy. Am J Dis Child 1963;106:586–90.
15. Bongiovanni AM, McFadden AJ. Steroids during pregnancy and possible fetal consequences. Fertil Steril 1960;11:181–4.
16. McConnell JB, Glasgow JF, McNair R. Effect on neonatal jaundice of oestrogens and progestogens taken before and after conception. Br Med J 1973;3:605–7.
17. Bracken MB, Srisuphan W. Oral contraception as a risk factor for preeclampsia. Am J Obstet Gynecol 1982;142:191–6.
18. Bacon JF, Shenfield GM. Pregnancy attributable to interaction between tetracycline and oral contraceptives. Br Med J 1980;1:283.
19. Stockley I. Interactions with oral contraceptives. Pharm J 1976;216:140.
20. Reiners D, Nockefinck L, Breurer H. Rifampin and the "pill" do not go well together. JAMA 1974;227:608.
21. Dosseter EJ. Drug interactions with oral contraceptives. Br Med J 1975;1:1967.
22. Pullskinnen MO, Williams K. Reduced maternal plasma and urinary estriol during ampicillin treatment. Am J Obstet Gynecol 1971;109:895–6.
23. Friedman GI, Huneke AL, Kim MH, Powell J. The effect of ampicillin on oral contraceptive effectiveness. Obstet Gynecol 1980;55:33–7.
24. Back DJ, Breckenridge AM. Drug interactions with oral contraceptives. IPFF Med Bull 1978;12:1–2.
25. Orme ML, Back DJ. Therapy with oral contraceptive steroids and antibiotics J Antimicrob Chemother 1979;5:124–6.
26. Miller GH, Hughes LR. Lactation and genital involution effects of a new low-dose oral contraceptive on breast-feeding mothers and their infants. Obstet Gynecol 1970;35:44–50.
27. Kora SJ. Effect of oral contraceptives on lactation. Fertil Steril 1969;20:419–23.
28. Guiloff E, Ibarra-Polo A, Zanartu J, Tuscanini C, Mischler TW, Gomez-Rodgers C. Effect of contraception on lactation. Am J Obstet Gynecol 1974;118:42–5.
29. Lonnerdal B, Forsum E. Hambraeus L. Effect of oral contraceptives on consumption and volume of breast milk. Am J Clin Nutr 1980;33:816–24.
30. Committee on Drugs, American Academy of Pediatrics. Breast-feeding and contraception. Pediatrics 1981;68:138–40.
31. Nilsson S, Nygren KC, Johansson EDB. D-Norgestrel concentrations in maternal plasma, milk, and child plasma during administration of oral contraceptives to nursing women. Am J Obstet Gynecol 1977;129:178–83.

32. van der Molen HJ, Hart PG, Wijmenga HG. Studies with 4-^{14}C-lynestrol in normal and lactating women. Acta Endocrinol 1969;61:255–74.
33. Committee on Drugs, American Academy of Pediatrics. Transfer of drugs and other chemicals into human milk. Pediatrics 1989;84:924–36.

Name: **ORPHENADRINE**

Class: **Parasympatholytic**   Risk Factor: **C**

Fetal Risk Summary

Orphenadrine is an anticholinergic agent used in the treatment of parkinsonism. No reports of its use in pregnancy have been located (see also Atropine).

Breast Feeding Summary

No data are available (see also Atropine).

Name: **OUABAIN**

Class: **Cardiac Glycoside**   Risk Factor: **B**

Fetal Risk Summary

See Digitalis.

Breast Feeding Summary

See Digitalis.

Name: **OXACILLIN**

Class: **Antibiotic**   Risk Factor: **B$_M$**

Fetal Risk Summary

Oxacillin is a penicillin antibiotic (see also Penicillin G). The drug crosses the placenta in low concentrations. Cord serum and amniotic fluid levels were less than 0.3 μg/ml in 15 of 18 patients given 500 mg orally 0.5–4 hours prior to cesarean section (1). No effects were seen in the infants.

No reports linking the use of oxacillin with congenital defects have been located. The Collaborative Perinatal Project monitored 50,282 mother-child pairs, 3,546 of which had 1st trimester exposure to penicillin derivatives (2, pp. 297–313). For use anytime during pregnancy, 7,171 exposures were recorded (2, p. 435). In neither case was evidence found to suggest a relationship to large categories of major or minor malformations or to individual defects.

An interaction between oxacillin and oral contraceptives resulting in pregnancy has been reported (3). Other penicillins (e.g., see Ampicillin) have been suspected of this interaction, but not all investigators believe it occurs. Although controversial, an alternate means of contraception may be a practical solution if both drugs are consumed at the same time.

Breast Feeding Summary

Oxacillin is excreted in breast milk in low concentrations. Although no adverse effects have been reported, three potential problems exist for the nursing infant: modification of bowel flora, direct effects on the infant (e.g., allergic response), and interference with the interpretation of culture results if a fever workup is required.

References

1. Prigot A, Froix C, Rubin E. Absorption, diffusion, and excretion of new penicillin, oxacillin. Antimicrob Agents Chemother 1962:402–10.
2. Heinonen OP, Slone D, Shapiro S. *Birth Defects and Drugs in Pregnancy*. Littleton:Publishing Sciences Group, 1977.
3. Silber TJ. Apparent oral contraceptive failure associated with antibiotic administration. J Adolesc Health Care 1983;4:287–9.

Name: **OXAZEPAM**

Class: **Sedative**   Risk Factor: **D**

Fetal Risk Summary

Oxazepam is an active metabolite of diazepam (see also Diazepam). It is a member of the benzodiazepine group. The drug, both free and conjugated forms, crosses the placenta achieving average cord:maternal serum ratios during the 2nd trimester of 0.6 and at term of 1.1 (1). Large variations between patients for placental transfer have been observed (1–3). Passage of oxazepam is slower than diazepam, but the clinical significance of this is unknown (4). Two reports have suggested that the use of oxazepam in preeclampsia would be safer for the newborn infant than diazepam (5, 6). However, it is doubtful if either drug is indicated for this condition.

A 1989 report described characteristic dysmorphic features, growth retardation, and central nervous system defects in eight infants exposed either to oxazepam, 75 mg or more/day, or diazepam, 30 mg or more/day (7). See Diazepam for a detailed description of the infants. The authors concluded that the clinical characteristics observed in the infants probably represented a teratogenic syndrome due to benzodiazepines (7).

Breast Feeding Summary

Specific data relating to oxazepam usage in lactating women have not been located. Oxazepam, an active metabolite of diazepam, was detected in the urine of an infant exposed to high doses of diazepam during lactation (8). The infant was lethargic and demonstrated an EEG pattern compatible with sedative medication (see Diazepam).

References

1. Kangas L, Erkkola R, Kanto J, Eronen M. Transfer of free and conjugated oxazepam across the human placenta. Eur J Clin Pharmacol 1980;17:301–4.
2. Kanto J, Erkkola R, Sellman R. Perinatal metabolism of diazepam. Br Med J 1974;1:641–2.
3. Mandelli M, Morselli PL, Nordio S, Pardi G, Principi N, Seveni F, Tognoni G. Placental transfer of diazepam and its disposition in the newborn. Clin Pharmacol Ther 1975;17:564–72.
4. Kanto JH. Use of benzodiazepines during pregnancy, labour and lactation, with particular reference to pharmacokinetic considerations. Drugs 1982;23:354–80.
5. Gillberg C. "Floppy infant syndrome" and maternal diazepam. Lancet 1977;2:612–3.
6. Drury KAD, Spalding E, Donaldson D, Rutherford D. Floppy-infant syndrome: is oxazepam the answer? Lancet 1977;2:1126–7.
7. Laegreid L, Olegard R, Walstrom J, Conradi N. Teratogenic effects of benzodiazepine use during pregnancy. J Pediatr 1989;114:126–31.
8. Patrick MJ, Tilstone WJ, Reavey P. Diazepam and breast-feeding. Br Med J 1972;1:542–3.

Name: **OXPRENOLOL**

Class: **Sympatholytic (β-Adrenergic Blocker)**   Risk Factor: **C**

Fetal Risk Summary

Oxprenolol, a nonselective β-adrenergic blocking agent, has been used for the treatment of hypertension occurring during pregnancy (1–4). Oxprenolol and other β-blockers are generally considered safe and effective for this purpose by some reviewers (5, 6). However, one reviewer recommended that agents with either cardioselectivity or α-blocking activity may be preferred to the nonselective blockers because these agents would be less likely to interfere with uterine perfusion (5). Other suggested guidelines governing the use of β-blockers in pregnancy were: (*a*) if possible, avoid use in the 1st trimester, (*b*) use the lowest possible dose, and (*c*) if possible, discontinue the drugs 2–3 days prior to delivery (5). Oxprenolol crosses the placenta, but mean fetal serum levels at term are only about 25–37% of maternal concentrations (4, 6).

No fetal malformations or other fetal adverse effects attributable to oxprenolol have been reported, but experience during the 1st trimester is lacking. The drug has been compared with methyldopa in two studies of pregnant hypertensive women (1, 2). In one of these studies, oxprenolol-exposed infants were significantly larger, 3051 g vs. 2654 g, than offspring of methyldopa-treated mothers (1). The difference was thought to be due to the greater maternal plasma volume expansion and placental growth observed in the β-blocker group (1). In a follow-up report, the investigators noted that the differences between the two groups disappeared after 10 weeks of treatment (7). A 1983 study found no difference between oxprenolol- and methyldopa-treated groups in birth weight, placental weight, head circumference, and Apgar scores (2). In a third study, the combination of oxprenolol and prazosin (an α-adrenergic blocking agent) was effective for the control of severe essential hypertension in 25 pregnant women but not effective in 19 patients with pregnancy-induced hypertension (3).

Although β-blockade of the newborn has not been reported in the offspring of oxprenolol-treated mothers, this complication has occurred with other members of this class (see Acebutolol, Atenolol, and Nadolol). Thus, close observation of the newborn for bradycardia and other symptoms of β-blockade is recommended during the first 24–48 hours after birth. Long-term effects of *in utero* exposure to β-blockers have not been studied but warrant evaluation.

Breast Feeding Summary

Oxprenolol is excreted into breast milk (8, 9). In nine lactating women given 80 mg twice daily, the mean milk concentration of oxprenolol 105–135 minutes after a dose was 118 ng/ml (9). When a dose of 160 mg twice daily was given to three women, mean milk levels were 160 ng/ml. Finally, one woman was treated with 320 mg twice daily, producing a milk level of 470 ng/ml. The milk:plasma ratios for the three regimens were 0.14, 0.16, and 0.43, respectively. The mean milk:plasma ratio in another study was 0.45 (8). These low ratios, relative to other β-blockers, may be due to the high maternal serum protein binding (80%) which negates trapping of the weakly basic drug in the relatively acidic milk (8). Based on calculations, a mother ingesting 240 mg/day would provide a 3-kg infant with a dose of 0.07 mg/kg in 500 ml of milk (8). This amount is probably clinically insignificant.

Although no adverse reactions have been noted in nursing infants of mothers treated with oxprenolol, infants should be closely observed for bradycardia and other symptoms of β-blockade. Long-term effects of exposure to β-blockers from milk have not been studied but warrant evaluation. The American Academy of Pediatrics considers oxprenolol to be compatible with breast feeding (10).

References

1. Gallery EDM, Saunders DM, Hunyor SN, Gyory AZ. Randomized comparison of methyldopa and oxprenolol for treatment of hypertension in pregnancy. Br Med J 1979;1:1591–4.
2. Fidler J, Smith V, Fayers P, DeSwiet M. Randomized controlled comparative study of methyldopa and oxprenolol in treatment of hypertension in pregnancy. Br Med J 1983;286:1927–30.
3. Lubbe WF, Hodge JV. Combined α- and β-adrenoceptor antagonism with prazosin and oxprenolol in control of severe hypertension in pregnancy. NZ Med J 1981;94:169–72.
4. Lubbe WF. More on beta-blockers in pregnancy. N Engl J Med 1982;307:753.
5. Frishman WH, Chesner M. Beta-adrenergic blockers in pregnancy. Am Heart J 1988;115:147–52.
6. Gallery EDM. Hypertension in pregnant women. Med J Aust 1985;143:23–7.
7. Gallery EDM, Ross MR, Gyory AZ. Antihypertensive treatment in pregnancy: analysis of different responses to oxprenolol and methyldopa. Br Med J 1985;291:563–6.
8. Sioufi A, Hillion D, Lumbroso P, Wainer R, Olivier-Martin M, Schoeller JP, Colussi D, Leroux F, Mangoni P. Oxprenolol placental transfer, plasma concentrations in newborns and passage into breast milk. Br J Clin Pharmacol 1984;18:453–6.
9. Fidler J, Smith V, DeSwiet M. Excretion of oxprenolol and timolol in breast milk. Br J Obstet Gynaecol 1983;90:961–5.
10. Committee on Drugs, American Academy of Pediatrics. Transfer of drugs and other chemicals into human milk. Pediatrics 1989;84:924–36.

Name: **OXTRIPHYLLINE**

Class: **Spasmolytic/Vasodilator**   Risk Factor: **C**

Fetal Risk Summary

Oxtriphylline is a methylxanthine that is metabolized to theophylline. Theophylline has been found in cord blood but not in the serum of an infant whose mother had taken oxtriphylline during pregnancy (1). No adverse effects in the infant were observed (see also Theophylline).

Breast Feeding Summary

No data are available. See also Theophylline.

Reference

1. Labovitz E, Spector S. Placental theophylline transfer in pregnant asthmatics. JAMA 1982;247:786–8.

Name: **OXYCODONE**

Class: **Narcotic Analgesic**   Risk Factor: **B***

Fetal Risk Summary

No reports linking the use of oxycodone with congenital defects have been located. The drug is rarely used in pregnancy.

[*Risk Factor D if used for prolonged periods or in high doses at term.]

Breast Feeding Summary

Oxycodone is excreted into human breast milk (1). Six healthy postpartum women received a combination product of oxycodone and acetaminophen, one or two capsules every 4–7 hours, while breast feeding their newborn infants (1). Maternal plasma levels were in the expected range of 14–35 ng/ml, and milk concentrations ranged from <5–226 ng/ml. Peak milk concentrations occurred 1.5–2.0 hours after the first dose, then at variable times after multiple doses. Although a large degree of variability was present, the mean milk:plasma ratio was 3.4:1. No mention was made of any effects observed in the nursing infants.

Reference

1. Marx CM, Pucino F, Carlson JD, Driscoll JW, Ruddock V. Oxycodone excretion in human milk in the puerperium. Drug Intell Clin Pharm 1986;20:474 (Abstract).

Name: **OXYMORPHONE**

Class: **Narcotic Analgesic**   Risk Factor: **B***

Fetal Risk Summary

No reports linking the use of oxymorphone with congenital defects have been located. Use of this drug during labor produces neonatal respiratory depression to the same degree as other narcotic analgesics (1–4).

[*Risk Factor D if used for prolonged periods or in high doses at term.]

Breast Feeding Summary

No data are available.

References

1. Simeckova M, Shaw W, Pool E, Nichols EE. Numorphan in labor—a preliminary report. Obstet Gynecol 1960;16:119–23.
2. Sentnor MH, Solomons E, Kohl SG. An evaluation of oxymorphone in labor. Am J Obstet Gynecol 1962;84:956–61.
3. Eames GM, Pool KRS. Clinical trial of oxymorphone in labor. Br Med J 1964; 2:353–5.
4. Ransom S. Oxymorphone as an obstetric analgesic—a clinical trial. Anesthesia 1966;21:464–71.

Name: **OXYPHENBUTAZONE**

Class: **Nonsteroidal Anti-inflammatory**   Risk Factor: **D**

Fetal Risk Summary

See Phenylbutazone.

Breast Feeding Summary

See Phenylbutazone.

Name: **OXYPHENCYCLIMINE**

Class: **Parasympatholytic (Anticholinergic)**   Risk Factor: **C**

Fetal Risk Summary

Oxyphencyclimine is an anticholinergic agent. In a large prospective study, 2323 patients were exposed to this class of drugs during the 1st trimester, 1 of whom took oxyphencyclimine (1). A possible association was found between the total group and minor malformations.

Breast Feeding Summary

No data are available (see also Atropine).

Reference

1. Heinonen OP, Slone D, Shapiro S. *Birth Defects and Drugs in Pregnancy*. Littleton:Publishing Sciences Group, 1977:346–53.

Name: **OXYPHENONIUM**

Class: **Parasympatholytic (Anticholinergic)**   Risk Factor: **C**

Fetal Risk Summary

Oxyphenonium is an anticholinergic quaternary ammonium bromide. No reports of its use in pregnancy have been located (see also Atropine).

Breast Feeding Summary

No data are available (see also Atropine).

Name: **OXYTETRACYCLINE**

Class: **Antibiotic**   Risk Factor: **D**

Fetal Risk Summary

See Tetracycline.

Breast Feeding Summary

See Tetracycline.

Name: **PANTOTHENIC ACID**

Class: **Vitamin**   Risk Factor: **A***

Fetal Risk Summary

Pantothenic acid, a water-soluble B complex vitamin, acts as a coenzyme in the metabolism or synthesis of a number of carbohydrates, proteins, lipids, and steroid hormones (1). The American recommended daily allowance (RDA) for pantothenic acid or its derivatives (dexpanthenol and calcium pantothenate) in pregnancy is 10.0 mg (2).

No reports of maternal or fetal complications associated with pantothenic acid have been located. Deficiency of this vitamin was not found in two studies evaluating maternal vitamin levels during pregnancy (3, 4). Like other B complex vitamins, newborn pantothenic acid levels are significantly greater than maternal levels (3–6). At term, mean pantothenate levels in 174 mothers were 430 ng/ml (range 250–710) and in their newborns 780 ng/ml (range 400–1480) (3). Placental transfer of pantothenate to the fetus is by active transport, but it is slower than transfer of other B complex vitamins (7, 8). In one report, low-birth-weight infants had significantly lower levels of pantothenic acid than did normal weight infants (6).

[*Risk Factor C in amounts above the RDA.]

Breast Feeding Summary

Pantothenic acid is excreted in human breast milk with concentrations directly proportional to intake (9, 10). With a dietary intake of 8–15 mg/day, mean milk concentrations average 1.93–2.35 μg/ml (9). In a group of mothers who had delivered premature babies (28–34 weeks gestational age), pantothenic acid milk levels were significantly greater than a comparable group with term babies (39–41 weeks) (10). Milk levels in the preterm group averaged 3.91 μg/ml up to 40 weeks gestational age and then fell to 3.16 μg/ml. For the term group, levels at 2 and 12 weeks postpartum were 2.57 and 2.55 μg/ml, respectively. A 1983 English study measured pantothenic acid levels in pooled human milk obtained from preterm (26 mothers—29–34 weeks) and term (35 mothers—39 weeks or longer) patients (11). Preterm milk rose from 1.29 μg/ml (colostrum) to 2.27 μg/ml (16–196 days), while term milk increased over the same period from 1.26 μg/ml to 2.61 μg/ml.

An RDA for pantothenic acid during lactation has not been established. However, since this vitamin is required for good health, amounts at least equal to the RDA for pregnancy are recommended. If the diet of the lactating woman adequately supplies this amount, maternal supplementation with pantothenic acid is probably not required. Supplementation with the pregnancy RDA for pantothenic acid is recommended for those women with inadequate nutritional intake.

References

1. American Hospital Formulary Service. *Drug Information 1990*. Bethesda:American Society of Hospital Pharmacists, 1990:2115–6.
2. *Recommended Dietary Allowances*, 9th ed. Washington:National Academy of Sciences, 1980:122–4.
3. Baker H, Frank O, Thomson AD, Langer A, Munves ED, De Angelis B, Kaminetzky HA. Vitamin profile of 174 mothers and newborns at parturition. Am J Clin Nutr 1975;28:59–65.
4. Baker H, Frank O, Deangelis B, Feingold S, Kaminetzky HA. Role of placenta in maternal-fetal vitamin transfer in humans. Am J Obstet Gynecol 1981;141:792–6.
5. Cohenour SH, Calloway DH. Blood, urine, and dietary pantothenic acid levels of pregnant teenagers. Am J Clin Nutr 1972;25:512–7.
6. Baker H, Thind IS, Frank O, DeAngelis B, Caterini H, Louria DB. Vitamin levels in low-birth-weight newborn infants and their mothers. Am J Obstet Gynecol 1977;129:521–4.
7. Hill EP, Longo LD. Dynamics of maternal-fetal nutrient transfer. Fed Proc 1980;39:239–44.
8. Kaminetsky HA, Baker H, Frank O, Langer A. The effects of intravenously administered water-soluble vitamins during labor in normovitaminemic and hypovitaminemic gravidas on maternal and neonatal blood vitamin levels at delivery. Am J Obstet Gynecol 1974;120:697–703.
9. Deodhar AD, Rajalakshmi R, Ramakrishnan CV. Studies on human lactation. Part III. Effect of dietary vitamin supplementation on vitamin contents of breast milk. Acta Paediatr Scand 1964;53:42–8.
10. Song WO, Chan GM, Wyse BW, Hansen RG. Effect of pantothenic acid status on the content of the vitamin in human milk. Am J Clin Nutr 1984;40:317–24.
11. Ford JE, Zechalko A, Murphy J, Brooke OG. Comparison of the B vitamin composition of milk from mothers of preterm and term babies. Arch Dis Child 1983;58:367–72.

Name: **PARAMETHADIONE**

Class: **Anticonvulsant**   Risk Factor: D_M

Fetal Risk Summary

Paramethadione is an oxazolidinedione anticonvulsant used in the treatment of petit mal epilepsy. There have been three families (10 pregnancies) in which an increase in spontaneous abortion or abnormalities have been reported (1, 2). Paramethadione is considered equivalent to trimethadione in regard to its fetal effects. In fact, one of the families described by German was included in the fetal trimethadione syndrome (see Trimethadione) (3). This patient had one normal infant after anticonvulsant medications were withdrawn. Malformations reported in two additional families by Rutman are consistent with fetal paramethadione/trimethadione syndrome (2). The malformations included tetralogy of Fallot, mental retardation, failure to thrive, and increased incidence of spontaneous abortions (2). Because paramethadione has demonstrated both clinical and experimental fetal risk greater than other anticonvulsants, its use should be abandoned in favor of other anticonvulsants for the treatment of petit mal epilepsy (see also Ethosuximide, Phensuximide, Methsuximide) (4–6).

Breast Feeding Summary

No data are available.

References

1. German J, Ehlers KH, Kowal A, DeGeorge PU, Engle MA, Passarge E. Possible teratogenicity of trimethadione and paramethadione. Lancet 1970;2:261–2.
2. Rutman JT. Anticonvulsants and fetal damage. N Engl J Med 1973;189:696–7.
3. German J, Kowal A, Ehlers KH. Trimethadione and human teratogenesis. Teratology 1970;3:349–62.
4. National Institute of Health. Anticonvulsants found to have teratogenic potential. JAMA 1981;245:36.
5. Fabro S, Brown NA. Teratogenic potential of anticonvulsants. N Engl J Med 1979; 300:1280–1.
6. Hill RM. Managing the epileptic patient during pregnancy. Drug Ther 1976:204–5.

Name: **PAREGORIC**

Class: **Antidiarrheal**   Risk Factor: **B***

Fetal Risk Summary

Paregoric is a mixture of opium powder, anise oil, benzoic acid, camphor, glycerin, and ethanol. Its action is mainly due to morphine (see also Morphine). The Collaborative Perinatal Project monitored 50,282 mother-child pairs, 90 of which had 1st trimester exposure to paregoric (1, pp. 287–295). For use anytime during pregnancy, 562 exposures were recorded (1, p. 434). No evidence was found to suggest a relationship to large categories of major or minor malformations or to individual defects.

[*Risk Factor D if used for prolonged periods in high doses at term.]

Breast Feeding Summary

See Morphine.

Reference

1. Heinonen OP, Slone D, Shapiro S. *Birth Defects and Drugs in Pregnancy*. Littleton:Publishing Sciences Group, 1977.

Name: **PARGYLINE**

Class: **Antihypertensive**   Risk Factor: **C$_M$**

Fetal Risk Summary

No data are available.

Breast Feeding Summary

No data are available.

Name: **PAROMOMYCIN**

Class: **Antibiotic**   Risk Factor: **C**

Fetal Risk Summary

Paromomycin is an aminoglycoside antibiotic used for intestinal amebiasis. No reports linking this agent with congenital malformations have been located. Since it is poorly absorbed, with almost 100% of an oral dose excreted unchanged in the feces, little if any of the drug will reach the fetus.

Two women, one at 13 weeks' gestation and the other at 23 weeks, were treated for a symptomatic intestinal infection due to *Giardia lamblia* (1). Both delivered normal female infants at term. A 1985 review of intestinal parasites and pregnancy concluded that treatment of the pregnant patient should only be considered if the "parasite is causing clinical disease or may cause public health problems" (2). When indicated, paromomycin was recommended for the treatment of protozoan infections due to *Giardia lamblia* and *Entamoeba histolytica*, and for tapeworm infestations occurring during pregnancy (2).

Breast Feeding Summary

Paromomycin excretion in human milk is not expected since the drug is not absorbed into the systemic circulation after oral dosing. Following parenteral administration to lactating ewes, only 0.018% of the dose was recovered from the milk over a 12-hour period (3). The poor lipid solubility of the antibiotic limited its passage into milk (3).

References

1. Kreutner AK, Del Bene VE, Amstey MS. Giardiasis in pregnancy. Am J Obstet Gynecol 1981;140:895–901.
2. D'Alauro F, Lee RV, Pao-In K, Khairallah M. Intestinal parasites and pregnancy. Obstet Gynecol 1985;66:639–43.
3. Ziv G, Sulman FG. Distribution of aminoglycoside antibiotics in blood and milk. Res Vet Sci 1974;17:68–74.

Name: **PENICILLAMINE**

Class: **Heavy Metal Antagonist**   Risk Factor: **D**

Fetal Risk Summary

The use of penicillamine during pregnancy has been observed in approximately 100 pregnancies (1–14; G.G. Briggs, unpublished data, 1982). The mothers were treated for rheumatoid arthritis, cystinuria, or Wilson's disease. From these pregnancies, anomalies were observed in eight infants:

Cutis laxa, hypotonia, hyperflexion of hips and shoulders, pyloric stenosis, vein fragility, varicosities, impaired wound healing, death (2)
Cutis laxa, growth retardation, inguinal hernia, simian crease, perforated bowel, death (6)
Cutis laxa (3)

Cutis laxa, mild micrognathia, low-set ears, inguinal hernia (11)

Cutis laxa, inguinal hernia (12)

Marked flexion deformities of extremities, dislocated hips, hydrocephalus, intraventricular hemorrhage, death (13)

Cerebral palsy, blindness, bilateral club feet, sudden infant death at 3 months (13)

Hydrocephalus (13)

The relationship of the last three cases listed above to penicillamine is controversial since they did not include connective tissue anomalies. The drug may be partially responsible, but other factors, such as maternal infections and surgery, may have a stronger association with the defects (13). A small ventricular septal defect was observed in another newborn but this was probably not related to penicillamine (8).

Penicillamine crosses the placenta to the fetus. A mother was treated for cystinuria throughout gestation with penicillamine hydrochloride 1050 mg/day (843 mg of penicillamine base) (1). The drug was found in the urine of her newborn infant. The baby's physical and mental development was normal at 3 months.

Although the evidence is incomplete, maintaining the daily dose at 500 mg or less may reduce the incidence of penicillamine-induced toxicity in the newborn (5, 10). However, authors of one review believe the drug should be avoided during pregnancy (15).

Breast Feeding Summary

No reports that describe the use of penicillamine during lactation or if the drug is excreted in milk have been located. Authors of one review recommend avoiding penicillamine during lactation (15).

References

1. Crawhall JC, Scowen EF, Thompson CJ, Watts RWE. Dissolution of cystine stones during d-penicillamine treatment of a pregnant patient with cystinuria. Br Med J 1967;2:216–8.
2. Mjolnerod OK, Rasmussen K, Dommerud SA, Gjeruldsen ST. Congenital connective-tissue defect probably due to d-penicillamine treatment in pregnancy. Lancet 1971;1:673–5.
3. Laver M, Fairley KF. D-penicillamine treatment in pregnancy. Lancet 1971;1:1019–20.
4. Scheinberg IH, Sternlieb I. Pregnancy in penicillamine-treated patients with Wilson's disease. N Engl J Med 1975;293:1300–3.
5. Marecek Z, Graf M. Pregnancy in penicillamine-treated patients with Wilson's disease. N Engl J Med 1976;295:841–2.
6. Solomon L, Abrams G, Dinner M, Berman L. Neonatal abnormalities associated with d-penicillamine treatment during pregnancy. N Engl J Med 1977;296:54–5.
7. Walshe JM. Pregnancy in Wilson's disease. Q J Med 1977;46:73–83.
8. Lyle WH. Penicillamine in pregnancy. Lancet 1978;1:606–7.
9. Linares A, Zarranz JJ, Rodriguez-Alarcon J, Diaz-Perez JL. Reversible cutis laxa due to maternal d-penicillamine treatment. Lancet 1979;2:43.
10. Endres W. D-penicillamine in pregnancy—to ban or not to ban? Klin Wochenschr 1981;59:535–7.
11. Harpey JP, Jaudon MC, Clavel JP, Galli A, Darbois Y. Cutis laxa and low serum zinc after antenatal exposure to penicillamine. Lancet 1983;2:858.
12. Beck RB, Rosenbaum KN, Byers PH, Holbrook KA, Perry LW. Ultrastructural findings in the fetal penicillamine syndrome (Abstr). Presented at the 13th Annual Birth Defects Conference, March of Dimes and University of California, San Diego, June, 1980.
13. Gal P, Ravenel SD. Contractures and hydrocephalus with penicillamine and maternal hypotension. J Clin Dysmorphol 1984;2:9–12.
14. Gregory MC, Mansell MA. Pregnancy and cystinuria. Lancet 1983;2:1158–60.

15. Ostensen M, Husby G. Antirheumatic drug treatment during pregnancy and lactation. Scand J Rheumatol 1985;14:1–7.

Name: **PENICILLIN G**

Class: **Antibiotic**   Risk Factor: **B**

Fetal Risk Summary

Penicillin G is used routinely for maternal infections during pregnancy. Several investigators have documented its rapid passage into the fetal circulation and amniotic fluid (1–5). Therapeutic levels are reached in both sites except for the amniotic fluid during the 1st trimester (5). At term, maternal serum and amniotic fluid concentrations are equal 60–90 minutes after intravenous (IV) administration (2). Continuous IV infusions (10,000 units/hour) produced equal concentrations of penicillin G at 20 hours in maternal serum, cord serum, and amniotic fluid (2).

The early use of penicillin G was linked to increased uterine activity and abortion (6–10). It is not known if this was due to impurities in the drug or to penicillin itself. No reports of this effect have appeared since a reference in 1950 (10). An anaphylactic reaction in a pregnant patient reportedly led to the death of her fetus *in utero* (11).

Only one reference has linked the use of penicillin G with congenital abnormalities (12). An examination of hospital records indicated that in three of four cases the administration of penicillin G had been followed by the birth of a malformed baby. A retrospective review of additional patients exposed to antibiotics in the 1st trimester indicated an increase in congenital defects. Unfortunately, the authors did not analyze their data for each antibiotic, so no causal relationship to penicillin G could be shown (12, 13). In another case, a patient was treated in early pregnancy with high doses of penicillin G procaine IV (?), cortisone, and sodium salicylate (14). A cyclopic male was delivered at term but died 5 minutes later. The defect was attributed to salicylates, cortisone, or maternal viremia. (Penicillin G procaine should not be given IV. The Editors are assuming the drug was either given intramuscularly (IM) or the procaine form was not used. We have not been able to contact the authors to clarify these assumptions.)

In a controlled study, 110 patients received one to three antibiotics during the 1st trimester for a total of 589 weeks (15). Penicillin G was given for a total of 107 weeks. The incidence of birth defects was no different than in a nontreated control group.

The Collaborative Perinatal Project monitored 50,282 mother-child pairs, 3,546 of which had 1st trimester exposure to penicillin derivatives (16, pp. 297–313). For use anytime during pregnancy, 7,171 exposures were recorded (16, p. 435). In neither case was evidence found to suggest a relationship to large categories of major or minor malformations or to individual defects. Based on these data, it is unlikely that penicillin G is teratogenic.

Breast Feeding Summary

Penicillin G is excreted into breast milk in low concentrations. Milk:plasma ratios following intramuscular doses of 100,000 units in 11 patients varied between

0.02–0.13 (17). The maximum concentration measured in milk was 0.6 unit/ml after this dose. Although no adverse effects were reported, three potential problems exist for the nursing infant: modification of bowel flora, direct effects on the infant (e.g., allergic response), and interference with the interpretation of culture results if a fever workup is required.

References

1. Herrel W, Nichols D, Heilman D. Penicillin. Its usefulness, limitations, diffusion and detection, with analysis of 150 cases in which it was employed. JAMA 1944;125:1003–11.
2. Woltz J, Zintel H. The transmission of penicillin to amniotic fluid and fetal blood in the human. Am J Obstet Gynecol 1945;50:338–40.
3. Hutter A, Parks J. The transmission of penicillin through the placenta. A preliminary report. Am J Obstet Gynecol 1945;49:663–5.
4. Woltz J, Wiley M. The transmission of penicillin to the previable fetus. JAMA 1946;131:969–70.
5. Wasz-Hockert O, Nummi S, Vuopala S, Jarvinen P. Transplacental passage of azidocillin, ampicillin and penicillin G during early and late pregnancy. Acta Paediatr Scand (Suppl) 1970;206:109–10.
6. Lentz J, Ingraham N Jr, Beerman H, Stokes J. Penicillin in the prevention and treatment of congenital syphilis. JAMA 1944;126:408–13.
7. Leavitt H. Clinical action of penicillin on the uterus. J Vener Dis Inf 1945;26:150–3.
8. McLachlan A, Brown D. The effects of penicillin administration on menstrual and other sexual functions. Br J Vener Dis 1947;23:1–10.
9. Mazingarbe A. Le penciline possede-t-elle une action abortive? Gynecol Obstet 1946;45:487.
10. Perin L, Sissmann R, Detre F, Chertier A. La penciline a-t-elle une action abortive? Bull Soc Fr Dermatol 1950;57:534–8.
11. Kosim H. Intrauterine fetal death as a result of anaphylactic reaction to penicillin in a pregnant woman. Dapim Refuiim 1959;18:136–7.
12. Carter M, Wilson F. Antibiotics and congenital malformations. Lancet 1963;1:1267–8.
13. Carter M, Wilson F. Antibiotics in early pregnancy and congenital malformations. Dev Med Child Neurol 1965;7:353–9.
14. Khudr G, Olding L. Cyclopia. Am J Dis Child 1973;125:120–2.
15. Ravid R, Toaff R. On the possible teratogenicity of antibiotic drugs administered during pregnancy-a prospective study. In Klingberg M, Abramovici A, Chemki J, eds. *Drugs and Fetal Development*. New York:Plenum Press, 1972:505–10.
16. Heinonen OP, Slone D, Shapiro S. *Birth Defects and Drugs in Pregnancy*. Littleton:Publishing Sciences Group, 1977.
17. Greene H, Burkhart B, Hobby G. Excretion of penicillin in human milk following parturition. Am J Obstet Gynecol 1946;51:732–3.

Name: **PENICILLIN G, BENZATHINE**

Class: **Antibiotic**   Risk Factor: **B**

Fetal Risk Summary

Benzathine penicillin G is a combination of an ammonium base and penicillin G suspended in water. See Penicillin G.

Breast Feeding Summary

See Penicillin G.

Name: **PENICILLIN G, PROCAINE**

Class: **Antibiotic**   Risk Factor: **B**

Fetal Risk Summary

Procaine penicillin G is an equimolar combination of procaine and penicillin G suspended in water (1). The combination is broken down *in vivo* into the two components. See also Penicillin G.

A case report described the use of high doses of penicillin G procaine intravenously (IV) (?), cortisone, and sodium salicylate in early pregnancy followed by the delivery at term of a cyclopic male infant (2). The lethal defect was attributed to salicylates, cortisone, or maternal viremia. (Note: Penicillin G procaine should not be given IV. The Editors are assuming the drug was either given intramuscularly or the procaine form was not used. We have been unable to contact the authors of the paper to clarify these assumptions.)

Breast Feeding Summary

See Penicillin G.

References

1. Mandel G, Sande M. Antimicrobial agents (continued). Penicillins and cephalosporins. In Gilman AG, Goodman LS, Gilman A, eds. *The Pharmacological Basis of Therapeutics*, ed 6. New York:MacMillan, 1980:1137.
2. Khudr G, Olding L. Cyclopia. Am J Dis Child 1973;125:120–2.

Name: **PENICILLIN V**

Class: **Antibiotic**   Risk Factor: **B**

Fetal Risk Summary

No reports linking the use of penicillin V with congenital defects have been located. The Collaborative Perinatal Project monitored 50,282 mother-child pairs, 3,546 of which had 1st trimester exposure to penicillin derivatives (1, pp. 297–313). For use anytime during pregnancy, 7,171 exposures were recorded (1, p. 435). In neither case was evidence found to suggest a relationship to large categories of major or minor malformations or to individual defects.

Penicillin V depresses both plasma-bound and urinary excreted estriol (2). Urinary estriol was formerly used to assess the condition of the fetoplacental unit, depressed levels being associated with fetal distress. This assessment is now made by measuring plasma-unconjugated estriol, which is not usually affected by penicillin V.

Breast Feeding Summary

No data are available (see Penicillin G).

References

1. Heinonen OP, Slone D, Shapiro S. *Birth Defects and Drugs in Pregnancy*. Littleton:Publishing Sciences Group, 1977.

2. Pulkkinen M, Willman K. Maternal oestrogen levels during penicillin treatment. Br Med J 1971;4:48.

Name: **PENTAERYTHRITOL TETRANITRATE**

Class: **Vasodilator** Risk Factor: **C**

Fetal Risk Summary

Pentaerythritol tetranitrate is a long-acting agent used for the prevention of angina pectoris. Due to the nature of its indication, experience in pregnancy is limited. The Collaborative Perinatal Project recorded 3 1st trimester exposures to pentaerythritol tetranitrate plus 12 other patients exposed to other vasodilators (1). From this small sample, four malformed children were produced, a statistically significant incidence ($p < 0.02$). It was not reported if pentaerythritol tetranitrate was taken by any of the mothers of the affected infants. Although these data serve as a warning, the number of patients is so small that conclusions as to the relative safety of this drug cannot be made.

Breast Feeding Summary

No data are available.

Reference

1. Heinonen OP, Slone D, Shapiro S. *Birth Defects and Drugs in Pregnancy*. Littleton:Publishing Sciences Group, 1977.

Name: **PENTAZOCINE**

Class: **Analgesic** Risk Factor: **B***

Fetal Risk Summary

No reports linking the use of pentazocine with congenital defects have been located. The drug rapidly crosses the placenta resulting in cord blood levels of 40–70% of maternal serum (1). Withdrawal has been reported in infants exposed *in utero* to chronic maternal ingestion of pentazocine (2–6). Symptoms, presenting within 24–48 hours of birth, consist of trembling and jitteriness, marked hyperirritability, hyperactivity with hypertonia, high-pitched cry, diaphoresis, diarrhea, vomiting, and opisthotonic posturing.

During labor, increased overall uterine activity has been observed after pentazocine, but without changes in fetal heart rate (7). In equianalgesic doses, most studies report no significant differences between meperidine and pentazocine in pain relief, length of labor, or Apgar scores (8–13). However, meperidine in one study was observed to produce significantly lower Apgar scores than pentazocine, especially in repeated doses (14). Severe neonatal respiratory depression may also occur with pentazocine (8, 14).

A 1982 report from New Orleans described 24 infants born of mothers using the intravenous combination of pentazocine/tripelennamine (T's and Blue's) (15). Doses were unknown but probably ranged from 200–600 mg of pentazocine and 100–250 mg of tripelennamine. Six of the newborns were exposed early in pregnancy. Birth weights for 11 of the infants were less than 2500 g; nine of these were premature (less than 37 weeks) and two were small for gestational age. Daily or weekly exposure throughout pregnancy produced withdrawal symptoms, occurring within 7 days of birth, in 15 of 16 infants. Withdrawal was thought to be due to pentazocine, but antihistamine withdrawal has been reported (see Diphenhydramine). Thirteen of 15 infants became asymptomatic 3–11 days following onset of withdrawal, but symptoms persisted for up to 6 months in two.

Three cases of maternal bacterial endocarditis were observed following intravenous drug abuse, one of which involved the injection of pentazocine/tripelennamine intermittently throughout pregnancy (16). Following satisfactory antibiotic treatment for the infection, the mother gave birth at term to a healthy, male infant.

In a study published in 1983, three groups of pregnant women were evaluated in a perinatal addiction program in the Chicago area (17). One group ($N = 13$) was composed of women addicted to pentazocine/tripelennamine. A second group consisted of women who conceived while self-administering heroin, and who were then converted to low-dose (5–40 mg/day) methadone ($N = 46$). The third group consisted of drug-free controls ($N = 27$). The three groups were statistically similar as to mean maternal age, educational level, gravidity, cigarette smoking, and mean weight gain during pregnancy. Heavy alcohol users were excluded. All infants were delivered at term. Apgar scores were similar among the three groups of newborns, and no significant perinatal complications were observed. Mean birth weight, length, and head circumference were similar between the two drug groups. Compared to the drug-free controls, the pentazocine/tripelennamine-exposed infants weighed less (2799 vs. 3479 g, $p < 0.0001$), were shorter (48.1 vs. 51.1 cm, $p < 0.002$), and had smaller heads (32.9 vs. 34.7 cm, $p < 0.003$). Neonatal withdrawal was observed in both drug-exposed infant groups. Withdrawal characteristics observed in the pentazocine/tripelennamine infants were similar to those seen in the methadone group, consisting of irritability, voracious sucking, and feeding difficulties (17). However, none of these infants required therapy for their symptoms. Neonatal behavior was evaluated using the Brazelton Neonatal Behavioral Assessment Scale. Results of these tests indicated that the infants exposed to the drug combination had interactive deficits and withdrawal similar to the methadone-addicted babies (17).

Another study described the effects of pentazocine/tripelennamine abuse in 50 pregnancies identified retrospectively from a total of 23,779 deliveries occurring between January 1, 1981, and June 30, 1983 (18). Compared to matched controls, users of the combination were more likely to have no prenatal care ($p < 0.005$), to be anemic ($p < 0.001$), and to have syphilis ($p < 0.001$), gonorrhea ($p < 0.01$), or hepatitis ($p < 0.005$). Moreover, their infants were more likely to be small for gestational age ($p < 0.01$), to have lower birth weights (3260 g vs. 2592 g, $p < 0.01$), to have a 1-minute Apgar score less than 7 ($p < 0.025$), and to have neonatal withdrawal ($p < 0.001$). No congenital abnormalities were observed in the infants exposed to the drug combination.

[*Risk Factor D if used for prolonged periods in high doses at term.]

Breast Feeding Summary

No data are available.

References

1. Beckett AH, Taylor JF. Blood concentrations of pethidine and pentazocine in mother and infant at time of birth. J Pharm Pharmacol 1967;19(Suppl):50s–2s.
2. Goetz RL, Bain RV. Neonatal withdrawal symptoms associated with maternal use of pentazocine. J Pediatr 1974;84:887–8.
3. Scanlon JW. Pentazocine and neonatal withdrawal symptoms. J Pediatr 1974;85:735–6.
4. Kopelman AE. Fetal addiction to pentazocine. Pediatrics 1975;55:888–9.
5. Reeds TO. Withdrawal symptoms in a neonate associated with maternal pentazocine abuse. J Pediatr 1975;87:324.
6. Preis O, Choi SJ, Rudolph N. Pentazocine withdrawal syndrome in the newborn infant. Am J Obstet Gynecol 1977;127:205–6.
7. Filler WW, Filler NW. Effect of a potent non-narcotic analgesic agent (pentazocine) on uterine contractility and fetal heart rate. Obstet Gynecol 1966;28:224–32.
8. Freedman H, Tafeen CH, Harris H. Parenteral Win 20,228 as analgesic in labor. NY State J Med 1967;67:2849–51.
9. Duncan SLB, Ginsburg J, Morris NF. Comparison of pentazocine and pethidine in normal labor. Am J Obstet Gynecol 1969;105:197–202.
10. Moore J, Hunter RJ. A comparison of the effects of pentazocine and pethidine administered during labor. J Obstet Gynaecol Br Commonw 1970;77:830–6.
11. Mowat J, Garrey MM. Comparison of pentazocine and pethidine in labour. Br Med J 1970;2:757–9.
12. Levy DL. Obstetric analgesia. Pentazocine and meperidine in normal primiparous labor. Obstet Gynecol 1971;38:907–11.
13. Moore J, Ball HG. A sequential study of intravenous analgesic treatment during labour. Br J Anaesth 1974;46:365–72.
14. Refstad SO, Lindbaek E. Ventilatory depression of the newborn of women receiving pethidine or pentazocine. Br J Anaesth 1980;52:265–70.
15. Dunn DW, Reynolds J. Neonatal withdrawal symptoms associated with "T's and Blue's" (pentazocine and tripelennamine). Am J Dis Child 1982;136:644–5.
16. Pastorek JG, Plauche WC, Faro S. Acute bacterial endocarditis in pregnancy: a report of three cases. J Reprod Med 1983;28:611–4.
17. Chasnoff IJ, Hatcher R, Burns WJ, Schnoll SH. Pentazocine and tripelennamine ("T's and blue's"): effects on the fetus and neonate. Dev Pharmacol Ther 1983;6:162–9.
18. von Almen WF II, Miller JM Jr. "Ts and Blues" in pregnancy. J Reprod Med 1986;31:236–9.

Name: **PENTOBARBITAL**

Class: **Sedative/Hypnotic**   Risk Factor: **D_M**

Fetal Risk Summary

No reports linking the use of pentobarbital with congenital defects have been located. The Collaborative Perinatal Project monitored 50,282 mother-child pairs, 250 of which had 1st trimester exposure to pentobarbital (1). No evidence was found to suggest a relationship to large categories of major or minor malformations or to individual defects. Hemorrhagic disease and barbiturate withdrawal in the newborn are theoretical possibilities (see also Phenobarbital).

Breast Feeding Summary

Pentobarbital is excreted into breast milk (2). Breast milk levels of 0.17 μg/ml have been detected 19 hours after a dose of 100 mg daily for 32 days. The effect on the nursing infant is not known.

References

1. Heinonen OP, Slone D, Shapiro S. *Birth Defects and Drugs in Pregnancy*. Littleton:Publishing Sciences Group, 1977:336–7.
2. Wilson JT, Brown RD, Cherek DR, Dailey JW, Hilman B, Jobe PC, Manno BR, Manno JE, Redetzki HM, Stewart JJ. Drug excretion in human breast milk: principles, pharmacokinetics and projected consequences. Clin Pharmacokinet 1980;5:1–66.

Name: **PENTOXIFYLLINE**

Class: **Hemorrheologic Agent**   Risk Factor: C_M

Fetal Risk Summary

Pentoxifylline is a synthetic xanthine derivative used to lower blood viscosity in peripheral vascular and cerebrovascular diseases. No reports of its use in human pregnancy have been located. Animal studies have not shown a teratogenic effect (1, 2).

Breast Feeding Summary

Pentoxifylline is excreted into human milk. Five healthy women, who had been breast feeding for at least 6 weeks, were given a single 400-mg sustained-release tablet of pentoxifylline (commercially available formulation) after a 4-hour fast (3). The mean milk:plasma ratio of unmetabolized pentoxifylline at 4 hours was 0.87. Mean milk:plasma ratios for the three major metabolites at 4 hours were 0.76, 0.54, and 1.13, respectively. Mean milk concentrations of pentoxifylline at 2 hours (73.9 ng/ml) were approximately twice as much as those occurring at 4 hours (35.7 ng/ml) (3). Pentoxifylline and its metabolites are stable in breast milk for 3 weeks when stored at $-15°$ (4).

References

1. Product information. Trental. Hoechst-Roussel Pharmaceuticals, 1990.
2. Shepard TH. *Catalog of Teratogenic Agents*, ed 5. Baltimore: The Johns Hopkins University Press, 1986:444.
3. Witter FR, Smith RV. The excretion of pentoxifylline and its metabolites into human breast milk. Am J Obstet Gynecol 1985;151:1094–7.
4. Bauza MT, Smith RV, Knutson DE, Witter FR. Gas chromatographic determination of pentoxifylline and its major metabolites in human breast milk. J Chromatogr 1984;310:61–9.

Name: **PERPHENAZINE**

Class: **Tranquilizer**   Risk Factor: **C**

Fetal Risk Summary

Perphenazine is a piperazine phenothiazine in the same group as prochlorperazine (see Prochlorperazine). The phenothiazines readily cross the placenta (1).
The Collaborative Perinatal Project monitored 50,282 mother-child pairs, 63 of
which had 1st trimester exposure to perphenazine (2). For use anytime during
pregnancy, 166 exposures were recorded. No evidence was found in either group
to suggest a relationship to malformations, nor an effect on perinatal mortality
rates, birth weight, or intelligence quotient scores at 4 years of age. Perphenazine
has been used as an antiemetic during normal labor without producing any observable effect on the newborn (3). Although occasional reports have attempted
to link various phenothiazine compounds with congenital defects, the bulk of the
evidence indicates that these drugs are safe for the mother and fetus (see also
Chlorpromazine).

Breast Feeding Summary

No data are available.

References

1. Moya F, Thorndike V. Passage of drugs across the placenta. Am J Obstet Gynecol
   1962;84:1778–98.
2. Slone D, Siskind V, Heinonen OP, Monson RR, Kaufman DW, Shapiro S. Antenatal exposure to
   the phenothiazines in relation to congenital malformations, perinatal mortality rate, birth weight,
   and intelligence quotient score. Am J Obstet Gynecol 1977;128:486–8.
3. McGarry JM. A double-blind comparison of the anti-emetic effect during labour of metoclopramide
   and perphenazine. Br J Anaesth 1971;43:613–5.

Name: **PHENACETIN**

Class: **Analgesic/Antipyretic**   Risk Factor: **B**

Fetal Risk Summary

Phenacetin, in combination products, is routinely used during pregnancy. It is metabolized mainly to acetaminophen (see also Acetaminophen). The Collaborative
Perinatal Project monitored 50,282 mother-child pairs, 5,546 of which had 1st trimester exposure to phenacetin (1, pp. 286–295). Although no evidence was
found to suggest a relationship to large categories of major or minor malformations, possible associations were found with several individual defects (1, p. 471).
The statistical significance of these associations is unknown and independent
confirmation is required. Further, phenacetin is rarely used alone, being consumed usually in combination with aspirin and caffeine.

Craniosynostosis (six cases)
Adrenal syndromes (five cases)

Anal atresia (seven cases)
Accessory spleen (five cases)

For use anytime during pregnancy, 13,031 exposures were recorded (1, p. 434). With the same qualifications, possible associations with individual defects were found (1, p. 483).

Musculoskeletal (six cases)
Hydronephrosis (eight cases)
Adrenal anomalies (eight cases)

Breast Feeding Summary

Phenacetin is excreted into breast milk, appearing along with its major metabolite, acetaminophen (2). A patient who consumed two tablets of Empirin Compound with Codeine No. 3 (aspirin-phenacetin-caffeine-codeine) produced an average phenacetin milk concentration of 71 ng/ml (2). Milk:plasma ratios in this and a second patient varied from 0.16–0.90 (2).

References

1. Heinonen OP, Slone D, Shapiro S. *Birth Defects and Drugs in Pregnancy*. Littleton:Publishing Sciences Group, 1977.
2. Findlay JWA, DeAngelis RL, Kearney MF, Welch RM, Findlay JM. Analgesic drugs in breast milk and plasma. Clin Pharmacol Ther 1981;29:625–33.

Name: **PHENAZOCINE**

Class: **Narcotic Analgesic**   Risk Factor: **B***

Fetal Risk Summary

No reports linking the use of phenazocine with congenital defects have been located. The drug is not commercially available in the United States. Withdrawal could theoretically occur in infants exposed *in utero* to prolonged maternal ingestion of phenazocine. Phenazocine may cause neonatal respiratory depression when used in labor (1, 2).

[*Risk Factor D if used for prolonged periods in high doses at term.]

Breast Feeding Summary

No data are available.

References

1. Sadove M, Balagot R, Branion J Jr, Kobak A. Report on the use of a new agent, phenazocine, in obstetric analgesia. Obstet Gynecol 1960;16:448–53.
2. Corbit J, First S. Clinical comparison of phenazocine and meperidine in obstetric analgesia. Obstet Gynecol 1961;18:488–91.

Name: **PHENAZOPYRIDINE**

Class: **Urinary Tract Analgesic** Risk Factor: **B$_M$**

Fetal Risk Summary

No reports linking the use of phenazopyridine with congenital defects have been located. The Collaborative Perinatal Project monitored 50,282 mother-child pairs, 219 of which had 1st trimester exposure to phenazopyridine (1, pp. 299–308). For use anytime during pregnancy, 1,109 exposures were recorded (1, p. 435). In neither case was evidence found to suggest a relationship to large categories of major or minor malformations or to individual defects.

Breast Feeding Summary

No data are available.

Reference

1. Heinonen OP, Slone D, Shapiro S. *Birth Defects and Drugs in Pregnancy*. Littleton:Publishing Sciences Group, 1977.

Name: **PHENCYCLIDINE**

Class: **Hallucinogen** Risk Factor: **X**

Fetal Risk Summary

Phencyclidine (PCP) is an illicit drug used for its hallucinogenic effects. Transfer to the fetus has been demonstrated in humans with placental metabolism of the drug (1–7). Qualitative analysis of the urine from two newborns revealed phencyclidine levels of 75 ng/ml or greater up to 3 days after birth (2). In 24 (12%) of 200 women evaluated at a Los Angeles hospital, cord blood PCP levels ranged from 0.10–5.80 ng/ml (3). Cord blood concentrations were twice as high as maternal serum—1215 vs. 514 pg/ml in one woman who allegedly consumed her last dose approximately 53 days before delivery (4). PCP in the newborn's urine was found to be 5,841 pg/ml (4).

Relatively few studies have appeared on the use of phencyclidine during pregnancy, but fetal exposure may be more common than this lack of reporting indicates. During a 9-month period of 1980–1981 in a Cleveland hospital, 30 of 519 (5.8%) consecutively screened pregnant patients were discovered to have PCP exposure (8). In a subsequent report from this same hospital, 2,327 pregnant patients were screened for PCP exposure between 1981–1982 (6). Only 19 patients (0.8%) had positive urine samples, but up to 256 (11%) or more may have tested positive with more frequent checking (6). In the Los Angeles study cited above, 12% were exposed (3). However, the specificity of the chemical screening methods used in this latter report have been questioned (7).

Most pregnancies in which the mother used phencyclidine apparently end with healthy newborns (3, 4, 9). However, case reports involving four newborns indicate that the use of this agent may result in long-term damage (2, 9, 10):

Depressed at birth, jittery, hypertonic, poor feeding (2) (two infants)

Irritable, poor feeding and sucking reflex (9) (one infant)

Triangular-shaped face with pointed chin, narrow mandibular angle, antimongo-
loid slanted eyes, poor head control, nystagmus, inability to track visually,
respiratory distress, hypertonic, jitteriness (10) (one infant)

Irritability, jitteriness, hypertonicity, and poor feeding were common features in the
affected infants. In three of the neonates, most of the symptoms had persisted at
the time of the report. In the case with the malformed child, no causal relationship
with PCP could be established. Marijuana was also taken and it is a known teratogen in some animal species (11). However, marijuana is not considered to be
a human teratogen (see Marijuana).

Breast Feeding Summary

Phencyclidine (PCP) is excreted into breast milk (12). One lactating mother, who
took her last dose 40 days previously, excreted 3.90 ng/ml in her milk. In animal
studies, milk concentrations of PCP were 10 times that of plasma (1). Women
consuming PCP should not breast feed. The American Academy of Pediatrics
considers the drug to be contraindicated during breast feeding (13).

References

1. Nicholas JM, Lipshitz J, Schreiber EC. Phencyclidine: its transfer across the placenta as well as
   into breast milk. Am J Obstet Gynecol 1982;143:143–6.
2. Strauss AA, Modanlou HD, Bosu SK. Neonatal manifestations of maternal phencyclidine (PCP)
   abuse. Pediatrics 1981;68:550–2.
3. Kaufman KR, Petrucha RA, Pitts FN Jr, Kaufman ER. Phencyclidine in umbilical cord blood: preliminary data. Am J Psychiatry 1983;140:450–2.
4. Petrucha RA, Kaufman KR, Pitts FN. Phencyclidine in pregnancy: a case report. J Reprod Med
   1982;27:301–3.
5. Rayburn WF, Holsztynska EF, Domino EF. Phencyclidine: biotransformation by the human placenta. Am J Obstet Gynecol 1984;148:111–2.
6. Golden NL, Kuhnert BR, Sokol RJ, Martier S, Bagby BS. Phencyclidine use during pregnancy. Am
   J Obstet Gynecol 1984;148:254–9.
7. Lipton MA. Phencyclidine in umbilical cord blood: some cautions. Am J Psychiatry 1983;140:449.
8. Golden NL, Sokol RJ, Martier S, Miller SI. A practical method for identifying angel dust abuse
   during pregnancy. Am J Obstet Gynecol 1982;142:359–61.
9. Lerner SE, Burns RS. Phencyclidine use among youth: history, epidemiology, and acute and
   chronic intoxication. In Petersen R, Stillman R, eds. Phencyclidine (PCP) Abuse: An Appraisal.
   National Institute on Drug Abuse Research Monograph No. 21, US Government Printing Office,
   1978.
10. Golden NL, Sokol RJ, Rubin IL. Angel dust: possible effects on the fetus. Pediatrics 1980;65:18–
    20.
11. Persaud TVN, Ellington AC. Teratogenic activity of cannabis resin. Lancet 1968;2:406–7.
12. Kaufman KR, Petrucha RA, Pitts FN Jr, Weekes ME. PCP in amniotic fluid and breast milk: case
    report. J Clin Psychiatry 1983;44:269–70.
13. Committee on Drugs, American Academy of Pediatrics. Transfer of drugs and other chemicals
    into human milk. Pediatrics 1989;84:924–36.

Name: **PHENDIMETRAZINE**
Class: **Central Stimulant/Anorectant**   Risk Factor: **C**

Fetal Risk Summary

No data are available (see Phentermine or Dextroamphetamine).

Breast Feeding Summary

No data are available.

Name: **PHENELZINE**
Class: **Antidepressant**   Risk Factor: **C**

Fetal Risk Summary

Phenelzine is a monoamine oxidase inhibitor. The Collaborative Perinatal Project monitored 21 mother-child pairs exposed to these drugs during the 1st trimester, three of which were exposed to phenelzine (1). An increased risk of malformations was found. Details of the three cases with phenelzine exposure are not available.

Breast Feeding Summary

No data are available.

Reference

1. Heinonen OP, Slone D, Shapiro S. *Birth Defects and Drugs in Pregnancy*. Littleton:Publishing Sciences Group, 1977:336–7.

Name: **PHENINDIONE**
Class: **Anticoagulant**   Risk Factor: **D**

Fetal Risk Summary

See Coumarin Derivatives.

Breast Feeding Summary

See Coumarin Derivatives.

Name: **PHENIRAMINE**

Class: **Antihistamine**   Risk Factor: **C**

Fetal Risk Summary

The Collaborative Perinatal Project monitored 50,282 mother-child pairs, 831 of whom were exposed to pheniramine during the 1st trimester (1, pp. 322–334). A possible relationship between this use and respiratory malformations and eye/ear defects was found, but the statistical significance of these findings is unknown. Independent confirmation is required to determine the actual risk. For use anytime during pregnancy, 2,442 exposures were recorded (1, pp. 436–437). No evidence was found in this group to suggest a relationship to congenital anomalies.

An association between exposure during the last 2 weeks of pregnancy to antihistamines in general and retrolental fibroplasia in premature infants has been reported. See Brompheniramine for details.

Breast Feeding Summary

No data are available.

Reference

1. Heinonen OP, Slone D, Shapiro S. *Birth Defects and Drugs in Pregnancy*. Littleton:Publishing Sciences Group, 1977.

Name: **PHENOBARBITAL**

Class: **Sedative/Anticonvulsant**   Risk Factor: **D**

Fetal Risk Summary

Phenobarbital has been used widely in clinical practice as a sedative and anticonvulsant since 1912 (1). The potential teratogenic effects of phenobarbital were recognized in 1964 along with phenytoin (2). Since this report, there have been numerous reviews and studies on the teratogenic effects of phenobarbital either alone or in combination with phenytoin and other anticonvulsants. Based on this literature, the epileptic pregnant woman taking phenobarbital in combination with other antiepileptics has a two to three times greater risk for delivering a child with congenital defects over the general population (3–10). It is not known if this increased risk is due to antiepileptic drugs, the disease itself, genetic factors, or a combination of these, although some evidence indicates that drugs are the causative factor (10). A phenotype, as described for phenytoin in the fetal hydantoin syndrome (FHS), apparently does not occur with phenobarbital (see Phenytoin for details of FHS). However, as summarized by Janz (11), some of the minor malformations composing the FHS have been occasionally observed in infants of epileptic mothers treated only with phenobarbital.

The Collaborative Perinatal Project monitored 50,282 mother-child pairs, 1,415 of which had 1st trimester exposure to phenobarbital (12, pp. 336–339). For use anytime during pregnancy, 8,037 exposures were recorded (12, p. 438). In neither case was evidence found to suggest a relationship to large categories of major or minor malformations, although a possible association with Down's syndrome was shown statistically. However, a relationship between phenobarbital and Down's syndrome is unlikely.

Phenobarbital and other anticonvulsants (e.g., phenytoin) may cause early hemorrhagic disease of the newborn (13–22). Hemorrhage occurs during the first 24 hours after birth and may be severe or even fatal. The exact mechanism of the defect is unknown but may involve phenobarbital induction of fetal liver microsomal enzymes that deplete the already low reserves of fetal vitamin K (22). This results in suppression of the vitamin K-dependent coagulation factors, II, VII, IX, and X. A 1985 review summarized the various prophylactic treatment regimens that have been proposed (see Phenytoin for details) (22).

Barbiturate withdrawal has been observed in newborns exposed to phenobarbital *in utero* (23). The average onset of symptoms in 15 addicted infants was 6 days (range 3–14 days). These infants had been exposed during gestation to doses varying from 64–300 mg/day with unknown amounts in four patients.

Phenobarbital may induce folic acid deficiency in the pregnant woman (24–26). A discussion of this effect and the possible consequences for the fetus are presented under Phenytoin.

High-dose phenobarbital, contained in an anti-asthmatic preparation, was reported in a mother giving birth to a stillborn full-term female infant with complete triploidy (27). The authors speculated on the potential for phenobarbital-induced chromosome damage. However, an earlier *in vitro* study found no effect of phenobarbital on the incidence of chromosome gaps, breaks, or abnormal forms (28). Any relationship between the drug and the infant's condition is probably coincidental.

Phenobarbital and/or cholestyramine have been used to treat cholestasis of pregnancy (29, 30). Although no drug-induced fetal complications were noted, the therapy was ineffective for this condition.

In summary, phenobarbital therapy in the epileptic pregnant woman presents a risk to the fetus in terms of minor congenital defects, hemorrhage at birth, and addiction. The risk to the mother, however, is greater if the drug is withheld and seizure control is lost. The benefit:risk ratio, in this case, favors continued use of the drug during pregnancy at the lowest possible level to control seizures. Use of the drug in nonepileptic patients does not seem to pose a significant risk for congenital defects, but hemorrhage and addiction in the newborn are still concerns.

Breast Feeding Summary

Phenobarbital is excreted into breast milk (31–35). The milk:plasma ratio varies between 0.4–0.6 (32, 33). The amount of phenobarbital ingested by the nursing infant has been estimated to reach 2–4 mg/day (34). The pharmacokinetics of phenobarbital during lactation have been reviewed (33). Due to slower elimination in the nursing infant, accumulation may occur to the point that blood levels in the infant may actually exceed those of the mother (33). Phenobarbital-induced sedation has been observed in three nursing infants probably caused by this accumulation (31). Women consuming phenobarbital during breast feeding, especially those on high doses, should be instructed to observe their infants for sedation. Phenobarbital levels in the infant should also be monitored to avoid toxic concentrations (33, 36). The American Academy of Pediatrics classifies phenobarbital as a drug that has caused major adverse effects in some nursing infants, and it should be given to nursing women with caution (36).

References

1. Hauptmann A. Luminal bei epilepsie. Munchen Med Wochenschr 1912;59:1907–8.
2. Janz D, Fuchs V. Are anti-epileptic drugs harmful when given during pregnancy? German Med Monogr 1964;9:20–3.
3. Hill RB. Teratogenesis and anti-epileptic drugs. N Engl J Med 1973;289:1089–90.
4. Bodendorfer TW. Fetal effects of anticonvulsant drugs and seizure disorders. Drug Intell Clin Pharm 1978;12:14–21.
5. Committee on Drugs, American Academy of Pediatrics. Anticonvulsants and pregnancy. Pediatrics 1977;63:331–3.
6. Nakane Y, Okoma T, Takahashe R, et al. Multi-institutional study of the teratogenicity and fetal toxicity of anti-epileptic drugs: a report of a collaborative study group in Japan. Epilepsia 980;21:633–80.
7. Andermann E, Dansky L, Andermann F, Loughnan PM, Gibbons J. Minor congenital malformations and dermatoglyphic alterations in the offspring of epileptic women; a clinical investigation of the teratogenic effects of anticonvulsant medication. In *Epilepsy, Pregnancy and the Child*. Proceedings of a Workshop in Berlin, September 1980. New York:Raven Press, 1981.
8. Dansky L, Andermann E, Andermann F. Major congenital malformations in the offspring of epileptic patients. In *Epilepsy, Pregnancy and the Child*. Proceedings of a Workshop in Berlin, September 1980. New York:Raven Press, 1981.
9. Janz D. The teratogenic risks of antiepileptic drugs. Epilepsia 1975;16:159–69.
10. Hanson JW, Buehler BA. Fetal hydantoin syndrome: current status. J Pediatr 1982;101:816–8.
11. Janz D. Antiepileptic drugs and pregnancy: altered utilization patterns and teratogenesis. Epilepsia 1982;23(Suppl 1):S53–S63.
12. Heinonen OP, Slone D, Shapiro S. *Birth Defects and Drugs in Pregnancy.* Littleton:Publishing Sciences Group, 1977.
13. Spiedel BD, Meadow SR. Maternal epilepsy and abnormalities of the fetus and the newborn. Lancet 1972;2:839–43.
14. Bleyer WA, Skinner AL. Fatal neonatal hemorrhage after maternal anticonvulsant therapy. JAMA 1976;235:826–7.
15. Lawrence A. Anti-epileptic drugs and the foetus. Br Med J 1963;2:1267.
16. Kohler HG. Haemorrhage in the newborn of epileptic mothers. Lancet 1966;1:267.
17. Mountain KR, Hirsh J, Gallus AS. Neonatal coagulation defect due to anticonvulsant drug treatment in pregnancy. Lancet 1970;1:265–8.
18. Evans AR, Forrester RM, Discombe C. Neonatal haemorrhage during anticonvulsant therapy. Lancet 1970;1:517–8.
19. Margolin FG, Kantor NM. Hemorrhagic disease of the newborn. An unusual case related to maternal ingestion of an anti-epileptic drug. Clin Pediatr (Phila) 1972;11:59–60.
20. Srinivasan G, Seeler RA, Tiruvury A, Pildes RS. Maternal anticonvulsant therapy and hemorrhagic disease of the newborn. Obstet Gynecol 1982;59:250–2.
21. Payne NR, Hasegawa DK. Vitamin K deficiency in newborns: a case report in α-1-antitrypsin deficiency and a review of factors predisposing to hemorrhage. Pediatrics 1984;73:712–6.
22. Lane PA, Hathaway WE. Vitamin K in infancy. J Pediatr 1985;106:351–9.
23. Desmond MM, Schwanecke RP, Wilson GS, Yasunaga S, Burgdorff I. Maternal barbiturate utilization and neonatal withdrawal symptomatology. J Pediatr 1972;80:190–7.
24. Pritchard JA, Scott DE, Whalley PJ. Maternal folate deficiency and pregnancy wastage. IV. Effects of folic acid supplements, anticonvulsants, and oral contraceptives. Am J Obstet Gynecol 1971;109:341–6.
25. Hiilesmaa VK, Teramo K, Granstrom ML, Bardy AH. Serum folate concentrations during pregnancy in women with epilepsy: relation to antiepileptic drug concentrations, number of seizures, and fetal outcome. Br Med J 1983;287:577–9.
26. Biale Y, Lewenthal H. Effect of folic acid supplementation on congenital malformations due to anticonvulsive drugs. Eur J Obstet Reprod Biol 1984;18:211–6.
27. Halbrecht I, Komlos L, Shabtay F, Solomon M, Book JA. Triploidy 69, XXX in a stillborn girl. Clin Genet 1973;4:210–2.

28. Stenchever MA, Jarvis JA. Effect of barbiturates on the chromosomes of human cells in vitro—a negative report. J Reprod Med 1970;5:69–71.
29. Heikkinen J, Maentausta O, Ylostalo P, Janne O. Serum bile acid levels in intrahepatic cholestasis of pregnancy during treatment with phenobarbital or cholestyramine. Eur J Obstet Reprod Biol 1982;14:153–62.
30. Shaw D, Frohlich J, Wittmann BAK, Willms M. A prospective study of 18 patients with cholestasis of pregnancy. Am J Obstet Gynecol 1982;142:621–5.
31. Tyson RM, Shrader EA, Perlman HN. Drugs transmitted through breast-milk. II. Barbiturates. J Pediatr 1938;13:86–90.
32. Kaneko S, Sata T, Suzuki K. The levels of anticonvulsants in breast milk. Br J Clin Pharmacol 1979;7:624–7.
33. Nau H, Kuhnz, Egger HJ, Rating D, Helge H. Anticonvulsants during pregnancy and lactation: transplacental, maternal and neonatal pharmacokinetics. Clin Pharmacokinet 1982;7:508–43.
34. Horning MG, Stillwell WG, Nowlin J, Lertratanangkoon K, Stillwell RN, Hill RM. Identification and quantification of drugs and drug metabolites in human breast milk using GC-MS-COM methods. Mod Probl Paediatr 1975;15:73–9.
35. Reith H, Schafer H. Antiepileptic drugs during pregnancy and the lactation period. Pharmacokinetic data. Dtsch Med Wochenschr 1979;104:818–23.
36. Committee on Drugs, American Academy of Pediatrics. Transfer of drugs and other chemicals into human breast milk. Pediatrics 1989;84;924–36.

Name: **PHENPROCOUMON**

Class: **Anticoagulant**   Risk Factor: **D**

Fetal Risk Summary

See Coumarin Derivatives.

Breast Feeding Summary

See Coumarin Derivatives.

Name: **PHENSUXIMIDE**

Class: **Anticonvulsant**   Risk Factor: **D**

Fetal Risk Summary

The use of phensuximide, the first succinimide anticonvulsant used in the treatment of petit mal epilepsy, has been reported in three pregnancies (1, 2). Due to multiple drug therapy and difference in study methodology, conclusions linking the use of phensuximide with congenital defects are difficult. Fetal abnormalities identified with the three pregnancies include ambiguous genitalia, inquinal hernia, and pyloric stenosis. Phensuximide has a much lower teratogenic potential than the oxazolidinedione class of anticonvulsants (see Trimethadione) (3, 4). Due to a high incidence of toxic effects, the new succinimides should be considered in favor of phensuximide for the treatment of petit mal epilepsy (see Ethosuximide, Methsuximide) (5).

Breast Feeding Summary

No data are available.

References

1. Fedrick J. Epilepsy and pregnancy: a report from the Oxford Record Linkage Study. Br Med J 1973;2:442–8.
2. McMullin GP. Teratogenic effects of anticonvulsants. Br Med J 1971;2:430.
3. Fabro S, Brown NA. Teratogenic potential of anticonvulsants. New Engl J Med 1979;300:1280–1.
4. The National Institutes of Health. Anticonvulsants found to have teratogenic potential. JAMA 1981;241:36.
5. Schmidt RP, Wilder BJ. Epilepsy. In *Contemporary Neurology Series*, No. 2. Philadelphia:FA Davis, 1968;159.

Name: **PHENTERMINE**

Class: **Central Stimulant**   Risk Factor: **C**

Fetal Risk Summary

No data are available (see Diethylpropion or Dextroamphetamine).

Breast Feeding Summary

No data are available.

Name: **PHENYLBUTAZONE**

Class: **Nonsteroidal Anti-Inflammatory Analgesic**   Risk Factor: **D**

Fetal Risk Summary

Two reports have been located that describe congenital defects in the offspring of mothers consuming phenylbutazone during pregnancy (1, 2). A cause-and-effect relationship was not established in either case. One review on the use of antirheumatic drug treatment during pregnancy stated that phenylbutazone is nonteratogenic in humans (3). Possible embryotoxicity has been demonstrated in animals, and the drug crosses the placenta to the human fetus (4–7).

Theoretically, phenylbutazone, a prostaglandin synthetase inhibitor, could cause constriction of the ductus arteriosus *in utero* (8). Persistent pulmonary hypertension of the newborn should also be considered (8). Drugs in this class have been shown to inhibit labor and prolong pregnancy (9). The manufacturer recommends that the drug not be used in pregnancy (4).

Breast Feeding Summary

Phenylbutazone is excreted into breast milk in low concentrations, although some investigators failed to detect the drug 3 hours after maternal administration (8–10). The drug has been measured in infant serum after breast feeding, but no adverse effects in the nursing infant have been reported. The American Academy of Pediatrics considers phenylbutazone to be compatible with breast feeding (11).

References

1. Tuchmann-Duplessis H. Medication in the course of pregnancy and teratogenic malformation. Concours Med 1967;89:2119–20.
2. Kullander S, Kallen B. A prospective study of drugs in pregnancy. Acta Obstet Gynecol Scand 1976;55:289–95.
3. Ostensen M, Husby G. Antirheumatic drug treatment during pregnancy and lactation. Scand J Rheumatol 1985;14:1–7.
4. Product information. Butazolidin. Geigy Pharmaceuticals, 1985.
5. Leuxner E, Pulver R. Verabreichung von irgapryin bei schwangeren und wochnerinnen. Munchen Med Wochenschr 1956;98:84–6.
6. Strobel S, Leuxner E. Uber die zullassigkeit der verabreichung von butazolidin bei schwangeren und wochnerinnen. Med Klin 1957;39:1708–10.
7. Akbaraly R, Leng JJ, Brachet-Liermain A, White P, Laclau-Lacrouts B. Trans-placental transfer of four anti-inflammatory agents. A study carried out by *in vitro* perfusion. J Gynecol Obstet Biol Reprod (Paris) 1981;10:7–11.
8. Levin DL. Effects of inhibition of prostaglandin synthesis on fetal development, oxygenation, and the fetal circulation. Semin Perinatol 1980;4:35–44.
9. Fuchs F. Prevention of prematurity. Am J Obstet Gynecol 1976;126:809–20.
10. Wilson JT. Milk/plasma ratios and contraindicated drugs. In Wilson JT, ed. *Drugs in Breast Milk.* Australia:ADIS Press, 1981:78–9.
11. Committee on Drugs, American Academy of Pediatrics. Transfer of drugs and other chemicals into human milk. Pediatrics 1989;84:924–36.

Name: **PHENYLEPHRINE**

Class: **Sympathomimetic (Adrenergic)**   Risk Factor: **C**

Fetal Risk Summary

Phenylephrine is a sympathomimetic used in emergency situations to treat hypotension and to alleviate allergic symptoms of the eye and ear. Uterine vessels are normally maximally dilated and they have only α-adrenergic receptors (1). Use of the predominantly α-adrenergic stimulant, phenylephrine, could cause constriction of these vessels and reduce uterine blood flow, thereby producing fetal hypoxia (bradycardia). Phenylephrine may also interact with oxytocics or ergot derivatives to produce severe persistent maternal hypertension (1). Rupture of a cerebral vessel is possible. If a pressor agent is indicated, other drugs such as ephedrine should be considered. Sympathomimetic amines are teratogenic in some animal species, but human teratogenicity has not been suspected (2, 3).

The Collaborative Perinatal Project monitored 50,282 mother-child pairs, 1,249 of which had 1st trimester exposure to phenylephrine (4, pp. 345–356). For use anytime during pregnancy, 4,194 exposures were recorded (4, p. 439). An association was found between 1st trimester use of phenylephrine and malformations; association with minor defects was greater than with major defects (4, pp. 345–356). For individual malformations, several possible associations were found (4, pp. 345–356, 476, 491):

First trimester
    Eye and ear (eight cases)
    Syndactyly (six cases)
    Pre-auricular skin tag (four cases)
    Clubfoot (three cases)
Anytime use
    Congenital dislocation of hip (15 cases)
    Other musculoskeletal defects (four cases)
    Umbilical hernia (six cases)

The statistical significance of these associations is not known and independent confirmation is required. For the sympathomimetic class of drugs as a whole, an association was found between 1st trimester use and minor malformations (not life-threatening or major cosmetic defects), inguinal hernia, and clubfoot (4, pp. 345–356).

Sympathomimetics are often administered in combination with other drugs to alleviate the symptoms of upper respiratory infections. Thus, the fetal effects of sympathomimetics, other drugs, and viruses cannot be totally separated. However, indiscriminate use of this class of drugs, especially in the 1st trimester, is not without risk.

Phenylephrine has been used as a stress test to determine fetal status in high-risk pregnancies (5). In the United States, however, this test is normally conducted with oxytocin.

Breast Feeding Summary

No data are available.

References

1. Smith NT, Corbascio AN. The use and misuse of pressor agents. Anesthesiology 1970;33:58–101.
2. Nashimura H, Tanimura T. *Clinical Aspects of the Teratogenicity of Drugs*. Amsterdam:Excerpta Medica, 1976:231.
3. Shepard TH. *Catalog of Teratogenic Agents*, ed. 3. Baltimore:Johns Hopkins University Press, 1980:134–5.
4. Heinonen OP, Slone D, Shapiro S. *Birth Defects and Drugs in Pregnancy*. Littleton:Publishing Sciences Group, 1977.
5. Eguchi K, Yonezawa M, Hagegawa T, Lin TT, Ejiri K, Kudo T, Sekiba K, Takeda Y. Fetal activity determination and Neosynephrine test for evaluation of fetal well-being in high risk pregnancies. Nippon Sanka Fujinka Gakkai Zasshi 1980;32:663–8.

Name: **PHENYLPROPANOLAMINE**

Class: **Sympathomimetic (Adrenergic)**   Risk Factor: **C**

Fetal Risk Summary

Phenylpropanolamine is a sympathomimetic used for anorexia and to alleviate the symptoms of allergic disorders or upper respiratory infections. Uterine vessels are normally maximally dilated and they have only α-adrenergic receptors (1). Use of the α- and β-adrenergic stimulant, phenylpropanolamine, could cause constriction of these vessels and reduce uterine blood flow, thereby producing fetal hypoxia (bradycardia). This drug is a common component of proprietary mixtures containing antihistamines and other drugs. Thus, it is difficult to separate the effects of phenylpropanolamine on the fetus from other drugs, disease states, and viruses.

Sympathomimetic amines are teratogenic in some animal species, but human teratogenicity has not been suspected (2, 3). The Collaborative Perinatal Project monitored 50,282 mother-child pairs, 726 of which had 1st trimester exposure to phenylpropanolamine (4, pp. 345–356). For use anytime during pregnancy, 2,489 exposures were recorded (4, p. 439). An association was found between 1st trimester use of phenylpropanolamine and malformations; association with minor defects was greater than with major defect (4, pp. 345–356). For individual malformations, several possible associations were found (4, pp. 345–356, 477, 491):

First trimester
  Hypospadias (four cases)
  Eye and ear (seven cases) (statistically significant)
  Polydactyly (six cases)
  Cataract (three cases)
  Pectus excavatum (seven cases)
Anytime use
  Congenital dislocation of hip (12 cases)

Except for eye and ear defects, the statistical significance of these associations is not known and independent confirmation is required. For the sympathomimetic class of drugs as a whole, an association was found between 1st trimester use and minor malformations (not life-threatening or major cosmetic defects), inguinal hernia, and clubfoot (4, pp. 345–356). Indiscriminate use of this class of drugs, especially in the 1st trimester, is not without risk.

A case of infantile malignant osteopetrosis was described in a 4-month-old boy exposed *in utero* on several occasions to Contac (chlorpheniramine, phenylpropanolamine, and belladonna alkaloids) but this is a known genetic defect (5). The infant also had a continual "stuffy" nose.

Breast Feeding Summary

No data are available.

References

1. Smith NT, Corbascio AN. The use and misuse of pressor agents. Anesthesiology 1970;33:58–101.
2. Nishimura H, Tanimura T. *Clinical Aspects of the Teratogenicity of Drugs*. Amsterdam:Excerpta Medica, 1976:231.
3. Shepard TH. *Catalog of Teratogenic Drugs*, 3rd ed. Baltimore:Johns Hopkins University Press, 1980:134–5.
4. Heinonen OP, Slone D, Shapiro S. *Birth Defects and Drugs in Pregnancy*. Littleton:Publishing Sciences Group, 1977.
5. Golbus MS, Koerper MA, Hall BD. Failure to diagnose osteopetrosis in utero. Lancet 1976;2:1246.

Name: **PHENYLTOLOXAMINE**

Class: **Antihistamine**   Risk Factor: **C**

Fetal Risk Summary

No data are available.

Breast Feeding Summary

No data are available.

Name: **PHENYTOIN**

Class: **Anticonvulsant**   Risk Factor: **D**

Fetal Risk Summary

Phenytoin is a hydantoin anticonvulsant introduced in 1938. The teratogenic effects of phenytoin were recognized in 1964 (1). Since this report there have been numerous reviews and studies on the teratogenic effects of phenytoin and other anticonvulsants. Based on this literature, the epileptic pregnant woman taking phenytoin, either alone or in combination with other anticonvulsants, has a two to three times greater risk for delivering a child with congenital defects over the general population (2–9). It is not known if this increased risk is due to antiepileptic drugs, the disease itself, genetic factors, or a combination of these, although some evidence indicates that drugs are the causative factor (9). Fifteen epidemiologic studies cited by reviewers in 1982 found an incidence of defects in treated epileptics varying from 2.2%–26.1% (9). In each case, the rate for treated patients was higher than untreated epileptics or normal controls. Animal studies have also implicated drugs and have suggested that a dose-related response may occur (9).

A recognizable pattern of malformations, now known as the fetal hydantoin syndrome (FHS), was partially described in 1968 when Meadow (10) observed distinct facial abnormalities in infants exposed to phenytoin and other anticonvulsants. In 1973, two groups of investigators, in independent reports, described unusual anomalies of the fingers and toes in exposed infants (11, 12). The basic syndrome consists of variable degrees of hypoplasia and ossification of the distal phalanges and craniofacial abnormalities. Clinical features of the FHS, not all of which are apparent in every infant, are (10–12):

Craniofacial
    Broad nasal bridge
    Wide fontanel
    Low-set hairline
    Broad alveolar ridge
    Metopic ridging
    Short neck
    Ocular hypertelorism
    Microcephaly
    Cleft lip/palate

Abnormal or low-set ears
Epicanthal folds
Ptosis of eyelids
Coloboma
Coarse scalp hair
Limbs
Small or absent nails
Hypoplasia of distal phalanges
Altered palmar crease
Digital thumb
Dislocated hip

Impaired growth, both physical and mental, congenital heart defects and cleft lip and/or palate are often observed in conjunction with the FHS.

Numerous other defects have been reported to occur after phenytoin exposure in pregnancy. Janz, in a 1982 review (13), stated that nearly all possible types of malformations may be observed in the offspring of epileptic mothers. This statement is supported by the large volume of literature describing various anomalies that have been attributed to phenytoin with or without other anticonvulsants (1–49).

Eleven case reports have been located that, taken in sum, suggest phenytoin is a human transplacental carcinogen (14–24). Tumors reported to occur in infants after *in utero* exposure to phenytoin include:

Neuroblastoma (five cases) (14–18)
Ganglioneuroblastoma (one case) (19)
Melanotic neuroectodermal tumor (one case) (20)
Extrarenal Wilms' tumor (one case) (21)
Mesenchymoma (one case) (22)
Lymphangioma (one case) (23)
Ependymoblastoma (one case) (24)

Children exposed *in utero* to phenytoin should be closely observed for several years since tumor development may take that long to express itself.

Phenytoin and other anticonvulsants (e.g., phenobarbital) may cause early hemorrhagic disease of the newborn (14, 50–64). Hemorrhage occurs during the first 24 hours after birth and may be severe or even fatal. The exact mechanism of the defect is unknown but may involve phenytoin induction of fetal liver microsomal enzymes that deplete the already low reserves of fetal vitamin K (64). This results in suppression of the vitamin K-dependent coagulation factors, II, VII, IX, and X. Phenytoin-induced thrombocytopenia has also been reported as a mechanism for hemorrhage in the newborn (61). In a 1985 review, Lane and Hathaway (64) summarized the various prophylactic treatment regimens that have been proposed:

Administering 10 mg of oral vitamin K daily during the last 2 months of pregnancy
Administering 20 mg of oral vitamin K daily during the last 2 weeks of pregnancy
Avoiding salicylates and administering vitamin K during labor

Caesarean section if a difficult or traumatic delivery is anticipated
Administering intravenous vitamin K to the newborn in the delivery room plus
  cord blood clotting studies

Although all of the above suggestions are logical, none has been tested in controlled trials (64). Lane and Hathaway (64) recommend immediate intramuscular
vitamin K and close observation of the infant (see also Phytonadione).

Liver damage was observed in an infant exposed during gestation to phenytoin
and valproic acid (65). Although they were unable to demonstrate which anticonvulsant caused the injury, the authors concluded that valproic acid was the more
likely offending agent.

Phenytoin may induce folic acid deficiency in the epileptic patient by impairing
gastrointestinal absorption or by increasing hepatic metabolism of the vitamin
(66–68). Whether phenytoin also induces folic acid deficiency in the fetus is less
certain since the fetus seems to be efficient in drawing on available maternal
stores of folic acid (see Folic Acid). Low maternal folate levels, however, have
been proposed as one possible mechanism for the increased incidence of defects
observed in infants exposed in utero to phenytoin. In a 1984 report, two investigators studied the relationship between folic acid, anticonvulsants, and fetal defects
(66). In the retrospective part of this study, a group of 24 women treated with
phenytoin and other anticonvulsants produced 66 infants, 10 (15%) with major
anomalies. Two of the mothers with affected infants had markedly low red blood
cell folate concentrations. A second group of 22 epileptic women was then supplemented with daily folic acid, 2.5–5.0 mg, starting before conception in 26 pregnancies and within the first 40 days in six. This group produced 33 newborns (32
pregnancies—1 set of twins) with no defects, a significant difference from the unsupplemented group. Loss of seizure control caused by folic acid lowering of
phenytoin serum levels, which is known to occur, was not a problem in this small
series.

Negative associations between phenytoin-induced folate deficiency have been
reported (67, 68). In one study, mothers were given supplements with an average
folic acid dose of 0.5 mg/day from the 6th–16th week of gestation until delivery
(68). Defects were observed in 20 infants (15%) from the 133 women taking anticonvulsants, which is similar to the reported frequency in pregnant patients not
given supplements. Folate levels were usually within the normal range for pregnancy.

The pharmacokinetics and placental transport of phenytoin have been extensively studied and reviewed (69–71). Plasma concentrations of phenytoin may fall
during pregnancy. Animal studies and recent human reports suggest a dose-
related teratogenic effect of phenytoin (72, 73). While these results are based on
a small series of patients, it is reasonable to avoid excessively high plasma concentrations of phenytoin. Close monitoring of plasma phenytoin concentrations is
recommended to maintain adequate seizure control and prevent potential fetal
hypoxia.

Placental function in women taking phenytoin has been evaluated (74). No effect was detected from phenytoin as measured by serum human placental
lactogen, 24-hour urinary total estriol excretion, placental weight, and birth weight.

In a study evaluating thyroid function, no differences were found between
treated epileptic pregnant women and normal pregnant controls (75). Thyroxine

levels in the cord blood of anticonvulsant-exposed infants were significantly lower than in controls, but this was shown to be due to altered protein binding and not to altered thyroid function. Other parameters studied—thyrotropin, free thyroxine, and triiodothyronine—were similar in both groups.

The effect of phenytoin on maternal and fetal vitamin D metabolism was examined in a 1984 study (76). In comparison to normal controls, several significant differences were found in the level of various vitamin D compounds and in serum calcium, but the values were still within normal limits. No alterations were found in alkaline phosphatase and phosphate concentrations. The authors doubted if the observed differences were of major clinical significance.

Phenytoin may be used for the management of digitalis-induced arrhythmias that are unresponsive to other agents and for refractory ventricular tachyarrhythmias (77–79). This short-term use has not been reported to cause problems in the exposed fetuses. The drug has also been used for anticonvulsant prophylaxis in severe preeclampsia (80).

In summary, the use of phenytoin during pregnancy involves significant risk to the fetus in terms of major and minor congenital abnormalities and hemorrhage at birth. The risk to the mother, however, is also great if the drug is not used to control her seizures. The benefit:risk ratio, in this case, favors continued use of the drug during pregnancy. Frequent determinations of phenytoin levels are recommended to maintain the lowest level required to prevent seizures and possibly to lessen the likelihood of fetal anomalies. Based on recent research, consideration should also be given to monitoring folic acid levels simultaneously with phenytoin determinations and administering folic acid very early in pregnancy or before conception to those women shown to have low folate concentrations.

Breast Feeding Summary

Phenytoin is excreted into breast milk. Milk:plasma ratios range from 0.18–0.54 (69, 81–84). The pharmacokinetics of phenytoin during lactation have been reviewed (69). The reviewers concluded that little risk to the nursing infant was present if maternal levels were kept in the therapeutic range. However, methemoglobinemia, drowsiness, and decreased sucking activity have been reported in one infant (85). Except for this one case, no other reports of adverse effects with the use of phenytoin during lactation have been located. The American Academy of Pediatrics considers phenytoin to be compatible with breast feeding (86).

References

1. Janz D, Fuchs V. Are anti-epileptic drugs harmful when given during pregnancy? German Med Monogr 1964;9:20–3.
2. Hill RB. Teratogenesis and antiepileptic drugs. N Engl J Med 1973;289:1089–90.
3. Janz D. The teratogenic risk of antiepileptic drugs. Epilepsia 1975;16:159–69.
4. Bodendorfer TW. Fetal effects of anticonvulsant drugs and seizure disorders. Drug Intell Clin Pharm 1978;12:14–21.
5. Committee on Drugs, American Academy of Pediatrics. Anticonvulsants and pregnancy. Pediatrics 1977;63:331–3.
6. Nakane Y, Okuma T, Takahashi R, et al. Multi-institutional study of the teratogenicity and fetal toxicity of antiepileptic drugs: a report of a collaborative study group in Japan. Epilepsia 1980;21:663–80.
7. Andermann E, Dansky L, Andermann F, Loughnan PM, Gibbons J. Minor congenital malformations and dermatoglyphic alterations in the offspring of epileptic women: a clinical investigation of

the teratogenic effects of anticonvulsant medication. In *Epilepsy, Pregnancy and the Child*. Proceedings of a Workshop in Berlin, September 1980. New York:Raven Press, 1981.

8. Dansky L, Andermann E, Andermann F. Major congenital malformations in the offspring of epileptic patients. In *Epilepsy, Pregnancy and the Child*. Proceedings of a Workshop in Berlin, September 1980. New York:Raven Press, 1981.

9. Hanson JW, Buehler BA. Fetal hydantoin syndrome: current status. J Pediatr 1982;101:816–8.

10. Meadow SR. Anticonvulsant drugs and congenital abnormalities. Lancet 1968;2:1296.

11. Loughnan PM, Gold H, Vance JC. Phenytoin teratogenicity in man. Lancet 1973;1:70–2.

12. Hill RM, Horning MG, Horning EC. Antiepileptic drugs and fetal well-being. In Boreus L, ed. *Fetal Pharmacology*. New York:Raven Press, 1973:375–9.

13. Janz D. Antiepileptic drugs and pregnancy: altered utilization patterns and teratogenesis. Epilepsia 1982;23(Suppl 1):S53–S63.

14. Allen RW Jr, Ogden B, Bentley FL, Jung AL. Fetal hydantoin syndrome, neuroblastoma, and hemorrhagic disease in a neonate. JAMA 1980;244:1464–5.

15. Ramilo J, Harris VJ. Neuroblastoma in a child with the hydantoin and fetal alcohol syndrome. The radiographic features. Br J Radiol 1979;52:993–5.

16. Pendergrass TW, Hanson JW. Fetal hydantoin syndrome and neuroblastoma. Lancet 1976;2:150.

17. Sherman S, Roizen N. Fetal hydantoin syndrome and neuroblastoma. Lancet 1976;2:517.

18. Ehrenbard LT, Chagantirs K. Cancer in the fetal hydantoin syndrome. Lancet 1981;1:197.

19. Seeler RA, Israel JN, Royal JE, Kaye CI, Rao S, Abulaban M. Ganglioneuroblastoma and fetal hydantoin-alcohol syndromes. Pediatrics 1979;63:524–7.

20. Jimenez JF, Seibert RW, Char F, Brown RE, Seibert JJ. Melanotic neuroectodermal tumor of infancy and fetal hydantoin syndrome. Am J Pediatr Hematol Oncol 1981;3:9–15.

21. Taylor WF, Myers M, Taylor WR. Extrarenal Wilms' tumour in an infant exposed to intrauterine phenytoin. Lancet 1980;2:481–2.

22. Blattner WA, Hanson DE, Young EC, Fraumeni JF. Malignant mesenchymoma and birth defects. JAMA 1977;238:334–5.

23. Kousseff BG. Subcutaneous vascular abnormalities in fetal hydantoin syndrome. Birth Defects 1982;18:51–4.

24. Lipson A. Bale P. Ependymoblastoma associated with prenatal exposure to diphenylhydantoin and methylphenobarbitone. Cancer 1985;55:1859–62.

25. Corcoran R, Rizk MW. VACTERL congenital malformation and phenytoin therapy? Lancet 1976;2:960.

26. Pinto W Jr, Gardner LI, Rosenbaum P. Abnormal genitalia as a presenting sign in two male infants with hydantoin embryopathy syndrome. Am J Dis Child 1977;131:452–5.

27. Hoyt CS, Billson FA. Maternal anticonvulsants and optic nerve hypoplasia. Br J Ophthalmol 1978;62:3–6.

28. Wilson RS, Smead W, Char F. Diphenylhydantoin teratogenicity: ocular manifestations and related deformities. J Pediatr Ophthalmol Strabismus 1970;15:137–40.

29. Dabee V, Hart AG, Hurley RM. Teratogenic effects of diphenylhydantoin. Can Med Assoc J 1975;112:75–7.

30. Anderson RC. Cardiac defects in children of mothers receiving anticonvulsant therapy during pregnancy. J Pediatr 1976;89:318–9.

31. Hill RM, Verniaud WM, Horning MG, McCulley LB, Morgan NF. Infants exposed in utero to antiepileptic drugs. A prospective study. Am J Dis Child 1974;127:645–53.

32. Stankler L, Campbell AGM. Neonatal acne vulgaris: a possible feature of the fetal hydantoin syndrome. Br J Dermatol 1980;103:453–5.

33. Ringrose CAD. The hazard of neurotropic drugs in the fertile years. Can Med Assoc J 1972;106:1058.

34. Pettifor JM, Benson R. Congenital malformations associated with the administration of oral anticoagulants during pregnancy. J Pediatr 1975;86:459–61.

35. Biale Y, Lewenthal H, Aderet NB. Congenital malformations due to anticonvulsant drugs and congenital abnormalities. Obstet Gynecol 1975;45:439–42.

36. Aase JM. Anticonvulsant drugs and congenital abnormalities. Am J Dis Child 1974;127:758.

37. Lewin PK. Phenytoin associated congenital defects with Y-chromosome variant. Lancet 1973;l:559.

38. Yang TS, Chi CC, Tsai CJ, Chang MJ. Diphenylhydantoin teratogenicity in man. Obstet Gynecol 1978;52:682–4.

39. Mallow DW, Herrick MK, Gathman G. Fetal exposure to anticonvulsant drugs. Arch Pathol Lab Med 1980;104:215–8.
40. Hirschberger M, Kleinberg F. Maternal phenytoin ingestion and congenital abnormalities: report of a case. Am J Dis Child 1975;129:984.
41. Hanson JW, Myrianthopoulos NC, Sedgwick Harvey MA, Smith DW. Risks to the offspring of women treated with hydantoin anticonvulsants, with emphasis on the fetal hydantoin syndrome. J Pediatr 1976;89:662–8.
42. Shakir RA, Johnson RH, Lambie DG, Melville ID, Nanda RN. Comparison of sodium valproate and phenytoin as single drug treatment in epilepsy. Epilepsia 1981;22:27–33.
43. Michalodimitrakis M, Parchas S, Coutselinis A. Fetal hydantoin syndrome: congenital malformation of the urinary tract—a case report. Clin Toxicol 1981;18:1095–7.
44. Phelan MC, Pellock JM, Nance WE. Discordant expression of fetal hydantoin syndrome in heteropaternal dizygotic twins. N Engl J Med 1982;307:99–101.
45. Kousseff BG, Root ER. Expanding phenotype of fetal hydantoin syndrome. Pediatrics 1982;70:328–9.
46. Wilker R, Nathenson G. Combined fetal alcohol and hydantoin syndromes. Clin Pediatr 1982;21:331–4.
47. Kogutt MS. Fetal hydantoin syndrome. South Med J 1984;77:657–8.
48. Krauss CM, Holmes LB, VanLang, QN, Keith DA. Four siblings with similar malformations after exposure to phenytoin and primidone. J Pediatr 1984;105:750–5.
49. Pearl KN, Dickens S, Latham P. Functional palatal incompetence in the fetal anticonvulsant syndrome. Arch Dis Child 1984;59:989–90.
50. Lawrence A. Antiepileptic drugs and the foetus. Br Med J 1963;2:1267.
51. Kohler HG. Haemorrhage in newborn of epileptic mothers. Lancet 1966;1:267.
52. Douglas H. Haemorrhage in the newborn. Lancet 1966;1:816–7.
53. Monnet P, Rosenberg D, Bovier-Lapierre M. Terapeutique anticomitale administree pendant la grosses et maladie hemorragique du nouveau-ne. Cited in Bleyer WA, Skinner AL. Fetal neonatal hemorrhage after maternal anticonvulsant therapy. JAMA 1976;235:626–7.
54. Davis PP. Coagulation defect due to anticonvulsant drug treatment in pregnancy. Lancet 1970;1:413.
55. Evans AR, Forrester RM, Discombe C. Neonatal hemorrhage following maternal anticonvulsant therapy. Lancet 1970;1:517–8.
56. Stevensom MM, Bilbert EF. Anticonvulsants and hemorrhagic diseases of the newborn infant. J Pediatr 1970;77:516.
57. Speidel BD, Meadow SR. Maternal epilepsy and abnormalities of the fetus and newborn. Lancet 1972;2:839–40.
58. Truog WE, Feusner JH, Baker DL. Association of hemorrhagic disease and the syndrome of persistent fetal circulation with the fetal hydantoin syndrome. J Pediatr 1980;96:112–4.
59. Solomon GE, Hilgartner MW, Kutt H. Coagulation defects caused by diphenylhydantoin. Neurology 1972;22:1165–71.
60. Griffiths AD. Neonatal haemorrhage associated with maternal anticonvulsant therapy. Lancet 1981;2:1296–7.
61. Page TE, Hoyme HE, Markarian M, Jones KL. Neonatal hemorrhage secondary to thrombocytopenia: an occasional effect of prenatal hydantoin exposure. Birth Defects 1982;18:47–50.
62. Srinivasan G, Seeler RA, Tiruvury A, Pildes RS. Maternal anticonvulsant therapy and hemorrhagic disease of the newborn. Obstet Gynecol 1982;59:250–2.
63. Payne NR, Hasegawa DK. Vitamin K deficiency in newborns: a case report in α-1-antitrypsin deficiency and a review of factors predisposing to hemorrhage. Pediatrics 1984;73:712–6.
64. Lane PA, Hathaway WE. Vitamin K in infancy. J Pediatr 1985;106:351–9.
65. Felding I, Rane A. Congenital liver damage after treatment of mother with valproic acid and phenytoin? Acta Paediatr Scand 1984;73:565–8.
66. Biale Y, Lewenthal H. Effect of folic acid supplementation on congenital malformations due to anticonvulsive drugs. Eur J Obstet Reprod Biol 1984;18:211–6.
67. Pritchard JA, Scott DE, Whalley PJ. Maternal folate deficiency and pregnancy wastage. IV. Effects of folic acid supplements, anticonvulsants, and oral contraceptives. Am J Obstet Gynecol 1971;109:341–6.
68. Hiilesmaa VK, Teramo K, Granstrom ML, Bardy AH. Serum folate concentrations during pregnancy in women with epilepsy: relation to antiepileptic drug concentrations, number of seizures, and fetal outcome. Br Med J 1983;287:577–9.

69. Nau H, Kuhnz W, Egger HJ, Rating D, Helge H. Anticonvulsants during pregnancy and lactation: transplacental, maternal and neonatal pharmacokinetics. Clin Pharmacokinet 1982;7:508–43.

70. Chen SS, Perucca E, Lee JN, Richens A. Serum protein binding and free concentrations of phenytoin and phenobarbitone in pregnancy. Br J Clin Pharmacol 1982;13:547–52.

71. van der Klign E, Schobben F, Bree TB. Clinical pharmacokinetics of antiepileptic drugs. Drug Intell Clin Pharm 1980;14:674–85.

72. Dansky L, Andermann E, Sherwin AL, Andermann F. Plasma levels of phenytoin during pregnancy and the puerperium. In *Epilepsy, Pregnancy and the Child*. Proceedings of a Workshop held in Berlin, September 1980. New York:Raven Press, 1981.

73. Dansky L, Andermann E, Andermann F, Sherwin AL, Kinch RA. Maternal epilepsy and congenital malformation: correlation with maternal plasma anticonvulsant levels during pregnancy. In *Epilepsy, Pregnancy and the Child*. Proceedings of a Workship held in Berlin, September 1980. New York:Raven Press, 1981.

74. Hiilesmaa VK. Evaluation of placental function in women on antiepileptic drugs. J Perinat Med 1983;11:187–92.

75. Carriero R, Andermann E, Chen MF, Eeg-Oloffson O, Kinch RAH, Klein G, Pearson Murphy BE. Thyroid function in epileptic mothers and their infants at birth. Am J Obstet Gynecol 1985;151:641–4.

76. Markestad T, Ulstein M, Strandjord RE, Aksnes L, Aarskog D. Anticonvulsant drug therapy in human pregnancy: effects on serum concentrations of vitamin D metabolites in maternal and cord blood. Am J Obstet Gynecol 1984;150:254–8.

77. Tamari I, Eldar M, Rabinowitz B, Neufeld HN. Medical treatment of cardiovascular disorders during pregnancy. Am Heart J 1982;104:1357–63.

78. Rotmensch HH, Elkayam U, Frishman W. Antiarrhythmic drug therapy during pregnancy. Ann Intern Med 1983;98:487–497.

79. Rotmensch HH, Rotmensch S, Elkayam U. Management of cardiac arrhythmias during pregnancy: current concepts. Drugs 1987;33:623–33.

80. Ryan G, Lange IR, Naugler MA. Clinical experience with phenytoin prophylaxis in severe preeclampsia. Am J Obstet Gynecol 1989;161:1297–304.

81. Horning MG, Stillwell WG, Nowling J, Lertratanangkoon K, Stillwell RN, Hill RM. Identification and quantification of drugs and drug metabolites in human breast milk using GC-MS-COM methods. Mod Probl Pediatr 1975;15:73–9.

82. Svensmark O, Schiller PJ. 5-5-Diphenylhydantoin (Dilantin) blood level after oral or intravenous dosage in man. Acta Pharmacol Toxicol 1960;16:331–46.

83. Kok THHG, Taitz LS, Bennett MJ, Holt DW. Drowsiness due to clemastine transmitted in breast milk. Lancet 1982;1:914–5.

84. Steen B, Rane A, Lonnerholm G, Falk O, Elwin CE, Sjoqvist F. Phenytoin excretion in human breast milk and plasma levels in nursed infants. Ther Drug Monit 1982;4:331–4.

85. Finch E, Lorber J. Methaemoglobinaemia in the newborn: probably due to phenytoin excreted in human milk. J Obstet Gynaecol Br Emp 1954;61:833.

86. Committee on Drugs, American Academy of Pediatrics. Transfer of drugs and other chemicals into human milk. Pediatrics 1989;84:924–36.

Name: **PHYSOSTIGMINE**

Class: **Parasympathomimetic (Cholinergic)**   Risk Factor: **C**

Fetal Risk Summary

Physostigmine is rarely used in pregnancy. No reports linking its use with congenital defects have appeared. One report described its use in 15 women at term to reverse scopolamine-induced twilight sleep (1). Apgar scores of 14 of the newborns ranged from 7–9 at 1 minute and 8–10 at 5 minutes. One infant was depressed at birth and required resuscitation, but the mother had also received meperidine and diazepam. No other effects in the infants were mentioned.

Physostigmine is an anticholinesterase agent, but it does not contain a quaternary ammonium element. It crosses the blood-brain barrier and should be expected to cross the placenta (2).

Transient muscular weakness has been observed in about 20% of newborns of mothers with myasthenia gravis (3–5). The neonatal myasthenia is due to transplacental passage of anti-acetylcholine receptor immunoglobulin G antibodies (5).

Breast Feeding Summary

No data are available.

References

1. Smiller BG, Bartholomew EG, Sivak BJ, Alexander GD, Brown EM. Physostigmine reversal of scopolamine delirium in obstetric patients. Am J Obstet Gynecol 1973;116:326–9.
2. Taylor P. Anticholinesterase agents. In Gilman AG, Goodman LS, Gilman A, eds. *The Pharmacological Basis of Therapeutics*, ed. 6. New York:MacMillan, 1980:100–19.
3. McNall PG, Jafarnia MR. Management of myasthenia gravis in the obstetrical patient. Am J Obstet Gynecol 1965;92:518–25.
4. Blackhall MI, Buckley GA, Roberts DV, Roberts JB, Thomas BH, Wilson A. Drug-induced neonatal myasthenia. J Obstet Gynaecol Br Commonw 1969;76:157–62.
5. Plauche WG. Myasthenia gravis in pregnancy: an update. Am J Obstet Gynecol 1979;135:691–7.

Name: **PHYTONADIONE**

Class: **Vitamin**   Risk Factor: **C**

Fetal Risk Summary

Phytonadione is a synthetic, fat-soluble substance identical to vitamin K_1, the natural vitamin found in a variety of foods (1). It is used for the prevention and treatment of hypoprothrombinemia due to vitamin K deficiency (1).

The use of phytonadione (vitamin K_1) during pregnancy and in the newborn has been the subject of several large reviews (2–5). Administration of vitamin K during pregnancy is usually not required due to the abundance of natural sources in food and the synthesis of the vitamin by the normal intestinal flora. Vitamin K_1 is indicated for maternal hypoprothrombinemia and for the prevention of hemorrhagic disease of the newborn (HDN) induced by maternal drugs, such as anticonvulsants, warfarin, rifampin, and isoniazid (2–5).

The placental transfer of vitamin K_1 is poor. A 1982 study found no detectable vitamin K (<0.10 ng/ml) in the cord blood of nine term infants, although adequate levels (mean 0.20 ng/ml) were present in eight of the nine mothers (6). Vitamin K_1, 1 mg intravenously (IV), was then given to six additional mothers shortly before delivery (11–47 minutes) resulting in plasma K_1 values of 45–93 ng/ml. K_1 was detected in only four of the six cord blood samples (ranging from 0.10–0.14 ng/ml), and its appearance did not seem to be time dependent.

Vitamin K_1 is nontoxic in doses less than 20 mg (3). In a double blind trial, 933 women at term were given 20 mg of either K_1 or K_2, the naturally occurring vitamins (7). No toxicity from either vitamin was found, including any association with low birth weight, asphyxia, neonatal jaundice, or perinatal mortality.

Oral vitamin K_1 has been suggested during the last 2 weeks of pregnancy for women taking anticonvulsants to prevent hypoprothrombinemia and hemorrhage in their newborns, but the effectiveness of this therapy has not been proven (2, 3). In a group of mothers receiving phenindione, an oral anticoagulant, 10–30 mg of K_1 were given either IV or intra-amniotically 2–4 days prior to delivery (8). In a separate group, 2.5–3.0 mg of K_1 were injected intramuscularly into the fetuses at the same interval before delivery. Only in this latter group were coagulation factors significantly improved.

In summary, phytonadione (vitamin K_1) is the treatment of choice for maternal hypoprothrombinemia and for the prevention of HDN. Maternal supplements are not needed except for those patients deemed at risk for vitamin K deficiency.

Breast Feeding Summary

Levels of phytonadione (vitamin K_1) in breast milk are naturally low with most samples having less than 20 ng/ml and many less than 5 ng/ml (2, 3). In 20 lactating women, colostrum and mature milk concentrations were 2.3 and 2.1 ng/ml, less than half that found in cow's milk (9). Administration of a single 20-mg oral dose of phytonadione to one mother produced a concentration of 140 ng/ml at 12 hours with levels at 48 hours still about double normal values (9). In another study, 40 mg orally of K_1 or K_3 (menadione) were given to mothers within 2 hours after delivery (10). Effects from either vitamin on the prothrombin time of the breast-fed newborns were nil to slight during the first 3 days.

Natural levels of K_1 or K_2 in milk will not provide adequate supplies of the vitamin for the breast-fed infant (2, 3). The vitamin K_1-dependent coagulation factors, II, VII, IX, and X, are dependent on gestational age (2). In the newborn, these factors are approximately 30–60% of normal and do not reach adult levels until about 6 weeks (2). While not all newborns are vitamin K_1 deficient, many are, due to poor placental transfer of the vitamin. Exclusive breast feeding will not prevent further decline of these already low stores and the possible development of deficiency in 48–72 hours (2, 3). In addition, the intestinal flora of breast-fed infants may produce less vitamin K than the flora of formula-fed infants (2). The potential consequence of this deficiency is hemorrhagic disease of the newborn.

The American Academy of Pediatrics has suggested that HDN be defined as "a hemorrhagic disorder of the first days of life caused by a deficiency of vitamin K and characterized by deficiency of prothrombin and proconvertin (stable factor, factor VII), and probably of other factors" (11). The hemorrhage is frequently life threatening with intracranial bleeds common. In a 1985 review, Lane and Hathaway (2) identified three types of HDN:

Early HDN (onset 0–24 hours)
Classic HDN (onset 2–5 days)
Late HDN (onset 1–12 months)

The maternal ingestion of certain drugs, such as anticonvulsants, warfarin, or antituberculous agents, is one of the known causes of early and classic HDN, while breast feeding has been shown to be a cause of classic and late HDN (2). The administration of phytonadione to the newborn prevents HDN by preventing further decline of factors II, VII, IX, and X (2).

The use of prophylactic vitamin K_1 in all newborns is common in the United States but is controversial in other countries (2). The Committee on Nutrition, American Academy of Pediatrics, recommended in 1961 and again in 1980 that all newborns receive 0.5–1.0 mg of parenteral vitamin K_1 (11, 12). The Committee recommended that administration to the mother prenatally should not be substituted for newborn prophylaxis (11). The bleeding risk in breast-fed infants who did not receive prophylactic K_1 is 15–20 times greater than in infants fed cow's milk, given K_1, or both (2). In spite of this evidence, new cases of HDN are still reported (3, 13). In a recent report, 10 breast-fed infants with intracranial hemorrhage due to vitamin K deficiency were described (13). Onset of the bleeding was between 27 and 47 days of age with three infants dying and three having permanent brain injury. Milk levels of total vitamin K (K_1 + K_2) varied between 1.36–9.17 ng/ml. None of the infants had been given prophylactic therapy at birth.

In summary, the natural vitamin K content of breast milk is too low to protect the newborn from vitamin K deficiency and resulting hemorrhagic disease. The administration of vitamin K to the mother to increase milk concentrations may be possible but needs further study. All newborns should receive parenteral prophylactic therapy at birth consisting of 0.5–1.0 mg of phytonadione. Larger and/or repeat doses may be required for infants whose mothers are consuming anticonvulsants or oral anticoagulants (2, 11). The American Academy of Pediatrics considers the maternal use of vitamin k_1 to be compatible with breast feeding (14).

References

1. American Hospital Formulary Service. *Drug Information 1990*. Bethesda:American Society of Hospital Pharmacists, 1990:2136–38.
2. Lane PA, Hathaway WE. Vitamin K in infancy. J Pediatr 1985;106:351–9.
3. Payne NR, Hasegawa DK. Vitamin K deficiency in newborns: a case report in α-1-antitrypsin deficiency and a review of factors predisposing to hemorrhage. Pediatrics 1984;73:712–6.
4. Wynn RM. The obstetric significance of factors affecting the metabolism of bilirubin, with particular reference to the role of vitamin K. Obstet Gynecol Surv 1963;18:333–54.
5. Finkel MJ. Vitamin K_1 and the vitamin K analogues. J Clin Pharmacol Therap 1961;2:795–814.
6. Shearer MJ, Rahim S, Barkhan P, Stimmler L. Plasma vitamin K_1 in mothers and their newborn babies. Lancet 1982;2:460–3.
7. Blood Study Group of Gynecologists. Effect of vitamins K_2 and K_1 on the bleeding volume during parturition and the blood coagulation disturbance of newborns by a double blind controlled study. Igaku no Ayumi 1971;76:818. As cited in Nishimura H, Tanimura T. *Clinical Aspects of the Teratogenicity of Drugs*. New York:American Elsevier, 1976:253.
8. Larsen JF, Jacobsen B, Holm HH, Pedersen JF, Mantoni M. Intrauterine injection of vitamin K before delivery during anticoagulant therapy of the mother. Acta Obstet Gynecol Scand 1978;57:227–30.
9. Haroon Y, Shearer MJ, Rahim S, Gunn WG, McEnery G, Barkhan P. The content of phylloquinone (vitamin K_1) in human milk, cows' milk and infant formula foods determined by high-performance liquid chromatography. J Nutr 1982;112:1105–17.
10. Dyggve HV, Dam H, Sondergaard E. Influence on the prothrombin time of breast-fed newborn babies of one single dose of vitamin K_1 or Synkavit given to the mother within 2 hours after birth. Acta Obstet Gynecol Scand 1956;35:440–4.
11. Committee on Nutrition, American Academy of Pediatrics. Vitamin K compounds and the water-soluble analogues. Pediatrics 1961;28:501–7.
12. Committee on Nutrition, American Academy of Pediatrics. Vitamin and mineral supplement needs in normal children in the United States. Pediatrics 1980;66:1015–21.
13. Motohara K, Matsukura M, Matsuda I, Iribe K, Ikeda T, Kondo Y, Yonekubo A, Yamamoto Y, Tsuchiya F. Severe vitamin K deficiency in breast-fed infants. J Pediatr 1984;105:943–5.

14. Committee on Drugs, American Academy of Pediatrics. Transfer of drugs and other chemicals into human milk. Pediatrics 1989;84:924–36.

Name: **PILOCARPINE**

Class: **Parasympathomimetic (Cholinergic)**   Risk Factor: **C**

Fetal Risk Summary

Pilocarpine is used in the eye. No reports of its use in pregnancy have been located.

Breast Feeding Summary

No data are available.

Name: **PINDOLOL**

Class: **Sympatholytic (β-Adrenergic Blocker)**   Risk Factor: **B$_M$**

Fetal Risk Summary

Pindolol, a nonselective β-adrenergic blocking agent, has been used for the treatment of hypertension occurring during pregnancy (1–4). A 1988 review compared the effects of β-blockers, including pindolol, in pregnancy and concluded that these agents are relatively safe (5).

Pindolol crosses the placenta to the fetus with maternal serum levels higher than cord concentrations (6). Cord:maternal serum ratios at 2 and 6 hours after the last dose were 0.37 and 0.67, respectively. Elimination half-lives in fetal and maternal serum were 1.6 hours and 2.2 hours, respectively.

No fetal malformations attributable to pindolol have been reported, but experience in the 1st trimester is lacking. In a study comparing three β-blockers for the treatment of hypertension during pregnancy, the mean birth weight of pindolol-exposed babies was slightly higher than the acebutolol group and much higher than the offspring of atenolol-treated mothers (3375 g vs. 3160 g vs. 2745 g) (2). It is not known if these differences were due to the degree of maternal hypertension, the potency of the drugs used, or a combination of these and other factors.

The preliminary results of another study found over a third of the infants delivered from hypertensive women treated with pindolol were of low birth weight, but the authors thought this did not differ significantly from the expected rate for this population (3). In mothers treated with pindolol or atenolol, a decrease in the basal fetal heart rate was noted only in the atenolol-exposed fetuses (4).

β-blockade in the newborn has not been reported in the offspring of pindolol-treated mothers. However, since this complication has been observed in infants exposed to other β-blockers (see Acebutolol, Atenolol, and Nadolol), close observation of the newborn is recommended during the first 24–48 hours after birth.

Long-term effects of *in utero* exposure to β-blockers have not been studied but warrant evaluation.

Breast Feeding Summary

No reports have been located describing the excretion of pindolol into breast milk. Other members of this class are excreted into milk and the passage of pindolol should be anticipated. Although milk levels of other beta-blockers are apparently too small to produce adverse reactions, nursing infants should be closely observed for bradycardia and other symptoms of beta-blockade. Long-term effects of exposure to beta-blockers from milk have not been studied but warrant evaluation.

References

1. Dubois D, Petitcolas J, Temperville B, Klepper A. Beta blockers and high-risk pregnancies. Int J Biol Res Pregnancy 1980;1:141–5.
2. Dubois D, Petitcolas J, Temperville B, Klepper A, Catherine PH. Treatment of hypertension in pregnancy with β-adrenoceptor antagonists. Br J Clin Pharmacol 1982;13(Suppl):375S-8S.
3. Sukerman-Voldman E. Pindolol therapy in pregnant hypertensive patients. Br J Clin Pharmacol 1982;13(Suppl):379S.
4. Ingemarsson I, Liedholm H, Montan S, Westgren M, Melander A. Fetal heart rate during treatment of maternal hypertension with beta-adrenergic antagonists. Acta Obstet Gynecol Scand 1984;118(Suppl):95–7.
5. Frishman WH, Chesner M. Beta-adrenergic blockers in pregnancy. Am Heart J 1988; 115:147–52.
6. Grunstein S, Ellenbogen A, Anderman S, Davidson A, Jaschevatsky O. Transfer of pindolol across the placenta in hypertensive pregnant women. Curr Ther Res 1985;37:587–91.

Name: **PIPERACETAZINE**

Class: **Tranquilizer**   Risk Factor: **C**

Fetal Risk Summary

Piperacetazine is a piperidyl phenothiazine. The phenothiazines readily cross the placenta (1). No specific information on the use of piperacetazine in pregnancy has been located. Although occasional reports have attempted to link various phenothiazine compounds with congenital malformations, the bulk of the evidence indicates that these drugs are safe for the mother and fetus (see also Chlorpromazine).

Breast Feeding Summary

No reports describing the excretion of piperacetazine into breast milk have been located. The American Academy of Pediatrics considered the drug to be compatible with breast feeding in a 1983 statement (2), but the drug was not included in the 1989 revision.

References

1. Moya F, Thorndike V. Passage of drugs across the placenta. Am J Obstet Gynecol 1962;84:1778–98.
2. Committee on Drugs, American Academy of Pediatrics. The transfer of drugs and other chemicals into human breast milk. Pediatrics 1983;72:375–83.

Name: **PIPERACILLIN**

Class: **Antibiotic**   Risk Factor: **B$_M$**

Fetal Risk Summary

Piperacillin, a piperazine derivative of ampicillin, is a broad-spectrum penicillin (see also Ampicillin). No reports linking the use of piperacillin with congenital defects have been located. Animal reproduction studies have not shown any evidence of fetal harm (1).

Breast Feeding Summary

Piperacillin is excreted in small amounts in human breast milk. Although concentrations are low, three potential problems exist for the nursing infant: modification of bowel flora, direct effects on the infant, and interference with the interpretation of culture results if a fever workup is required.

Reference

1. Product information. Pipracil. Lederle Laboratories, 1990.

Name: **PIPERAZINE**

Class: **Anthelmintic**   Risk Factor: **B**

Fetal Risk Summary

No reports linking the use of piperazine with congenital defects have been located. Animal data have also failed to demonstrate any teratogenic effect. The Collaborative Perinatal Project monitored 50,282 mother-child pairs, 3 of which had 1st trimester exposure to piperazine. No evidence was found to suggest a relationship to malformations (1).

Breast Feeding Summary

No data are available.

Reference

1. Heinonen OP, Slone D, Shapiro S. *Birth Defects and Drugs in Pregnancy*. Littleton:Publishing Sciences Group, 1977:299.

Name: **PIPERIDOLATE**

Class: **Parasympatholytic (Anticholinergic)**   Risk Factor: **C**

Fetal Risk Summary

Piperidolate is an anticholinergic agent. In a large prospective study, 2323 patients were exposed to this class of drugs during the 1st trimester, 16 of whom took piperadolate (1). A possible association was found between the total group and minor malformations.

Breast Feeding Summary

No data are available (see also Atropine).

Reference

1. Heinonen OP, Slone D, Shapiro S. *Birth Defects and Drugs in Pregnancy*. Littleton:Publishing Sciences Group, 1977:346–53.

Name: **PLICAMYCIN**

Class: **Antineoplastic**   Risk Factor: **D**

Fetal Risk Summary

No reports on the use of plicamycin (formerly named mithramycin) during pregnancy have been located. Occupational exposure of the mother to antineoplastic agents during pregnancy may present a risk to the fetus. A position statement from the National Study Commission on Cytotoxic Exposure and a research article involving some antineoplastic agents are presented in the monograph for cyclophosphamide (see Cyclophosphamide).

Breast Feeding Summary

No data are available.

Name: **POLYMYXIN B**

Class: **Antibiotic**   Risk Factor: **B**

Fetal Risk Summary

No reports linking the use of polymyxin B with congenital defects have been located. Although available for injection, polymyxin B is used almost exclusively by topical administration. In one study, seven exposures were recorded in the 1st trimester (1). No association with congenital defects was observed.

Breast Feeding Summary

No data are available.

Reference

1. Heinonen OP, Slone D, Shapiro S. *Birth Defects and Drugs in Pregnancy*. Littleton:Publishing Sciences Group, 1977:297.

Name: **POLYTHIAZIDE**

Class: **Diuretic**   Risk Factor: **D**

Fetal Risk Summary

See Chlorothiazide.

Breast Feeding Summary

See Chlorothiazide.

Name: **POTASSIUM CHLORIDE**

Class: **Electrolyte**   Risk Factor: **A**

Fetal Risk Summary

Potassium chloride is a natural constituent of human tissues and fluids. Exogenous potassium chloride may be indicated as replacement therapy for pregnant women with low potassium serum levels, such as those receiving diuretics. Since high or low levels are detrimental to maternal and fetal cardiac function, serum levels should be closely monitored.

Breast Feeding Summary

Human milk is naturally low in potassium (1). If maternal serum levels are maintained in a physiologic range, no harm will result in the nursing infant from the administration of potassium chloride to the mother.

Reference

1. Wilson JT. Production and characteristics of breast milk. In Wilson JT, ed. *Drugs in Breast Milk*. Australia:ADIS Press, 1981:12.

Name: **POTASSIUM CITRATE**

Class: **Electrolyte**   Risk Factor: **A**

Fetal Risk Summary

See Potassium Chloride.

Breast Feeding Summary

See Potassium Chloride.

Name: **POTASSIUM GLUCONATE**

Class: **Electrolyte**   Risk Factor: **A**

Fetal Risk Summary

See Potassium Chloride.

Breast Feeding Summary

See Potassium Chloride.

Name: **POTASSIUM IODIDE**

Class: **Expectorant**   Risk Factor: **D**

Fetal Risk Summary

The primary concern with the use of potassium iodide during pregnancy relates to the effect of iodide on the fetal thyroid gland. Since aqueous solutions of iodine are in equilibrium with the ionized form, all iodide or iodine products are considered as one group.

Iodide readily crosses the placenta to the fetus (1). When used for prolonged periods or close to term, iodide may cause hypothyroidism and goiter in the fetus and newborn. Short-term use, such as a 10-day preparation course for maternal thyroid surgery, does not carry this risk and is apparently safe (2, 3). A 1983 review tabulated 49 cases of congenital iodide goiter dating back to 1940 (66 references) (4). In 14 cases, the goiter was large enough to cause tracheal compression resulting in death. Cardiomegaly was present in three surviving newborns and in one of the fatalities. In a majority of the cases, exposure to the iodide was due to maternal asthma treatment.

Three recent studies have shown the potential hazard resulting from the use of povidone-iodine during pregnancy (5–7). In each case, significant absorption of iodine occurred in the mother and fetus following vaginal or perineal use before delivery. Transient hypothyroidism was demonstrated in some newborns (5).

Since a large number of prescription and over-the-counter medications contain iodide or iodine, pregnant patients should consult with their physician prior to using these products. The American Academy of Pediatrics considers the use of iodides as expectorants during pregnancy to be contraindicated (8).

Breast Feeding Summary

Iodide is concentrated in breast milk (4, 9). In one report, a breast feeding mother used povidone-iodine vaginal gel daily for 6 days without douching (9). Two days after stopping the gel, the mother noted an odor of iodine on the 7 1/2-month-old baby. The free iodide serum:milk ratio 1 day later was approximately 23:1. By day 7, the ratio had fallen to about 4:1 but then rose again on day 8 to 10:1. Serum and urine iodide levels in the infant were grossly elevated. No problems or alterations in thyroid tests were noted in the baby.

The normal iodine content of human milk has been recently assessed (10). Mean iodide levels in 37 lactating women were 178 µg/L. This is approximately four times the recommended daily allowance (RDA) for infants. The RDA for iodine was based on the amount of iodine found in breast milk in earlier studies (10). The higher levels now are probably due to dietary supplements of iodine (e.g., salt, bread, cow's milk). The significance to the nursing infant from the chronic ingestion of higher levels of iodine is not known. The American Academy of Pediatrics, although recognizing that the maternal use of iodides during lactation may affect the infant's thyroid activity by producing elevated iodine levels in breast milk, considers the agents to be compatible with breast feeding (11).

References

1. Wolff J. Iodide goiter and the pharmacologic effects of excess iodide. Am J Med 1969; 47:101–24.
2. Herbst AL, Selenkow HA. Hyperthyroidism during pregnancy. N Engl J Med 1965; 273:627–33.
3. Selenkow HA, Herbst AL. Hyperthyroidism during pregnancy. N Engl J Med 1966; 274:165–6.
4. Mehta PS, Mehta SJ, Vorherr H. Congenital iodide goiter and hypothyroidism: a review. Obstet Gynecol Surv 1983;38:237–47.
5. l'Allemand D, Gruters A, Heidemann P, Schurnbrand P. Iodine-induced alterations of thyroid function in newborn infants after prenatal and perinatal exposure to povidone iodine. J Pediatr 1983;102:935–8.
6. Bachrach LK, Burrow GN, Gare DJ. Maternal-fetal absorption of povidone-iodine. J Pediatr 1984;104:158–9.
7. Jacobson JM, Hankins GV, Young RL, Hauth JC. Changes in thyroid function and serum iodine levels after prepartum use of a povidone-iodine vaginal lubricant. J Reprod Med 1984; 29:98–100.
8. Committee on Drugs. American Academy of Pediatrics. Adverse reactions to iodide therapy of asthma and other pulmonary diseases. Pediatrics 1976;57:272–4.
9. Postellon DC, Aronow R. Iodine in mother's milk. JAMA 1982;247:463.
10. Gushurst CA, Mueller JA, Green JA, Sedor F. Breast milk iodide: reassessment in the 1980s. Pediatrics 1984;73:354–7.
11. Committee on Drugs, American Academy of Pediatrics. Transfer of drugs and other chemicals into human milk. Pediatrics 1989;84:924–36.

Name: **POVIDONE-IODINE**

Class: **Anti-infective**   Risk Factor: **D**

Fetal Risk Summary

See Potassium Iodide.

Breast Feeding Summary

See Potassium Iodide.

Name: **PRAZOSIN**

Class: **Antihypertensive**   Risk Factor: **C**

Fetal Risk Summary

Prazosin is an α-adrenergic blocking agent used for hypertension. In two studies, prazosin was combined with oxprenolol or atenolol, β-adrenergic blockers, in the treatment of pregnant women with severe essential hypertension or pregnancy-induced hypertension (PIH) (1, 2). The combinations were effective in the first group but less so in the PIH patients. No adverse effects attributable to the drugs were noted. Prazosin, 20 mg/day, was combined with minoxidil and metoprolol throughout gestation to treat severe maternal hypertension secondary to chronic nephritis (3). The child, normal except for hypertrichosis due to minoxidil, was doing well at 2 years of age.

Prazosin has been used during the 3rd trimester in a patient with pheochromocytoma (4). Blood pressure was well controlled, but maternal tachycardia required the addition of a β-blocker. A healthy male infant was delivered by cesarean section.

Breast Feeding Summary

No data are available.

References

1. Lubbe WF, Hodge JV. Combined alpha- and beta-adrenoceptor antagonism with prazosin and oxprenolol in control of severe hypertension in pregnancy. NZ Med J 1981;94:169–72.
2. Lubbe WF. More on beta-blockers in pregnancy. N Engl J Med 1982;307:753.
3. Rosa FW, Idanpaan-Heikkila J, Asanti R. Fetal minoxidil exposure. Pediatrics 1987;80:120.
4. Venuto R, Burstein P, Schneider R. Pheochromocytoma: antepartum diagnosis and management with tumor resection in the puerperium. Am J Obstet Gynecol 1984;150:431–2.

Name: **PREDNISOLONE**

Class: **Corticosteroid**   Risk Factor: **B**

Fetal Risk Summary

Prednisolone is the biologically active form of prednisone (see Prednisone). The placenta can oxidize prednisolone to inactive prednisone or less active cortisone (see Cortisone).

Breast Feeding Summary

See Prednisone.

Name: **PREDNISONE**

Class: **Corticosteroid**   Risk Factor: **B**

Fetal Risk Summary

Prednisone is metabolized to prednisolone. There are a number of studies in which pregnant patients received either prednisone or prednisolone (see also various antineoplastic agents for additional references) (1–14). These corticosteroids apparently have little, if any, effect on the developing fetus.

Immunosuppression was observed in a newborn exposed to high doses of prednisone with azathioprine throughout gestation (15). The newborn had lymphopenia, decreased survival of lymphocytes in culture, absence of IgM, and reduced levels of IgG. Recovery occurred at 15 weeks of age. However, these effects were not observed in a larger group of similarly exposed newborns (16). A 1968 study reported an increase in the incidence of stillbirths following prednisone therapy during pregnancy (7). Increased fetal mortality has not been confirmed by other investigators.

An infant exposed to prednisone throughout pregnancy was born with congenital cataracts (1). The eye defect was consistent with reports of subcapsular cataracts observed in adults receiving corticosteroids. However, in this case, the relationship between the cataracts and prednisone is doubtful because of the lack of similar reports.

In a 1970 case report, a female infant with multiple deformities was described (17). Her father had been treated several years prior to conception with prednisone, azathioprine and radiation for a kidney transplant. The authors speculated that the child's defects may have been related to the father's immunosuppressive therapy. A relationship to prednisone seems remote since previous studies have shown that the drug has no effect on chromosome number or morphology (18). High, prolonged doses of prednisolone (30 mg/day for at least 4 weeks) may damage spermatogenesis (19). Recovery may require 6 months after the drug is stopped.

Prednisone has been used successfully to prevent neonatal respiratory distress syndrome when premature delivery occurs between 28 and 36 weeks of gestation (20). Therapy between 16 and 25 weeks of gestation had no effect on lecithin:sphingomyelin ratios (21).

In summary, prednisone and prednisolone apparently pose a very small risk to the developing fetus. The available evidence supports their use to control various maternal diseases.

Breast Feeding Summary

Trace amounts of prednisone and prednisolone have been measured in breast milk (22–24). Following a 10-mg oral dose of prednisone, milk concentrations of prednisone and prednisolone at 2 hours were 0.03 and 0.002 μg/ml, respectively (22). In a second study utilizing radioactive-labeled prednisolone in seven patients, a mean of 0.14% of a 5-mg oral dose was recovered/L of milk over 48–61 hours (23). This is equivalent to 0.007 μg/ml.

In six lactating women, prednisolone doses of 10–80 mg/day resulted in milk concentrations ranging from 5–25% of maternal serum levels (24). The milk:plasma ratio increased with increasing serum concentrations. For maternal doses of 20 mg once or twice daily, the authors concluded that the nursing infant would be exposed to minimal amounts of steroid. At higher doses, they recommended waiting at least 4 hours after a dose before nursing was performed. However, even at 80 mg/day, the nursing infant would ingest <0.1% of the dose, which corresponds to <10% of the infant's endogenous cortisol production (24).

Although nursing infants were not involved in either study, it is doubtful if these amounts are clinically significant. The American Academy of Pediatrics considers prednisone and prednisolone to be compatible with breast feeding (25).

References

1. Kraus AM. Congenital cataract and maternal steroid injection. J Pediatr Ophthalmol 1975;12:107–8.
2. Durie BGM, Giles HR. Successful treatment of acute leukemia during pregnancy: combination therapy in the third trimester. Arch Intern Med 1977;137:90–1.
3. Nolan GH, Sweet RL, Laros RK, Roure CA. Renal cadaver transplantation followed by successful pregnancies. Obstet Gynecol 1974;43:732–9.
4. Grossman JH III, Littner MR. Severe sarcoidosis in pregnancy. Obstet Gynecol 1977;50(Suppl):81s-4s.
5. Cutting HO, Collier TM. Acute lymphocytic leukemia during pregnancy: report of a case. Obstet Gynecol 1964;24:941–5.
6. Hanson GC, Ghosh S. Systemic lupus erythematosus and pregnancy. Br Med J 1965;2:1227–8.
7. Warrell DW, Taylor R. Outcome for the foetus of mothers receiving prednisolone during pregnancy. Lancet 1968;1:117–8.
8. Walsh SD, Clark FR. Pregnancy in patients on long-term corticosteroid therapy. Scott Med J 1967;12:302–6.
9. Zulman JI, Talal N, Hoffman GS, Epstein WV. Problems associated with the management of pregnancies in patients with systemic lupus erythematosus. J Rheumatol 1980;7:37–49.
10. Hartikainen-Sorri AL, Kaila J. Systemic lupus erythematosus and habitual abortion: case report. Br J Obstet Gynaecol 1980;87:729–31.
11. Minchinton RM, Dodd NJ, O'Brien H, Amess JAL, Waters AH. Autoimmune thrombocytopenia in pregnancy. Br J Haematol 1980;44:451–9.
12. Tozman ECS, Urowitz MB, Gladman DD. Systemic lupus erythematosus and pregnancy. J Rheumatol 1980;7:624–32.
13. Karpatkin M, Porges RF, Karpatkin S. Platelet counts in infants of women with autoimmune thrombocytopenia: effect of steroid administration to the mother. N Engl J Med 1981;305:936–9.
14. Pratt WR. Allergic diseases in pregnancy and breast feeding. Ann Allergy 1981;47:355–60.
15. Cote CJ, Meuwissen HJ, Pickering RJ. Effects on the neonate of prednisone and azathioprine administered to the mother during pregnancy. J Pediatr 1974;85:324–8.
16. Cederqvist LL, Merkatz IR, Litwin SD. Fetal immunogloblin synthesis following maternal immunosuppression. Am J Obstet Gynecol 1977;129:687–90.
17. Tallent MB, Simmons RL, Najarian JS. Birth defects in child of male recipient of kidney transplant. JAMA 1970;211:1854–5.
18. Jensen MK. Chromosome studies in patients treated with azathioprine and amethopterin. Acta Med Scand 1967;182:445–55.
19. Mancini RE, Larieri JC, Muller F, Andrada JA, Saraceni DJ. Effect of prednisolone upon normal and pathologic human spermatogenesis. Fertil Steril 1966;17:500–13.
20. Szabo I, Csaba I, Novak P, Drozgyik I. Single-dose glucocorticoid for prevention of respiratory-distress syndrome. Lancet 1977;2:243.
21. Szabo I, Csaba I, Bodis J, Novak P, Drozgyik J, Schwartz J. Effect of glucocorticoid on fetal lecithin and sphingomyelin concentrations. Lancet 1980;1:320.
22. Katz FH, Duncan BR. Entry of prednisone into human milk. N Engl J Med 1975;293:1154.
23. McKenzie SA, Selley JA, Agnew JE. Secretion of prednisone into breast milk. Arch Dis Child 1975;50:894–6.
24. Ost L, Wettrell G, Bjorkhem I, Rane A. Prednisolone excretion in human milk. J Pediatr 1985;106:1008–11.
25. Committee on Drugs, American Academy of Pediatrics. Transfer of drugs and other chemicals into human milk. Pediatrics 1989;84:924–36.

Name: **PRIMAQUINE**

Class: **Plasmodicide**   Risk Factor: **C**

Fetal Risk Summary

No reports linking the use of primaquine with congenital defects have been located. Primaquine may cause hemolytic anemia in patients with glucose-6-phosphate dehydrogenase deficiency. Pregnant patients at risk for this disorder should be tested accordingly (1). If possible, the drug should be withheld until after delivery (2). However, if prophylaxis or treatment is required, primaquine should not be withheld (3).

Breast Feeding Summary

No data are available.

References

1. Trenholme GM, Parson PE. Therapy and prophylaxis of malaria. JAMA 1978;240:2293–5.
2. Anonymous. Chemoprophylaxis of malaria. MMWR 1978;27:81–90.
3. Diro M, Beydoun SN. Malaria in pregnancy. South Med J 1982;75:959–62.

Name: **PRIMIDONE**

Class: **Anticonvulsant**   Risk Factor: **D**

Fetal Risk Summary

Primidone, a structural analogue of phenobarbital, is effective against generalized convulsive seizures and psychomotor attacks. It is clear that the epileptic patient on anticonvulsant medication is at a higher risk for having a child with congenital defects than the general population (1–7). The difficulty in evaluating the increased malformation rate in epileptic patients lies in attempting to disentangle the effects of multiple drug therapy, the effects of the disease itself on the fetal outcome, and any pattern of malformations associated with the drug. The literature describes 323 infants who were exposed to primidone during the 1st trimester (4, 8–17). Of the 41 malformed infants described in these reports, only three infants were exposed to primidone and no other anticonvulsants during gestation (8, 15, 16). The anomalies observed in these three infants were similar to those observed in the fetal hydantoin syndrome (see Phenytoin).

There are other potential complications associated with the use of primidone during pregnancy. Neurologic manifestations in the newborn, such as overactivity and tumors, have been associated with use of primidone in pregnancy (16, 18). Neonatal hemorrhagic disease with primidone alone or in combination with other anticonvulsants has been reported (14, 19–23). Suppression of vitamin K_1-dependent clotting factors is the proposed mechanism of the hemorrhagic effect (14, 19). Administration of prophylatic vitamin K_1 to the infant immediately after birth is recommended (see Phytonadione, Phenytoin, and Phenobarbital).

Breast Feeding Summary

Primidone is excreted into breast milk (24). Because primidone undergoes limited conversion to phenobarbital, breast milk concentrations of phenobarbital should also be anticipated (see Phenobarbital). A milk:plasma ratio of 0.8 for primidone has been reported (24). The amount of primidone available to the nursing infant is small with milk concentrations of 2.3 μg/ml. No reports linking adverse effects to the nursing infant have been located, however, patients that breast feed should be instructed to watch for potential sedative effects in the infant. In the American Academy of Pediatrics' 1989 statement, primidone is classified as an agent that may produce significant adverse effects in the nursing infant, and, thus, should be used with caution in the lactating woman (25).

References

1. Hill RB. Teratogenesis and antiepileptic drugs. N Engl J Med 1973;289:1089–90.
2. Bodendorfer TW. Fetal effect of anticonvulsant drugs and seizure disorders. Drug Intell Clin Pharm 1978;12:14–21.
3. Committee on Drugs, American Academy of Pediatrics. Anticonvulsants and pregnancy. Pediatrics 1977;63:331–3.
4. Nakane Y, Okoma T, Takahashe R, et al. Multiple-institutional study of the teratogenicity and fetal toxicity of antiepileptic drugs: a report of a collaborative study group in Japan. Epilepsia 1980;21:663–80.
5. Andermann E, Dansky L, Andermann F, Loughnan PM, Gibbons J. Minor congenital malformations and dermatoglyphic alterations in the offspring of epileptic women: a clinical investigation of the teratogenic effects of anticonvulsant medication. In *Epilepsy, Pregnancy and the Child*. Proceedings of a Workshop held in Berlin September 1980. New York:Raven Press, 1981.
6. Dansky L, Andermann F. Major congenital malformations in the offspring of epileptic patients. In *Epilepsy, Pregnancy and the Child*. Proceedings of a Workshop held in Berlin September 1980. New York:Raven Press, 1981.
7. Janz D. The teratogenic risks of antiepileptic drugs. Epilepsia 1975;16:159–69.
8. Lowe CR. Congenital malformations among infants born to epileptic women. Lancet 1973;1:9–10.
9. Lander CM, Edwards BE, Eadie MJ, Tyrer JH. Plasma anticonvulsants concentrations during pregnancy. Neurology 1977;27:128–31.
10. Speidel BD, Meadow SR. Maternal epilepsy and abnormalities of the fetus and newborn. Lancet 1972;2:839–43.
11. McMullin GP. Teratogenic effects of anticonvulsants. Br Med J 1971;4:430.
12. Fedrick J. Epilepsy and pregnancy: a report from the Oxford Record Linkage Study. Br Med J 1973;2:442–8.
13. Biale Y, Lewenthal H, Aderet NB. Congenital malformations due to anticonvulsant drugs. Obstet Gynecol 1975;45:439–42.
14. Thomas P, Buchanan N. Teratogenic effect of anticonvulsants. J Pediatr 1981;99:163.
15. Myhree SA, Williams R. Teratogenic effects associated with maternal primidone therapy. J Pediatr 1981;99:160–2.
16. Rudd NL, Freedom RM. A possible primidone embryopathy. J Pediatr 1979;94:835–7.
17. Heinonen OP, Slone D, Shapiro S. *Birth Defects and Drugs in Pregnancy*. Littleton:Publishing Sciences Group, 1977:358.
18. Martinez G, Snyder RD. Transplacental passage of primidone. Neurology 1973;23:381–3.
19. Kohler HG. Haemorrhage in the newborn of epileptic mothers. Lancet 1966;1:267.
20. Bleyer WA, Skinner AL. Fatal neonatal hemorrhage after maternal anticonvulsant therapy. JAMA 1976;235:826–7.
21. Mountain KR, Hirsh J, Gallus AS. Neonatal coagulation defect due to anticonvulsant drug treatment in pregnancy. Lancet 1970;1:265–8.
22. Evans AR, Forrester RM, Discombe C. Neonatal hemorrhage following maternal anticonvulsant therapy. Lancet 1970;1:517–8.
23. Margolin DO, Kantor NM. Hemorrhagic disease of the newborn: an unusual case related to maternal ingestion of antiepileptic drug. Clin Pediatr (Phila) 1972;11:59–60.

24. Kaneko S, Sato T, Suzuki K. The levels of anticonvulsants in breast milk. Br J Clin Pharmacol 1979;7:624–7.
25. Committee on Drugs, American Academy of Pediatrics. Transfer of drugs and other chemicals into human milk. Pediatrics 1989;84:924–36.

Name: **PROBENECID**

Class: **Uricosuric/Renal Tubular Blocking Agent**   Risk Factor: **B**

Fetal Risk Summary

No reports linking the use of probenecid with congenital defects have been located. Probenecid has been used during pregnancy without producing adverse effects in the fetus or in the infant (1–3).

Breast Feeding Summary

No data are available.

References

1. Beidleman B. Treatment of chronic hypoparathyroidism with probenecid. Metabolism 1958;7:690–8.
2. Lee FI, Loeffler FE. Gout and pregnancy. J Obstet Gynaecol Br Commonw 1962;69:299.
3. Batt RE, Cirksena WJ, Lebhertz TB. Gout and salt-wasting renal disease during pregnancy. Diagnosis, management and follow-up. JAMA 1963;186:835–8.

Name: **PROCAINAMIDE**

Class: **Antiarrhythmic**   Risk Factor: **C$_M$**

Fetal Risk Summary

Procainamide is a cardiac drug used for the termination and prophylaxis of atrial and ventricular tachyarrhythmias (1). The use of procainamide during pregnancy has not been associated with congenital anomalies or other adverse fetal effects (1–6).

Successful cardioversion with procainamide of a fetal supraventricular tachycardia presenting at 30 weeks' gestation has been reported (4). Therapy with digoxin alone and digoxin combined with propranolol failed to halt the arrhythmia. Procainamide was then combined with digoxin, resulting in cardioversion to a sinus rhythm and resolution of fetal ascites and pericardial effusion. During the following 3 weeks, the mother was maintained on oral procainamide, 1 g every 6 hours, and digoxin. Maternal serum levels of procainamide varied from 2.4–4.1 μg/ml. The abnormal rhythm returned at 33 weeks' gestation, and control became increasingly difficult. Additional therapy with procainamide increased the maternal serum concentration to 6.8 μg/ml. Over the last 24 hours, four intravenous bolus doses of procainamide (700 mg three times, 650 mg once) were administered plus a maintenance dose of 3 mg/minute. Three hours after the last bolus dose, a 2650-g female infant was delivered by cesarean section. Serum procainamide concentrations in the newborn and mother were 4.3 and 15.6 µg/ml, respectively, a ratio of 0.28. During the subsequent neonatal course, the infant was successfully treated for congestive heart failure and persistent supraventricular tachycardia. The ECG was normal at 6 months of age.

In a case similar to the one described above, therapy with digoxin, verapamil, and procainamide failed to control fetal supraventricular tachycardia presenting at 24 weeks' gestation (5). At cordocentesis, procainamide concentrations in the fetus and mother were 11.7 and 12.8 µg/ml (ratio 0.91), respectively. Levels of the active metabolite, N-acetylprocainamide, were 3.0 and 3.5 µg/ml (ratio 0.86), respectively. Cardioversion was eventually accomplished with direct fetal digitalization by periodic intramuscular injection.

Breast Feeding Summary

Procainamide and its active metabolite, N-acetylprocainamide, are accumulated in breast milk (7). A woman was treated with procainamide, 375 mg four times daily, for premature ventricular contractions during the 3rd trimester (7). The dose was increased to 500 mg four times daily 1 week prior to delivery at 39 weeks' gestation. Simultaneous serum and milk samples were obtained in the postpartum period (exact time not specified) every 3 hours for a total of 15 hours. Procainamide (500 mg) was administered orally at hours 0, 6, and 12 immediately after samples were obtained. Mean serum concentrations of procainamide and N-acetylprocainamide were 1.1 and 1.6 µg/ml, respectively, while the concentrations in the milk were 5.4 and 3.5 µg/ml, respectively. The mean milk:serum ratios for the parent drug and the metabolite were 4.3 (range 1.0–7.3) and 3.8 (range 1.0–6.2), respectively. The amount of drug available to the nursing infant based on a hypothetical serum level of 8 µg/ml was estimated to be 64.8 µg/ml (procainamide plus metabolite). Assuming the infant could ingest 1000 ml of milk/day (thought to be unlikely), this would only provide about 65 mg of total active drug. This amount was not expected to yield clinically significant serum concentrations (7). The American Academy of Pediatrics considers procainamide to be compatible with breast feeding (8). However, the long-term effects of exposure in the nursing infant to procainamide and its metabolites are unknown, particularly in regard to potential drug toxicity (e.g., development of antinuclear antibodies and lupus-like syndrome).

References

1. Rotmensch HH, Elkayam U, Frishman W. Antiarrhythmic drug therapy during pregnancy. Ann Intern Med 1983;98:487–97.
2. Mendelson CL. Disorders of the heartbeat during pregnancy. Am J Obstet Gynecol 1956;72:1268–301.
3. Tamari I, Eldar M, Rabinowitz B, Neufeld HN. Medical treatment of cardiovascular disorders during pregnancy. Am Heart J 1982;104:1357–63.
4. Dumesic DA, Silverman NH, Tobias S, Golbus MS. Transplacental cardioversion of fetal supraventricular tachycardia with procainamide. N Engl J Med 1982;307:1128–31.
5. Weiner CP, Thompson MIB. Direct treatment of fetal supraventricular tachycardia after failed transplacental therapy. Am J Obstet Gynecol 1988;158:570–3.
6. Little BB, Gilstrap LC III. Cardiovascular drugs during pregnancy. Clin Obstet Gynecol 1989;32:13–20.
7. Pittard WB III, Glazier H. Procainamide excretion in human milk. J Pediatr 1983;102:631–3.
8. Committee on Drugs, American Academy of Pediatrics. Transfer of drugs and other chemicals into human milk. Pediatrics 1989;84:924–36.

Name: **PROCARBAZINE**
Class: **Antineoplastic**   Risk Factor: **D**

Fetal Risk Summary

The use of procarbazine, in combination with other antineoplastic agents, during pregnancy has been described in nine patients, five during the 1st trimester (1–8). One of the 1st trimester exposures was electively terminated, but no details on the fetus were given (5). Congenital malformations were observed in the remaining four 1st trimester exposures (1–4):

Multiple hemangiomas (1)
Oligodactyly of both feet with webbing of third and fourth toes, four metatarsals on left, three on right, bowing of right tibia, cerebral hemorrhage, spontaneously aborted at 24 weeks' gestation (2)
Malformed kidneys — markedly reduced size and malposition (3)
Small secundum atrial septal defect, intrauterine growth retardation (4)

A patient in her 12th week of pregnancy received procarbazine, 50 mg daily, in error for 30 days when she was given the drug instead of an iron/vitamin supplement (6). A normal 3575-g male infant was delivered at term.

Long-term studies of growth and mental development in offspring exposed to procarbazine during the 2nd trimester, the period of neuroblast multiplication, have not been conducted (9). Data from one review indicated that 40% of the infants exposed to anticancer drugs were of low birth weight (10). This finding was not related to the timing of exposure.

Procarbazine is mutagenic and carcinogenic in animals (11). In combination with other antineoplastic drugs, procarbazine may produce gonadal dysfunction in males and females (12–17). Ovarian and testicular function may return to normal, with successful pregnancies possible, depending on the patient's age at the time of therapy and the total dose of chemotherapy received (16–20).

Occupational exposure of the mother to antineoplastic agents during pregnancy may present a risk to the fetus. A position statement from the National Study Commission on Cytotoxic Exposure and a research article involving some antineoplastic agents are presented in the monograph for cyclophosphamide (see Cyclophosphamide).

Breast Feeding Summary

No data are available.

References

1. Wells JH, Marshall JR, Carbone PP. Procarbazine therapy for Hodgkin's disease in early pregnancy. JAMA 1968;205:935–7.
2. Garrett MJ. Teratogenic effects of combination chemotherapy. Ann Intern Med 1974;80:667.
3. Mennuti MT, Shepard TH, Mellman WJ. Fetal renal malformation following treatment of Hodgkin's disease during pregnancy. Obstet Gynecol 1975;46:194–6.
4. Thomas PRM, Peckham MJ. The investigation and management of Hodgkin's disease in the pregnant patient. Cancer 1976;38:1443–51.
5. Daly H, McCann SR, Hanratty TD, Temperley IJ. Successful pregnancy during combination chemotherapy for Hodgkin's disease. Acta Haematol (Basel) 1980;64:154–6.
6. Daw EG. Procarbazine in pregnancy. Lancet 1970;2:984.

7. Johnson IR, Filshie GM. Hodgkin's disease diagnosed in pregnancy: case report. Br J Obstet Gynaecol 1977;84:791–2.
8. Jones RT, Weinerman ER. MOPP (nitrogen mustard, vincristine, procarbazine, and prednisone) given during pregnancy. Obstet Gynecol 1979;54:477–8.
9. Dobbing J. Pregnancy and leukaemia. Lancet 1977;1:1155.
10. Nicholson HO. Cytotoxic drugs in pregnancy: review of reported cases. J Obstet Gynecol Br Commonw 1968;75:307–12.
11. Lee IP, Dixon RL. Mutagenicity, carcinogenicity and teratogenicity of procarbazine. Mutat Res 1978;55:1–14.
12. Sherins RJ, DeVita VT Jr. Effect of drug treatment for lymphoma on male reproductive capacity: studies of men in remission after therapy. Ann Intern Med 1973;79:216–20.
13. Sherins RJ, Olweny CLM, Ziegler JL. Gynecomastia and gonadal dysfunction in adolescent boys treated with combination chemotherapy for Hodgkin's disease. N Engl J Med 1978;299:12–6.
14. Johnson SA, Goldman JM, Hawkins DF. Pregnancy after chemotherapy for Hodgkin's disease. Lancet 1979;2:93.
15. Card RT, Holmes IH, Sugarman RG, Storb R, Thomas ED. Successful pregnancy after high dose chemotherapy and marrow transplantation for treatment of aplastic anemia. Exp Hematol 1980;8:57–60.
16. Schilsky RL, Sherins RJ, Hubbard SM, Wesley MN, Young RC, DeVita VT Jr. Long-term follow-up of ovarian function in women treated with MOPP chemotherapy for Hodgkin's disease. Am J Med 1981;71:552–6.
17. Shalet SM, Vaughan Williams CA, Whitehead E. Pregnancy after chemotherapy induced ovarian failure. Br Med J 1985;290:898.
18. Whitehead E, Shalet SM, Blackledge G, Todd I, Crowther D, Beardwell CG. The effect of combination chemotherapy on ovarian function in women treated for Hodgkin's disease. Cancer 1983;52:988–93.
19. Andrieu JM, Ochoa-Molina ME. Menstrual cycle, pregnancies and offspring before and after MOPP therapy for Hodgkin's disease. Cancer 1983;52:435–8.
20. Schapira DV, Chudley AE. Successful pregnancy following continuous treatment with combination chemotherapy before conception and throughout pregnancy. Cancer 1984;54:800–3.

Name: **PROCHLORPERAZINE**

Class: **Tranquilizer**   Risk Factor: **C**

Fetal Risk Summary

Prochlorperazine is a piperazine phenothiazine. The drug readily crosses the placenta (1). Prochlorperazine has been used to treat nausea and vomiting of pregnancy. Most studies have found the drug to be safe for this indication (see also Chlorpromazine) (2–4). The Collaborative Perinatal Project monitored 50,282 mother-child pairs, 877 of which had 1st trimester exposure to prochlorperazine (4). For use anytime during pregnancy, 2,023 exposures were recorded. No evidence was found in either group to suggest a relationship to malformations or an effect on perinatal mortality rate, birth weight, or intelligence quotient scores at 4 years of age. Two infants exposed to prochlorperazine during the 1st trimester are described below:

Cleft palate, micrognathia, congenital heart defects, skeletal defects (5)
Thanatophoric dwarfism (short limb anomaly (6)

The relationship between prochlorperazine and the above defects is unknown. The case of dwarfism may be due to genetic factors. A third report provided brief data on 14 infants, half of whom were exposed to the drug before embryologic timing of their malformations (7).

In summary, although there are isolated reports of congenital defects in children exposed to prochlorperazine *in utero*, the majority of the evidence indicates that this drug and the general class of phenothiazines are safe for both mother and fetus if used occasionally in low doses. Other reviewers have also concluded that the phenothiazines are not teratogenic (8, 9).

Breast Feeding Summary

No reports describing the excretion of prochlorperazine into breast milk have been located. Although prochlorperazine was listed as compatible with breast feeding in the American Academy of Pediatrics' 1983 statement (10), the agent was not included in the 1989 revision.

References

1. Moya F, Thornidke V. Passage of drugs across the placenta. Am J Obstet Gynecol 1962;84:1778–98.
2. Reider RO, Rosenthal D. Wender P, Blumenthal H. The offspring of schizophrenics. Fetal and neonatal deaths. Arch Gen Psychiatry 1975;32:200–11.
3. Milkovich L, Van den Berg BJ. An evaluation of the teratogenicity of certain antinauseant drugs. Am J Obstet Gynecol 1976;125:244–8.
4. Slone D, Siskind V, Heinonen OP, Monson RR, Kaufman DW, Shapiro S. Antenatal exposure to the phenothiazines in relation to congenital malformations, perinatal mortality rate, birth weight, and intelligence quotient score. Am. J Obstet Gynecol 1977;128:486–8.
5. Ho CK, Kaufman RL, McAlister WH. Congenital malformations. Cleft palate, congenital heart disease, absent tibiae, and polydactyly. Am J Dis Child 1975;129:714–6.
6. Farag RA, Ananth J. Thanatophoric dwarfism associated with prochlorperazine administration. NY State J Med 1978;78:279–82.
7. Mellin GW. Report of prochlorperazine during pregnancy from the fetal life study bank. Teratology 1975;11:28A (Abstract).
8. Ayd FJ Jr. Children born of mothers treated with chlorpromazine during pregnancy. Clin Med 1964;71:1758–63.
9. Ananth J. Congenital malformations with psychopharmacologic agents. Compr Psychiatry 1975;16:437–45.
10. Committee on Drugs, American Academy of Pediatrics. The transfer of drugs and other chemicals into human breast milk. Pediatrics 1983;72:375–83.

Name: **PROCYCLIDINE**

Class: **Parasympatholytic (Anticholinergic)**   Risk Factor: **C**

Fetal Risk Summary

Procyclidine is an anticholinergic agent used in the treatment of parkinsonism. No reports of its use in pregnancy have been located (see also Atropine).

Breast Feeding Summary

No data are available (see also Atropine).

Name: **PROMAZINE**

Class: **Tranquilizer**   Risk Factor: **C**

Fetal Risk Summary

Promazine is a propylamino phenothiazine structurally related to chlorpromazine. The drug readily crosses the placenta (1, 2). A possible relationship between the use of promazine (100 mg or more) in labor and neonatal hyperbilirubinemia was reported in 1975 (3). The Collaborative Perinatal Project monitored 50,282 mother-child pairs, 50 of which had 1st trimester exposure to promazine (4). For use anytime during pregnancy, 347 exposures were recorded. No evidence was found in either group to suggest a relationship to malformations or an effect on perinatal mortality rate, birth weight, or intelligence quotient scores at 4 years of age. Although occasional reports have attempted to link various phenothiazine compounds with congenital defects, the bulk of the evidence indicates that these drugs are safe for mother and fetus (see also Chlorpromazine).

Breast Feeding Summary

No data are available.

References

1. Moya F, Thorndike V. Passage of drugs across the placenta. Am J Obstet Gynecol 1962;84:1778–98.
2. O'Donoghue SEF. Distribution of pethidine and chlorpromazine in maternal, foetal and neonatal biological fluids. Nature 1971;229:124–5.
3. John E. Promazine and neonatal hyperbilirubinemia. Med J Aust 1975;2:342–4.
4. Slone D, Siskind V, Heinonen OP, Monson RR, Kaufman DW, Shapiro S. Antenatal exposure to the phenothiazines in relation to congenital malformations, perinatal mortality rate, birth weight, and intelligence quotient score. Am J Obstet Gynecol 1977;128:486–8.

Name: **PROMETHAZINE**

Class: **Antihistamine**   Risk Factor: **C**

Fetal Risk Summary

Promethazine is a phenothiazine antihistamine that is sometimes used as an antiemetic in pregnancy and as an adjunct to narcotic analgesics during labor. The Collaborative Perinatal Project monitored 50,282 mother-child pairs, 114 of which had promethazine exposure in the 1st trimester (1, pp. 323–324). For use anytime during pregnancy, 746 exposures were recorded (1, p. 437). In neither case was evidence found to suggest a relationship to large categories of major or minor malformations or to individual defects. A 1964 report also failed to show an association between 165 cases of promethazine exposure in the 1st trimester and malformations (2). Finally, in a 1971 reference, infants of mothers who had ingested antiemetics during the 1st trimester actually had significantly fewer abnormalities when compared to controls (3). Promethazine was the most commonly used antiemetic in this latter study.

At term, the drug rapidly crosses the placenta, appearing in cord blood within 1 1/2 minutes of an intravenous dose (4). Fetal and maternal blood concentrations are at equilibrium in 15 minutes with infant levels persisting for at least 4 hours.

Several investigators have studied the effect of promethazine on labor and the newborn (5–12). Significant neonatal respiratory depression was seen in a small group of patients (5). However, in three large series, no clinical evidence of promethazine-induced respiratory depression was found (6–8). In a series of 33 mothers at term, 28 received either promethazine alone (one patient) or a combination of meperidine with promethazine or phenobarbital (27 patients). Transient behavioral and EEG changes, persisting for less than 3 days, were seen in all newborns (10).

Maternal tachycardia due to promethazine (mean increase 30 beats/minute) or promethazine-meperidine (mean increase 42 beats/minute) was observed in one series (9). The maximum effect occurred about 10 minutes after injection. The fetal heart rate did not change significantly.

Fatal shock was reported in a pregnant woman with an undiagnosed pheochromocytoma given promethazine (13). A precipitous drop in blood pressure resulted from administration of the drug, probably secondary to unmasking of hypovolemia (13).

Effects on the uterus have been mixed, with both increases and decreases in uterine activity reported (8, 9, 11).

Promethazine used during labor has been shown to markedly impair platelet aggregation in the newborn but less so in the mother (12, 14). While the clinical significance of this is unknown, the degree of impairment in the newborn is comparable to those disorders associated with a definite bleeding state.

Promethazine has been used to treat hydrops fetalis in cases of anti-erythrocytic isoimmunization (15). Six patients were treated with 150 mg orally/day between the 26th and 34th weeks of gestation while undergoing intraperitoneal transfusions. No details on the infants' conditions were given except that all were born alive. Other authors have reported similarly successful results in Rh-sensitized pregnancies (16, 17). As described by some authors, doses up to 6.5 mg/kg/day may be required (16).

Two female anencephalic infants were born to mothers after ovulatory stimulation with clomiphene (18). One of the mothers had taken promethazine for morning sickness. No association between promethazine and this defect has been suggested.

Breast Feeding Summary

Available laboratory methods for the accurate detection of promethazine in breast milk are not clinically useful due to the rapid metabolism of phenothiazines (M. Lipshutz, personal communication, Wyeth Laboratories, 1981). Passage of the drug into breast milk, however, should be expected.

References

1. Heinonen OP, Slone D, Shapiro S. *Birth Defects and Drugs in Pregnancy.* Littleton:Publishing Sciences Group, 1977.
2. Wheatley D. Drugs and the embryo. Br Med J 1964;1:630.
3. Nelson MM, Forfar JO. Association between drugs administered during pregnancy and congenital abnormalities of the fetus. Br Med J 1971;1:523–7.

4. Moya F, Thorndike V. The effects of drugs used in labor on the fetus and newborn. Clin Pharmacol Ther 1963;4:628–53.
5. Crawford JS, as quoted by Moya F, Thorndike V. The effects of drugs used in labor on the fetus and newborn. Clin Pharmacol Ther 1963;4:628–53.
6. Powe CE, Kiem IM, Fromhagen C, Cavanagh D. Propiomazine hydrochloride in obstetrical analgesia. JAMA 1962;181:290–4.
7. Potts CR, Ullery JC. Maternal and fetal effects of obstetric analgesia. Am J Obstet Gynecol 1961;81:1253–9.
8. Carroll JJ, Moir RS. Use of promethazine (Phenergan) hydrochloride in obstetrics. JAMA 1958;168:2218–24.
9. Riffel HD, Nochimson DJ, Paul RH, Hon EH. Effects of meperidine and promethazine during labor. Obstet Gynecol 1973;42:738–45.
10. Borgstedt AD, Rosen MG. Medication during labor correlated with behavior and EEG of the newborn. Am J Dis Child 1968;115:21–4.
11. Zakut H, Mannor SM, Serr DM. Effect of promethazine on uterine contractions. Harefuah 1970;78:61–2. As reported in JAMA 1970; 211:1572.
12. Corby DG, Shulman I. The effects of antenatal drug administration on aggregation of platelets of newborn infants. J Pediatr 1971;79:307–13.
13. Montminy M, Teres D. Shock after phenothiazine administration in a pregnant patient with a pheochromocytoma: a case report and literature review. J Reprod Med 1983;28:159–62.
14. Whaun JM, Smith GR, Sochor VA. Effect of prenatal drug administration on maternal and neonatal platelet aggregation and PF$_4$ release. Haemostasis 1980;9:226–37.
15. Bierme S, Bierme R. Antihistamines in hydrops foetalis. Lancet 1967;1:574.
16. Gusdon JP Jr. The treatment of erythroblastosis with promethazine hydrochloride. J Reprod Med 1981;26:454–8.
17. Charles AG, Blumenthal LS. Promethazine hydrochloride therapy in severely Rh-sensitized pregnancies. Obstet Gynecol 1982;60:627–30.
18. Dyson JL, Kohler HC. Anecephaly and ovulation stimulation. Lancet 1973;1:1256–7.

Name: **PROPANTHELINE**

Class: **Parasympatholytic (Anticholinergic)**   Risk Factor: **C$_M$**

Fetal Risk Summary

Propantheline is an anticholinergic quaternary ammonium bromide. The Collaborative Perinatal Project monitored 50,282 mother-child pairs, 33 of which used propantheline in the 1st trimester (1). No evidence was found for an association with congenital malformations. However, when the group of parasympatholytics were taken as a whole (2,323 exposures), a possible association with minor malformations was found (1).

Breast Feeding Summary

No data are available (see also Atropine).

Reference

1. Heinonen OP, Slone D, Shapiro S. *Birth Defects and Drugs in Pregnancy*. Littleton:Publishing Sciences Group, 1977:346–53.

Name: **PROPOXYPHENE**

Class: **Analgesic**   Risk Factor: **C***

Fetal Risk Summary

Three case reports, involving four patients, have linked the use of propoxyphene during pregnancy to congenital abnormalties (1–3). However, other drugs were used in each case and any association may be fortuitous:

Pierre Robin syndrome, arthrogryposis, severe mental and growth retardation (1) (one infant)

Absence of left forearm and radial two digits, syndactyly of ulnar three digits and left fourth and fifth toes, hypoplastic left femur (2) (one infant)

Omphalocele, defective anterior left wall, diaphragmatic defect, congenital heart disease with partial ectopic cordis due to sternal cleft, dysplastic hips (2) (one infant)

Micrognathia, widely spaced sutures, beaked nose, bifid uvula, defects of toes, withdrawal seizures (3) (one infant)

The Collaborative Perinatal Project monitored 50,282 mother-child pairs, 686 of which had 1st trimester exposure to propoxyphene (4, pp. 287–295). For use any-time during pregnancy, 2,914 exposures were recorded (4, p. 434). No evidence was found in either case to suggest a relationship to large categories of major or minor malformations or, in the 1st trimester, to individual defects. Five possible associations with individual defects after anytime use were observed (4, p. 484). The statistical significance of these associations is unknown and independent confirmation is required:

Microcephaly (6 cases)
Ductus arteriosus persistens (5 cases)
Cataract (5 cases)
Benign tumors (12 cases)
Clubfoot (18 cases)

Neonatal withdrawal has been reported in five infants (3, 5–8). The relationship between heavy maternal ingestion of this drug and neonatal withdrawal seems clear. The infants were asymptomatic with normal Apgar scores until 3 1/2–14 hours after delivery. Withdrawal was marked by the onset of irritability, tremors, diarrhea, fever, high-pitched cry, hyperactivity, hypertonicity, diaphoresis, and, in two cases, seizures. Symptoms began to subside by day 4, usually without spe-cific therapy. Examinations after 2–3 months were normal.

Propoxyphene has been used in labor without causing neonatal respiratory de-pression (9). However, a significant shortening of the first stage of labor occurred without an effect on uterine contractions.

[*Risk Factor D if used for prolonged periods.]

Breast Feeding Summary

Propoxyphene passes into breast milk, but the amounts and clinical significance are unknown. In one case, a nursing mother attempted suicide with propoxyphene

(10). The concentration of the drug in her breast milk was found to be 50% of her plasma level. By calculation, the authors predicted a mother consuming a maximum daily dose of the drug would provide her infant with 1 mg/day. The American Academy of Pediatrics considers propoxyphene to be compatible with breast feeding (11).

References

1. Barrow MV, Souder DE. Propoxyphene and congenital malformations. JAMA 1971;217:1551–2.
2. Ringrose CAD. The hazard of neurotrophic drugs in the fertile years. Can Med Assoc J 1972;106:1058.
3. Golden NL, King KC, Sokol RJ. Propoxyphene and acetaminophen: possible effects on the fetus. Clin Pediatr 1982;21:752–4.
4. Heinonen OP, Slone D, Shapiro S. *Birth Defects and Drugs in Pregnancy*. Littleton:Publishing Sciences Group, 1977.
5. Tyson HK. Neonatal withdrawal symptoms associated with maternal use of propoxyphene hydrochloride (Darvon). J Pediatr 1974;85:684–5.
6. Klein RB, Blatman S, Little GA. Probable neonatal propoxyphene withdrawal: a case report. Pediatrics 1975;55:882–4.
7. Quillan WW, Dunn CA. Neonatal drug withdrawal from propoxyphene. JAMA 1976;235:2128.
8. Ente G, Mehra MC. Neonatal drug withdrawal from propoxyphene hydrochloride. NY State J Med 1978;78:2084–5.
9. Eddy NB, Friebel H, Hahn KJ, Halbach H. Codeine and its alternatives for pain and cough relief. 2. Alternates for pain relief. Bull WHO 1969;40:1–53.
10. Catz C, Giacoia G. Drugs and breast milk. Pediatr Clin North Am 1972;19:151–66.
11. Committee on Drugs, American Academy of Pediatrics. Transfer of drugs and other chemicals into human milk. Pediatrics 1989;84:924–36.

Name: **PROPRANOLOL**

Class: **Sympatholytic (β-Adrenergic Blocker)**   Risk Factor: **C$_M$**

Fetal Risk Summary

Propranolol, a nonselective β-adrenergic blocking agent, has been used for various indications in pregnancy:

Maternal hyperthyroidism (1–7)
Pheochromocytoma (8)
Maternal cardiac disease (6, 7, 9–20)
Fetal tachycardia/arrhythmia (21, 22)
Maternal hypertension (7, 20, 23–30)
Dysfunctional labor (31)
Termination of pregnancy (32)

The drug readily crosses the placenta (2, 6, 12, 16, 22, 29, 33, 34). Cord serum levels varying between 19–127% of maternal serum have been reported (2, 16, 22, 29). Oxytocic effects have been demonstrated following intravenous, extra-amniotic injections, and high oral dosing (17, 31, 32, 35, 36). Intravenous propranolol has been shown to block or decrease the marked increase in maternal plasma progesterone induced by vasopressin or theophylline (37). The pharmacokinetics of propranolol in pregnancy have been described (38). Plasma levels and elimination were not significantly altered by pregnancy.

A number of fetal/neonatal adverse effects have been reported following the use of propranolol in pregnancy. Whether these effects are due to propranolol, maternal disease, other drugs consumed concurrently, or a combination of these factors is not always clear. Daily doses of 160 mg or higher seem to produce the more serious complications, but lower doses have also resulted in toxicity. Analysis of 23 reports involving 167 liveborn infants exposed to chronic propranolol *in utero* is shown below (1–4, 6, 7, 9, 11–14, 20, 22–24, 26–29, 39–42):

	No. Cases	%
Intrauterine growth retardation	23	14
Hypoglycemia	16	10
Bradycardia	12	7
Respiratory depression at birth	6	4
Hyperbilirubinemia	6	4
Small placenta (size not always noted)	4	2
Polycythemia	2	1
Thrombocytopenia (40,000/mm^3)	1	0.6
Hyperirritability	1	0.6
Hypocalcemia with convulsions	1	0.6
Blood coagulation defect	1	0.6

Two infants were reported to have anomalies (pyloric stenosis; crepitus of hip), but the authors did not relate these to propranolol (27, 39). In another case, a malformed fetus was spontaneously aborted from a 30-year-old woman with chronic renovascular hypertension (43). The patient had been treated with propranolol, amiloride, and captopril for her severe hypertension. Malformations included absence of the left leg below the midthigh and no obvious skull formation above the brain tissue. The authors attributed the defect either to captopril alone or to a combination effect of the three drugs.

Respiratory depression was noted in four of five infants whose mothers were given 1 mg of propranolol intravenously just prior to cesarean section (44). None of the five controls in the double blind study was depressed at birth. The author suggested the mechanism may have been β-adrenergic blockade of the cervical sympathetic discharge which occurs at cord clamping.

Fetal bradycardia was observed in 2 of 10 patients treated with propranolol, 1 mg/minute for 4 minutes, for dysfunctional labor (31). No lasting effects were seen in the babies. In a retrospective study, eight markedly hypertensive patients (nine pregnancies) treated with propranolol were compared with 15 hypertensive controls not treated with propranolol (25). Other antihypertensives were used in both groups. A significant difference was found between the perinatal mortality rates, with seven deaths in the propranolol group (78%) and only five deaths in the controls (33%). However, a possible explanation for the difference may have been the more severe hypertension and renal disease in the propranolol group than in the controls (45).

Intrauterine growth retardation may be related to propranolol. Several possible mechanisms for this effect, if indeed it is associated with the drug, have been reviewed (46). Premature labor has been suggested as a possible complication of propranolol therapy in patients with pregnancy-induced hypertension (PIH) (41). In nine women treated with propranolol for PIH, three delivered prematurely. The author speculated that these patients were relatively hypovolemic and when a compensatory increase in cardiac output failed to occur, premature delivery resulted. However, another report on chronic propranolol use in 14 women did not observe premature labor (42).

In a randomized, double blind trial, 36 patients at term were given either 80 mg of propranolol or placebo (47). Fetal heart rate reaction to a controlled sound stimulus was then measured at 1, 2, and 3 hours. The heart rate reaction in the propranolol group was significantly depressed, compared to placebo, at all three time intervals.

The reactivity of nonstress tests (NSTs) was affected by propranolol in two hypertensive women in the 2nd and 3rd trimesters (48). One woman was taking 20 mg every 6 hours and the other 10 mg three times daily. Repeated NST were nonreactive in both women, but immediate follow-up contraction stress tests were negative. The NSTs became reactive 2 and 10 days, respectively, after propranolol was discontinued.

In summary, propranolol has been used during pregnancy for maternal and fetal indications. The drug is apparently not a teratogen, but fetal and neonatal toxicity may occur. A 1988 review on the use of β-blockers, including propranolol, during pregnancy concluded that these agents are relatively safe (49). However, newborn infants of women consuming the drug near delivery should be closely observed during the first 24–48 hours after birth for bradycardia, hypoglycemia and other symptoms of β-blockade. Long-term effects of *in utero* exposure to β-blockers have not been studied but warrant evaluation.

Breast Feeding Summary

Propranolol is excreted into breast milk. Peak concentrations occur 2–3 hours after a dose (12, 20, 42, 50). Milk levels have ranged from 4–64 ng/ml with milk:plasma ratios of 0.2–1.5 (12, 20, 29, 49). Although such adverse effects as respiratory depression, bradycardia, and hypoglycemia have not been reported, nursing infants exposed to propranolol in breast milk should be closely observed for these symptoms of β-blockade. Long-term effects of exposure to β-blockers from milk have not been studied but warrant evaluation. The American Academy of Pediatrics considers propranolol to be compatible with breast feeding (51).

References

1. Jackson GL. Treatment of hyperthyroidism in pregnancy. Pa Med 1973;76:56–7.
2. Langer A, Hung CT, McA'Nulty JA, Harrigan JT, Washington E. Adrenergic blockade: a new approach to hyperthyroidism during pregnancy. Obstet Gynecol 1974;44:181–6.
3. Bullock JL, Harris RE, Young R. Treatment of thyrotoxicosis during pregnancy with propranolol. Am J Obstet Gynecol 1975;121:242–5.
4. Lightner ES, Allen HD, Loughlin G. Neonatal hyperthyroidism and heart failure: a different approach. Am J Dis Child 1977;131:68–70.
5. Levy CA, Waite JH, Dickey R. Thyrotoxicosis and pregnancy. Use of preoperative propranolol for thyroidectomy. Am J Surg 1977;133:319–21.
6. Habib A, McCarthy JS. Effects on the neonate of propranolol administered during pregnancy. J Pediatr 1977;91:808–11.
7. Pruyn SC, Phelan JP, Buchanan GC. Long-term propranolol therapy in pregnancy: maternal and fetal outcome. Am J Obstet Gynecol 1979;135:485–9.
8. Leak D, Carroll JJ, Robinson DC, Ashworth EJ. Management of pheochromocytoma during pregnancy. Can Med Assoc J 1977;116:371–5.
9. Turner GM, Oakley CM, Dixon HG. Management of pregnancy complicated by hypertrophic obstructive cardiomyopathy. Br Med J 1968;4:281–4.

10. Barnes AB. Chronic propranolol administration during pregnancy: a case report. J Reprod Med 1970;5:79–80.

11. Schroeder JS, Harrison DC. Repeated cardioversion during pregnancy. Am J Cardiol 1971;27:445–6.

12. Levitan AA, Manion JC. Propranolol therapy during pregnancy and lactation. Am J Cardiol 1973;32:247.

13. Reed RL, Cheney CB, Fearon RE, Hook R, Hehre FW. Propranolol therapy throughout pregnancy: a case report. Anesth Analg (Cleve) 1974;53:214–8.

14. Fiddler GI. Propranolol pregnancy. Lancet 1974;2:722–3.

15. Kolibash AE, Ruiz DE, Lewis RP. Idiopathic hypertrophic subaortic stenosis in pregnancy. Ann Intern Med 1975;82:791–4.

16. Cottrill CM, McAllister RG Jr, Gettes L, Noonan JA. Propranolol therapy during pregnancy, labor, and delivery: evidence for transplacental drug transfer and impaired neonatal drug disposition. J Pediatr 1977;91:812–4.

17. Datta S, Kitzmiller JL, Ostheimer GW, Schoenbaum SC. Propranolol and parturition. Obstet Gynecol 1978;51:577–81.

18. Diaz JH, McDonald JS. Propranolol and induced labor: anesthetic implications. Anesth Rev 1979;6:29–32.

19. Oakley GDG, McGarry K, Limb DG, Oakley CM. Management of pregnancy in patients with hypertrophic cardiomyopathy. Br Med J 1979;1:1749–50.

20. Bauer JH, Pape B, Zajicek J, Groshong T. Propranolol in human plasma and breast milk. Am J Cardiol 1979;43:860–2.

21. Eibschitz I, Abinader EG, Klein A, Sharf M. Intrauterine diagnosis and control of fetal ventricular arrhythmia during labor. Am J Obstet Gynecol 1975;122:597–600.

22. Teuscher A, Boss E, Imhof P, Erb E, Stocker FP, Weber JW. Effect of propranolol on fetal tachycardia in diabetic pregnancy. Am J Cardiol 1978;42:304–7.

23. Gladstone GR, Hordof A, Gersony WM. Propranolol administration during pregnancy: effects on the fetus. J Pediatr 1975;86:962–4.

24. Tcherdakoff PH, Colliard M, Berrard E, Kreft C, Dupry A, Bernaille JM. Propranolol in hypertension during pregnancy. Br Med J 1978;2:670.

25. Lieberman BA, Stirrat GM, Cohen SL, Beard RW, Pinker GD, Belsey E. The possible adverse effect of propranolol on the fetus in pregnancies complicated by severe hypertension. Br J Obstet Gynaecol 1978;85:678–83.

26. Eliahou HE, Silverberg DS, Reisin E, Romen I, Mashiach S, Serr DM. Propranolol for the treatment of hypertension in pregnancy. Br J Obstet Gynaecol 1978;85:431–6.

27. Bott-Kanner G, Schweitzer A, Schoenfeld A, Joel-Cohen J, Rosenfeld JB. Treatment with propranolol and hydralazine throughout pregnancy in a hypertensive patient: a case report. Isr J Med Sci 1978;14:466–8.

28. Bott-Kanner G, Reisner SH, Rosenfeld JB. Propranolol and hydralazine in the management of essential hypertension in pregnancy. Br Obstet Gynaecol 1980;87:110–4.

29. Taylor EA, Turner P. Anti-hypertensive therapy with propranolol during pregnancy and lactation. Postgrad Med J 1981;57:427–30.

30. Serup J. Propranolol for the treatment of hypertension in pregnancy. Acta Med Scand 1979;206:333.

31. Mitrani A, Oettinger M, Abinader EG, Sharf M, Klein A. Use of propranolol in dysfunctional labour. Br J Obstet Gynaecol 1975;82:651–5.

32. Amy JJ, Karim SMM. Intrauterine administration of 1-noradrenaline and propranolol during the second trimester of pregnancy. J Obstet Gynaecol Br Commonw 1974;81:75–83.

33. Smith MT, Livingstone I, Eadie MJ, Hooper WD, Triggs EJ. Metabolism of propranolol in the human maternal-placental-foetal unit. Eur J Clin Pharmacol 1983;24:727–32.

34. Erkkola R, Lammintausta R, Liukko P, Anttila M. Transfer of propranolol and sotalol across the human placenta. Acta Obstet Gynecol Scand 1982;61:31–4.

35. Barden TP, Stander RW. Myometrial and cardiovascular effects of an adrenergic blocking drug in human pregnancy. Am J Obstet Gynecol 1968;101:91–9.

36. Wansbrough H, Nakanishi H, Wood C. The effect of adrenergic receptor blocking drugs on the human fetus. J Obstet Gynaecol Br Commonw 1968;75:189–98.

37. Fylling P. Dexamethasone or propranolol blockade of induced increase in plasma progesterone in early human pregnancy. Acta Endocrinol (Copenh) 1973;72:569–72.

38. Smith MT, Livingstone I, Eadie MJ, Hooper WD, Triggs EJ. Chronic propranolol administration during pregnancy: maternal pharmacokinetics. Eur J Clin Pharmacol 1983;25:481–90.
39. O'Connor PC, Jick H, Hunter JR, Stergachis A, Madsen S. Propranolol and pregnancy outcome. Lancet 1981;2:1168.
40. Caldroney RD. Beta-blockers in pregnancy. N Engl J Med 1982;306:810.
41. Goodlin RC. Beta blocker in pregnancy-induced hypertension. Am J Obstet Gynecol 1982;143:237.
42. Livingstone I, Craswell PW, Bevan EB, Smith MT, Eadie MJ. Propranolol in pregnancy: three year prospective study. Clin Exp Hypertens (B) 1983;2:341–50.
43. Duminy PC, Burger P du T. Fetal abnormality associated with the use of captopril during pregnancy. S Afr Med J 1981;60:805.
44. Tunstall ME. The effect of propranolol on the onset of breathing at birth. Br J Anaesth 1969;41:792.
45. Rubin PC. Beta-blockers in pregnancy. N Engl J Med 1981;305:1323–6.
46. Redmond GP. Propranolol and fetal growth retardation. Semin Perinatol 1982;6:142–7.
47. Jensen OH. Fetal heart rate response to a controlled sound stimulus after propranolol administration to the mother. Acta Obstet Gynecol Scand 1984;63:199–202.
48. Margulis E, Binder D, Cohen AW. The effect of propranolol on the nonstress test. Am J Obstet Gynecol 1984;148:340–1.
49. Frishman WH, Chesner M. Beta-adrenergic blockers in pregnancy. Am Heart J 1988;115:147–52.
50. Karlberg B, Lundberg O, Aberg H. Excretion of propranolol in human breast milk. Acta Pharmacol Toxicol (Copenh) 1974;34:222–4.
51. Committee on Drugs, American Academy of Pediatrics. Transfer of drugs and other chemicals into human milk. Pediatrics 1989;84:924–36.

Name: **PROPYLTHIOURACIL**

Class: **Antithyroid**   Risk Factor: **D**

Fetal Risk Summary

Propylthiouracil (PTU) has been used for the treatment of hyperthyroidism during pregnancy since its introduction in the 1940s (1–37). The drug prevents synthesis of thyroid hormones and inhibits peripheral deiodination of levothyroxine (T4) to liothyronine (T3) (38).

PTU crosses the placenta. Four patients undergoing therapeutic abortion were given a single 15-mg ^{35}S-labeled oral dose 2 hours before pregnancy termination (39). Serum could not be obtained from two 8-week-old fetuses, but 0.0016–0.0042% of the given dose was found in the fetal tissues. In two other fetuses at 12 and 16 weeks of age, the fetal:maternal serum ratios were 0.27 and 0.35, with 0.020% and 0.025% of the dose in the fetuses. A 1986 report descibed the pharmacokinetics of PTU in six pregnant, hyperthyroid women (40). Serum concentrations of PTU consistently decreased during the 3rd trimester. At delivery in five patients, 1–9 hours after the last dose of 100–150 mg, the mean maternal serum concentration of PTU was 0.19 μg/ml (range <0.02–0.52 μg/ml) compared to a mean cord blood level of 0.36 μg/ml (range 0.03–0.67). The cord:maternal serum ratio was 1.9:1.

The primary effect on the fetus from transplacental passage of PTU is the production of a mild hypothyroidism when the drug is used close to term. This usually resolves within a few days without treatment (34). Clinically, the hypothyroid state may be observed as a goiter in the newborn and is the result of increased levels of fetal pituitary thyrotropin (24). The incidence of fetal goiter after PTU treatment in reported cases is approximately 12% (29 goiters/241 patients) (1–37, 41). Some of these cases may have been due to co-administration of iodides (9, 11, 18, 22). Use of PTU early in pregnancy does not produce fetal goiter since the fetal thyroid does not begin hormone production until approximately the 11th or 12th week of gestation (42). Goiters from PTU exposure are usually small and do not obstruct the airway as do iodide-induced goiters (see also Potassium Iodide) (41–43). However, two reports have been located that described PTU-induced goiters in newborns that were sufficiently massive to produce tracheal compression resulting in death in one infant and moderate respiratory distress in the second (7, 10). In two other PTU-exposed fetuses, clinical hypothyroidism was evident at birth with subsequent retarded mental and physical development (10–12). One of these infants was also exposed to high doses of iodide during gestation (12). PTU-induced goiters are not predictable or dose dependent, but the smallest possible dose of PTU should be used, especially during the 3rd trimester (19, 33, 42–44). No effect on intellectual or physical development from PTU-induced hypothyroxinemia was observed in comparison studies between exposed and nonexposed siblings (19, 45).

Congenital anomalies have been reported in seven newborns exposed to PTU *in utero* (14, 17, 21, 27, 34). This incidence is well within the expected rate of malformations. Maternal hyperthyroidism itself has been shown to be a cause of malformations (46). No association between PTU and defects has been suggested. The reported defects are:

Congenital dislocation of hip (14)
Cryptorchidism (17)
Muscular hypotonicity (17)
Syndactyly of hand/foot (I^{131} also used) (21)
Hypospadias (27)
Aortic atresia (27)
Choanal atresia (34)

In a large prospective study, 25 patients were exposed to one or more noniodide thyroid suppressants during the 1st trimester, 16 of whom took PTU (47). From the total group, four children with nonspecified malformations were found, suggesting that this group of drugs may be teratogenic. However, because of the maternal disease and the use of other drugs (i.e., methimazole in nine women and other thiouracil derivatives in two), the relationship between PTU and the anomalies cannot be determined. This study also noted that independent confirmation of the data was required (47).

In comparison with other antithyroid drugs, propylthiouracil is considered the drug of choice for the medical treatment of hyperthyroidism during pregnancy (see also Carbimazole, Methimazole, Potassium Iodide) (34, 36, 42–44). Combination therapy with thyroid-antithyroid drugs was advocated at one time but is now considered inappropriate (25, 26, 34, 36, 42–44, 48). Two reasons contributed to this change: (*a*) use of thyroid hormones may require higher doses of PTU to be used, and (*b*) placental transfer of T4 and T3 is minimal and not sufficient to reverse fetal hypothyroidism (see also Levothyroxine and Liothyronine).

Breast Feeding Summary

Propylthiouracil (PTU) is excreted into breast milk in low amounts. In a patient given 100 mg of radiolabeled PTU, the milk:plasma ratio was a constant 0.55 over a 24-hour period, representing about 0.077% of the given radioactive dose (49). In a second study, nine patients were given an oral dose of 400 mg (50). Mean serum and milk levels at 90 minutes were 7.7 μg/ml and 0.7 μg/ml, respectively. The average amount excreted in milk during 4 hours was 99 μg, about 0.025% of the total dose. One mother took 200–300 mg daily while breast feeding (50). No changes in any of the infant's thyroid parameters were observed.

Based on these two reports, PTU does not seem to pose a significant risk to the breast-fed infant. However, periodic evaluation of the infant's thyroid function may be prudent. The American Academy of Pediatrics considers propylthiouracil to be compatible with breast feeding (51).

References

1. Astwood EB, VanderLaan WP. Treatment of hyperthyroidism with propylthiouracil. Ann Intern Med 1946;25:813–21.
2. Bain L. Propylthiouracil in pregnancy: report of a case. South Med J 1947;40:1020–1.
3. Lahey FH, Bartels EC. The use of thiouracil, thiobarbital and propylthiouracil in patients with hyperthyroidism. Ann Surg 1947;125:572–81.
4. Reveno WS. Propylthiouracil in the treatment of toxic goiter. J Clin Endocrinol Metab 1948;8:866–74.
5. Eisenberg L. Thyrotoxicosis complicating pregnancy. NY State J Med 1950;50:1618–9.
6. Astwood EB. The use of antithyroid drugs during pregnancy. J Clin Endocrinol Metab 1951;11:1045–56.
7. Aaron HH, Schneierson SJ, Siegel E. Goiter in newborn infant due to mother's ingestion of propylthiouracil. JAMA 1955;159:848–50.
8. Waldinger C, Wermer OS, Sobel EH. Thyroid function in infant with congenital goiter resulting from exposure to propylthiouracil. J Am Med Wom Assoc 1955;10:196–7.
9. Bongiovanni AM, Eberlein WR, Thomas PZ, Anderson WB. Sporadic goiter of the newborn. J Clin Endocrinol Met 1956;16:146–52.
10. Krementz ET, Hooper RG, Kempson RL. The effect on the rabbit fetus of the maternal administration of propylthiouracil. Surgery 1957;41:619–31.
11. Branch LK, Tuthill SW. Goiters in twins resulting from propylthio-uracil given during pregnancy. Ann Intern Med 1957;46:145–8.
12. Man EB, Shaver BA Jr, Cooke RE. Studies of children born to women with thyroid disease. Am J Obstet Gynecol 1958;75:728–41.
13. Becker WF, Sudduth PG. Hyperthyroidism and pregnancy. Ann Surg 1959;149:867–74.
14. Greenman GW, Gabrielson MO, Howard-Flanders J, Wessel MA. Thyroid dysfunction in pregnancy. N Engl J Med 1962;267:426–31.
15. Herbst AL, Selenkow HA. Combined antithyroid-thyroid therapy of hyperthyroidism in pregnancy. Obstet Gynecol 1963;21:543–50.
16. Reveno WS, Rosenbaum H. Observations on the use of antithyroid drugs. Ann Intern Med 1964;60:982–9.
17. Herbst AL, Selenkow HA. Hyperthyroidism during pregnancy. N Engl J Med 1965;273:627–33.
18. Burrow GN. Neonatal goiter after maternal propylthiouracil therapy. J Clin Endocrinol Metab 1965;25:403–8.
19. Burrow GN, Bartsocas C, Klatskin EH, Grunt JA. Children exposed in utero to propylthiouracil. Am J Dis Child 1968;116:161–5.
20. Talbert LM, Thomas CG Jr, Holt WA, Rankin P. Hyperthyroidism during pregnancy. Obstet Gynecol 1970;36:779–85.
21. Hollingsworth DR, Austin E. Thyroxine derivatives in amniotic fluid. J Pediatr 1971;79:923–9.
22. Ayromlooi J. Congenital goiter due to maternal ingestion of iodides. Obstet Gynecol 1972;39:818–22.
23. Worley RJ, Crosby WM. Hyperthyroidism during pregnancy. Am J Obstet Gynecol 1974;119:150–5.

24. Refetoff S, Ochi Y, Selenkow HA, Rosenfield RL. Neonatal hypothyroidism and goiter in one infant of each of two sets of twins due to maternal therapy with antithyroid drugs. J Pediatr 1974;85:240–4.
25. Mestman JH, Manning PR, Hodgman J. Hyperthyroidism and pregnancy. Arch Intern Med 1974;134:434–9.
26. Goluboff LG, Sisson JC, Hamburger JI. Hyperthyroidism associated with pregnancy. Obstet Gynecol 1974;44:107–16.
27. Mujtaba Q, Burrow GN. Treatment of hyperthyroidism in pregnancy with propylthiouracil and methimazole. Obstet Gynecol 1975;46:282–6.
28. Serup J, Petersen S. Hyperthyroidism during pregnancy treated with propylthiouracil. Acta Obstet Gynecol Scand 1977;56:463–6.
29. Petersen S, Serup J. Case report: neonatal thyrotoxicosis. Acta Paediatr Scand 1977;66:639–42.
30. Serup J. Maternal propylthiouracil to manage fetal hyperthyroidism. Lancet 1978;2:896.
31. Wallace EZ, Gandhi VS. Triiodothyronine thyrotoxicosis in pregnancy. Am J Obstet Gynecol 1978;130:106–7.
32. Weiner S, Scharf JI, Bolognese RJ, Librizzi RJ. Antenatal diagnosis and treatment of a fetal goiter. J Reprod Med 1980;24:39–42.
33. Sugrue D, Drury MI. Hyperthyroidism complicating pregnancy: results of treatment by antithyroid drugs in 77 pregnancies. Br J Obstet Gynaecol 1980;87:970–5.
34. Cheron RG, Kaplan MM, Larsen PR, Selenkow HA, Crigler JF Jr. Neonatal thyroid function after propylthiouracil therapy for maternal Graves' disease. N Engl J Med 1981;304:525–8.
35. Check JH, Rezvani I, Goodner D, Hopper B. Prenatal treatment of thyrotoxicosis to prevent intrauterine growth retardation. Obstet Gynecol 1982;60:122–4.
36. Kock HCLV, Merkus JMWM. Graves' disease during pregnancy. Eur J Obstet Gynecol Reprod Biol 1983;14:323–30.
37. Hollingsworth DR, Austin E. Observations following I[131] for Graves disease during first trimester of pregnancy. South Med J 1969;62:1555–6.
38. American Hospital Formulary Service. Drug Information 84. Bethesda:American Society of Hospital Pharmacists, 1984:1318.
39. Marchant B, Brownlie EW, Hart DM, Horton PW, Alexander WD. The placental transfer of propylthiouracil, methimazole and carbimazole. J Clin Endocrinol Metab 1977;45:1187–93.
40. Gardner DF, Cruikshank DP, Hays PM, Cooper DS. Pharmacology of propylthiouracil (PTU) in pregnant hyperthyroid women: correlation of maternal PTU concentrations with cord serum thyroid function tests. J Clin Endocrinol Metab 1986;62:217–20.
41. Ramsay I, Kaur S, Krassas G. Thyrotoxicosis in pregnancy: results of treatment by antithyroid drugs combined with T4. Clin Endocrinol (Oxf) 1983;18:73–85.
42. Burr WA. Thyroid disease. Clin Obstet Gynecol 1981;8:341–51.
43. Burrow GN. Hyperthyroidism during pregnancy. N Engl J Med 1978; 298:150–3.
44. Burrow GN. Maternal-fetal considerations in hyperthyroidism. Clin Endocrinol Metab 1978;7:115–25.
45. Burrow GN, Klatskin EH, Genel M. Intellectual development in children whose mothers received propylthiouracil during pregnancy. Yale J Biol Med 1978;51:151–6.
46. Momotani N, Ito K, Hamada N, Ban Y, Nishikawa Y, Mimura T. Maternal hyperthyroidism and congenital malformations in the offspring. Clin Endocrinol (Oxf) 1984;20:695–700.
47. Heinonen OP, Slone D, Shapiro S. Birth Defects and Drugs in Pregnancy. Littleton:Publishing Sciences Group, 1977:388–400.
48. Anonymous. Transplacental passage of thyroid hormones. N Engl J Med 1967;277:486–7.
49. Low LCK, Lang J, Alexander WD. Excretion of carbimazole and propylthiouracil in breast milk. Lancet 1979;2:1011.
50. Kampmann JP, Johansen K, Hansen JM, Helweg J. Propylthiouracil in human milk. Lancet 1980;1:736–8.
51. Committee on Drugs, American Academy of Pediatrics. Transfer of drugs and other chemicals into human milk. Pediatrics 1989;84:924–36.

Name: **PROTAMINE**

Class: **Antiheparin** Risk Factor: **C**

Fetal Risk Summary

Protamine is used to neutralize the anticoagulant effect of heparin. No reports of its use in pregnancy have been located. Reproduction studies in animals have not been conducted (1).

Breast Feeding Summary

No data are available.

Reference

1. Product information. Protamine sulfate. Eli Lilly, 1985.

Name: **PROTRIPTYLINE**

Class: **Antidepressant** Risk Factor: **C**

Fetal Risk Summary

No data are available.

Breast Feeding Summary

No data are available.

Name: **PSEUDOEPHEDRINE**

Class: **Sympathomimetic (Adrenergic)** Risk Factor: **C**

Fetal Risk Summary

Pseudoephedrine is a sympathomimetic used to alleviate the symptoms of allergic disorders or upper respiratory infections. It is a common component of proprietary mixtures containing antihistamines and other ingredients. Thus, it is difficult to separate the effects of pseudoephedrine on the fetus from those of other drugs, disease states, and viruses.

Sympathomimetic amines are teratogenic in some animal species, but human teratogenicity has not been suspected (1). The Collaborative Perinatal Project monitored 50,282 mother-child pairs, 3,082 of which had 1st trimester exposure to sympathomimetic drugs (2, pp. 345–356). For use anytime during pregnancy, 9,719 exposures were recorded (2, p. 439). An association in the 1st trimester was found between the sympathomimetic class of drugs as a whole and minor malformations (not life-threatening or major cosmetic defects), inguinal hernia, and clubfoot (2, pp. 345–356). However, independent confirmation of these results is required (2, pp. 345–356).

A 1981 report described a woman who consumed, throughout pregnancy, 480–840 ml/day of a cough syrup (3). The potential maximum daily doses based on 840 ml of syrup were 5.0 g of pseudoephedrine, 16.8 g of guaifenesin, 1.68 g of dextromethorphan, and 79.8 ml of ethanol. The infant had features of the fetal alcohol syndrome (see Ethanol) and displayed irritability, tremors, and hypertonicity. It is not known if the ingredients, other than the ethanol, were associated with the adverse effects observed in the infant.

Breast Feeding Summary

Pseudoephedrine is excreted into breast milk (4). Three mothers, who were nursing healthy infants, were given an antihistamine-decongestant preparation containing 60 mg of pseudoephedrine and 2.5 mg of triprolidine as the hydrochloride salts. Two of the mothers had been nursing for 14 weeks, and one had been nursing for 18 months. Milk concentrations of pseudoephedrine were higher than plasma levels in all three patients, with peak milk concentrations occurring at 1.0–1.5 hours. The milk:plasma ratios at 1, 3, and 12 hours in one subject were 3.3, 3.9, and 2.6, respectively. The investigators calculated that 1000 ml of milk produced over 24 hours would contain 0.25–0.33 mg of pseudoephedrine base, approximately 0.5–0.7% of the maternal dose (4). The American Academy of Pediatrics considers the drug to be compatible with breast feeding (5).

References

1. Nishimura H, Tanimura T. *Clinical Aspects of the Teratogenicity of Drugs*. Amsterdam:Excerpta Medica, 1976:231.
2. Heinonen OP, Slone D, Shapiro S. *Birth Defects and Drugs in Pregnancy*. Littleton:Publishing Sciences Group, 1977.
3. Chasnoff IJ, Diggs G. Fetal alcohol effects and maternal cough syrup abuse. Am J Dis Child 1981;135:968.
4. Findlay JWA, Butz RF, Sailstad JM, Warren JT, Welch RM. Pseudoephedrine and triprolidine in plasma and breast milk of nursing mothers. Br J Clin Pharmacol 1984;18:901–6.
5. Committee on Drugs, American Academy of Pediatrics. Transfer of drugs and other chemicals into human milk. Pediatrics 1989;84:924–36.

Name: **PYRANTEL PAMOATE**

Class: **Anthelmintic**   Risk Factor: **C**

Fetal Risk Summary

No data are available.

Breast Feeding Summary

No data are available.

Name: **PYRAZINAMIDE**

Class: **Antituberculosis Agent** Risk Factor: **C**

Fetal Risk Summary

Pyrazinamide is a synthetic antituberculosis agent derived from niacinamide. No reports of its use in pregnancy have been located.

Breast Feeding Summary

Pyrazinamide is excreted into human milk. In one non-breast-feeding patient given an oral 1-g dose of pyrazinamide, the peak concentration of the drug, 1.5 μg/ml, was measured in the milk at 3 hours (1). The peak concentration in the maternal plasma, 42.0 μg/ml, occurred at 2 hours.

Reference

1. Holdiness MR. Antituberculosis drugs and breast-feeding. Arch Intern Med 1984;144:1888.

Name: **PYRETHRINS WITH PIPERONYL BUTOXIDE**

Class: **Pediculicide** Risk Factor: **C**

Fetal Risk Summary

Pyrethrins with piperonyl butoxide is a synergistic combination product used topically for the treatment of lice infestations. It is not effective for the treatment of scabies (mite infestations). Pyrethrins with piperonyl butoxide is considered the drug of choice for lice (1). Although no reports of its use in pregnancy have been located, topical absorption is poor, so potential toxicity should be less than that of lindane (see also Lindane) (2). For this reason, use of the combination is probably preferred over lindane in the pregnant patient.

Breast Feeding Summary

No data are available.

References

1. Anonymous. Drugs for parasitic infections. In: *Handbook for Antimicrobial Therapy*. New Rochelle:The Medical Letter, Inc, 1984:100.
2. Robinson DH, Shepherd DA. Control of head lice in schoolchildren. Curr Ther Res 1980;27:1–6.

Name: **PYRIDOSTIGMINE**

Class: **Parasympathomimetic (Cholinergic)** Risk Factor: **C**

Fetal Risk Summary

Pyridostigmine is a quaternary ammonium compound with anticholinesterase activity used in the treatment of myasthenia gravis. The drug has been used in pregnancy without producing fetal malformations (1–13). Because it is ionized at physiologic pH, pyridostigmine would not be expected to cross the placenta in significant amounts. Caution has been advised against the use in pregnancy of intravenous anticholinesterases since they may cause premature labor (1, 2). This effect on the pregnant uterus increases near term.

Transient muscular weakness has been observed in about 20% of newborns of mothers with myasthenia gravis (9). The neonatal myasthenia is due to transplacental passage of anti-acetylcholine receptor immunoglobulin G antibodies (9).

Breast Feeding Summary

Pyridostigmine is excreted into breast milk (13). Levels in two women receiving 120–300 mg/day were 2–25 ng/ml, representing milk:plasma ratios of 0.36–1.13. Because it is an ionized quaternary ammonium compound, these values were surprisingly high. The drug was not detected in the infants nor were any adverse effects noted. The authors estimated that the two infants were ingesting 0.1% or less of the maternal doses (13). The American Academy of Pediatrics considers pyridostigmine to be compatible with breast feeding (14).

References

1. Foldes FF, McNall PG. Myasthenia gravis: a guide for anesthesiologists. Anesthesiology 1962;23:837–72.
2. McNall PG, Jafarnia MR. Management of myasthenia gravis in the obstetric patient. Am J Obstet Gynecol 1965;92:518–25.
3. Plauche WC. Myasthenia gravis in pregnancy. Am J Obstet Gynecol 1964;88:404–9.
4. Chambers DC, Hall JE, Boyce J. Myasthenia gravis and pregnancy. Obstet Gynecol 1967;29:597–603.
5. Hay DM. Myasthenia gravis and pregnancy. J Obstet Gynaecol Br Commonw 1969;76:323–9.
6. Heinonen OP, Slone D, Shapiro S. *Birth Defects and Drugs in Pregnancy*. Littleton:Publishing Sciences Group, 1977:345–56.
7. Blackhall MI, Buckley GA, Roberts DV, Roberts JB, Thomas BH, Wilson A. Drug-induced neonatal myasthenia. J Obstet Gynaecol Br Commonw 1969;76:157–62.
8. Rolbin SH, Levinson G, Shnider SM, Wright RG. Anesthetic considerations for myasthenia gravis and pregnancy. Anesth Analg (Cleve) 1978;57:441–7.
9. Plauche WC. Myasthenia gravis in pregnancy: an update. Am J Obstet Gynecol 1979;135:691–7.
10. Eden RD, Gall SA. Myasthenia gravis and pregnancy: a reappraisal of thymectomy. Obstet Gynecol 1983;62:328–33.
11. Cohen BA, London RS, Goldstein PJ. Myasthenia gravis and preeclampsia. Obstet Gynecol 1976;48(Suppl):35S–7S.
12. Catanzarite VA, McHargue AM, Sandberg EC, Dyson DC. Respiratory arrest during therapy for premature labor in a patient with myasthenia gravis. Obstet Gynecol 1984;64:819–22.
13. Hardell LI, Lindstrom B, Lonnerholm G, Osterman PO. Pyridostigmine in human breast milk. Br J Clin Pharmacol 1982;14:565–7.
14. Committee on Drugs, American Academy of Pediatrics. Transfer of drugs and other chemicals into human milk. Pediatrics 1989;84:924–36.

Name: **PYRIDOXINE**

Class: **Vitamin**   Risk Factor: **A***

Fetal Risk Summary

Pyridoxine (vitamin B_6), a water-soluble B complex vitamin, acts as an essential coenzyme involved in the metabolism of amino acids, carbohydrates, and lipids (1). The American recommended dietary allowance (RDA) for pyridoxine in pregnancy is 2.4–2.6 mg (2).

Pyridoxine is actively transported to the fetus (3–5). Like other B complex vitamins, concentrations of pyridoxine in the fetus and newborn are higher than in the mother and are directly proportional to maternal intake (6–17). Actual pyridoxine levels vary from report to report due to the nutritional status of the populations studied and the microbiologic assays used, but usually indicate an approximate newborn:maternal ratio of 2:1 with levels ranging from 22–87 ng/ml for newborns and 13–51 ng/ml for mothers (5, 15–17).

Pyridoxine deficiency without clinical symptoms is common during pregnancy (11, 17–35). Clinical symptoms consisting of oral lesions have been reported, however, in severe B_6 deficiency (36). Supplementation with multivitamin products reduces, but does not always eliminate, the incidence of pyridoxine hypovitaminemia (17).

Severe vitamin B_6 deficiency is teratogenic in experimental animals (37). No reports of human malformations linked to B_6 deficiency have been located. A brief report in 1976 described an anencephalic fetus resulting from a woman treated with high doses of pyridoxine and other vitamins and nutrients for psychiatric reasons, but the relationship between the defect and the vitamins is unknown (38).

The effects on the mother and fetus resulting from pyridoxine deficiency or excess are controversial. These effects can be summarized as:

Pregnancy-induced hypertension (PIH, toxemia, preeclampsia, eclampsia)
Gestational diabetes mellitus
Infantile convulsions
Hyperemesis gravidarum
Congenital malformations
Miscellaneous

Several researchers have claimed that pyridoxine deficiency is associated with the development of PIH (13, 39–41). Others have not found this relationship (11, 20, 42, 43). One group of investigators demonstrated that women with PIH excreted larger amounts of xanthurenic acid in their urine after a loading dose of dl-tryptophan than did normal pregnant women (39). Although the test was not totally specific for PIH, they theorized that it could be of value for early detection of the disease and was indicative of abnormal pyridoxine-niacin-protein metabolism. In another study, 410 women treated with 10 mg of pyridoxine daily were compared to 410 controls (40). PIH occurred in 18 (4.4%) of the untreated controls and in 7 (1.7%) of the pyridoxine-supplemented patients, a significant difference. In an earlier report, no significant differences were found between women with PIH and normal controls in urinary excretion of 4-pyridoxic acid, a pyridoxine metabolite, after a loading dose of the vitamin (20). Some investigators have measured lower levels of pyridoxine in mothers with PIH than in mothers without PIH (13). The difference in levels between the newborns of PIH and normal mothers was more than 2-fold and highly significant. In a 1961 Swedish report, pyridoxine levels in 10 women with PIH were compared to those in 26 women with uncomplicated pregnancies (42). The difference between the mean levels of the two groups, 25 and 33 ng/ml, respectively, was not significant. Similarly, others have been unable to find a correlation between pyridoxine levels and PIH (11, 43).

Pyridoxine levels were studied in 14 pregnant women with an abnormal glucose tolerance test (GTT), and 13 of these patients were shown to be pyridoxine deficient (44). All were placed on a diet and given 100 mg of pyridoxine/day for 14 days, after which only two were diagnosed as having gestational diabetes mellitus. The effect of the diet on the GTT was said to be negligible, although a control group was not used. Other investigators duplicated these results in 13 women using the same dose of pyridoxine but without mentioning any dietary manipulation and without controls (45). However, a third study was unable to demonstrate a beneficial effect in four patients with an abnormal GTT using 100 mg of B_6 for 21 days (46). Moreover, all of the mothers had large-for-gestational-age infants, an expected complication of diabetic pregnancies. In 13 gestational diabetic women treated with the doses of pyridoxine described above, an improvement was observed in the GTT in two patients, a worsening was seen in six, and no significant change occurred in the remaining five (47).

An association between pyridoxine and infantile convulsions was first described in the mid-1950s (48–52). Some infants fed a diet deficient in this vitamin developed intractable seizures that responded only to pyridoxine. A 1967 publication reviewed this complication in infants and differentiated between the states of pyridoxine deficiency and dependency (53). Whether or not these states can be induced *in utero* is open to question. As noted earlier, pyridoxine deficiency is common during pregnancy, even in well-nourished women, but the fetus accumulates the vitamin, although at lower levels, even in the face of maternal hypovitaminemia. Reports of seizures in newborn infants delivered from mothers with pyridoxine deficiency have not been located. On the other hand, high doses of pyridoxine early in gestation in one patient were suspected of altering the normal metabolism of pyridoxine leading to intractable convulsions in the newborn (54). The woman, in whom two pregnancies were complicated by hyperemesis gravidarum, was treated with frequent injections of pyridoxine and thiamine, 50 mg each (54). The first newborn began convulsing 4 hours after birth and died within 30 hours. The second infant began mild twitching at 3 hours of age and progressed to severe generalized convulsions on the 5th day. Successful treatment was eventually accomplished with pyridoxine but not before marked mental retardation had occurred. The authors of this report postulated that the fetus, exposed to high doses of pyridoxine, developed an adaptive enzyme system that was capable of rapidly metabolizing the vitamin; following delivery, this adaptation was manifested by pyridoxine dependency and convulsions (54). Since this case, more than 50 additional cases of pyridoxine dependency have been reported, and the disease is now thought to be an inherited autosomal recessive disorder (55). *In utero* dependency-induced convulsions in three successive pregnancies have been reported in one woman (56). The first two newborns died—one during the 7th week and one on day 2—as a result of intractable convulsions. During the third pregnancy, *in utero* convulsions stopped after the mother was treated with

110 mg/day of pyridoxine 4 days before delivery. Following birth, the newborn was treated with pyridoxine. Convulsions occurred on three separate occasions when vitamin therapy was withheld and then abated when therapy was restarted.

The first use of pyridoxine for severe nausea and vomiting of pregnancy (hyperemesis gravidarum) was reported in 1942 (57). Individual injections ranged from 10–100 mg with total doses up to 1500 mg being given. Satisfactory relief was obtained in most cases. In one study, patients were successfully treated with intramuscular doses of 50–100 mg three times weekly (58). Another report described a single patient with hyperemesis who responded to an intravenous mixture of high-dose B complex vitamins, including 50 mg of pyridoxine, each day for 3 days (59). Much smaller doses were used in a study of 17 patients (60). Intramuscular doses of 5 mg every 2–4 days were administered to these patients with an immediate response observed in 12 women and all responding by the second dose. Oral doses of 60–80 mg/day up to a total dose of 2500 mg gave partial or complete relief from nausea and vomiting in 68 patients; an additional 10 patients required oral plus injectable pyridoxine (61). A success rate of 95% was claimed in a study of 62 women treated with a combination of pyridoxine and suprarenal cortex (adrenal cortex extract) (62). None of the preceding six studies was double blind or controlled. The effect of pyridoxine on blood urea concentrations in hyperemesis has been investigated (63). Blood urea was decreased below normal adult levels in pregnant women and even lower in patients with hyperemesis. Pyridoxine, 40 mg orally/day for 3 days, significantly increased blood urea only in women suffering from hyperemesis. In another measure of the effect of pyridoxine on hyperemesis, elevated serum glutamic acid levels observed with this condition were returned to normal pregnant values after pyridoxine therapy (64). However, another investigator could not demonstrate any value from pyridoxine therapy in 16 patients (65). Placebos were used but the study was not blinded. In addition, only 1 of 16 patients had hyperemesis gravidarum with the remaining 15 presenting with lesser degrees of nausea and vomiting. Based on the above studies, it is impossible to judge the effectiveness of the vitamin in allaying true hyperemesis gravidarum. More than likely, the effect of hydration, possibly improved prenatal care, the attention of health care personnel, the transitory nature of hyperemesis, the lack of strict diagnostic criteria in classifying patients with the disease, and other factors were the primary reasons for the reversal of the symptoms of the women involved in these studies.

A recent case report suggested a link between high doses of pyridoxine and phocomelia (66). The mother, who weighed only 47 kg, took 50 mg of pyridoxine daily plus unknown doses of lecithin and vitamin B_{12} through the first 7 months of pregnancy. The full-term female infant was born with a near-total amelia of her left leg at the knee. A relationship between any of the drugs and the defect is doubtful.

The combination of doxylamine and pyridoxine (Bendectin, others) has been the focus of considerable debate in the past. The debate centered on whether the preparation was teratogenic. The combination had been used by millions of women for pregnancy-induced nausea and vomiting but was removed from the market by the manufacturer because of a number of large legal awards against the company. Jury decisions notwithstanding, the available scientific evidence indicates the combination is not teratogenic (see Doxylamine).

Among miscellaneous effects, two studies were unable to associate low maternal concentrations of pyridoxine with premature labor (30, 43). Similarly, no correlation was found between low levels and stillbirths (11, 40). However, 1-minute Apgar scores were significantly related to low maternal and newborn pyridoxine concentrations (15, 67). The effects of pyridoxine supplementation in black pregnant women have been studied (68). Lower maternal serum lipid, fetal weight, and placental weight, and the frequency of placental vascular sclerosis were observed. Others have not found a correlation between pyridoxine levels and birth weight (16, 43, 67). In an unusual report, pregnant women given daily 20-mg supplements of pyridoxine by either lozenges or capsules had less dental disease than untreated controls (69). The best cariostatic effect was seen in patients in the lozenge group.

In summary, pyridoxine deficiency during pregnancy is a common problem in unsupplemented women. Supplementation with oral pyridoxine reduces but does not eliminate the frequency of deficiency. No definitive evidence has appeared that indicates mild to moderate deficiency of this vitamin is a cause of maternal or fetal complications. Most of the studies with this vitamin have been open and uncontrolled. If a relationship does exist with poor pregnancy outcome, it is probable that a number of factors, of which pyridoxine may be one, contribute to the problem.

Severe deficiency or abnormal metabolism is related to fetal and infantile convulsions and possibly to other conditions. High doses apparently pose little risk to the fetus. The available evidence does not support a teratogenic risk either alone or in combination with doxylamine. Double blind, randomized trials are needed to determine if pyridoxine is effective for severe nausea and vomiting of pregnancy.

Since pyridoxine is required for good maternal and fetal health, and an increased demand for the vitamin occurs during pregnancy, supplementation of the pregnant woman with the RDA for pyridoxine is recommended.

[*Risk Factor C if used in doses above RDA.]

Breast Feeding Summary

Pyridoxine (vitamin B_6) is excreted in human breast milk (15, 70–76). Concentrations in milk are directly proportional to intake (70–76). In well nourished women, pyridoxine levels varied, depending on intake, from 123–314 ng/ml (70–72). Peak pyridoxine milk levels occurred 3–8 hours after ingestion of a vitamin supplement (70, 72, 73). A 1983 study measured pyridoxine levels in pooled human milk obtained from preterm (26 mothers: 29–34 weeks) and term (35 mothers: 39 weeks or longer) patients (74). Preterm milk rose from 11.1 ng/ml (colostrum) to 62.2 ng/ml (16–196 days) while term milk increased over the same period from 17.0–107.1 ng/ml. In a 1985 study, daily supplements of 0–20 mg resulted in milk concentrations of 93–413 ng/ml, corresponding to an infant intake of 0.06–0.28 mg/day (73). A significant correlation was found between maternal intake and infant intake. Most infants, however, did not receive the RDA for infants (0.3 mg) even when the mother was consuming eight times the RDA for lactating women (2.5 mg) (73). In lactating women with low nutritional status, supplementation with pyridoxine, 0.4–40.0 mg/day, resulted in mean milk concentrations of 80–158 ng/ml (75).

Convulsions have been reported in infants fed a pyridoxine-deficient diet (see discussion under "Fetal Risk Summary") (48–53). Seizures were described in two breast-fed infants, one of whom was receiving only 67 μg/day in the milk (77).

Intake in the second infant was not determined. A similar report involved three infants whose mothers had levels less than 20 ng/ml (at 7 days postpartum) or less than 60 ng/ml (at 4 weeks) of pyridoxine in their milk (78). The convulsions responded promptly to B_6 therapy in all five of these infants.

Very large doses of pyridoxine have been reported to have a lactation-inhibiting effect (79). Using oral doses of 600 mg/day, lactation was successfully inhibited in 95% of patients within 1 week as compared to only 17% of placebo-treated controls. Very high intravenous doses of pyridoxine, 600 mg infused over 1 hour in healthy, nonlactating young adults, successfully suppressed the rise in prolactin induced by exercise (80). However, since use of this dose and method of administration in lactating women would be unusual, the relevance of these data to breast feeding is limited. With dosage much closer to physiologic levels, such as 20 mg/day, no effect on lactation has been observed (73). In addition, two separate trials, utilizing 450 mg and 600 mg/day in divided oral doses, failed to reproduce the lactation-inhibiting effect observed earlier or to show any suppression of serum prolactin levels (81, 82). One writer, however, has suggested that pyridoxine be removed from multivitamin supplements intended for lactating women (83). This proposal has invoked sharp opposition from other correspondents who claimed the available evidence does not support a milk-inhibiting property for pyridoxine (84, 85). Moreover, a study published in 1985 examined the effects of pyridoxine supplements, 0.5 or 4.0 mg/day started 24 hours after delivery, on lactation (86). Women receiving the higher dose of pyridoxine had significantly higher concentrations of plasma pyridoxal phosphate ($p < 0.01$) and milk total vitamin B_6 ($p < 0.05$) at 1, 3, 6, and 9 months. Plasma prolactin concentrations were similar between the two groups throughout the study. The American Academy of Pediatrics considers pyridoxine to be compatible with breast feeding (87).

In summary, the American RDA for pyridoxine during lactation is 2.3–2.5 mg (2). If the diet of the lactating woman adequately supplies this amount, maternal supplementation with pyridoxine is not required (76). Supplementation with the RDA for pyridoxine is recommended for those women with inadequate nutritional intake.

References

1. American Hospital Formulary Service. *Drug Information 1990*. Bethesda:American Society of Hospital Pharmacists, 1990:2116–8.
2. *Recommended Dietary Allowances*, 9th ed. Washington:National Academy of Sciences, 1980.
3. Frank O, Walbroehl G, Thomson A, Kaminetzky H, Kubes Z, Baker H. Placental transfer: fetal retention of some vitamins. Am J Clin Nutr 1970;23:662–3.
4. Hill EP, Longo LD. Dynamics of maternal-fetal nutrient transfer. Fed Proc 1980;39:239–44.
5. Baker H, Frank O, Deangelis B, Feingold S, Kaminetzky HA. Role of placenta in maternal-fetal vitamin transfer in humans. Am J Obstet Gynecol 1981;141:792–6.
6. Wachstein M, Moore C, Graffeo LW. Pyridoxal phosphate (B_6-al-PO_4) levels of circulating leukocytes in maternal and cord blood. Proc Soc Exp Biol Med 1957;96:326–8.
7. Wachstein M, Kellner JD, Ortiz JM. Pyridoxal phosphate in plasma and leukocytes of normal and pregnant subjects following B_6 load tests. Proc Soc Exp Biol Med 1960;103:350–3.
8. Brin M. Thiamine and pyridoxine studies of mother and cord blood. Fed Proc 1966;25:245.
9. Contractor SF, Shane B. Blood and urine levels of vitamin B_6 in the mother and fetus before and after loading of the mother with vitamin B_6. Am J Obstet Gynecol 1970;107:635–40.
10. Brin M. Abnormal tryptophan metabolism in pregnancy and with the oral contraceptive pill. II. Relative levels of vitamin B_6-vitamers in cord and maternal blood. Am J Clin Nutr 1971;24:704–8.
11. Heller S, Salkeld RM, Korner WF. Vitamin B_6 status in pregnancy. Am J Clin Nutr 1973;26:1339–48.

12. Kaminetzky HA, Baker H, Frank O, Langer A. The effects of intravenously administered water-soluble vitamins during labor in normovitaminemic and hypovitaminemic gravidas on maternal and neonatal blood vitamin levels at delivery. Am J Obstet Gynecol 1974;120:697–703.
13. Brophy MH, Siiteri PK. Pyridoxal phosphate and hypertensive disorders of pregnancy. Am J Obstet Gynecol 1975;121:1075–9.
14. Bamji MS. Enzymic evaluation of thiamin, riboflavin and pyridoxine status of parturient women and their newborn infants. Br J Nutr 1976;35:259–65.
15. Roepke JLB, Kirksey A. Vitamin B$_6$ nutriture during pregnancy and lactation. I. Vitamin B$_6$ intake, levels of the vitamin in biological fluids, and condition of the infant at birth. Am J Clin Nutr 1979;32:2249–56.
16. Baker H, Thind IS, Frank O, DeAngelis B, Caterini H, Lquria DB. Vitamin levels in low-birth-weight newborn infants and their mothers. Am J Obstet Gynecol 1977;129:521–4.
17. Baker H, Frank O, Thomason AD, Langer A, Munves ED, De Angelis B, Kaminetzky HA. Vitamin profile of 174 mothers and newborns at parturition. Am J Clin Nutr 1975;28:59–65.
18. Wachstein M, Gudaitis A. Disturbance of vitamin B$_6$ metabolism in pregnancy. J Lab Clin Med 1952;40:550–7.
19. Wachstein M, Gudaitis A. Disturbance of vitamin B$_6$ metabolism in pregnancy. II. The influence of various amounts of pyridoxine hydrochloride upon the abnormal tryptophane load test in pregnant women. J Lab Clin Med 1953;42:98–107.
20. Wachstein M, Gudaitis A. Disturbance of vitamin B$_6$ metabolism in pregnancy. III. Abnormal vitamin B$_6$ load test. Am J Obstet Gynecol 1953;66:1207–13.
21. Wachstein M, Lobel S. Abnormal tryptophan metabolites in human pregnancy and their relation to deranged vitamin B$_6$ metabolism. Proc Soc Exp Biol Med 1954;86:624–7.
22. Zartman ER, Barnes AC, Hicks DJ. Observations on pyridoxine metabolism in pregnancy. Am J Obstet Gynecol 1955;70:645–9.
23. Turner ER, Reynolds MS. Intake and elimination of vitamin B$_6$ and metabolites by women. J Am Diet Assoc 1955;31:1119–20.
24. Page EW. The vitamin B$_6$ requirement for normal pregnancy. West J Surg Obstet Gynecol 1956;64:96–103.
25. Coursin DB, Brown VC. Changes in vitamin B$_6$ during pregnancy. Am J Obstet Gynecol 1961;82:1307–11.
26. Brown RR, Thornton MJ, Price JM. The effect of vitamin supplementation on the urinary excretion of tryptophan metabolites by pregnant women. J Clin Invest 1961;40:617–23.
27. Hamfelt A, Hahn L. Pyridoxal phosphate concentration in plasma and tryptophan load test during pregnancy. Clin Chim Acta 1969;25:91–6.
28. Rose DP, Braidman IP. Excretion of tryptophan metabolites as affected by pregnancy, contraceptive steroids, and steroid hormones. Am J Clin Nutr 1971;24:673–83.
29. Kaminetzky HA, Langer A, Baker H, Frank O, Thomson AD, Munves ED, Opper A, Behrle FC, Glista B. The effect of nutrition in teen-age gravidas on pregnancy and the status of the neonate. I. A nutritional profile. Am J Obstet Gynecol 1973;115:639–46.
30. Shane B, Contractor SF. Assessment of vitamin B$_6$ status. Studies on pregnant women and oral contraceptive users. Am J Clin Nutr 1975;28:739–47.
31. Cleary RE, Lumeng L, Li TK. Maternal and fetal plasma levels of pyridoxal phosphate at term: adequacy of vitamin B$_6$ supplementation during pregnancy. Am J Obstet Gynecol 1975;121:25–8.
32. Lumeng L, Cleary RE, Wagner R, Yu PL, Li TK. Adequacy of vitamin B$_6$ supplementation during pregnancy: a prospective study. Am J Clin Nutr 1976;29:1376–83.
33. Anonymous. Requirement of vitamin B$_6$ during pregnancy. Nutr Rev 1976;34:15–6.
34. Dostalova L. Correlation of the vitamin status between mother and newborn during delivery. Dev Pharmacol Ther 1982;4(Suppl I):45–57.
35. Hunt IF, Murphy NJ, Martner-Hewes PM, Faraji B, Swendseid ME, Reynolds RD, Sanchez A, Mejia A. Zinc, vitamin B-6, and other nutrients in pregnant women attending prenatal clinics in Mexico. Am J Clin Nutr 1987;46:563–9.
36. Bapurao S, Raman L, Tulpule PG. Biochemical assessment of vitamin B$_6$ nutritional status in pregnant women with orolingual manifestations. Am J Clin Nutr 1982;36:581–6.
37. Shepard TH. Catalog of Teratogenic Agents, 3rd ed. Baltimore:Johns Hopkins University Press, 1980:279.
38. Averback P. Anencephaly associated with megavitamin therapy. Can Med Assoc J 1976;114:995.
39. Sprince H, Lowy RS, Folsome CE, Behrman J. Studies on the urinary excretion of "xanthurenic acid" during normal and abnormal pregnancy: a survey of the excretion of "xanthurenic acid" in

normal nonpregnant, normal pregnant, preeclamptic, and eclamptic women. Am J Obstet Gynecol 1951;62:84–92.

40. Wachstein M, Graffeo LW. Influence of vitamin B₆ on the incidence of preeclampsia. Obstet Gynecol 1956;8:177–80.
41. Kaminetzky HA, Baker H. Micronutrients in pregnancy. Clin Obstet Gynecol 1977;20:363–80.
42. Diding NA, Melander SEJ. Serum vitamin B₆ level in normal and toxaemic pregnancy. Acta Obstet Gynecol Scand 1961;40:252–61.
43. Hillman RW, Cabaud PG, Nilsson DE, Arpin PD, Tufano RJ. Pyridoxine supplementation during pregnancy. Clinical and laboratory observations. Am J Clin Nutr 1963;12:427–30.
44. Coelingh Bennink HJT, Schreurs WHP. Improvement of oral glucose tolerance in gestational diabetes by pyridoxine. Br Med J 1975;3:13–5.
45. Spellacy WN, Buhi WC, Birk SA. Vitamin B₆ treatment of gestational diabetes mellitus. Studies of blood glucose and plasma insulin. Am J Obstet Gynecol 1977;127:599–602.
46. Perkins RP. Failure of pyridoxine to improve glucose tolerance in gestational diabetes mellitus. Obstet Gynecol 1977;50:370–2.
47. Gillmer MDG, Mazibuko D. Pyridoxine treatment of chemical diabetes in pregnancy. Am J Obstet Gynecol 1979;133:499–502.
48. Snyderman SE, Holt LE, Carretero R, Jacobs K. Pyridoxine deficiency in the human infant. J Clin Nutr 1953;1:200–7.
49. Molony CJ, Parmalee AH. Convulsions in young infants as a result of pyridoxine (vitamin B₆) deficiency. JAMA 1954;154:405–6.
50. Coursin DB. Vitamin B₆ deficiency in infants. Am J Dis Child 1955;90:344–8.
51. Coursin DB. Effects of vitamin B₆ on the central nervous activity in childhood. Am J Clin Nutr 1956;4:354–63.
52. Molony CJ, Parmelee AH. Convulsions in young infants as a result of pyridoxine (vitamin B₆) deficiency. JAMA 1954;154:405–6.
53. Scriver CR. Vitamin B₆ deficiency and dependency in man. Am J Dis Child 1967;113:109–14.
54. Hunt AD Jr, Stokes J Jr, McCrory WW, Stroud HH. Pyridoxine dependency: report of a case of intractable convulsions in an infant controlled by pyridoxine. Pediatrics 1954;13:140–5.
55. Bankier A, Turner M, Hopkins IJ. Pyridoxine dependent seizures—a wider clinical spectrum. Arch Dis Child 1983;58:415–8.
56. Bejsovec MIR, Kulenda Z, Ponca E. Familial intrauterine convulsions in pyridoxine dependency. Arch Dis Child 1967;42:201–7.
57. Willis RS, Winn WW, Morris AT, Newsom AA, Massey WE. Clinical observations in treatment of nausea and vomiting in pregnancy with vitamins B₁ and B₆. A preliminary report. Am J Obstet Gynecol 1942;44:265–71.
58. Weinstein BB, Mitchell GJ, Sustendal GF. Clinical experiences with pyridoxine hydrochloride in treatment of nausea and vomiting of pregnancy. Am J Obstet Gynecol 1943;46:283–5.
59. Hart BF, McConnell WT. Vitamin B factors in toxic psychosis of pregnancy and the puerperium. Am J Obstet Gynecol 1943;46:283.
60. Varas O. Treatment of nausea and vomiting of pregnancy with vitamin B₆. Bol Soc Chilena Obstet Ginecol 1943;8:404. As abstracted in Am J Obstet Gynecol 1945;50:347–8.
61. Weinstein BB, Wohl Z, Mitchell GJ, Sustendal GF. Oral administration of pyridoxine hydrochloride in the treatment of nausea and vomiting of pregnancy. Am J Obstet Gynecol 1944;47:389–94.
62. Dorsey CW. The use of pyridoxine and suprarenal cortex combined in the treatment of the nausea and vomiting of pregnancy. Am J Obstet Gynecol 1949;58:1073–8.
63. McGanity WJ, McHenry EW, Van Wyck HB, Watt GL. An effect of pyridoxine on blood urea in human subjects. J Biol Chem 1949;178:511–6.
64. Beaton JR, McHenry EW. Observations on plasma glutamic acid. Fed Proc 1951;10:161.
65. Hesseltine HC. Pyridoxine failure in nausea and vomiting of pregnancy. Am J Obstet Gynecol 1946;51:82–6.
66. Gardner LI, Welsh-Sloan J, Cady RB. Phocomelia in infant whose mother took large doses of pyridoxine during pregnancy. Lancet 1985;1:636.
67. Schuster K, Bailey LB, Mahan CS. Vitamin B₆ status of low-income adolescent and adult pregnant women and the condition of their infants at birth. Am J Clin Nutr 1981;34:1731–5.
68. Swartwout JR, Unglaub WG, Smith RC. Vitamin B₆, serum lipids and placental arteriolar lesions in human pregnancy. A preliminary report. Am J Clin Nutr 1960;8:434–44.
69. Hillman RW, Cabaud PG, Schenone RA. The effects of pyridoxine supplements on the dental caries experience of pregnant women. Am J Clin Nutr 1962;10:512–5.

70. West KD, Kirksey A. Influence of vitamin B_6 intake on the content of the vitamin in human milk. Am J Clin Nutr 1976;29:961–9.
71. Thomas MR, Kawamoto J, Sneed SM, Eakin R. The effects of vitamin C, vitamin B_6, and vitamin B_{12} supplementation on the breast milk and maternal status of well-nourished women. Am J Clin Nutr 1979;32:1679–85.
72. Sneed SM, Zane C, Thomas MR. The effects of ascorbic acid, vitamin B_6, vitamin B_{12}, and folic acid supplementation on the breast milk and maternal nutritional status of low socioeconomic lactating women. Am J Clin Nutr 1981;34:1338–46.
73. Styslinger L, Kirksey A. Effects of different levels of vitamin B-6 supplementation on vitamin B-6 concentrations in human milk and vitamin B-6 intakes of breastfed infants. Am J Clin Nutr 1985;41:21–31.
74. Ford JE, Zechalko A, Murphy J, Brooke OG. Comparison of the B vitamin composition of milk from mothers of preterm and term babies. Arch Dis Child 1983;58:367–72.
75. Deodhar AD, Rajalakshmi R, Ramakrishnan CV. Studies on human lactation. Part III. Effect of dietary vitamin supplementation vitamin contents of breast milk. Acta Pediatr 1964;53:42–8.
76. Thomas MR, Sneed SM, Wei C, Nail PA, Wilson M, Sprinkle EE III. The effects of vitamin C, vitamin B_6, vitamin B_{12}, folic acid, riboflavin, and thiamin on the breast milk and maternal status of well-nourished women at 6 months postpartum. Am J Clin Nutr 1980;33:2151–6.
77. Bessey OA, Adam DJD, Hansen AE. Intake of vitamin B_6 and infantile convulsions: a first approximation of requirements of pyridoxine in infants. Pediatrics 1957;20:33–44.
78. Kirksey A, Roepke JLB. Vitamin B-6 nutriture of mothers of three breast-fed neonates with central nervous system disorders. Fed Proc 1981;40:864.
79. Foukas MD. An antilactogenic effect of pyridoxine. J Obstet Gynaecol Br Commonw 1973;80:718–20.
80. Moretti C, Fabbri A, Gnessi L, Bonifacio V, Fraioli F, Isidori A. Pyridoxine (B6) suppresses the rise in prolactin and increases the rise in growth hormone induced by exercise. N Engl J Med 1982;307:444–5.
81. MacDonald HN, Collins YD, Tobin MJW, Wijayaratne, DN. The failure of pyridoxine in suppression of puerperal lactation. Br J Obstet Gynaecol 1976;83:54–5.
82. Canales ES, Soria J, Zarate A, Mason M, Molina M. The influence of pyridoxine on prolactin secretion and milk production in women. Br J Obstet Gynaecol 1976;83:387–8.
83. Greentree LB.Dangers of vitamin B_6 in nursing mothers. N Engl J Med 1979;300:141–2.
84. Lande NI. More on dangers of vitamin B_6 in nursing mothers. N Engl J Med 1979;300:926–7.
85. Rivlin RS. More on dangers of vitamin B_6 in nursing mothers. N Engl J Medi 1979;300:927.
86. Andon MB, Howard MP, Moser PB, Reynolds RD. Nutritionally relevant supplementation of vitamin B6 in lactating women: effect on plasma prolactin. Pediatrics 1985;76:769–73.
87. Committee on Drugs, American Academy of Pediatrics. Transfer of drugs and other chemicals into human milk. Pediatrics 1989;84:924–36.

Name: **PYRILAMINE**

Class: **Antihistamine**   Risk Factor: **C**

Fetal Risk Summary

Pyrilamine is used infrequently during pregnancy. The Collaborative Perinatal Project monitored 50,282 mother-child pairs, 121 of which had pyrilamine exposure in the 1st trimester (1, pp. 323–324). No evidence was found to suggest a relationship to large categories of major or minor malformations. For use anytime during pregnancy, 392 exposures were recorded (1, pp. 436–437). A possible association with malformations was found based on 12 defects, 6 of which involved benign tumors (1, p. 489).

An association between exposure during the last 2 weeks of pregnancy to antihistamines in general and retrolental fibroplasia in premature infants has been reported. See Brompheniramine for details.

Breast Feeding Summary

No data are available.

Reference

1. Heinonen OP, Slone D, Shapiro S. *Birth Defects and Drugs in Pregnancy*. Littleton:Publishing Sciences Group, 1977.

Name: **PYRIMETHAMINE**

Class: **Antimalarial**   Risk Factor: **C**

Fetal Risk Summary

Pyrimethamine is a folic acid antagonist used as an antimalarial agent. Although some folic acid antagonists are teratogenic (see Methotrexate), no malformations attributable to pyrimethamine have been reported. One case report described gastroschisis in an infant exposed to the drug early in gestation (1). An association between the drug and the defect, however, is questionable (2, 3).

Most studies have found pyrimethamine to be safe during pregnancy (3–11). Folic acid supplementation should be given to prevent folate deficiency.

Breast Feeding Summary

Pyrimethamine is excreted into breast milk (12, 13). Mothers treated with 25–75 mg orally produced peak concentrations of 3.1–3.3 µg/ml at 6 hours (12). The drug was detectable up to 48 hours after a dose. Malaria parasites were completely eliminated in infants up to 6 months of age who were entirely breast fed. In a 1986 study, three women were treated with a combination tablet containing 100 mg of dapsone and 12.5 mg of pyrimethamine at 2–5 days postpartum (13). Blood and milk samples were collected up to 227 hours after the dose. The milk:plasma area under the concentration-time curve ratios ranged from 0.46–0.66. Based on an estimated ingestion of 1000 ml of milk/day, the infants would have consumed between 16.8 and 45.6% of the maternal doses over a 9-day period. The American Academy of Pediatrics considers pyrimethamine to be compatible with breast feeding (14).

References

1. Harpey J-P, Darbois Y, Lefebvre G. Teratogenicity of pyrimethamine. Lancet 1983;2:399.
2. Smithells RW, Sheppard S. Teratogenicity of Debendox and pyrimethamine. Lancet 1983;2:623–4.
3. Anonymous. Pyrimethamine combinations in pregnancy. Lancet 1983;2:1005–7.
4. Morley D, Woodland M, Cuthbertson WFJ. Controlled trial of pyrimethamine in pregnant women in an African village. Br Med J 1964;1:667–8.
5. Gilles HM, Lawson JB, Sibelas M, Voller A, Allan N. Malaria, anaemia and pregnancy. Ann Trop Med Parasitol 1969;63:245–63.
6. Heinonen OP, Slone D, Shapiro S. *Birth Defects and Drugs in Pregnancy*. Littleton:Publishing Sciences Group, 1977;299,302.

7. Bruce-Chwatt LJ. Malaria and pregnancy. Br Med J 1983;286:1457–8.
8. Anonymous. Malaria in pregnancy. Lancet 1983;2:84–5.
9. Strang A, Lachman E, Pitsoe SB, Marszalek A, Philpott RH. Malaria in pregnancy with fatal complications. Case report. Br J Obstet Gynaecol 1984;91:399–403.
10. Main EK, Main DM, Krogstad DJ. Treatment of chloroquine-resistant malaria during pregnancy. JAMA 1983;249:3207–9.
11. Nahlen BL, Akintunde A, Alakija T, Nguyen-Dinh P, Ogunbode O, Edungbola LD, Adetoro O, Breman JG. Lack of efficacy of pyrimethamine prophylaxis in pregnant Nigerian women. Lancet 1989;2:830–4.
12. Clyde DF, Shute GT, Press J. Transfer of pyrimethamine in human milk. J Trop Med Hyg 1956;59:277–84.
13. Edstein MD. Veerendaal JR, Newman K, Hyslop R. Excretion of chloroquine, dapsone and pyrimethamine in human milk. Br J Clin Pharmacol 1986;22:733–5.
14. Committee on Drugs, American Academy of Pediatrics. Transfer of drugs and other chemicals into human milk. Pediatrics 1989;84:924–36.

Name: **PYRVINIUM PAMOATE**

Class: **Anthelmintic**   Risk Factor: **C**

Fetal Risk Summary

No data are available.

Breast Feeding Summary

No data are available.

Name: **QUINACRINE**

Class: **Antimalarial/Anthelmintic**   Risk Factor: **C**

Fetal Risk Summary

A newborn with renal agenesis, hydronephrosis, spina bifida, megacolon, and hydrocephalus whose mother received quinacrine 0.1 g/day during the 1st trimester has been reported (1). Animal data do not support a teratogenic effect. Topical application of solutions containing 125 mg/ml of quinacrine directly into the uterine cavity has resulted in tubal occlusion and infertility (2).

Breast Feeding Summary

No data are available.

References

1. Vevera J, Zatlovkal F. Pfipad uruzenych malformact zpusobenych pravdepodobne atebrinem-ym uranem tehotenstui. In Nishmura H, Tanimura T, eds. *Clinical Aspects of the Teratogenicity of Drugs*. New York:American Elsevier, 1976:145.
2. Zipper JA, Stachetti E, Medel M. Human fertility control by transvaginal application of quinacrine on the fallopian tube. Fertil Steril 1970;21:581–9.

Name: **QUINETHAZONE**

Class: **Diuretic**   Risk Factor: **D**

Fetal Risk Summary

Quinethazone is structurally related to the thiazide diuretics. See Chlorothiazide.

Breast Feeding Summary

See Chlorothiazide.

Name: **QUINIDINE**

Class: **Antiarrhythmic**   Risk Factor: **C**

Fetal Risk Summary

No reports linking the use of quinidine with congenital defects have been located. Quinidine has been in use as an antiarrhythmic drug for over a 100 years (1), and in pregnancy, at least back to the 1920s (2–8). Eighth cranial nerve damage has been associated with high doses of the optical isomer, quinine, but not with quinidine (4). Neonatal thrombocytopenia has been reported after maternal use of quinidine (5).

Quinidine crosses the placenta and achieves fetal serum levels similar to maternal levels (1, 6–8). In a 1979 case, a woman taking 600 mg every 8 hours plus an additional dose of 300 mg (2100 mg/day) had serum and amniotic fluid levels of 5.8 and 10.6 μg/ml, respectively, 10 days prior to term (6). Three days later, 10 hours after the last dose, a healthy male infant was delivered by elective cesarean section. Quinidine concentrations in the serum, cord blood, and amniotic fluid were 3.4, 2.8, and 9.3 μg/ml, respectively (6). The cord blood:serum ratio was 0.82. The cord blood levels were greater than those measured in three other reports (1, 7, 8). In a 1984 study, three women maintained on quinidine, 300 mg every 6 hours, and digoxin had serum levels of quinidine at delivery ranging from 0.7–2.1 μg/ml (7). A quinidine level in one amniotic fluid sample was 0.9 μg/ml, while cord blood levels ranged from <0.5–1.6 μg/ml. In two of the three cases, cord blood:serum ratios were 0.2 and 0.9. In a 1985 report, a woman taking quinidine, 400 mg every 6 hours, plus digoxin and propranolol was electively delivered by cesarean section 18 hours after the last dose (8). The quinidine concentration in the cord blood was 0.8 μg/ml. The last case involved a woman in whom quinidine doses were escalated over a 6-day interval from 300 mg every 6 hours to 1500 mg every 6 hours (1). On day 8, dosage was reduced to 1500 mg every 8 hours, then to 1200 mg every 8 hours on day 9, and then stopped on day 10. Amniotic fluid levels of quinidine and the metabolite, 3-hydroxyquinidine, on day 10 were 2.2 and 9.7 μg/ml, respectively. At delivery 2 days later, cord blood contained 0.5 μg/ml of quinidine and 0.7 μg/ml of the metabolite.

The drug has been used in combination with digoxin to treat fetal supraventricular and reciprocating atrioventricular tachycardia (7, 8). The authors of one of these reports consider quinidine to be the drug of choice after digoxin for the treatment of persistent fetal tachyrhythmias (8).

A mother treated with quinidine for a fetal supraventricular tachycardia developed symptoms of quinidine toxicity consisting of severe nausea and vomiting, diarrhea, light-headedness, and tinnitus (1). ECG changes were consistent with quinidine toxicity. Her dosage had been increased over an interval of 6 days in a manner described above producing serum quinidine levels of 1.4–3.3 μg/ml (therapeutic range in the author's laboratory was 1.5–5.0 μg/ml) (1). At the highest dose, her serum level was 2.3 μg/ml. Levels of the metabolite, 3-hydroxyquinidine, rose from 1.1 μg/ml to 6.8 μg/ml over the 6-day interval, eventually reaching 9.7 μg/ml 1 day after quinidine was discontinued. The 3-hydroxyquinidine:quinidine ratio varied from 0.8 (on day 2) to 3.7 (on day 10). These ratios were much higher than those observed in previously reported patients (1). Since the fetal heart rate continued to be elevated, with only occasional reductions to 120–130 beats/minute, and fetal lung maturity had been demonstrated, labor was induced, resulting in the delivery of a 3540-g infant with hydrops fetalis. The infant required pharmacologic therapy to control the supraventricular tachycardia. The maternal toxicity was attributed to the elevated levels of 3-hydroxyquinidine, since concentrations of quinidine were in the low to mid-therapeutic range (1).

In an *in vitro* study using plasma from 16 normal pregnant women, quinidine concentrations between 0.5–5.0 µg/ml were shown to inhibit plasma pseudocholinesterase activity (9). Inhibition varied from 29% (0.5 µg/ml) to 71% (5.0 µg/ml). Pseudocholinesterase is responsible for the metabolism of succinylcholine and ester-type local anesthetics (e.g., procaine, tetracaine, cocaine, and chloroprocaine) (9). The quinidine-induced inhibition of this enzyme, which is already significantly decreased by pregnancy itself, could potentially result in toxicity if these agents were used in a mother maintained on quinidine.

The use of quinidine during pregnancy has been classified in reviews of cardiovascular drugs as relatively safe for the fetus (10–12). The oxytocic properties of quinidine have not been observed in gravid patients, but high doses may produce this effect (13).

Breast Feeding Summary

Quinidine is excreted into breast milk (6). A woman taking 600 mg every 8 hours had milk and serum concentrations determined on the 5th postpartum day, 3 hours after a dose (6). Levels in the two samples were 6.4 and 9.0 µg/ml, respectively, a milk:serum ratio of 0.71. A quinidine level of 8.2 µg/ml was noted in a milk sample on the preceding day (time relationship to the dose not specified) but a simultaneous serum concentration was not determined. The infant in this case did not breast feed. The American Academy of Pediatrics considers quinidine to be compatible with breast feeding (14).

References

1. Killeen AA, Bowers LD. Fetal supraventricular tachycardia treated with high-dose quinidine: toxicity associated with marked elevation of the metabolite, 3(S)-3-hydroxyquinidine. Obstet Gynecol 1987;70:445–9.
2. Meyer J, Lackner JE, Schochet SS. Paroxysmal tachycardia in pregnancy. JAMA 1930;94:1901–4.
3. McMillan TM, Bellet S. Ventricular paroxysmal tachycardia: report of a case in a pregnant girl of sixteen years with an apparently normal heart. Am Heart J 1931;7:70–8.
4. Mendelson CL. Disorders of the heartbeat during pregnancy. Am J Obstet Gynecol 1956;72:1268–1301.
5. Domula VM, Weissach G, Lenk H. Uber die auswirkung medikamentoser behandlung in der schwangerschaft auf das gerennungspotential des neugeborenen. Zentralbl Gynaekol 1977;99:473.
6. Hill LM, Malkasian GD Jr. The use of quinidine sulfate throughout pregnancy. Obstet Gynecol 1979;54:366–8.
7. Spinnato JA, Shaver DC, Flinn GS, Sibai BM, Watson DL, Marin-Garcia J. Fetal supraventricular tachycardia: in utero therapy with digoxin and quinidine. Obstet Gynecol 1984;64:730–5.
8. Guntheroth WG, Cyr DR, Mack LA, Benedetti T, Lenke RR, Petty CN. Hydrops from reciprocating atrioventricular tachycardia in a 27-week fetus requiring quinidine for conversion. Obstet Gynecol 1985;66(Suppl):29S–33S.
9. Kambam JR, Franks JJ, Smith BE. Inhibitory effect of quinidine on plasma pseudocholinesterase activity in pregnant women. Am J Obstet Gynecol 1987;157:897–9.
10. Rotmensch HH, Elkayam U, Frishman W. Antiarrhythmic drug therapy during pregnancy. Ann Intern Med 1983;98:487–97.
11. Tamari I, Eldar M, Rabinowitz B, Neufeld HN. Medical treatment of cardiovascular disorders during pregnancy. Am Heart J 1982;104:1357–63.
12. Rotmensch HH, Rotmensch S, Elkayam U. Management of cardiac arrhythmias during pregnancy: current concepts. Drugs 1987;33:623–33.
13. Bigger JT, Hoffman BF. Antiarrythmic drugs. In Gilman AG, Goodman LS, Gilman A eds. *The Pharmacological Basis of Therapeutics*, 6th ed. New York:MacMillan, 1980:768.

14. Committee on Drugs, American Academy of Pediatrics. Transfer of drugs and other chemicals into human milk. Pediatrics 1989;84:924–36.

Name: **QUININE**

Class: **Plasmodicide**   Risk Factor: **D***

Fetal Risk Summary

Nishimura and Tanimura (1) summarized the human case reports of teratogenic effects linked with quinine in 21 infants who were exposed during the 1st trimester after unsuccessful abortion attempts (some infants had multiple defects and are listed more than once):

Central nervous system anomalies (CNS) (6 with hydrocephalus) (10 cases)
Limb defects (3 dysmelias) (8 cases)
Facial defects (7 cases)
Heart defects (6 cases)
Digestive organ anomalies (5 cases)
Urogenital anomalies (3 cases)
Hernias (3 cases)
Vertebral anomaly (1 case)

The malformations noted are varied, although CNS anomalies and limb defects were the most frequent. Auditory defects and optic nerve damage have also been reported (1–5). These reports usually concern the use of quinine in toxic doses as an abortifacient. Quinine has also been used for the induction of labor in women with intrauterine fetal death (6). Epidemiologic observations do not support an increased teratogenic risk or increased risk of congenital deafness over non-quinine-exposed patients (1, 7). Neonatal and maternal thrombocytopenia purpura and hemolysis in glucose-6-phosphate dehydrogenase-deficient newborns has been reported (8, 9).

Quinine has effectively been replaced by newer agents for the treatment of malaria. Although no increased teratogenic risk can be documented, its use during pregnancy should be avoided. One manufacturer considers the drug to be contraindicated in pregnancy (10). However, some investigators believe quinine should be used for the treatment of chloroquine-resistant *Plasmodium falciparum* malaria (11).

[*Risk Factor X according to manufacturer — Merrell Dow, 1990.]

Breast Feeding Summary

Quinine is excreted into breast milk. Following 300- and 640-mg oral doses in six patients, milk concentrations varied up to 2.2 μg/ml with an average level of 1 μg/ml at 3 hours (12). No adverse effects were reported in the nursing infants. Patients at risk for glucose-6-phosphate dehydrogenase deficiency should not be breast fed until this disease can be ruled out. The American Academy of Pediatrics considers quinine to be compatible with breast feeding (13).

References

1. Nishimura H, Tanimura T. *Clinical Aspects of the Teratogenicity of Drugs.* Amsterdam:Excerpta Medica, 1976:140–3.
2. Robinson GC, Brummitt JR, Miller JR. Hearing loss in infants and preschool children. II. Etiological considerations. Pediatrics 1963;32:115–24.
3. West RA. Effect of quinine upon auditory nerve. Am J Obstet Gynecol 1938;36:241–8.
4. McKinna AJ. Quinine induced hypoplasia of the optic nerve. Can J Ophthalmol 1966;1:261.
5. Morgon A, Charachon D, Brinquier N. Disorders of the auditory apparatus caused by embryopathy or foetopathy. Prophylaxis and treatment. Acta Otolaryngol (Stockh) 1971;291(Suppl):5.
6. Mukherjee S, Bhose LN. Induction of labor and abortion with quinine infusion in intrauterine fetal deaths. Am J Obstet Gynecol 1968;101:853–4.
7. Heinonen OP, Slone D, Shapiro S. *Birth Defects and Drugs in Pregnancy.* Littleton:Publishing Sciences Group, 1977:299,302,333.
8. Mauer MA, DeVaux W, Lahey ME. Neonatal and maternal thrombocytopenic purpura due to quinine. Pediatrics 1957;19:84–7.
9. Glass L, Rajegowda BK, Bowne E, Evans HE. Exposure to quinine and jaundice in a glucose-6-phosphate dehydrogenase-deficient newborn infant. Pediatrics 1973;82:734–5.
10. Product information. Quinamm. Merrell Dow, 1990.
11. Strang A, Lachman E, Pitsoe SB, Marszalek A, Philpott RH. Malaria in pregnancy with fatal complications: case report. Br J Obstet Gynaecol 1984;91:399–403.
12. Terwilliger WG, Hatcher RA. The elimination of morphine and quinine in human milk. Surg Gynecol Obstet 1934;58:823–6.
13. Committee on Drugs, American Academy of Pediatrics. Transfer of drugs and other chemicals into human milk. Pediatrics 1989;84:924–36.

Name: **RANITIDINE**

Class: **Histamine (H$_2$) Receptor Antagonist**   Risk Factor: **B$_M$**

Fetal Risk Summary

The use of ranitidine in the 1st trimester has not been reported. Ranitidine crosses the placenta at term to produce a cord blood:maternal serum ratio of 0.9 (1). The drug has been used alone and in combination with antacids to prevent gastric acid aspiration (Mendelson's syndrome) prior to vaginal delivery or cesarean section (1–3). No effect was observed in the frequency and strength of uterine contractions, in fetal heart rate pattern, or in Apgar scores (1). Neonatal gastric acidity was not affected at 24 hours (1). No problems in the newborn attributable to ranitidine were reported in these studies.

Breast Feeding Summary

Following a single oral dose of 150 mg in six subjects, ranitidine milk concentrations increased with time, producing mean milk:plasma ratios at 2, 4, and 6 hours of 1.9, 2.8, and 6.7, respectively (4). The effect of these concentrations on the nursing infant is not known. Ranitidine decreases gastric acidity, but this effect has not been studied in nursing infants. However, cimetidine, an agent with similar activity, is considered to be compatible during breast feeding by the American Academy of Pediatrics (5).

References

1. McAuley DM, Moore J, Dundee JW, McCaughey W. Preliminary report on the use of ranitidine as an antacid in obstetrics. Ir J Med Sci 1982;151:91–2.
2. Gillett GB, Watson JD, Langford RM. Prophylaxis against acid aspiration syndrome in obstetric practice. Anesthesiology 1984;60:525.
3. Mathews HML, Wilson CM, Thompson EM, Moore J. Combination treatment with ranitidine and sodium bicarbonate prior to obstetric anaesthesia. Anaesthesia 1986;41:1202–6.
4. Riley AJ, Crowley P, Harrison C. Transfer of ranitidine to biological fluids: milk and semen. In Misiewicz JJ, Wormsley KG, eds. *Proceedings of the 2nd International Symposium on Ranitidine,* London. Oxford:Medicine Publishing Foundation, 1981:78–81.
5. Committee on Drugs, American Academy of Pediatrics. Transfer of drugs and other chemicals into human milk. Pediatrics 1989;84:924–36.

Name: **RESERPINE**

Class: **Antihypertensive**   Risk Factor: **D**

Fetal Risk Summary

The Collaborative Perinatal Project monitored 50,282 mother-child pairs, 48 of which had 1st trimester exposure to reserpine (1, p. 376). There were four defects with 1st trimester use. Although this incidence (8%) is greater than the expected frequency of occurrence, no major category or individual malformations were identified. For use anytime in pregnancy, 475 exposures were recorded (1, p. 441). Malformations included:

Microcephaly (7 cases)
Hydronephrosis (3 cases)
Hydroureter (3 cases)
Inguinal hernia (12 cases)

Incidence of these latter malformations was not found to be statistically significant (1, p. 495). Reserpine crosses the placenta. Use of reserpine near term has resulted in nasal discharge, retraction, lethargy, and anorexia in the newborn (2). Concern over the ability of reserpine to deplete catecholamine levels has appeared (3). The significance of this is not known.

Breast Feeding Summary

Reserpine is excreted into breast milk (4). No clinical reports of adverse effects in the nursing infant have been located.

References

1. Heinonen OP, Slone D, Shapiro S. *Birth Defects and Drugs in Pregnancy.* Littleton:Publishing Sciences Group, 1977.
2. Budnick IS, Leikin S, Hoeck LE. Effect in the newborn infant to reserpine administration ante partum. Am J Dis Child 1955;90:286–9.
3. Towell ME, Hyman AI. Catecholamine depletion in pregnancy. J Obstet Gynaecol Br Commonw 1966;73:431–8.
4. Product information. Diupres. Merck Sharpe & Dohme, 1990.

Name: **RIBAVIRIN**

Class: **Antiviral**   Risk Factor: X_M

Fetal Risk Summary

Ribavirin is teratogenic and/or embryolethal in nearly all animal species tested (1). According to the manufacturer, ribavirin is still present in human blood 4 weeks after dosing (1). Only a single case of human pregnancy exposure has been located (2). A 34-year-old woman, at 33 weeks' gestation, was treated with ribavirin inhalation therapy for influenza pneumonia complicated by respiratory failure. Shortly after treatment, a cesarean section was performed because of worsening maternal cardiopulmonary function. A normal female infant was delivered, who is alive and well at 1 year of age.

The Centers for Disease Control and the manufacturer consider the use of ribavirin during pregnancy to be contraindicated (1, 3). In a 1988 statement addressing the issue of ribavirin exposure among health care personnel, the CDC commented: ". . . health-care workers who are pregnant, or may become pregnant should be advised of the potential risks of exposure during direct patient care when patients are receiving ribavirin through oxygen tent or mist mask and should be counseled about risk-reduction strategies, including alternative job responsibilities" (3).

Breast Feeding Summary

No data are available.

References

1. Product information. Virazole. ICN Pharmaceuticals, 1990.
2. Kirshon B, Faro S, Zurawin RK, Samo TC, Carpenter RJ. Favorable outcome after treatment with amantadine and ribavirin in a pregnancy complicated by influenza pneumonia: a case report. J Reprod Med 1988;33:399–401.
3. Centers for Disease Control. Assessing exposures of health-care personnel to aerosols of ribavirin-California. MMWR 1988;37:560–3.

Name: **RIBOFLAVIN**

Class: **Vitamin**   Risk Factor: **A***

Fetal Risk Summary

Riboflavin (Vitamin B_2), a water-soluble B complex vitamin, acts as a coenzyme in humans and is essential for tissue respiration systems (1). The American recommended daily allowance (RDA) for riboflavin in pregnancy is 1.5–1.6 mg (2).

The vitamin is actively transferred to the fetus, resulting in higher concentrations of riboflavin in the newborn than in the mother (3–13). The placenta converts flavin-adenine dinucleotide existing in the maternal serum to free riboflavin found in the fetal circulation (6, 7). This allows retention of the vitamin by the fetus since the transfer of free riboflavin back to the mother is inhibited (7, 13). At term, mean riboflavin values in 174 mothers were 184 ng/ml (range 80–390) and in their newborns 318 ng/ml (range 136–665) (8). In a more recent study, the cord serum concentration was 158 nmol/L compared to 113 nmol/L in the maternal serum (12).

The incidence of riboflavin deficiency in pregnancy is low (8, 14). In two studies, no correlation was discovered between the riboflavin status of the mother and the outcome of pregnancy even when riboflavin deficiency was present (15, 16). A 1977 study found no difference in riboflavin levels between infants of low and normal birth weight (11).

Riboflavin deficiency is teratogenic in animals (17). Although human teratogenicity has not been reported, low riboflavin levels were found in six mothers who had given birth to infants with neural tube defects (18). Other vitamin deficiencies present in these women were thought to be of more significance (see Folic Acid and Vitamin B_{12}).

A mother has been described with multiple acylcoenzyme A dehydrogenase deficiency probably related to riboflavin metabolism (19). The mother had given birth to a healthy child followed by one stillbirth and six infants who had been breast fed and died in early infancy after exhibiting a strong sweaty foot odor. In her 9th and 10th pregnancies, she was treated with 20 mg/day of riboflavin during the 3rd trimesters and delivered healthy infants. The authors thought the maternal symptoms were consistent with a mild form of acute fatty liver of pregnancy.

[*Risk Factor C if used in doses above the RDA.]

Breast Feeding Summary

Riboflavin (Vitamin B_2) is excreted in human breast milk (20–24). Well-nourished lactating women were given supplements of a multivitamin preparation containing 2.0 mg of riboflavin (20). At 6 months postpartum, milk concentrations of riboflavin did not differ significantly from those in control patients not receiving supplements. In a study of lactating women with low nutritional status, supplementation with riboflavin in doses of 0.10–10.0 mg/day resulted in mean milk concentrations of 200–740 ng/ml (21). Milk concentrations were directly proportional to dietary intake. A 1983 English study measured riboflavin levels in pooled human milk obtained from preterm (26 mothers: 29–34 weeks) and term (35 mothers: 39 weeks or longer) patients (22). Preterm milk rose from 276 ng/ml (colostrum) to 360 ng/ml (6–15 days) and then fell to 266 ng/ml (16–196 days). Over approximately the same time frame, term milk levels were 288, 279, and 310 ng/ml. In a Finnish study, premature infants (mean gestational age 30.1 weeks) fed human milk, but without riboflavin supplementation, became riboflavin deficient by 6 weeks of age (25).

The American RDA for riboflavin during lactation is 1.7–1.8 mg (2). If the diet of the lactating woman adequately supplies this amount, supplementation with riboflavin is not needed (23). Maternal supplementation with the RDA for riboflavin is recommended for those women with inadequate nutritional intake. The American Academy of Pediatrics considers maternal consumption of riboflavin to be compatible with breast feeding (26).

References

1. American Hospital Formulary Service. *Drug Information 1990*. Bethesda:American Society of Hospital Pharmacists, 1990:2118–20.
2. *Recommended Dietary Allowances*, 9th ed. Washington:National Academy of Sciences, 1980.
3. Hill EP, Longo LD. Dynamics of maternal-fetal nutrient transfer. Fed Proc 1980;39:239–44.
4. Lust JE, Hagerman DD, Villee CA. The transport of riboflavin by human placenta. J Clin Invest 1954;33:38–40.
5. Frank O, Walbroehl G, Thomason A, Kaminetzky H, Kubes Z, Baker H. Placental transfer: fetal retention of some vitamins. Am J Clin Nutr 1970;23:662–3.
6. Kaminetzky HA, Baker H, Frank O, Langer A. The effects of intravenously administered water-soluble vitamins during labor in normovitaminemic and hypovitaminemic gravidas on maternal and neonatal blood vitamin levels at delivery. Am J Obstet Gynecol 1974;120:697–703.
7. Kaminetzky HA, Baker H. Micronutrients in pregnancy. Clin Obstet Gynecol 1977;20:363–80.
8. Baker H, Frank O, Thomason AD, Langer A, Munves ED, De Angelis B, Kaminetzky HA. Vitamin profile of 174 mothers and newborns at parturition. Am J Clin Nutr 1975;28:59–65.
9. Baker H, Frank O, Deangelis B, Feingold S, Kaminetzky HA. Role of placenta in maternal-fetal vitamin transfer in humans. Am J Obstet Gynecol 1981;141:792–6.
10. Bamji MS. Enzymic evaluation of thiamin, riboflavin and pyridoxine status of parturient women and their newborn infants. Br J Nutr 1976;35:259–65.
11. Baker H, Thind IS, Frank O, DeAngelis B, Caterini H, Lquria DB. Vitamin levels in low-birth-weight newborn infants and their mothers. Am J Obstet Gynecol 1977;129:521–4.
12. Kirshenbaum NW, Dancis J, Levitz M, Lehanka J, Young BK. Riboflavin concentration in maternal and cord blood in human pregnancy. Am J Obstet Gynecol 1987;157:748–52.
13. Dancis J, Lehanka J, Levitz M. Placental transport of riboflavin: differential rates of uptake at the maternal and fetal surfaces of the perfused human placenta. Am J Obstet Gynecol 1988;158:204–10.

14. Dostalova L. Correlation of the vitamin status between mother and newborn during delivery. Dev Pharmacol Ther 1982;4(Suppl 1):45–57.

15. Vir SC, Love AHG, Thompson W. Riboflavin status during pregnancy. Am J Clin Nutr 1981;34:2699–2705.

16. Heller S, Salkeld RM, Korner WF. Riboflavin status in pregnancy. Am J Clin Nutr 1974;27:1225–30.

17. Shepard TH. Catalog of Teratogenic Agents, ed. 3. Baltimore:The Johns Hopkins University Press, 1980:288–9.

18. Smithells RW, Sheppard S, Schorah CJ. Vitamin deficiencies and neural tube defects. Arch Dis Child 1976;51:944–50.

19. Harpey JP, Charpentier C. Acute fatty liver of pregnancy. Lancet 1983;1:586–7.

20. Thomas MR, Sneed SM, Wei C, Nail PA, Wilson M, Sprinkle EE III. The effects of vitamin C, vitamin B$_6$, vitamin B$_{12}$, folic acid, riboflavin, and thiamin on the breast milk and maternal status of well-nourished women at 6 months postpartum. Am J Clin Nutr 1980;33:2151–6.

21. Deodhar AD, Rajalakshmi R, Ramakrishnan CV. Studies on human lactation. Part III. Effect of dietary vitamin supplementation on vitamin contents of breast milk. Acta Paediatr Scand 1964;53:42–8.

22. Ford, JE, Zechalko A, Murphy J, Brooke OG. Comparison of the B vitamin composition of milk from mothers of preterm and term babies. Arch Dis Child 1983;58:367–72.

23. Nail PA, Thomas MR, Eakin R. The effect of thiamin and riboflavin supplementation on the level of those vitamins in human breast milk and urine. Am J Clin Nutr 1980;33:198–204.

24. Gunther M. Diet and milk secretion in women. Proc Nutr Soc 1968;27:77–82.

25. Ronnholm KAR. Need for riboflavin supplementation in small prematures fed human milk. Am J Clin Nutr 1986;43:1–6.

26. Committee on Drugs, American Academy of Pediatrics. Transfer of drugs and other chemicals into human milk. Pediatrics 1989;84:924–36.

Name: **RIFAMPIN**

Class: **Antituberculosis Agent**   Risk Factor: **C**

Fetal Risk Summary

No controlled studies have linked the use of rifampin with congenital defects (1, 2). One report described nine malformations in 204 pregnancies that went to term (3). This incidence, 4.4%, is similar to the expected frequency of defects in a healthy nonexposed population but higher than the 1.8% rate noted in other tuberculosis patients (3):

Anencephaly (one case)
Hydrocephalus (two cases)
Limb malformations (four cases)
Renal tract defects (one case)
Congenital hip dislocation (one case)

Several reviews have evaluated the available treatment of tuberculosis during pregnancy (4–6). All concluded that rifampin was not a proven teratogen and recommended use of the drug with isoniazid and ethambutol if necessary. Other reports on the use of the agent in pregnancy have observed no fetal harm (7, 8).

Rifampin crosses the placenta to the fetus (9–11). At term, the cord:maternal serum ratio ranged from 0.12–0.33 (10). In a second case involving pregnancy termination at 13 weeks' gestation, the fetal:maternal ratio 4 hours after a 300-mg dose was 0.23 (9).

Rifampin has been implicated as one of the agents responsible for hemorrhagic disease of the newborn (12). In one of the three infants affected, only laboratory evidence of hemorrhagic disease of the newborn was present, but in the other two, clinically evident bleeding was observed. Prophylactic vitamin K_1 is recommended to prevent this serious complication (see Phytonadione).

Rifampin may interfere with oral contraceptives, resulting in unplanned pregnancies (see Oral Contraceptives) (13).

Breast Feeding Summary

Rifampin is excreted into human milk. In one report, the concentrations were 1–3 μg/ml with about 0.05% of the daily dose appearing in the milk (14). In another study, milk levels were 3.4–4.9 μg/ml, 12 hours after a single 450-mg oral dose (15). Maternal plasma samples averaged 21.3 μg/ml, indicating a milk:plasma ratio of about 0.20. These amounts were thought to represent a very low risk to the nursing infant (16). No reports describing adverse effects in nursing infants have been located. The American Academy of Pediatrics considers rifampin to be compatible with breast feeding (17).

References

1. Reimers D. Missbildungen durch Rifampicin. Bericht ueber 2 faelle von normaler fetaler entwicklung nach rifampicin-therapie in der fruehsch wangerschaft. Munchen Med Wochenschr 1971;113:1690.
2. Warkany J. Antituberculous drugs. Teratology 1979;20:133–8.
3. Steen JSM, Stainton-Ellis DM. Rifampicin in pregnancy. Lancet 1977;2:604–5.
4. Snider DE, Layde PM, Johnson MW, Lyle MA. Treatment of tuberculosis during pregnancy. Am Rev Respir Dis 1980;122:65–79.
5. American Thoracic Society. Treatment of tuberculosis and tuberculosis infection in adults and children. Am Rev Respir Dis 1986;134:355–63.
6. Medchill MT, Gillum M. Diagnosis and management of tuberculosis during pregnancy. Obstet Gynecol Surv 1989;44:81–4.
7. Shneerson JM, Frances RS. Ethambutol in pregnancy: foetal exposure. Tubercle 1979;60:167–9.
8. Kingdon JCP, Kennedy DH. Tuberculosis meningitis in pregnancy. Br J Obstet Gynaecol 1989;96:233–5.
9. Rocker I. Rifampicin in early pregnancy. Lancet 1977;2:48.
10. Kenny MT, Strates B. Metabolism and pharmacokinetics of the antibiotic rifampin. Drug Metab Rev 1981;12:159–218.
11. Holdiness MR. Transplacental pharmacokinetics of the antituberculosis drugs. Clin Pharmacokinet 1987;13:125–9.
12. Eggermont E, Logghe N, Van De Casseye W, Casteels-Van Daele M, Jaeken J, Cosemans J, Verstraete M, Renaer M. Haemorrhagic disease of the newborn in the offspring of rifampicin and isoniazid treated mothers. Acta Paediatr Belg 1976;29:87–90.
13. Gupta KC, Ali MY. Failure of oral contraceptives with rifampicin. Med J Zambia 1980;15:23.
14. Vorherr H. Drug excretion in breast milk. Postgrad Med J 1974;56:97–104.
15. Lenzi E, Santuari S. Preliminary observations on the use of a new semi-synthetic rifamycin derivative in gynecology and obstetrics. Atti Accad Lancisiana Roma 1969;13(suppl 1):87–94. As cited in Snider DE Jr, Powell KE. Should women taking antituberculosis drugs breast-feed? Arch Intern Med 1984;144:589–90.
16. Snider DE Jr, Powell KE. Should women taking antituberculosis drugs breast-feed? Arch Intern Med 1984;144:589–90.
17. Committee on Drugs, American Academy of Pediatrics. Transfer of drugs and other chemicals into human milk. Pediatrics 1989;84:924–36.

Name: **RITODRINE**

Class: **Sympathomimetic (Adrenergic)**   Risk Factor: **B$_M$**

Fetal Risk Summary

Ritodrine is a β-sympathomimetic agent approved for the management of preterm labor. Although congenital malformations due to ritodrine have not been observed, experience with the drug prior to the 20th week of gestation is very limited and no reports of 1st trimester use have been located. The manufacturer considers ritodrine to be contraindicated before the 20th week of gestation (1).

Ritodrine rapidly crosses the placenta, appearing in cord blood in amounts ranging from 26–117% of the maternal level (2–5). The mean cord:maternal venous blood ratio in eight of nine women delivering at a gestational length of 32 weeks' or greater was 0.67 (2). In experiments utilizing an *in vitro* perfused lobe of human placental tissue, ritodrine was shown to diffuse freely to the fetal side (3). Maternal and fetal plasma concentrations were determined in 28 women-infant pairs who had been treated with intravenous ritodrine for preterm labor but who progressed to delivery in spite of the therapy (4). A mean cord:maternal venous ratio of 1.17 (range 0.79–2.24) was measured. In addition, ritodrine levels greater than 10 ng/ml in both maternal and fetal venous samples were present up to 5 hours after cessation of ritodrine therapy with detectable concentrations present up to 16.5 hours. Umbilical cord vein ritodrine levels up to 7 ng/ml were measured at this latter time. Fetal concentrations were closely correlated with maternal dose and the time interval between cessation of intravenous therapy and delivery (4). In a study of the placental passage of ritodrine utilizing seven healthy women undergoing elective cesarean section at 39–40 weeks' gestation, ritodrine was infused at a rate of 72–149 μg/minute for 161–335 minutes (5). The mean umbilical:maternal venous blood ratio in this study was only 0.263 (range 0.066–0.544). The mean ritodrine concentrations (approximately 21–24 ng/ml) in umbilical vein, umbilical artery, and amniotic fluid were similar. In an investigation of the effects of ritodrine on fetal and placental blood flow, no significant changes in either intervillous or umbilical vein blood flows were noted at 1 hour in 14 women with premature uterine contractions at 31–36 weeks of gestation given ritodrine at 200 μg/minute (6). A comparison of the pharmacokinetics of orally administered ritodrine in pregnant and nonpregnant women has been published (7).

The effects of ritodrine on the mother, the fetus, and the newborn have been the subject of several reviews (8–11). Maternal complications may occur frequently with intravenous therapy, especially when the dose is rapidly increased. The more serious adverse effects include tachycardia, pulmonary edema, myocardial ischemia, cardiac arrhythmias, hyperglycemia followed by a rise in serum insulin levels, and hypokalemia. Severe maternal hypoglycemia secondary to hyperinsulinemia has been reported in a woman following a cesarean section for triplets (12). The woman had been treated prophylactically with oral ritodrine from 15–32 weeks' gestation and then with intravenous ritodrine or high dose oral therapy for another 12 days. Delivery occurred at approximately 34 weeks' gestation. Symptoms of hypoglycemia, including unconsciousness, occurred slightly more than 24 hours after delivery with blood glucose levels as low as 20 mg/100 ml and plasma insulin levels up to 19.4 mU/L. Normal glucose levels finally returned about 5 days later. Other causes of the hyperinsulinemia were excluded, and the investigators concluded that the condition was most likely due to prolonged ritodrine therapy.

Severe fetal and neonatal complications of ritodrine therapy occur infrequently. Increases in fetal heart rate are the most commonly observed manifestation of toxicity. Fetal heart rates up to 200 beats/minute have been recorded (1, 8–10). Neonatal cardiac arrhythmias have been reported in three newborns exposed in utero to intravenous ritodrine (13–15). One infant presented with paroxysmal supraventricular tachycardia involving short bursts up to 300 beats/minute with cyanosis and right cardiac failure occurring 10 minutes, 42 hours, and 60 hours after birth (13). The heart rate converted spontaneously to sinus rhythm a minute after each occurrence. Digitalization, continued until age 2 months, may have prevented further episodes of the arrhythmia in this infant, but therapy was not required in a second case. In this newborn, the episodes of tachyarrhythmias first presented at 11 hours of age and then decreased in frequency until 24 hours of age, after which no further episodes were observed (14). A third case involved a newborn twin with hydrops fetalis who experienced atrial fibrillation at birth with tachycardia and congestive heart failure most likely due to maternal treatment with intravenous ritodrine (15).

Disproportionate septal hypertrophy (DSH), defined as an interventricular septal thickness/posterior left ventricular wall thickness ratio (ST/PW) of greater than 1.3, was observed in infants exposed in utero to ritodrine for 2 weeks or longer (16). Compared to 22 control infants matched for gestational age, the mean ST/PW ratios for all ritodrine-exposed newborns ($N = 41$) and for a subset of infants exposed for 2 weeks or longer ($N = 22$) were significantly ($p < 0.05$) increased. Ritodrine exposure of less than 2 weeks did not cause DSH. However, significant posterior wall thinning was observed in all exposed infants (mean duration of therapy was 16.2 days, range 1–49 days). In those infants exposed for 2 weeks or longer, DSH was due to an increasing interventricular septal thickness and a thinning posterior wall thickness. Both the ST/PW ratio and the septal thickness were highly correlated with duration of ritodrine exposure (16). The right systolic time interval was also significantly higher in the exposed infants compared to controls. The echocardiographic changes lasted for less than 3 months. Since there were no statistical differences in the mortality rates between the ritodrine and control groups, the clinical significance of these findings is unknown. Possible mechanisms for the defects were thought to include chronic fetal tachycardia, increased glycogen deposition, pulmonary hypertension, or genetic factors (16).

Use of ritodrine may result in transient maternal and fetal hyperglycemia followed by increases in levels of serum insulin. If delivery occurs before these effects have terminated (usually 48–72 hours), hypoglycemia in the newborn may occur (17). Severe maternal ketoacidosis with fetal death has been reported (18). An insulin-dependent diabetic was treated with intravenous ritodrine up to 0.3 mg/min for preterm labor at 28 weeks of gestation. Fetal heart patterns were normal prior to therapy. Maternal hyperglycemia with ketoacidosis developed after 26 hours of therapy and 6 hours later fetal heart activity was undetectable. She was subsequently delivered of a stillborn 970-g fetus with cheilognathouranoschisis but no other abnormalities either in the fetus or the placenta.

A 1989 study compared indomethacin, administered for 48 hours, with intravenous ritodrine (initiated at 50 μg/minute, then titrated, based on response, to a maximum of 350 μg/minute) in 106 women in preterm labor with intact membranes who were at a gestational age of 32 weeks or less (19). Fifty-four women received ritodrine and 52 received indomethacin. Thirteen (24%) of the ritodrine group developed adverse drug reactions severe enough to require discontinuance of the drug and a change to magnesium sulfate: cardiac arrhythmia (one), chest pain (two), tachycardia (three), and hypotension (seven). None of the indomethacin cases developed drug intolerance ($p < 0.01$). For all maternal adverse drug reactions, 39 (72%) of those treated with ritodrine had a side effect versus six (11.5%) of the indomethacin group ($p < 0.01$). The outcomes of the pregnancies were similar, regardless of whether delivery occurred close to or remote from therapy. Of those delivered within 48 hours of initiation of therapy, the mean glucose level in the ritodrine-exposed newborns ($N = 9$) was significantly higher than that in those exposed to indomethacin ($N = 8$), 198 mg/dL vs. 80 mg/dL ($p < 0.05$), respectively. No cases of premature closure of the ductus arteriosus or pulmonary hypertension were observed. A reduction in amniotic fluid volume was noted in three (5.6%) of the ritodrine group and in six (11.5%) of those treated with indomethacin. On a cost basis, tocolysis with indomethacin was 17 times less costly than tocoloysis with ritodrine (19).

Ritodrine-induced neonatal hypoglycemia appears to be related to the route of drug administration. In a double blind comparison of 17 mothers treated with intravenous, followed by oral, ritodrine for a mean duration of 9 days vs. 18 control mothers treated with placebo for 10 days, no significant differences between the groups were measured up to 12 hours of age in terms of heart rate, blood pressure, blood volume (measured at 12–24 hours of age), arterial or venous pH, plasma insulin, or blood glucose (20). In contrast, neonatal hypoglycemia (defined as less than 45 mg/100 ml) was found in 32% (17 of 53) of newborns exposed to intravenous ritodrine within 12 hours of birth compared to 15% (8 of 54) of controls matched for gestational age and birth weight ($p < 0.05$) (21). The mean onset of hypoglycemia was at 1.0 hour of age. Neither gestational age nor maternal ritodrine dose nor the interval between cessation of therapy and delivery correlated well with the onset. Other parameters not significantly different between the groups were Apgar scores, neonatal pH, plasma bicarbonate, hypotension, respiratory distress syndrome, and neonatal mortality. This lack of neonatal toxicity (other than hypoglycemia) has been confirmed by other studies. In a report involving 82 infants whose mothers had been treated with parenteral ritodrine, with or without oral therapy, for an average of 28.5 days compared to a similar number of matched controls, umbilical pH, Apgar scores, head circumference, and neurologic condition were statistically similar (22). Five study infants had neonatal jaundice compared to none of the controls, but the groups were statistically similar in the number of infants with bilirubin values above 5.2 mg/100 ml (28 and 23, respectively) (22). The investigators were unable to determine if ritodrine caused the increased incidence of jaundice.

Neonatal renal function was evaluated in 15 infants exposed in utero to ritodrine for at least 12 of the 24 hours prior to delivery compared to 15 matched controls (23). On day 1 (12–36 hours of age), exposed infants had significantly decreased glomerular filtration rates (as measured by inulin clearances), higher plasma renin activity, and higher urinary arginine vasopressin excretion than controls. These parameters were not statistically different between the groups on day 6. Both plasma renin activity and urinary arginine vasopressin excretion were statistically associated with plasma ritodrine levels (mean 16.6 ng/ml on day 1) but not inulin clearance. Correlations were not conducted on day 6 due to the low ritodrine levels (mean 1.0 ng/ml in six infants; less than 0.3 ng/ml in nine). The clinical significance of these findings is unknown since clinical signs of renal failure were not observed in any infant. Furthermore, serum and urine electrolyte values, osmolality, fractional sodium excretion, and urine flow rate were similar in treated and control infants.

In a 1988 review of 12 published and 4 unpublished "methodologically acceptable" controlled trials of β-sympatholytic tocolytic therapy, ritodrine was used in 12 (8 published/4 unpublished) (24). The total number of women involved in the ritodrine trials consisted of 412 treated and 329 controls. The outcomes analyzed, not all of which were available in each trial, were (a) delivery within 24 hours of trial entry; (b) delivery within 48 hours of trial entry; (c) delivery before 37 completed weeks; (d) birth weight below 2500 g; (e) respiratory distress syndrome or severe respiratory problems; and (f) perinatal death. The reviewers confirmed that ritodrine was effective in delaying delivery after preterm labor in comparison to placebo or other, nontocolytic therapy. The frequencies of both preterm birth and low birth weight were reduced. However, in contrast to the prevailing view that ritodrine decreases the incidence of neonatal death and respiratory distress syndrome (25–27), neither perinatal mortality nor severe neonatal respiratory problems were reduced. This raised important questions as to the clinical significance of the positive benefits (24). In attempting to explain their findings, the investigators speculated that the trials may have included too many women in whom tocolytic therapy was unlikely to benefit their fetuses. In addition, they concluded that only a small percentage of perinatal mortality resulted from pregnancies that might benefit from tocolytic therapy. The primary benefit of tocolytic therapy, in their opinion, was the attainment of short-term delay of delivery to allow transfer of the patient to medical centers with obstetric and neonatal intensive care facilities and to allow time for the beneficial effects of glucocorticoids on fetal lung development to appear.

Two-year follow-up studies of infants exposed in utero to ritodrine have failed to detect harmful effects on growth, incidence of disease, development, or functional maturation (28, 29). More recent studies have also failed to detect statistical evidence of adverse effects of ritodrine exposure (30, 31). In a study of 20 children examined at 7–9 years of age who had been exposed between 24–34 weeks' gestation, no significant differences were found compared to controls in physical growth (height and weight), neurologic parameters (motor, sensory, and cerebellar function), and psychometric testing (30). However, scores and measurements were consistently poorer, although not significantly, in the exposed group, even after correction for socioeconomic status. Most of the controls, however, had not experienced preterm labor, which may have affected the findings (30). A group of 78 6-year-old children exposed in utero at a mean gestational age of 32.1 weeks (range 12–37 weeks) for a mean duration of 28.2 days (range 7–163 days) was compared to two control groups composed of 78 children each (31). No significant differences between the three groups were discovered in urinalysis (including no glucosuria in any child), body length and weight, head circumference, neurologic findings, and general behavior as judged by their parents and teachers. The teachers, however, felt the exposed group did worse in school performance (motor and social skills, emotional and cognitive development). As in previous studies, the authors could not determine if the latter assessment was due to ritodrine exposure, an unfavorable obstetric situation, or other factors.

Breast Feeding Summary

No data are available.

References

1. Product information. Yutopar, Astra Pharmaceutical Products, 1990.
2. Gandar R, de Zoeten LW, van der Schoot JB. Serum level of ritodrine in man. Eur J Clin Pharmacol 1980;17:117–22.
3. Sodha RJ, Schneider H. Transplacental transfer of beta-adrenergic drugs studied by an in vitro perfusion method of an isolated human placental lobule. Am J Obstet Gynecol 1983;147:303–10.
4. Gross TL, Kuhnert BR, Kuhnert PM, Rosen MG, Kazzi NJ. Maternal and fetal plasma concentrations of ritodrine. Obstet Gynecol 1985;65:793–7.
5. Fujimoto S, Akahane M, Sakai A. Concentrations of ritodrine hydrochloride in maternal and fetal serum and amniotic fluid following intravenous administration in late pregnancy. Eur J Obstet Reprod Biol 1986;23:145–52.
6. Jouppila P, Kirkinen P, Koivula A, Ylikorkala O. Ritodrine infusion during late pregnancy: effects on fetal and placental blood flow, prostacyclin, and thromboxane. Am J Obstet Gynecol 1985;151:1028–32.
7. Cartis SN, Venkataramanan R, Cotroneo M, Chiao J-P. Pharmacokinetics of orally administered ritodrine. Am J Obstet Gynecol 1989;161:32–5.
8. Barden TP, Peter JB, Merkatz IR. Ritodrine hydrochloride: a betamimetic agent for use in preterm labor. I. Pharmacology, clinical history, administration, side effects, and safety. Obstet Gynecol 1980;56:1–6.
9. Anonymous. Ritodrine for inhibition of preterm labor. Med Lett Drugs Ther 1980;22:89–90.
10. Finkelstein BW. Ritodrine (Yutopar, Merrell Dow Pharmaceuticals Inc.). Drug Intell Clin Pharm 1981;15:425–33.
11. Benedetti TJ. Maternal complications of parenteral β-sympathomimetic therapy for premature labor. Am J Obstet Gynecol 1983;145:1–6.
12. Caldwell G, Scougall I, Boddy K, Toft AD. Fasting hyperinsulinemic hypoglycemia after ritodrine therapy for premature labor. Obstet Gynecol 1987;70:478–80.
13. Brosset P, Ronayette D, Pierre MC, Lorier BLE, Bouquier JJ. Cardiac complications of ritodrine in mother and baby. Lancet 1982;1:1468.
14. Hermansen MC, Johnson GL. Neonatal supraventricular tachycardia following prolonged maternal ritodrine administration. Am J Obstet Gynecol 1984;149:798–9.
15. Beitzke A, Winter R, Zach M, Grubbauer HM. Kongenitales vorhofflattern mit hydrops fetalis durch mutterliche tokolytikamedikation. Klin Paediatr 1979;191:410–7.
16. Nuchpuckdee P, Brodsky N, Porat R, Hurt H. Ventricular septal thickness and cardiac function in neonates after in utero ritodrine exposure. J Pediatr 1986;109:687–91.
17. Leake RD, Hobel CJ, Oh W, Thiebeault DW, Okada DM, Williams PR. A controlled, prospective study of the effects of ritodrine hydrochloride for premature labor. Clin Res 1980;28:90A (abstr).
18. Schilthuis MS, Aarnoudse JG. Fetal death associated with severe ritodrine induced ketoacidosis. Lancet 1980;1:1145.
19. Morales WJ, Smith SG, Angel JL, O'Brien WF, Knuppel RA. Efficacy and safety of indomethacin versus ritodrine in the management of preterm labor: a randomized study. Obstet Gynecol 1989;74:567–72.
20. Leake RD, Hobel CJ, Okada DM, Ross MG, Williams PR. Neonatal metabolic effects of oral ritodrine hydrochloride administration. Pediatr Pharmacol 1983;3:101–6.
21. Kazzi NJ, Gross TL, Kazzi GM, Williams TG. Neonatal complications following in utero exposure to intravenous ritodrine. Acta Obstet Gynecol Scand 1987;66:65–9.
22. Huisjes HJ, Touwen BCL. Neonatal outcome after treatment with ritodrine: a controlled study. Am J Obstet Gynecol 1983;147:250–3.
23. Hansen NB, Oh W, LaRochelle F, Stonestreet BS. Effects of maternal ritodrine administration on neonatal renal function. J Pediatr 1983;103:774–80.
24. King JF, Grant A, Keirse MJNC, Chalmers I. Beta-mimetics in preterm labour: an overview of the randomized controlled trials. Br J Obstet Gynaecol 1988;95:211–22.

25. Boog G, Ben Brahim M, Gandar R. Beta-mimetic drugs and possible prevention of respiratory distress syndrome. Br J Obstet Gynaecol 1975;82:285–8.

26. Merkatz IR, Peter JB, Barden TP. Ritodrine hydrochloride: a betamimetic agent for use in preterm labor. II. Evidence of efficacy. Obstet Gynecol 1980;56:7–12.

27. Laursen NH, Merkatz IR, Tejani N, et al. Inhibition of premature labor: a multicenter comparison of ritodrine and ethanol. Am J Obstet Gynecol 1977;127:837–45.

28. Freysz H, Willard D, Lehr A, Messer J, Boog G. A long term evaluation of infants who received a beta-mimetic drug while in utero. J Perinat Med 1977;5:94–9.

29. Product information and clinical summary of Yutopar. Merrell National Laboratories, Inc., Cincinnati, 1980.

30. Polowczyk D, Tejani N, Laursen N, Siddiq F. Evaluation of seven- to nine-year-old children exposed to ritodrine in utero. Obstet Gynecol 1984;64:485–8.

31. Hadders-Algra M, Touwen BCL, Huisjes HJ. Long-term follow-up of children prenatally exposed to ritodrine. Br J Obstet Gynaecol 1986;93:156–61.

Name: **SCOPOLAMINE**

Class: **Parasympatholytic (Anticholinergic)**   Risk Factor: **C**

Fetal Risk Summary

Scopolamine is an anticholinergic agent. The Collaborative Perinatal Project monitored 50,282 mother-child pairs, 309 of which used scopolamine in the 1st trimester (1, pp. 346–353). For anytime use, 881 exposures were recorded (1, p. 439). In neither case was evidence found for an association with malformations. However, when the group of parasympatholytics was taken as a whole (2,323 exposures), a possible association with minor malformations was found (1, pp. 346–353). Scopolamine readily crosses the placenta (2). When administered to the mother at term, fetal effects include tachycardia, decreased heart rate variability, and decreased heart rate deceleration (3–5). Maternal tachycardia is comparable to that with other anticholinergic agents, such as atropine or glycopyrrolate (6). Scopolamine toxicity in a newborn has been described (7). The mother had received six doses of scopolamine (1.8 mg total) with several other drugs during labor. Symptoms in the female infant consisted of fever, tachycardia, and lethargy; she was also "barrel chested" without respiratory depression. Therapy with physostigmine reversed the condition.

Breast Feeding Summary

See Atropine.

References

1. Heinonen OP, Slone D, Shapiro S. *Birth Defects and Drugs in Pregnancy*. Littleton:Publishing Sciences Group, 1977.
2. Moya F, Thorndike V. The effects of drugs used in labor on the fetus and newborn. Clin Pharmacol Ther 1963;4:628–53.
3. Shenker L. Clinical experiences with fetal heart rate monitoring of one thousand patients in labor. Am J Obstet Gynecol 1973;115:1111–6.
4. Boehm FH, Growdon JH Jr. The effect of scopolamine on fetal heart rate baseline variability. Am J Obstet Gynecol 1974;120:1099–1104.
5. Ayromlooi J, Tobias M, Berg P. The effects of scopolamine and ancillary analgesics upon the fetal heart rate recording. J Reprod Med 1980;25:323–6.
6. Diaz DM, Diaz SF, Marx GF. Cardiovascular effects of glycopyrrolate and belladonna derivatives in obstetric patients. Bull NY Acad Med 1980;56:245–8.
7. Evens RP, Leopold JC. Scopolamine toxicity in a newborn. Pediatrics 1980;329–30.

Name: **SECOBARBITAL**

Class: **Sedative/Hypnotic** Risk Factor: **D**$_M$

Fetal Risk Summary

No reports linking the use of secobarbital with congenital defects have been located. The Collaborative Perinatal Project monitored 50,282 mother-child pairs, 378 of which had 1st trimester exposure to secobarbital (1). No evidence was found to suggest a relationship to large categories of major or minor malformations or to individual defects. Hemorrhagic disease of the newborn and barbiturate withdrawal are theoretical possibilities (see also Phenobarbital).

An *in vitro* study found no evidence of chromosome changes on exposure to secobarbital (2).

Breast Feeding Summary

Secobarbital is excreted into breast milk (3). The amount and effects on the nursing infant are not known. The American Academy of Pediatrics considers secobarbital to be compatible with breast feeding (4).

References

1. Heinonen OP, Slone D, Shapiro S. *Birth Defects and Drugs in Pregnancy*. Littleton:Publishing Sciences Group, 1977:336–7.
2. Stenchever MA, Jarvis JA. Effect of barbiturates on the chromosomes of human cells in vitro—a negative report. J Reprod Med 1970;5:69–71.
3. Wilson JT, Brown RD, Cherek DR, Dailey JW, Hilman B, Jobe PC, Manno BR, Manno JE, Redetzki HM, Stewart JJ. Drug excretion in human breast milk: principles, pharmacokinetics and projected consequences. Clin Pharmacokinet 1980;5:1–66.
4. Committee on Drugs, American Academy of Pediatrics. Transfer of drugs and other chemicals into human milk. Pediatrics 1989;84:924–36.

Name: **SENNA**

Class: **Laxative** Risk Factor: **C**

Fetal Risk Summary

Senna, a naturally occurring laxative, contains the stereoisomeric glucosides, sennosides A and B. These anthraquinone glucosides are the main active cathartic agents of senna. Senna is not teratogenic in animals (1). No reports of human teratogenicity or other fetal toxicity have been located.

Breast Feeding Summary

Sennosides A and B are apparently not excreted into human breast milk. A 1973 study using colorimetric analysis (sensitivity limit 0.34 µg/ml) failed to detect the natural agents (2). This is compatible with the fact that the anthraquinone laxatives are absorbed only slightly after oral administration (3). Use of the laxative during lactation has been reported in three studies (2, 4, 5). Although diarrhea occurred in some of the infants, this was probably due to other causes, not to senna. In one of these studies, mothers who ingested a single 100-mg dose of senna (containing 8.6 mg of sennosides A and B) and whose infants developed diarrhea, were later given a double dose of the laxative (2). No diarrhea was observed in the infants after the higher dose. The American Academy of Pediatrics considers senna to be compatible with breast feeding (6).

References

1. Shepard TH. *Catalog of Teratogenic Agents*, ed 6. Baltimore:Johns Hopkins University Press, 1989:574–5.
2. Werthmann MW Jr, Krees SV. Quantitative excretion of Senokot in human breast milk. Med Ann Dist Col 1973;42:4–5.
3. American Hospital Formulary Service. *Drug Information 1990*. Bethesda:American Society of Hospital Pharmacists, 1990:1635.
4. Baldwin WF. Clinical study of senna administration to nursing mothers: assessment of effects on infant bowel habits. Can Med Assoc J 1963;89:566–8.
5. Greenhalf JO, Leonard HSD. Laxatives in the treatment of constipation in pregnant and breast-feeding mothers. Practitioner 1973;210:259–63.
6. Committee on Drugs, American Academy of Pediatrics. Transfer of drugs and other chemicals into human milk. Pediatrics 1989;84:924–36.

Name: **SIMETHICONE**

Class: **Antiflatulent/Defoaming Agent**   Risk Factor: **C**

Fetal Risk Summary

Simethicone is a silicone product that is used as an antiflatulent. No reports linking the use of this agent with congenital defects have been located.

Breast Feeding Summary

No data are available.

Name: **SODIUM IODIDE**

Class: **EXPECTORANT**   Risk Factor: **D**

Fetal Risk Summary

See Potassium Iodide.

Breast Feeding Summary

See Potassium Iodide.

Name: **SODIUM IODIDE I125**

Class: **Radiopharmaceutical**   Risk Factor: **X**

Fetal Risk Summary

See Sodium Iodide I131.

Breast Feeding Summary

See Sodium Iodide I131.

Name: **SODIUM IODIDE I131**

Class: **Radiopharmaceutical**   Risk Factor: **X**

Fetal Risk Summary

Sodium iodide I131 (^{131}I) is a radiopharmaceutical agent used for diagnostic procedures and for therapeutic destruction of thyroid tissue. The diagnostic dose is approximately one-thousandth of the therapeutic dose. Like all iodides, the drug concentrates in the thyroid gland. ^{131}I readily crosses the placenta. The fetal thyroid is able to accumulate ^{131}I by about the 12th week of gestation (1–3). At term, the maternal serum:cord blood ratio is 1 (4).

As suggested by the above studies on uptake of ^{131}I in fetal thyroids, maternal treatment with radioiodine early in the 1st trimester should not pose a significant danger to the fetus. Two reports describing ^{131}I therapy at 4 and 8 weeks' gestation resulting in normal infants seemingly confirmed the lack of risk (5, 6). However, a newborn has been described with a large head, exophthalmia, and thick, myxedematous-like skin who was exposed to ^{131}I at about 2 weeks' gestation (7). The infant died shortly after birth. In another early report, exposure to a diagnostic dose of ^{131}I during the middle of the 1st trimester was considered the cause of anomalies observed in the newborn including microcephaly, hydrocephaly, dysplasia of the hip joints, and clubfoot (8). Finally, ^{131}I administered 1–3 days prior to conception was suggested as the cause of a spontaneous abortion at the end of the 1st trimester (9). All three of these latter reports must be viewed with caution due to the uniqueness of the effects and/or the timing of the exposure. Factors other than radioiodine may have been involved.

Therapeutic doses of radioiodine administered near the end of the 1st trimester (12 weeks) or beyond usually result in partial or complete abolition of the fetal thyroid gland (10–20). This effect is dose dependent, however, as one mother was treated at 19 weeks' gestation with 6.1 mCi of ^{131}I apparently without causing fetal harm (2). In the pregnancies terminating with a hypothyroid infant, ^{131}I doses ranged from 10–225 mCi (10–20). Clinical features observed at or shortly after birth in 10 of the 12 newborns were consistent with congenital hypothyroidism. One of these infants was also discovered to have hypoparathyroidism (20). In one child, exposed *in utero* to repeated small doses over a 5-week period (total dose 12.2 mCi), hypothyroidism did not become evident until 4 years of age (17). Unusual anomalies observed in another infant included hydrocephaly, cardiopathy, genital hypotrophy, and a limb deformity (15).

In summary, sodium iodide I131 is a proven human teratogen. Because the effects of even small doses are not predictable, the use of the drug for diagnostic and therapeutic purposes should be avoided during pregnancy.

Breast Feeding Summary

Sodium iodide I131 is concentrated in breast milk (21–24). [125]I also appears in milk in significant quantities (25, 26). Uptake of ^{131}I contained in milk by an infant's thyroid gland has been observed (21). The time required for elimination of radioiodine from the milk may be as long as 14 days. Since this exposure may result in damage to the nursing infant's thyroid, including an increased risk of thyroid cancer, breast feeding should be stopped until radioactivity is no longer present in the milk (27).

References

1. Chapman EM, Corner GW Jr, Robinson D, Evans RD. The collection of radioactive iodine by the human fetal thyroid. J Clin Endocrinol Metab 1948;8:717–20.
2. Hodges RE, Evans TC, Bradbury JT, Keettel WC. The accumulation of radioactive iodine by human fetal thyroids. J Clin Endocrinol Metab 1955;15:661–7.
3. Shepard TH. Onset of function in the human fetal thyroid: biochemical and radioautographic studies from organ culture. J Clin Endocrinol Metab 1967;27:945–58.
4. Kearns JE, Hutson W. Tagged isomers and analogues of thyroxine (their transmission across the human placenta and other studies). J Nucl Med 1963;4:453–61.
5. Hollingsworth DR, Austin E. Observations following I[131] for Graves' disease during first trimester of pregnancy. South Med J 1969;62:1555–6.
6. Talbert LM, Thomas CG Jr, Holt WA, Rankin P. Hyperthyroidism during pregnancy. Obstet Gynecol 1970;36:779–85.
7. Valensi G, Nahum A. Action de l'iode radio-actif sur le foetus humain. Tunisie med 1958;36:69. As cited in Nishimura H, Tanimura T. *Clinical Aspects of the Teratogenicity of Drugs*. New York:American Elsevier, 1976:260.
8. Falk W. Beitrag zur Frage der menschlichen Fruchtschadigung durch kunstliche radioaktive Isotope. Medizinische 1959;22:1480. As cited in Nishimura H, Tanimura T. *Clinical Aspects of the Teratogenicity of Drugs*. New York:American Elsevier, 1976:260.
9. Berger M, Briere J. Les dangers de la therapeutique par l'iode radioactif au debut d'une grossesse ignoree. Bull Med leg Toxicol med 1967;10:37. As cited in Nishimura H, Tanimura T. *Clinical Aspects of the Teratogenicity of Drugs*. New York:American Elsevier, 1976:260.
10. Russell KP, Rose H, Starr P. The effects of radioactive iodine on maternal and fetal thyroid function during pregnancy. Surg Gynecol Obstet 1957;104:560–4.
11. Ray EW, Sterling K, Gardner LI. Congenital cretinism associated with I[131] therapy of the mother. Am J Dis Child 1959;98:506–7.
12. Hamill GC, Jarman JA, Wynne MD. Fetal effects of radioactive iodine therapy in a pregnant woman with thyroid cancer. Am J Obstet Gynecol 1961;81:1018–23.
13. Fisher WD, Voorhess ML, Gardner LI. Congenital hypothyroidism in infant following maternal I[131] therapy. J Pediatr 1963;62:132–46.
14. Pfannenstiel P, Andrews GA, Brown DW. Congenital hypothyroidism from intrauterine ^{131}I damage. In Cassalino C, Andreoli M, eds. *Current Topics in Thyroid Research*. New York:Academic Press, 1965:749. As cited in Nishimura H, Tanimura T. *Clinical Aspects of the Teratogenicity of Drugs*. New York:American Elsevier, 1976:260.
15. Sirbu P, Macarie E, Isaia V, Zugravesco A. L'influence de l'iode radio-actif sur le foetus. Bull Fed Soc Gynecol Obstet Franc 1968;20: Suppl 314. As cited in Nishimura H, Tanimura T. *Clinical Aspects of the Teratogenicity of Drugs*. New York:American Elsevier, 1976:260.
16. Hollingsworth DR, Austin E. Thyroxine derivatives in amniotic fluid. J Pediatr 1971;79:923–9.
17. Green HG, Gareis FJ, Shepard TH, Kelley VC. Cretinism associated with maternal sodium iodide I 131 therapy during pregnancy. Am J Dis Child 1971;122:247–9.

18. Jafek BW, Small R, Lillian DL. Congenital radioactive iodine-induced stridor and hypothyroidism. Arch Otolaryng 1974;99:369–71.
19. Exss R, Graewe B. Congenital athyroidism in the newborn infant from intra-uterine radioiodine action. Biol Neonate 1974;24:289–91.
20. Richards GE, Brewer ED, Conley SB, Saldana LR. Combined hypothyroidism and hypoparathyroidism in an infant after maternal ^{131}I administration. J Pediatr 1981;99:141–43.
21. Nurnberger CE, Lipscomb A. Transmission of radioiodine (I^{131}) to infants through human maternal milk. JAMA 1952;150:1398–1400.
22. Miller H, Weetch RS. The excretion of radioactive iodine in human milk. Lancet 1955;2:1013.
23. Weaver JC, Kamm ML, Dobson RL. Excretion of radioiodine in human milk. JAMA 1960;173:872–5.
24. Karjalainen P, Penttila IM, Pystynen P. The amount and form of radioactivity in human milk after lung scanning, renography and placental localization by ^{131}I labelled tracers. Acta Obstet Gynecol Scand 1971;50:357–61.
25. Bland EP, Crawford JS, Docker MF, Farr RF. Radioactive iodine uptake by thyroid of breast-fed infants after maternal blood-volume measurements. Lancet 1969;2:1039–41.
26. Palmer KE. Excretion of ^{125}I in breast milk following administration of labelled fibinogen. Br J Radiol 1979;52:672–3.
27. Committee on Drugs, American Academy of Pediatrics. Transfer of drugs and other chemicals into human milk. Pediatrics 1989;84:924–36.

Name: **SODIUM NITROPRUSSIDE**

Class: **Antihypertensive**   Risk Factor: **C**

Fetal Risk Summary

No reports linking the use of sodium nitroprusside with congenital defects have been located. Nitroprusside has been used in pregnancy to produce deliberate hypotension during aneurysm surgery or to treat severe hypertension (1–8). Transient fetal bradycardia was the only adverse effect noted (1). One advantage of nitroprusside is the very rapid onset of action and the return to pretreatment blood pressure levels when the drug is stopped (8). Balanced against this is the potential accumulation of cyanide in the fetus.

Sodium nitroprusside crosses the placenta and produces fetal cyanide concentrations higher than maternal levels in animals (9). This effect has not been studied in humans. A 1984 article reviewed the potential fetal toxicity of sodium nitroprusside (6). Avoidance of prolonged use and the monitoring of serum pH, plasma cyanide, red blood cell cyanide, and methemoglobin levels in the mother were recommended. Standard doses of nitroprusside apparently do not pose a major risk of excessive accumulation of cyanide in the fetal liver (6).

Breast Feeding Summary

No data are available.

References

1. Donchin Y, Amirav B, Sahar A, Yarkoni S. Sodium nitroprusside for aneurysm surgery in pregnancy. Br J Anaesth 1978;50:849–51.
2. Paull J. Clinical report of the use of sodium nitroprusside in severe pre-eclampsia. Anesth Intensive Care 1975;3:72.

3. Rigg D, McDonogh A. Use of sodium nitroprusside for deliberate hypotension during pregnancy. Br J Anaesth 1981;53:985–7.
4. Willoughby JS. Case reports: Sodium nitroprusside, pregnancy and multiple intracranial aneurysms. Anaesth Intensive Care 1984;12:358–60.
5. Stempel JE, O'Grady JP, Morton MJ, Johnson KA. Use of sodium nitroprusside in complications of gestational hypertension. Obstet Gynecol 1982;60:533–8.
6. Shoemaker CT, Meyers M. Sodium nitroprusside for control of severe hypertensive disease of pregnancy: a case report and discussion of potential toxicity. Am J Obstet Gynecol 1984;149:171–3.
7. Willoughby JS. Review article: sodium nitroprusside, pregnancy and multiple intracranial aneurysms. Anaesth Intensive Care 1984;12:351–7.
8. de Swiet M. Antihypertensive drugs in pregnancy. Br Med J 1985;291:365–6.
9. Lewis PE, Cefalo RC, Naulty JS, Rodkey RL. Placental transfer and fetal toxicity of sodium nitroprosside. Gynecol Invest 1977;8:46.

Name: **SOMATOSTATIN**

Class: **Pituitary Hormone**   Risk Factor: **B**

Fetal Risk Summary

No data are available.

Breast Feeding Summary

No data are available.

Name: **SPECTINOMYCIN**

Class: **Antibiotic**   Risk Factor: **B**

Fetal Risk Summary

No reports linking the use of spectinomycin with congenital defects have been located. The drug has been used to treat gonorrhea in pregnant patients allergic to penicillin. Available data do not suggest a threat to mother or fetus (1, 2).

Breast Feeding Summary

No data are available.

References

1. McCormack WM, Finland M. Spectinomycin. Ann Intern Med 1976;84:712–6.
2. Anonymous. Treatment of syphilis and gonorrhea. Med Lett Drugs Ther 1977;19:105–7.

Name: **SPIRONOLACTONE**

Class: **Diuretic** Risk Factor: **D**

Fetal Risk Summary

Spironolactone is a potassium-conserving diuretic. No reports linking it with congenital defects have been located. Some have commented, however, that spironolactone may be contraindicated during pregnancy based on the known antiandrogenic effects in humans and the feminization observed in male rat fetuses (1). Other investigators consider diuretics in general to be contraindicated in pregnancy, except for patients with cardiovascular disorders, since they do not prevent or alter the course of toxemia and they may decrease placental perfusion (2–4).

Breast Feeding Summary

It is not known if unmetabolized spironolactone is excreted in breast milk. Canrenone, the principal metabolite, was found with milk:plasma ratios of 0.72 (2 hours) and 0.51 (14.5 hours) (5). These amounts would provide an estimated maximum of 0.2% of the mother's daily dose to the infant (5). The effects on the infant from this ingestion are unknown. The American Academy of Pediatrics considers spironolactone to be compatible with breast feeding (6).

References

1. Messina M, Biffignandi P, Ghiga E, Jeantet MG, Molinatti GM. Possible contraindication of spironolactone during pregnancy. J Endocrinol Invest 1979;2:222.
2. Pitkin RM, Kaminetzky HA, Newton M, Pritchard JA. Maternal nutrition: a selective review of clinical topics. Obstet Gynecol 1972;40:773–85.
3. Lindheimer MD, Katz AI. Sodium and diuretics in pregnancy. N Engl J Med 1973;288:891–4.
4. Christianson R, Page EW. Diuretic drugs and pregnancy. Obstet Gynecol 1976;48:647–52.
5. Phelps DL, Karim A. Spironolactone: relationship between concentrations of dethioacetylated metabolite in human serum and milk. J Pharm Sci 1977;66:1203.
6. Committee on Drugs, American Academy of Pediatrics. Transfer of drugs and other chemicals into human milk. Pediatrics 1989;84:924–36.

Name: **STREPTOKINASE**

Class: **Thrombolytic** Risk Factor: **C**

Fetal Risk Summary

No reports linking the use of streptokinase with congenital defects have been located. Only minimal amounts cross the placenta and are not sufficient to cause fibrinolytic effects in the fetus (1–7). Although the passage of streptokinase is blocked by the placenta, streptokinase antibodies do cross to the fetus (5). This passive sensitization would have clinical importance only if the neonate required streptokinase therapy. Ludwig has treated 24 patients in the 2nd and 3rd trimesters without fetal complications (5). Use in the 1st trimester for maternal thrombophlebitis has also been reported (6). No adverse effects were observed in the infant born at term.

Breast Feeding Summary

No data are available.

References

1. Pfeifer GW. Distribution and placental transfer of 131–I streptokinase. Aust Ann Med 1970;19(Suppl):17–8.
2. Hall RJC, Young C, Sutton GC, Campbell S. Treatment of acute massive pulmonary embolism by streptokinase during labour and delivery. Br Med J 1972;4:647–9.
3. McTaggart DR, Ingram TG. Massive pulmonary embolism during pregnancy treated with streptokinase. Med J Aust 1977;1:18–20.
4. Benz JJ, Wick A. The problem of fibrinolytic therapy in pregnancy. Schweiz Med Wochenschr 1973;103:1359–63.
5. Ludwig H. Results of streptokinase therapy in deep venous thrombosis during pregnancy. Postgrad Med J 1973;49(Suppl 5):65–7.
6. Walter C, Koestering H. Therapeutische thrombolyse in der neunten schwangerschalftswoche. Dtsch Med Wochenschr 1969;94:32–4.
7. Witchitz S, Veyrat C, Moisson P, Scheinman N, Rozenstajn L. Fibrinolytic treatment of thrombus on prosthetic heart valves. Br Heart J 1980;44:545–54.

Name: **STREPTOMYCIN**

Class: **Antibiotic**   Risk Factor: **D**

Fetal Risk Summary

Streptomycin is an aminoglycoside antibiotic. The drug rapidly crosses the placenta into the fetal circulation and amniotic fluid, obtaining concentrations usually less than 50% of the maternal serum level (1, 2). Early investigators, well aware of streptomycin-induced ototoxicity, were unable to observe this defect in infants exposed *in utero* to the agent (3–5). Eventually, ototoxicity was described in a 2 1/2-month-old infant whose mother had been treated for tuberculosis with 30 g of streptomycin during the last month of pregnancy (6). The infant was deaf with a negative cochleopalpebral reflex. Several other case reports and small surveys describing similar toxicity followed this initial report (7, 8). In general, however, the incidence of congenital ototoxicity, cochlear or vestibular, from streptomycin is low, especially with careful dosage calculations and if the duration of fetal exposure is limited (9).

Except for eighth cranial nerve damage, no reports of congenital defects due to streptomycin have been located. The Collaborative Perinatal Project monitored 50,282 mother-child pairs, 135 of which had 1st trimester exposure to streptomycin (10, pp. 297–301). For use anytime during pregnancy, 355 exposures were recorded (10, p. 435). In neither case was evidence found to suggest a relationship to large categories of major or minor malformations or to individual defects.

In a group of 1619 newborns whose mothers were treated for tuberculosis during pregnancy with multiple drugs, including streptomycin, the incidence of congenital defects was the same as in a healthy control group (2.34% vs. 2.56%) (11). Other investigators had previously concluded that the use of streptomycin in pregnant tuberculosis patients was not teratogenic (12).

Breast Feeding Summary

Streptomycin is excreted into breast milk. Milk:plasma ratios of 0.5–1.0 have been reported (13). Since the oral absorption of this antibiotic is poor, ototoxicity in the infant would not be expected. However, three potential problems exist for the nursing infant: modification of bowel flora, direct effects on the infant, and interference with the interpretation of culture results if a fever workup is required. The American Academy of Pediatrics considers the drug to be compatible with breast feeding (14).

References

1. Woltz J, Wiley M. Transmission of streptomycin from maternal blood to the fetal circulation and the amniotic fluid. Proc Soc Exp Biol Med 1945;60:106–7.
2. Heilman D, Heilman F, Hinshaw H, Nichols D, Herrell W. Streptomycin: absorption, diffusion, excretion and toxicity. Am J Med Sci 1945;210:576–84.
3. Watson E, Stow R. Streptomycin therapy: effects on fetus. JAMA 1948;137:1599–1600.
4. Rubin A, Winston J, Rutledge M. Effects of streptomycin upon the human fetus. Am J Dis Child 1951;82:14–6.
5. Kistner R. The use of streptomycin during pregnancy. Am J Obstet Gynecol 1950;60:422–6.
6. Lerox M. Existe-t-il une surdite congenitale acquise due a la streptomycine? Am Otolaryngol 1950;67:194–6.
7. Nishimura H, Tanimura T. *Clinical Aspects of the Teratogenicity of Drugs*. Amsterdam:Excerpta Medica, 1976:130.
8. Donald PR, Sellars SL. Streptomycin ototoxicity in the unborn child. S Afr Med J 1981;60:316–8.
9. Mann J, Moskowitz R. Plaque and pregnancy. A case report. JAMA 1977;237:1854–5.
10. Heinonen OP, Slone D, Shapiro S. *Birth Defects and Drugs in Pregnancy*. Littleton:Publishing Sciences Group, 1977.
11. Marynowski A, Sianozecka E. Comparison of the incidence of congenital malformations in neonates from healthy mothers and from patients treated because of tuberculosis. Ginekol Pol 1972;43:713–5.
12. Lowe C. Congenital defects among children born under supervision or treatment for pulmonary tuberculosis. Br J Prev Soc Med 1964;18:14–6.
13. Wilson JT. Milk/plasma ratios and contraindicated drugs. In Wilson JT, ed. *Drugs in Breast Milk*. Australia:ADIS Press, 1981:79.
14. Committee on Drugs, American Academy of Pediatrics. Transfer of drugs and other chemicals into human milk. Pediatrics 1989;84:924–36.

Name: SULFASALAZINE

Class: **Anti-infective** Risk Factor: **B***

Fetal Risk Summary

Sulfasalazine is a compound composed of 5-aminosalicylic acid (5-ASA) joined to sulfapyridine by an azo-linkage (refer to Sulfonamides for a complete review of this class of agents). Sulfasalazine is used for the treatment of ulcerative colitis and Crohn's disease. No increase in congenital defects or newborn toxicity has been observed from its use in pregnancy (1–11). However, three reports, involving five infants (two stillborn), have described congenital malformations after exposure to this drug (12–14). It cannot be determined if the observed defects were related to the therapy, the disease, or a combination of these or other factors:

Bilateral cleft lip/palate, severe hydrocephalus, death (12)

Ventricular septal defect, coarctation of aorta (13)

Potter-type IIa polycystic kidney, rudimentary left uterine cornu, stillborn (first twin) (13)

Potter's facies, hypoplastic lungs, absent kidneys and ureters, talipes equinovarus, stillborn (second twin) (13)

Ventricular septal defect, coarctation of aorta, macrocephaly; gingival hyperplasia, small ears (both thought to be inherited) (14)

Sulfasalazine and its metabolite, sulfapyridine, readily cross the placenta to the fetal circulation (5, 6). Fetal concentrations are approximately the same as maternal concentrations. Placental transfer of 5-aminosalicylic acid is limited since only negligible amounts are absorbed from the cecum and colon, and these are rapidly excreted in the urine (15).

At birth, concentrations of sulfasalazine and sulfapyridine in 11 infants were 4.6 and 18.2 μg/ml, respectively (6). Neither of these levels was sufficient to cause significant displacement of bilirubin from albumin (6). Kernicterus and severe neonatal jaundice have not been reported following maternal use of sulfasalazine, even when the drug was given up to the time of delivery (6, 7). Caution is advised, however, since other sulfonamides have caused jaundice in the newborn when given near term (see Sulfonamides).

Sulfasalazine may adversely affect spermatogenesis in male patients with inflammatory bowel disease (16, 17). Sperm counts and motility are both reduced and require 2 months or longer after the drug is stopped to return to normal levels (16).

[*Risk Factor D if administered near term.]

Breast Feeding Summary

Sulfapyridine is excreted into breast milk (see also Sulfonamides) (5, 15, 18). Milk concentrations were approximately 40–60% of maternal serum levels. One of the infant's urine contained 3–4 μg/ml of the drug (1.2–1.6 mg/24 hours), representing about 30–40% of the total dose excreted in the milk. Unmetabolized sulfasalazine was detected in only one of the studies (milk:plasma ratio of 0.3) (5). Levels of 5-aminosalicylic acid were undetectable. No adverse effects were observed in the 16 nursing infants exposed in these reports (5, 15, 18). However, bloody diarrhea in an infant exclusively breast fed, occurring first at 2 months of age, and then recurring 2 weeks later and persisting until 3 months of age, was attributed to the mother's sulfasalazine therapy (3 g/day) (19). The mother was a slow acetylator with a blood concentration of sulfapyridine of 42.4 μg/ml (therapeutic range 20–50 μg/ml) (19). The acetylation phenotype of the infant was not determined, but his blood level of sulfapyridine was 5.3 μg/ml. A diagnostic workup of the infant was negative. The bloody diarrhea did stop, however, 48–72 hours after discontinuance of the mother's therapy. A repeat colonoscopy of the infant 1.5 months later was normal. Based on this report, the American Academy of Pediatrics classifies sulfasalazine as a drug that should be given to nursing women with caution because significant adverse effects may occur in some nursing infants (20).

References

1. McEwan HP. Anorectal conditions in obstetric practice. Proc R Soc Med 1972;65:279–81.

2. Willoughby CP, Truelove SC. Ulcerative colitis and pregnancy. Gut 1980;21:469–74.
3. Levy N, Roisman I, Teodor I. Ulcerative colitis in pregnancy in Israel. Dis Colon Rectum 1981;24:351–4.
4. Mogadam M, Dobbins WO III, Korelitz BI, Ahmed SW. Pregnancy in inflammatory bowel disease: effect of sulfasalazine and corticosteroids on fetal outcome. Gastroenterology 1981;80:72–6.
5. Azad Khan AK, Truelove SC. Placental and mammary transfer of sulphasalazine. Br Med J 1979;2:1553.
6. Jarnerot G, Into-Malmberg MB, Esbjorner E. Placental transfer of sulphasalazine and sulphapyridine and some of its metabolites. Scand J Gastroenterol 1981;16:693–7.
7. Modadam M. Sulfasalazine, IBD, and pregnancy: reply. Gastroenterology 1981;81:194.
8. Fielding JF. Pregnancy and inflammatory bowel disease. J Clin Gastroenterol 1983;5:107–8.
9. Sorokin JJ, Levine SM. Pregnancy and inflammatory bowel disease: a review of the literature. Obstet Gynecol 1983;62:247–52.
10. Baiocco PJ, Korelitz BI. The influence of inflammatory bowel disease and its treatment on pregnancy and fetal outcome. J Clin Gastroenterol 1984;6:211–6.
11. Fedorkow DM, Persaud D, Nimrod CA. Inflammatory bowel disease: a controlled study of late pregnancy outcome. Am J Obstet Gynecol 1989;160:998–1001.
12. Craxi A, Pagliarello F. Possible embryotoxicity of sulfasalazine. Arch Intern Med 1980;140:1674.
13. Newman NM, Correy JF. Possible teratogenicity of sulphasalazine. Med J Aust 1983;1:528–9.
14. Hoo JJ, Hadro TA, Von Behren P. Possible teratogenicity of sulfasalazine. N Engl J Med 1988;318:1128.
15. Berlin CM Jr, Yaffe SJ. Disposition of salicylazosulfapyridine (Azulfidine) and metabolites in human breast milk. Dev Pharmacol Ther 1980;1:31–9.
16. Toovey S, Hudson E, Hendry WF, Levi AJ. Sulphasalazine and male infertility: reversibility and possible mechanism. Gut 1981;22:445–51.
17. Freeman JG, Reece VAC, Venables CW. Sulphasalazine and spermatogenesis. Digestion 1982;23:68–71.
18. Jarnerot G, Into-Malmberg MB. Sulphasalazine treatment during breast feeding. Scand J Gastroenterol 1979;14:869–71.
19. Branski D, Kerem E, Gross-Kieselstein E, Hurvitz H, Litt R, Abrahamov A. Bloody diarrhea—a possible complication of sulfasalazine transferred through human breast milk. J Pediatr Gastroenterol Nutr 1986;5:316–7.
20. Committee on Drugs, American Academy of Pediatrics. Transfer of drugs and other chemicals into human milk. Pediatrics 1989;84:924–36.

Name: **SULFONAMIDES**

Class: **Anti-infective**   Risk Factor: **B***

Fetal Risk Summary

Sulfonamides are a large class of antibacterial agents. While there are differences in their bioavailability, all share similar actions in the fetal and newborn periods, and they will be considered as a single group. The sulfonamides readily cross the placenta to the fetus during all stages of gestation (1–9). Equilibrium with maternal blood is usually established after 2–3 hours, with fetal levels averaging 70–90% of maternal. Significant levels may persist in the newborn for several days after birth when given near term. The primary danger of sulfonamide administration during pregnancy is manifested when these agents are given close to delivery. Toxicities that may be observed in the newborn include jaundice, hemolytic anemia and, theoretically, kernicterus. Severe jaundice in the newborn has been related to maternal sulfonamide ingestion at term by several authors (10–15). Premature infants seem especially prone to development of hyperbilirubinemia (14).

However, a study of 94 infants exposed to sulfadiazine *in utero* for maternal prophylaxis of rheumatic fever failed to show an increase in prematurity, hyperbilirubinemia or kernicterus (16). Hemolytic anemia has been reported in two newborns and in a fetus following *in utero* exposure to sulfonamides (10, 11, 15). Both newborns survived. In the case involving the fetus, the mother had homozygous glucose-6-phosphate dehydrogenase deficiency (15). She was treated with sulfisoxazole for a urinary tract infection 2 weeks prior to delivery of a stillborn male infant. Autopsy revealed a 36-week infant with maceration, severe anemia, and hydrops fetalis.

Sulfonamides compete with bilirubin for binding to plasma albumin. *In utero*, the fetus clears free bilirubin by the placental circulation, but after birth, this mechanism is no longer available. Unbound bilirubin is free to cross the blood-brain barrier and may result in kernicterus. While this toxicity is well known when sulfonamides are administered directly to the neonate, kernicterus in the newborn following *in utero* exposure has not been reported. Most reports of sulfonamide exposure during gestation have failed to demonstrate an association with congenital malformations (9, 10, 17–23). Offspring of patients treated throughout pregnancy with sulfasalazine (sulfapyridine plus 5-aminosalicylic acid) for ulcerative colitis or Crohn's disease have not shown an increase in adverse effects (see also Sulfasalazine) (9, 20, 22). In contrast, a retrospective study of 1369 patients found that significantly more mothers of 458 infants with congenital malformations took sulfonamides than did mothers in the control group (24). A 1975 study examined the *in utero* drug exposures of 599 children born with oral clefts (25). A significant difference ($p < 0.05$), as compared with matched controls, was found with 1st and 2nd trimester sulfonamide use only when other defects, in addition to the clefts, were present.

Sulfonamides are teratogenic in some species of animals, a finding which has prompted warnings of human teratogenicity (26, 27). In two reports, investigators associated *in utero* sulfonamide exposure with tracheoeosophageal fistula and cataracts, but additional descriptions of these effects have not appeared (28, 29). A mother treated for food poisoning with sulfaguanidine in early pregnancy delivered a child with multiple anomalies (30). The author attributed the defects to use of the drug, but a relationship is doubtful.

The Collaborative Perinatal Project monitored 50,282 mother-child pairs, 1,455 of which had 1st trimester exposure to sulfonamides (31, pp. 296–313). For use anytime during pregnancy, 5,689 exposures were reported (31, p. 435). In neither case was evidence found to suggest a relationship to large categories of major or minor malformations. Several possible associations were found with individual defects after anytime use, but the statistical significance of these are unknown (31, pp. 485–6). Independent confirmation is required.

Ductus arteriosus persistens (8 cases)
Coloboma (4 cases)
Hypoplasia of limb or part thereof (7 cases)
Miscellaneous foot defects (4 cases)
Urethral obstruction (13 cases)
Hypoplasia/atrophy of adrenals (6 cases)
Benign tumors (12 cases)

Taken in sum, sulfonamides do not appear to pose a significant teratogenic risk. Due to the potential toxicity to the newborn, these agents should be avoided near term.

[*Risk Factor D if administered near term.]

Breast Feeding Summary

Sulfonamides are excreted into breast milk in low concentrations. Milk levels of sulfanilamide (free and conjugated) are reported to range from 6–94 μg/ml (3, 32–37). Up to 1.6% of the total dose could be recovered from the milk (32, 35). Milk levels often exceeded serum levels and persisted for several days after maternal consumption of the drug was stopped. Milk:plasma ratios during therapy with sulfanilamide were 0.5–0.6 (36). Reports of adverse effects in nursing infants are rare. One author found reports of diarrhea and rash in breast-fed infants whose mothers were receiving sulfapyridine or sulfathiazole (6). (See Sulfasalazine for another report of bloody diarrhea.) Milk levels of sulfapyridine, the active metabolite of sulfasalazine, were 10.3 μg/ml, a milk:plasma ratio of 0.5 (9). Based on these data, the nursing infant would receive approximately 3–4 mg/kg/day of sulfapyridine, an apparently nontoxic amount for a healthy neonate (16). Sulfisoxazole, a very water-soluble drug, was reported to produce a low milk:plasma ratio of 0.06 (38). The conjugated form achieved a ratio of 0.22. The total amount of sulfisoxazole recovered in milk over 48 hours after a 4-g divided dose was only 0.45%. Although controversial, breast feeding during maternal administration of sulfisoxazole seems to present a very low risk for the healthy neonate (39, 40).

In summary, sulfonamide excretion into breast milk apparently does not pose a significant risk for the healthy, full-term neonate. Exposure to sulfonamides via breast milk should be avoided in ill, stressed, or premature infants and in infants with hyperbilirubinemia or glucose-6-phosphate dehydrogenase deficiency. With these latter precautions, the American Academy of Pediatrics considers sulfonamides to be compatible with breast feeding (41).

References

1. Barker RH. The placental transfer of sulfanilamide. N Engl J Med 1938;219:41.
2. Speert H. The passage of sulfanilamide through the human placenta. Bull Johns Hopkins Hosp 1938;63:337–9.
3. Stewart HL Jr, Pratt JP. Sulfanilamide excretion in human breast milk and effect on breast-fed babies. JAMA 1938;111:1456–8.
4. Speert H. The placental transmission of sulfanilamide and its effects upon the fetus and newborn. Bull Johns Hopkins Hosp 1940;66:139–55.
5. Speert H. Placental transmission of sulfathiazole and sulfadiazine and its significance for fetal chemotherapy. Am J Obstet Gynecol 1943;45:200–7.
6. von Freisen B. A study of small dose sulphamerazine prophylaxis in obstetrics. Acta Obstet Gynecol Scand 1951;31(Suppl):75–116.
7. Sparr RA, Pritchard JA. Maternal and newborn distribution and excretion of sulfamethoxypyridine (Kynex). Obstet Gynecol 1958;12:131–4.
8. Nishimura H, Tanimura T. Clinical Aspects of the Teratogenicity of Drugs. Amsterdam:Excerpta Medica, 1976:88.
9. Azad Khan AK, Truelove SC. Placental and mammary transfer of sulphasalazine. Br Med J 1979;2:1553.
10. Heckel GP. Chemotherapy during pregnancy. Danger of fetal injury from sulfanilamide and its derivatives. JAMA 1941;117:1314–6.

11. Ginzler AM, Cherner C. Toxic manifestations in the newborn infant following placental transmission of sulfanilamide. With a report of 2 cases simulating erythroblastosis fetalis. Am J Obstet Gynecol 1942;44:46–55.

12. Lucey JF, Driscoll TJ Jr. Hazard to newborn infants of administration of long-acting sulfonamides to pregnant women. Pediatrics 1959;24:498–9.

13. Kantor HI, Sutherland DA, Leonard JT, Kamholz FH, Fry ND, White WL. Effect on bilirubin metabolism in the newborn of sulfisoxazole administration to the mother. Obstet Gynecol 1961;17:494–500.

14. Dunn PM. The possible relationship between the maternal administration of sulphamethoxypyridazine and hyperbilirubinaemia in the newborn. J Obstet Gynaecol Br Commonw 1964;71:128–31.

15. Perkins RP. Hydrops fetalis and stillbirth in a male glucose-6-phosphate dehydrogenase-deficient fetus possibly due to maternal ingestion of sulfisoxazole. Am J Obstet Gynecol 1971;111:379–81.

16. Baskin CG, Law S, Wenger NK. Sulfadiazine rheumatic fever prophylaxis during pregnancy: does it increase the risk of kernicterus in the newborn? Cardiology 1980;65:222–5.

17. Bonze EJ, Fuerstner PG, Falls FH. Use of sulfanilamide derivative in treatment of gonorrhea in pregnant and nonpregnant women. Am J Obstet Gynecol 1939;38:73–9.

18. Carter MP, Wilson F. Antibiotics and congenital malformations. Lancet 1963;1:1267–8.

19. Little PJ. The incidence of urinary infection in 5000 pregnant women. Lancet 1966;2:925–8.

20. McEwan HP. Anorectal conditions in obstetric patients. Proc R Soc Med 1972;65:279–81.

21. Williams JD, Smith EK. Single-dose therapy with streptomycin and sulfametopyrazine for bacteriuria during pregnancy. Br Med J 1970;4:651–3.

22. Mogadam M, Dobbins WO III, Korelitz BI, Ahmed SW. Pregnancy in inflammatory bowel disease: effect of sulfasalazine and corticosteroids on fetal outcome. Gastroenterology 1981;80:72–6.

23. Richards IDG. A retrospective inquiry into possible teratogenic effects of drugs in pregnancy. Adv Exp Med Biol 1972;27:441–55.

24. Nelson MM, Forfar JO. Association between drugs administered during pregnancy and congenital abnormalities of the fetus. Br Med J 1971;1:523–7.

25. Saxen I. Associations between oral clefts and drugs taken during pregnancy. Int J Epidemiol 1975;4:37–44.

26. Anonymous. Teratogenic effects of sulphonamides. Br Med J 1965;1:142.

27. Green KG. "Bimez" and teratogenic action. Br Med J 1963;2:56.

28. Ingalls TH, Prindle RA. Esophageal atresia with tracheoeosophageal fistula. Epidemiologic and teratologic implications. N Engl J Med 1949;240:987–95.

29. Harly JD, Farrar JF, Gray JB, Dunlop IC. Aromatic drugs and congenital cataracts. Lancet 1964;1:472–3.

30. Pogorzelska E. A case of multiple congenital anomalies in a child of a mother treated with sulfaguanidine. Patol Pol 1966;17:383–6.

31. Heinonen OP, Slone D, Shapiro S. Birth Defects and Drugs in Pregnancy. Littleton:Publishing Sciences Group, 1977.

32. Adair FL, Hesseltine HC, Hac LR. Experimental study of the behavior of sulfanilamide. JAMA 1938;111:766–70.

33. Hepburn JS, Paxson NF, Rogers AN. Secretion of ingested sulfanilamide in breast milk and in the urine of the infant. J Biol Chem 1938;123:liv-lv.

34. Pinto SS. Excretion of sulfanilamide and acetylsulfanilamide in human milk. JAMA 1938;111:1914–6.

35. Hac LR, Adair FL, Hesseltine HC. Excretion of sulfanilamide and acetylsulfanilamide in human breast milk. Am J Obstet Gynecol 1939;38:57–66.

36. Foster FP. Sulfanilamide excretion in breast milk: report of a case. Proc Staff Meet Mayo Clin 1939;14:153–5.

37. Hepburn JS, Paxson NF, Rogers AN. Secretion of ingested sulfanilamide in human milk and in the urine of the nursing infant. Arch Pediatr 1942;59:413–8.

38. Kauffman RE, O'Brien C, Gilford P. Sulfisoxazole secretion into human milk. J Pediatr 1980;97:839–41.

39. Elliott GT, Quinn SI. Sulfisoxazole in human milk. J Pediatr 1981;99:171–2.

40. Kauffman RE. Reply. J Pediatr 1981;99:172.

41. Committee on Drugs, American Academy of Pediatrics. Transfer of drugs and other chemicals into human milk. Pediatrics 1989;84:924–36.

Name: **SULINDAC**

Class: **Nonsteroidal Anti-inflammatory**   Risk Factor: **B***

Fetal Risk Summary

No reports linking the use of sulindac with congenital defects have been located. Theoretically, sulindac, a prostaglandin synthetase inhibitor, could cause constriction of the ductus arteriosus *in utero* (1). Persistent pulmonary hypertension of the newborn should also be considered (2). Drugs in this class have been shown to inhibit labor and prolong pregnancy (2).

[*Risk Factor D if used in the 3rd trimester or near delivery.]

Breast Feeding Summary

No data are available (J.J. Whalen, personal communication, Merck Sharpe & Dohme, 1981).

References

1. Levin DL. Effects of inhibition of prostaglandin synthesis on fetal development, oxygenation, and the fetal circulation. Semin Perinatol 1980;4:35–44.
2. Fuchs F. Prevention of prematurity. Am J Obstet Gynecol 1976;126:809–20.

Name: **TEMAZEPAM**

Class: **Hypnotic**   Risk Factor: **X_m**

Fetal Risk Summary

Temazepam is a benzodiazepine that is used as a hypnotic for the short-term management of insomnia. The manufacturer considers the drug to be contraindicated during pregnancy (1).

A potential drug interaction between temazepam and diphenhydramine, resulting in the stillbirth of a term female infant, has been reported (1). The mother had taken diphenhydramine 50 mg for mild itching of the skin and approximately 1.5 hours later, took 30 mg of temazepam for sleep. Three hours later she awoke with violent intrauterine fetal movements, which lasted several minutes and then abruptly stopped. The stillborn infant was delivered approximately 4 hours later. Autopsy revealed no gross or microscopic anomalies. In an experiment with pregnant rabbits, neither of the drugs alone caused fetal mortality but when combined, 51 (81%) of 63 fetuses were stillborn or died shortly after birth (1). No definite mechanism could be established for the apparent interaction.

Breast Feeding Summary

No reports on the use of temazepam during lactation have been located. The drug should be expected to pass into breast milk since other benzodiazepines and their metabolites are found in milk (see also Diazepam).

Reference

1. Kargas GA, Kargas SA, Bruyere HJ Jr, Gilbert EF, Opitz JM. Perinatal mortality due to interaction of diphenhydramine and temazepam. N Engl J Med 1985;313:1417.

Name: **TENIPOSIDE**

Class: **Antineoplastic**   Risk Factor: **D**

Fetal Risk Summary

Teniposide, a podophyllin derivative, has been used in the 2nd and 3rd trimesters of one pregnancy (1). An apparently normal infant was delivered at 37 weeks of gestation.

Long-term studies of growth and mental development in offspring exposed to antineoplastic agents during the 2nd trimester, the period of neuroblast multiplication, have not been conducted (2).

Occupational exposure of the mother to antineoplastic agents during pregnancy may present a risk to the fetus. A position statement from the National Study Commission on Cytotoxic Exposure and a research article involving some antineoplastic agents are presented in the monograph for cyclophosphamide (see Cyclophosphamide).

Breast Feeding Summary

No data are available.

References

1. Lowenthal RM, Funnell CF, Hope DM, Stewart IG, Humphrey DC. Normal infant after combination chemotherapy including teniposide for Burkitt's lymphoma in pregnancy. Med Pediatr Oncol 1982;10:165–9.
2. Dobbing J. Pregnancy and leukaemia. Lancet 1977;1:1155.

Name: **TERBUTALINE**

Class: **Sympathomimetic (Adrenergic)**   Risk Factor: **B$_M$**

Fetal Risk Summary

Terbutaline is a β-sympathomimetic used during pregnancy primarily to prevent or treat premature labor (i.e., tocolysis). No reports linking the use of terbutaline with congenital defects have been located. However, the tocolytic use of this drug is confined to the late 2nd and early 3rd trimesters. Reports describing the use of terbutaline as a bronchodilator in pregnant asthmatic patients during early pregnancy have not been found.

Terbutaline rapidly crosses the placenta to the fetus (1). In seven women given 0.25 mg intravenously (IV) during the second stage of labor, cord blood levels 7–60 minutes after the dose ranged from 12–55% (mean 36%) of maternal serum.

Terbutaline has been used as a tocolytic agent since the early 1970s (2, 3). The incidence of maternal side effects is usually low (e.g., 5% or less) but may be severe (2, 4–8). A 1983 review listed the more serious side effects of parenteral β-sympathomimetic therapy (e.g., terbutaline, ritodrine, etc.) as pulmonary edema, myocardial ischemia, cardiac arrhythmias, cerebral vasospasm, hypotension, hyperglycemia, and miscellaneous metabolic alterations (hypokalemia, increased serum lactate, and a decrease in measured hemoglobin concentration) (9). The more serious adverse effects are seen with continuous infusions of these drugs. Avoidance of this route of administration as well as careful selection of patients, appropriate dosing, and close monitoring of patient status may help to prevent serious maternal effects.

Terbutaline may cause fetal and maternal tachycardia (2, 4–6). Fetal rates are usually less than 175 beats/minute (5). As mentioned previously, maternal hypotension may occur, especially in the bleeding patient (9). More commonly, increases in systolic pressure and decreases in diastolic pressure occur with no reduction in mean arterial pressure and, thus, do not adversely effect the fetus (6, 9, 10).

Like all β-mimetics, terbutaline may cause transient maternal hyperglycemia followed by an increase in serum insulin levels (2, 11, 12). Sustained neonatal hypoglycemia may be observed if maternal effects have not terminated prior to delivery (11). Maternal glucose intolerance was observed at 1 hour in 19 of 30 patients receiving oral terbutaline for at least 1 week (13). Although macrosomia was not observed, the birth weights (after adjustment for gestational age) of infants from terbutaline-treated mothers had a tendency to be greater than those of babies from comparable controls (13).

Sudden, unexplained intrapartum death in a 30-gestational-week-old fetus occurred 5 hours after the start of an IV infusion of terbutaline for premature labor (14). No evidence of uterine, placental, or fetal anomalies was discovered. Maternal liver impairment was reported in a patient after 1 week of continuous IV administration of terbutaline (15). Therapy was stopped and 1 week later a healthy newborn was delivered without signs of liver toxicity. A paradoxical reaction to terbutaline was observed in a patient after 0.25 mg IV produced marked uterine hypertonus and subsequent severe fetal bradycardia (<50 beats/minute) (16). A healthy baby was delivered by emergency cesarean section.

Terbutaline has been used frequently to treat intrapartum fetal distress (17–21). The mechanism of the beneficial effects on fetal pH and heart rate are thought to be due to relief of the ischemia produced by uterine contractions on the placental circulation.

Although maternal complications may occur, few direct adverse effects, other than transient tachycardia and hypoglycemia, have been observed in the fetus or newborn. In many studies, neonatal complications are minimal or nonexistent (22–26). Compared to controls, prophylactic terbutaline in low-risk patients with twin gestations has produced significant gains in birth weights due to longer gestational times (25). In addition, terbutaline decreases the incidence of neonatal respiratory distress syndrome similar to other β-mimetics (27). Long-term evaluation of infants exposed to terbutaline *in utero* has been reported (28–30). No harmful effects in the infants (2–24 months) have been found.

In summary, terbutaline has been used as a tocolytic for approximately 17 years. Only rare reports of serious toxicity in the fetus/newborn have appeared and, although maternal adverse effects are much more common, toxicity in both are no more frequent than with other β-mimetics used for the treatment of premature labor. Avoidance of continuous terbutaline infusions lessens the chance of serious maternal effects. The manufacturer has now categorized the drug as "not indicated for the management of preterm labor," but this was apparently done for regulatory concerns since published information does not support the reclassification.

Breast Feeding Summary

Terbutaline is excreted into breast milk (31, 32). In two mothers with chronic asthma about 6–8 weeks postpartum, 5 mg three times daily produced mean maternal plasma levels of 1.9–4.8 ng/ml, while milk concentrations ranged between 2.5–3.8 ng/ml (31). The nursing infants ingested approximately 0.2% of the maternal dose, and the drug could not be detected in their plasma. In the second report, two mothers, both at 3 weeks postpartum and both with chronic asthma, were treated with 2.5 mg three times a day (32). Plasma levels varied between 0.97–3.07 ng/ml while mean milk levels were 2.76–3.91 ng/ml. Peak milk concentrations occurred at about 4 hours. The milk:plasma ratios of 1.4–2.9 are indicative of ionic trapping in the milk (32). Concentrations of terbutaline were highest in the fat fraction of the milk. Based on calculations, the infants were ingesting approximately 0.7% of the maternal dose.

No symptoms of adrenergic stimulation were observed in the four infants and all exhibited normal development. Long-term effects of this exposure, however, have not been studied. The American Academy of Pediatrics considers terbutaline to be compatible with breast feeding (33).

References

1. Ingemarsson I, Westgren M, Lindberg C, Ahren B, Lundquist I, Carlsson C. Single injection of terbutaline in term labor: placental transfer and effects on maternal and fetal carbohydrate metabolism. Am J Obstet Gynecol 1981;139:697–701.
2. Haller DL. The use of terbutaline for premature labor. Drug Intell Clin Pharm 1980;14:757–64.
3. Ingemarsson I. Cardiovasuclar complications of terbutaline for preterm labor. Am J Obstet Gynecol 1982;142:117.
4. Andersson KE, Bengtsson LP, Gustafson I, Ingermarsson I. The relaxing effect of terbutaline on the human uterus during term labor. Am J Obstet Gynecol 1975;121:602–9.
5. Ingermarrson I. Effect of terbutaline on premature labor. A double-blind placebo-controlled study. Am J Obstet Gynecol 1976;125:520–4.
6. Ravindran R, Viegas OJ, Padilla LM, LaBlonde P. Anesthetic considerations in pregnant patients receiving terbutaline therapy. Anesth Analg (Cleve) 1980;59:391–2.
7. Katz M, Robertson PA, Creasy RK. Cardiovascular complications associated with terbutaline treatment for preterm labor. Am J Obstet Gynecol 1981;139:605–8.
8. Ingemarsson I, Bengtsson B. A five-year experience with terbutaline for preterm labor: low rate of severe side effects. Obstet Gynecol 1985;66:176–80.
9. Benedetti TJ. Maternal complications of parenteral β-sympathomimetic therapy for premature labor. Am J Obstet Gynecol 1983;145:1–6.
10. Vargas GC, Macedo GJ, Amved AR, Lowenberg FE. Terbutaline, a new uterine inhibitor. Ginecol Obstet Mex 1974;36:75–88.
11. Epstein MF, Nicholls RN, Stubblefield PG. Neonatal hypoglycemia after beta-sympathomimetic tocolytic therapy. J Pediatr 1979;94:449–53.
12. Westgren M, Carlsson C, Lindholm T, Thysell H, Ingemarsson I. Continuous maternal glucose measurements and fetal glucose and insulin levels after administration of terbutaline in term labor. Acta Obstet Gynecol Scand 1982;Suppl 108:63–5.
13. Main EK, Main DM, Gabbe SG. Chronic oral terbutaline tocolytic therapy is associated with maternal glucose intolerance. Am J Obstet Gynecol 1987;157:644–7.
14. Lenke RR, Trupin S. Sudden, unforeseen fetal death in a woman being treated for premature labor: a case report. J Reprod Med 1984;29:872–4.
15. Suzuki M, Inagaki K, Kihira M, Matsuzawa K, Ishikawa K, Ishizuka T. Maternal liver impairment associated with prolonged high-dose administration of terbutaline for premature labor. Obstet Gynecol 1985;66:14S-15S.
16. Bhat N, Seifer D, Hensleigh P. Paradoxical response to intravenous terbutaline. Am J Obstet Gynecol 1985;153:310–1.
17. Tejani NA, Verma UL, Chatterjee S, Mittelmann S. Terbutaline in the management of acute intrapartum fetal acidosis. J Reprod Med 1983;28:857–61.
18. Barrett JM. Fetal resuscitation with terbutaline during eclampsia-induced uterine hypertonus. Am J Obstet Gynecol 1984;150:895.
19. Ingemarsson I, Arulkumaran S, Ratnam SS. Single injection of terbutaline in term labor. I. Effect on fetal pH in cases with prolonged bradycardia. Am J Obstet Gynecol 1985;153:859–65.
20. Ingemarsson I, Arulkumaran S, Ratnam SS. Single injection of terbutaline in term labor. II. Effect on uterine activity. Am J Obstet Gynecol 1985;153:865–9.
21. Mendez-Bauer C, Shekarloo A, Cook V, Freese U. Treatment of acute intrapartum fetal distress by β2-sympathomimetics. Am J Obstet Gynecol 1987;156:638–42.
22. Stubblefield PG, Heyl PS. Treatment of premature labor with subcutaneous terbutaline. Obstet Gynecol 1982;59:457–62.

23. Caritis SN, Carson D, Greebon D, McCormick M, Edelstone DI, Mueller-Heubach E. A comparison of terbutaline and ethanol in the treatment of preterm labor. Am J Obstet Gynecol 1982;142:183–90.
24. Kaul AF, Osathanondy R, Safon LE, Frigoletto FD Jr, Friedman PA. The management of preterm labor with the calcium channel-blocking agent nifedipine combined with the β-mimetic terbutaline. Drug Intell Clin Pharm 1985;19:369–71.
25. O'Leary JA. Prophylactic tocolysis of twins. Am J Obstet Gynecol 1986;154:904–5.
26. Arias F, Knight AB, Tomich PB. A retrospective study on the effects of steroid administration and prolongation of the latent phase in patients with preterm premature rupture of the membranes. Am J Obstet Gynecol 1986;154:1059–63.
27. Bergman B, Hedner T. Antepartum administration of terbutaline and the incidence of hyaline membrane disease in preterm infants. Acta Obstet Gynecol Scand 1978;57:217–21.
28. Wallace R, Caldwell D, Ansbacher R, Otterson W. Inhibition of premature labor by terbutaline. Obstet Gynecol 1978;51:387–93.
29. Svenningsen NW. Follow-up studies on preterm infants after maternal β-receptor agonist treatment. Acta Obstet Gynecol Scand 1982;Suppl 108:67–70.
30. Karlsson K, Krantz M, Hamberger L. Comparison of various beta-mimetics on preterm labor, survival and development of the child. J Perinat Med 1980;8:19–26.
31. Lonnerholm G, Lindstrom B. Terbutaline excretion into breast milk. Br J Clin Pharmacol 1982;13:729–30.
32. Boreus LO, de Chateau P, Lindberg C, Nyberg L. Terbutaline in breast milk. Br J Clin Pharmacol 1982;13:731–2.
33. Committee on Drugs, American Academy of Pediatrics. Transfer of drugs and other chemicals into human milk. Pediatrics 1989;84:924–36.

Name: TETANUS/DIPHTHERIA TOXOIDS (ADULT)

Class: **Toxoid**   Risk Factor: **C**

Fetal Risk Summary

Tetanus/diphtheria toxoids for adult use are the specific toxoids of *Clostridium tetani* and *Corynebacterium diphtheriae* adsorbed onto aluminum compounds. Tetanus and diphtheria produce severe morbidity and mortality in the mother and a newborn tetanus mortality rate of 60% (2, 3). The risk to the fetus from tetanus/diphtheria toxoids is unknown (1, 2). The American College of Obstetricians and Gynecologists Technical Bulletin No. 64 recommends the use of tetanus/diphtheria toxoids in pregnancy for those women at risk who lack the primary series of immunizations or in whom no booster has been given within the past 10 years (1).

Breast Feeding Summary

No data are available.

References

1. American College of Obstetricians and Gynecologists. *Technical Bulletin*, Number 64, May 1982.
2. Amstey MS. Vaccination in pregnancy. Clin Obstet Gynaecol 1983;10:13–22.

Name: **TETRABENAZINE**

Class: **Tranquilizer** Risk Factor: **C**

Fetal Risk Summary

Tetrabenazine has been used in pregnancy for the treatment of chorea gravidarum (1). Therapy was started late in the 2nd trimester in one patient. No drug-induced fetal or newborn effects were observed. A small ventricular septal defect was probably not due to tetrabenazine exposure.

Breast Feeding Summary

No data are available.

Reference

1. Lubbe WF, Walker EB. Chorea gravidarum associated with circulating lupus anticoagulant: successful outcome of pregnancy with prednisone and aspirin therapy. Case report. Br J Obstet Gynaecol 1983;90:487–90.

Name: **TETRACYCLINE**

Class: **Antibiotic** Risk Factor: **D**

Fetal Risk Summary

Tetracyclines are a class of antibiotics that should be used with extreme caution, if at all, in pregnancy. The following discussion, unless otherwise noted, applies to all members of this class. Problems attributable to the use of the tetracyclines during or around the gestational period can be classified into four areas:

Adverse effects on fetal teeth and bones
Maternal liver toxicity
Congenital defects
Miscellaneous effects

Placental transfer of a tetracycline was first demonstrated in 1950 (1). The tetracyclines were considered safe for the mother and fetus and were routinely used for maternal infections during the following decade (2–5). It was not until 1961 that an intense yellow-gold fluorescence was observed in the mineralized structures of a fetal skeleton whose mother had taken tetracycline just prior to delivery (6). Following this report, a 2-year-old child was described whose erupted deciduous teeth formed normally but were stained a bright yellow due to tetracycline exposure *in utero* (7). Fluorescence under ultraviolet light and yellow-colored deciduous teeth that eventually changed to yellow-brown were associated with maternal tetracycline ingestion during pregnancy by several other investigators (8–22). An increase in enamel hypoplasia and caries was initially suspected but later shown not to be related to *in utero* tetracycline exposure (14, 15, 22). Newborn growth and development were normal in all of these reports, although tetracycline has been shown to cause inhibition of fibula growth in premature infants (6). The mechanism for the characteristic dental defect produced by tetracycline is due to the potent chelating ability of the drug (13). Tetracycline forms a complex with calcium orthophosphate and becomes incorporated into bones and teeth undergoing calcification. In the latter structure, this complex causes a permanent discoloration, as remodeling and calcium exchange do not occur after calcification is completed. Since the deciduous teeth begin to calcify at around 5 or 6 months *in utero*, use of tetracycline after this time will result in staining.

The first case linking tetracycline with acute fatty metamorphosis of the liver in a pregnant woman was described in 1963 (23), although two earlier papers reported the disease without associating it with the drug (24, 25). This rare but often fatal syndrome usually follows intravenous dosing of more than 2 g/day. Many of the pregnant patients were being treated for pyelonephritis (24–37). Tetracycline-induced hepatotoxicity differs from acute fatty liver of pregnancy in that it is not unique to pregnant women and reversal of the disease does not occur with pregnancy termination (38). The symptoms include jaundice, azotemia, acidosis, and terminal, irreversible shock. Pancreatitis and nonoliguric renal failure are often related findings. The fetus may not be affected directly, but as a result of the maternal pathology, stillborns and premature births are common. In an experimental study, increasing doses of tetracycline caused increasing fatty metamorphosis of the liver (39). The possibility that chronic maternal use of tetracycline before conception could result in fatal hepatotoxicity of pregnancy was recently raised (36). The authors speculated that tetracycline deposited in the bone of a 21-year-old patient was released during pregnancy, resulting in liver damage.

The Collaborative Perinatal Project monitored 50,282 mother-child pairs, 341 of which had 1st trimester exposure to tetracycline, 14 to chlortetracycline, 90 to demeclocycline, and 119 to oxytetracycline (40, pp. 297–313). For use anytime in pregnancy, 1,336 exposures were recorded for tetracycline, 0 for chlortetracycline, 280 for demeclocycline, and 328 for oxytetracycline (40, p. 435). The findings of this study were as follows:

Tetracycline: Evidence was found to suggest a relationship to minor, but not major, malformations. Three possible associations were found with individual defects, but the statistical significance of these is unknown (40, pp. 472, 485). Independent confirmation is required to determine the actual risk.

    Hypospadias (1st trimester only) (5 cases)
    Inguinal hernia (25 cases)
    Hypoplasia of limb or part thereof (6 cases)

Chlortetracycline: No evidence was found to suggest a relationship to large categories of major or minor malformations or to individual defects. However, the sample size is extremely small, and safety should not be inferred from these negative results.

Demeclocycline: Evidence was found to suggest a relationship to major or minor malformations, but the sample size is small (40, pp. 297–313). Two possible associations were found with individual defects, but the statistical significance of these is unknown (40, pp. 472, 485). Independent confirmation is required to determine the actual risk.

    Clubfoot (1st trimester only) (3 cases)
    Inguinal hernia (8 cases)

Oxytetracycline: Evidence was found to suggest a relationship to major and minor malformations (40, pp. 297–313). One possible association was found with individual defects, but the statistical significance of this is unknown (40, pp. 472, 485). Independent confirmation is required to determine the actual risk.

Inguinal hernia (14 cases)

In 1962, a woman treated with tetracycline in the 1st trimester for acute bronchitis delivered an infant with congenital defects of both hands (41, 42). The mother had a history of minor congenital defects on her side of the family and doubt was cast on the role of the drug in this anomaly (43). A possible association between the use of tetracyclines in pregnancy or during lactation and congenital cataracts has been reported in four patients (44). The effects of other drugs, including several antibiotics and maternal infection, could not be determined and a causal relationship to the tetracyclines seems remote. An infant with multiple anomalies whose mother had been treated with clomocycline for acne daily during the first 8 weeks of pregnancy has been described (45). Some of the defects, particularly the incomplete fibrous ankylosis and bone changes, made the authors suspect this tetracycline as the likely cause.

Doxycycline has been used for 10 days very early in the 1st trimester for the treatment of *Mycoplasma* infection in a group of previously infertile women (46). Dosage was based on the patient's weight, varying from 100–300 mg/day. All 43 of the exposed liveborns were normal at 1 year of age. Bubonic plague occurring in a woman at 22 weeks' gestation was successfully treated with tetracycline and streptomycin (47). Long-term evaluation of the infant was not reported.

Under miscellaneous effects, two reports have appeared which, although they do not directly relate to effects on the fetus, do directly affect pregnancy. In 1974, a researcher observed that a 1-week administration of 500 mg of chlortetracycline/day to male subjects was sufficient to produce sperm levels of the drug averaging 4.5 μg/ml (48). He theorized that tetracycline overdose could modify the fertilizing capacity of human sperm by inhibiting capacitation. Finally, a possible interaction between oral contraceptives and tetracycline resulting in pregnancy has been reported (49). The mechanism for this interaction may involve the interruption of enterohepatic circulation of contraceptive steroids by inhibiting gut bacterial hydrolysis of steroid conjugates resulting in a lower concentration of circulating steroids.

Breast Feeding Summary

Tetracycline is excreted into breast milk in low concentrations. Milk:plasma ratios vary between 0.25–1.5 (4, 50, 51). Theoretically, dental staining and inhibition of bone growth could occur in breast-fed infants whose mothers were consuming tetracycline. However, this theoretical possibility seems remote, since tetracycline serum levels in infants exposed in such a manner were undetectable (less than 0.05 μg/ml) (4). Three potential problems may exist for the nursing infant even though there are no reports in this regard: modification of bowel flora, direct effects on the infant, and interference with the interpretation of culture results if a fever workup is required. The American Academy of Pediatrics considers tetracycline to be compatible with breast feeding (52).

References

1. Guilbeau JA, Schoenbach EG, Schaub IG, Latham DV. Aureomycin in obstetrics: therapy and prophylaxis. JAMA 1950;143:520–6.
2. Charles D. Placental transmission of antibiotics. J Obstet Gynaecol Br Emp 1954;61:750–7.
3. Gibbons RJ, Reichelderfer TE. Transplacental transmission of demethylchlortetracycline and toxicity studies in premature and full term, newly born infants. Antibiot Med Clin Ther 1960;7:618–22.
4. Posner AC, Prigot A, Konicoff NG. Further observations on the use of tetracycline hydrochloride in prophylaxis and treatment of obstetric infections. In *Antibiotics Annual, 1954–55*, New York:Medical Encyclopedia, 1955:594–8.
5. Posner AC, Konicoff NG, Prigot A. Tetracycline in obstetric infections. In *Antibiotics Annual, 1955–56*. New York:Medical Encyclopedia, 1956:345–8.
6. Cohlan SQ, Bevelander G, Bross S. Effect of tetracycline on bone growth in the premature infant. Antimicrob Agents Chemother 1961:340–7.
7. Harcourt JK, Johnson NW, Storey E. In vivo incorporation of tetracycline in the teeth of man. Arch Oral Biol 1962;7:431–7.
8. Rendle-Short TJ. Tetracycline in teeth and bone. Lancet 1962;1:1188.
9. Douglas AC. The deposition of tetracycline in human nails and teeth: a complication of long term treatment. Br J Dis Chest 1963;57:44–7.
10. Kutscher AH, Zegarelli EV, Tovell HM, Hochberg B. Discoloration of teeth induced by tetracycline. JAMA 1963;184:586–7.
11. Kline AH, Blattner RJ, Lunin M. Transplacental effect of tetracyclines on teeth. JAMA 1964;188:178–80.
12. Macaulay JC, Leistyna JA. Preliminary observations on the prenatal administration of demethyl-chlortetracycline HCl. Pediatrics 1964;34:423–4.
13. Stewart DJ. The effects of tetracyclines upon the dentition. Br J Dermatol 1964;76:374–8.
14. Swallow JN. Discoloration of primary dentition after maternal tetracycline ingestion in pregnancy. Lancet 1964;2:611–2.
15. Porter PJ, Sweeney EA, Golan H, Kass EH. Controlled study of the effect of prenatal tetracycline on primary dentition. Antimicrob Agents Chemother 1965:668–71.
16. Toaff R, Ravid R. Tetracyclines and the teeth. Lancet 1966;2:281–2.
17. Kutscher AH, Zegarelli EV, Tovell HM, Hochberg B, Hauptman J. Discoloration of deciduous teeth induced by administrations of tetracycline antepartum. Am J Obstet Gynecol 1966;96:291–2.
18. Brearley LJ, Stragis AA, Storey E. Tetracycline-induced tooth changes. Part 1. Prevalence in pre-school children. Med J Aust 1968;2:653–8.
19. Brearley LJ, Storey E. Tetracycline-induced tooth changes. Part 2. Prevalence, localization and nature of staining in extracted deciduous teeth. Med J Aust 1968;2:714–9.
20. Baker KL, Storey E. Tetracycline-induced tooth changes. Part 3. Incidence in extracted first permanent molar teeth. Med J Aust 1970;1:109–13.
21. Anthony JR. Effect on deciduous and permanent teeth of tetracycline deposition in utero. Postgrad Med 1970;48:165–8.
22. Genot MT, Golan HP, Porter PJ, Kass EH. Effect of administration of tetracycline in pregnancy on the primary dentition of the offspring. J Oral Med 1970;25:75–9.
23. Schultz JC, Adamson JS Jr, Workman WW, Normal TD. Fatal liver disease after intravenous administration of tetracycline in high dosage. N Engl J Med 1963;269:999–1004.
24. Bruno M, Ober WB. Clinicopathologic conference: jaundice at the end of pregnancy. NY State J Med 1962;62:3792–800.
25. Lewis PL, Takeda M, Warren MJ. Obstetric acute yellow atrophy. Report of a case. Obstet Gynecol 1963;22:121–7.
26. Briggs RC. Tetracycline and liver disease. N Engl J Med 1963;269:1386.
27. Leonard GL. Tetracycline and liver disease. N Engl J Med 1963;269:1386.
28. Gough GS, Searcy RL. Additional case of fatal liver disease with tetracycline therapy. N Engl J Med 1964;270:157–8.
29. Whalley PJ, Adams RH, Combes B. Tetracycline toxicity in pregnancy. JAMA 1964;189:357–62.
30. Kunelis CT, Peters JL, Edmondson HA. Fatty liver of pregnancy and its relationship to tetracycline therapy. Am J Med 1965;38:359–77.
31. Lew HT, French SW. Tetracycline nephrotoxicity and nonoliguric acute renal failure. Arch Intern Med 1966;118:123–8.

32. Meihoff WE, Pasquale DN, Jacoby WJ Jr. Tetracycline-induced hepatic coma, with recovery. A report of a case. Obstet Gynecol 1967;29:260–5.
33. Aach R, Kissane J. Clinicopathologic conference: a seventeen year old girl with fatty liver of pregnancy following tetracycline therapy. Am J Med 1967;43:274–83.
34. Whalley PJ, Martin FG, Adams RH, Combes B. Disposition of tetracycline by pregnant women with acute pyelonephritis. Obstet Gynecol 1970;36:821–6.
35. Pride GL, Cleary RE, Hamburger RJ. Disseminated intravascular coagulation associated with tetracycline-induced hepatorenal failure during pregnancy. Am J Obstet Gynecol 1973;115:585–6.
36. Wenk RE, Gebhardt FC, Behagavan BS, Lustgarten JA, McCarthy EF. Tetracycline-associated fatty liver of pregnancy, including possible pregnancy risk after chronic dermatologic use of tetracycline. J Reprod Med 1981;26:135–41.
37. King TM, Bowe ET, D'Esopo DA. Toxic effects of the tetracyclines. Bull Sloane Hosp Women 1964;10:35–41.
38. Kaplan MM. Acute fatty liver of pregnancy. N Engl J Med 1985;313:367–70.
39. Allen ES, Brown WE. Hepatic toxicity of tetracycline in pregnancy. Am J Obstet Gynecol 1966;95:12–8.
40. Heinonen O, Slone D, Shaprio S. *Birth Defects and Drugs in Pregnancy*. Littleton:Publishing Sciences Group, 1977.
41. Wilson F. Congenital defects in the newborn. Br Med J 1962;2:255.
42. Carter MP, Wilson F. Tetracycline and congenital limb abnormalities. Br Med J 1962;2:407–8.
43. Mennie AT. Tetracycline and congenital limb abnormalities. Br Med J 1962;2:480.
44. Harley JD, Farrar JF, Gray JB, Dunlop IC. Aromatic drugs and congenital cataracts. Lancet 1964;1:472.
45. Corcoran R, Castles JM. Tetracycline for acne vulgaris and possible teratogenesis. Br Med J 1977;2:807–8.
46. Horne HW Jr, Kundsin RB. The role of mycoplasma among 81 consecutive pregnancies: a prospective study. Int J Fertil 1980;25:315–7.
47. Coppes JB. Bubonic plague in pregnancy. J Reprod Med 1980;25:91–5.
48. Briggs M. Tetracycline and steroid hormone binding to human spermatozoa. Acta Endocrinol 1974;75:785–92.
49. Bacon JF, Shenfield GM. Pregnancy attributable to interaction between tetracycline and oral contraceptives. Br Med J 1980;1:283.
50. Knowles JA. Drugs in milk. Pediatr Curr 1972;21:28–32.
51. Graf VH, Reimann S. Untersuchungen uber die konzentration von pyrrolidino-methyl-tetracycline in der muttermilch. Dtsch Med Wochenschr 1959;84:1694.
52. Committee on Drugs, American Academy of Pediatrics. Transfer of drugs and other chemicals into human milk. Pediatrics 1989;84;924–36.

Name: **THEOPHYLLINE**

Class: **Spasmolytic/Vasodilator** Risk Factor: **C**

Fetal Risk Summary

Theophylline is the bronchodilator of choice for asthma and chronic obstructive pulmonary disease in the pregnant patient (1–6). No reports linking the use of theophylline with congenital defects have been located.

Theophylline crosses the placenta, and newborn infants may have therapeutic serum levels (7–11). Transient tachycardia, irritability, and vomiting have been reported in newborns delivered from mothers consuming theophylline (7, 8). These effects are more likely to occur when maternal serum levels at term are in the high therapeutic range or above (therapeutic range 8–20 μg/ml) (9). Cord blood levels are approximately 100% of the maternal serum concentration (10, 11).

In patients at risk for premature delivery, aminophylline (theophylline ethylenediamine) was found to exert a beneficial effect by reducing the perinatal death rate and the frequency of respiratory distress syndrome (12, 13). In a nonrandomized study, aminophylline 250 mg intramuscularly every 12 hours up to a maximum of 3 days was compared to betamethasone, 4 mg intramuscularly every 8 hours for 2 days (13). Patients in the aminophylline group were excluded from receiving corticosteroids because of diabetes (4 patients), hypertension (10 patients), and ruptured membranes for more than 24 hours (4 patients). The aminophylline and steroid groups were comparable in length of gestation (32.5 weeks vs. 32.1 weeks), male/female infant sex ratio (10/8 vs. 8/8), Apgar scores (7.6 vs. 7.7), birth weight (1720 g vs. 1690 g) and hours between treatment and delivery (73 vs. 68). Respiratory distress syndrome occurred in 11% (2 of 18) of the aminophylline group compared to 0% (0 of 16) of the corticosteroid group. The difference was not statistically significant. A significant difference (p = 0.01) was found in the incidence of neonatal infection with 8 of 16 (50%) of the betamethasone group having signs of infection and none in the aminophylline group. The mechanism proposed for aminophylline-induced fetal lung maturation is similar to that observed with betamethasone: enhancement of tissue cyclic AMP by inhibition of cyclic AMP phosphodiesterase and a corresponding increased production and/or release of phosphatidylcholine (13).

An intravenous infusion of aminophylline has been tested for its tocolytic effects on oxytocin-induced uterine contractions (14). A slight decrease in uterine activity occurred in the first 15 minutes, but this was due to the effect on contraction intensity, not frequency. The author concluded that aminophylline was a poor tocolytic agent. However, a more recent *in vitro* study examined the effect of increasing concentrations of aminophylline on pregnant human myometrium (15). Aminophylline produced a dose-related decrease in contraction strength and a non-dose-dependent lengthening of the period of contraction. In this study, the authors concluded that aminophylline may be a clinically useful tocolytic agent (15).

A reduction in the occurrence of preeclampsia among pregnant asthmatic women treated with theophylline has been reported (16). Preeclampsia occurred in 1.2% (1 of 85) of patients treated with theophylline compared to 8.8% (6 of 68) (*p* < 0.05) of asthmatic patients not treated with the drug. Although the results were significant, the small numbers indicate that the results must be interpreted cautiously (16). The authors proposed a possible mechanism for the protective effect, if indeed it does occur, involving the inhibition of platelet aggregation and the altering of vascular tone, two known effects of theophylline (16).

The Collaborative Perinatal Project monitored 193 mother-child pairs with 1st trimester exposure to theophylline or aminophylline (17). No evidence was found for an association with malformations.

Concern over the depressant effects of methylxanthines on lipid synthesis in developing neural systems has been reported (18). Recent observations that infants treated with theophylline for apnea exhibit no overt neurologic deficits at 9–27 months of age are encouraging (19, 20). However, the long term effects of these drugs on human brain development are not known (18).

Frequent, high-dose asthmatic medication containing theophylline, ephedrine, phenobarbital, and diphenhydramine was used by one woman throughout pregnancy who delivered a stillborn girl with complete triploidy (21). Although drug-induced chromosome damage could not be proven, theophylline has been shown in *in vitro* tests to cause breakage in chromosomes of human lymphocytes (22). However, the clinical significance of this breakage is doubtful.

Theophylline withdrawal in a newborn exposed throughout gestation has been reported (10). Apneic spells developed at 28 hours after delivery and became progressively worse over the next 4 days. Therapy with theophylline resolved the spells.

The pharmacokinetics of theophylline during pregnancy have been studied (23, 24). One report suggested that plasma concentrations of theophylline fall during the 3rd trimester due to an increased maternal volume of distribution (23). However, a more recent study found a significantly lower clearance of theophylline during the 3rd trimester, ranging in some cases between 20–53% less (24). Two women had symptoms of toxicity requiring a dosage reduction.

Breast Feeding Summary

Theophylline is excreted into breast milk (25, 26). A milk:plasma ratio of 0.7 has been measured (26). Estimates indicate that less than 1% of the maternal dose is excreted into breast milk (25, 26). However, one infant became irritable secondary to a rapidly absorbed oral solution of aminophylline taken by the mother (25). Because very young infants may be more sensitive to levels that would be nontoxic in older infants, less rapidly absorbed theophylline preparations may be advisable for nursing mothers (8, 27). Except for the precaution that theophylline may cause irritability in the nursing infant, the American Academy of Pediatrics considers the drug to be compatible with breast feeding (28).

References

1. Greenberger P, Patterson R. Safety of therapy for allergic symptoms during pregnancy. Ann Intern Med 1978;89:234–7.
2. Weinstein AM, Dubin BD, Podleski WK, Spector SL, Farr RS. Asthma and pregnancy. JAMA 1979;241:1161–5.
3. Hernandez E, Angell CS, Johnson JWC. Asthma in pregnancy: current concepts. Obstet Gynecol 1980;55:739–43.
4. Turner ES, Greenberger PA, Patterson R. Management of the pregnant asthmatic patient. Ann Intern Med 1980;93:905–18.
5. Pratt WR. Allergic diseases in pregnancy and breast feeding. Ann Allergy 1981;47:355–60.
6. Lalli CM, Raju L. Pregnancy and chronic obstructive pulmonary disease. Chest 1981;80:759–61.
7. Arwood LL, Dasta JF, Friedman C. Placental transfer of theophylline: two case reports. Pediatrics 1979;63:844–6.
8. Yeh TF, Pildes RS. Transplacental aminophylline toxicity in a neonate. Lancet 1977;1:910.
9. Labovitz E, Spector S. Placental theophylline transfer in pregnant asthmatics. JAMA 1982;247:786–8.
10. Horowitz DA, Jablonski W, Mehta KA. Apnea associated with theophylline withdrawal in a term neonate. Am J Dis Child 1982;136:73–4.
11. Ron M, Hochner-Celnikier D, Menczel J, Palti Z, Kidroni G. Maternal-fetal transfer of aminophylline. Acta Obstet Gynecol Scand 1984;63:217–8.
12. Hadjigeorgiou E, Kitsiou S, Psaroudakis A, Segos C, Nicolopoulos D, Kaskarelis D. Antepartum aminophylline treatment for prevention of the respiratory distress syndrome in premature infants. Am J Obstet Gynecol 1979;135:257–60.
13. Granati B, Grella PV, Pettenazzo A, Di Lenardo L, Rubaltelli FF. The prevention of respiratory distress syndrome in premature infants: efficacy of antenatal aminophylline treatment versus prenatal glucocorticoid administration. Pediatr Pharmacol 1984;4:21–4.
14. Lipshitz J. Uterine and cardiovasuclar effects of aminophylline. Am J Obstet Gynecol 1978;131:716–8.
15. Bird LM, Anderson NC Jr, Chandler ML, Young RC. The effects of aminophylline and nifedipine on contractility of isolated pregnant human myometrium. Am J Obstet Gynecol 1987;157:171–7.

16. Dombrowski MP, Bottoms SF, Boike GM, Wald J. Incidence of preeclampsia among asthmatic patients lower with theophylline. Am J Obstet Gynecol 1986;155:265–7.
17. Heinonen OP, Slone D, Shapiro S. *Birth Defects and Drugs in Pregnancy*. Littleton:Publishing Sciences Group, 1977:367,370.
18. Volpe JJ. Effects of methylxanthines on lipid synthesis in developing neural systems. Semin Perinatol 1981;5:395–405.
19. Aranda JV, Dupont C. Metabolic effects of methylxanthines in premature infants. J Pediatr 1976;89:833–4.
20. Nelson RM, Resnick MB, Holstrum WJ, Eitzman DV. Development outcome of premature infants treated with theophylline. Dev Pharmacol Ther 1980;1:274–80.
21. Halbrecht I, Komlos L, Shabtay F, Solomon M, Book JA. Triploidy 69, XXX in a stillborn girl. Clin Genet 1973;4:210–2.
22. Weinstein D, Mauer I, Katz ML, Kazmer S. The effect of methylxanthines on chromosomes of human lymphocytes in culture. Mutat Res 1975;31:57–61.
23. Sutton PL, Koup JR, Rose JQ, Middleton E. The pharmacokinetics of theophylline in pregnancy. J Allergy Clin Immunol 1978;61:174.
24. Carter BL, Driscoll CE, Smith GD. Theophylline clearance during pregnancy. Obstet Gynecol 1986;68:555–9.
25. Yurchak AM, Jusko WJ. Theophylline secretion into breast milk. Pediatrics 1976;57:518–25.
26. Stec GP, Greenberger P, Ruo TI, Henthorn T, Morita Y, Atkinson AJ Jr, Patterson R. Kinetics of theophylline transfer to breast milk. Clin Pharmacol Ther 1980;28:404–8.
27. Berlin CM. Excretion of methylxanthines in human milk. Semin Perinatol 1981;5:389–94.
28. Committee on Drugs, American Academy of Pediatrics. Transfer of drugs and other chemicals into human milk. Pediatrics 1989;84:924–36.

Name:. **THIABENDAZOLE**

Class: **Anthelmintic**   Risk Factor: **C$_M$**

Fetal Risk Summary

Thiabendazole is an anthelmintic agent. Although an animal teratogen in some species, no reports of human teratogenicity due to thiabendazole have been located. No adverse fetal effects were encountered when a single or divided dose of 50 mg/kg body weight was given to a group of pregnant women with intestinal parasites, although maternal side effects such as nausea and vomiting were common (1). The period of gestation was not specified in this report except that many of the pregnant patients received the drug just prior to delivery.

A 1985 review of intestinal parasites and pregnancy concluded that treatment of the pregnant patient should only be considered if the "parasite is causing clinical disease or may cause public health problems" (2). That review, and a similar article published in 1986 (3), recommended thiabendazole, when indicated, for the treatment of *Strongyloides stercoralis* infection occurring during pregnancy.

Breast Feeding Summary

No data are available.

References

1. Chari MV, Hiremath RS. Thiabendazole (a new broadspectrum anthelmintic) in intestinal helminthiasis. J Assoc Phys India 1967;15:93–6.
2. D'Alauro F, Lee RV, Pao-In K, Khairallah M. Intestinal parasites and pregnancy. Obstet Gynecol 1985;66:639–43.
3. Ellis CJ. Antiparasitic agents in pregnancy. Clin Obstet Gynecol 1986;13:269–75.

Name: **THIAMINE**

Class: **Vitamin**   Risk Factor: **A***

Fetal Risk Summary

Thiamine (vitamin B_1), a water-soluble B complex vitamin, is an essential nutrient required for carbohydrate metabolism (1). The American recommended daily allowance (RDA) for thiamine in pregnancy is 1.4–1.5 mg (2).

Thiamine is actively transported to the fetus (3–6). Like other B complex vitamins, concentrations of thiamine in the fetus and newborn are higher than in the mother (5–12).

Maternal thiamine deficiency is common during pregnancy (11–13). Supplementation with multivitamin products reduces the thiamine hypovitaminemia only slightly (10). Since 1938, several authors have attempted to link this deficiency to toxemia of pregnancy (14–17). In a 1945 paper, King and Ride (15) summarized the early work published in this area. All of the reported cases, however, involved patients with poor nutrition and pregnancy care in general. More recent investigations have failed to find any relationship between maternal thiamine deficiency and toxemia, fetal defects, or other outcome of pregnancy (9, 18).

No association was found between low birth weight and thiamine levels in a 1977 report (8). Roecklein and co-workers (19) have shown experimentally, though, that the characteristic intrauterine growth retardation of the fetal alcohol syndrome may be due to ethanol-induced thiamine deficiency.

Thiamine has been used to treat hyperemesis gravidarum although pyridoxine (vitamin B_6) was found to be more effective (see Pyridoxine) (20–22). In one early report, thiamine was effective in reversing severe neurologic complications associated with hyperemesis (20). A mother treated with frequent injections of thiamine and pyridoxine, 50 mg each/dose, for hyperemesis during the first half of two pregnancies delivered two infants with severe convulsions, one of whom died within 30 hours of birth (22). The convulsions in the mentally retarded second infant were eventually controlled with pyridoxine. Pyridoxine dependency-induced convulsions are rare. The authors speculated that the defect was caused by *in utero* exposure to high circulating levels of the vitamin. Thiamine was not thought to be involved (see Pyridoxine).

An isolated case report described an anencephalic fetus whose mother was under psychiatric care (23). She had been treated with very high doses of vitamins B_1, B_6, C and folic acid. The relationship between the vitamins and the defect is unknown. Also unproven is the speculation by one writer than an association exists between thiamine deficiency and Down's syndrome (trisomy 21) or preleukemic bone marrow changes (24).

[*Risk Factor C if used in doses above the RDA.]

Breast Feeding Summary

Thiamine (vitamin B_1) is excreted into breast milk (25–28). One group of investigators supplemented well-nourished lactating women with a multivitamin preparation containing 1.7 mg of thiamine (25). At 6 months postpartum, milk concentrations of thiamine did not differ significantly from those of control patients not receiving supplements. In a study of lactating women with low nutritional status, supplementation with thiamine, 0.2–20.0 mg/day, resulted in mean milk concentrations of 125–268 ng/ml (26). Milk concentrations were directly proportional to dietary intake. A 1983 English study measured thiamine levels in pooled human milk obtained from preterm (26 mothers: 29–34 weeks) and term (35 mothers: 39 weeks or longer) patients (27). Preterm milk rose from 23.7 ng/ml (colostrum) to 89.3 ng/ml (16–196 days), while term milk increased over the same period from a level of 28.4 to 183 ng/ml.

In Asian mothers with severe thiamine deficiency, including some with beriberi, infants have become acutely ill after breast feeding, leading in some cases to convulsions and sudden death (29–32). Pneumonia was usually a characteristic finding. One author thought the condition was related to toxic intermediary metabolites, such as methylglyoxal, passing to the infant via the milk (29). Although a cause and effect relationship has not been proven, one report suggested that thiamine deficiency may aggravate the condition (30). Indian investigators measured very low thiamine milk levels in mothers of children with convulsions of unknown etiology (33). Mean milk thiamine concentrations in mothers of healthy children were 111 ng/ml, whereas those in mothers of children with convulsions were 29 ng/ml. The authors were unable to establish an association between the low thiamine content in milk and infantile convulsions. (see Pyridoxine for correlation between low levels of vitamin B_6 and convulsions).

The American RDA for thiamine during lactation is 1.5–1.6 mg (2). If the diet of the lactating woman adequately supplies this amount, maternal supplementation with thiamine is not needed (28). Supplementation with the RDA for thiamine is recommended for those women with inadequate nutritional intake. The American Academy of Pediatrics considers the maternal consumption of thiamine to be compatible with breast feeding (34).

References

1. American Hospital Formulary Service. *Drug Information 1990*. Bethesda:American Society of Hospital Pharmacists, 1990:2120–1.
2. *Recommended Dietary Allowances*, ed. 9th. Washington, DC:National Academy of Sciences, 1980.
3. Frank O, Walbroehl G, Thomson A, Kaminetzky H, Kubes Z, Baker H. Placental transfer:fetal retention of some vitamins. Am J Clin Nutr 1970;23:662–3.
4. Hill EP, Longo LD. Dynamics of maternal-fetal nutrient transfer. Fed Proc 1980;39:239–44.
5. Kaminetzky HA, Baker H, Frank O, Langer A. The effects of intravenously administered water-soluble vitamins during labor in normovitaminemic and hypovitaminemic gravidas on maternal and neonatal blood vitamin levels at delivery. Am J Obstet Gynecol 1974;120:697–703.
6. Baker H, Frank O, Deangelis B, Feingold S, Kaminetzky HA. Role of placenta in maternal-fetal vitamin transfer in humans. Am J Obstet Gynecol 1981;141:792–6.
7. Slobody LB, Willner MM, Mestern J. Comparison of vitamin B_1 levels in mothers and their newborn infants. Am J Dis Child 1949;77:736–9.
8. Baker H, Thind IS, Frank O, DeAngelis B, Caterini H, Louria DB. Vitamin levels in low-birth-weight newborn infants and their mothers. Am J Obstet Gynecol 1977;129:521–4.
9. Heller S, Salkeld RM, Korner WF. Vitamin B_1 status in pregnancy. Am J Clin Nutr 1974;27:1221–4.
10. Baker H, Frank O, Thomson AD, Langer A, Munves ED, De Angelis B, Kaminetzky HA. Vitamin profile of 174 mothers and newborns at parturition. Am J Clin Nutr 1975;28:59–65.
11. Tripathy K. Erythrocyte transketolase activity and thiamine transfer across human placenta. Am J Clin Nutr 1968;21:739–42.
12. Bamji MS. Enzymic evaluation of thiamin, riboflavin and pyridoxine status of parturient women and their newborn infants. Br J Nutr 1976;35:259–65.
13. Dostalova L. Correlation of the vitamin status between mother and newborn during delivery. Dev Pharmacol Ther 1982;4(Suppl 1):45–57.

14. Siddall AC. Vitamin B_1 deficiency as an etiologic factor in pregnancy toxemias. Am J Obstet Gynecol 1938;35:662–7.
15. King G, Ride LT. The relation of vitamin B_1 deficiency to the pregnancy toxaemias: a study of 371 cases of beri-beri complicating pregnancy. J Obstet Gynaecol Br Emp 1945;52:130–47.
16. Chaudhuri SK, Halder K, Chowdhury SR, Bagchi K. Relationship between toxaemia of pregnancy and thiamine deficiency. J Obstet Gynaecol Br Commonw 1969;76:123–6.
17. Chaudhuri SK. Role of nutrition in the etiology of toxemia of pregnancy. Am J Obstet Gynecol 1971;110:46–8.
18. Thomson AM. Diet in pregnancy. 3. Diet in relation to the course and outcome of pregnancy. Br J Nutr 1959;13:509–25.
19. Roecklein B, Levin SW, Comly M, Mukherjee AB. Intrauterine growth retardation induced by thiamine deficiency and pyrithiamine during pregnancy in the rat. Am J Obstet Gynecol 1985;151:455–60.
20. Fouts PJ, Gustafson GW, Zerfas LG. Successful treatment of a case of polyneuritis of pregnancy. Am J Obstet Gynecol 1934;28:902–7.
21. Willis RS, Winn WW, Morris AT, Newsom AA, Massey WE. Clinical observations in treatment of nausea and vomiting in pregnancy with vitamins B_1 and B_6: a preliminary report. Am J Obstet Gynecol 1942;44:265–71.
22. Hunt AD Jr, Stokes J Jr, McCrory WW, Stroud HH. Pyridoxine dependency: report of a case of intractable convulsions in an infant controlled by pyridoxine. Pediatrics 1954;13:140–5.
23. Averback P. Anencephaly associated with megavitamin therapy. Can Med Assoc J 1976;114:995.
24. Reading C. Down's syndrome, leukaemia and maternal thiamine deficiency. Med J Aust 1976;1:505.
25. Thomas MR, Sneed SM, Wei C, Nail P, Wilson M, Sprinkle EE III. The effects of vitamin C, vitamin B_6, vitamin B_{12}, folic acid, riboflavin, and thiamin on the breast milk and maternal status of well-nourished women at 6 months postpartum. Am J Clin Nutr 1980;33:2151–6.
26. Deodhar AD, Rajalakshmi R, Ramakrishnan CV. Studies on human lactation. Part III. Effect of dietary vitamin supplementation on vitamin contents of breast milk. Acta Paediatr Scand 1964;53:42–8.
27. Ford JE, Zechalko A, Murphy J, Brooke OG. Comparison of the B vitamin composition of milk from mothers of preterm and term babies. Arch Dis Child 1983;58:367–72.
28. Nail PA, Thomas MR, Eakin R. The effect of thiamin and riboflavin supplementation on the level of those vitamins in human breast milk and urine. Am J Clin Nutr 1980;33:198–204.
29. Fehily L. Human-milk intoxication due to B_1 avitaminosis. Br Med J 1944;2:590–2.
30. Cruickshank JD, Trimble AP, Brown JAH. Interstitial mononuclear pneumonia: a cause of sudden death in Gurkha infants in the Far East. Arch Dis Child 1957;32:279–84.
31. Mayer J. Nutrition and lactation. Postgrad Med 1963;33:380–5.
32. Gunther M. Diet and milk secretion in women. Proc Nutr Soc 1968;27:77–82.
33. Rao RR, Subrahmanyam I. An investigation on the thiamine content of mother's milk in relation to infantile convulsions. Ind J Med Res 1964;52:1198–201.
34. Committee on Drugs, American Academy of Pediatrics. Transfer of drugs and other chemicals into human milk. Pediatrics 1989;84:924–36.

Name: **THIOGUANINE**

Class: **Antineoplastic**　　　　　　　　　　　　　　　　Risk Factor: **D$_M$**

Fetal Risk Summary

The use of thioguanine in pregnancy has been reported in 26 patients, four during the 1st trimester (1–18). An elective abortion, resulting in a normal fetus, was performed at 21 weeks' gestation in one pregnancy after 4 weeks of chemotherapy (16). Use in the 1st and 2nd trimesters has been associated with chromosomal abnormalities in one infant (relationship to antineoplastic therapy unknown) and congenital malformations in another: trisomy for group C autosomones with mosaicism (1); two medial digits of both feet missing, distal phalanges of both thumbs missing with hypoplastic remnant of right thumb (2). In a third case, a fetus, who was not exposed to antineoplastic agents until the 23rd week, long after development of the affected extremity, was delivered at 42 weeks' gestation with polydactyly (six toes on the right foot), a condition that had occurred previously in this family (17).

Two cases of intrauterine fetal death have occurred after antineoplastic therapy with thioguanine and other agents (14, 17). In one case, a mother, whose antileukemic chemotherapy was initiated at 15 weeks' gestation, developed severe pregnancy-induced hypertension in the 29th week of pregnancy (14). Prior to this time, fetal well-being had been continuously documented. One week after onset of the preeclampsia, intrauterine fetal death was confirmed by ultrasound. In the second case, a woman, with a history of two previous 1st trimester spontaneous abortions, was treated for acute myeloblastic leukemia and ulcerative colitis beginning at 15 weeks' gestation (17). Intrauterine fetal death occurred at 20 weeks. No congenital abnormalities were found at autopsy in either of the fetuses.

Data from one review indicated that 40% of the infants exposed to anticancer drugs were of low birth weight (19). This finding was not related to the timing of exposure. Long-term studies of growth and mental development in offspring exposed to thioguanine during the 2nd trimester, the period of neuroblast multiplication, have not been conducted (20). However, individual children have been followed for periods ranging from a few months to 5 years and, in each case, normal development was documented (13, 14, 16, 17).

Although abnormal chromosomal changes were observed in one aborted fetus, the clinical significance of this observation and the relationship to antineoplastic therapy are unknown. In two other newborns, karyotyping of cultured cells did not show anomalies (1, 4). Paternal use of thioguanine with other antineoplastic agents prior to conception has been suggested as a cause of congenital defects observed in three infants: anencephalic stillborn (21), tetralogy of Fallot with syndactyly of the first and second toes (21), and multiple anomalies (22). However, confirmation of these data has not been forthcoming, and any such relationship is probably tenuous at best. Exposed men have also fathered normal children (22, 23).

Occupational exposure of the mother to antineoplastic agents during pregnancy may present a risk to the fetus. A position statement from the National Study Commission on Cytotoxic Exposure and a research article involving some antineoplastic agents are presented in the monograph for cyclophosphamide (see Cyclophosphamide).

Breast Feeding Summary

No data are available.

References

1. Maurer LH, Forcier RJ, McIntyre OR, Benirschke K. Fetal group C trisomy after cytosine arabinoside and thioguanine. Ann Intern Med 1971;75:809–10.
2. Schafer AI. Teratogenic effects of antileukemic chemotherapy. Arch Intern Med 1981;141:514–5.
3. Au-Yong R, Collins P, Young JA. Acute myeloblastic leukaemia during pregnancy. Br Med J 1972;4:493–4.
4. Raich PC, Curet LB. Treatment of acute leukemia during pregnancy. Cancer 1975;36:861–2.
5. Gokal R, Durrant J, Baum JD, Bennett MJ. Successful pregnancy in acute monocytic leukaemia. Br J Cancer 1976;34:299–302.

6. Lilleyman JS, Hill AS, Anderton KJ. Consequences of acute myelogenous leukemia in early pregnancy. Cancer 1977;40:1300–3.
7. Moreno H, Castleberry RP, McCann WP. Cytosine arabinoside and 6-thioguanine in the treatment of childhood acute myeloblastic leukemia. Cancer 1977;40:998–1004.
8. Manoharan A, Leyden MJ. Acute non-lymphocytic leukaemia in the third trimester of pregnancy. Aust NZ J Med 1979;9:71–4.
9. Taylor G, Blom J. Acute leukemia during pregnancy. South Med J 1980;73:1314–5.
10. Tobias JS, Bloom HJG. Doxorubicin in pregnancy. Lancet 1980;1:776.
11. Pawliger DF, McLean FW, Noyes WD. Normal fetus after cytosine arabinoside therapy. Ann Intern Med 1971;74:1012.
12. Plows CW. Acute myelomonocytic leukemia in pregnancy: report of a case. Am J Obstet Gynecol 1982;143:41–3.
13. Lowenthal RM, Marsden KA, Newman NM, Baikie MJ, Campbell SN. Normal infant after treatment of acute myeloid leukaemia in pregnancy with daunorubicin. Aust NZ J Med 1978;8:431–2.
14. O'Donnell R, Costigan C, O'Connell LG. Two cases of acute leukaemia in pregnancy. Acta Haematol 1979;61:298–300.
15. Hamer JW, Beard MEJ, Duff GB. Pregnancy complicated by acute myeloid leukaemia. NZ Med J 1979;89:212–3.
16. Doney KC, Kraemer KG, Shepard TH. Combination chemotherapy for acute myelocytic leukemia during pregnancy: three case reports. Cancer Treat Rep 1979;63:369–71.
17. Volkenandt M, Buchner T, Hiddemann W, Van De Loo J. Acute leukaemia during pregnancy. Lancet 1987;2:1521–2.
18. Feliu J, Juarez S, Ordonez A, Garcia-Paredes ML, Gonzalez-Baron M, Montero JM. Acute leukemia and pregnancy. Cancer 1988;61:580–4.
19. Nicholson HO. Cytotoxic drugs in pregnancy: review of reported cases. J Obstet Gynaecol Br Commonw 1968;75:307–12.
20. Dobbing J. Pregnancy and leukaemia. Lancet 1977;1:1155.
21. Russell JA, Powles RL, Oliver RTD. Conception and congenital abnormalities after chemotherapy of acute myelogenous leukaemia in two men. Br Med J 1976;1:1508.
22. Evenson DP, Arlin Z, Welt S, Claps ML, Melamed MR. Male reproductive capacity may recover following drug treatment with the L-10 protocol for acute lymphocytic leukemia. Cancer 1984;53:30–6.
23. Matthews JH, Wood JK. Male fertility during chemotherapy for acute leukemia. N Engl J Med 1980;303:1235.

Name: **THIOPROPAZATE**

Class: **Tranquilizer**   Risk Factor: **C**

Fetal Risk Summary

Thiopropazate is a piperazine phenothiazine in the same group as prochlorperazine (see Prochlorperazine). Phenothiazines readily cross the placenta (1). No specific information on the use of thiopropazate in pregnancy has been located. Although occasional reports have attempted to link various phenothiazine compounds with congenital malformations, the bulk of the evidence indicates that these drugs are safe for the mother and fetus (see also Chlorpromazine).

Breast Feeding Summary

No data are available.

Reference

1. Moya F, Thorndike V. Passage of drugs across the placenta. Am J Obstet Gynecol 1962;84:1778–98.

Name: **THIORIDAZINE**

Class: **Tranquilizer**   Risk Factor: **C**

Fetal Risk Summary

Thioridazine is a piperidyl phenothiazine. The phenothiazines readily cross the placenta (1). Extrapyramidal symptoms were seen in a newborn exposed to thioridazine *in utero*, but the reaction was probably due to chlorpromazine (2). A case of a congenital heart defect was described in 1969 (3). However, one investigator found no anomalies in the offspring of 23 patients exposed throughout gestation to thioridazine (4). Twenty of the infants were evaluated for up to 13 years. Although occasional reports have attempted to link various phenothiazine compounds with congenital malformations, the bulk of the evidence indicates that these drugs are safe for the mother and fetus (see Chlorpromazine).

Breast Feeding Summary

No data are available.

References

1. Moya F, Thorndike V. Passage of drugs across the placenta. Am J Obstet Gynecol 1962;84:1778–98.
2. Hill RM, Desmond MM, Kay JL. Extrapyramidal dysfunction in an infant of a schizophrenic mother. J Pediatr 1966;69:589–95.
3. Vince DJ. Congenital malformations following phenothiazine administration during pregnancy. Can Med Assoc J 1969;100:223.
4. Scanlan FJ. The use of thioridazine (Mellaril) during the first trimester. Med J Aust 1972;1:1271–2.

Name: **THIOTEPA**

Class: **Antineoplastic**   Risk Factor: **D**

Fetal Risk Summary

Thiotepa has been used during the 2nd and 3rd trimesters in one patient without apparent fetal harm (1). Long-term studies of growth and mental development in offspring exposed to antineoplastic agents during the 2nd trimester, the period of neuroblast multiplication, have not been conducted (2).

Occupational exposure of the mother to antineoplastic agents during pregnancy may present a risk to the fetus. A position statement from the National Study Commission on Cytotoxic Exposure and a research article involving some antineoplastic agents are presented in the monograph for cyclophosphamide (see Cyclophosphamide).

Breast Feeding Summary

No data are available.

References

1. Gililland J, Weinstein L. The effects of cancer chemotherapeutic agents on the developing fetus. Obstet Gynecol Surv 1983;38:6–13.
2. Dobbing J. Pregnancy and leukaemia. Lancet 1977;1:1155.

Name: **THIOTHIXENE**

Class: **Tranquilizer**   Risk Factor: **C**

Fetal Risk Summary

Thiothixene is structurally and pharmacologically related to trifluoperazine and chlorprothixene. No specific data on its use in pregnancy have been located (see also Trifluoperazine).

Breast Feeding Summary

No data are available.

Name: **THIPHENAMIL**

Class: **Parasympatholytic (Anticholinergic)**   Risk Factor: **C**

Fetal Risk Summary

Thiphenamil is an anticholinergic agent used in the treatment of parkinsonism. No reports of its use in pregnancy have been located (see also Atropine).

Breast Feeding Summary

No data are available (see also Atropine).

Name: **THYROGLOBULIN**

Class: **Thyroid**   Risk Factor: **A**

Fetal Risk Summary

See Thyroid.

Breast Feeding Summary

See Thyroid.

Name: **THYROID**

Class: **Thyroid**   Risk Factor: **A**

Fetal Risk Summary

Thyroid contains the two thyroid hormones levothyroxine (T4) and liothyronine (T3) plus other materials peculiar to the thyroid gland. It is used during pregnancy for the treatment of hypothyroidism. Neither T4 or T3 crosses the placenta when physiologic serum concentrations are present in the mother (see Levothyroxine

and Liothyronine). In one report, however, two patients, each of whom had produced two cretins in previous pregnancies, were given huge amounts of thyroid,
up to 1600 mg or more/day (1). Both newborns were normal at birth even though
one was found to be athyroid. The authors concluded that sufficient hormone was
transported to the fetuses to prevent hypothyroidism.

Congenital defects have been reported with the use of thyroid but are thought to
be due to maternal hypothyroidism or other factors (see Levothyroxine and
Liothyronine).

Combination therapy with thyroid-antithyroid drugs was advocated at one time
for the treatment of hyperthyroidism but is now considered inappropriate (see
Propylthiouracil).

Breast Feeding Summary

See Levothyroxine and Liothyronine.

Reference

1. Carr EA Jr, Beierwaltes WH, Raman G, Dodson VN, Tanton J, Betts JS, Stambaugh RA. The
   effect of maternal thyroid function on fetal thyroid function and development. J Clin Endocrinol
   Metab 1959;19:1–18.

Name: **THYROTROPIN**

Class: **Thyroid**   Risk Factor: **C$_M$**

Fetal Risk Summary

Thyrotropin (thyroid-stimulating hormone, TSH) does not cross the placenta (1).
No correlation exists between maternal and fetal concentrations of TSH at any
time during gestation (2).

Breast Feeding Summary

No reports describing the excretion of thyrotropin in human milk have been located.
Levels of this hormone have been measured and compared in breast-fed and bottle-
fed infants (3–7). Breast milk does not provide sufficient levothyroxine (T4) or
liothyronine (T3) to prevent the effects of congenital hypothyroidism (see Levothyroxine and Liothyronine). As a consequence, serum levels of TSH in breast-fed hypothyroid infants are markedly elevated (3, 4). In euthyroid babies, no differences in TSH
levels have been discovered between breast-fed and bottle-fed groups (5–7).

References

1. Cohlan SQ. Fetal and neonatal hazards from drugs administered during pregnancy. NY State J
   Med 1964;64:493–9.
2. Feely J. The physiology of thyroid function in pregnancy. Postgrad Med J 1979;55:336–9.
3. Abbassi V, Steinour TA. Successful diagnosis of congenital hypothyroidism in four breast-fed neonates. J Pediatr 1980;97:259–61.
4. Letarte J, Guyda H, Dussault JH, Glorieux J. Lack of protective effect of breast-feeding in congenital hypothyroidism: report of 12 cases. Pediatrics 1980;65:703–5.
5. Mizuta H, Amino N, Ichihara K, Harada T, Nose O, Tanizawa O, Miyai K. Thyroid hormones in
   human milk and their influence on thyroid function of breast-fed babies. Pediatr Res 1983;17:468–
   71.

6. Hahn HB Jr, Spiekerman M, Otto WR, Hossalla DE. Thyroid function tests in neonates fed human milk. Am J Dis Child 1983;137:220–2.
7. Franklin R, O'Grady C, Carpenter L. Neonatal thyroid function: comparison between breast-fed and bottle-fed infants. J Pediatr 1985;106:124–6.

Name: **TICARCILLIN**

Class: **Antibiotic**   Risk Factor: **B**

Fetal Risk Summary

Ticarcillin is a penicillin antibiotic. The drug rapidly crosses the placenta to the fetal circulation and amniotic fluid (1). Following a 1-g intravenous dose, single determinations of the amniotic fluid from six patients, 15–76 minutes after injection, yielded levels ranging from 1.0–3.3 μg/ml. Similar measurements of ticarcillin in cord serum ranged from 12.6–19.2 μg/ml.

No reports linking the use of ticarcillin with congenital defects have been located. The Collaborative Perinatal Project monitored 50,282 mother-child pairs, 3,546 of which had 1st trimester exposure to penicillin derivatives (2, pp. 297–313). For use anytime during pregnancy, 7,171 exposures were recorded (2, p. 435). In neither case was evidence found to suggest a relationship to large categories of major or minor malformations or to individual defects.

Breast Feeding Summary

Ticarcillin is excreted into breast milk in low concentrations. After a 1-g intravenous dose given to five' patients, only trace amounts of drug were measured at intervals up to 6 hours (1). Although these amounts are probably not significant, three potential problems exist for the nursing infant: modification of bowel flora, direct effects on the infant (e.g., allergic response), and interference with the interpretation of culture results if a fever workup is required. The American Academy of Pediatrics considers ticarcillin to be compatible with breast feeding (3).

References

1. Cho N, Nakayama T, Vehara K, Kunii K. Laboratory and clinical evaluation of ticarcillin in the field of obstetrics and gynecology. Chemotherapy (Tokyo) 1977;25:2911–23.
2. Heinonen OP, Slone, D, Shapiro S. *Birth Defects and Drugs in Pregnancy*. Littleton:Publishing Sciences Group, 1977.
3. Committee on Drugs, American Academy of Pediatrics. Transfer of drugs and other chemicals into human milk. Pediatrics 1989;84:924–36.

Name: **TIMOLOL**

Class: **Sympatholytic (β-Adrenergic Blocker)**   Risk Factor: **C$_M$**

Fetal Risk Summary

Timolol is a nonselective β-adrenergic blocking agent. No reports of its use in pregnancy have been located. The use near delivery of some agents in this class has resulted in persistent β-blockade in the newborn (see Acebutolol, Atenolol, and Nadolol). Thus, newborns exposed *in utero* to timolol should be closely observed during the first 24–48 hours after birth for bradycardia and other symptoms. The long-term effects of *in utero* exposure to β-blockers have not been studied but warrant evaluation.

Breast Feeding Summary

Timolol is excreted into breast milk (1, 2). In nine lactating women given 5 mg orally three times daily, the mean milk concentration of timolol 105–135 minutes after a dose was 15.9 ng/ml (1). When a dose of 10 mg three times daily was given to four patients, mean milk levels of 41 ng/ml were measured. The milk:plasma ratios for the two regimens were 0.80 and 0.83, respectively.

A woman with elevated intraocular pressure applied ophthalmic 0.5% timolol drops to the right eye twice daily, resulting in excretion of the drug in her breast milk (2). Maternal timolol levels in milk and plasma were 5.6 ng/ml and 0.93 ng/ml, respectively, about 1.5 hours after a dose. A milk sample taken 12 hours after the last dose contained 0.5 ng/ml of timolol. Assuming that the infant nursed every 4 hours and received 75 ml at each feeding, the daily dose would be below that expected to produce cardiac effects in the infant (2).

No adverse reactions were noted in the nursing infants described in the above reports. However, infants exposed to timolol via breast milk should be closely observed for bradycardia and other signs or symptoms of β-blockade. Long-term effects of exposure to β-blockers from milk have not been studied but warrant evaluation. The American Academy of Pediatrics considers timolol to be compatible with breast feeding (3).

References

1. Fidler J, Smith V, DeSwiet M. Excretion of oxprenolol and timolol in breast milk. Br J Obstet Gynaecol 1983;90:961–5.
2. Lustgarten JS, Podos SM. Topical timolol and the nursing mother. Arch Ophthalmol 1983;101:1381–2.
3. Committee on Drugs, American Academy of Pediatrics. Transfer of drugs and other chemicals into human milk. Pediatrics 1989;84:924–36.

Name: **TOBRAMYCIN**

Class: **Antibiotic**   Risk Factor: D_M

Fetal Risk Summary

Tobramycin is an aminoglycoside antibiotic. The drug crosses the placenta into the fetal circulation and amniotic fluid (1). Studies in patients undergoing elective abortions in the 1st and 2nd trimesters indicate that tobramycin distributes to most fetal tissues except the brain and cerebrospinal fluid. Amniotic fluid levels generally did not occur until the 2nd trimester. The highest fetal concentrations were found in the kidneys and urine. Reports measuring the passage of tobramycin in the 3rd trimester and at term are lacking.

No reports linking the use of tobramycin with congenital defects have been located. Ototoxicity, which is known to occur after tobramycin therapy, has not been reported as an effect of *in utero* exposure. However, eighth cranial nerve toxicity in the fetus is well known following exposure to other aminoglycosides (see Kanamycin and Streptomycin) and may potentially occur with tobramycin.

A potentially serious drug interaction may occur in newborns treated with aminoglycosides who were also exposed *in utero* to magnesium sulfate (see Gentamicin).

Breast Feeding Summary

Tobramycin is excreted into breast milk. Following an 80-mg intramuscular dose given to five patients, milk levels varied from trace to 0.52 μg/ml over 8 hours (2). Peak levels occurred at 4 hours postinjection. Since oral absorption of this antibiotic is poor, ototoxicity in the infant would not be expected. However, three potential problems exist for the nursing infant: modification of bowel flora, direct effects on the infant, and interference with the interpretation of culture results if a fever workup is required.

References

1. Bernard B, Garcia-Cazares S, Ballard C, Thrupp L, Mathies A, Wehrle P. Tobramycin: maternal-fetal pharmacology. Antimicrob Agents Chemother 1977;11:688–94.
2. Takase Z. Laboratory and clinical studies on tobramycin in the field of obstetrics and gynecology. Chemotherapy (Tokyo) 1975;23:1402.

Name: **TOLAZAMIDE**

Class: **Oral Hypoglycemic**   Risk Factor: **D***

Fetal Risk Summary

Tolazamide is a sulfonylurea used for the treatment of adult-onset diabetes mellitus. It is not indicated for the pregnant diabetic since tolazamide will not provide good control in patients who cannot be controlled by diet alone. Oral hypoglycemics may cause prolonged symptomatic hypoglycemia in newborns if exposed near term (see Chlorpropamide).

[*Risk Factor C according to manufacturer—Upjohn, 1990.]

Breast Feeding Summary

No data are available.

Name: **TOLAZOLINE**

Class: **Vasodilator**   Risk Factor: **C**

Fetal Risk Summary

Tolazoline is structurally and pharmacologically related to phentolamine (see also Phentolamine). Experience with tolazoline in pregnancy is limited. The Collaborative Perinatal Project monitored two 1st trimester exposures to tolazoline plus 13 other patients exposed to other vasodilators (1). From this small group of 15 patients, four malformed children were produced, a statistically significant incidence ($p < 0.02$). It was not stated if tolazoline was taken by any of the mothers of the affected infants. Although the data serve as a warning, the number of patients is so small that conclusions as to the relative safety of this drug in pregnancy cannot be made.

Breast Feeding Summary

No data are available.

Reference

1. Heinonen OP, Slone D, Shapiro S. *Birth Defects and Drugs in Pregnancy.* Littleton:Publishing Sciences Group, 1977:371–3.

Name: **TOLBUTAMIDE**

Class: **Oral Hypoglycemic**   Risk Factor: **D***

Fetal Risk Summary

Tolbutamide is a sulfonylurea used for the treatment of adult-onset diabetes mellitus. It is not indicated for the pregnant diabetic. When administered near term, the drug crosses the placenta (1, 2). Neonatal serum levels are higher than corresponding maternal concentrations. In one infant whose mother took 500 mg/day, serum levels at 27 hours were 7.2 mg/100 ml (maternal 2.7 mg/100 ml) (2). Prolonged symptomatic hypoglycemia has not been reported with tolbutamide but has been observed with other oral hypoglycemics (see also Acetohexamide and Chlorpropamide). If used during pregnancy, tolbutamide should be stopped at least 48 hours before delivery to avoid this potential complication (3).

Although teratogenic in animals, an increased incidence of congenital defects, other than those expected in diabetes mellitus, has not been found with tolbutamide (4–14). Four malformed infants have been attributed to tolbutamide but the relationship is unclear (2, 15–17):

Hand/foot anomalies, finger/toe syndactyly, external ear defect, atresia of external auditory canal, gastrointestinal, heart, and renal anomalies (15)
Grossly malformed (16)
Severe talipes, absent left toe (17)
Right-sided preauricular skin tag, accessory right thumb, thrombocytopenia (nadir 19,000 mm^3 on 4th day) (2)

Maternal diabetes is known to increase the rate of malformations by 2-4-fold, but the mechanism(s) are not fully understood (see also Insulin). The neonatal thrombocytopenia, persisting for about 2 weeks, may have been induced by tolbutamide (2).

In spite of this relative lack of teratogenicity, tolbutamide should be avoided in pregnancy since the drug will not provide good control in patients who cannot be controlled by diet alone (3).

[*Risk Factor C according to manufacturer—Upjohn, 1990.]

Breast Feeding Summary

Tolbutamide is excreted into breast milk. Following long-term dosing with 500 mg orally twice daily, milk levels 4 hours after a dose in two patients averaged 3 and 18 µg/ml, respectively (18). Milk:plasma ratios were 0.09 and 0.40, respectively. The effect on an infant from these levels is unknown. The American Academy of Pediatrics, although noting the possibility of jaundice in the nursing infant, considers tolbutamide to be compatible with breast feeding (19).

References

1. Miller DI, Wishinsky H, Thompson G. Transfer of tolbutamide across the human placenta. Diabetes 1962;11(Suppl):93–7.
2. Schiff D, Aranda J, Stern L. Neonatal thrombocytopenia and congenital malformation associated with administration of tolbutamide to the mother. J Pediatr 1970; 77:457–8.
3. Friend JR. Diabetes. Clin Obstet Gynaecol 1981; 8:353–82.
4. Ghanem MH. Possible teratogenic effect of tolbutamide in the pregnant prediabetic. Lancet 1961;1:1227.
5. Dolger H, Bookman JJ, Nechemias C. The diagnostic and therapeutic value of tolbutamide in pregnant diabetics. Diabetes 1962;11(Suppl):97–8.
6. Jackson WPU, Campbell GD, Notelovitz M, Blumsohn D. Tolbutamide and chlorpropamide during pregnancy in human diabetes. Diabetes 1962; 11(Suppl):98–101.
7. Campbell GD. Chlorpropamide and foetal damage. Br Med J 1963;1:59–60.
8. Macphail I. Chlorpropamide and foetal damage. Br Med J 1963; 1:192.
9. Jackson WPU, Campbell GD. Chlorpropamide and perinatal mortality. Br Med J 1963;2:1652.
10. Malins JM, Cooke AM, Pyke DA, Fitzgerald MG. Sulphonylurea drugs in pregnancy. Br Med J 1964;2:187.
11. Moss JM, Connor EJ. Pregnancy complicated by diabetes. Report of 102 pregnancies including eleven treated with oral hypoglycemic drugs. Med Ann Dist Col 1965;34:253–60.
12. Adam PAJ, Schwartz R. Diagnosis and treatment: should oral hypoglycemic agents be used in pediatric and pregnant patients? Pediatrics 1968;42:819–23.
13. Dignan PSJ. Teratogenic risk and counseling in diabetes. Clin Obstet Gynecol 1981;24:149–59.
14. Burt RL. Reactivity to tolbutamide in normal pregnancy. Obstet Gynecol 1958;12:447–53.
15. Larsson Y, Sterky G. Possible teratogenic effect of tolbutamide in a pregnant prediabetic. Lancet 1960;2:1424–6.
16. Campbell GD. Possible teratogenic effect of tolbutamide in pregnancy. Lancet 1961;1:891–2.
17. Soler NG, Walsh CH, Malins JM. Congenital malformations in infants of diabetic mothers. QJ Med 1976;45:303–13.
18. Moiel RH, Ryan JR. Tolbutamide (Orinase) in human breast milk. Clin Pediatr 1967;6:480.
19. Committee on Drugs, American Academy of Pediatrics. Transfer of drugs and other chemicals into human milk. Pediatrics 1989;84:924–36.

Name: **TOLMETIN**

Class: **Nonsteroidal Anti-inflammatory**   Risk Factor: **B***

Fetal Risk Summary

No reports linking the use of tolmetin with congenital defects have been located. Theoretically, tolmetin, a prostaglandin synthetase inhibitor, could cause constriction of the ductus arteriosus *in utero* (1). Persistent pulmonary hypertension of the newborn should also be considered (2). Drugs in this class have been shown to inhibit labor and prolong pregnancy (2).

[*Risk Factor D if used in 3rd trimester or near delivery.]

Breast Feeding Summary

Tolmetin is excreted into breast milk (3). In the 4 hours following a single 400-mg oral dose, milk levels varied from 0.06–0.18 μg/ml with the highest concentration occurring at 0.67 hour. Milk:plasma ratios were 0.005–0.007. The significance of these levels to the nursing infant is unknown. The American Academy of Pediatrics considers tolmetin to be compatible with breast feeding (4).

References

1. Levin DL. Effects of inhibition of prostaglandin synthesis on fetal development, oxygenation, and the fetal circulation. Semin Perinatol 1980;4:35–44.
2. Fuchs F. Prevention of prematurity. Am J Obstet Gynecol 1976;126:809–20.
3. Sagraves R, Waller ES, Goehrs HR. Tolmetin in breast milk. Drug Intell Clin Pharm 1985;19:55–6.
4. Committee on Drugs, American Academy of Pediatrics. Transfer of drugs and other chemicals into breast milk. Pediatrics 1989;84:924–36.

Name: **TRANYLCYPROMINE**

Class: **Antidepressant**   Risk Factor: **C**

Fetal Risk Summary

Tranylcypromine is a monoamine oxidase inhibitor. The Collaborative Perinatal Project monitored 21 mother-child pairs exposed to these drugs during the 1st trimester, 13 of which were exposed to tranylcypromine (1). An increased risk of malformations was found. Details of the 13 cases with exposure to tranylcypromine are not available.

Breast Feeding Summary

No reports describing the excretion of tranylcypromine into breast milk have been located.

Reference

1. Heinonen OP, Slone D, Shapiro S. *Birth Defects and Drugs in Pregnancy*. Littleton:Publishing Sciences Group, 1977:336–7.

Name: **TRETINOIN**

Class: **Vitamin**   Risk Factor: **B$_M$**

Fetal Risk Summary

Tretinoin (retinoic acid) is a retinoid and vitamin A derivative used topically for the treatment of acne vulgaris. Like other retinoids, the drug is a potent teratogen when taken systemically (see also Etretinate, Isotretinoin, and Vitamin A). However, since tretinoin is only used topically, the teratogenic risk is thought to be close to zero (1). According to one source, no cases have been reported after nearly 20 years of use (1). It has been estimated that even if maximal absorption (approximately 33%) occurred from a 1-g daily application of a 0.1% preparation, this would only result in about one-seventh of the vitamin A activity received from a typical prenatal vitamin supplement (2).

Breast Feeding Summary

No data are available on the excretion of tretinoin into human milk. Although other retinoids are excreted (see Vitamin A), the minimal absorption that occurs after topical application of tretinoin probably precludes the detection of clinically significant amounts in milk.

References

1. Kligman AM. Question and answers: is topical tretinoin teratogenic? JAMA 1988;259:2918.
2. Zbinden G. Investigations on the toxicity of tretinoin administered systemically to animals. Acta Derm Venereol (Stockh) 1975;Suppl 74:36–40.

Name: **TRIAMTERENE**

Class: **Diuretic** Risk Factor: **D***

Fetal Risk Summary

Triamterene is a potassium-conserving diuretic. No reports linking it with congenital efects have been located. The drug crosses to the fetus in animals, but this has not been studied in humans (1). No defects were observed in five infants exposed to triamterene in the 1st trimester (2, p. 372). For use anytime during pregnancy, 271 exposures were recorded without an increase in malformations (2, p. 441). Many investigators consider diuretics to be contraindicated in pregnancy, except for patients with heart disease, since they do not prevent or alter the course of toxemia, and they may decrease placental perfusion (3–5).

[Risk Factor M according to Manufacturer—Smith Kline & French, 1990.]

Breast Feeding Summary

Triamterene is excreted into cow's milk (1). Human data are not available.

References

1. Product information. Dyrenium. Smith Kline & French Laboratories, 1990.
2. Heinonen OP, Slone D, Shapiro S. *Birth Defects and Drugs in Pregnancy*. Littleton:Publishing Sciences Group, 1977.
3. Pitkin RM, Kaminetzky HA, Newton M, Pritchard JA. Maternal nutrition: a selective review of clinical topics. Obstet Gynecol 1972;40:773–85.
4. Lindheimer MD, Katz AI. Sodium and diuretics in pregnancy. N Engl J Med 1973;288:891–4.
5. Christianson R, Page EW. Diuretic drugs and pregnancy. Obstet Gynecol 1976;48:647–52.

Name: **TRICHLORMETHIAZIDE**

Class: **Diuretic**   Risk Factor: **D**

Fetal Risk Summary

See Chlorothiazide.

Breast Feeding Summary

See Chlorothiazide.

Name: **TRIDIHEXETHYL**

Class: **Parasympatholytic (Anticholinergic)**   Risk Factor: **C**

Fetal Risk Summary

Tridihexethyl is an anticholinergic quaternary ammonium chloride. In a large prospective study, 2,323 patients were exposed to this class of drugs during the 1st trimester, six of whom took tridihexethyl (1). A possible association was found between the total group and minor malformations, but the significance of this is unknown. Independent confirmation is required (1).

Breast Feeding Summary

No data are available (see also Atropine).

Reference

1. Heinonen OP, Slone D, Shapiro S. *Birth Defects and Drugs in Pregnancy*. Littleton:Publishing Sciences Group, 1977:346–53.

Name: **TRIFLUOPERAZINE**

Class: **Tranquilizer**   Risk Factor: **C**

Fetal Risk Summary

Trifluoperazine is a piperazine phenothiazine. The drug readily crosses the placenta (1). Trifluoperazine has been used for the treatment of nausea and vomiting of pregnancy, but it is primarily used as a psychotropic agent. In 1962, the Canadian Food and Drug Directorate released a warning that eight cases of congenital defects had been associated with trifluoperazine therapy (2). This correlation was refuted in a series of articles from the medical staff of the manufacturer of the drug (3–5). In 480 trifluoperazine-treated pregnant women, the incidence of liveborn infants with congenital malformations was 1.1%, as compared to 8,472 non-treated controls with an incidence of 1.5% (4). Two reports of phocomelia appeared in 1962–1963 and a case of a congenital heart defect in 1969 (6–8):

   Twins, both with phocomelia of all four limbs (6)

Phocomelia of upper limbs (7)
Complete transposition of great vessels in heart (8)

In none of these cases is there a clear relationship between use of the drug and the defect. Extrapyramidal symptoms have been described in a newborn exposed to trifluoperazine *in utero*, but the reaction was probably due to chlorpromazine (see Chlorpromazine) (9).

The Collaborative Perinatal Project monitored 50,282 mother-child pairs, 42 of which had 1st trimester exposure to trifluoperazine (10). No evidence was found to suggest a relationship to malformations or an effect on perinatal mortality rate, birth weight, or intelligence quotient scores at 4 years of age.

In summary, although some reports have attempted to link trifluoperazine with congenital defects, the bulk of the evidence indicates that the drug is safe for mother and fetus. Other reviewers have also concluded that the phenothiazines are not teratogenic (11, 12).

Breast Feeding Summary

No data are available.

References

1. Moya F, Thorndike V. Passage of drugs across the placenta. Am J Obstet Gynecol 1962;84:1778–98.
2. Canadian Department of National Health and Welfare, Food and Drug Directorate. Letter of notification to Canadian physicians. Ottawa, December 7, 1962.
3. Moriarity AJ. Trifluoperazine and congenital malformations. Can Med Assoc J 1963;88:97.
4. Moriarty AJ, Nance MR. Trifluoperazine and pregnancy. Can Med Assoc J 1963; 88:375–6.
5. Schrire I. Trifluoperazine and foetal abnormalities. Lancet 1963;1:174.
6. Corner BD. Congenital malformations. Clinical considerations. Med J Southwest 1962;77:46–52.
7. Hall G. A case of phocomelia of the upper limbs. Med J Aust 1963;1:449–50.
8. Vince DJ. Congenital malformations following phenothiazine administration during pregnancy. Can Med Assoc J 1969;100:223.
9. Hill RM, Desmond MM, Kay JL. Extrapyramidal dysfunction in an infant of a schizophrenic mother. J Pediatr 1966;69:589–95.
10. Slone D, Siskind V, Heinonen OP, Monson RR, Kaufman DW, Shapiro S. Antenatal exposure to the phenothiazines in relation to congenital malformations, perinatal mortality rate, birth weight, and intelligence quotient score. Am J Obstet Gynecol 1977;128:486–8.
11. Ayd FJ Jr. Children born of mothers treated with chlorpromazine during pregnancy. Clin Med 1964;71:1758–63.
12. Ananth J. Congenital malformations with psychopharmacologic agents. Compr Psychiatry 1975;16:437–45.

Name: **TRIFLUPROMAZINE**

Class: **Tranquilizer** Risk Factor: **C**

Fetal Risk Summary

Triflupromazine is a propylamino phenothiazine in the same class as chlorpromazine. The phenothiazines readily cross the placenta (1). The Collaborative Perinatal Project monitored 50,282 mother-child pairs, 36 of which had 1st trimester exposure to triflupromazine (2). No evidence was found to suggest a relationship to malformations or an effect on perinatal mortality rates, birth weight, or intelligence quotient scores at 4 years of age. Although occasional reports have attempted to link various phenothiazine compounds with congenital defects, the bulk of the evidence indicates that these drugs are safe for the mother and fetus (see also Chlorpromazine).

Breast Feeding Summary

No data are available.

References

1. Moya F, Thorndike V. Passage of drugs across the placenta. Am J Obstet Gynecol 1962;84:1778–98.
2. Slone D, Siskind V, Heinonen OP, Monson RR, Kaufman DW, Shapiro S. Antenatal exposure to the phenothiazines in relation to congenital malformations, perinatal mortality rate, birth weight, and intelligence quotient score. Am J Obstet Gynecol 1977;128:486–8.

Name: **TRIHEXYPHENIDYL**

Class: **Parasympatholytic (Anticholinergic)**   Risk Factor: **C**

Fetal Risk Summary

Trihexyphenidyl is an anticholinergic agent used in the treatment of parkinsonism. In a large prospective study, 2,323 patients were exposed to this class of drugs during the 1st trimester, nine of whom took trihexyphenidyl (1). A possible association was found between the total group and minor malformations.

Breast Feeding Summary

No data are available (see also Atropine).

Reference

1. Heinonen OP, Slone D, Shapiro S. *Birth Defects and Drugs in Pregnancy*. Littleton:Publishing Sciences Group, 1977:346–53.

Name: **TRIMEPRAZINE**

Class: **Antihistamine**   Risk Factor: **C**

Fetal Risk Summary

Trimeprazine is a phenothiazine antihistamine that is primarily used as an antipruritic. The Collaborative Perinatal Project monitored 50,282 mother-child pairs, 14 of which had 1st trimester exposure to trimeprazine (1, p. 323). From this small sample, no evidence was found to suggest a relationship to large categories of major or minor malformations or to individual malformations. For use anytime in pregnancy, 140 exposures were recorded (1, p. 437). Based on defects in five children, a possible association with malformations was found, but the significance of this is unknown.

In a 1971 study, infants of mothers who had ingested antihistamines during the 1st trimester actually had significantly fewer abnormalities when compared to controls (2). Trimeprazine was the eighth most commonly used antihistamine.

Breast Feeding Summary

Trimeprazine is excreted into human milk but the levels are too low to produce effects in the infant (3).

References

1. Heinonen OP, Slone D, Shapiro S. *Birth Defects and Drugs in Pregnancy.* Littleton:Publishing Sciences Group, 1977.
2. Nelson MM, Forfar JO. Associations between drugs administered during pregnancy and congenital abnormalities. Br Med J 1971;1:523–7.
3. O'Brien TE. Excretion of drugs in human milk. Am J Hosp Pharm 1974;31:844–54.

Name: **TRIMETHADIONE**

Class: **Anticonvulsant** Risk Factor: **D**

Fetal Risk Summary

Trimethadione is an oxazolidinedione anticonvulsant used in the treatment of petit mal epilepsy. Several case histories have suggested a phenotype for a fetal trimethadione syndrome of congenital malformations (1–7). The use of trimethadione in nine families was associated with a 69% incidence of congenital defects— 25 malformed children from 36 pregnancies. Three of these families reported five normal births after the anticonvulsant medication was stopped (1, 4). The incidence of fetal loss in these families was also increased over that seen in the general epileptic population. Because trimethadione has demonstrated both clinical and experimental fetal risk greater than other anticonvulsants, its use should be abandoned in favor of other medications used in the treatment of petit mal epilepsy (8–11). Features of Fetal Trimethadione Syndrome (25 Cases)

Features of Fetal Trimethadione Syndrome (25 Cases)

Feature	No.*	%	Feature	No.*	%
Growth:			Cardiac:		
Prenatal deficiency	8	32	Septal defect	5	20
Postnatal deficiency	6	24	Not stated	4	16
Performance (19 cases):			Patent ductus arteriosus	4	16
Mental retardation	7	28	Limb:		
Vision (myopia)	5	20	Simian crease	7	28
Speech disorder	4	16	Malformed hand	2	8
Impaired hearing	2	8	Clubfoot	1	4
Craniofacial:			Genitourinary:		
Low-set, cupped, or			Kidney and ureter		
abnormal ears	18	72	abnormalities	5	20
High arched or cleft			Inguinal hernia(s)	3	12
lip and/or palate	16	64	Hypospadias	3	12
Microcephaly	6	24	Ambiguous genitalia	2	8
Irregular teeth	4	16	Clitoral hypertrophy	1	4
Epicanthic folds	3	12	Imperforate anus	1	4

Features of Fetal Trimethadione Syndrome (25 Cases) Cont.

Feature	No.*	%	Feature	No.*	%
Broad nasal bridge	3	12	Other:		
Strabismus	3	12	Tracheoesophageal		
Low hairline	2	8	fistula	3	12
Facial hemangiomata	1	4	Esophageal atresia	2	8
(details not given)	3	12			

*Not mutually exclusive

Breast Feeding Summary

No data are available.

References

1. German J, Kowan A, Ehlers KH. Trimethadione and human teratogenesis. Teratology 1970;3:349–62.
2. Zackae EH, Mellman WJ, Neiderer B, Hanson JW. The fetal trimethadione syndrome. J Pediatr 1975;87:280–4.
3. Nichols MM. Fetal anomalies following maternal trimethadione ingestion. J Pediatr 1973;82:885–6.
4. Feldman GL, Weaver DD, Lourien EW. The fetal trimethadione syndrome. Report of an additional family and further delineation of this syndrome. Am J Dis Child 1977;131:1389–92.
5. Rosen RC, Lightner ES. Phenotypic malformations in association with maternal trimethadione therapy. J Pediatr 1978;92:240–4.
6. Zellweger H. Anticonvulsants during pregnancy: a danger to the developing fetus? Clin Pediatr 1974;13:338–45.
7. Rischbieth RH. Troxidone (trimethadione) embryopathy: case report with review of the literature. Clin Exp Neurol 1979;16:251–6.
8. Fabro S, Brown NA. Teratogenic potential of anticonvulsants. N Engl J Med 1979;300:1280–1.
9. National Institute of Health. Anticonvulsants found to have teratogenic potential. JAMA 1981;245:36.
10. Dansky L, Andermann E, Andermann F. Major congenital malformations in the offspring of epileptic patients. Genetic and environmental risk factors. In *Epilepsy, Pregnancy and the Child*. Proceedings of a Workshop held in Berlin, September 1980. New York:Raven Press, 1981.
11. Nakane Y, Okuma T, Takahashi R, et al. Multi-institutional study on the teratogenicity and fetal toxicity of antiepileptic drugs: a report of a collaborative study group in Japan. Epilepsia 1980;21:663–80.

Name: **TRIMETHAPHAN**

Class: **Antihypertensive**   Risk Factor: **C**

Fetal Risk Summary

No reports linking the use of trimethaphan with congenital defects have been located. Trimethaphan, a short-acting ganglionic blocker that requires continuous infusion for therapeutic effect, has been studied in pregnant patients (1, 2). It is not recommended for use in pregnancy because of adverse hemodynamic effects (3). The drug is not effective in the control of hypertension in toxemic patients (1–3).

Breast Feeding Summary

No data are available.

References

1. Assali NS, Douglas RA Jr, Suyemoto R. Observations on the hemodynamic properties of a thiophanium derivative, Ro 2–2222 (Arfonad), in human subjects. Circulation 1953;8:62–9.
2. Assali NS, Suyemoto R. The place of the hydrazinophthalazine and thiophanium compounds in the management of hypertensive complications of pregnancy. Am J Obstet Gynecol 1952;64:1021–36.
3. Assali NS. Hemodynamic effects of hypotensive drugs used in pregnancy. Obstet Gynecol Surv 1954;9:776–94.

Name: **TRIMETHOBENZAMIDE**

Class: **Antiemetic**   Risk Factor: **C**

Fetal Risk Summary

Trimethobenzamide has been used in pregnancy to treat nausea and vomiting (1, 2). No adverse effects in the fetus were observed. In a third study, 193 patients were treated with trimethobenzamide in the 1st trimester (3). The incidences of severe congenital defects at 1 month, 1 year, and 5 years were 2.6%, 2.6%, and 5.8%, respectively. The 5.8% incidence was increased over nontreated controls (3.2%) ($p < 0.05$), but other factors, including the use of other antiemetics in some patients, may have contributed to the results. The authors concluded that the risk of congenital malformations with trimethobenzamide was low.

Breast Feeding Summary

No data are available.

References

1. Breslow S, Belafsky HA, Shangold JE, Hirsch LM, Stahl MB. Antiemetic effect of trimethobenzamide in pregnant patients. Clin Med 1961;8:2153–5.
2. Winters HS. Antiemetics in nausea and vomiting of pregnancy. Obstet Gynecol 1961;18:753–6.
3. Milkovich L, van den Berg BJ. An evaluation of the teratogenicity of certain antinauseant drugs. Am J Obstet Gynecol 1976;125:244–8.

Name: **TRIMETHOPRIM**

Class: **Anti-infective**   Risk Factor: **C$_M$**

Fetal Risk Summary

Trimethoprim is available as a single agent and in combination with various sulfonamides (see also Sulfonamides). The drug crosses the placenta, producing similar levels in fetal and maternal serum and in amniotic fluid (1–3). Because trimethoprim is a folate antagonist, caution has been advocated for its use in pregnancy (4, 5). However, case reports and placebo-controlled trials involving several hundred patients have failed to demonstrate an increase in fetal abnormalities (6–13).

A case of Niikawa-Kuroki syndrome has been described in a non-Japanese girl whose mother had a viral and bacterial infection during the 2nd month of pregnancy (14). The bacterial infection was treated with trimethoprim-sulfamethoxazole. The syndrome is characterized by mental and growth retardation and craniofacial malformations (14). The etiology of the defects in this patient was unknown.

Sulfa-trimethoprim combinations have been shown to cause a drop in the sperm count after 1 month of continuous treatment in males (15). Decreases varied between 7–88%. The authors theorized that trimethoprim deprived the spermatogenetic cells of active folate by inhibiting dihydrofolate reductase.

No interaction between trimethoprim-sulfamethoxazole and oral contraceptives was found in one study (16). Short courses of the anti-infective combination are unlikely to affect contraceptive control.

Breast Feeding Summary

Trimethoprim is excreted into breast milk in low concentrations. Following 160 mg twice daily for 5 days, milk concentrations varied between 1.2–2.4 μg/ml (average 1.8) with peak levels occurring at 2–3 hours (17). No adverse effects were reported in the infants. Nearly identical results were found in a study with 50 patients (18). Mean milk levels were 2.0 μg/ml, representing a milk:plasma ratio of 1.25:1. The authors concluded that these levels represented a negligible risk to the suckling infant. The American Academy of Pediatrics considers the combination of trimethoprim-sulfamethoxazole to be compatible with breast feeding (19).

References

1. Ylikorkala O, Sjostedt E, Jarvinen PA, Tikkanen R, Raines T. Trimethoprim-sulfonamide combination administered orally and intravaginally in the 1st trimester of pregnancy: its absorption into serum and transfer to amniotic fluid. Acta Obstet Gynecol Scand 1973;52:229–34.
2. Reid DWJ, Caille G, Kaufmann NR. Maternal and transplacental kinetics of trimethoprim and sulfamethoxazole, separately and in combination. Can Med Assoc J 1975;112:67s–72s.
3. Reeves DS, Wilkinson PJ. The pharmacokinetics of trimethoprim and trimethoprim/sulfonamide combinations, including penetration into body tissues. Infection 1979;7(Suppl 4):S330–41.
4. McEwen LM. Trimethoprim/sulphamethoxazole mixture in pregnancy. Br Med J 1971;4:490–1.
5. Smithells RW. Co-trimoxazole in pregnancy. Lancet 1983;2:1142.
6. Williams JD, Condie AP, Brumfitt W, Reeves DS. The treatment of bacteriuria in pregnant women with sulphamethoxazole and trimethoprim. Postgrad Med J 1969;45(Suppl):71–6.
7. Ochoa AG. Trimethoprim and sulfamethoxazole in pregnancy. JAMA 1971;217:1244.
8. Brumfitt W, Pursell R. Double-blind trial to compare ampicillin, cephalexin, co-trimoxazole, and trimethoprim in treatment of urinary infection. Br Med J 1972;2:673–6.
9. Brumfitt W, Pursell R. Trimethoprim/sulfamethoxazole in the treatment of bacteriuria in women. J Infect Dis 1973;128(Suppl):S657–63.
10. Brumfitt W, Pursell R. Trimethoprim/sulfamethoxazole in the treatment of urinary infection. Med J Aust 1973;1(Suppl):44–8.
11. Bailey RR. Single-dose antibacterial treatment for bacteriuria in pregnancy. Drugs 1984;27:183–6.
12. Soper DE, Merrill-Nach S. Successful therapy of penicillinase-producing Neisseria gonorrhoeae pharyngeal infection during pregnancy. Obstet Gynecol 1986;68:290–1.
13. Cruikshank DP, Warenski JC. First-trimester maternal Listeria monocytogenes sepsis and chorioamnionitis with normal neonatal outcome. Obstet Gynecol 1989;73:469–71.
14. Koutras A, Fisher S. Niikawa-Kuroki syndrome: a new malformation syndrome of postnatal dwarfism, mental retardation, unusual face, and protruding ears. J Pediatr 1982;101:417–9.
15. Murdia A, Mathur V, Kothari LK, Singh KP. Sulpha-trimethoprim combinations and male fertility. Lancet 1978;2:375–6.

16. Grimmer SFM, Allen WL, Back DJ, Breckenridge AM, Orme M, Tjia J. The effect of cotrimoxazole on oral contraceptive steroids in women. Contraception 1983;28:53–9.
17. Arnauld R, Soutoul JH, Gallier J, Borderon JC, Borderon E. A study of the passage of trimethoprim into the maternal milk. Quest Med 1972;25:959–64.
18. Miller RD, Salter AJ. The passage of trimethoprim/sulphamethoxazole into breast milk and its significance. In Daikos GK, ed. *Progress in Chemotherapy*, Proceedings of the Eighth International Congress of Chemotherapy, Athens, 1973. Athens:Hellenic Society for Chemotherapy, 1974:687–91.
19. Committee of Drugs, American Academy of Pediatrics. Transfer of drugs and other chemicals into human milk. Pediatrics 1989;84:924–36.

Name: **TRIPELENNAMINE**

Class: **Antihistamine**   Risk Factor: **B**

Fetal Risk Summary

The Collaborative Perinatal Project monitored 50,282 mother-child pairs, 100 of which were exposed to tripelennamine in the 1st trimester (1, pp. 323–324). For use anytime during pregnancy, 490 exposures were recorded (1, pp. 436–437). In neither case was evidence found to suggest a relationship to major or minor malformations.

The illicit use of pentazocine and tripelennamine ("T's and Blue's") has been described in a number of cases (2–5). These cases are discussed in detail under the monograph for pentazocine (see Pentazocine).

Breast Feeding Summary

Tripelennamine is excreted into bovine milk but human studies have not been reported (6). The manufacturer considers the drug to be contraindicated in the nursing mother, possibly due to the increased sensitivity of newborn or premature infants to antihistamines (7).

References

1. Heinonen OP, Slone D, Shapiro S. *Birth Defects and Drugs in Pregnancy.* Littleton:Publishing Sciences Group 1977.
2. Dunn DW, Reynolds J. Neonatal withdrawal symptoms associated with "T's and Blue's" (pentazocine and tripelennamine). Am J Dis Child 1982;136:644–5.
3. Pastorek JG II, Plauche WC, Faro S. Acute bacterial endocarditis in pregnancy: a report of three cases. J Reprod Med 1983;28:611–4.
4. Chasnoff IJ, Hatcher R, Burns WJ, Schnoll SH. Pentazocine and tripelennamine ("T's and Blue's"): effects on the fetus and neonate. Dev Phamacol Ther 1983;6:162–9.
5. von Almen WF II, Miller JM Jr. "Ts and Blues" in pregnancy. J Reprod Med 1986; 31:236–9.
6. O'Brien TE. Excretion of drugs in human milk. Am J Hosp Pharm 1974;31:844–54.
7. Product information. PBZ. Geigy Pharmaceuticals, 1990.

Name: **TRIPROLIDINE**

Class: **Antihistamine**   Risk Factor: **C$_M$**

Fetal Risk Summary

No reports linking the use of triprolidine with congenital defects have been located. The Collaborative Perinatal Project monitored 50,282 mother-child pairs, 16 of which had 1st trimester exposure to triprolidine (1). From this small sample, no evidence was found to suggest a relationship to large categories of major or minor malformations or to individual malformations.

In a 1971 study, infants and mothers who had ingested antihistamines during the 1st trimester actually had fewer abnormalities when compared to controls (2). Triprolidine was the third most commonly used antihistamine. The manufacturer claims that in over 20 years of marketing the drug no reports of triprolidine teratogenicity have been received (M.F. Frosolono, personal communication, Burroughs Wellcome, 1980). Their animal studies have also been negative.

Breast Feeding Summary

Triprolidine is excreted into human breast milk (3). Three mothers, who were nursing healthy infants, were given an antihistamine-decongestant preparation containing 2.5 mg of triprolidine and 60 mg of pseudoephedrine. The women had been nursing their infants for 14 weeks, 14 weeks, and 18 months, respectively. Triprolidine was found in the milk of all three subjects, with milk:plasma ratios in one woman at 1, 3, and 12 hours of 0.5, 1.2, and 0.7, respectively. Using area under the concentration-time curves in the other two women gave more reliable results of 0.56 and 0.50, respectively (3). The authors calculated that a milk production of 1000 ml/24 hours would contain 0.001–0.004 mg of triprolidine base, or about 0.06–0.2% of the maternal dose. The American Academy of Pediatrics considers triprolidine to be compatible with breast feeding (4).

References

1. Heinonen OP, Slone D, Shapiro S. *Birth Defects and Drugs in Pregnancy*. Littleton:Publishing Sciences Group, 1977:323.
2. Nelson MM, Forfar JO. Associations between drugs administered during pregnancy and congenital abnormalities of the fetus. Br Med J 1971;1:523–7.
3. Findlay JWA, Butz RF, Sailstad JM, Warren JT, Welch RM. Pseudoephedrine and triprolidine in plasma and breast milk of nursing mothers. Br J Clin Pharmac 1984;18:901–6.
4. Committee on Drugs, American Academy of Pediatrics. Transfer of drugs and other chemicals into human milk. Pediatrics 1989;84:924–36.

Name: **TROLEANDOMYCIN**

Class: **Antibiotic**   Risk Factor: **C**

Fetal Risk Summary

Troleandomycin is the triacetyl ester of oleandomycin (see Oleandomycin).

Breast Feeding Summary

See Oleandomycin.

Name: **TYROPANOATE**

Class: **Diagnostic**   Risk Factor: **D**

Fetal Risk Summary

Tyropanoate contains a high concentration of organically bound iodine. See Diatrizoate for possible effects on the fetus and newborn.

Breast Feeding Summary

See Potassium Iodide.

Name: **UREA**

Class: **Diuretic**

Risk Factor: **C**

Fetal Risk Summary

Urea is an osmotic diuretic that is used primarily to treat cerebral edema. Topical formulations for skin disorders are also available. No reports of its use in pregnancy following intravenous, oral, or topical administration have been located. Urea, given by intra-amniotic injection, has been used for the induction of abortion (1).

Breast Feeding Summary

No data are available.

Reference

1. Ware A, ed. *Martindale: The Extra Pharmacopoeia*, ed 27. London:The Pharmaceutical Press, 1977:572.

Name: **UROKINASE**

Class: **Thrombolytic**

Risk Factor: **B$_M$**

Fetal Risk Summary

Urokinase is not teratogenic in rats or mice (1). Only one report of its use in human pregnancy has been located. A woman, at 28 weeks' gestation, was treated with urokinase, 4400 IU/kg over 10 minutes followed by 4400 IU/kg/hour for 12 hours, for hemodynamically significant pulmonary thromboemboli (2). Heparin therapy was then administered, first intravenously then subcutaneously, for the remainder of the pregnancy. A healthy term infant was delivered 2 months after initiation of therapy.

Breast Feeding Summary

No data are available.

References

1. Shepard TH. *Catalog of Teratogenic Agents*, ed 6. Baltimore:Johns Hopkins University Press, 1989:655.
2. Delclos GL, Davila F. Thrombolytic therapy for pulmonary embolism in pregnancy: a case report. Am J Obstet Gynecol 1986;155:375–6.

Name: **VACCINE, BCG**

Class: **Vaccine**   Risk Factor: **C**

Fetal Risk Summary

BCG vaccine is a live, attenuated bacteria vaccine used to provide immunity to tuberculosis (1, 2). The risk to the fetus from maternal vaccination is unknown. However, since it is a live preparation, the vaccine should probably not be used during pregnancy (2).

Breast Feeding Summary

No data are available.

References

1. American Hospital Formulary Service. *Drug Information 1990*. Bethesda:American Society of Hospital Pharmacists, 1990:1921–24.
2. Amstey MS. Vaccination in pregnancy. Clin Obstet Gynaecol 1983;10:13–22.

Name: **VACCINE, CHOLERA**

Class: **Vaccine**   Risk Factor: **C**

Fetal Risk Summary

Cholera vaccine is a killed bacteria vaccine (1, 2). Cholera during pregnancy may result in significant morbidity and mortality to the mother and the fetus, particularly during the 3rd trimester (1). The risk to the fetus from maternal vaccination is unknown. The American College of Obstetricians and Gynecologists *Technical Bulletin* No. 64 recommends that the vaccine be given during pregnancy to meet international travel requirements (1).

Breast Feeding Summary

Maternal vaccination with cholera vaccine has increased specific IgA antibody titers in breast milk (3). In a second study, cholera vaccine (whole cell plus toxoid) was administered to six lactating mothers, resulting in a significant rise in milk anti-cholera toxin IgA titers in five of the patients (4). Milk from three of these five mothers also had a significant increase in anti-cholera toxin IgG titers.

References

1. American College of Obstetricians and Gynecologists. *Technical Bulletin*, No. 64, May 1982.
2. Amstey MS. Vaccination in pregnancy. Clin Obstet Gynaecol 1983;10:13–22.

3. Svennerholm AM, Holmgren J, Hanson LA, Lindblad BS, Quereshi F, Rahimtoola RJ. Boosting of secretory IgA antibody responses in man by parenteral cholera vaccination. Scand J Immunol 1977;6:1345–49.
4. Merson MH, Black RE, Sack DA, Svennerholm AM, Holmgren J. Maternal cholera immunisation and secretory IgA in breast milk. Lancet 1980;1:931–2.

Name: **VACCINE, *ESCHERICHIA COLI***

Class: **Vaccine**   Risk Factor: **C**

Fetal Risk Summary

Escherichia coli (*E. coli*) vaccine is a nonpathogenic strain of bacteria used experimentally as a vaccine. Two reports of its use (strains O111 and 083) in pregnant women in labor or waiting for the onset of labor have been located (1, 2). The vaccines were given to these patients in an attempt to produce antimicrobial activity in their colostrum. No adverse effects in the newborn were noted.

Breast Feeding Summary

Escherichia coli (*E. coli* strains O111 and 083) vaccines were given to mothers in labor or waiting for the onset of labor (1, 2). Antibodies against E. coli were found in the colostrum of 7 of 47 (strain 0111) and 3 of 3 (strain 083) treated mothers but in only 1 of 101 controls. No adverse effects were noted in the nursing infants.

References

1. Dluholucky S, Siragy P, Dolezel P, Svac J, Bolgac A. Antimicrobial activity of colostrum after administering killed Escherichia coli O111 vaccine orally to expectant mothers. Arch Dis Child 1980;55:558–60.
2. Goldblum RM, Ahlstedt S, Carlsson B, Hanson LA, Jodal U, Lidin-Janson G, Sohl-Akerlund A. Antibody-forming cells in human colostrum after oral immunisation. Nature 1975;257:797–9.

Name: **VACCINE, HEPATITIS B**

Class: **Vaccine**   Risk Factor: **C$_M$**

Fetal Risk Summary

Hepatitis B vaccine is a killed virus (surface antigen HBsAg) vaccine (1, 2). The risk to the fetus from maternal vaccination is unknown. Pre-exposure prophylaxis is indicated for persons at high risk for exposure to the disease (1). Pregnancy probably does not change this recommendation.

Breast Feeding Summary

No data are available.

References

1. American Hospital Formulary Service. *Drug Information 1990*. Bethesda:American Society of Hospital Pharmacists, 1990:1931–8.

2. Amstey MS. Vaccination in pregnancy. Clin Obstet Gynaecol 1983;10:13–22.

Name: **VACCINE, INFLUENZA**

Class: **Vaccine** Risk Factor: **C**

Fetal Risk Summary

Influenza vaccine is an inactivated virus vaccine (1). Influenza during pregnancy may potentially result in an increased rate of spontaneous abortions (1). The risk to the fetus from maternal vaccination is unknown. The American College of Obstetricians and Gynecologists *Technical Bulletin* No. 64 recommends that the vaccine be given only to pregnant women with serious underlying diseases (1). Public health officials should be consulted for current recommendations (1).

Breast Feeding Summary

No data are available. Maternal vaccination is not thought to present any risk to the nursing infant (2).

References

1. American College of Obstetricians and Gynecologists. *Technical Bulletin,* No. 64, May 1982.
2. Kilbourne ED. Questions and answers. Artificial influenza immunization of nursing mothers not harmful. JAMA 1973;226:87.

Name: **VACCINE, MEASLES**

Class: **Vaccine** Risk Factor: **X**

Fetal Risk Summary

Measles (rubeola) vaccine is a live attenuated virus vaccine (1, 2). Measles occurring during pregnancy may result in significant maternal morbidity, an increased abortion rate, and congenital malformations (1). Although a fetal risk from the vaccine has not been confirmed, the vaccine should not be used during pregnancy because fetal infection with the attenuated viruses may occur (1, 2). The American College of Obstetricians and Gynecologists Technical Bulletin No. 64 lists the vaccine as contraindicated in pregnancy (1). (See also Vaccine, Rubella).

Breast Feeding Summary

No data are available.

References

1. American College of Obstetricians and Gynecologists. *Technical Bulletin*, No. 64, May 1982.
2. Amstey MS. Vaccination in pregnancy. Clin Obstet Gynaecol 1983;10:13–22.

Name: VACCINE, MENINGOCOCCUS

Class: **Vaccine**   Risk Factor: **C**

Fetal Risk Summary

Meningococcus vaccine is a killed bacteria (cell wall) vaccine (1, 2). The risk to the fetus from vaccination during pregnancy is unknown (1). In one study, vaccination resulted in transfer of maternal antibodies to the fetus, but the transfer was irregular and was not dependent on maternal titer or the period in pregnancy when vaccination occurred (3). The American College of Obstetricians and Gynecologists *Technical Bulletin* No. 64 recommends that the vaccine be used during pregnancy only when the risk of maternal infection is high (1).

Breast Feeding Summary

No data are available.

References

1. American College of Obstetricians and Gynecologists. *Technical Bulletin*, No. 64, May 1982.
2. Amstey MS. Vaccination in pregnancy. Clin Obstet Gynaecol 1983;10:13–22.
3. Carvalho ADA, Giampaglia CMS, Kimura H, Pereira OADC, Farhat CK, Neves JC, Prandini R, Carvalho EDS, Zarvos AM. Maternal and infant antibody response to meningococcal vaccination in pregnancy. Lancet 1977;2:809–11.

Name: VACCINE, MUMPS

Class: **Vaccine**   Risk Factor: **X**

Fetal Risk Summary

Mumps vaccine is a live attenuated virus vaccine (1, 2). Mumps occurring during pregnancy may result in an increased rate of 1st trimester abortion, and there is a questionable association with fibroelastosis in the newborn (1). Although a fetal risk from the vaccine has not been confirmed, the vaccine should not be used during pregnancy because fetal infection with the attenuated viruses may occur (1, 2). The American College of Obstetricians and Gynecologists *Technical Bulletin* No. 64 lists the vaccine as contraindicated in pregnancy (1).

Breast Feeding Summary

No data are available.

References

1. American College of Obstetricians and Gynecologists. *Technical Bulletin*, No. 64, May 1982.
2. Amstey MS. Vaccination in pregnancy. Clin Obstet Gynaecol 1983;10:13–22.

Name: **VACCINE, PLAGUE**

Class: **Vaccine**   Risk Factor: **C**

Fetal Risk Summary

Plague vaccine is a killed bacteria vaccine (1, 2). The risk to the fetus from vaccination during pregnancy is unknown (1). The American College of Obstetricians and Gynecologists *Technical Bulletin* No. 64 recommends that the vaccine be used in pregnancy only for exposed persons (1).

Breast Feeding Summary

No data are available.

References

1. American College of Obstetricians and Gynecologists. *Technical Bulletin*, No. 64, May 1982.
2. Amstey MS. Vaccination in pregnancy. Clin Obstet Gynaecol 1983;10:13–22.

Name: **VACCINE, PNEUMOCOCCAL POLYVALENT**

Class: **Vaccine**   Risk Factor: **C**

Fetal Risk Summary

Pneumococcal vaccine is a killed bacteria (cell wall) vaccine (1, 2). The risk to the fetus from vaccination during pregnancy is unknown (1). The American College of Obstetricians and Gynecologists *Technical Bulletin* No. 64 recommends the vaccine be used in pregnancy only for high-risk patients (1). The American College of Physicians concurs with this recommendation (3).

Breast Feeding Summary

No data are available.

References

1. American College of Obstetricians and Gynecologists. *Technical Bulletin*, No. 64, May 1982.
2. Amstey MS. Vaccination in pregnancy. Clin Obstet Gynaecol 1983;10:13–22.
3. Health and Public Policy Committee, American College of Physicians. Pneumococcal vaccine. Ann Intern Med 1986;104:118–20.

Name: **VACCINE, POLIOVIRUS INACTIVATED**

Class: **Vaccine**   Risk Factor: **C**

Fetal Risk Summary

Poliovirus vaccine inactivated (Salk vaccine, IPV) is an inactivated virus vaccine administered by injection (1, 2). Although fetal damage may occur when the mother contracts the disease during pregnancy, the risk to the fetus from the vaccine is unknown (1). The American College of Obstetricians and Gynecologists *Technical Bulletin* No. 64 recommends use of the vaccine during pregnancy only if an increased risk of exposure exists (1). The oral vaccine (Sabin vaccine, OPV) is a live, attenuated virus strain and probably should not be used in the pregnant woman (2). However, if immediate protection against poliomyelitis is needed, the Immunization Practices Advisory Committee (ACIP) recommends the oral vaccine (3).

Breast Feeding Summary

No data are available.

References

1. American College of Obstetricians and Gynecologists. *Technical Bulletin*, No. 64, May 1982.
2. Amstey MS. Vaccination in pregnancy. Clin Obstet Gynaecol 1983;10:13–22.
3. Recommendation of the Immunization Practices Advisory Committee (ACIP); Poliomyelitis prevention. MMWR 1982;31:22–6, 31–4.

Name: **VACCINE, POLIOVIRUS LIVE**

Class: **Vaccine**   Risk Factor: **C**

Fetal Risk Summary

Poliovirus vaccine live (Sabin vaccine, OPV) is a live, attenuated virus strain vaccine administered orally (1, 2). Although fetal damage may occur when the mother contracts the disease during pregnancy, the risk to the fetus from the vaccine is unknown (1). If vaccination is required during pregnancy, one author has recommended use of the inactivated virus vaccine (Salk vaccine) to reduce the risk of potential fetal and neonatal infection (2). When immediate protection is needed, the Immunization Practices Advisory Committee (ACIP) recommends the oral (OPV) vaccine (3).

Breast Feeding Summary

Human milk contains poliovirus antibodies in direct relation to titers found in the mother's serum. When oral poliovirus vaccine (Sabin vaccine, OPV) is administered to the breast-fed infant in the immediate neonatal period, these antibodies, which are highest in colostrum, may prevent infection and development of subsequent immunity to wild poliovirus (4–15). To prevent inhibition of the vaccine, breast feeding should be withheld 6 hours before and after administration of the vaccine, although some authors recommend shorter times (10–14).

In the United States, the ACIP and the Committee on Infectious Diseases of the American Academy of Pediatrics do not recommend vaccination before 6 weeks of age (3, 16). At this age or older, the effect of the oral vaccine is not inhibited by breast feeding and no special instructions or planned feeding schedules are required (3, 16–20).

References

1. American College of Obstetricians and Gynecologists. *Technical Bulletin*, No. 64, May 1982.
2. Amstey MS. Vaccination in pregnancy. Clin Obstet Gynaecol 1983;10:13–22.
3. Recommendation of the Immunization Practices Advisory Committee (ACIP); Poliomyelitis prevention. MMWR 1982;31:22–6, 31–4.
4. Lepow ML, Warren RJ, Gray N, Ingram VG, Robbins FC. Effect of Sabin type I poliomyelitis vaccine administered by mouth to newborn infants. N Engl J Med 1961;264:1071–8.
5. Holguin AH, Reeves JS, Gelfand HM. Immunization of infants with the Sabin oral poliovirus vaccine. Am J Public Health 1962;52:600–10.
6. Sabin AB, Fieldsteel AH. Antipoliomyelitic activity of human and bovine colostrum and milk. Pediatrics 1962;29:105–15.
7. Sabin AB, Michaels RH, Krugman S, Eiger ME, Berman PH, Warren J. Effect of oral poliovirus vaccine in newborn children. I. Excretion of virus after ingestion of large doses of type I or of mixture of all three types, in relation to level of placentally transmitted antibody. Pediatrics 1963;31:623–40.
8. Warren RJ, Lepow ML, Bartsch GE, Robbins FC. The relationship of maternal antibody, breast feeding, and age to the susceptibility of newborn infants to infection with attenuated polioviruses. Pediatrics 1964;34:4–13.
9. Plotkin SA, Katz M, Brown RE, Pagano JS. Oral poliovirus vaccination in newborn African infants. The inhibitory effect of breast feeding. Am J Dis Child 1966;111:27–30.
10. Katz M, Plotkin SA. Oral polio immunization of the newborn infant; a possible method for overcoming interference by ingested antibodies. J Pediatr 1968;73:267–70.
11. Adcock E, Greene H. Poliovirus antibodies in breast-fed infants. Lancet 1971;2:662–3.
12. Anonymous. Sabin vaccine in breast-fed infants. Med J Aust 1972;2:175.
13. John TJ. The effect of breast-feeding on the antibody response of infants to trivalent oral poliovirus vaccine. J Pediatr 1974;84:307.
14. Plotkin SA, Katz M. Administration of oral polio vaccine in relation to time of breast feeding. J Pediatr 1974;84:309.
15. Deforest A, Smith DS. Reply. J Pediatr 1974;84:308.
16. Kelein JO, Brunell PA, Cherry JD, Fulginiti VA, eds. *Report of the Committee on Infectious Diseases*, 19th ed. Evanston:American Academy of Pediatrics, 1982:208.
17. Kim-Farley R, Brink E, Orenstein W, Bart K. Vaccination and breast-feeding. JAMA 1982;248:2451–2.
18. Deforest A, Parker PB, DiLiberti JH, Yates HT Jr, Sibinga MS, Smith DS. The effect of breast-feeding on the antibody response of infants to trivalent oral poliovirus vaccine. J Pediatr 1973;83:93–5.
19. John TJ, Devarajan LV, Luther L, Vijayarathnam P. Effect of breast-feeding on seroresponse of infants to oral poliovirus vaccination. Pediatrics 1976;57:47–53.
20. Welsh J, May JT. Breast-feeding and trivalent oral polio vaccine. J Pediatr 1979;95:333.

Name: VACCINE, RABIES (HUMAN)

Class: **Vaccine**   Risk Factor: **C**

Fetal Risk Summary

Rabies vaccine (human) is an inactivated virus vaccine (1, 2). Since rabies is nearly 100% fatal if contracted, the vaccine should be given for postexposure prophylaxis (1, 2). Fetal risk from the vaccine is unknown (1). Two reports that described the use of rabies vaccine (human) during pregnancy have been located (3, 4). Passive immunity was found in one newborn (titer >1:50) but was lost by 1 year of age (3). No adverse effects from the vaccine were noted in the newborn. The mother had not delivered at the time of the report in the second case (4).

Two other reports of the use in pregnancy of duck embryo cultured vaccine have also been located (5, 6). In 1974 a report appeared describing the use of rabies vaccine (duck embryo) in a woman in her 7th month of pregnancy (5). She was given a 21-day treatment course of the vaccine. She subsequently delivered a healthy term male infant who was developing normally at 9 months of age. A second case was described in 1975 involving a woman exposed to rabies at 35 weeks' gestation (6). She was treated with a 14-day course of vaccine (duck embryo) followed by three booster injections. She gave birth at 39 weeks' gestation to a healthy male infant. Cord blood rabies neutralizing antibody titer was 1:30, indicative of passive immunity, compared to a titer of 1:70 in maternal serum. Titers in the infant fell to 1:5 at 3 weeks of age, then to <1:5 at 6 weeks. Development was normal at 9 months of age.

Breast Feeding Summary

No data are available.

References

1. American College of Obstetricians and Gynecologists. *Technical Bulletin*, No. 64, May 1982.
2. Amstey MS. Vaccination in pregnancy. Clin Obstet Gynaecol 1983;10:13–22.
3. Varner MW, McGuinness GA, Galask RP. Rabies vaccination in pregnancy. Am J Obstet Gynecol 1982;143:717–8.
4. Klietmann W, Domres B, Cox JH. Rabies post-exposure treatment and side-effects in man using HDC (MRC 5) vaccine. Dev Biol Stand 1978;40:109–13.
5. Cates W Jr. Treatment of rabies exposure during pregnancy. Obstet Gynecol 1974; 44:893–6.
6. Spence MR, Davidson DE, Dill GS Jr, Boonthai P, Sagartz JW. Rabies exposure during pregnancy. Am J Obstet Gynecol 1975;123:655–6.

Name: **VACCINE, RUBELLA**

Class: **Vaccine**   Risk Factor: **X**

Fetal Risk Summary

Rubella (German measles) vaccine is a live, attenuated virus vaccine (1, 2). Rubella occurring during pregnancy may result in the congenital rubella syndrome (CRS). The greatest risk period for viremia and fetal defects is 1 week prior to 4 weeks after conception (3). The United States Department of Health and Human Services Centers for Disease Control (CDC) defines CRS as any two complications from list A or one complication from list A plus one from list B (3):

LIST A
  Cataracts/congenital glaucoma
  Congenital heart disease
  Loss of hearing
  Pigmentary retinopathy

LIST B
  Purpura
  Splenomegaly
  Jaundice (onset within 24 hours of birth)
  Microcephaly
  Mental retardation
  Meningoencephalitis
  Radiolucent bone disease

Prior to April 1979, the CDC collected data on 538 women vaccinated within 3 months before or after conception with either the Cendehill or HPV-77 vaccines (3). A total of 149 of these women were known to be susceptible at the time of vaccination and the outcome of pregnancy was known for 143 (96%). No evidence of CRS or other maternal/fetal complication was found in any of these cases or in an additional 196 infants exposed during pregnancy (3). Eight infants had serologic evidence of intrauterine infection after maternal vaccination, but follow-up for 2–7 years revealed no problems attributable to CRS.

Since January 1979, only RA 27/3 rubella vaccine has been available in the United States. In the United States between January 1979 and December 1988, a total of 683 women vaccinated within the time frame stated above with RA 27/3 have been reported to the CDC (4). The outcomes of these pregnancies were:

Total vaccinated (1/79–12/88)	683	
Susceptible at vaccination	272	
Live births	212	(2 sets of twins)
Spontaneous abortions/stillbirths	13	
Induced abortions	31	
Outcome unknown	18	
Immune/unknown at vaccination	411	
Live births	350	(1 set of twins)
Spontaneous abortions/stillbirths	9	
Induced abortions	24	
Outcome unknown	29	

Evidence of subclinical infection was found in 3 (2%) of the 154 liveborn infants from susceptible mothers who were serologically evaluated (4). However, no evidence of defects compatible with CRS was found in the total sample of 212 liveborn infants. Two infants did have asymptomatic glandular hypospadias, but both mothers had negative rubella-specific IgM titers in the cord blood at birth (4). In a 1985 evaluation of earlier CDC data, no defects compatible with CRS were found in any of the fetuses/infants where the outcome was known (5). Examinations up to 29 months after birth have revealed normal growth and development (4, 5).

Although no defects attributable to rubella vaccine have been reported, the CDC calculates the theoretical risk of CRS following vaccination to be as high as 4.9% (for those vaccinated within 1 week before to 4 weeks after conception), still considerably lower than the 20% or greater risk associated with wild rubella virus infection during the 1st trimester (4). Because a risk does exist, the use of the vaccine in pregnancy is contraindicated (1–5). However, if vaccination does occur within 3 months of conception or during pregnancy, the actual risk is considered to be negligible and, in itself, should not be an indication to terminate the pregnancy (3–5).

Breast Feeding Summary

Vaccination of susceptible women with rubella vaccine in the immediate postpartum period is recommended by the American College of Obstetricians and Gynecologists *Technical Bulletin* No. 64 and the United States Public Health Service Immunization Practices Advisory Committee (1, 6). A large number of these women will breast feed their newborns. Although two studies failed to find evidence of the attenuated virus in milk, subsequent reports have demonstrated transfer (7–11).

In one case, the mother noted rash and adenopathy 12 days after vaccination with the HPV-77 vaccine on the 1st postpartum day (8). Rubella virus was isolated from her breast milk and from the infant's throat (9). A significant level of rubella-specific cell-mediated immunity was found in the infant, but there was no detectable serologic response as measured by rubella hemagglutination inhibition antibody titers (9). No adverse effects were noted in the infant. In a second case report, a 13-day-old breast-fed infant developed rubella about 11 days after maternal vaccination with HPV-77 (12). It could not be determined if the infant was infected by virus transmission via the milk (13, 14). Nine (69%) of 13 lactating women given either HPV-77 or RA 27/3 vaccine in the immediate postpartum period shed virus in their milk (10). In another report by these same researchers, 11 (68%) of 16 vaccinated women shed rubella virus or virus antigen in their milk (11). No adverse effects or symptoms of clinical disease were observed in the infants.

References

1. American College of Obstetricians and Gynecologists. *Technical Bulletin*, No. 64, May 1982.
2. Amstey MS. Vaccination in pregnancy. Clin Obstet Gynaecol 1983;10:13–22.
3. Centers For Disease Control, U.S. Department of Health and Human Services. Rubella vaccination during pregnancy—United States, 1971–1982. MMWR 1983;32:429–32.
4. Centers For Disease Control, U.S. Department of Health and Human Services. Rubella vaccination during pregnancy—United States, 1971–1988. MMWR 1989;38:289–93.
5. Preblud SR, Williams NM. Fetal risk associated with rubella vaccine: implications for vaccination of susceptible women. Obstet Gynecol 1985;66:121–3.
6. American Hospital Formulary Service. *Drug Information 1985*. Bethesda:American Society of Hospital Pharmacists, 1985:1560–3.
7. Isacson P, Kehrer AF, Wilson H, Williams S. Comparative study of live, attenuated rubella virus vaccines during the immediate puerperium. Obstet Gynecol 1971;37:332–7.
8. Grillner L, Hedstrom CE, Bergstrom H, Forssman L, Rigner A, Lycke E. Vaccination against rubella of newly delivered women. Scand J Infect Dis 1973;5:237–41.
9. Buimovici-Klein E, Hite RL, Byrne T, Cooper LZ. Isolation of rubella virus in milk after postpartum immunization. J Pediatr 1977;91:939–41.
10. Losonsky GA, Fishaut JM, Strussenberg J, Ogra PL. Effect of immunization against rubella on lactation products. I. Development and characterization of specific immunologic reactivity in breast milk. J Infect Dis 1982;145:654–60.
11. Losonsky GA, Fishaut JM, Strussenberg J, Ogra PL. Effect of immunization against rubella on lactation products. II. Maternal-neonatal interactions. J Infect Dis 1982;145:661–6.
12. Landes RD, Bass JW, Millunchick EW, Oetgen WJ. Neonatal rubella following postpartum maternal immunization. J Pediatr 1980;97:465–7.
13. Lerman SJ. Neonatal rubella following maternal immunization. J Pediatr 1981;98:668.

14. Bass JW, Landes RD. Neonatal rubella following maternal immunization. Reply. J Pediatr 1981;98:668–9.

Name: **VACCINE, SMALLPOX**

Class: **Vaccine**   Risk Factor: **X**

Fetal Risk Summary

Smallpox vaccine is a live, attenuated virus vaccine (1, 2). Although smallpox infection had a high mortality rate, the disease has been largely eradicated from the world (1, 3). Vaccination during pregnancy between 3 and 24 weeks has resulted in fetal death (2, 3). Based on the above information, smallpox vaccine is contraindicated during pregnancy (1–3).

Breast Feeding Summary

No data are available.

References

1. Amstey MS. Vaccination in pregnancy. Clin Obstet Gynaecol 1983;10:13–22.
2. American Hospital Formulary Service. *Drug Information 1990*. Bethesda:American Society of Hospital Pharmacists, 1990:1965–7.
3. Hart RJC. Immunization. Clin Obstet Gynaecol 1981;8:421–30.

Name: **VACCINE, TULAREMIA**

Class: **Vaccine**   Risk Factor: **C**

Fetal Risk Summary

Tularemia vaccine is a live, attenuated bacteria vaccine (1, 2). Tularemia is a serious infectious disease occurring primarily in laboratory personnel, rabbit handlers, and forest workers (1). The risk to the fetus from the vaccine is unknown. One report described vaccination in a woman early in the 1st trimester (2). No adverse effects were observed in the term infant or at 1 year follow-up. Since tularemia is a severe disease, pre-exposure prophylaxis of indicated persons should occur regardless of pregnancy (1).

Breast Feeding Summary

No data are available.

References

1. Amstey MS. Vaccination in pregnancy. Clin Obstet Gynaecol 1983;10:13–22.
2. Albrecht RC, Cefalo RC, O'Brien WF. Tularemia immunization in early pregnancy. Am J Obstet Gynecol 1980;138:1226–7.

Name: **VACCINE, TYPHOID**

Class: **Vaccine**   Risk Factor: **C**

Fetal Risk Summary

Typhoid vaccine is a killed bacteria vaccine (1, 2). Typhoid is a serious infectious disease with high morbidity and mortality. The risk to the fetus from the vaccine is unknown (1). The American College of Obstetricians and Gynecologists *Technical Bulletin* No. 64 recommends vaccination during pregnancy only for close, continued exposure or travel to endemic areas (1).

Breast Feeding Summary

No data are available.

References

1. American College of Obstetricians and Gynecologists. *Technical Bulletin*, No. 64, May 1982.
2. Amstey MS. Vaccination in pregnancy. Clin Obstet Gynaecol 1983;10:13–22.

Name: **VACCINE, YELLOW FEVER**

Class: **Vaccine**   Risk Factor: **D**

Fetal Risk Summary

Yellow fever vaccine is a live, attenuated virus vaccine (1, 2). Yellow fever is a serious infectious disease with high morbidity and mortality. The risk to the fetus from the vaccine is unknown (1, 2). The American College of Obstetricians and Gynecologists *Technical Bulletin* No. 64 lists the vaccine as contraindicated in pregnancy except if exposure is unavoidable (1).

Breast Feeding Summary

No data are available.

References

1. American College of Obstetricians and Gynecologists. *Technical Bulletin*, No. 64, May 1982.
2. Amstey MS. Vaccination in pregnancy. Clin Obstet Gynaecol 1983;10:13–22.

Name: **VALPROIC ACID**

Class: **Anticonvulsant**   Risk Factor: **D**

Fetal Risk Summary

Valproic acid and its salt form, sodium valproate, are anticonvulsants used in the treatment of seizure disorders. The drugs readily cross the placenta to the fetus. At term, the range of cord blood:maternal serum ratios of total valproic acid (protein bound and unbound) has been reported to be 0.52–4.6 (1–13). More recent studies have reported mean ratios of 1.4–2.4 (4, 7, 9–13). In contrast, the mean cord blood:maternal serum ratio of free (unbound) valproic acid was 0.82 (10). Two mechanisms have been proposed to account for the accumulation of total valproic acid in the fetus: partial displacement of the drug from maternal binding sites by increased free fatty acid concentrations in maternal blood at the time of birth (10), and increased protein binding of valproic acid in fetal serum (11). Increased unbound valproic acid in the maternal serum may also be partially a result of decreased serum albumin (14). Although one study measured a mean serum half-life for valproic acid in the newborn of 28.3 hours (9), other studies have reported values of 43–47 hours, approximately four times the adult value (2, 4, 8, 10, 13). In agreement with these data, valproic acid has been shown to lack fetal hepatic enzyme induction activity when used alone and will block the enzyme induction activity of primidone when the two anticonvulsants are combined during pregnancy (15).

In published reports, doses of valproic acid in pregnancy have ranged from 300–3000 mg (1–3, 8, 12, 16–28). Although a good correlation between serum levels and seizure control is not always observed, most patients will respond when levels are in the range of 50–100 µg/ml (29). In early pregnancy, high (i.e., >1000 mg) daily doses of valproic acid may produce maternal serum concentrations that are much greater than 100 µg/ml (8). However, as pregnancy progresses and without dosage adjustment, valproic acid levels fall steadily so that in the 3rd trimester, maternal levels are often less than 50 µg/ml (8). One study concluded that the decreased serum concentrations were a result of increased hepatic clearance and an increased apparent volume of distribution (8).

Fetal/newborn consequences resulting from the use of valproic acid and sodium valproate during pregnancy have been reported to include: major and minor congenital abnormalities, intrauterine growth retardation, hyperbilirubinemia, hepatotoxicity (which may be fatal), transient hyperglycinemia, afibrinogenemia (one case), and fetal/neonatal distress.

Prior to 1981, the maternal use of valproic acid was not thought to present a risk to the fetus. A 1981 editorial recommended sodium valproate or carbamazepine as anticonvulsants of choice in appropriate types of epilepsy for women who may become pregnant (30). Although the drug was known to be a potent animal teratogen (31), more potent than phenytoin and at least as potent as trimethadione (32), only a single unconfirmed case of human teratogenicity (in a fetus exposed to at least two other anticonvulsants) had been published between 1969 and 1976 (33). (An editorial comment in that report noted that subsequent investigation had failed to confirm the defect.) In other published cases, both before and after 1980, healthy term infants resulted after in utero exposure to valproic acid (1–3, 12, 19, 27, 28, 32, 34–38). Moreover, a committee of the American Academy of Pediatrics stated in 1982 that the data for a teratogenic potential in humans for valproic acid were inadequate and that recommendations for or against its use in pregnancy could not be given (39).

The first confirmed report of an infant with congenital defects after valproic acid exposure during pregnancy appeared in 1980 (16). The mother, who took 1000 mg of valproic acid daily throughout gestation, delivered a growth-retarded infant with facial dysmorphism and heart and limb defects. The infant expired at age 19 days. Since this initial report, several studies and case reports have described newborns with malformations after *in utero* exposure to either valproic acid monotherapy or combination therapy (4, 17–26, 36, 40–58).

The most serious abnormalities observed with valproic acid (or sodium valproate) exposure are defects in neural tube closure. The absolute risk of this defect is approximately 1–2%, about the same risk for a familial occurrence of this anomaly (37, 40, 59, 60). No cases of anencephaly have been associated with valproic acid (21, 60, 61). Exposure to valproic acid between the 17th and 30th day after fertilization must occur before the drug can be considered a cause of neural tube defects (62). Other predominant defects involve the heart, face, and limbs. A characteristic pattern of minor facial abnormalities has been attributed to valproic acid (60). Cardiac anomalies and cleft lip/palate occur with most anticonvulsants and a causal relationship with valproic acid has not been established (37, 46). In addition, almost all types of congenital malformations have been observed after treatment of epilepsy during pregnancy (see Janz 1982, Phenytoin). Consequently, the list below, while abstracting the cited references, is not meant to be inclusive and, at times, reflects multiple anticonvulsant therapy.

NEURAL TUBE DEFECTS
Defects in neural tube closure (17, 19, 21, 22, 24, 26, 40–42, 44–46, 53–58)   (includes entire spectrum from spina bifida occulta to meningomyelocele)

CARDIAC DEFECTS
Multiple (not specified) (21, 24, 26, 37, 42, 44, 51)
Levocardia (16)
Patent ductus arteriosus (4, 26, 48, 50, 52)

Valvular aortic stenosis (23, 48)
Ventricular septal defect (4, 20, 48)
Tetralogy of Fallot (18, 51)
Partial right bundle branch block (16)
Anomalies of great vessels (51)

FACIAL DEFECTS
Facial dysmorphism (4, 26, 42, 46, 50, 53)
Small nose (16, 20, 24, 26, 50, 53)
Depressed nasal bridge (18, 20, 26, 50)
Flat orbits (26)
Protruding eyes (16)
Hypertelorism (4, 26)
Low-set/rotated ears (4, 16, 24, 26, 50)
Micrognathia/retrognathia (16, 23, 26)
Thin upper vermilion border (24, 26, 48, 50, 53)
Down-turned angles of mouth (50)

High forehead (24, 26)
Bulging frontal eminences (16, 20)
Strabismus (50)
Nystagmus (50)
Epicanthal folds (4, 26, 50, 53)
Coarsened facies (20)
Cleft lip/palate (18, 37, 42, 44, 51)
Microstomia (24, 26, 48, 50)
Esotropia (50)
Depigmentation of eyelashes and brow (16, 25)
Short palpebral fissure (26, 48, 50)
Long upper lip (26, 50)
Agenesis of lacrimal ducts (51)

HEAD/NECK DEFECTS
Brachycephaly (24, 26)
Hydrocephaly (19, 21, 42, 46)
Wide anterior fontanelle (18)
Abnormal or premature stenosis of metopic suture (24, 26, 50)

Microcephaly (4, 21, 24, 38, 50, 63, 64)
Short neck (20)
Craniostenosis (26)

UROGENITAL DEFECTS

Bilateral duplication of caliceal collecting systems (25)
Bilateral undescended testes (23)

Nonspecified (26)
Hypospadias (21, 23, 26, 46, 50)
Bilateral renal hypoplasia (23)

SKELETAL/LIMB DEFECTS

Aplasia of radius (23, 26)
Dislocated hip (16, 26, 35)
Hypoplastic thumb (20)
Hemifusion of second and third lumbar vertebrae (25)
Scoliosis (25)
Broad or asymmetric chest (16, 26)
Multiple (not specified) (24)
Talipes equinovarus (53)

Rib defects (24, 26)
Foot deformity (17, 23, 24, 50)
Abnormal digits (23, 26, 37, 42)
Shortened fingers and toes (4, 20)
Abnormal sternum (16, 26)
Arachnodactyly (24, 26)
Overlapping fingers/toes (24, 26)
Clinodactyly of fingers (26)
Tracheomalacia (53)

SKIN/MUSCLE DEFECTS

Accessory, wide-spaced, or inverted nipples (20, 26)
Diastasis recti abdominis (4, 25)
Syndactyly of toes (16, 23, 50)
Hyperconvex fingernails (24, 26)
Hemangioma (4, 25, 26, 50)
Sacral dimple (43)
Telangiectasia (4)

Cutis aplasia of scalp (50)
Weak abdominal walls (4)
Hirsutism (26)
Abnormal palmar creases (16, 18, 50)
Hypoplastic nails (4, 18)
Umbilical hernias (4, 26)
Linea alba hernia (47)
Inguinal hernia (4, 26, 50)

OTHER DEFECTS

Multiple defects (not specified) (24, 51)
Mental retardation (4, 20, 50, 51, 53)
Withdrawal/irritation (4, 50)

Duodenal atresia (25)
Single umbilical artery (50)

Although a wide variety of minor anomalies, many of which are similar in nature, occurs in infants of epileptic mothers, three groups of investigators have concluded that the deformities associated with valproic acid are distinctly different from those associated with other anticonvulsants and may constitute a valproic acid syndrome (26, 50, 53). The combined features cited in the three reports were: neural tube defects; craniofacial: brachycephaly, high forehead, epicanthal folds, strabismus, nystagmus, shallow orbits, flat nasal bridge, small up-turned nose, hypertelorism, long upper lip, thin upper vermilion border, microstomia, down-turned angles of mouth, low-set/rotated ears; digits: long, thin, partly overlapping fingers and toes, hyperconvex nails; urogenital: hypospadias (in about 50% of males); other: retarded psychomotor development, low birth weight. Normal psychomotor development has been observed, however, in follow-up studies of children up to 4 years of age after *in utero* exposure to either mono- or combination therapy with valproic acid (3, 34, 63, 65).

A correlation between valproic acid dosage and the number of minor anomalies in an infant has been proposed (26). Such a correlation has not been observed with other anticonvulsants (26). The conclusion was based on the high concentrations of valproic acid that occur in the 1st trimester after large doses (i.e., 1500–2000 mg/day).

Intrauterine growth retardation (IUGR) and/or small-for-gestational-age infants have been noted in several reports (4, 16, 19, 23, 24, 47, 48, 50, 63, 64). Both monotherapy and combination therapy with valproic acid were involved in these cases. However, normal birth weights, heights, and head circumferences have been reported with valproic acid monotherapy (25, 50, 53, 63). Growth impairment is a common problem with some anticonvulsant therapy (e.g., see Phenytoin), but the relationship between this problem and valproic acid needs further clarification.

A 1983 letter correspondence proposed that the mechanism for valproic acid-induced teratogenicity involved zinc deficiency (66). From in vitro studies, the authors had previously shown that valproic acid readily binds zinc. Low zinc serum levels potentiated the teratogenicity of certain drugs in animals and produced adverse effects similar to valproic acid-induced human toxicity (66). Another proposed mechanism, especially when valproic acid is combined with other anticonvulsants, involves the inhibition of liver microsomal epoxide hydrolase, the enzyme responsible for the biotransformation of reactive epoxide metabolites (67). The inhibition of the detoxifying enzyme could result in enhanced fetal exposure to reactive epoxide metabolites, such as carbamazepine epoxide, by preventing its biotransformation to a trans-dihydrodiol metabolite (67). Based on these findings, the authors recommended that combination drug therapy with valproic acid be avoided during pregnancy (67).

Three reports have observed hyperbilirubinemia in nine newborns exposed in utero to valproic acid monotherapy and in one infant exposed to combination therapy (4, 25, 48). A causal relationship is uncertain since other studies have not reported this problem.

Liver toxicity has been observed in three infants after in utero exposure to valproic acid (47, 48). In the first report, a growth-retarded female infant, exposed to valproic acid and phenytoin, had a linea alba hernia noted at birth but liver function tests were normal (47). The mother breast fed the child for the first several weeks. At 2.5 months of age, the infant presented with an enlarged liver, slight icterus, vomiting, and failure to thrive. Liver function tests indicated a cholestatic type of hyperbilirubinemia, and liver biopsy demonstrated fibrosis with ongoing necrosis of liver cells. Although they were unable to determine which anticonvulsant caused the injury, the authors concluded that valproic acid was the more likely offending agent. The second report described two siblings born of a mother treated with valproic acid monotherapy during two pregnancies (48). A male infant, exposed in utero to 300 mg/day, was normal at birth but expired at age 5 months of liver failure. Autopsy revealed liver atrophy, necrosis, and cholestasis. The female infant, exposed in utero to 500 mg/day, expired at age 6 weeks of liver failure. At birth, the infant was noted to have defects characteristic of valproic acid exposure (defects described in list above), intrauterine growth retardation, hyperbilirubinemia, hypoglycemia, hypocalcemia, and seizures. Liver atrophy and cholestasis were noted at autopsy.

Nondetectable fibrinogen levels resulting in fatal hemorrhage in a full-term 2-day-old infant were attributed to in utero sodium valproate exposure (68). The mother had taken daily doses of sodium valproate 600 mg, phenytoin 375 mg, and lorazepam 1 mg throughout pregnancy. In a subsequent pregnancy, the measurement of slightly decreased maternal fibrinogen levels in late gestation caused the authors to discontinue the sodium valproate while continuing the other two agents. Oral vitamin K was also administered to the mother. A healthy infant without bleeding problems resulted.

Transient hyperglycinemia has been observed in two newborns exposed *in utero* to sodium valproate combination therapy (combined with phenytoin in one; phenytoin, carbamazepine, and clonazepam in the other) (3). Similar increases of glycine have been observed in epileptic adults treated with valproic acid (3). No adverse effects in the newborns resulted from the amino acid alteration.

Fetal distress during labor (late decelerations, silent or accelerated beat-to-beat variations) was observed in 6 (43%) of 14 cases exposed to valproic acid monotherapy (26). Two of the newborns plus two others had low Apgar scores (0–3 after 1 minute or 0–6 after 5 minutes). Maternal doses were 1500–1800 mg/day in three cases and 600 mg/day in one case. Low Apgar scores were not observed in 12 infants whose mothers had been treated with valproic acid combination therapy. Other studies and case reports have not mentioned this complication. The fetal and newborn depression was thought to have resulted from a 3-fold increase in the maternal serum of valproic acid free fraction (26). A similar increase had been measured in an earlier study (10).

No decreases in adrenocorticotropic hormone (ACTH) or cortisol levels were measured in a mother or her newborn after the use of valproic acid 3000 mg/day during the last 3 months of pregnancy (28). The mother had received combination anticonvulsant therapy during the first 6 months of gestation.

Valproic acid has been measured in the semen of two healthy males (69). Following oral doses of 500 mg, semen levels ranged from 0.53–3.26 μg/ml up to 39 hours after the dose. Simultaneous serum levels were 11–17 times those measured in the semen. No effect on sperm motility was suggested based on animal experiments.

In summary, valproic acid and the salt form, sodium valproate, should be considered human teratogens. The absolute risk of producing a child with neural tube defects when these agents are used between the 17th and 30th day after fertilization is 1–2%. A characteristic pattern of minor facial defects is apparently also associated with valproic acid. Other major and minor abnormalities may be related to valproic acid therapy, but since an epileptic woman has a 2–3 times greater risk for delivering a child with congenital defects over the general population (see Phenytoin), these associations are difficult to establish. Two studies have suggested that a distinct constellation of defects may exist for infants exposed *in utero* to the anticonvulsant. These defects involve the head and face, digits, urogenital tract, and mental and physical growth. A correlation between maternal dose and major and minor anomalies has been reported, but additional studies are needed for confirmation. Other problems, such as intrauterine growth retardation, hyperbilirubinemia, hepatotoxicity, and fetal/newborn distress, also need additional investigation. Because of the risk for neural tube defects, women exposed during the critical period of gestation should consult their physician about prenatal testing (37, 70, 71).

Breast Feeding Summary

Valproic acid and its salt, sodium valproate, are excreted into human milk in low concentrations (1, 2, 4, 5, 8, 10, 12, 72). Milk concentrations have been measured up to 15% of the corresponding level in the mother's serum. No adverse effects in the nursing infant from this exposure have been reported. The American Academy of Pediatrics considers valproic acid to be compatible with breast feeding (73).

References

1. Alexander FW. Sodium valproate and pregnancy. Arch Dis Child 1979;54:240.
2. Dickinson RG, Harland RC, Lynn RK, Smith WB, Gerber N. Transmission of valproic acid (Depakene) across the placenta: half-life of the drug in mother and baby. J Pediatr 1979;94:832–5.
3. Simila S, von Wendt L, Hartikainen-Sorri A-L, Kaapa P, Saukkonen A-L. Sodium valproate, pregnancy, and neonatal hyperglycinaemia. Arch Dis Child 1979;54:985–6.
4. Nau H, Rating D, Koch S, Hauser I, Helge H. Valproic acid and its metabolites: placental transfer, neonatal pharmacokinetics, transfer via mother's milk and clinical status in neonates of epileptic mothers. J Pharmacol Exp Ther 1981;219:768–77.
5. Froescher W, Eichelbaum M, Niesen M, Altmann D, von Unruh GE. Antiepileptic therapy with carbamazepine and valproic acid during pregnancy and lactation period. In Dam M, Gram L, Penry JK, eds. *Advances in Epileptology: the XIIth Epilepsy International Symposium.* New York:Raven Press, 1981;581–8. As cited in Froescher W, Gugler R, Niesen M, Hoffmann F. Protein binding of valproic acid in maternal and umbilical cord serum. Epilepsia 1984;25:244–9.
6. Froescher W, Niesen M, Altmann D, Eichelbaum M, Gugler R, Hoffmann F, Penin H. Antiepileptika-therapie wahrend schwangerschaft und geburt. In Remschmidt H, Rentz R, Jungmann J, eds. *Epilepsie* 1980. Stuttgart: Georg Thieme Publishers, 1981:152–63. As cited in Froescher W, Gugler R, Niesen M, Hoffman F. Protein binding of valproic acid in maternal and umbilical cord serum. Epilepsia 1984;25:244–9.
7. Iskizaki T, Yokochi K, Chiba K, Tabuchi T, Wagatsuma T. Placental transfer of anticonvulsants (phenobarbital, phenytoin, valproic acid) and the elimination from neonates. Pediatr Pharmacol 1981;1:291–303.
8. Nau H, Kuhnz W, Egger H-J, Rating D, Helge H. Anticonvulsants during pregnancy and lactation: transplacental, maternal and neonatal pharmacokinetics. Clin Pharmacokinet 1982;7:508–43.
9. Kaneko S, Otani K, Fukushima Y, Sato T, Nomura Y, Ogawa Y. Transplacental passage and half-life of sodium valproate in infants born to epileptic mothers. Br J Clin Pharmacol 1983;15:503–6.
10. Nau H, Helge H, Luck W. Valproic acid in the perinatal period: decreased maternal serum protein binding results in fetal accumulation and neonatal displacement of the drug and some metabolites. J Pediatr 1984;104:627–34.
11. Froescher W, Gugler R, Niesen M, Hoffmann F. Protein binding of valproic acid in maternal and umbilical cord serum. Epilepsia 1984;25:244–9.
12. Philbert A, Pedersen B, Dam M. Concentration of valproate during pregnancy, in the newborn and in breast milk. Acta Neurol Scand 1985;72:460–3.
13. Nau H, Schafer H, Rating D, Jakobs C, Helge H. Placental transfer and neonatal pharmacokinetics of valproic acid and some of its metabolites. In Janz D, Bossi L, Dam M, Helge H, Richens A, Schmidt D, eds. *Epilepsy, Pregnancy, and the Child.* New York:Raven Press, 1982:367–72.
14. Perucca E, Ruprah M, Richens A. Altered drug binding to serum proteins in pregnant women: therapeutic relevance. J R Soc Med 1981;74:422–6.
15. Rating D, Jager-Roman E, Koch S, Nau H, Klein PD, Helge H. Enzyme induction in neonates due to antiepileptic therapy during pregnancy. In Janz D, Bossi L, Dam M, Helge H, Richens A, Schmidt D, eds. *Epilepsy, Pregnancy, and the Child.* New York:Raven Press, 1982:349–55.
16. Dalens B, Raynaud E-J, Gaulme J. Teratogenicity of valproic acid. J Pediatr 1980;97:332–3.
17. Gomez MR. Possible teratogenicity of valproic acid. J Pediatr 1981;98:508–9.
18. Thomas D, Buchanan N. Teratogenic effects of anticonvulsants. J Pediatr 1981;99:163.
19. Weinbaum PJ, Cassidy SB, Vintzileos AM, Campbell WA, Ciarleglio L, Nochimson DJ. Prenatal detection of a neural tube defect after fetal exposure to valproic acid. Obstet Gynecol 1986;67:31S-3S.
20. Clay SA, McVie R, Chen H. Possible teratogenic effect of valproic acid. J Pediatr 1981;99:828.
21. Robert E, Guibaud P. Maternal valproic acid and congenital neural tube defects. Lancet 1982;2:937.
22. Blaw ME, Woody RC. Valproic acid embryopathy? Neurology 1983;33:255.
23. Bailey CJ, Pool RW, Poskitt EME, Harris F. Valproic acid and fetal abnormality. Br Med J 1983;286:190.

24. Koch S, Jager-Roman E, Rating D, Helge H. Possible teratogenic effect of valproate during pregnancy. J Pediatr 1983;103:1007–8.
25. Bantz EW. Valproic acid and congenital malformations: a case report. Clin Pediatr 1984;23:353–4.
26. Jager-Roman E, Deichl A, Jakob S, Hartmann A-M, Koch S, Rating D, Steldinger R, Nau H, Helge H. Fetal growth, major malformations, and minor anomalies in infants born to women receiving valproic acid. J Pediatr 1986;108:997–1004.
27. Shakir RA, Johnson RH, Lambie DG, Melville ID, Nanda RN. Comparison of sodium valproate and phenytoin as single drug treatment in epilepsy. Epilepsia 1981;22:27–33.
28. Hatjis CG, Rose JC, Pippitt C, Swain M. Effect of treatment with sodium valproate on plasma adrenocorticotropic hormone and cortisol concentrations in pregnancy. Am J Obstet Gynecol 1985;152:315–6.
29. Product information. Depakene. Abbott Laboratories, 1988.
30. Anonymous. Teratogenic risks of antiepileptic drugs. Br Med J 1981;283;515–6.
31. Paulson GW, Paulson RR. Teratogenic effects of anticonvulsants. Arch Neurol 1981;38:140–43.
32. Brown NA, Kao J, Fabro S. Teratogenic potential of valproic acid. Lancet 1980;1:660–1.
33. Whittle BA. Pre-clinical teratological studies on sodium valproate (Epilim) and other anticonvulsants. In Legg NJ, ed. Clinical and Pharmacological Aspects of Sodium Valproate (Epilim) in the Treatment of Epilepsy. Tunbridge Wells:MCS Consultants, 1976:105–11.
34. Hiilesmaa VK, Bardy AH, Granstrom M-L, Teramo KAW. Valproic acid during pregnancy. Lancet 1980;1:883.
35. Nakane Y, Okuma T, Takahashi R, Sato Y, Wada T, Sato T, Fukushima Y, Kumashiro H, Ono T, Takahashi T, Aoki Y, Kazamatsuri H, Inami M, Komai S, Seino M, Miyakoshi M, Tanimura T, Hazama H, Kawahara R, Otsuki S, Hosokawa K, Inanaga K, Nakazawa Y, Yamamoto K. Multi-institutional study on the teratogenicity and fetal toxicity of antiepileptic drugs: a report of a collaborative study group in Japan. Epilepsia 1980;21:663–80.
36. Jeavons PM. Non-dose-related side effects of valproate. Epilepsia 1984;25(Suppl 1):S50–S5.
37. Centers For Disease Control, U.S. Department of Health and Human Services. Valpoate: a new cause of birth defects—report from Italy and follow-up from France. MMWR 1983;32:438–9.
38. Bossi L, Battino D, Boldi B, Caccamo ML, Ferraris, G, Latis GO, Simionato L. Anthropometric data and minor malformations in newborns of epileptic mothers. In Janz D, Bossi L, Dam M, Helge H, Richens A, Schmidt D, eds. Epilepsy, Pregnancy, and the Child. New York:Raven Press, 1982:299–301.
39. Committee on Drugs, American Academy of Pediatrics. Valproic acid: benefits and risks. Pediatrics 1982;70:316–9.
40. Bjerkedal T, Czeizel A, Goujard J, Kallen B, Mastroiacova P, Nevin N, Oakley G Jr, Robert E. Valproic acid and spina bifida. Lancet 1982;2:1096, 1172.
41. Stanely OH, Chambers TL. Sodium valproate and neural tube defects. Lancet 1982;2:1282.
42. Jeavons PM. Sodium valproate and neural tube defects. Lancet 1982;2:1282–3.
43. Castilla E. Valproic acid and spina bifida. Lancet 1983;2:683.
44. Robert E, Rosa F. Valproate and birth defects. Lancet 1983;2:1142.
45. Mastroiacovo P, Bertollini R, Morandini S, Segni G. Maternal epilepsy, valproate exposure, and birth defects. Lancet 1983;2:1499.
46. Lindhout D, Meinardi H. Spina bifida and in-utero exposure to valproate. Lancet 1984;2:396.
47. Felding I, Rane A. Congenital liver damage after treatment of mother with valproic acid and phenytoin? Acta Paediatr Scand 1984;73:565–8.
48. Legius E, Jaeken J, Eggermont E. Sodium valproate, pregnancy, and infantile fatal liver failure. Lancet 1987;2:1518–9.
49. Rating D, Jager-Roman E, Koch S, Gopfert-Geyer I, Helge H. Minor anomalies in the offspring of epileptic parents. In Janz D, Bossi L, Dam M, Helge H, Richens A, Schmidt D, eds. Epilepsy, Pregnancy, and the Child. New York:Raven Press, 1982:283–8.
50. DiLiberti JH, Farndon PA, Dennis NR, Curry CJR. The fetal valproate syndrome. Am J Med Genet 1984;19:473–81.
51. Lindhout D, Meinardi H, Barth PG. Hazards of fetal exposure to drug combinations. In Janz D, Bossi L, Dam M, Helge H, Richens A, Schmidt D, eds. Epilepsy, Pregnancy, and the Child. New York:Raven Press, 1982:275–81.
52. Koch S, Hartmann A, Jager-Roman E, Rating D, Helge H. Major malformations in children of epileptic parents-due to epilepsy or its therapy? In Janz D, Bossi L, Dam M, Helge H, Richens A, Schmidt D, eds. Epilepsy, Pregnancy, and the Child. New York:Raven Press, 1982:313–5.

53. Ardinger HH, Atkin JF, Blackston RD, Elsas LJ, Clarren SK, Livingstone S, Flannery DB, Pellock JM, Harrod MJ, Lammer EJ, Majewski F, Schinzel A, Toriello HV, Hanson JW. Verification of the fetal valproate syndrome phenotype. Am J Med Genet 1988;29:171–85.
54. Staunton H. Valproate, spina bifida, and birth defect registries. Lancet 1989;1:381.
55. Oakeshott P, Hunt GM. Valproate and spina bifida. Br Med J 1989;298:1300–1.
56. Oakeshott P, Hunt G. Valproate and spina bifida. Lancet 1989;1:611.
57. Martinez-Frias ML, Rodriguez-Pinilla E, Salvador J. Valproate and spina bifida. Lancet 1989;1:611–2.
58. Carter BS, Stewart JM. Valproic acid prenatal exposure: association with lipomyelomeningocele. Clin Pediatr 1989;28:81–5.
59. Centers For Disease Control, U.S. Department of Health and Human Services. Valproic acid and spina bifida: a preliminary report — France. MMWR 1982;31:565–6.
60. Lammer EJ, Sever LE, Oakley GP Jr. Teratogen update: valproic acid. Teratology 1987;35:465–73.
61. Anonymous. Valproate and malformations. Lancet 1982;2:1313–4.
62. Lemire RJ. Neural tube defects. JAMA 1988;259:558–62.
63. Jager-Roman E, Rating D, Koch S, Gopfert-Geyer I, Jacob S, Helge H. Somatic parameters, diseases, and psychomotor development in the offspring of epileptic parents. In Janz D, Bossi L, Dam M, Helge H, Richens A, Schmidt D, eds. *Epilepsy, Pregnancy, and the Child*. New York:Raven Press, 1982:425–32.
64. Granstrom M-L, Hiilesmaa VK. Physical growth of the children of epileptic mothers: preliminary results from the prospective Helsinki study. In Janz D, Bossi L, Dam M, Helge H, Richens A, Schmidt D, eds. *Epilepsy, Pregnancy, and the Child*. New York:Raven Press, 1982:397–401.
65. Granstrom M-L. Development of the children of epileptic mothers: preliminary results from the prospective Helsinki study. In Janz D, Bossi L, Dam M, Helge H, Richens A, Schmidt D, eds. *Epilepsy, Pregnancy, and the Child*. New York:Raven Press, 1982;403–8.
66. Hurd RW, Wilder BJ, Van Rinsvelt HA. Valproate, birth defects, and zinc. Lancet 1983;1:181.
67. Kerr BM, Levy RH. Inhibition of epoxide hydrolase by anticonvulsants and risk of teratogenicity. Lancet 1989;1:610–1.
68. Majer RV, Green PJ. Neonatal afibrinogenaemia due to sodium valproate. Lancet 1987;2:740–1.
69. Swanson BN, Harland RC, Dickinson RG, Gerber N. Excretion of valproic acid into semen of rabbits and man. Epilepsia 1978;19:541–6.
70. Frew J. Valproate link to spina bifida. Med J Aust 1983;1:150.
71. Committee on Drugs, American Academy of Pediatrics. Valproate teratogenicity. Pediatrics 1983;71:980.
72. Bardy AH, Granstrom M-L, Hiilesmaa VK. Valproic acid and breast-feeding. In Janz D, Bossi L, Dam M, Helge H, Richens A, Schmidt D, eds. *Epilepsy, Pregnancy, and the Child*. New York:Raven Press, 1982:359–60.
73. Committee on Drugs, American Academy of Pediatrics. Transfer of drugs and other chemicals into human milk. Pediatrics 1989;84:924–36.

Name: **VANCOMYCIN**

Class: **Antibiotic**   Risk Factor: **C$_M$**

Fetal Risk Summary

Vancomycin is an antibiotic that is used for Gram-positive bacteria when either the organisms are resistant to less toxic anti-infectives (e.g., penicillins and cephalosporins) or the patient is sensitive to these agents. No cases of congenital defects attributable to vancomycin have been located. The manufacturer has received reports on the use of vancomycin in pregnancy without adverse fetal effects (A.F. Crumley, personal communication, 1983).

Vancomycin was used for subacute bacterial endocarditis prophylaxis in a penicillin-allergic woman at term with mitral valve prolapse (1). One hour prior to vaginal delivery, a 1-g intravenous dose was given over 3 minutes (recommended infusion time is 60 minutes (2, 3)). Immediately after the dose, maternal blood pressure fell from 130/74 to 80/40 torr and then recovered in 3 minutes. Fetal bradycardia, 90 beats/minute, persisted for 4 minutes. No adverse effects of the hypotension-induced fetal distress were observed in the newborn. The Apgar scores were 9 and 10 at 1 and 5 minutes, respectively.

A 1989 report examined the effects of multiple dose vancomycin on newborn hearing and renal function (4). Ten pregnant, drug-dependent women were treated with intravenous vancomycin (1 g every 12 hours for at least 1 week) for suspected or documented infections due to methicillin-resistant *Staphylococcus aureus*. Four of the 10 women also received concomitant gentamicin. Two control groups, neither of which received antibiotics, were formed: 10 infants from non-drug-dependent mothers (group II), and 10 infants from drug-dependent mothers (group III). Auditory brainstem response testing was conducted on the infants at birth and at 3 months of age, and blood urea nitrogen and serum creatinine were measured at birth. The placental transfer of vancomycin was measured in two patients with cord blood levels of 16.7 and 13.2 µg/ml, 6 and 2.5 hours postinfusion, respectively. At birth, abnormal auditory brainstem responses were measured in a total of six infants: two infants from the study group (neither was exposed to gentamicin), three from control group II, and one from control group III. The hearing defect in all six infants was an absent wave V at 40 dB (the average behavioral threshold of adult listeners) in one or both ears. Repeat testing at 3 months in five infants was normal, indicating that the initial tests were falsely positive (4). In the sixth infant (one from the study group), the tests at 3 months again showed no response in either ear at 40 dB. This infant's mother had received a 2-g vancomycin dose after initial dosing had produced low serum levels (<20 µg/ml) of the antibiotic. The peak serum level obtained following the double dose was 65.7 µg/ml, a potentially toxic level if it was maintained. Following this, the mother was treated with the same regimen as the other women. On further examination, however, reduced compliance was discovered in both ears and the loss of hearing was diagnosed as a conduction defect, rather than sensorineural. Tests at 12 months, following improved compliance in both ears, were normal. Renal function studies in all 30 infants were also normal.

Breast Feeding Summary

Vancomycin is excreted into breast milk. In one woman treated with intravenous vancomycin (1 g every 12 hours for at least 1 week), a milk level 4 hours after a dose was 12.7 µg/ml (4). This value was nearly identical to the serum trough concentration measured at 12 hours in the mother during pregnancy. The effect of vancomycin in milk on the nursing infant is unknown. Vancomycin is poorly absorbed from the normal, intact gastrointestinal tract, and, thus, systemic absorption would not be expected (3). However, three potential problems exist for the nursing infant: modification of bowel flora, direct effects on the infant (e.g., allergic response/sensitization), and interference with the interpretation of culture results if a fever workup is required.

References

1. Hill LM. Fetal distress secondary to vancomycin-induced maternal hypotension. Am J Obstet Gynecol 1985;153:74–5.
2. Product information. Vancocin. Eli Lilly and Company, 1989.
3. Vancomycin. *AHFS Drug Information 1989*. Bethesda:American Society of Hospital Pharmacists, 1989:331–4.
4. Reyes MP, Ostrea EM Jr, Cabinian AE, Schmitt C, Rintelmann W. Vancomycin during pregnancy: does it cause hearing loss or nephrotoxicity in the infant? Am J Obstet Gynecol 1989;161:977–81.

Name: **VASOPRESSIN**

Class: **Pituitary Hormone**   Risk Factor: **B**

Fetal Risk Summary

No reports linking the use of vasopressin with congenital defects have been located. Vasopressin and the structurally related synthetic polypeptides, desmopressin and lypressin, have been used during pregnancy to treat diabetes insipidus, a rare disorder (1–8). No adverse effects on the newborns were reported.

A 3-fold increase of circulating levels of endogenous vasopressin has been reported for women in the last trimester and in labor as compared to nonpregnant women (9). Although infrequent, the induction of uterine activity in the 3rd trimester has been reported after intramuscular and intranasal vasopressin (10). The intravenous use of desmopressin, which is normally given intranasally, has also been reported to cause uterine contractions (4).

Two investigators speculated that raised levels of vasopressin resulted from hypoxemia and acidosis and could produce signs of fetal distress (bradycardia and meconium staining) (11).

Breast Feeding Summary

Patients receiving vasopressin, desmopressin, or lypressin for diabetes insipidus have been reported to breast feed without apparent problems in the infant (1, 2). Experimental work in lactating women suggests that suckling almost doubles the maternal blood concentration of vasopressin (9).

References

1. Hime MC, Richardson JA. Diabetes insipidus and pregnancy. Obstet Gynecol Surv 1978;33:375–9.
2. Hadi HA, Mashini IS, Devoe LD. Diabetes insipidus during pregnancy complicated by preeclampsia. A case report. J Reprod Med 1985;30:206–8.
3. Phelan JP, Guay AT, Newman C. Diabetes insipidus in pregnancy: a case review. Am J Obstet Gynecol 1978;130:365–6.
4. van der Wildt B, Drayer JIM, Eske TKAB. Diabetes insipidus in pregnancy as a first sign of a craniopharyngioma. Eur J Obstet Gynecol Reprod Biol 1980;10:269–74.
5. Ford SM Jr. Transient vasopressin-resistant diabetes insipidus of pregnancy. Obstet Gynecol 1986;68:288–9.
6. Ford SM Jr, Lumpkin HL III. Transient vasopressin-resistant diabetes insipidus of pregnancy. Obstet Gynecol 1986;68:726–8.
7. Rubens R, Thiery M. Case report: diabetes insipidus and pregnancy. Eur J Obstet Gynecol Reprod Biol 1987;26:265–70.

8. Hughes JM, Barron WM, Vance ML. Recurrent diabetes insipidus associated with pregnancy: pathophysiology and therapy. Obstet Gynecol 1989;73:462–4.
9. Robinson KW, Hawker RW, Robertson PA. Antidiuretic hormone (ADH) in the human female. J Clin Endocrinol Metab 1957;17:320–2.
10. Oravec D, Lichardus B. Management of diabetes insipidus in pregnancy. Br Med J 1972;4:114–5.
11. Gaffney PR, Jenkins DM. Vasopressin: mediator of the clinical signs of fetal distress. Br J Obstet Gynaecol 1983;90:987.

Name: **VERAPAMIL**

Class: **Cardiac**   Risk Factor: **C$_M$**

Fetal Risk Summary

Verapamil is a calcium channel inhibitor used as an antiarrhythmic agent. Clinically, verapamil can be classified as a type 1 calcium blocking agent whose predominant actions involve electrophysiologic and vascular effects on myocardium (1). Verapamil-induced vasodilatory effects are moderate, as opposed to the marked peripheral vasodilation caused by another calcium channel inhibitor, nifedipine (see also Nifepidine) (1). No reports linking the use of verapamil with congenital defects have been located.

Placental passage of verapamil has been demonstrated in two of six patients given 80 mg orally at term (2). Cord levels were 15.4 and 24.5 ng/ml (17 and 26% of maternal serum) in two newborns delivered at 49 and 109 minutes after verapamil administration, respectively. Verapamil could not be detected in the cord blood of four infants delivered 173–564 minutes after the dose. Intravenous (IV) verapamil was administered to patients in labor at a rate of 2 μg/kg/minute for 60–110 minutes (3). The serum concentrations of the infants averaged 8.5 ng/ml (44% of maternal serum).

A 33-week fetus with a tachycardia of 240–280 beats/minute was treated *in utero* for 6 weeks with β-acetyldigoxin and verapamil (80 mg three times daily) (2). The fetal heart rate returned to normal 5 days after initiation of therapy, but the authors could not determine if verapamil had produced the beneficial effect. At birth, no signs of cardiac hypertrophy or disturbances in repolarization were observed. Several other reports have described successful *in utero* treatment of supraventricular tachycardia with verapamil in combination with other agents (4–6). In one case, indirect therapy via the mother with verapamil, digoxin, and procainamide failed to control the fetal arrhythmia and direct fetal digitalization was required (7). In another case, verapamil, 120 mg three times daily, and digoxin were used successfully to control a fetal supraventricular tachycardia at 32 weeks' gestation (8). At 36 weeks' gestation, after 4 weeks of therapy, ultrasound examination showed complete resolution of both the hydropic changes and polyhydramnios, but the fetus died within 2 days. No autopsy was permitted. The authors speculated that the drug combination may have caused complete heart block (8). Maternal supraventricular tachycardia occurring in the 3rd trimester has been treated with a single 5-mg IV dose of verapamil (9). Other than the single case of fetal death in which the etiology is not certain, no adverse fetal or newborn effects attributable to verapamil have been noted in the above reports.

Verapamil has been used to lower blood pressure in a woman with severe pregnancy-induced hypertension in labor (10). Fifteen milligrams were given by rapid IV injection followed by an infusion of 185 mg over 6 hours. Fetal heart rate increased from 60 to 110 beats/minute, and a normal infant was delivered without signs or symptoms of toxicity. Tocolysis with verapamil, either alone or in combination with β-mimetics, has also been described (11–15).

The manufacturer has reports of patients treated with verapamil during the 1st trimester without production of fetal problems (M.S. Anderson, personal communication, GD Searle & Co., 1981). However, hypotension (systolic and diastolic) has been observed in patients after rapid intravenous bolus (16). Because of this, reduced uterine blood flow with fetal hypoxia is a potential risk.

Breast Feeding Summary

Verapamil is excreted into breast milk (17, 18). A daily dose of 240 mg produced milk levels that were approximately 23% of maternal serum (17). Serum levels in the infant were 2.1 ng/ml but could not be detected (<1 ng/ml) 38 hours after treatment was stopped. No effects of this exposure were observed in the infant. In a second case, a mother was treated with 80 mg three times daily for hypertension for 4 weeks prior to the determination of serum and milk concentrations (18). Steady-state concentrations of verapamil and the metabolite, norverapamil, in milk were 25.8 and 8.8 ng/ml, respectively. These values were 60% and 16% of the concentrations in plasma. The investigators estimated that the breast-fed child received less than 0.01% of the mother's dose. Neither verapamil nor the metabolite could be detected in the plasma of the child. The American Academy of Pediatrics considers verapamil to be compatible with breast feeding (19).

References

1. Raehl CL, Nolan PE Jr. Angina pectoris. In Young LY, Koda-Kimble MA, eds. *Applied Therapeutics. The Clinical Use of Drugs,* ed 4. Vancouver, WA:Applied Therapeutics, 1988:283–4.
2. Wolff F, Breuker KH, Schlensker KH, Bolte A. Prenatal diagnosis and therapy of fetal heart rate anomalies: with a contribution on the placental transfer of verapamil. J Perinat Med 1980;8:203–8.
3. Strigl R, Gastroph G, Hege HG, et al. Nachweis von verapamil in mutterlichen und fetalen blut des menschen. Geburtshilfe Frauenheilkd 1980;40:496–9.
4. Lilja H, Karlsson K, Lindecrantz K, Sabel KG. Treatment of intrauterine supraventricular tachycardia with digoxin and verapamil. J Perinat Med 1984;12:151–4.
5. Rey E, Duperron L, Gauthier R, Lemay M, Grignon A, LeLorier J. Transplacental treatment of tachycardia-induced fetal heart failure with verapamil and amiodarone: a case report. Am J Obstet Gynecol 1985;153:311–2.
6. Maxwell DJ, Crawford DC, Curry PVM, Tynan MJ, Allan LD. Obstetric importance, diagnosis, and management of fetal tachycardias. Br Med J 1988;297:107–10.
7. Weiner CP, Thompson MIB. Direct treatment of fetal supraventricular tachycardia after failed transplacental therapy. Am J Obstet Gynecol 1988;158:570–3.
8. Owen J, Colvin EV, Davis RO. Fetal death after successful conversion of fetal supraventricular tachycardia with digoxin and verapamil. Am J Obstet Gynecol 1988;158:1169–70.
9. Klein V, Repke JT. Supraventricular tachycardia in pregnancy: cardioversion with verapamil. Obstet Gynecol 1984;63:16S-8S.
10. Brittinger WD, Schwarzbeck A, Wittenmeier KW, et al. Klinisch-experimentelle untersuchungen uber die blutdruckendende wirkung von verapamil. Dtsch Med Wochenschr 1970;95:1871–7.
11. Mosler KH, Rosenboom HG. Neuere moglichkeiten einer tokolytischen behandlung in de geburtschilfe. Z Geburtschilfe Perinatol 1972;176:85–96.
12. Gummerus M. Prevention of premature birth with nylidrin and verapamil. Z Geburtschilfe Perinatol 1975;179:261–6.
13. Gummerus M. Treatment of premature labor and antagonization of the side effects of tocolytic therapy with verapamil. Z Geburtschilfe Perinatol 1977;181:334–40.

14. Gummerus M. Prevention of premature birth with nylidrin and verapamil. Z Geburtshilfe Perinatol 1975;179:261–6.
15. Gummerus M. Treatment of premature labour and antagonization of the side effects of tocolytic therapy with verapamil. Z Geburtshilfe Perinatol 1977;181:334–40.
16. Rotmensch HH, Rotmensch S, Elkayam U. Management of cardiac arrhythmias during pregnancy: current concepts. Drugs 1987;33:623–33.
17. Andersen HJ. Excretion of verapamil in human milk. Eur J Clin Pharmacol 1983;25:279–80.
18. Anderson P, Bondesson U, Mattiasson I, Johansson BW. Verapamil and norverapamil in plasma and breast milk during breast feeding. Eur J Clin Pharmacol 1987;31:625–7.
19. Committee on Drugs, American Academy of Pediatrics. Transfer of drugs and other chemicals into human milk. Pediatrics 1989;84;924–36.

Name: **VIDARABINE**

Class: **Antiviral**   Risk Factor: **C$_M$**

Fetal Risk Summary

Vidarabine has not been studied in human pregnancy. The drug is a potent teratogen in some species of animals after topical and intramuscular administration (1, 2). Daily instillations of a 10% solution into the vaginas of pregnant rats in late gestation had no effect on the offspring (2).

Vidarabine was used for disseminated herpes simplex in one woman at about 28 weeks' gestation (3, 4). Spontaneous rupture of the membranes occurred 48 hours after initiation of therapy, and a premature infant was delivered. The infant died on the 13th day of life from complications of prematurity. In a second case, a woman at 32 weeks' gestation with herpes simplex type II encephalitis was treated with vidarabine, 10 mg/kg/day, and acyclovir (5). A female infant with culture-documented herpes neonatorum was delivered by cesarean section 13 days later. The infant responded to further treatment with acyclovir and is alive and well at 2 months of age, but the mother died 2 days after delivery.

Vidarabine, 10 mg/kg/day (800 mg/day), was administered to a woman at 26 weeks' gestation with varicella pneumonitis (6). Peak and trough levels of the agent were 12.8 and 2.7 μg/ml, respectively. She delivered a healthy female infant at 38 weeks' gestation who is developing normally at 12 months of age. In a similar case, another woman with varicella pneumonitis at 27 weeks' gestation was treated with vidarabine (6). Except for a delay in speech at age 3 years which responded to special education, the child has done well and was considered normal at 5 years.

Breast Feeding Summary

No reports involving the use of vidarabine in lactating women have been located.

References

1. Pavan-Langston D, Buchanan RA, Alford CA Jr, eds. *Adenine Arabinoside: An Antiviral Agent.* New York:Raven Press, 1975:153.
2. Schardein JL, Hertz DL, Petretre JA, Fitzgerald JE, Kurtz SM. The effect of vidarabine on the development of the offspring of rats, rabbits and monkeys. Teratology 1977;15:213–42.
3. Hillard P, Seeds J, Cefalo R. Disseminated herpes simplex in pregnancy: two cases and a review. Obstet Gynecol Surv 1982;37:449–53.

4. Peacock JE Jr, Sarubbi FA. Disseminated herpes simplex virus infection during pregnancy. Obstet Gynecol 1983;61:13S-8S.
5. Berger SA, Weinberg M, Treves T, Sorkin P, Geller E, Yedwab G, Tomer A, Rabey M, Michaeli D. Herpes encephalitis during pregnancy: failure of acyclovir and adenine arabinoside to prevent neonatal herpes. Isr J Med Sci 1986;22:41–4.
6. Landsberger EJ, Hager WD, Grossman JH III. Successful management of varicella pneumonia complicating pregnancy: a report of three cases. J Reprod Med 1986;31:311–4.

Name: **VINBLASTINE**

Class: **Antineoplastic**   Risk Factor: **D**

Fetal Risk Summary

Vinblastine is an antimitotic antineoplastic agent. The drug has been used in pregnancy, including the 1st trimester, without producing malformations (1–8). Two cases of malformed infants have been reported following 1st trimester exposure to vinblastine (8, 9). In 1974, a case of a 27-year-old woman with Hodgkin's disease who was given vinblastine, mechlorethamine, and procarbazine during the 1st trimester was described (9). At 24 weeks of gestation, she spontaneously aborted a male fetus with oligodactyly of both feet with webbing of the third and fourth toes. These defects were attributed to mechlorethamine therapy. A mother with Hodgkin's disease treated with vinblastine, vincristine, and procarbazine in the 1st trimester (3 weeks after the last menstrual period) delivered a 1900-g male infant at about 37 weeks of gestation (10). The newborn developed fatal respiratory distress syndrome. At autopsy, a small secundum atrial septal defect was found.

Vinblastine in combination with other antineoplastic agents may produce gonadal dysfunction in men and women (11–14). Alkylating agents are the most frequent cause of this problem (13). Although total aspermia may result, return of fertility has apparently been documented in at least two cases (14). Ovarian function may return to normal with successful pregnancies possible, depending on the patient's age at the time of therapy and the total dose of chemotherapy received (12, 15). The long-term effects of combination chemotherapy on menstrual and reproductive function were described in a 1988 report (16). Only 5 of 40 women treated for malignant ovarian germ cell tumors received vinblastine. The results of this study are discussed in the monograph for cyclophosphamide (see Cyclophosphamide).

In 436 long-term survivors treated with chemotherapy for gestational trophoblastic tumors between 1958–1978, 11 (2.5%) received vinblastine as part of their treatment regimens (17). Of the 11 women, 2 (18%) had at least one live birth (mean and maximum vinblastine dose 20 mg), and 9 (82%) did not try to conceive (mean dose 37 mg, maximum dose 80 mg). Additional details, including congenital anomalies observed, are described in the monograph for vincristine (see Vincristine).

Data from one review indicated that 40% of infants exposed to anticancer drugs were of low birth weight (18). This finding was not related to the timing of exposure. Long-term studies of growth and mental development in offspring exposed to vinblastine during the 2nd trimester, the period of neuroblast multiplication, have not been conducted (19). However, two children, exposed throughout gestation beginning with the 3rd–4th week of gestation, were normal at 2 and 5 years of age, respectively (8).

Occupational exposure of the mother to antineoplastic agents during pregnancy may present a risk to the fetus. A position statement from the National Study Commission on Cytotoxic Exposure and a research article involving some antineoplastic agents are presented in the monograph for cyclophosphamide (see Cyclophosphamide).

Breast Feeding Summary

No data are available.

References

1. Armstrong JG, Dyke RW, Fouts PJ, Jansen CJ. Delivery of a normal infant during the course of oral vinblastine sulfate therapy for Hodgkin's disease. Ann Intern Med 1964;61:106–7.
2. Rosenzweig AI, Crews QE Jr, Hopwood HG. Vinblastine sulfate in Hodgkin's disease in pregnancy. Ann Intern Med 1964;61:108–12.
3. Lacher MJ. Use of vinblastine sulfate to treat Hodgkin's disease during pregnancy. Ann Intern Med 1964;61:113–5.
4. Lacher MJ, Geller W. Cyclophosphamide and vinblastine sulfate in Hodgkin's disease during pregnancy. JAMA 1966;195:192–4.
5. Nordlund JJ, DeVita VT Jr, Carbone PP. Severe vinblastine-induced leukopenia during late pregnancy with delivery of a normal infant. Ann Intern Med 1968;69:581–2.
6. Goguei A. Hodgkin's disease and pregnancy. Nouv Presse Med 1970;78:1507–10.
7. Johnson IR, Filshie GM. Hodgkin's disease diagnosed in pregnancy: case report. Br J Obstet Gynaecol 1977;84:791–2.
8. Nisce LZ, Tome MA, He S, Lee BJ III, Kutcher GJ. Management of coexisting Hodgkin's disease and pregnancy. Am J Clin Oncol 1986;9:146–51.
9. Garrett MJ. Teratogenic effects of combination chemotherapy. Ann Intern Med 1974;80:667.
10. Thomas RPM, Peckham MJ. The investigation and management of Hodgkin's disease in the pregnant patient. Cancer 1976;38:1443–51.
11. Morgenfeld MC, Goldberg V, Parisier H, Bugnard SC, Bur GE. Ovarian lesions due to cytostatic agents during the treatment of Hodgkin's disease. Surg Gynecol Obstet 1972;134:826–8.
12. Ross GT. Congenital anomalies among children born of mothers receiving chemotherapy for gestational trophoblastic neoplasms. Cancer 1976;37:1043–7.
13. Schilsky RL, Lewis BJ, Sherins RJ, Young RC. Gonadal dysfunction in patients receiving chemotherapy for cancer. Ann Intern Med 1980;93:109–14.
14. Rubery ED. Return of fertility after curative chemotherapy for disseminated teratoma of testis. Lancet 1983;1:186.
15. Shalet SM, Vaughan Williams CA, Whitehead E. Pregnancy after chemotherapy induced ovarian failure. Br Med J 1985;290:898.
16. Gershenson DM. Menstrual and reproductive function after treatment with combination chemotherapy for malignant ovarian germ cell tumors. J Clin Oncol 1988;6:270–5.
17. Rustin GJS, Booth M, Dent J, Salt S, Rustin F, Bagshawe KD. Pregnancy after cytotoxic chemotherapy for gestational trophoblastic tumours. Br Med J 1984;288:103–6.
18. Nicholson HO. Cytotoxic drugs in pregnancy: review of reported cases. J Obstet Gynaecol Br Commonw 1968;75:307–12.
19. Dobbing J. Pregnancy and leukaemia. Lancet 1977;1:1155.

Name: **VINCRISTINE**

Class: **Antineoplastic**   Risk Factor: **D**

Fetal Risk Summary

Vincristine is an antimitotic antineoplastic agent. The use of vincristine has been described in at least 34 pregnancies (one with twins), eight during the 1st trimester (1–29).

A mother with Hodgkin's disease treated with vincristine, vinblastine, and procarbazine in the 1st trimester (3 weeks after the last menstrual period) delivered a 1900-g male infant at about 37 weeks' gestation (9). Neonatal death occurred due to respiratory distress syndrome. At autopsy, a small secundum atrial septal defect was found. In a Hodgkin's case treated with vincristine, mechlorethamine, and procarbazine during the 1st trimester, the electively aborted fetus had malformed kidneys (markedly reduced size and malpositioned) (15). Other adverse fetal outcomes observed following vincristine use include a 1000-g male infant born with pancytopenia who was exposed to six different antineoplastic agents in the 3rd trimester (1), and transient severe bone marrow hypoplasia in another newborn that was most likely due to mercaptopurine (18). Intrauterine fetal death occurred in a 1200 g-female fetus 36 hours after maternal treatment with vincristine, doxorubicin, and prednisone for diffuse, undifferentiated lymphoma of T-cell origin at 31 weeks' gestation (21). The fetus was macerated, but no other abnormalities were observed at autopsy. In another case, a 34-year-old woman with acute lymphoblastic leukemia was treated with multiple antineoplastic agents from 22 weeks' gestation until delivery of a healthy female infant 18 weeks later (24). Vincristine was administered four times between 22–25 weeks' gestation. Chromosome analysis of the newborn revealed a normal karyotype (46,XX) but with gaps and a ring chromosome. The clinical significance of these findings is unknown, but since these abnormalities may persist for several years, the potential existed for an increased risk of cancer, as well as for a risk of genetic damage in the next generation (24).

Data from one review indicated that 40% of the infants exposed to anticancer drugs were of low birth weight (30). This finding was not related to the timing of exposure. Long-term studies of growth and mental development in offspring exposed to these drugs during the 2nd trimester, the period of neuroblast multiplication, have not been conducted (31). However, individual infants have been evaluated for periods ranging from a few weeks up to 7 years and all have had normal growth and development (16–19, 21–23, 25, 26, 28).

Vincristine, in combination with other antineoplastic agents, may produce gonadal dysfunction in men and women (32–39). Alkylating agents are the most frequent cause of this problem (36). Ovarian and testicular function may return to normal with successful pregnancies possible, depending on the patient's age at time of treatment and the total dose of chemotherapy received (32). In a 1989 case report, a woman with an immature teratoma of the ovary was treated with conservative surgery and chemotherapy consisting of six courses of vincristine, dactinomycin, and cyclophosphamide (40). She conceived 20 months after her last chemotherapy and eventually delivered a normal 3340-g male infant. The long-term effects of combination chemotherapy on menstrual and reproductive function have been described in a 1988 report (41). Twenty-nine of 40 women treated for malignant ovarian germ cell tumors received vincristine. The results of this study are discussed in the monograph for cyclophosphamide (see Cyclophosphamide).

In 436 long-term survivors treated with chemotherapy between 1958–1978 for gestational trophoblastic tumors, 132 (30%) received vincristine in combination with other antineoplastic agents (42). The mean duration of chemotherapy was 4 months with a mean interval from completion of therapy to the first pregnancy of 2.7 years. Conception occurred within 1 year of therapy completion in 45 women (antineoplastic agents used in these women were not specified), resulting in 31 live births, one anencephalic stillbirth, seven spontaneous abortions, and six elective abortions. Of the 132 women treated with vincristine, 37 (28%) had at least one live birth (numbers in parentheses refer to mean/maximum vincristine dose in milligrams) (7.4/17.0), 8 (6%) had no live births (7.1/22.0), 4 (3%) failed to conceive (7.3/18.0), and 83 (63%) did not try to conceive (11.3/46.0). The average ages at the end of treatment in the four groups were 24.9, 24.4, 24.4, and 31.5 years, respectively. Congenital abnormalities noted in the total group (368 conceptions) were anencephaly (two), spina bifida (one), tetralogy of Fallot (one), talipes equinovarus (one), collapsed lung (one), umbilical hernia (one), desquamative fibrosing alveolitis (one), asymptomatic heart murmur (one), and mental retardation (one). Another child had tachycardia but developed normally after treatment. One case of sudden infant death syndrome occurred in a female infant at 4 weeks of age. None of these outcomes differed statistically from that expected in a normal population (42).

Occupational exposure of the mother to antineoplastic agents during pregnancy may present a risk to the fetus. A position statement from the National Study Commission on Cytotoxic Exposure and a research article involving some antineoplastic agents are presented in the monograph for cyclophosphamide (see Cyclophosphamide).

Breast Feeding Summary

No data are available.

References

1. Pizzuto J, Aviles A, Noriega L, Niz J, Morales M, Romero F. Treatment of acute leukemia during pregnancy: presentation of nine cases. Cancer Treat Rep 1980;64:679–83.
2. Colbert N, Najman A, Gorin NC, et al. Acute leukaemia during pregnancy: favourable course of pregnancy in two patients treated with cytosine arabinoside and anthracyclines. Nouv Presse Med 1980;9:175–8.
3. Daly H, McCann SR, Hanratty TD, Temperley IJ. Successful pregnancy during combination chemotherapy for Hodgkin's disease. Acta Haematol (Basel) 1980;64:154–6.
4. Tobias JS, Bloom HJG. Doxorubicin in pregnancy. Lancet 1980;1:776.
5. Garcia V, San Miguel J, Borrasea AL. Doxorubicin in the first trimester of pregnancy. Ann Intern Med 1981;94:547.
6. Dara P, Slater LM, Armentrout SA. Successful pregnancy during chemotherapy for acute leukemia. Cancer 1981;47:845–6.
7. Burnier AM. Discussion. In Plows CW. Acute myelomonocytic leukemia in pregnancy: report of a case. Am J Obstet Gynecol 1982;143:41–3.
8. Lilleyman JS, Hill AS, Anderton KJ. Consequences of acute myelogenous leukemia in early pregnancy. Cancer 1977;40:1300–3.
9. Thomas PRM, Peckham MJ. The investigation and management of Hodgkin's disease in the pregnant patient. Cancer 1976;38:1443–51.

10. Pawliger DF, McLean FW, Noyes WD. Normal fetus after cytosine arabinoside therapy. Ann Intern Med 1971;74:1012.

11. Lowenthal RM, Funnell CF, Hope DM, Stewart IG, Humphrey DC. Normal infant after combination chemotherapy including teniposide for Burkitt's lymphoma in pregnancy. Med Pediatr Oncol 1982;10:165–9.

12. Sears HF, Reid J. Granulocytic sarcoma: local presentation of a systemic disease. Cancer 1976;37:1808–13.

13. Durie BGM, Giles HR. Successful treatment of acute leukemia during pregnancy: combination therapy in the third trimester. Arch Intern Med 1977;137:90–1.

14. Newcomb M, Balducci L, Thigpen JT, Morrison FS. Acute leukemia in pregnancy: successful delivery after cytarabine and doxorubicin. JAMA 1978;239:2691–2.

15. Mennuti MT, Shepard TH, Mellman WJ. Fetal renal malformation following treatment of Hodgkin's disease during pregnancy. Obstet Gynecol 1975;46:194–6.

16. Coopland AT, Friesen WJ, Galbraith PA. Acute leukemia in pregnancy. Am J Obstet Gynecol 1969;105:1288–9.

17. Doney KC, Kraemer KG, Shepard TH. Combination chemotherapy for acute myelocytic leukemia during pregnancy: three case reports. Cancer Treat Rep 1979;63:369–71.

18. Okun DB, Groncy PK, Sieger L, Tanaka KR. Acute leukemia in pregnancy: transient neonatal myelosuppression after combination chemotherapy in the mother. Med Pediatr Oncol 1979;7:315–9.

19. Weed JC Jr, Roh RA, Mendenhall HW. Recurrent endodermal sinus tumor during pregnancy. Obstet Gynecol 1979;54:653–6.

20. Kim DS, Park MI. Maternal and fetal survival following surgery and chemotherapy of endodermal sinus tumor of the ovary during pregnancy: a case report. Obstet Gynecol 1989;73:503–7.

21. Karp GI, von Oeyen P, Valone F, Khetarpal VK, Israel M, Mayer RJ, Frigoletto FD, Garnick MB. Doxorubicin in pregnancy: possible transplacental passage. Cancer Treat Rep 1983;67:773–7.

22. Haerr RW, Pratt AT. Multiagent chemotherapy for sarcoma diagnosed during pregnancy. Cancer 1985;56:1028–33.

23. Volkenandt M, Buchner T, Hiddemann W, Van De Loo J. Acute leukaemia during pregnancy. Lancet 1987;2:1521–2.

24. Schleuning M, Clemm C. Chromosomal aberrations in a newborn whose mother received cytotoxic treatment during pregnancy. N Engl J Med 1987;317:1666–7.

25. Feliu J, Juarez S, Ordonez A, Garcia-Paredes ML, Gonzalez-Baron M, Montero JM. Acute leukemia and pregnancy. Cancer 1988;61:580–4.

26. Turchi JJ, Villasis C. Anthracyclines in the treatment of malignancy in pregnancy. Cancer 1988;61:435–40.

27. Weinrach RS. Leukemia in pregnancy. Ariz Med 1972;29:326–9.

28. Ortega J. Multiple agent chemotherapy including bleomycin of non-Hodgkin's lymphoma during pregnancy. Cancer 1977;40:2829–35.

29. Jones RT, Weinerman ER. MOPP (nitrogen mustard, vincristine, procarbazine, and prednisone) given during pregnancy. Obstet Gynecol 1979;54:477–8.

30. Nicholson HO. Cytotoxic drugs in pregnancy: review of reported cases. J Obstet Gynaecol Br Commonw 1968;75:307–12.

31. Dobbing J. Pregnancy and leukaemia. Lancet 1977;1:1155.

32. Schilsky RL, Sherins RJ, Hubbard SM, Wesley MN, Young RC, DeVita VT Jr. Long-term follow-up of ovarian function in women treated with MOPP chemotherapy for Hodgkin's disease. Am J Med 1981;71:552–6.

33. Schwartz PE, Vidone RA. Pregnancy following combination chemotherapy for a mixed germ cell tumor of the ovary. Gynecol Oncol 1981;12:373–8.

34. Estiu M. Successful pregnancy in leukaemia. Lancet 1977;1:433.

35. Johnson SA, Goldman JM, Hawkins DF. Pregnancy after chemotherapy for Hodgkin's disease. Lancet 1979;2:93.

36. Schilsky RL, Lewis BJ, Sherins RJ, Young RC. Gonadal dysfunction in patients receiving chemotherapy for cancer. Ann Intern Med 1980;93:109–14.

37. Sherins RJ, DeVita VT Jr. Effect of drug treatment for lymphoma on male reproductive capacity. Ann Intern Med 1973;79:216–20.

38. Sherins RJ, Olweny CLM, Ziegler JL. Gynecomastia and gonadal dysfunction in adolescent boys treated with combination chemotherapy for Hodgkin's disease. N Engl J Med 1978;299:12–6.

39. Lendon PRM, Peckham MJ. The investigation and management of Hodgkin's disease in the pregnant patient. Cancer 1976;38:1944–51.
40. Lee RB, Kelly J, Elg SA, Benson WL. Pregnancy following conservative surgery and adjunctive chemotherapy for stage III immature teratoma of the ovary. Obstet Gynecol 1989;73:853–5.
41. Gershenson DM. Menstrual and reproductive function after treatment with combination chemotherapy for malignant ovarian germ cell tumors. J Clin Oncol 1988;6:270–5.
42. Rustin GJS, Booth M, Dent J, Salt S, Rustin F, Bagshawe KD. Pregnancy after cytotoxic chemotherapy for gestational trophoblastic tumours. Br Med J 1984;288:103–6.

Name: **VITAMIN A**

Class: **Vitamin** Risk Factor: **A***

Fetal Risk Summary

Vitamin A (retinol; vitamin A[1]) is a fat-soluble essential nutrient that occurs naturally in a variety of foods. Vitamin A is required for the maintenance of normal epithelial tissue and for growth and bone development, vision and reproduction (1). The recommended daily allowance (RDA) for normal pregnant women in America is 1000 retinol equivalents/day (3300 IU of vitamin A obtained from a supplement as retinol, or 5000 IU obtained from a combination of a typical American diet in the forms of retinol and various precursors such as β-carotene) (2–4). The Food and Drug Administration's RDA (i.e., U.S. RDA) for pregnant women is 8000 IU (3, 4). These recommendations were made in 1980 and 1976, respectively. Based on more recent data, some authors are now citing evidence for consumption of lower daily amounts by healthy pregnant women, such as 2000 IU (5).

The teratogenicity of vitamin A in animals is well known. Both high and low levels of the vitamin result in defects (6–14). In the past, various authors have speculated on the teratogenic effect of the vitamin in humans (6, 15–17). A 1983 case report suggested that the vitamin A contained in a multivitamin product may have caused a cleft palate in one infant; however, the mother had a family history of cleft palate and had produced a previous infant with a malformation (17). Another case report, this one published in 1987, described an infant with multiple defects whose mother had consumed a vitamin preparation containing 2000 IU/day of vitamin A (18). The authors thought the phenotype of their patient was similar to the one observed with isotretinoin, but they could not exclude other causes of the defect, including a phenocopy of the isotretinoin syndrome (18). Therefore, in both cases, no definite association between the defects and vitamin A can be established, and the possibility that other etiologies were involved is high.

In response to the 1983 case report cited above, one investigator wrote in 1983 that there was no acceptable evidence of human vitamin A teratogenicity and none at all with doses less than 10,000 IU/day (19). Since that time, however, two synthetic isomers of vitamin A, isotretinoin and etretinate, have been shown to be powerful human teratogens (see Isotretinoin and Etretinate). Although only a few cases are available, the effects of deficiencies and excesses of vitamin A (retinol) in human pregnancy are summarized below. Because of these cases and supporting animal data for vitamin A, and because of the human experience with isotretinoin and etretinate, large doses or severe shortages of vitamin A must be viewed as harmful to the human fetus.

Severe human vitamin A deficiency has been cited as the cause of three malformed infants (20–22). In the first case, a mother with multiple vitamin deficiencies produced a baby with congenital xerophthalmia and bilateral cleft lip (20). The defects may have been due to vitamin A deficiency because of their similarity to anomalies seen in animals deprived of this nutrient. The second report involved a malnourished pregnant woman with recent onset of blindness whose symptoms were the result of vitamin A deficiency (21). The mother gave birth to a premature male child with microcephaly and what appeared to be anophthalmia. The final case described a blind, mentally retarded girl with bilateral microphthalmia, coloboma of the iris and choroid, and retinal aplasia (22). During pregnancy, the mother was suspected of having vitamin A deficiency manifested by night blindness.

In 1986, investigators from the United States Food and Drug Administration reviewed 18 cases of suspected vitamin A-induced teratogenicity (23). Some of these cases had been reviewed in previous communications by the FDA investigators (24, 25). Six of the cases (26–31) had been previously published and 12 represented unpublished reports. All of the cases, except one, involved long-term, high-dose (>25,000 IU/day) consumption continuing past conception. The exception involved a woman who accidentally consumed 500,000 IU, as a single dose, during the 2nd month of pregnancy (30). Twelve of the infants had malformations similar to those seen in animal and human retinoid syndromes (i.e., central nervous system and cardiovascular anomalies, microtia, and clefts) (23). The defects observed in the 18 infants were microtia ($N = 4$), craniofacial ($N = 4$), brain ($N = 4$), facial palsy ($N = 1$), micro/anophthalmia ($N = 2$), facial clefts ($N = 4$), cardioaortic ($N = 2$), limb reduction ($N = 4$), gastrointestinal atresia ($N = 1$), and urinary ($N = 4$) (23).

The Centers for Disease Control (CDC) reported in 1987 the results of an epidemiologic study conducted by the New York State Department of Health from April 1983 through February 1984 (3). The mothers of 492 liveborn infants without congenital defects were interviewed to obtain their drug histories. Vitamin A supplements were taken by 81.1% (399/492) of the women. Of this group, 0.6% (3/492) took 25,000 IU or more/day, and 2.6% (13/492) consumed 15,000–24,999 IU/day (3). In an editorial comment, the CDC noted that the excessive vitamin A consumption by some of the women was a public health concern (3).

Preliminary results of a Spanish epidemiologic case-control study conducted between 1976–1987 were reported in 1988 (32). A total of 12,315 cases of malformed infants were compared to 12,206 normal controls. Nineteen of the case mothers (1.5/1,000) used vitamin A either alone or in combination with other vitamins during their pregnancies compared to 14 (1.1/1,000) of the controls, an odds ratio of 1.4 (difference not significant). Five of the case infants and 10 of the controls were exposed to high doses (<40,000 IU) (odds ratio 0.5, $p = 0.15$). In contrast, 11 of the case infants and four controls were exposed to 40,000 IU or more (odds ratio 2.7, $p = 0.06$). The data suggested a dose-effect relationship and provided support for earlier statements that doses lower than 10,000 IU were not teratogenic (32).

Several investigators have studied maternal and fetal vitamin A levels during various stages of gestation (6, 33–44). Transport to the fetus is by passive diffusion (45). Maternal vitamin A concentrations are slightly greater than those found in either premature or term infants (33–35). In women with normal levels of vitamin A, maternal and newborn levels were 270 and 220 ng/ml, respectively (34). In 41 women not given supplements of vitamin A, a third of whom had laboratory evidence of hypovitaminemia A, mean maternal levels exceeded those in the newborn by almost a 2:1 ratio (34). In two reports, maternal serum levels were dependent on the length of gestation with concentrations decreasing during the 1st trimester, then increasing during the remainder of pregnancy until about the 38th week when they began to decrease again (6, 36). A more recent study found no difference in serum levels between 10 and 33 weeks' gestation, even though amniotic fluid vitamin A levels at 20 weeks onward were significantly greater than at 16–18 weeks (37). Premature infants (36 weeks or less) have significantly lower serum retinol and retinol-binding protein concentrations than do term neonates (33, 38–40).

Mild to moderate deficiency is common during pregnancy (34, 41). A 1984 report concluded that vitamin A deficiency in poorly nourished mothers was one of the features associated with an increased incidence of prematurity and intrauterine growth retardation (33). An earlier study, however, found no difference in vitamin A levels between low-birth-weight (<2500 g) and normal-birth-weight (>2500 g) infants (35). Maternal vitamin A concentrations of the low-birth-weight group were lower than those of normals, 211 vs. 273 ng/ml, but not significantly. An investigation in premature infants revealed that infants developing bronchopulmonary dysplasia had significantly lower serum retinol levels as compared to infants who did not develop this disease (40).

Relatively high liver vitamin A stores were found in the fetuses of women younger than 18 and older than 40 years of age, two groups that produce a high incidence of fetal anomalies (6). Low fetal liver concentrations were measured in two infants with hydrocephalus and high levels in 14 infants with neural tube defects (NTDs) (6). In another report relating to NTDs, a high liver concentration occurred in an anencephalic infant (42). Significantly higher vitamin A amniotic fluid concentrations were discovered in 12 pregnancies from which infants with NTDs were delivered as compared with 94 normal pregnancies (43). However, attempts to use this measurement as an indicator of anencephaly or other fetal anomalies failed because the values for abnormal and normal fetuses overlapped (37, 43).

The effect of stopping oral contraceptives shortly before conception on vitamin A levels has been studied (44). Since oral contraceptives had been shown to increase serum levels of vitamin A, it was postulated that early conception might involve a risk of teratogenicity. However, no difference was found in early pregnancy vitamin A levels between users and nonusers. The results of this study have been challenged based on the methods used to measure vitamin A (46).

In summary, excessive doses of vitamin A are teratogenic, as may be severe maternal deficiency. β-Carotene, a vitamin A precursor, has not been associated with either human or animal toxicity (see also β-Carotene). Doses exceeding the RDA (5,000 IU/day) should be avoided by women who are, or who may become, pregnant. Moreover, the U.S. RDA established by the Food and Drug Administration should be considered the maximum dose (4). Although the minimum teratogenic dose has not yet been defined, doses of 25,000 IU/day or more, in the form of retinol or retinyl esters, should be considered potentially teratogenic (3, 4, 23).

One of the recommendations of the Teratology Society, published in a 1987 position paper, states: "Women in their reproductive years should be informed that the excessive use of vitamin A shortly before and during pregnancy could be harmful to their babies" (4). The Teratology Society also noted that the average balanced diet contains approximately 7,000–8,000 IU of vitamin A from various sources, and this should be considered prior to additional supplementation (4).

[*Risk Factor X if used in doses above the RDA.]

Breast Feeding Summary

Vitamin A is naturally present in breast milk. Deficiency of this vitamin in breast-fed infants is rare (47). The RDA of vitamin A during lactation is 6000 IU (2). It is not known if high maternal doses of vitamin A present a danger to the nursing infant.

References

1. American Hospital Formulary Service. *Drug Information 1990.* Bethesda:American Society of Hospital Pharmacists, 1990:2109–11.
2. *Recommended Dietary Allowances,* 9th ed. Washington:National Academy of Sciences, 1980.
3. Centers for Disease Control, U.S. Department of Health and Human Services. Use of supplements containing high-dose vitamin A—New York state, 1983–1984. 1987;36.
4. Public Affairs Committee, the Teratology Society. Teratology Society position paper: recommendations for vitamin A use during pregnancy. Teratology 1987;35:269–75.
5. Olson JA. Recommended dietary intakes (RDI) of vitamin A in humans. Am J Clin Nutr 1987;45:704–16.
6. Gal I, Sharman IM, Pryse-Davies J. Vitamin A in relation to human congenital malformations. Adv Teratol 1972;5:143–58.
7. Cohlan SQ. Excessive intake of vitamin A as a cause of congenital anomalies in the rat. Science 1953;117:535–6.
8. Muenter MD. Hypervitaminosis A. Ann Intern Med 1974;80:105–6.
9. Morriss GM. Vitamin A and congenital malformations. Int J Vitam Nutr Res 1976;46:220–2.
10. Fantel AG, Shepard TH, Newell-Morris LL, Moffett BC. Teratogenic effects of retinoic acid in pigtail monkeys (Macaca nemestrina). Teratology 1977;15:65–72.
11. Vorhees CV, Brunner RL, McDaniel CR, Butcher RE. The relationship of gestational age to vitamin A induced postnatal dysfunction. Teratology 1978;17:271–6.
12. Ferm VH, Ferm RR. Teratogenic interaction of hyperthermia and vitamin A. Biol Neonate 1979;36:168–72.
13. Geelen JAG. Hypervitaminosis A induced teratogenesis. CRC Crit Rev Toxicol 1979;6:351–75.
14. Kamm JJ. Toxicology, carcinogenicity, and teratogenicity of some orally administered retinoids. J Am Acad Dermatol 1982;6:652–9.
15. Muenter MD. Hypervitaminosis A. Ann Intern Med 1974;80:105–6.
16. Read AP, Harris R. Spina bifida and vitamins. Br Med J 1983;286:560–1.
17. Bound JP. Spina bifida and vitamins. Br Med J 1983;286:147.
18. Lungarotti MS, Marinelli D, Mariani T, Calabro A. Multiple congenital anomalies associated with apparently normal maternal intake of vitamin A: a phenocopy of the isotretinoin syndrome? Am J Med Genet 1987;27:245–8.
19. Smithells RW. Spina bifida and vitamins. Br Med J 1983;286:388–9.
20. Houet R, Ramioul-Lecomte S. Repercussions sur l'enfant des avitaminoses de la mere pendant la grossesse. Ann Paediatr 1950;175:378. As cited in Warkany J. *Congenital Malformations. Notes and Comments.* Chicago:Year Book Medical Publishers, 1971:127–8.
21. Sarma V. Maternal vitamin A deficiency and fetal microcephaly and anophthalmia. Obstet Gynecol 1959;13:299–301.
22. Lamba PA, Sood NN. Congenital microphthalmus and colobomata in maternal vitamin A deficiency. J Pediatr Ophthalmol 1968;115–7. As cited in Warkany J. *Congenital Malformations. Notes and Comments.* Chicago:Year Book Medical Publishers, 1971:127–8.

23. Rosa FW, Wilk AL, Kelsey FO. Teratogen update: vitamin A congeners. Teratology 1986;33:355–64.
24. Rosa FW. Teratogenicity of isotretinoin. Lancet 1983;2:513.
25. Rosa FW. Retinoic acid embryopathy. N Engl J Med 1986;315:262.
26. Pilotti G, Scorta A. Ipervitaminosi A gravidica e malformazioni neonatali dell'apparato urinaria. Minerva Ginecol 1965;17:1103–8. As cited in Nishimura H, Tanimura T. *Clinical Aspects of the Teratogenicity of Drugs.* New York:American Elsevier, 1976:251–2.
27. Bernhardt IB, Dorsey DJ. Hypervitaminosis A and congenital renal anomalies in a human infant. Obstet Gynecol 1974;43:750–5.
28. Stange L, Carlstrom K, Eriksson M. Hypervitaminosis A in early human pregnancy and malformations of the central nervous system. Acta Obstet Gynecol Scand 1978;57:289–91.
29. Morriss GM, Thomson AD. Vitamin A and rat embryos. Lancet 1974;2:899–900.
30. Mounoud RL, Klein D, Weber F. A propos d'un cas de syndrome de Goldenhar: intoxication aigue a la vitamine A chez la mere pendant la grossesse. J Genet Hum 1975;23:135–54.
31. Von Lennep E, El Khazen N, De Pierreux G, Amy JJ, Rodesch F, Van Regemorter N. A case of partial sirenomelia and possible vitamin A teratogenesis. Prenat Diagn 1985;5:35–40.
32. Martinez-Frias ML, Salvador J. Megadose vitamin A and teratogenicity. Lancet 1988;1:236.
33. Shah RS, Rajalakshmi R. Vitamin A status of the newborn in relation to gestational age, body weight, and maternal nutritional status. Am J Clin Nutr 1984;40:794–800.
34. Baker H, Frank O, Thomson AD, Langer A, Munves ED, De Angelis B, Kaminetzky HA. Vitamin profile of 174 mothers and newborns at parturition. Am J Clin Nutr 1975;28:59–65.
35. Baker H, Thind IS, Frank O, DeAngelis B, Caterini H, Lquria DB. Vitamin levels in low-birth-weight newborn infants and their mothers. Am J Obstet Gynecol 1977;129:521–4.
36. Gal I, Parkinson CE. Effects of nutrition and other factors on pregnant women's serum vitamin A levels. Am J Clin Nutr 1974;27:688–95.
37. Wallingford JC, Milunsky A, Underwood BA. Vitamin A and retinol-binding protein in amniotic fluid. Am J Clin Nutr 1983;38:377–81.
38. Brandt RB, Mueller DG, Schroeder JR, Guyer KE, Kirkpatrick BV, Hutcher NE, Ehrlich FE. Serum vitamin A in premature and term neonates. J Pediatr 1978;92:101–4.
39. Shenai JP, Chytil F,.Jhaveri A, Stahlman MT. Plasma vitamin A and retinol-binding protein in premature and term neonates. J Pediatr 1981:99:302–5.
40. Hustead VA, Gutcher GR, Anderson SA, Zachman RD. Relationship of vitamin A (retinol) status to lung disease in the preterm infant. J Pediatr 1984;105:610–5.
41. Kaminetzky HA, Langer A, Baker H, Frank O, Thomson AD, Munves ED, Opper A, Behrle FC, Glista B. The effect of nutrition in teen-age gravidas on pregnancy and the status of the neonate. I. A nutritional profile. Am J Obstet Gynecol 1973;115:639–46.
42. Gal I, Sharman IM, Pryse-Davies J, Moore T. Vitamin A as a possible factor in human teratology. Proc Nutr Soc 1969;28:9A-10A.
43. Parkinson CE, Tan JCY. Vitamin A concentrations in amniotic fluid and maternal serum related to neural-tube defects. Br J Obstet Gynaecol 1982;89:935–9.
44. Wild J, Schorah CJ, Smithells RW. Vitamin A, pregnancy, and oral contraceptives. Br Med J 1974;1:57–9.
45. Hill EP, Longo LD. Dynamics of maternal-fetal nutrient transfer. Fed Proc 1980;39:239–44.
46. Bubb FA. Vitamin A, pregnancy, and oral contraceptives. Br Med J 1974;1:391–2.
47. Committee on Nutrition, American Academy of Pediatrics. Vitamin and mineral supplement needs in normal children in the United States. Pediatrics 1980;66:1015–21.

Name: **VITAMIN B$_{12}$**

Class: **Vitamin**   Risk Factor: **A***

Fetal Risk Summary

Vitamin B$_{12}$ (cyanocobalamin), a water-soluble B complex vitamin, is an essential nutrient required for nucleoprotein and myelin synthesis, cell reproduction, normal growth, and the maintenance of normal erythropoiesis (1). The American recommended daily allowance (RDA) for vitamin B$_{12}$ in pregnancy is 4 μg (2). A slightly lower recommended dietary intake of 2.5 μg/day (1.8 nmol/day) has been suggested as adequate to meet both maternal and fetal demands (3).

Vitamin B$_{12}$ is actively transported to the fetus (4–8). This process is responsible for the progressive decline of maternal levels that occurs during pregnancy (8–16). Fetal demands for the vitamin have been estimated to be approximately 0.3 μg/day (0.2 nmol/day) (3). Similar to other B complex vitamins, higher concentrations of B$_{12}$ are found in the fetus and newborn than in the mother (3, 7–11, 17–25). At term, mean vitamin B$_{12}$ levels in 174 mothers were 115 pg/ml and in their newborns 500 pg/ml, a newborn:maternal ratio of 4.3 (17). Comparable values have been observed by others (7, 9, 22–24). Mean levels in 51 Brazilian women, in their newborns, and in the intervillous space of their placentas were approximately 340, 797, and 1074 pg/ml, respectively (25). The newborn:maternal ratio in this report was 2.3. The high levels in the placenta may indicate a mechanism by which the fetus can accumulate the vitamin against a concentration gradient. This study also found a highly significant correlation between vitamin B$_{12}$ and folate concentrations. This is in contrast to an earlier report that did not find such a correlation in women with megaloblastic anemia (26).

Maternal deficiency of vitamin B$_{12}$ is common during pregnancy (17, 18, 27, 28). Tobacco smoking reduces maternal levels of the vitamin even further (29). Megaloblastic anemia may result when the deficiency is severe, but it responds readily to therapy (30–33). On the other hand, tropical macrocytic anemia during pregnancy responds erratically to B$_{12}$ therapy and is better treated with folic acid (33, 34).

Megaloblastic (pernicious) anemia may be a cause of infertility (31, 32, 35). One report described a mother with undiagnosed pernicious anemia who had lost her 3rd, 9th, and 10th pregnancies (31). A healthy child resulted from her 11th pregnancy following treatment with B$_{12}$. In another study, eight infertile women with pernicious anemia were treated with B$_{12}$ and seven became pregnant within 1 year of therapy (32). One of three patients in still another report may have had infertility associated with very low B$_{12}$ levels (35).

Vitamin B$_{12}$ deficiency was associated with prematurity (as defined by a birth weight of 2500 g or less) in a 1968 paper (11). However, many of the patients who delivered prematurely had normal or elevated B$_{12}$ levels. No correlation between B$_{12}$ deficiency and abruptio placentae was found in two studies published in the 1960s (36, 37). Two reports found a positive association between low birth weight and low B$_{12}$ levels (22, 38). In both instances, however, folate levels were also low and iron was deficient in one. Others could not correlate low B$_{12}$ concentrations with the weight at delivery (13, 27). Based on these reports, it is doubtful if vitamin B$_{12}$ deficiency is associated with any of the conditions.

In experimental animals, vitamin B$_{12}$ deficiency is teratogenic (9, 39). Investigators studying the etiology of neural tube defects measured very low B$_{12}$ levels in three of four mothers of anencephalic fetuses (40). Additional evidence led them to conclude that the low B$_{12}$ resulted in depletion of maternal folic acid and involvement in the etiology of the defects. In contrast, two other reports have shown no relationship between low levels of vitamin B$_{12}$ and congenital malformations (11, 20).

No reports linking high doses of vitamin B$_{12}$ with maternal or fetal complications have been located. B$_{12}$ administration at term has produced maternal levels approaching 50,000 pg/ml with corresponding cord blood levels of approximately 15,000 pg/ml (6, 7). In fetal methylmalonic acidemia, large doses of B$_{12}$, 10 mg orally initially then changed to 5 mg intramuscularly, were administered daily to a mother to treat the affected fetus (41). On this dosage regimen, maternal levels rose as high as 18,000 pg/ml shortly after a dose. This metabolic disorder is not always treatable with B$_{12}$: one study reported a newborn with the B$_{12}$-unresponsive form of methylmalonic acidemia (42).

In summary, severe maternal vitamin B$_{12}$ deficiency may result in megaloblastic anemia with subsequent infertility and poor pregnancy outcome. Less severe maternal deficiency apparently is common and does not pose a significant risk to the mother or fetus. Ingestion of vitamin B$_{12}$ during pregnancy up to the RDA either via the diet or by supplementation is recommended.

[*Risk Factor C if used in doses above the RDA.]

Breast Feeding Summary

Vitamin B$_{12}$ is excreted into human breast milk. In the first 48 hours after delivery, mean colostrum levels were 2431 pg/ml and then fell rapidly to concentrations comparable to those of normal serum (43). One group of investigators also observed very high colostrum levels ranging from 6–17.5 times that of milk (4). Milk:plasma ratios are approximately 1.0 during lactation (20). Reported milk concentrations of B$_{12}$ vary widely (44–47). Mothers supplemented with daily doses of 1–200 μg had milk levels increase from a level of 79 to a level of 100 pg/ml (44). Milk concentrations were directly proportional to dietary intake. In a study using 8-μg/day supplements, mean milk levels of 1650 pg/ml at 1 week and 1100 pg/ml at 6 weeks were measured (45). Corresponding levels in unsupplemented mothers were significantly different at 1220 and 610 pg/ml, respectively. Other investigators also used 8-μg/day supplements and found significantly different levels compared to women not receiving supplements: 910 vs. 700 pg/ml at 1 week and 790 vs. 550 pg/ml at 6 weeks (46). In contrast, others found no difference between supplemented and unsupplemented well-nourished women with 5–100 μg/day (47). The mean B$_{12}$ concentration in these latter patients was 970 pg/ml. A 1983 English study measured B$_{12}$ levels in pooled human milk obtained from preterm (26 mothers: 29–34 weeks) and term (35 mothers: 39 weeks or longer) patients (48). Preterm milk decreased from 920 pg/ml (colostrum) to 220 pg/ml (16–196 days), while term milk decreased over the same period from a level of 490 to a level of 230 pg/ml.

Vitamin B$_{12}$ deficiency in the lactating mother may cause severe consequences in the nursing infant. Several reports have described megaloblastic anemia in infants exclusively breast fed by B$_{12}$-deficient mothers (49–53). Many of these mothers were vegetarians whose diets provided low amounts of the vitamin (50–53). The adequacy of vegetarian diets in providing sufficient B$_{12}$ has been debated (54–56). However, a recent report measured only 1.4 μg of B$_{12}$ intake/day in lactovegetarians (57). This amount is approximately 35% of the RDA for lactating women in America (2). Moreover, a 1986 case of vitamin B$_{12}$-induced anemia supports the argument that the low B$_{12}$ intake of some vegetarian diets is inadequate to meet the total needs of a nursing infant for this vitamin (58). The case involved a 7-month-old male infant, exclusively breast fed by a strict vegetarian mother, who was diagnosed as suffering from macrocytic anemia. The infant was lethargic, irritable, and failing to thrive. His vitamin B$_{12}$ level was less than 100 pg/ml (normal 180–960 pg/ml), but iron and folate levels were both within normal limits. The anemia responded rapidly to administration of the vitamin, and he was developing normally at 11 months of age (58).

The American RDA for vitamin B$_{12}$ during lactation is 4 µg (2). If the diet of the lactating woman adequately supplies this amount, maternal supplementation with B$_{12}$ is not needed. Supplementation with the RDA for B$_{12}$ is recommended for those women with inadequate nutritional intake. The American Academy of Pediatrics considers maternal consumption of the vitamin to be compatible with breast feeding (59).

References

1. American Hospital Formulary Service. *Drug Information 1990*. Bethesda:American Society of Hospital Pharmacists, 1990:2121–4.
2. *Recommended Dietary Allowances*, ed 9. Washington, DC:National Academy of Sciences, 1980.
3. Herbert V. Recommended dietary intakes (RDI) of vitamin B-12 in humans. Am J Clin Nutr 1987;45:671–8.
4. Luhby AL, Cooperman JM, Donnenfeld AM, Herrero JM, Teller DN, Wenig JB. Observations on transfer of vitamin B$_{12}$ from mother to fetus and newborn. Am J Dis Child 1958;96:532–3.
5. Hill EP, Longo LD. Dynamics of maternal-fetal nutrient transfer. Fed Proc 1980;39:239–44.
6. Kaminetzky HA, Baker H, Frank O, Langer A. The effects of intravenously administered water-soluble vitamins during labor in normovitaminemic and hypovitaminemic gravidas on maternal and neonatal blood vitamin levels at delivery. Am J Obstet Gynecol 1974;120:697–703.
7. Frank O, Walbroehl G, Thomson A, Kaminetzky H, Kubes Z, Baker H. Placental transfer: fetal retention of some vitamins. Am J Clin Nutr 1970;23:662–3.
8. Luhby AL, Cooperman JM, Stone ML, Slobody LB. Physiology of vitamin B$_{12}$ in pregnancy, the placenta, and the newborn. Am J Dis Child 1961;102:753–4.
9. Baker H, Ziffer H, Pasher I, Sobotka H. A Comparison of maternal and foetal folic acid and vitamin B$_{12}$ at parturition. Br Med J 1958;1:978–9.
10. Boger WP, Bayne GM, Wright LD, Beck GD. Differential serum vitamin B$_{12}$ concentrations in mothers and infants. N Engl J Med 1957;256:1085–7.
11. Temperley IJ, Meehan MJM, Gatenby PBB. Serum vitamin B12 levels in pregnant women. J Obstet Gynaecol Br Commonw 1968;75:511–6.
12. Boger WP, Wright LD, Beck GD, Bayne GM. Vitamin B$_{12}$: correlation of serum concentrations and pregnancy. Proc Soc Exp Biol Med 1956;92:140–3.
13. Martin JD, Davis RE, Stenhouse N. Serum folate and vitamin B12 levels in pregnancy with particular reference to uterine bleeding and bacteriuria. J Obstet Gynaecol Br Commonw 1967;74:697–701.
14. Ball EW, Giles C. Folic acid and vitamin B$_{12}$ levels in pregnancy and their relation to megaloblastic anaemia. J Clin Pathol 1964;17:165–74.
15. Izak G, Rachmilewitz M, Stein Y, Berkovici B, Sadovsky A, Aronovitch Y, Grossowicz N. Vitamin B$_{12}$ and iron deficiencies in anemia of pregnancy and puerperium. Arch Intern Med 1957;99:346–55.
16. Edelstein T, Metz J. Correlation between vitamin B12 concentration in serum and muscle in late pregnancy. J Obstet Gynaecol Br Commonw 1969;76:545–8.
17. Baker H, Frank O, Thomson AD, Langer A, Munves ED, De Angelis B, Kaminetzky HA. Vitamin profile of 174 mothers and newborns at parturition. Am J Clin Nutr 1975;28:59–65.
18. Kaminetzky HA, Baker H. Micronutrients in pregnancy. Clin Obstet Gynecol 1977;20:363–80.
19. Lowenstein L, Lalonde M, Deschenes EB, Shapiro L. Vitamin B$_{12}$ in pregnancy and the puerperium. Am J Clin Nutr 1960;8:265–75.
20. Baker SJ, Jacob E, Rajan KT, Swaminathan SP. Vitamin-B$_{12}$ deficiency in pregnancy and the puerperium. Br Med J 1962;1:1658–61.
21. Killander A, Vahlquist B. The vitamin B$_{12}$ concentration in serum from term and premature infants. Nord Med 1954;51:777–9.

22. Baker H, Thind IS, Frank O, DeAngelis B, Caterini H, Lquria DB. Vitamin levels in low-birth-weight newborn infants and their mothers. Am J Obstet Gynecol 1977;129:521–4.
23. Okuda K, Helliger AE, Chow BF. Vitamin B$_{12}$ serum level and pregnancy. Am J Clin Nutr 1956;4:440–3.
24. Baker H, Frank O, Deangelis B, Feingold S, Kaminetzky HA. Role of placenta in maternal-fetal vitamin transfer in humans. Am J Obstet Gynecol 1981;141:792–6.
25. Giugliani ERJ, Jorge SM, Goncalves AL. Serum vitamin B$_{12}$ levels in parturients, in the intervillous space of the placenta and in full-term newborns and their interrelationships with folate levels. Am J Clin Nutr 1985;41:330–5.
26. Giles C. An account of 335 cases of megaloblastic anaemia of pregnancy and the puerperium. J Clin Pathol 1966;19:1–11.
27. Roberts PD, James H, Petrie A, Morgan JO, Hoffbrand AV. Vitamin B$_{12}$ status in pregnancy among immigrants to Britain. Br Med J 1973;3:67–72.
28. Dostalova L. Correlation of the vitamin status between mother and newborn during delivery. Dev Pharmacol Ther 1982;4(Suppl 1):45–57.
29. McGarry JM, Andrews J. Smoking in pregnancy and vitamin B$_{12}$ metabolism. Br Med J 1972;2:74–7.
30. Heaton D. Another case of megaloblastic anemia of infancy due to maternal pernicious anemia. N Engl J Med 1979;300:202–3.
31. Varadi S. Pernicious anaemia and infertility. Lancet 1967;2:1305.
32. Jackson IMD, Doig WB, McDonald G. Pernicious anaemia as a cause of infertility. Lancet 1967;2:1059–60.
33. Chaudhuri S. Vitamin B$_{12}$ in megaloblastic anaemia of pregnancy and tropical nutritional macrocytic anaemia. Br Med J 1951;2:825–8.
34. Patel JC, Kocher BR. Vitamin B$_{12}$ in macrocytic anaemia of pregnancy and the puerperium. Br Med J 1950;1:924–7.
35. Parr JH, Ramsay I. The presentation of osteomalacia in pregnancy. Case report. Br J Obstet Gynaecol 1984;91:816–8.
36. Streiff RR, Little AB. Folic acid deficiency as a cause of uterine hemorrhage in pregnancy. J Clin Invest 1965;44:1102.
37. Streiff RR, Little AB. Folic acid deficiency in pregnancy. N Engl J Med 1967;276:776–9.
38. Whiteside MG, Ungar B, Cowling DC. Iron, folic acid and vitamin B$_{12}$ levels in normal pregnancy, and their influence on birth-weight and the duration of pregnancy. Med J Aust 1968;1:338–42.
39. Shepard TH. *Catalog of Teratogenic Agents*, ed 3. Baltimore:Johns Hopkins University Press, 1980:348–9.
40. Schorah CJ, Smithells RW, Scott J. Vitamin B$_{12}$ and anencephaly. Lancet 1980;1:880.
41. Ampola MG, Mahoney MJ, Nakamura E, Tanaka K. Prenatal therapy of a patient with vitamin-B$_{12}$-responsive methylmalonic acidemia. N Engl J Med 1975;293:313–7.
42. Morrow G III, Schwarz RH, Hallock JA, Barness LA. Prenatal detection of methylmalonic acidemia. J Pediatr 1970;77:120–3.
43. Samson RR, McClelland DBL. Vitamin B$_{12}$ in human colostrum and milk. Acta Paediatr Scand 1980;69:93–9.
44. Deodhar AD, Rajalakshmi R, Ramakrishnan CV. Studies on human lactation. Part III. Effect of dietary vitamin supplementation on vitamin contents of breast milk. Acta Paediatr Scand 1964;53:42–8.
45. Thomas MR, Kawamoto J, Sneed SM, Eakin R. The effects of vitamin C, vitamin B$_6$, and vitamin B$_{12}$ supplementation on the breast milk and maternal status of well-nourished women. Am J Clin Nutr 1979;32:1679–85.
46. Sneed SM, Zane C, Thomas MR. The effects of ascorbic acid, vitamin B$_6$, vitamin B$_{12}$, and folic acid supplementation on the breast milk and maternal nutritional status of low socioeconomic lactating women. Am J Clin Nutr 1981;34:1338–46.
47. Sandberg DP, Begley JA, Hall CA. The content, binding, and forms of vitamin B$_{12}$ in milk. Am J Clin Nutr 1981;34:1717–24.
48. Ford JE, Zechalko A, Murphy J, Brooke OG. Comparison of the B vitamin composition of milk from mothers of preterm and term babies. Arch Dis Child 1983;58:367–72.
49. Lampkin BC, Shore NA, Chadwick D. Megaloblastic anemia of infancy secondary to maternal pernicious anemia. N Engl J Med 1966;274:1168–71.
50. Jadhav M, Webb JKG, Vaishnava S, Baker SJ. Vitamin-B$_{12}$ deficiency in Indian infants: a clinical syndrome. Lancet 1962;2:903–7.

51. Lampkin BC, Saunders EF. Nutritional vitamin B₁₂ deficiency in an infant. J Pediatr 1969;75:1053–5.
52. Higginbottom MC, Sweetman L, Nyhan WL. A syndrome of methylmalonic aciduria, homocystinuria, megaloblastic anemia and neurologic abnormalities in a vitamin B₁₂-deficient breast-fed infant of a strict vegetarian. N Engl J Med 1978;299:317–23.
53. Frader J, Reibman B, Turkewitz D. Vitamin B₁₂ deficiency in strict vegetarians. N Engl J Med 1978;299:1319.
54. Fleiss PM, Douglass JM, Wolfe L. Vitamin B₁₂ deficiency in strict vegetarians. N Engl J Med 1978;299:1319.
55. Hershaft A. Vitamin B₁₂ deficiency in strict vegetarians. N Engl J Med 1978;299:1319–20.
56. Nyhan WL. Vitamin B₁₂ deficiency in strict vegetarians. N Engl J Med 1978;299:1320.
57. Abdulla M, Aly KO, Andersson I, Asp NG, Birkhed D, Denker I, Johansson CG, Jagerstad M, Kolar K, Nair BM, Nilsson-Ehle P, Norden A, Rassner S, Svensson S, Akesson B, Ockerman PA. Nutrient intake and health status of lactovegetarians: chemical analyses of diets using the duplicate portion sampling technique. Am J Clin Nutr 1984;40:325–38.
58. Sklar R. Nutritional vitamin B12 deficiency in a breast-fed infant of a vegan-diet mother. Clin Pediatr 1986;25:219–21.
59. Committee on Drugs, American Academy of Pediatrics. Transfer of drugs and other chemicals into human milk. Pediatrics 1989;84:924–36.

Name: **VITAMIN C**

Class: **Vitamin**   Risk Factor: **A***

Fetal Risk Summary

Vitamin C (ascorbic acid) is a water-soluble essential nutrient required for collagen formation, tissue repair, and numerous metabolic processes including the conversion of folic acid to folinic acid and iron metabolism (1). The American recommended daily allowance (RDA) for vitamin C in pregnancy is 70–80 mg (2).

Vitamin C is actively transported to the fetus (3–6). When maternal serum levels are high, placental transfer changes to simple diffusion (6). During gestation, maternal serum vitamin C progressively declines (7, 8). As a consequence of this process, newborn serum vitamin C (9–22 µg/ml) is approximately 2–4 times that of the mother (4–10 µg/ml) (5–20).

Maternal deficiency of vitamin C without clinical symptoms is common during pregnancy (19–21). Most studies have found no association between this deficiency and maternal or fetal complications, including congenital malformations (12, 13, 22–25). When low vitamin C levels were found in women or fetuses with complications it was a consequence of the condition and not a cause. However, a 1971 retrospective study of 1369 mothers found that deficiency of vitamin C may have a teratogenic effect, although the authors advised caution in the interpretation of their results (26). In a later investigation, low 1st trimester white blood cell vitamin C levels were discovered in six mothers giving birth to infants with neural tube defects (27). Folic acid, vitamin B₁₂, and riboflavin were also low in serum or red blood cells. The low folic acid and B₁₂ levels were thought to be involved in the etiology of the defects (see also Folic Acid, Vitamin B₁₂, and Riboflavin).

A 1965 report suggested that high daily doses of vitamin C during pregnancy might have produced a "conditioned" scurvy in two infants (28). The mothers had apparent daily intakes of vitamin C in the 400 mg range throughout pregnancy, but both of their offspring had infantile scurvy. To study this condition, laboratory animals were given various doses of vitamin C throughout gestation. Two of 10 offspring exposed to the highest doses developed symptoms and histologic changes compatible with scurvy (28). The investigators concluded that the high *in utero* exposure may have induced ascorbic acid dependency. More recent reports of this condition have not been located; thus, the clinical significance is unknown.

Only one report has been found that potentially relates high doses of vitamin C with fetal anomalies. This was in a brief 1976 case report describing an anencephalic fetus delivered from a woman treated with high doses of vitamin C and other water-soluble vitamins and nutrients for psychiatric reasons (29). The relationship between the defect and the vitamins is unknown. In another study, no evidence of adverse effects was found with doses up to 2000 mg/day (30).

In summary, mild to moderate vitamin C deficiency or excessive doses do not seem to pose a major risk to the mother or fetus. Since vitamin C is required for good maternal and fetal health and an increased demand for the vitamin occurs during pregnancy, intake up to the RDA is recommended.

[*Risk Factor C if used in doses above the RDA.]

Breast Feeding Summary

Vitamin C (ascorbic acid) is excreted into human breast milk. Reported concentrations in milk vary from 24–158 μg/ml (31–39). In lactating women with low nutritional status, milk vitamin C is directly proportional to intake (32, 33). Supplementation with 4–200 mg/day of vitamin C produced milk levels of 24–61 μg/ml (32). Similarly, in another group of women with poor vitamin C intake, supplementation with 34–103 mg/day resulted in levels of 34–55 μg/ml (33). In contrast, studies in well-nourished women consuming the RDA or more of vitamin C in their diets indicate that ingestion of greater amounts does not significantly increase levels of the vitamin in their milk (34–38). Even consumption of total vitamin C exceeding 1000 mg/day, 10 times the RDA, did not significantly increase milk concentrations or vitamin C intake of the infants (37). However, maternal urinary excretion of the vitamin did increase significantly. These studies indicate that vitamin C excretion in human milk is regulated to prevent exceeding a saturation level (37).

Storage of human milk in the freezer for up to 3 months did not affect vitamin C concentrations of preterm milk but resulted in a significant decrease in term milk (40). Both types of milk, however, maintained sufficient vitamin C to meet the RDA for infants.

The RDA for vitamin C during lactation is 90–100 mg (2). Well-nourished lactating women consuming the RDA of vitamin C in their diets normally excrete sufficient vitamin C in their milk to reach a saturation level and additional supplementation is not required. Maternal supplementation up to the RDA is needed only in those women with poor nutritional status.

References

1. American Hospital Formulary Service. *Drug Information 1990*. Bethesda:American Society of Hospital Pharmacists, 1990:2124–6.
2. *Recommended Dietary Allowances*, ed 9. Washington, DC:National Academy of Sciences, 1980.
3. Hill EP, Longo LD. Dynamics of maternal-fetal nutrient transfer. Fed Proc 1980;39:239–44.
4. Streeter ML, Rosso P. Transport mechanisms for ascorbic acid in the human placenta. Am J Clin Nutr 1981;34:1706–11.
5. Hamil BM, Munks B, Moyer EZ, Kaucher M, Williams HH. Vitamin C in the blood and urine of the newborn and in the cord and maternal blood. Am J Dis Child 1947;74:417–33.

6. Kaminetzky HA, Baker H, Frank O, Langer A. The effects of intravenously administered water-soluble vitamins during labor in normovitaminemic and hypovitaminemic gravidas on maternal and neonatal blood vitamin levels at delivery. Am J Obstet Gynecol 1974;120:697–703.

7. Snelling CE, Jackson SH. Blood studies of vitamin C during pregnancy, birth, and early infancy. J Pediatr 1939;14:447–51.

8. Adlard BPF, De Souza SW, Moon S. Ascorbic acid in fetal human brain. Arch Dis Child 1974;49:278–82.

9. Braestrup PW. Studies of latent scurvy in infants. II. Content of ascorbic (cevitamic) acid in the blood-serum of women in labour and in children at birth. Acta Paediatr 1937;19:328–34.

10. Braestrup PW. The content of reduced ascorbic acid in blood plasma in infants, especially at birth and in the first days of life. J Nutr 1938;16:363–73.

11. Slobody LB, Benson RA, Mestern J. A comparison of the vitamin C in mothers and their newborn infants. J Pediatr 1946;29:41–4.

12. Teel HM, Burke BS, Draper R. Vitamin C in human pregnancy and lactation. I. Studies during pregnancy. Am J Dis Child 1938;56:1004–10.

13. Lund CJ, Kimble MS. Some determinants of maternal and plasma vitamin C levels. Am J Obstet Gynecol 1943;46:635–47.

14. Manahan CP, Eastman NJ. The cevitamic acid content of fetal blood. Bull Johns Hopkins Hosp 1938;62:478–81.

15. Raiha N. On the placental transfer of vitamin C. An experimental study on guinea pigs and human subjects. Acta Physiol Scand 1958;45:Suppl 155.

16. Khattab AK, Al Nagdy SA, Mourad KAH, El Azghal HI. Foetal maternal ascorbic acid gradient in normal Egyptian subjects. J Trop Pediatr 1970;16:112–5.

17. McDevitt E, Dove MA, Dove RF, Wright IS. Selective filtration of vitamin C by the placenta. Proc Soc Exp Biol Med 1942;51:289–90.

18. Sharma SC. Levels of total ascorbic acid, histamine and prostaglandins E_2 and $F_{2\alpha}$ in the maternal antecubital and foetal umbilical vein blood immediately following the normal human delivery. Int J Vitam Nutr Res 1982;52:320–5.

19. Dostalova L. Correlation of the vitamin status between mother and newborn during delivery. Dev Pharmacol Ther 1982;4(Suppl 1):45–57.

20. Baker H, Frank O, Thomson AD, Langer A, Munves ED, De Angelis B, Kaminetzky HA. Vitamin profile of 174 mothers and newborns at parturition. Am J Clin Nutr 1975;28:59–65.

21. Kaminetzky HA, Langer A, Baker H, Frank O, Thomson AD, Munves ED, Opper A, Behrle FC, Glista B. The effect of nutrition in teen-age gravidas on pregnancy and the status of the neonate. I. A nutritional profile. Am J Obstet Gynecol 1973;115:639–46.

22. Martin MP, Bridgforth E, McGanity WJ, Darby WJ. The Vanderbilt cooperative study of maternal and infant nutrition. X. Ascorbic acid. J Nutr 1957;62:201–24.

23. Chaudhuri SK. Role of nutrition in the etiology of toxemia of pregnancy. Am J Obstet Gynecol 1971;110:46–8.

24. Wilson CWM, Loh HS. Vitamin C and fertility. Lancet 1973;2:859–60.

25. Vobecky JS, Vobecky J, Shapcott D, Munan L. Vitamin C and outcome of pregnancy. Lancet 1974;1:630.

26. Nelson MM, Forfar JO. Associations between drugs administered during pregnancy and congenital abnormalities of the fetus. Br Med J 1971;1:523–7.

27. Smithells RW, Sheppard S, Schorah CJ. Vitamin deficiencies and neural tube defects. Arch Dis Child 1976;51:944–50.

28. Cochrane WA. Overnutrition in prenatal and neonatal life: a problem? Can Med Assoc J 1965;93:893–9.

29. Averback P. Anencephaly associated with megavitamin therapy. Can Med Assoc J 1976;114:995.

30. Korner WF, Weber F. Zur toleranz hoher Ascorbinsauredosen. Int J Vitam Nutr Res 1972;42:528–44.

31. Ingalls TH, Draper R, Teel HM. Vitamin C in human pregnancy and lactation. II. Studies during lactation. Am J Dis Child 1938;56:1011–19.

32. Deodhar AD, Rajalakshmi R, Ramakrishnan CV. Studies on human lactation. Part III. Effect of dietary vitamin supplementation on vitamin contents of breast milk. Acta Paediatr 1964;53:42–8.

33. Bates CJ, Prentice AM, Prentice A, Lamb WH, Whitehead RG. The effect of vitamin C supplementation on lactating women in Keneba, a West African rural community. Int J Vitam Nutr Res 1983;53:68–76.

34. Thomas MR, Kawamoto J, Sneed SM, Eakin R. The effects of vitamin C, vitamin B_6, and vitamin B_{12} supplementation on the breast milk and maternal status of well-nourished women. Am J Clin Nutr 1979;32:1679–85.

35. Thomas MR, Sneed SM, Wei C, Nail PA, Wilson M, Sprinkle EE III. The effects of vitamin C, vitamin B_6, vitamin B_{12}, folic acid, riboflavin, and thiamin on the breast milk and maternal status of well-nourished women at 6 months postpartum. Am J Clin Nutr 1980;33:2151–6.

36. Sneed SM, Zane C, Thomas MR. The effects of ascorbic acid, vitamin B_6, vitamin B_{12}. and folic acid supplementation on the breast milk and maternal nutritional status of low socioeconomic lactating women. Am J Clin Nutr 1981;34:1338–46.

37. Byerley LO, Kirksey A. Effects of different levels of vitamin C intake on the vitamin C concentration in human milk and the vitamin C intakes of breast-fed infants. Am J Clin Nutr 1985;41:665–71.

38. Salmenpera L. Vitamin C nutrition during prolonged lactation: optimal in infants while marginal in some mothers. Am J Clin Nutr 1984;40:1050–6.

39. Grewar D. Infantile scurvy. Clin Pediatr 1965;4:82–9.

40. Bank MR, Kirksey A, West K, Giacoia G. Effect of storage time and temperature on folacin and vitamin C levels in term and preterm human milk. Am J Clin Nutr 1985;41:235–42.

Name: **VITAMIN D**

Class: **Vitamin**   Risk Factor: **A***

Fetal Risk Summary

Vitamin D analogues are a group of fat-soluble nutrients essential for human life with antirachitic and hypercalcemic activity (1). The recommended daily allowance (RDA) for normal pregnant women in America is 400–600 IU (2).

The two natural biologically active forms of vitamin D are 1,25-dihydroxyergocalciferol and calcitriol (1,25-dihydroxyvitamin D_3) (1). A third active compound, 25-hydroxydihydrotachysterol, is produced in the liver from the synthetic vitamin D analogue, dihydrotachysterol.

Ergosterol (provitamin D_2) and 7-dehydrocholesterol (provitamin D_3) are activated by ultraviolet light to form ergocalciferol (vitamin D_2) and cholecalciferol (vitamin D_3), respectively. These, in turn, are converted in the liver to 25-hydroxyergocalciferol and calcifediol (25-hydroxyvitamin D_3), the major transport forms of vitamin D in the body. Activation of the transport compounds by enzymes in the kidneys results in the two natural active forms of vitamin D.

The commercially available forms of vitamin D are ergocalciferol, cholecalciferol, calcifediol, calcitriol, and dihydrotachysterol. Although differing in potency, all of these products have the same result in the mother and fetus. Thus, only the term vitamin D, unless otherwise noted, will be used in this monograph.

High doses of vitamin D are known to be teratogenic in experimental animals, but direct evidence for this is lacking in humans. Because of its action to raise calcium levels, vitamin D has been suspected in the pathogenesis of the supravalvular aortic stenosis syndrome, which is often associated with idiopathic hypercalcemia of infancy (3–5). The full features of this rare condition are characteristic elfin facies, mental and growth retardation, strabismus, enamel defects, craniosynostosis, supravalvular aortic and pulmonary stenosis, inguinal hernia, cryptorchidism in males, and early development of secondary sexual characteristics in females (3). Excessive intake or retention of vitamin D during pregnancy by mothers of infants who develop supravalvular aortic stenosis syndrome has not been consistently found (3, 4, 6). While the exact cause is unknown, it is possible that the syndrome results from abnormal vitamin D metabolism in the mother, the fetus, or both.

Very high levels of vitamin D have been used to treat maternal hypoparathyroidism during pregnancy (7–10). In two studies, 15 mothers were treated with doses averaging 107,000 IU/day throughout their pregnancies to maintain maternal calcium levels within the normal range (7, 8). All of the 27 children were normal at birth and during follow-up examinations ranging up to 16 years. Calcitriol, in doses up to 3 μg/day, was used to treat another mother with hypoparathyroidism (9). The high dose was required in the latter half of pregnancy to prevent hypocalcemia. The infant had no apparent adverse effects from this exposure. In a similar case, a mother received 100,000 IU/day throughout gestation resulting in a healthy, full-term infant (10). In contrast, a 1965 case report described a woman who received 600,000 IU of vitamin D and 40,000 IU of vitamin A daily for 1 month early in pregnancy (11). The resulting infant had a defect of the urogenital system, but this was probably due to ingestion of excessive vitamin A (see Vitamin A).

Vitamin D deficiency can be induced by decreased dietary intake or lack of exposure to sunlight. The conversion of provitamin D_3 to vitamin D_3 is catalyzed by ultraviolet light striking the skin (1). Severe deficiency during pregnancy, resulting in maternal osteomalacia, leads to significant morbidity in the mother and fetus (12–22). Pitkin (23), in a 1985 article, reviewed the relationship between vitamin D and calcium metabolism in pregnancy (23).

Although rare in America, the peak incidence of vitamin D deficiency occurs in the winter and early spring when exposure to sunlight is at a minimum. Certain ethnic groups, such as Asians, seem to be at greater risk for developing this deficiency because of their dietary and sun exposure habits (l2–22). In the pregnant woman, osteomalacia may cause, among other effects, decreased weight gain and pelvic deformities that prevent normal vaginal delivery (12, 13). For the fetus, vitamin D deficiency has been associated with:

Reduced fetal growth (12, 13)
Neonatal hypocalcemia without convulsions (13–15, 21)
Neonatal hypocalcemia with convulsions (tetany) (16–18)
Neonatal rickets (19, 20)
Defective tooth enamel (22, 24)

Long-term use of heparin may induce osteopenia by inhibiting renal activation of calcifediol to the active form of vitamin D_3 (calcitriol or 1,25-dihydroxyvitamin D_3) (23). The decreased levels of calcitriol prevent calcium uptake by bone and result in osteopenia (see reference 23 for detailed review of calcium metabolism in pregnancy). One investigator suggests that these patients may benefit from treatment with supplemental calcitriol (23).

A number of investigators have measured vitamin D levels in the mother during pregnancy and in the newborn (25–35). Although not universal, most studies have found a significant correlation between maternal serum and cord blood levels (25–29). In one study, a close association between both of the transport vitamin D forms in maternal and cord serum was discovered (30). No significant correlation could be demonstrated, however, between the two biologically active forms in maternal and cord blood.

Using a perfused human placenta, a 1984 report confirmed that calcifediol and calcitriol were transferred from the mother to the fetus, although at a very slow rate (36). Binding to vitamin D_3-binding protein was a major rate-limiting factor, especially for calcifediol, the transport form of vitamin D_3. The researchers concluded that placental metabolism of calcifediol was not a major source of fetal calcitriol (36).

Maternal levels at term are usually higher than those in the newborn since the fetus has no need for intestinal calcium absorption (25–31). Maternal levels are elevated in early pregnancy and continue to increase throughout pregnancy (33). During the winter months a weak correlation may exist between maternal vitamin D intake and serum levels, with exposure to ultraviolet light, the main determinant of maternal concentrations (34, 35). A Norwegian study, however, was able to increase maternal concentrations of active vitamin D significantly during all seasons with daily supplementation of 400 IU (30).

[*Risk Factor D if used in doses above the RDA.]

Breast Feeding Summary

Vitamin D is excreted into breast milk in limited amounts (37). A direct relationship exists between maternal serum levels of vitamin D and the concentration in breast milk (38). Chronic maternal ingestion of large doses may lead to greater than normal vitamin D activity in the milk and resulting hypercalcemia in the infant (39). In the lactating woman who is not receiving supplements, there is considerable controversy over whether her milk contains sufficient vitamin D to protect the infant from vitamin deficiency. Several studies have supported the need for infant supplementation during breast feeding (13, 37, 40–42). Other investigators have concluded that supplementation is not necessary if maternal vitamin D stores are adequate (29, 43–45).

A study published in 1977 measured high levels of a vitamin D metabolite in the aqueous phase of milk (46). Although two other studies supported these findings, the conclusions were in direct opposition to previous measurements and have been vigorously disputed (47, 48). The argument that human milk is low in vitamin D is supported by clinical reports of vitamin D deficiency-induced rickets and decreased bone mineralization in breast-fed infants (41, 42, 49–51). Moreover, one investigation measured the vitamin D activity of human milk and failed to find any evidence for significant activity of water-soluble vitamin D metabolites (52). Vitamin D activity in the milk was 40–50 IU/L with 90% of this accounted for by the usual fat-soluble components.

The American RDA for vitamin D in the lactating woman is 400–600 IU (2). The Committee on Nutrition, American Academy of Pediatrics, recommends vitamin D supplements for breast-fed infants if maternal vitamin D nutrition is inadequate or if the infant lacks sufficient exposure to ultraviolet light (53). A second committee of the American Academy of Pediatrics considers maternal consumption of vitamin D to be compatible with breast feeding (54). However, the serum calcium levels of the infant should be monitored if the mother is receiving pharmacologic doses (54).

References

1. American Hospital Formulary Service. *Drug Information 1990*. Bethesda:American Society of Hospital Pharmacists, 1990:2127–9.
2. *Recommended Dietary Allowances*, ed 9. Washington, DC:National Academy of Sciences, 1980.
3. Friedman WF, Mills LF. The relationship between vitamin D and the craniofacial and dental anomalies of the supravalvular aortic stenosis syndrome. Pediatrics 1969;43:12–8.
4. Rowe, RD, Cooke RE. Vitamin D and craniofacial and dental anomalies of supravalvular stenosis. Pediatrics 1969;43:1–2.
5. Taussig HB. Possible injury to the cardiovascular system from vitamin D. Ann Intern Med 1966;65:1195–1200.
6. Anita AU, Wiltse HE, Rowe RD, Pitt EL, Levin S, Ottesen OE, Cooke RE. Pathogenesis of the supravalvular aortic stenosis syndrome. J Pediatr 1967;71:431–41.
7. Goodenday LS, Gordan GS. Fetal safety of vitamin D during pregnancy. Clin Res 1971;19:200.
8. Goodenday LS, Gordan GS. No risk from vitamin D in pregnancy. Ann Intern Med 1971;75:807–8.
9. Sadeghi-Nejad A, Wolfsdorf JI, Senior B. Hypoparathyroidism and pregnancy: treatment with calcitriol. JAMA 1980;243:254–5.
10. Greer FR, Hollis BW, Napoli JL. High concentrations of vitamin D_2 in human milk associated with pharmacologic doses of vitamin D_2. J Pediatr 1984;105:61–4.
11. Pilotti G, Scorta A. Ipervitaminosi A gravidica e malformazioni neonatali dell'apparato urinaria. Minerva Ginecol 1965;17:1103–8. As cited in Nishimura H, Tanimura T. *Clinical Aspects of the Teratogenicity of Drugs*. New York:American Elsevier, 1976:251–2.
12. Parr JH, Ramsay I. The presentation of osteomalacia in pregnancy. Case report. Br J Obstet Gynaecol 1984;91:816–8.
13. Brooke OG, Brown IRF, Bone CDM, Carter ND, Cleeve HJW, Maxwell JD, Robinson VP, Winder SM. Vitamin D supplements in pregnant Asian women: effects on calcium status and fetal growth. Br Med J 1980;280:751–4.
14. Rosen JF, Roginsky M, Nathenson G, Finberg L. 25-Hydroxyvitamin D: plasma levels in mothers and their premature infants with neonatal hypocalcemia. Am J Dis Child 1974;127:220–3.
15. Watney PJM, Chance GW, Scott P, Thompson JM. Maternal factors in neonatal hypocalcaemia: a study in three ethnic groups. Br Med J 1971;2:432–6.
16. Heckmatt JZ, Peacock M, Davies AEJ, McMurray J, Isherwood DM. Plasma 25-hydroxyvitamin D in pregnant Asian women and their babies. Lancet 1979;2:546–9.
17. Roberts SA, Cohen MD, Forfar JO. Antenatal factors associated with neonatal hypocalcaemic convulsions. Lancet 1973;2:809–11.
18. Purvis RJ, Barrie WJM, MacKay GS, Wilkinson EM, Cockburn F, Belton NR, Forfar JO. Enamel hypoplasia of the teeth associated with neonatal tetany: a manifestation of maternal vitamin-D deficiency. Lancet 1973;2:811–4.
19. Ford JA, Davidson DC, McIntosh WB, Fyfe WM, Dunnigan MG. Neonatal rickets in Asian immigrant population. Br Med J 1973;3:211–2.
20. Moncrieff M, Fadahunsi TO. Congenital rickets due to maternal vitamin D deficiency. Arch Dis Child 1974;49:810–1.
21. Watney PJM. Maternal factors in the aetiology of neonatal hypocalcaemia. Postgrad Med J 1975;51(Suppl 3):14–7.
22. Cockburn F, Belton NR, Purvis RJ, Giles MM, Brown JK, Turner TL, Wilkinson EM, Forfar JO, Barrie WJM, McKay GS, Pocock SJ. Maternal vitamin D intake and mineral metabolism in mothers and their newborn infants. Br Med J 1980;2:11–4.
23. Pitkin RM. Calcium metabolism in pregnancy and the perinatal period: a review. Am J Obstet Gynecol 1985;151:99–109.
24. Stimmler L, Snodgrass GJAI, Jaffe E. Dental defects associated with neonatal symptomatic hypocalcaemia. Arch Dis Child 1973;48:217–20.
25. Hillman LS, Haddad JG. Human perinatal vitamin D metabolism. I: 25-hydroxyvitamin D in maternal and cord blood. J Pediatr 1974;84:742–9.
26. Dent CE, Gupta MM. Plasma 25-hydroxyvitamin-D levels during pregnancy in Caucasians and in vegetarian and non-vegetarian Asians. Lancet 1975;2:1057–60.
27. Weisman Y, Occhipinti M, Knox G, Reiter E, Root A. Concentrations of 24,25-dihydroxyvitamin D and 25-hydroxyvitamin D in paired maternal-cord sera. Am J Obstet Gynecol 1978;130:704–7.

28. Steichen JJ, Tsang RC, Gratton TL, Hamstra A, DeLuca HF. Vitamin D homeostasis in the perinatal period: 1,25-dihydroxyvitamin D in maternal, cord, and neonatal blood. N Engl J Med 1980;302:315–9.
29. Birkbeck JA, Scott HF. 25-Hydroxycholecalciferol serum levels in breast-fed infants. Arch Dis Child 1980;55:691–5.
30. Markestad T, Aksnes L, Ulstein M, Aarskog D. 25-Hydroxyvitamin D and 1,25-dihydroxyvitamin D of D_2 and D_3 origin in maternal and umbilical cord serum after vitamin D_2 supplementation in human pregnancy. Am J Clin Nutr 1984;40:1057–63.
31. Kumar R, Cohen WR, Epstein FH. Vitamin D and calcium hormones in pregnancy. N Engl J Med 1980;302:1143–5.
32. Hillman LS, Haddad JG. Perinatal vitamin D metabolism. II. Serial 25-hydroxyvitamin D concentrations in sera of term and premature infants. J Pediatr 1975;86:928–35.
33. Kumar R, Cohen WR, Silva P, Epstein FH. Elevated 1,25-dihydroxyvitamin D plasma levels in normal human pregnancy and lactation. J Clin Invest 1979;63:342–4.
34. Hillman LS, Haddad JG. Perinatal vitamin D metabolism. III. Factors influencing late gestational human serum 25-hydroxyvitamin D. Am J Obstet Gynecol 1976;125:196–200.
35. Turton CWG, Stanley P, Stamp TCB, Maxwell JD. Altered vitamin-D metabolism in pregnancy. Lancet 1977;1:222–5.
36. Ron M, Levitz M, Chuba J, Dancis J. Transfer of 25-hydroxyvitamin D_3 and 1,25-dihydroxyvitamin D_3 across the perfused human placenta. Am J Obstet Gynecol 1984;148:370–4.
37. Greer FR, Hollis BW, Cripps DJ, Tsang RC. Effects of maternal ultraviolet B irradiation on vitamin D content of human milk. J Pediatr 1984;105:431–3.
38. Rothberg AD, Pettifor JM, Cohen DF, Sonnendecker EWW, Ross FP. Maternal-infant vitamin D relationships during breast-feeding. J Pediatr 1982;101:500–3.
39. Goldberg LD. Transmission of a vitamin-D metabolite in breast milk. Lancet 1972;2:1258–9.
40. Greer FR, Ho M, Dodson D, Tsang RC. Lack of 25-hydroxyvitamin D and 1,25-dihydroxyvitamin D in human milk. J Pediatr 1981;99:233–5.
41. Greer FR, Searcy JE, Levin RS, Steichen JJ, Steichen-Asch PS, Tsang RC. Bone mineral content and serum 25-hydroxyvitamin D concentration in breast-fed infants with and without supplemental vitamin D. J Pediatr 1981;98:696–701.
42. Greer FR, Searcy JE, Levin RS, Steichen JJ, Steichen-Asche PS, Tsang RC. Bone mineral content and serum 25-hydroxyvitamin D concentrations in breast-fed infants with and without supplemental vitamin D: one-year follow-up. J Pediatr 1982;100:919–22.
43. Fairney A, Naughten E, Oppe TE. Vitamin D and human lactation. Lancet 1977;2:739–41.
44. Roberts CC, Chan GM, Folland D, Rayburn C, Jackson R. Adequate bone mineralization in breast-fed infants. J Pediatr 1981;99:192–6.
45. Chadwick DW. Commentary. Water-soluble vitamin D in human milk: a myth. Pediatrics 1982;70:499.
46. Lakdawala DR, Widdowson EM. Vitamin-D in human milk. Lancet 1977;1:167–8.
47. Greer FR, Reeve LE, Chesney RW, DeLuca HF. Water-soluble vitamin D in human milk: a myth. Pediatrics 1982;69:238.
48. Greer FR, Reeve LE, Chesney RW, DeLuca HF. Commentary. Water-soluble vitamin D in human milk: a myth. Pediatrics 1982;70:499–500.
49. Bunker JWM, Harris RS, Eustis RS. The antirachitic potency of the milk of human mothers fed previously on "vitamin D milk" of the cow. N Engl J Med 1933;208:313–5.
50. O'Connor P. Vitamin D-deficiency rickets in two breast-fed infants who were not receiving vitamin D supplementation. Clin Pediatr (Phila) 1977;16:361–3.
51. Little JA. Commentary. Water-soluble vitamin D in human milk: a myth. Pediatrics 1982;70:499.
52. Reeve LE, Chesney RW, DeLuca HF. Vitamin D of human milk: identification of biologically active forms. Am J Clin Nutr 1982;36:122–6.
53. Committee on Nutrition, American Academy of Pediatrics. Vitamin and mineral supplement needs in normal children in the United States. Pediatrics 1980;66:1015.
54. Committee on Drugs, American Academy of Pediatrics. Transfer of drugs and other chemicals into human milk. Pediatrics 1989;84:924–36.

Name: **VITAMIN E**

Class: **Vitamin**   Risk Factor: **A***

Fetal Risk Summary

Vitamin E (tocopherols) is comprised of a group of fat-soluble vitamins that are essential for human health, although their exact biologic function is unknown (1). The American recommended daily allowance (RDA) for vitamin E in pregnancy is 15 IU (about 15 mg) (2).

Vitamin E concentrations in mothers at term are approximately 4–5 times that of the newborn (3–9). Levels in the mother rise throughout pregnancy (4). Maternal blood vitamin E usually ranges between 9–19 μg/ml with corresponding newborn levels varying from 2–6 μg/ml (3–10). Supplementation of the mother with 15–30 mg/day had no effect on either maternal or newborn vitamin E concentrations at term (5). Use of 600 mg/day in the last 2 months of pregnancy produced about a 50% rise in maternal serum vitamin E (+8 μg/ml) but a much smaller increase in the cord blood (+1 μg/ml) (8). Although placental transfer is by passive diffusion, passage of vitamin E to the fetus is dependent upon plasma lipid concentrations (9–11). At term, cord blood is low in β-lipoproteins, the major carrier of vitamin E, in comparison to maternal blood; as a consequence, it is able to transport less of the vitamin (9). Since vitamin E is transported in the plasma by these lipids, recent investigations have focused on the ratio of vitamin E (in milligrams) to total lipids (in grams) rather than on blood vitamin E concentrations alone (10). Ratios above about 0.6–0.8 are considered normal depending on the author cited and the age of the patients (10, 12, 13).

Vitamin E deficiency is relatively uncommon in pregnancy, occurring in less than 10% of all patients (4, 5, 14). No maternal or fetal complications from deficiency or excess of the vitamin have been identified. Doses far exceeding the RDA have not proved to be harmful (8, 15, 16). Early studies used vitamin E in conjunction with other therapy in attempts to prevent abortion and premature labor, but no effect of the vitamin therapy was demonstrated (17, 18). Premature infants born with low vitamin E stores may develop hemolytic anemia, edema, reticulocytosis, and thrombocytosis if not given adequate vitamin E in the first months following birth (16, 19, 20). In two studies, supplementation of mothers with 500–600 mg of vitamin E during the last 1–2 months of pregnancy did not produce values significantly different from controls in the erythrocyte hemolysis test with hydrogen peroxide, a test used to determine adequate levels of vitamin E (8, 16).

In summary, neither deficiency nor excess of vitamin E has been associated with maternal or fetal complications during pregnancy. In well-nourished women, adequate vitamin E is consumed in the diet and supplementation is not required. If dietary intake is poor, supplementation up to the RDA for pregnancy is recommended.

[*Risk Factor C if used in doses above the RDA.]

Breast Feeding Summary

Vitamin E is excreted into human breast milk (12, 13, 21, 22). Human milk is more than five times richer in vitamin E than cow's milk and is more effective in maintaining adequate serum vitamin E and vitamin E/total lipid ratio in infants up to 1 year of age (12, 22). A 1985 study measured 2.3 μg/ml of the vitamin in mature milk (21). Preterm milk (gestational age 27–33 weeks) was significantly higher, 8.5 μg/ml, during the 1st week and then decreased progressively over the next 6 weeks to 3.7 μg/ml (21). The authors concluded that preterm milk plus multivitamin supplements would provide adequate levels of vitamin E for very-low-birth-weight infants (<1500 g and appropriate for gestational age).

Japanese researchers examined the pattern of vitamin E analogues (α-, γ-, δ-, and β-tocopherols) in plasma and red blood cells from breast-fed and bottle-fed infants (23). Several differences were noted, but the significance of these findings to human health is unknown.

Vitamin E applied for 6 days to the nipples of breast-feeding women resulted in a significant rise in infant serum levels of the vitamin (24). The study group, composed of 10 women, applied the contents of one 400-IU vitamin E capsule to both areolae and nipples after each nursing. Serum concentrations of the vitamin rose from 4 μg/ml to 17.5 μg/ml, and those in a similar group of untreated controls rose from 3.4 μg/ml to 12.2 μg/ml. The difference between the two groups was statistically significant ($p < 0.025$). Although no adverse effects were observed, the authors cautioned that the long-term effects were unknown.

The American RDA of vitamin E during lactation is 16 IU (about 16 mg) (2). Maternal supplementation is recommended only if the diet does not provide sufficient vitamin E to meet the RDA.

References

1. American Hospital Formulary Service. *Drug Information 1990*. Bethesda:American Society of Hospital Pharmacists, 1990:2133–4.
2. *Recommended Dietary Allowances*, ed 9. Washington, DC:National Academy of Sciences, 1980.
3. Moyer WT. Vitamin E levels in term and premature newborn infants. Pediatrics 1950;6:893–6.
4. Leonard PJ, Doyle E, Harrington W. Levels of vitamin E in the plasma of newborn infants and of the mothers. Am J Clin Nutr 1972;25:480–4.
5. Baker H, Frank O, Thomson AD, Langer A, Munves ED, De Angelis B, Kaminetzky HA. Vitamin profile of 174 mothers and newborns at parturition. Am J Clin Nutr 1975;28:59–65.
6. Dostalova L. Correlation of the vitamin status between mother and newborn during delivery. Dev Pharmacol Ther 1982;4(Suppl I):45–57.
7. Kaminetzky HA, Baker H. Micronutrients in pregnancy. Clin Obstet Gynecol 1977;20:363–80.
8. Mino M, Nishino H. Fetal and maternal relationship in serum vitamin E level. J Nutr Sci Vitaminol 1973;19:475–82.
9. Haga P, Ek J, Kran S. Plasma tocopherol levels and vitamin E/β-lipoprotein relationships during pregnancy and in cord blood. Am J Clin Nutr 1982;36:1200–4.
10. Martinez FE, Goncalves AL, Jorge SM, Desai ID. Vitamin E in placental blood and its interrelationship to maternal and newborn levels of vitamin E. J Pediatr 1981;99:298–300.
11. Hill EP, Longo LD. Dynamics of maternal-fetal nutrient transfer. Fed Proc 1980;39:239–44.
12. Martinez FE, Jorge SM, Goncalves AL, Desai ID. Evaluation of plasma tocopherols in relation to hematological indices of Brazilian infants on human milk and cows' milk regime from birth to 1 year of age. Am J Clin Nutr 1984;39:969–74.
13. Mino M, Kitagawa M, Nakagawa S. Red blood cell tocopherol concentrations in a normal population of Japanese children and premature infants in relation to the assessment of vitamin E status. Am J Clin Nutr 1985;41:631–8.
14. Kaminetzky HA, Langer A, Baker O, Frank O, Thomson AD, Munves ED, Opper A, Behrle FC, Glista B. The effect of nutrition in teen-age gravidas on pregnancy and the status of the neonate. I. A nutritional profile. Am J Obstet Gynecol 1973;115:639–46.
15. Hook EB, Healy KM, Niles AM, Skalko RG. Vitamin E: teratogen or anti-teratogen? Lancet 1974;1:809.

16. Gyorgy P, Cogan G, Rose CS. Availability of vitamin E in the newborn infant. Proc Soc Exp Biol Med 1952;81:536–8.
17. Kotz J, Parker E, Kaufman MS. Treatment of recurrent and threatened abortion. Report of two hundred and twenty-six cases. J Clin Endocrinol 1941;1:838–49.
18. Shute E. Vitamin E and premature labor. Am J Obstet Gynecol 1942;44:271–9.
19. Oski FA, Barness LA. Vitamin E deficiency: a previously unrecognized cause of hemolytic anemia in the premature infant. J Pediatr 1967;70:211–20.
20. Ritchie JH, Fish MB, McMasters V, Grossman M. Edema and hemolytic anemia in premature infants. A vitamin E deficiency syndrome. N Engl J Med 1968;279:1185–90.
21. Gross SJ, Gabriel E. Vitamin E status in preterm infants fed human milk or infant formula. J Pediatr 1985;106:635–9.
22. Friedman Z. Essential fatty acids revisited. Am J Dis Child 1980;134:397–408.
23. Mino M, Kijima Y, Nishida Y, Nakagawa S. Difference in plasma- and red blood cell-tocopherols in breast-fed and bottle-fed infants. J Nutr Sci Vitaminol 1980;26:103–12.
24. Marx CM, Izquierdo A, Driscoll JW, Murray MA, Epstein MF. Vitamin E concentrations in serum of newborn infants after topical use of vitamin E by nursing mothers. Am J Obstet Gynecol 1985;152:668–70.

Name: **VITAMINS, MULTIPLE**

Class: **Vitamins**   Risk Factor: **A***

Fetal Risk Summary

Vitamins are essential for human life. Preparations containing multiple vitamins (multivitamins) are routinely given to pregnant women. A typical product will contain the vitamins A, D, E, and C, plus the B complex vitamins thiamine (B_1), riboflavin (B_2), niacinamide (B_3), pantothenic acid (B_5), pyridoxine (B_6), B_{12}, and folic acid. Miscellaneous substances that may be included are iron, calcium, and other minerals. The practice of supplementation during pregnancy with multivitamins varies from country to country but is common in the United States. The American recommended daily allowance (RDA) for pregnant women are (1):

Vitamin A	5000 IU	Niacinamide (B_3)	15–17 mg
Vitamin D	400–600 IU	Pyridoxine (B_6)	2.4–2.6 mg
Vitamin C	70–80 mg	Folic acid	0.8 mg
Thiamine (B_1)	1.4–1.5 mg	Vitamin B_{12}	4 μg
Riboflavin (B_2)	1.5–1.6 mg	Vitamin E	15 IU

Although essential for health, vitamin K is normally not included in multivitamin preparations since it is adequately supplied from natural sources. The fat-soluble vitamins, A, D, and E, may be toxic or teratogenic in high doses. The water-soluble vitamins, C and the B complex group, are generally considered safe in amounts above the RDA, but there are exceptions. Deficiencies of vitamins may also be teratogenic (see individual vitamin monographs for further details).

The role of vitamins in the prevention of certain congenital defects continues to be a major area of controversy. Two different classes of anomalies, cleft lip and/or palate and neural tube defects, have been the focus of numerous investigations with multivitamins. An investigation into a third class of anomalies, limb reduction defects, has also appeared. The following sections will summarize the published work on these topics.

Animal research in the 1930s and 1940s had shown that both deficiencies and excesses of selected vitamins could result in fetal anomalies, but it was not until two papers in 1958 (2, 3) that attention was turned to humans. These investigations examined the role of environmental factors, in particular the B complex vitamins, as agents for preventing the recurrence of cleft lip and/or palate (CLP). In that same year, a study was published that involved 87 women who had previously given birth to infants with CLP (4). Although the series was too small to draw statistical conclusions, 48 women given no vitamin supplements had 78 pregnancies, resulting in four infants with CLP. The treated group, composed of 39 women, received multivitamins plus injectable B complex vitamins during the 1st trimester. This group had 59 pregnancies with none of the infants having CLP. A similar study found a CLP incidence of 1.9% (3 of 156) in treated pregnancies compared to 5.7% (22 of 383) in controls (5). The difference was not statistically significant. However, other researchers, in a 1964 survey, found no evidence that vitamins offered protection against CLP (6). Also in 1964, research was published involving 594 pregnant women who had previously given birth to an infant with CLP (7). This work was further expanded, and the total group involving 645 pregnancies was presented in a 1976 paper (8). Of the total group, 417 women were not given supplements during pregnancy, and they gave birth to 20 infants (4.8%) with CLP. In the treated group, 228 women were given B complex vitamins plus vitamin C before or during the 1st trimester. From this latter group, seven infants (3.1%) with CLP resulted. Although suggestive of a positive effect, the difference between the two groups was not significant. Another investigator found only one instance of CLP in his group of 85 supplemented pregnancies (9). These patients were given daily multivitamins plus 10 mg of folic acid. In 206 pregnancies in women not given supplements where the infants/fetuses were examined, 15 instances of CLP resulted. The difference between the two groups was significant ($p = 0.023$). In contrast, one author suggested that the vitamin A in the supplements caused a cleft palate in his patient (10). However, the conclusion of this report has been disputed (11). Thus, the published studies involving the role of multivitamins in the prevention of cleft lip and/or palate are inconclusive. No decisive benefit (or risk) of multivitamin supplementation has emerged from any of the studies.

The second part of the controversy surrounding multivitamins and the prevention of congenital defects involves their role in preventing neural tube defects (NTDs). (Three excellent reviews on the pathophysiology and various other aspects of NTDs, including discussions on the role that multivitamins might play in the etiology and prevention of these defects, have been recently published (12–14).) In a series of articles from 1976–1983, British investigators examined the effect of multivitamin supplements on a group of women who had previously given birth to one or more children with NTDs (15–19). For the purpose of their study, they defined NTDs to include anencephaly, encephalocele, cranial meningocele, iniencephaly, myelocele, myelomeningocele, and meningocele but excluded isolated hydrocephalus and spina bifida occulta (17). In their initial publication, they found that in six mothers who had given birth to infants with NTDs, there were lower 1st trimester levels of serum folate, red blood cell folate, white blood cell vitamin C, and riboflavin saturation index (15). The differences between the case mothers and the controls were significant for red blood cell folate ($p < 0.001$) and white blood cell vitamin C ($p < 0.05$). Serum vitamin A levels were comparable to those of controls. Based on this experience, a multicenter study was launched to compare mothers receiving full supplements with control patients not receiving supplements (16–19). The supplemented group received a multivitamin-iron-calcium preparation from 28 days before conception to the date of the second missed menstrual period, which is after the time of neural tube closure. The daily vitamin supplement provided:

Vitamin A	4000 IU	Nicotinamide	15 mg
Vitamin D	400 IU	Pyridoxine	1 mg
Vitamin C	40 mg	Folic acid	0.36 mg
Thiamine	1.5 mg	Ferrous sulfate	75.6 mg (as Fe)
Riboflavin	1.5 mg	Calcium phosphate	480 mg

Their findings, summarized in 1983, are shown below for the infants and fetuses who were examined (19):

One Previous NTD
    Supplemented   385
        Recurrences   2* (0.5%)
    Not supplemented   458
        Recurrences   19* (4.1%)   *p = 0.0004
Two or More Previous NTDs
    Supplemented   44
        Recurrences   1* (2.3%)
    Not supplemented   52
        Recurrences   5* (9.6%)   *p = 0.145
Total
    Supplemented   429
        Recurrences   3(0.7%)
    Not supplemented   510
        Recurrences   24(4.7%)

Although the numbers are suggestive of a protective effect offered by multivitamins, at least three other explanations were offered by the investigators (16):

1. A low-risk group had selected itself for supplementation.
2. The study group aborted more NTD fetuses than did controls.
3. Other factors were responsible for the reduction in NTDs.

A 1980 report found that women receiving well-balanced diets had a lower incidence and recurrence rate of infants with NTDs than did women receiving poor diets (20). Although multivitamin supplements were not studied, it was assumed that those patients who consumed adequate diets also consumed more vitamins from their food compared to those with poor diets. This study, then, added credibility to the thesis that good nutrition can prevent some NTDs. Other researchers, using Smithells' protocol, observed that fully supplemented mothers (N = 83) had no recurrences while an unsupplemented group (N = 141) had four recurrences of NTDs (21, 22). Interestingly, a short report that appeared 6 years before Smithells' work found that both vitamins and iron were consumed more by mothers who gave birth to infants with anencephalus and spina bifida (23).

The above investigations have generated a number of discussions, criticisms, and defenses (24–57). The primary criticism centered around the fact that the groups were not randomly assigned but were self-selected for supplementation or no supplementation. A follow-up study, in response to some of these objections, was published in 1986 (58). This study examined six factors that may have influenced the earlier results by increasing the risk of recurrence of NTDs: (a) two or more previous NTDs, (b) residence in Northern Ireland, (c) spontaneous abortions immediately prior to the studied pregnancy, (d) less than 12 months between studied pregnancy and abortion, (e) social class, and (f) therapeutic abortion immediately prior to the studied pregnancy. The relative risk was increased only for the first four factors, and only in those cases with two or more previous NTDs was the increase significant. In addition, none of the four factors would have predicted more than a 4% increase in the recurrence rate in unsupplemented mothers compared to those supplemented. The results indicated that none of these factors contributed significantly to the differential risk between supplemented and unsupplemented mothers, thus leading to the conclusion that the difference in recurrence rates was due to the multivitamin (58).

Several recent studies examining the effect of multivitamins on NTDs have been published. A case-control, population-based study evaluated the association between periconceptional (3 months before and after conception) multivitamin use and the occurrence of NTDs (59). The case group involved either liveborn or stillborn infants with anencephaly or spina bifida born during the years 1968–1980 in the Atlanta area. A total of 347 infants with NTDs were eligible for enrollment and became the case group, while 2829 infants without birth defects served as controls. Multivitamin usage and other factors were ascertained by interview 2–16 years after the pregnancies. This long time interval might have induced a recall problem into the study, even though the authors did take steps to minimize any potential bias (59). A protective effect of periconceptional multivitamin usage against having an infant with an NTD was found in comparison to controls with an estimated relative risk for all NTDs of 0.41 (95% confidence interval (CI) 0.26–0.66), anencephaly 0.47 (95% CI 0.25–0.91), and spina bifida 0.37 (95% CI 0.19–0.70). The odds ratios for whites, but not for other races, were statistically significant. Except for anencephaly among whites (odds ratio 0.68, 95% CI 0.35–1.34), similar results were obtained when infants with congenital defects other than NTDs were used as controls. Although the results indicated that periconceptional use of multivitamins did protect against NTDs, the authors could not determine if the effect was due to vitamins or to some unknown characteristic of vitamin users (59). In commenting on this study, one investigator speculated that if the lack of a statistical effect observed in black women was confirmed, it may be due to a different genetic makeup of the population (60). In other words, the gene(s) that cause NTDs are responsive to periconceptional multivitamins only in whites (60).

Three brief letter communications examined the effects of gastric or intestinal bypass surgery, performed for obesity, on the incidence of NTDs (61–63). The first report appeared in 1986 and described three births with NTDs occurring in Maine (61). During the interval 1980–1984, 261 gastric bypass procedures were performed in Maine, but only 133 were in women under the age of 35. One woman delivered an anencephalic fetus 2 years after her surgery. A second suffered a spontaneous abortion at 16 weeks' gestation, 6 years after a gastrojejunostomy. Her serum α-fetoprotein level 10 days prior to the abortion was 4.8

times the median. She became pregnant again 2 years later and eventually delivered a stillborn infant in the 3rd trimester. The infant had a midthoracic meningomyelocele, iniencephaly, absence of diaphragms, and hypoplastic lungs. During this latter pregnancy, she had intermittent heavy alcohol intake. In the third case, a woman, whose surgery had been done 7 years earlier, had an anencephalic fetus associated with a lumbar rachischisis diagnosed at 6 months' gestation. In response to this report, investigators in Denmark and Sweden could find no cases of NTDs in 77 infants born after their mothers had bypass operations for obesity (62). However, the procedures in these cases involved intestinal bypass, not gastric. Low birth weight and growth retardation were increased in 64 liveborn infants. Gastric bypass surgery is known to place recipients at risk for nutritional deficiencies, especially for iron, calcium, vitamin B_{12}, and folate (61, 63). In the third report, of a total of 908 women who underwent the procedure, 511 (57%) responded to a questionnaire (63). Of these, 87 (17%; 87 of 511) had been pregnant at least once after the surgery. The 87 women had 73 pregnancies (more than 20 weeks' gestation) before the operation with no cases of NTDs. After the surgery, these women had 110 pregnancies with two cases of NTDs. This represented a 12-fold increase in the risk for NTDs compared to the general population (incidence 0.15%) (63). A third case of an infant with an NTD born from a mother who had undergone the operation was identified later, but the mother was not part of the original group. In each of the three cases, the birth of the infant with an NTD had occurred more than 4 years after the bypass surgery. Moreover, the three mothers had not consumed vitamin supplements as prescribed by their physicians. Because of these findings, the authors recommended pregnancy counseling for any woman who has undergone this procedure and who then desires to become pregnant (63).

In another brief reference, the final results of a British clinical trial were presented in 1989 (64). Women who resided in the Yorkshire region were enrolled in the study if: (a) they had one or more previous NTD infants, (b) they were not pregnant at the time of enrollment, and (c) they were considering another pregnancy. Mothers were requested to take the vitamin formulation described above for at least 4 weeks before conception and until they had missed two menstrual periods (i.e., same as previously). The results of the study included three reporting intervals; 1977–1980, 1981–1984, and 1985–1987. The 148 fully supplemented mothers (those who took vitamins as prescribed or only missed taking vitamins on 1 day) had 150 infants/fetuses, only 1 (0.7%) of whom had an NTD. In contrast, 315 unsupplemented mothers had 320 infants/fetuses among whom there were 18 (5.6%) cases of NTDs. The difference between the groups was significant ($p = 0.006$). In addition, 37 partially supplemented (defined as mothers who took the prescribed vitamin for a shorter period of time than the fully supplemented group) women had 37 pregnancies with no cases of NTDs. The investigators concluded that the difference between the groups could not be attributed to declining NTD recurrence rates or to selection bias. Summarizing these and previously published results, only one NTD recurrence had been observed in 315 infants/fetuses born to 274 fully supplemented mothers, and no recurrences had been observed among 57 examined infants/fetuses born to 58 partially supplemented women (64).

A 1989 study conducted in California and Illinois examined three groups of patients to determine if multivitamins had a protective effect against NTDs (65). The groups were composed of women who had a conceptus with an NTD ($N = 571$) and two control groups: those who had a stillbirth or other defect ($N = 546$), and women who had delivered a normal child ($N = 573$). In this study, NTDs included anencephaly, meningocele, myelomeningocele, encephalocele, rachischisis, iniencephaly, and lipomeningocele. The periconceptional use of multivitamins, both in terms of vitamin supplements only and when combined with fortified cereals, was then evaluated for each of the groups. The outcome of this study, after appropriate adjustment for potential confounding factors, revealed an odds ratio of 0.95 (95% CI 0.78–1.14) for NTD-supplemented mothers (i.e., those who received the RDA of vitamins or more) compared to unsupplemented mothers of abnormal infants, and an odds ratio of 1.00 (95% CI 0.83–1.20) when the NTD group was compared to unsupplemented mothers of normal infants. Only slight differences from these values occurred when the data were evaluated by considering vitamin supplements only (no fortified cereals) or vitamin supplements of any amount (i.e., less than the RDA). Similarly, examination of the data for an effect of folate supplementation on the occurrence of NTDs did not change the results. Thus, this study could not show that the use of either multivitamin or folate supplements reduced the frequency of NTDs. However, the investigators cautioned that their results could not exclude the possibility that vitamins might be of benefit in a high-risk population. Several reasons were proposed by the authors to explain why their results were different than those obtained in the Atlanta study cited above: (a) recall bias, (b) a declining incidence of NTDs, (c) geographic differences such that a subset of vitamin-preventable NTDs was in the Atlanta region but not in the areas of the current study, and (d) the Atlanta study did not consider the vitamins contained in fortified cereals (65). However, others concluded that this study lead to a null result because: (a) the vitamin consumption history was obtained after delivery, (b) the history was obtained after the defect was identified, or (c) the study excluded those women taking vitamins after they knew they were pregnant (66).

In contrast to the above report, a Boston study published in 1989 found a significant effect of folic acid-containing multivitamins on the occurrence of NTDs (66). The study population comprised 22,715 women for whom complete information on vitamin consumption and pregnancy outcomes was available. Women were interviewed at the time of a maternal serum α-fetoprotein screen or an amniocentesis. Thus, in most cases, the interview was conducted before the results of the tests were known to either the patient or the interviewer. A total of 49 women had an NTD outcome (2.2/1,000). Among these, three cases occurred in 107 women with a history of previous NTDs (28.0/1,000), and two in 489 women with a family history of NTDs in someone other than an offspring (4.1/1,000). After excluding the 87 women whose family history of NTDs was unknown, the incidence of NTDs in the remaining women was 44 cases in 22,093 (2.0/1,000). Among the 3,157 women who did not use a folic acid-containing multivitamin, 11 cases of NTD occurred, a prevalence of 3.5/1,000. For those using the preparation during the first 6 weeks of pregnancy, 10 cases occurred from a total of 10,713 women (prevalence 0.9/1,000). The prevalence ratio estimate for these two groups was 0.27 (95% CI 0.12–0.59). For mothers who used vitamins during the first 6 weeks that did not contain folic acid, the prevalence was three cases in 926, a ratio of 3.2. The ratio, when compared to that of nonusers, was 0.93 (95% CI 0.26–3.3). When vitamin use was started in the 7th week of gestation, there were 25 cases of NTD from 7,795 mothers using the folic acid-multivitamin supplements (prevalence 3.2/1,000; prevalence ratio 0.92) and no cases in the 66 women who started consuming multivitamins without folate. This study, then, observed a markedly reduced risk of NTDs when folic acid-containing multivitamin preparations were consumed in the first 6 weeks of gestation.

A recent investigation into a third class of anomalies, limb reduction defects, was opened by a report that multivitamins may have caused this malformation in an otherwise healthy boy (52). The mother was taking the preparation because of a previous birth of a child with an NTD. A retrospective analysis of Finnish records, however, failed to show any association between 1st trimester use of multivitamins and limb reduction defects (67).

In summary, the use of multivitamins up to the RDA for pregnancy is recommended for the general good health of the mother and the fetus. There is no strong evidence to suggest that vitamin supplementation can prevent cleft lip and/or palate. However, a body of evidence is accumulating that supplementation during the first few weeks of gestation, especially when folic acid is included, may reduce the risk of neural tube defects. The evidence appears particularly strong for the prevention of NTD recurrences in England. Additional studies will be needed to establish if the protective effect includes only certain types of patients. Until that time, it seems prudent to recommend that folate-containing multivitamin preparations should be used immediately prior to and during at least the first few months of pregnancy. Women who have had gastric bypass surgery for obesity may be at increased risk for delivering offspring with NTDs, and pregnancy counseling to assure adequate nutritional intake may be of benefit.

[*Risk Factor varies for amounts exceeding RDA. See individual vitamins.]

Breast Feeding Summary

Vitamins are naturally present in breast milk (see individual vitamins). The recommended daily allowance of vitamins and minerals during lactation are (1):

Vitamin A	6000 IU
Vitamin D	400–600 IU
Vitamin E	16 IU
Vitamin C	90–100 mg
Folic acid	500 µg
Thiamine (B$_1$)	1.5–1.6 mg
Riboflavin (B$_2$)	1.7–1.8 mg
Niacinamide (B$_3$)	18–20 mg
Pyridoxine (B$_6$)	2.3–2.5 mg
Cyanocobalamin (B$_{12}$)	4 µg
Calcium	1200–1600 mg
Phosphorus	1200–1600 mg
Iodine	200 µg
Iron	18 mg
Magnesium	450 mg
Zinc	25 mg

References

1. *Recommended Dietary Allowances*, ed 9. Washington, DC:National Academy of Sciences, 1980.

2. Douglas B. The role of environmental factors in the etiology of "so-called" congenital malformations. I. Deductions from the presence of cleft lip and palate in one of identical twins, from embryology and from animal experiments. Plast Reconstr Surg 1958;22:94–108.

3. Douglas B. The role of environmental factors in the etiology of "so-called" congenital malformations. II. Approaches in humans; study of various extragenital factors, "theory of compensatory nutrients," development of regime for first trimester. Plast Reconstr Surg 1958;22:214–29.

4. Conway H. Effect of supplemental vitamin therapy on the limitation of incidence of cleft lip and cleft palate in humans. Plast Reconstr Surg 1958;22:450–3.

5. Peer LA, Gordon HW, Bernhard WG. Experimental production of congenital deformities and their possible prevention in man. J Int Coll Surg 1963;39:23–35.

6. Fraser FC, Warburton D. No association of emotional stress or vitamin supplement during pregnancy to cleft lip or palate in man. Plast Reconstr Surg 1964;33:395–9.

7. Peer LA, Gordon HW, Bernhard WG. Effect of vitamins on human teratology. Plast Reconstr Surg 1964;34:358–62.

8. Briggs RM. Vitamin supplementation as a possible factor in the incidence of cleft lip/palate deformities in humans. Clin Plast Surg 1976;3:647–52.

9. Tolarova M. Periconceptional supplementation with vitamins and folic acid to prevent recurrence of cleft lip. Lancet 1982;2:217.

10. Bound JP. Spina bifida and vitamins. Br Med J 1983;286:147.

11. Smithells RW. Spina bifida and vitamins. Br Med J 1983;286:388–9.

12. Main DM, Mennuti MT. Neural tube defects: issues in prenatal diagnosis and counselling. Obstet Gynecol 1986;67:1–16.

13. Rhoads GG, Mills JL. Can vitamin supplements prevent neural tube defects? Current evidence and ongoing investigations. Clin Obstet Gynecol 1986;29:569–79.

14. Lemire RJ. Neural tube defects. JAMA 1988;259:558–62.

15. Smithells RW, Sheppard S, Schorah CJ. Vitamin deficiencies and neural tube defects. Arch Dis Child 1976;51:944–50.

16. Smithells RW, Sheppard S, Schorah CJ, Seller MJ, Nevin NC, Harris R, Read AP, Fielding DW. Possible prevention of neural-tube defects by periconceptional vitamin supplementation. Lancet 1980;1:339–40.

17. Smithells RW, Sheppard S, Schorah CJ, Seller MJ, Nevin NC, Harris R, Read AP, Fielding DW. Apparent prevention of neural tube defects by periconceptional vitamin supplementation. Arch Dis Child 1981;56:911–8.

18. Smithells RW, Sheppard S, Schorah CJ, Seller MJ, Nevin NC, Harris R, Read AP, Fielding DW, Walker S. Vitamin supplementation and neural tube defects. Lancet 1981;2:1425.

19. Smithells RW, Nevin NC, Seller MJ, Sheppard S, Harris R, Read AP, Fielding DW, Walker S, Schorah CJ, Wild J. Further experience of vitamin supplementation for prevention of neural tube defect recurrences. Lancet 1983;1:1027–31.

20. Laurence KM, James N, Miller M, Campbell H. Increased risk of recurrence of pregnancies complicated by fetal neural tube defects in mothers receiving poor diets, and possible benefit of dietary counselling. Br Med J 1980;281:1592–4.

21. Holmes-Siedle M, Lindenbaum RH, Galliard A, Bobrow M. Vitamin supplementation and neural tube defects. Lancet 1982;1:276.

22. Holmes-Siedle M. Vitamin supplementation and neural tube defects. Lancet 1983;2:41.

23. Choi NW, Klaponski FA. On neural-tube defects: an epidemiological elicitation of etiological factors. Neurology 1970;20:399–400.

24. Stone DH. Possible prevention of neural-tube defects by periconceptional vitamin supplementation. Lancet 1980;1:647.

25. Smithells RW, Sheppard S. Possible prevention of neural-tube defects by periconceptional vitamin supplementation. Lancet 1980;1:647.

26. Fernhoff PM. Possible prevention of neural-tube defects by periconceptional vitamin supplementation. Lancet 1980;1:648.

27. Elwood JH. Possible prevention of neural-tube defects by periconceptional vitamin supplementation. Lancet 1980;1:648.

28. Anonymous. Vitamins, neural-tube defects, and ethics committees. Lancet 1980;1:1061–2.

29. Kirke PN. Vitamins, neural tube defects, and ethics committees. Lancet 1980;1:1300–1.

30. Freed DLJ. Vitamins, neural tube defects, and ethics committees. Lancet 1980;1:1301.

31. Raab GM, Gore SM. Vitamins, neural tube defects, and ethics committees. Lancet 1980;1:1301.

32. Hume K. Fetal defects and multivitamin therapy. Med J Aust 1980;2:731–2.

33. Edwards JH. Vitamin supplementation and neural tube defects. Lancet 1982;1:275–6.
34. Renwick JH. Vitamin supplementation and neural tube defects. Lancet 1982;1:748.
35. Chalmers TC, Sacks H. Vitamin supplements to prevent neural tube defects. Lancet 1982;1:748.
36. Stirrat GM. Vitamin supplementation and neural tube defects. Lancet 1982;1:625–6.
37. Kanofsky JD. Vitamin supplements to prevent neural tube defects. Lancet 1982;1:1075.
38. Walsh DE. Vitamin supplements to prevent neural tube defects. Lancet 1982;1:1075.
39. Meier P. Vitamins to prevent neural tube defects. Lancet 1982;1:859.
40. Smith DE, Haddow JE. Vitamins to prevent neural tube defects. Lancet 1982;1:859–60.
41. Smithells RW, Sheppard S, Schorah CJ, Seller MJ, Nevin NC, Harris R, Read AP, Fielding DW. Vitamin supplements and neural tube defects. Lancet 1982;1:1186.
42. Anonymous. Vitamins to prevent neural tube defects. Lancet 1982;2:1255–6.
43. Lorber J. Vitamins to prevent neural tube defects. Lancet 1982;2:1458–9.
44. Read AP, Harris R. Spina bifida and vitamins. Br Med J 1983;286:560–1.
45. Rose G, Cooke ID, Polani, Wald NJ. Vitamin supplementation for prevention of neural tube defect recurrences. Lancet 1983;1:1164–5.
46. Knox EG. Vitamin supplementation and neural tube defects. Lancet 1983;2:39.
47. Emanuel I. Vitamin supplementation and neural tube defects. Lancet 1983;2:39–40.
48. Smithells RW, Seller MJ, Harris R, Fielding DW, Schorah CJ, Nevin NC, Sheppard S, Read AP, Walker S, Wild J. Vitamin supplementation and neural tube defects. Lancet 1983;2:40.
49. Oakley GP Jr, Adams MJ Jr, James LM. Vitamins and neural tube defects. Lancet 1983;2:798–9.
50. Smithells RW, Seller MJ, Harris R, Fielding DW, Schorah CJ, Nevin NC, Sheppard S, Read AP, Walker S, Wild J. Vitamins and neural tube defects. Lancet 1983;2:799.
51. Elwood JM. Can vitamins prevent neural tube defects? Can Med Assoc J 1983;129:1088–92.
52. David TJ. Unusual limb-reduction defect in infant born to mother taking periconceptional multivitamin supplement. Lancet 1984;1:507–8.
53. Blank CE, Kumar D, Johnson M. Multivitamins and prevention of neural tube defects: a need for detailed counselling. Lancet 1984;1:291.
54. Smithells RW. Can vitamins prevent neural tube defects? Can Med Assoc J 1984;131:273–6.
55. Wald NJ, Polani PE. Neural-tube defects and vitamins: the need for a randomized clinical trial. Br J Obstet Gynecol 1984;91:516–23.
56. Seller MJ. Unanswered questions on neural tube defects. Br Med J 1987;294:1–2.
57. Harris R. Vitamins and neural tube defects. Br Med J 1988;296:80–1.
58. Wild J, Read AP, Sheppard S, Seller MJ, Smithells RW, Nevin NC, Schorah CJ, Fielding DW, Walker S, Harris R. Recurrent neural tube defects, risk factors and vitamins. Arch Dis Child 1986;61:440–4.
59. Mulinare J, Cordero JF, Erickson JD, Berry RJ. Periconceptional use of multivitamins and the occurrence of neural tube defects. JAMA 1988;260:3141–5.
60. Holmes LB. Does taking vitamins at the time of conception prevent neural tube defects? JAMA 1988;260:3181.
61. Haddow JE, Hill LE, Kloza EM, Thanhauser D. Neural tube defects after gastric bypass. Lancet 1986;1:1330.
62. Knudsen LB, Kallen B. Gastric bypass, pregnancy, and neural tube defects. Lancet 1986;2:227.
63. Martin L, Chavez GF, Adams MJ Jr, Mason EE, Hanson JW, Haddow JE, Currier RW. Gastric bypass surgery as maternal risk factor for neural tube defects. Lancet 1988;1:640–1.
64. Smithells RW, Sheppard S, Wild J, Schorah CJ. Prevention of neural tube defect recurrences in Yorkshire: final report. Lancet 1989;2:498–9.
65. Mills JL, Rhoads GG, Simpson JL, Cunningham GC, Conley MR, Lassman MR, Walden ME, Depp OR, Hoffman HJ. The absence of a relation between the periconceptional use of vitamins and neural-tube defects. N Engl J Med 1989;321:430–5.
66. Milunsky A, Jick H, Jick SS, Bruell CL, MacLaughlin DS, Rothman KJ, Willett W. Multivitamin/folic acid supplementation in early pregnancy reduces the prevalence of neural tube defects. JAMA 1989;262:2847–2852.
67. Aro T, Haapakoski J, Heinonen OP, Saxen L. Lack of association between vitamin intake during early pregnancy and reduction limb defects. Am J Obstet Gynecol 1984;150:433.

Name: **WARFARIN**

Class: **Anticoagulant**   Risk Factor: **D**

Fetal Risk Summary

See Coumarin Derivatives.

Breast Feeding Summary

See Coumarin Derivatives.

Z

Name: ZUCLOPENTHIXOL

Class: Tranquilizer　　　　　　　　　　　　　　　　Risk Factor: **C**

Fetal Risk Summary

Zuclopenthixol is a thioxanthene tranquilizer with properties similar to those of chlorpromazine. No reports of the use of zuclopenthixol in pregnancy have been located.

Breast Feeding Summary

Zuclopenthixol is excreted into human milk. In six women treated with the agent between 3 days and 10 months after delivery, the mean milk:serum ratio was 0.29 (range 0.12–0.56) (1). Maternal dosages were 72 mg (intramuscular depot injection) every 2 weeks in one patient and 4–50 mg/day orally in the other five women (time interval between oral dosing and sampling not specified). The milk concentrations were all less than 4 ng/ml, with the highest level occurring in the woman who received the injectable form. The authors estimated that an infant consuming 600 ml/day of milk would ingest 0.5–5 μg/day of zuclopenthixol. None of the nursing infants showed signs of sedation or other adverse effects.

In a 1988 study, zuclopenthixol was also measured in the milk of a woman who was being treated for puerperal psychosis 2 weeks after delivery of her first child (2). The mother was given 24 mg/day orally for 4 days, then 14 mg/day. Milk and serum samples were obtained on days 2, 3, 6, and 8 of therapy. The mean milk concentration while the mother was receiving 24 mg/day was 20 ng/ml, (milk:serum ratio 0.71–2.20); it fell to 5 ng/ml while she was receiving 14 mg/day (ratio of 0.24–0.66) (the time interval between dosing and sampling was not specified). No adverse effects were observed in the nursing infant.

Although no adverse effects were observed in the seven infants exposed via the milk to zuclopenthixol, the long-term effects of this exposure have not been studied. Caution is advised, especially during prolonged therapy, until additional studies have been conducted (2).

References

1. Aaes-Jorgensen T, Bjorndal F, Bartels U. Zuclopenthixol levels in serum and breast milk. Psychopharmacology 1986;90:417–8.
2. Matheson I, Skjaeraasen J. Milk concentrations of flupenthixol, nortriptyline and zuclopenthixol and between-breast differences in two patients. Eur J Clin Pharmacol 1988;35:217–20.

APPENDIX

A. ACIDIFYING AGENTS
Ammonium Chloride (B)

B. ANESTHETICS
1. Local
Lidocaine (C)

C. ANTIDIARRHEALS
Diphenoxylate (C_M)
Loperamide (B_M)
Paregoric (B/D)

D. ANTIHISTAMINES
Antazoline (C)
Azatadine (B_M)
Bromodiphenhydramine (C)
Brompheniramine (C_M)
Buclizine (C)
Carbinoxamine (C)
Chlorcyclizine (C)
Chlorpheniramine (B)
Cimetidine (B)
Cinnarizine (C)
Clemastine (C)
Cyclizine (B)
Cyproheptadine (B_M)
Dexbrompheniramine (C)
Dexchlorpheniramine (B_M)
Dimenhydrinate (B_M)
Dimethindene (C)
Dimethothiazine (C)
Diphenhydramine (C)
Doxylamine (B)
Hydroxyzine (C)
Meclizine (B_M)
Methdilazine (C)
Pheniramine (C)
Phenyltoloxamine (C)
Promethazine (C)
Pyrilamine (C)
Ranitidine (B_M)

Trimeprazine (C)
Tripelennamine (B)
Triprolidine (C_M)

E. ANTI-INFECTIVES
1. Amebicide
Carbarsone (D)
Iodoquinol (C)
2. Aminoglycosides
Amikacin (C)
Gentamicin (C)
Kanamycin (D)
Neomycin (C)
Streptomycin (D)
Tobramycin (D_M)
3. Anthelmintics
Gentian Violet (C)
Mebendazole (C_M)
Piperazine (B)
Pyrantel Pamoate (C)
Pyrvinium Pamoate (C)
Thiabendazole (C_M)
4. Antifungals
Amphotericin B (B)
Ciclopirox (B_M)
Clotrimazole (B)
Flucytosine (C)
Griseofulvin (C)
Miconazole (C_M)
Nystatin (B)
5. Antituberculosis
para-Aminosalicyclic Acid (C)
Cycloserine (C)
Ethambutol (B)
Isoniazid (C)
Pyrazinamide (C)
Rifampin (C)
6. Antivirals
Acyclovir (C_M)
Amantadine (C_M)
Idoxuridine (C)

Ribavirin (X$_M$)
Vidarabine (C$_M$)
7. Cephalosporins
Cefaclor (B$_M$)
Cefadroxil (B$_M$)
Cefamandole (B$_M$)
Cefatrizine (B)
Cefazolin (B$_M$)
Cefonicid (B$_M$)
Cefoperazone (B$_M$)
Ceforanide (B$_M$)
Cefotaxime (B$_M$)
Cefoxitin (B)
Ceftizoxime (B$_M$)
Ceftriaxone (B$_M$)
Cefuroxime (B)
Cephalexin (B$_M$)
Cephalothin (B$_M$)
Cephapirin (B$_M$)
Cephradine (B$_M$)
Moxalactam (C$_M$)
8. Iodine
Iodine (D)
Povidone-Iodine (D)
9. Other Anti-infectives
Bacitracin (C)
Chloramphenicol (C)
Clindamycin (B)
Colistimethate (B)
Erythromycin (B)
Furazolidone (C)
Lincomycin (B)
Novobiocin (C)
Oleandomycin (C)
Paromomycin (C)
Polymyxin B (B)
Spectinomycin (B)
Trimethoprim (C$_M$)
Troleandomycin (C)
Vancomycin (C$_M$)
10. Penicillins
Amoxicillin (B)
Ampicillin (B)
Bacampicillin (B$_M$)
Carbenicillin (B)
Cloxacillin (B$_M$)
Cyclacillin (B$_M$)
Dicloxacillin (B$_M$)
Hetacillin (B)
Methicillin (B$_M$)
Nafcillin (B)
Oxacillin (B$_M$)
Penicillin G (B)

Penicillin G, Benzathine (B)
Penicillin G, Procaine (B)
Penicillin V (B)
Piperacillin (B$_M$)
Ticarcillin (B)
11. Plasmodicides
Chloroquine (C)
Primaquine (C)
Pyrimethamine (C)
Quinacrine (C)
Quinine (D/X)
12. Scabicide/Pediculicide
Lindane (B$_M$)
Pyrethrins with Piperonyl Butoxide
    (C)
13. Sulfonamides
Sulfasalazine (B/D)
Sulfonamides (B/D)
14. Tetracyclines
Chlortetracycline (D)
Clomocycline (D)
Demeclocycline (D)
Doxycycline (D)
Methacycline (D)
Minocycline (D)
Oxytetracycline (D)
Tetracycline (D)
15. Trichomonacides
Metronidazole (B$_M$)
16. Urinary Germicides
Cinoxacin (B$_M$)
Mandelic Acid (C)
Methenamine (C$_M$)
Methylene Blue (C$_M$/D)
Nalidixic Acid (B)
Nitrofurantoin (B)

F. ANTINEOPLASTICS
    Aminopterin (X)
    Azathioprine (D)
    Bleomycin (D)
    Busulfan (D)
    Chlorambucil (D$_M$)
    Cisplatin (D)
    Cyclophosphamide (D)
    Cytarabine (D$_M$)
    Dacarbazine (C$_M$)
    Dactinomycin (C$_M$)
    Daunorubicin (D$_M$)
    Doxorubicin (D)
    Fluorouracil (D)
    Hydroxyurea (D)
    Laetrile (C)

Mechlorethamine (D)
Melphalan (D$_M$)
Mercaptopurine (D)
Methotrexate (D)
Plicamycin (Mithramycin) (D)
Procarbazine (D)
Teniposide (D)
Thioguanine (D$_M$)
Thiotepa (D)
Vinblastine (D)
Vincristine (D)

G. ANTITUSSIVES AND EXPECTORANTS

1. Antitussives
Codeine (C/D)

2. Expectorants
Guaifenesin (C)
Hydriodic Acid (D)
Iodinated Glycerol (X$_M$)
Potassium Iodide (D)
Sodium Iodide (D)

H. AUTONOMICS

1. Parasympathomimetics (Cholinergics)
Acetylcholine (C)
Ambenonium (C)
Bethanechol (C$_M$)
Carbachol (C)
Demecarium (C)
Echothiophate (C)
Edrophonium (C)
Isoflurophate (C)
Neostigmine (C$_M$)
Physostigmine (C)
Pilocarpine (C)
Pyridostigmine (C)

2. Parasympatholytics (Anticholinergic)
Anisotropine (C)
Atropine (C)
Belladonna (C)
Benztropine (C)
Biperiden (C$_M$)
Clidinium (C)
Cycrimine (C)
Dicyclomine (B)
Diphemanil (C)
Ethopropazine (C)
Glycopyrrolate (B$_M$)
Hexocyclium (C)
Homatropine (C)

l-Hyoscyamine (C)
Isopropamide (C)
Mepenzolate (C)
Methantheline (C)
Methixene (C)
Methscopolamine (C)
Orphenadrine (C)
Oxyphencyclimine (C)
Oxyphenonium (C)
Piperidolate (C)
Procyclidine (C)
Propantheline (C$_M$)
Scopolamine (C)
Thiphenamil (C)
Tridihexethyl (C)
Trihexyphenidyl (C)

3. Skeletal Muscle Relaxants
Chlorzoxazone (C)
Decamethonium (C)

4. Sympathomimetics (Adrenergic)
Albuterol (C$_M$)
Cocaine (C)
Dobutamine (C)
Dopamine (C)
Ephedrine (C)
Epinephrine (C)
Fenoterol (B)
Isoetharine (C)
Isoproterenol (C)
Isoxsuprine (C)
Levarterenol (D)
Mephentermine (C)
Metaproterenol (C$_M$)
Metaraminol (D)
Methoxamine (C$_M$)
Phenylephrine (C)
Phenylpropanolamine (C)
Pseudoephedrine (C)
Ritodrine (B$_M$/X)
Terbutaline (B)

5. Sympatholytics
Acebutolol (B$_M$)
Atenolol (C$_M$)
Esmolol (C$_M$)
Labetalol (C$_M$)
Mepindolol (C)
Metoprolol (B$_M$)
Nadolol (C$_M$)
Oxprenolol (C)
Pindolol (B$_M$)
Prazosin (C)
Propranolol (C$_M$)

Timolol (C_M)

I. CARDIOVASCULAR DRUGS
1. Antihypertensives
Acebutolol (B_M)
Atenolol (C_M)
Captopril (C_M)
Clonidine (C)
Diazoxide (C_M)
Enalapril (C_M)
Esmolol (C_M)
Hexamethonium (C)
Hydralazine (C_M)
Labetalol (C_M)
Mepindolol (C)
Methyldopa (C)
Metoprolol (B_M)
Minoxidil (C_M)
Nadolol (C_M)
Oxprenolol (C)
Pargyline (C_M)
Pindolol (B_M)
Prazosin (C)
Propranolol (C_M)
Reserpine (D)
Sodium Nitroprusside (C)
Timolol (C_M)
Trimethaphan (C)
2. Antilipemics
Cholestyramine (C)
Dextrothyroxine (C)
3. Cardiac Drugs
Acetyldigitoxin (C)
Amiodarone (C)
Amrinone (C_M)
Bretylium (C)
Deslanoside (C)
Digitalis (C)
Digitoxin (C_M)
Digoxin (C_M)
Disopyramide (C)
Encainide (B_M)
Flecainide (C_M)
Gitalin (C)
Lanatoside C (C)
Lidocaine (C)
Nifedipine (C_M)
Ouabain (B)
Procainamide (C_M)
Quinidine (C)
Verapamil (C_M)
4. Vasodilators
Amyl Nitrite (C)

Cyclandelate (C)
Dioxyline (C)
Dipyridamole (C)
Erythrityl Tetranitrate (C)
Isosorbide Dinitrate (C)
Isoxsuprine (C)
Nicotinyl Alcohol (C)
Nitroglycerin (C_M)
Nylidrin (C_M)
Pentaerythritol Tetranitrate (C)
Tolazoline (C)

J. CENTRAL NERVOUS SYSTEM DRUGS
1. Analgesics and Antipyretics
Acetaminophen (B)
Aspirin (C/D)
Aspirin, Buffered (C/D)
Ethoheptazine (C)
Phenacetin (B)
Propoxyphene (C/D)
2. Anticonvulsants
Aminoglutethimide (D_M)
Bromides (D)
Carbamazepine (C_M)
Clonazepam (C)
Ethosuximide (C)
Ethotoin (D)
Magnesium Sulfate (B)
Mephenytoin (C)
Mephobarbital (D)
Metharbital (B)
Methsuximide (C)
Paramethadione (D_M)
Phenobarbital (D)
Phensuximide (D)
Phenytoin (D)
Primidone (D)
Trimethadione (D)
Valproic Acid (D)
3. Antidepressants
Amitriptyline (D)
Amoxapine (C_M)
Butriptyline (D)
Clomipramine (D)
Desipramine (C)
Dibenzepin (D)
Dothiepin (D)
Doxepin (C)
Imipramine (D)
Iprindole (D)
Iproniazid (C)
Isocarboxazid (C)

Maprotiline (B_M)
Mebanazine (C)
Nialamide (C)
Nortriptyline (D)
Opipramol (D)
Phenelzine (C)
Protriptyline (C)
Tranylcypromine (C)

4. Hallucinogens

Lysergic Acid Diethylamide (C)
Marijuana (C)
Phencyclidine (X)

5. Narcotic Analgesics

Alphaprodine (C_M/D)
Anileridine (B/D)
Butorphanol (B/D)
Codeine (C/D)
Dihydrocodeine Bitartrate (B/D)
Fentanyl (B/D)
Heroin (B/D)
Hydrocodone (B/D)
Hydromorphone (B/D)
Levorphanol (B/D)
Meperidine (B/D)
Methadone (B/D)
Morphine (B/D)
Nalbuphine (B/D)
Opium (B/D)
Oxycodone (B/D)
Oxymorphone (B/D)
Pentazocine (B/D)
Phenazocine (B/D)

6. Narcotic Antagonists

Cyclazocine (D)
Levallorphan (D)
Nalorphine (D)
Naloxone (B_M)

7. Nonsteroidal Anti-inflammatory Drugs

Fenoprofen (B/D)
Ibuprofen (B/D)
Indomethacin (B/D)
Meclofenamate (B/D)
Naproxen (B_M/D)
Oxyphenbutazone (D)
Phenylbutazone (D)
Sulindac (B/D)
Tolmetin (C_M/D)

8. Sedatives and Hypnotics

Amobarbital (D/B)
Aprobarbital (C)
Butalbital (C/D)
Chloral Hydrate (C_M)

Chlordiazepoxide (D)
Diazepam (D)
Ethanol (D/X)
Ethchlorvynol (C_M)
Ethinamate (C_M)
Flunitrazepam (D)
Lorazepam (D_M)
Mephobarbital (D)
Meprobamate (D)
Methaqualone (D)
Metharbital (D)
Oxazepam (D)
Pentobarbital (D_M)
Phenobarbital (D)
Secobarbital (D_M)
Temazepam (X_M)

9. Stimulants

Amphetamine (C_M)
Caffeine (B)
Dextroamphetamine (C_M)
Diethylpropion (B)
Fenfluramine (C)
Mazindol (C)
Methamphetamine (C_M)
Methylphenidate (C)
Phendimetrazine (C)
Phentermine (C)

10. Tranquilizers

Acetophenazine (C)
Butaperazine (C)
Carphenazine (C)
Chlorpromazine (C)
Chlorprothixene (C)
Droperidol (C_M)
Flupenthixol (C)
Fluphenazine (C)
Haloperidol (C)
Hydroxyzine (C)
Lithium (D)
Loxapine (C)
Mesoridazine (C)
Methotrimeprazine (C)
Molindone (C)
Perphenazine (C)
Piperacetazine (C)
Prochlorperazine (C)
Promazine (C)
Tetrabenazine (C)
Thiopropazate (C)
Thioridazine (C)
Thiothixene (C)
Trifluoperazine (C)
Triflupromazine (C)

Zuclopenthixol (C)

**K. COAGULANTS/
ANTICOAGULANTS**
1. Anticoagulants
Anisindione (D)
Coumarin Derivatives (D)
Dicumarol (D)
Diphenadione (D)
Ethyl Biscoumacetate (D)
Heparin (C)
Nicoumalone (D)
Phenindione (D)
Phenprocoumon (D)
Warfarin (D)
2. Antiheparin
Protamine (C)
3. Hemorrheologic
Pentoxifylline (C_M)
4. Hemostatics
Aminocaproic Acid (C)
Aprotinin (C)
5. Thrombolytics
Streptokinase (C)
Urokinase (B_M)

L. DIAGNOSTIC AGENTS
Diatrizoate (D)
Ethiodized Oil (D)
Evans Blue (C)
Indigo Carmine (B)
Iocetamic Acid (D)
Iodamide (D)
Iodipamide (D)
Iodoxamate (D)
Iopanoic Acid (D)
Iothalamate (D)
Ipodate (D)
Methylene Blue (C_M/D)
Metrizamide (D)
Metrizoate (D)
Sodium Iodide I125 (X)
Sodium Iodide I131 (X)
Tyropanoate (D)

M. DIURETICS
Acetazolamide (C)
Amiloride (B_M)
Bendroflumethiazide (D/C)
Benzthiazide (D)
Chlorothiazide (D)
Chlorthalidone (D)
Cyclopenthiazide (D)

Cyclothiazide (D)
Ethacrynic Acid (D)
Furosemide (C_M)
Glycerin (C)
Hydrochlorothiazide (D)
Hydroflumethiazide (D)
Isosorbide (C)
Mannitol (C)
Methazolamide (C)
Methyclothiazide (D)
Metolazone (D)
Polythiazide (D)
Quinethazone (D)
Spironolactone (D)
Triamterene (D)
Trichlormethiazide (D)
Urea (C)

N. ELECTROLYTES
Potassium Chloride (A)
Potassium Citrate (A)
Potassium Gluconate (A)

O. GASTROINTESTINAL AGENTS
1. Antiemetics
Buclizine (C)
Cyclizine (B)
Dimenhydrinate (B)
Doxylamine (B)
Droperidol (C_M)
Meclizine (B_M)
Metoclopramide (B_M)
Prochlorperazine (C)
Trimethobenzamide (C)
2. Antiflatulents
Simethicone (C)
3. Laxatives/Purgatives
Casanthranol (C)
Cascara Sagrada (C)
Danthron (C)
Docusate Calcium (C)
Docusate Potassium (C)
Docusate Sodium (C)
Lactulose (C)
Mineral Oil (C)
Senna (C)

P. GOLD COMPOUNDS
Aurothioglucose (C)
Gold Sodium Thiomalate (C)

Q. HEAVY METAL ANTAGONISTS
Deferoxamine (C_M)

Penicillamine (D)

R. **HORMONES**
1. **Adrenal**
Beclomethasone (C)
Betamethasone (C)
Cortisone (D)
Dexamethasone (C)
Prednisolone (B)
Prednisone (B)
2. **Antidiabetic Agents**
Acetohexamide (D)
Chlorpropamide (D/C)
Insulin (B)
Tolazamide (D/C)
Tolbutamide (D/C)
3. **Antithyroid**
Carbimazole (D)
Methimazole (D)
Propylthiouracil (D)
Sodium Iodide I131 (X)
4. **Estrogens**
Chlorotrianisene (X_M)
Clomiphene (X_M)
Dienestrol (X)
Diethylstilbestrol (X_M)
Estradiol (X)
Estrogens, Conjugated (X_M)
Estrone (X)
Ethinyl Estradiol (X)
Hormonal Pregnancy Test
   Tablets (X)
Mestranol (X)
Oral Contraceptives (X)
5. **Pituitary**
Corticotropin/Cosyntropin (C)
Desmopressin (B_M)
Lypressin (C_M)
Somatostatin (B)
Vasopressin (B)
6. **Progestogens**
Ethisterone (D)
Ethynodiol (D)
Hydroxyprogesterone (D)
Lynestrenol (D)
Medroxyprogesterone (D)
Norethindrone (X_M)
Norethynodrel (X_M)
Norgestrel (X_M)
Oral Contraceptives (X)
7. **Thyroid**
Calcitonin (B)
Iodothyrin (A)

Levothyroxine (A_M)
Liothyronine (A_M)
Liotrix (A)
Thyroglobulin (A)
Thyroid (A)
Thyrotropin (C_M)

S. **NUTRIENTS**
Hyperalimentation, Parenteral (C)
Lipids (C)
l-Lysine (C)

T. **SERUMS, TOXOIDS, AND VACCINES**
1. **Serums**
Immune Globulin, Hepatitis B (B)
Immune Globulin, Rabies (B)
Immune Globulin, Tetanus (B)
2. **Toxoids**
Tetanus/Diphtheria Toxoids (Adult)
   (C)
3. **Vaccines**
BCG (C)
Cholera (C)
Escherichia coli (C)
Hepatitis B (C_M)
Influenza (C)
Measles (X)
Meningococcus (C)
Mumps (X)
Plague (C)
Pneumococcal Polyvalent (C)
Poliovirus Inactivated (C)
Poliovirus Live (C)
Rabies Human (C)
Rubella (X)
Smallpox (X)
Tularemia (C)
Typhoid (C)
Yellow Fever (D)

U. **SPASMOLYTICS**
Aminophylline (C)
Dyphylline (C_M)
Oxtriphylline (C)
Theophylline (C)

V. **VAGINAL SPERMICIDES**
Nonoxynol-9 (C)
Octooxynol-9 (C)

W. **VITAMINS**
β-Carotene (C)

Calcifediol (A/D)
Calcitriol (A/D)
Cholecalciferol (A/D)
Dihydrotachysterol (A/D)
Ergocalciferol (A/D)
Etretinate (X_M)
Folic Acid (A/C)
Isotretinoin (X)
Leucovorin (C_M)
Menadione (C_M/X)
Niacin (A/C)
Niacinamide (A/C)
Pantothenic Acid (A/C)
Phytonadione (C)
Pyridoxine (A/C)
Riboflavin (A/C)
Thiamine (A/C)
Vitamin A (A/X)

Vitamin B_{12} (A/C)
Vitamin C (A/C)
Vitamin D (A/D)
Vitamin E (A/C)
Vitamins, Multiple (A)

X.   MISCELLANEOUS
Bromocriptine (C_M)
Camphor (C)
Clofibrate (C)
Colchicine (C_M)
Cromolyn Sodium (B_M)
Cyclamate (C)
Cyclosporine (C_M)
Disulfiram (C)
Phenazopyridine (B_M)
Probenecid (B)

INDEX